Skin Signs of Systemic Disease

Second Edition

IRWIN M. BRAVERMAN, M.D.
Professor of Dermatology,
Yale University School of Medicine

1981 W. B. SAUNDERS COMPANY • PHILADELPHIA • LONDON • TORONTO • SYDNEY

W. B. Saunders Company: West Washington Square
Philadelphia, PA 19105

1 St. Anne's Road
Eastbourne, East Sussex BN21, 3UN, England

1 Goldthorne Avenue
Toronto, Ontario M8Z 5T9, Canada

9 Waltham Street
Artarmon, N.S.W. 2064, Australia

Library of Congress Cataloging in Publication Data

Braverman, Irwin M., 1929–

Skin signs of systemic disease.

Includes bibliographical references and index.

1. Cutaneous manifestations of general diseases. I. Title.
[DNLM: 1. Skin manifestations. WR 143 B826s]

RL100.B7 1981 616.07′2 80–53490

ISBN 0–7216–1927–4 AACR2

Listed here is the latest translated edition of this book together with the language of the translation and the publisher.

Spanish (1st Edition)—Ediciones Toray, S.A., Barcelona, Spain.

Skin Signs of Systemic Disease ISBN 0-7216-1927-4

Last digit is the print number: 9 8 7 6 5 4 3 2 1

to

MURIEL

and

PAULA, DAVID, *and* MICHAEL

Preface to Second Edition

The goals for this edition are the same as for the first. The major systemic diseases are discussed in terms of their cutaneous signs and clinical features. The spectrum of cutaneous lesions for each entity is illustrated or described so that recognition of the disorder can be made more easily. In many instances the relevant biochemical, immunologic, and histologic findings are also illustrated or discussed because they provide the basis for diagnosing, understanding, and treating these disorders. Many of the tests for obtaining these data are now readily available to physicians through clinical and surgical pathology laboratories and therefore have become part of the physician's diagnostic armamentarium.

New chapters have been added on infectious diseases, dermatoses associated with pregnancy and the menstrual cycle, and the neutrophilic dermatoses. Material dealing with the nervous system and connective tissue has been amplified. The entire text has been rewritten and in places reorganized. In some chapters, there has been a deliberate, but minor, duplication of text material in order to construct a coherent presentation. I have tried to correlate personal experience with that reported in the literature, and I have speculated on pathogenesis or etiology where I felt the evidence permitted. As before, this monograph is not intended to be all-inclusive. I have concentrated on those diseases which I considered most important or with which I have had the most experience. The bulk of the illustrations are of patients whom I have cared for or seen in consultation or who have been brought to my attention by my colleagues in the Department of Dermatology and at the Yale Medical Center.

I wish to thank my colleagues for their extremely helpful assistance in this revision. Drs. Ira Gouterman and Leonard Milstone gave generously of their time to read the manuscript and provide invaluable constructive criticisms. Drs. Thomas Lawley and Stephen Katz kindly allowed me to include their data on dermatitis herpetiformis and the PUPPP syndrome before they were published, as did Dr. Thomas Provost with his data on anti-Ro and anti-La antibodies in patients with lupus erythematosus. Dr. James Gilliam provided the opportunity for me to examine several of his patients with mixed connective tissue disease (MCTD) during a visit to Dallas. Dr. Jorge Sanchez arranged a similar opportunity for me with patients afflicted with Hansen's disease in San Juan. Dr. Michael Lerner provided me with his prepublication data on the nucleotide composition of SM and RNP antigens in MCTD. Dr. Jean Thivolet told me about the existence of Bazex's syndrome after reading about our "unique" case in the first edition. Dr. David McCallum graciously shared his personal experience relating to the skin lesions in Crohn's disease. Other colleagues provided me with illustrative material I did not have in my own collection, and I have acknowledged their contributions in the appropriate places in the text. I also want to thank my many colleagues who brought their interesting cases to my attention and, with the individuals' permission, allowed me to photograph the lesions for my use. I also wish to express my appreciation to Mr. Harry Hirsch, Jr., of the Davenport Photo Company, New Haven, for his superb skills in producing the new black and white photographs from color transparencies and to Eileen Fonferko for her assistance in preparing some of the illustrations. My appreciation is also extended to Mr. Donald Abbott and the team at W. B. Saunders Company for making this revision proceed so smoothly. I especially want to thank Mrs. Elena DiMassa for her dedication and skills in the preparation of this monograph.

New Haven, Connecticut IRWIN M. BRAVERMAN, M.D.

Preface to First Edition

The ability to diagnose systemic disorders by means of cutaneous signs has always fascinated physicians. In recent years there has been a renewed interest in this aspect of clinical diagnosis. Although the cutaneous manifestations of a few systemic diseases have been detailed in medical journals and monographs, currently there is no book that deals solely with this topic. This monograph combines a detailed atlas of the skin signs of the major systemic diseases with a discussion of their clinical features. Emphasis has been placed both on the criteria for accurate morphologic diagnosis and on the medical significance of these eruptions after they have been recognized. The disorders have been grouped in various ways: by pathogenetic mechanisms; by organ system involvement; by categories of disease; and on the basis of mutual, characteristic physical signs. These divisions reflect in part the types of broad clinical problems that physicians often face: e.g., cancer, angiitis, sarcoidosis, lymphomas, connective tissue diseases, and so forth.

The skin lesions are described in detail both in words and in pictures. The illustrations are mostly close-up views in black and white or in color and have been chosen to demonstrate the characteristic morphology and color necessary for correct clinical diagnosis. The morphologic detail in the figures can be enhanced with an ordinary reading glass. I have attempted to show the spectrum of cutaneous lesions encountered in medical practice in association with a given disease rather than as is often done in textbooks, to demonstrate a single "classic" eruption. The differential diagnosis of the cutaneous lesions is discussed and illustrated wherever possible. For example, the features of purpura caused by thrombocytopenia are distinguished from those produced by angiitis, avitaminosis C, meningococcemia, and Schamberg's disease. As another example, erythema multiforme is differentiated from urticaria, aphthous stomatitis, Behçet's syndrome, and bullous pemphigoid.

Over 95 per cent of the illustrations are photographs that I have taken of patients who have been under my care or whom I have seen in consultation during the past ten years.

The etiology and pathogenesis of most of the diseases have been discussed briefly in order to define the nature of the disorder and to relate etiology and pathogenesis to the cutaneous findings. The clinical features of the less frequently encountered diseases have been emphasized. It seemed unnecessarily repetitious to summarize the clinical manifestations of commonly encountered entities that are well known to physicians and amply discussed in available standard medical texts. Instead, the clinical features that are perhaps less well known and the recent observations in these diseases have been discussed.

This book is not meant to be merely a compilation of cutaneous findings in systemic diseases; the skin signs have been evaluated for relevancy and specificity. Some of the eruptions that are included have not been reported previously, and they represent personal observations. For several disorders, my clinical experiences have been compared with those reported in the literature. This monograph was also not meant to be all-inclusive. I have concentrated on those entities that I considered most important or with which I have had the most experience. There may be digressions into esoteric aspects of a few disorders, but this has been done only when a point needed reemphasis or had not been demonstrated previously.

I wish to express my appreciation for the extremely helpful assistance of my colleagues. Drs. Marguerite Lerner, Leonard Selsky, and James Herndon, Jr., gave generously of their time to read the entire manuscript and offer invaluable constructive criticisms. Drs. Ted Hersh, Fred Kantor, Sidney Klaus, Robert Rickert, and Robert Scheig reviewed selected portions of the manuscript that were related to their clinical and research interests. Drs. Dorothy Hollingsworth and Thomas Amatruda kindly allowed me to include their data on acanthosis nigricans and obesity before these data were published by them. Dr. Peter Pochi generously permitted me to include his unpublished data on sebum production in acromegaly. Dr. Herman Yannet, Director of the Southbury Training School, Southbury, Connecticut, and Dr. Peter Huttenlocher made arrangements for Dr. Sidney Hurwitz and me to examine and photograph their patients with tuberous sclerosis. Other colleagues graciously sent me photographs, both published and unpublished, to illustrate disorders for which I had no pictorial material in my own collection. Their contributions are acknowledged in the appropriate places in the text. I particularly want to thank Dr. Paul Beeson for his advice and assistance at the beginning of this undertaking.

This book was written during the tenure of a Career Research Development Award granted by the U.S. Public Health Service, No. AM 9631.

New Haven, Connecticut IRWIN M. BRAVERMAN, M.D.

Contents

List of Color Plates

1

Cancer

The skin markers of internal cancer are manifold. They include metastases to the skin, syndromes produced by humoral secretions from nonendocrine tumors, a variety of proliferative and inflammatory dermatoses, and disorders indicative of a systemic or organ-related carcinogenic process.

SKIN METASTASES AND RELATED DISORDERS

Tumor cells reach the skin through several routes: direct invasion from underlying structures, extension through lymphatics, embolization through lymphatics and blood vessels, and accidental implantation at surgery. The frequency of metastases to the skin varies from 1 to 4.5 per cent.[1, 2]

The carcinomas most frequently associated with cutaneous metastases originate in the breast, stomach, lung, uterus, kidney, ovary, colon, and urinary bladder. Skin metastases usually portend an extremely poor prognosis, and the patient often dies within three to six months. In malignant melanoma and cancers of the breast and kidney, the interval between the detection and treatment of the primary tumor and the appearance of distant metastases may be great. Metastases to the skin and bones may be delayed 15 years after surgical treatment of carcinoma of the breast. Six to ten years may elapse between the recognition and treatment of renal cancer and the subsequent development of cutaneous metastases. One individual with melanoma developed metastases 32 years after removal of the primary ocular tumor. Although much less frequent, delays of five to ten years between discovery of the primary tumor and the appearance of cutaneous metastases also have been observed in cases of carcinomas of the colon, larynx, ovary, and bladder.[4]

Certain areas of the skin are predisposed to metastases. The scalp is a favorite site for metastases from the breast, lung, and genitourinary system (Fig. 1–1); the chest wall from mammary carcinoma; the abdominal wall, especially around the umbilicus, from neoplasms in the stomach and in the remaining gastrointestinal tract; and the lower abdominal wall and external genitalia from cancers of the genitourinary system. Hypernephroma and carcinoma of the thyroid which metastasize to bone can produce a pulsating tumor mass with a bruit detectable through the

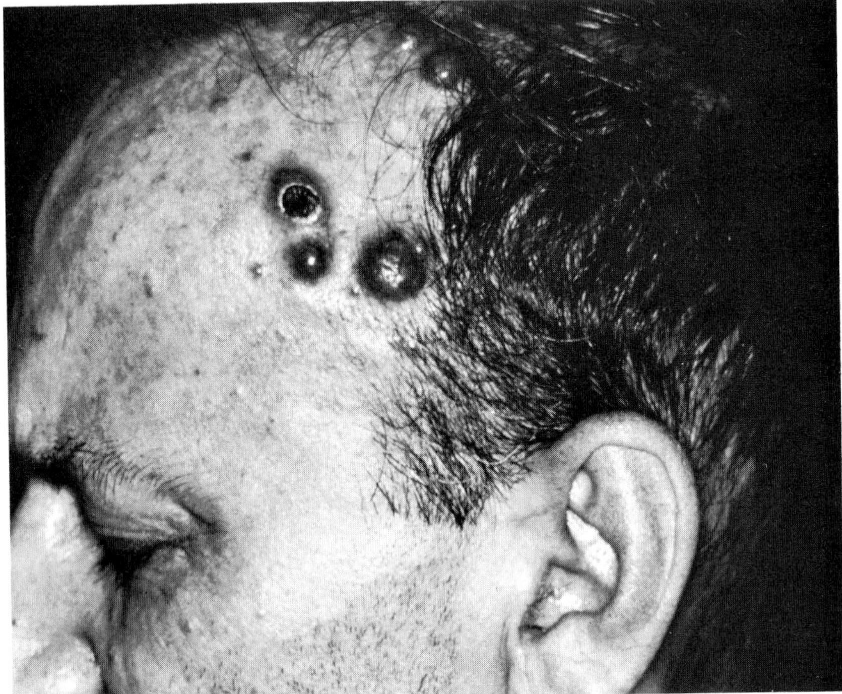

Figure 1–1. Cutaneous metastases from carcinoma of the larynx.

overlying skin.[5] Implantation of tumor cells in surgical scars is not uncommon.

Metastases form varied and at times bizarre clinical pictures.[6] Cancer of the prostate produces skin metastases in a zoster-like distribution over the flank because of perineural lymphatic spread. A 19-year-old man developed an ulcer, resembling a chancre, on his penis because of metastases from a transitional cell carcinoma of the nasopharynx.[7] Metastatic lesions can appear in the tongue and tonsils from melanoma and from cancers of the lung, kidney, breast, stomach, uterus, prostate, and pharynx. Renal cancer may produce lesions resembling an epulis or a cyst in the oral mucosa. Metastasis to the eyelid from an undifferentiated breast cancer has been reported, and an adenocarcinoma of the colon was first detected in a patient because of skin metastases to the sternum.

Skin metastases may be the first indication of an internal malignancy. In a study of 724 patients in whom both primary and metastatic sites of tumors were known, Brownstein and Helwig found that carcinomas of the lung, ovary, and kidney frequently declared their presence through cutaneous metastases. They also noted that it was unusual for carcinomas of the breast and oral cavity to do so.[8]

Metastatic carcinoma to the skin produces subcutaneous or intradermal nodules that vary from flesh color to pink, violaceous, and brown-black hues (Plate 1*A*); they are almost always stony-hard when palpated. Ulceration is an uncommon feature of cutaneous metastases. Any skin nodule or tumor which is atypical for known dermatologic disorders should be suspected of being a metastasis.

Histologic examination of a skin metastasis may indicate the site of the primary tumor. The presence of mucin in a glandular tumor suggests origin from the gastrointestinal tract. Hypernephroma, thyroid cancer,

PLATE 1

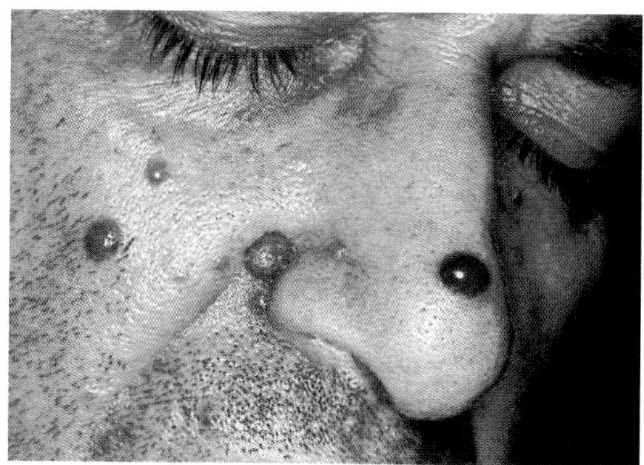

A, Metastases to skin from cancer of larynx. Note different colors of metastatic tumors.

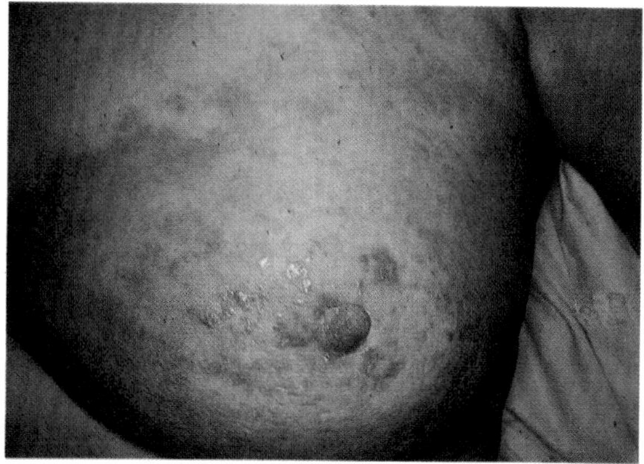

B, Carcinoma erysipelatoides caused by cancer of the breast.

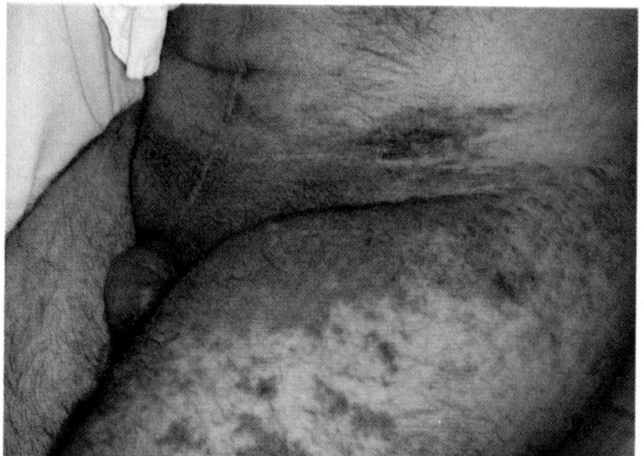

C, Carcinoma erysipelatoides on lower abdomen and thigh secondary to cancer of colon.

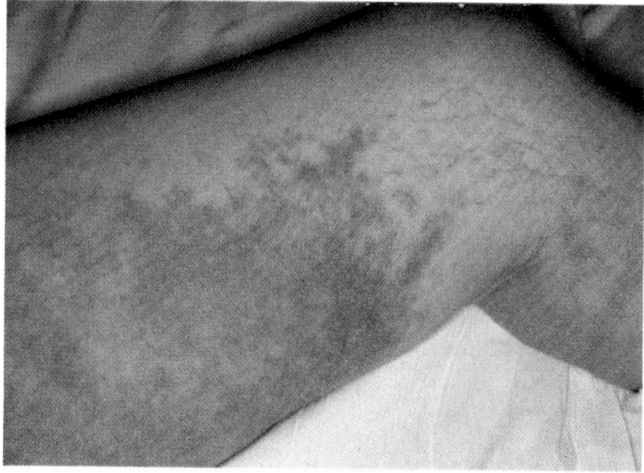

D, Carcinoma erysipelatoides. Upper thigh. Source was colonic cancer secondary to familial polyposis.

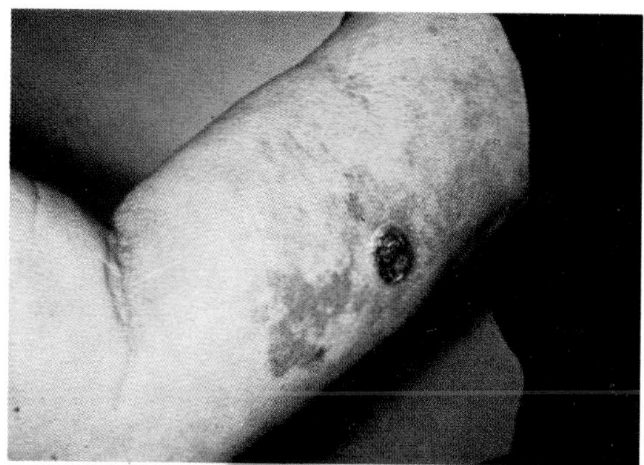

E, Lymphangiosarcoma of Stewart and Treves.

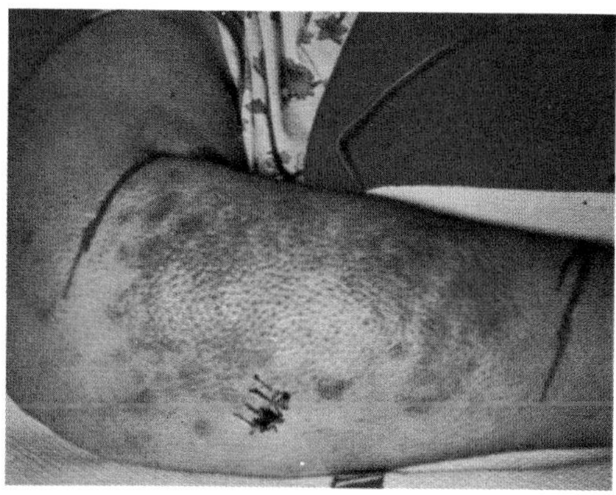

F, Lymphangiosarcoma of Stewart and Treves.

hepatoma, and seminoma may retain their characteristic histologic appearance in cutaneous metastases. Although it is generally believed that anaplastic and epidermoid cancers metastatic to skin do not reveal their sources on tissue examination, Brownstein and Helwig found that one can make reliable predictions about the origins of such metastases.[8] In their study of 724 patients, metastatic anaplastic cancers most commonly came from the lung; squamous cell carcinomas, excluding those from the oral cavity and esophagus, usually arose in the lung; and adenocarcinomas, poorly or moderately differentiated, were more likely to have come from the lung than from the gastrointestinal tract.

In women, cutaneous metastases in the anterior chest wall most frequently arose from cancer of the breast, and metastases in the abdominal wall, especially periumbilically, usually came from the ovary. In men, the sites of localization of metastases were not helpful in predicting the primary site of the malignancy.[8]

Although metastatic carcinoma usually produces nonspecific nodules and tumors in the skin, there are some characteristic pictures of metastatic disease. Metastases to the scalp simulate wens and turban tumors and may ulcerate.[9] They may also produce scarring alopecia with induration and atrophy of the scalp, even though such changes are associated more frequently with lupus erythematosus, sarcoidosis, or pseudopelade (an idiopathic noninflammatory scarring alopecia). Loss of hair resembling alopecia areata is an uncommon manifestation of metastases to the scalp.[10] Metastatic carcinoma should always be considered in the evaluation of an unusual alopecia.

Metastases from the breast, and less commonly from the stomach, kidney, and lung, can produce dramatic changes in the chest wall: carcinoma en cuirasse. Extensive thickening and fibrosis of the dermis and subcutaneous tissue result from lymphatic permeation by cancer cells. The chest and abdomen may be completely girdled by a thick rigid encasement which can inhibit respiration. Papules and nodules varying from flesh to pink and violaceous tones soon appear in the sclerotic plaque. Inflammation is usually not associated with this type of metastasis.

Inflammatory carcinoma (carcinoma erysipelatoides) is even more spectacular (Plate 1*B*, *C*). Although it is most commonly associated with carcinoma of the breast, it may also be seen with metastases from the uterus and lung. Plate 1*D* illustrates an example of inflammatory carcinoma produced by metastases from an adenocarcinoma arising in a polyp from a woman with familial polyposis. Initially, one sees a small area of inflammation with a sharply marginated and slightly elevated border. Tenderness and warmth may be present as well. Cellulitis or erysipelas is often diagnosed, and treatment with antibiotics begun. The correct diagnosis is made when tumor nodules appear in the erythematous lesion or when there is a lack of favorable response to antibiotic therapy.

Sometimes one sees fine telangiectasia and larger dilated vessels in association with small tumor nodules over the chest wall. A significant inflammatory reaction is absent. However, this telangiectatic variety of metastatic carcinoma is most uncommon.

The erysipelas-like lesions of metastatic breast carcinoma often begin in the surgical scar of the previous mastectomy, but lesions can develop as discrete patches distant from the surgical site, e.g., on the back.

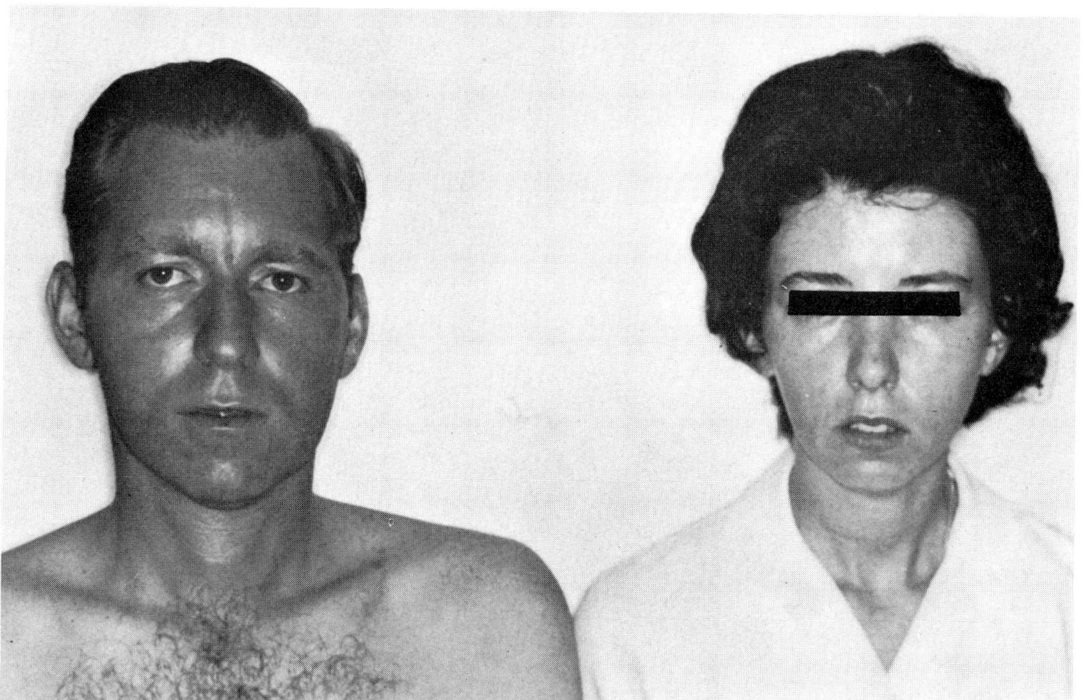

Figure 1-2. Melanin hyperpigmentation produced by disseminated malignant melanoma. Compare with normal pigmentation of healthy individual on right.

One of the complications of radical mastectomy for carcinoma of the breast is lymphedema of the arm. An unusual type of angiomatous malignancy that may develop in chronically lymphedematous limbs is lymphangiosarcoma of Stewart and Treves.[11, 12] Red to purplish firm nodules develop and slowly spread over the limb, at times coalescing into indurated plaques (Plate 1*E, F*). Ulcerations can occur. The interval between the onset of lymphedema and angiosarcoma has ranged from 2 to 24 years. Lymphedema is the common factor in all reported cases. Angiosarcoma has developed in cases of congenital lymphedema as well as in lymphedema of the legs following surgery for cancer of the cervix and melanoma.

In patients with malignant melanoma and widespread metastases, diffuse hyperpigmentation of the skin and mucous membranes can develop (Fig. 1–2).[13] The color varies from slate gray to deep blue-black pigmentation and may be accentuated in light-exposed areas. During the rapid production of melanin from tyrosine in the tumors, metabolic intermediates escape into the blood stream and are deposited in the tissues, where they become oxidized to melanin. These same intermediates are excreted in the urine which, upon standing in air, turns black. The brown-black melanin pigment in the dermis looks blue because of light scattering (Tyndall effect). Hyperpigmentation in melanoma is not common. Although malignant melanomas are usually pigmented, their metastases may be amelanotic (Fig. 1–3).

Konrad and Wolff described a patient with widespread metastatic melanoma and generalized hyperpigmentation in whom an additional

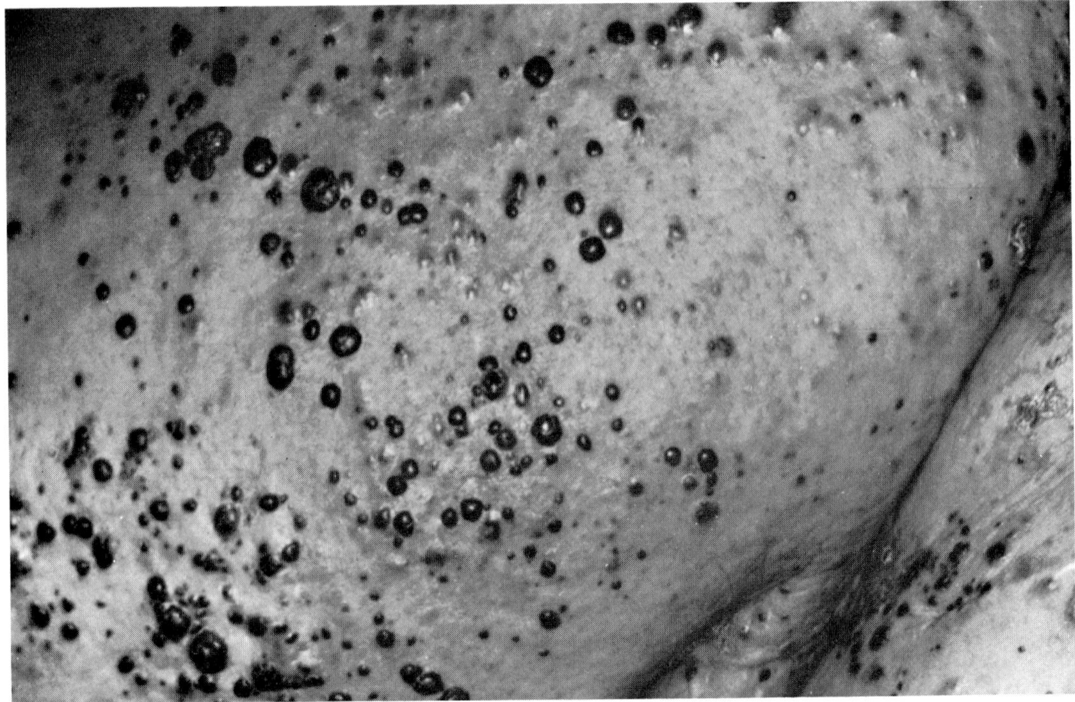

Figure 1–3. Cutaneous metastases of melanoma that display varied pigmentation.

factor appeared to be important in the development of the increased pigmentation.[14] Widespread metastases of individual melanoma cells were found within the dermis and the cutaneous blood vessels in the absence of microscopic and macroscopic tumor masses. The histologic evidence seemed to indicate that melanosomes from dying melanoma cells within the blood stream and dermis had been phagocytized by monocytes and macrophages, respectively, resulting in large accumulations of melanophages in the dermis. The melanophages, which considerably outnumbered the individual melanoma cells, made the major contribution to the patient's slate gray color.

Metastatic carcinoma to the liver may produce the stigmata associated with cirrhosis: palmar erythema, spider nevi, and jaundice.[15] Extensive invasion of the mediastinum by tumor produces the superior vena caval syndrome: edema of the face, conjunctivae, and neck, associated with a prominently distended venous pattern on the neck, chest, and upper extremities.

Paget's disease of the nipple and areola is a well-known indicator of underlying breast cancer. The clinical features are an eczematous weeping crusted lesion of the nipple with slow extension onto the areola (Fig. 1–4). The eruption does not respond to topical treatment. The differential diagnosis includes atopic eczema and contact dermatitis which improves with the administration of topical corticosteroids (Fig. 1–5). Eczematous lesions of the nipple that do not respond to topical therapy should be examined by biopsy. An underlying cancer is always found in the ipsilateral breast. The other breast should also be examined carefully because of the increased frequency of a second breast cancer in persons who already have one breast cancer.

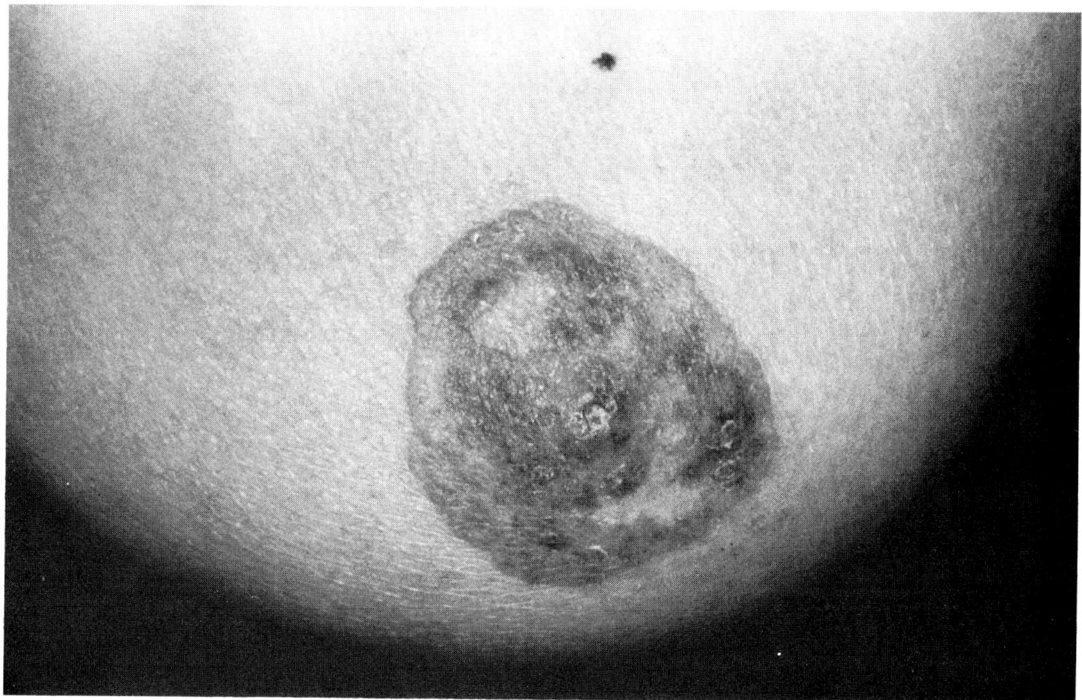

Figure 1–4. Paget's disease involving the nipple and areola.

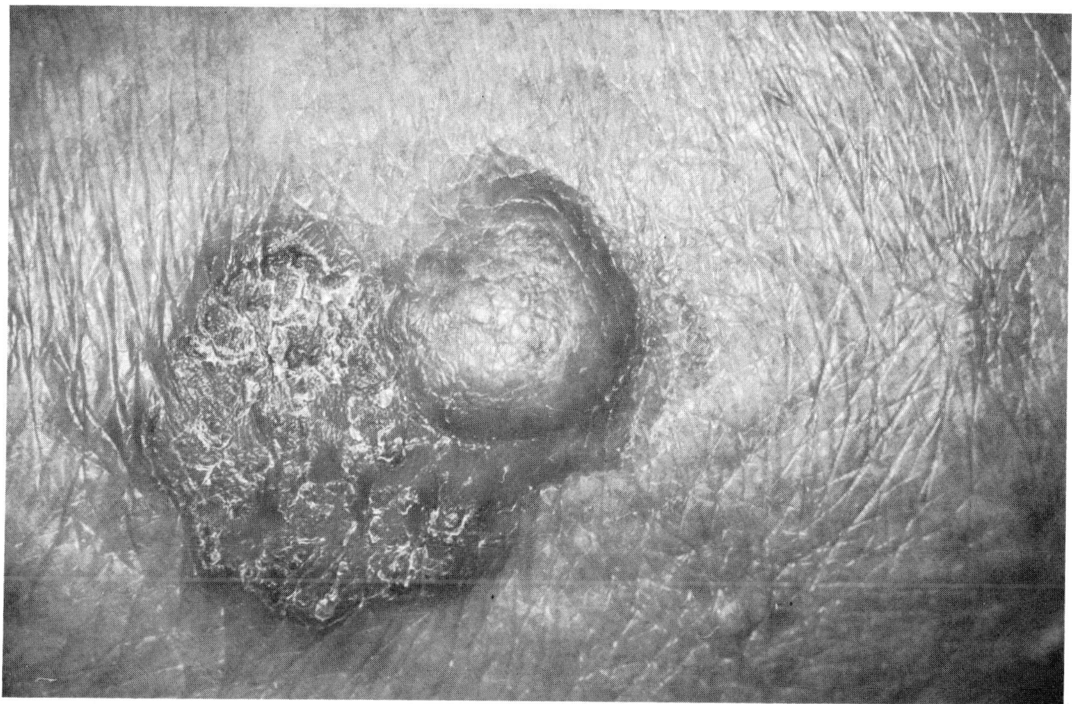

Figure 1–5. Eczema of areola simulating Paget's disease. However, absence of involvement of nipple excludes diagnosis of Paget's disease.

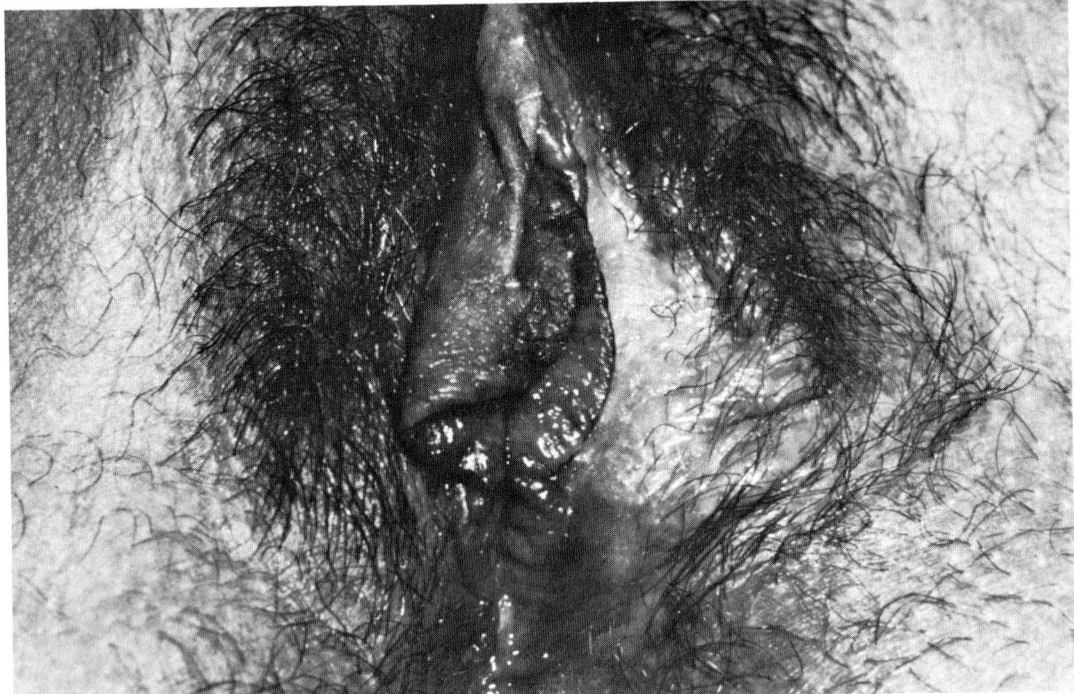

Figure 1–6. Extramammary Paget's disease associated with an underlying apocrine sweat gland carcinoma. (Courtesy of Dr. Irving Friedman.)

Extramammary (anogenital) Paget's disease has been appreciated only recently as a skin marker of internal malignancy (Fig. 1–6). In this disorder, found more often in women than in men and more commonly in those over the age of 50, lesions occur from the lower abdominal wall, inguinal regions, and buttocks to the genitalia, perianal area, and upper thighs. The axillae have been the sites of involvement in a few patients.[16, 17] The histopathology of extramammary Paget's disease is identical with that of mammary Paget's. The eruption is usually unilateral, pruritic, scaly, eczematous or lichenified, and well demarcated. Sometimes it may be exudative and have crusts or ulcerations, bleed, or be painful. The color varies from red to whitish gray. It is most often misdiagnosed as eczema, a fungal infection, candidiasis, leukoplakia, or lichen simplex chronicus. The lesion slowly increases in size over the course of its existence.

The man whose lesion is illustrated in Figures 1–7 and 1–8 had extramammary Paget's disease localized to the scrotum. The patch was eczematous with scale and lichenification and had a thinly elevated border similar to that seen in a superficial multicentric basal cell tumor. Figures 1–9 and 1–10 show the lesions in another man. In this patient, the Paget's disease extended from the perineum onto the left side of the scrotum to the penile shaft. There was an area of clinically normal appearing skin between the penis and the scrotum, but a biopsy of this area disclosed that it too was involved by Paget's disease. In both patients, the dermatoses had been present for at least five years. An associated cancer was not found regionally or in the surgically resected lesions of either patient.

In 50 per cent of the 40 patients in Helwig and Graham's series, an

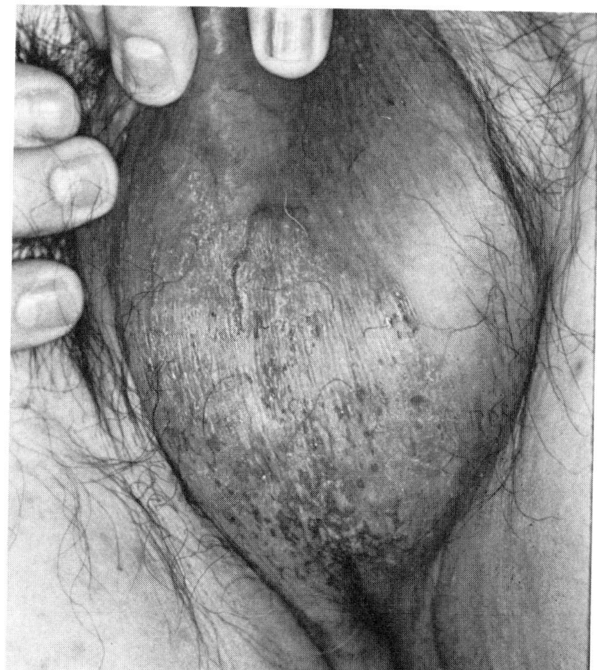

Figure 1–7. Paget's disease involving the scrotum simulating dermatitis.

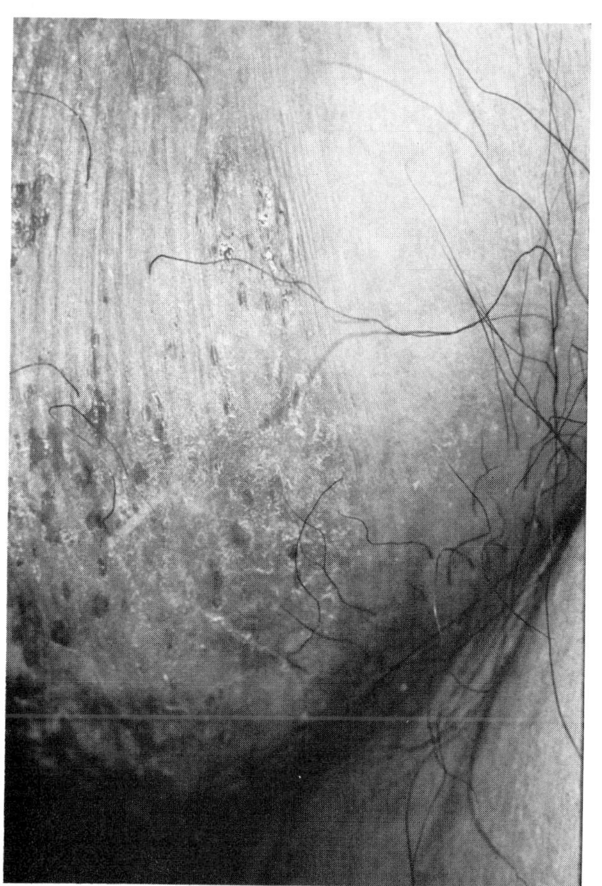

Figure 1–8. Close-up of scrotal Paget's diseae illustrated in Figure 1–7.

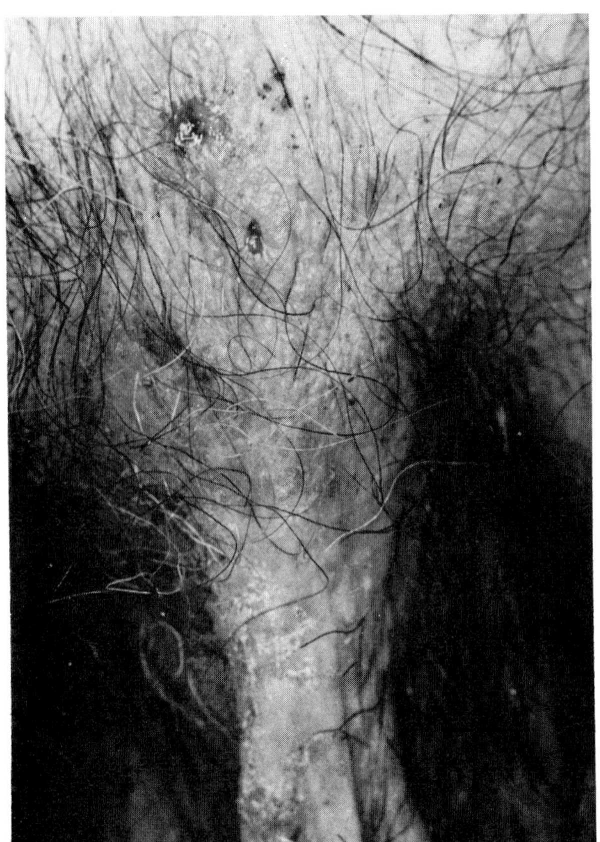

Figure 1–9. Paget's disease extending from the perineum onto the scrotum. Paget's lesion simulates chronic dermatitis.

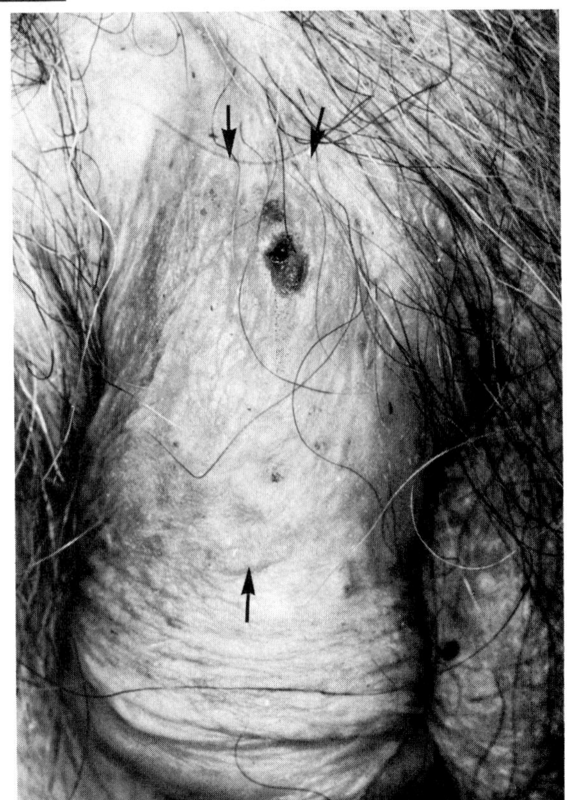

Figure 1–10. Paget's disease involved the entire area from the perineum onto the scrotum and penile shaft. Arrows indicate margin of lesion. Circular defects represent punch biopsy sites in both pictures. Same patient as in Figure 1–9.

underlying carcinoma was found.[18] Twelve of 14 patients with perianal lesions had an associated underlying carcinoma: four with rectal carcinoma, two with breast cancer, and six with apocrine gland carcinoma. Of the 26 remaining patients whose Paget's disease involved the genital, inguinal, pubic, and gluteal areas, only eight had an associated underlying carcinoma. In seven of the eight, an apocrine gland carcinoma was seen, and in one there was a primary mucinous adenocarcinoma of the urethra. It is clear that perianal Paget's disease is attended with a higher incidence of underlying cancer. Although apocrine gland cancer is the most common form of malignancy associated with extramammary Paget's disease, carcinomas of the urethra, eccrine sweat glands, prostate, Bartholin's glands, and breast have also been reported.[19-21] Friedrich et al. mentioned carcinoma of the cervix as an associated lesion without any further documentation.[19] Figure 1–11 shows an example of Paget's disease of the glans penis in one of our patients with a carcinoma of the prostate. In general, the cancers arising from the apocrine or eccrine sweat glands are small and may be missed if the surgically excised tissues are not examined by step-section technique. Regional and widespread metastases may develop from any of these associated malignancies.

Helwig and Graham found that there was no appreciable latent period between the establishment of the diagnosis of anogenital Paget's disease and the time an underlying carcinoma or internal cancer was detected. In almost all of their patients, the cancer was found at the same time or shortly after the diagnosis of anogenital Paget's disease was established. However, no quantitative data were presented for those patients in whom intervals did occur. Murrell and McMullen also concluded from their review of the literature that an associated cancer and metastases manifested themselves early in the course of the disorder, but again no data were given.[22] It appears that in the majority of patients the disease runs a course of many years without evidence of cancer or metastases. In some individuals, anogenital Paget's disease has been present for 19 to 30

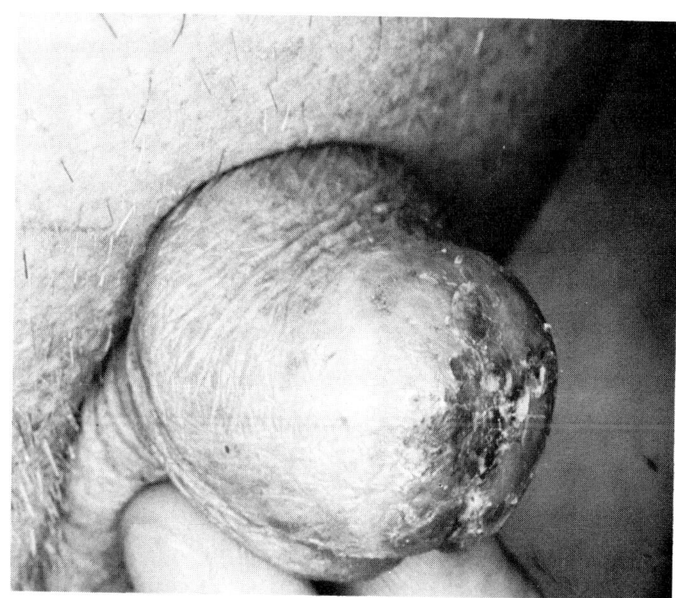

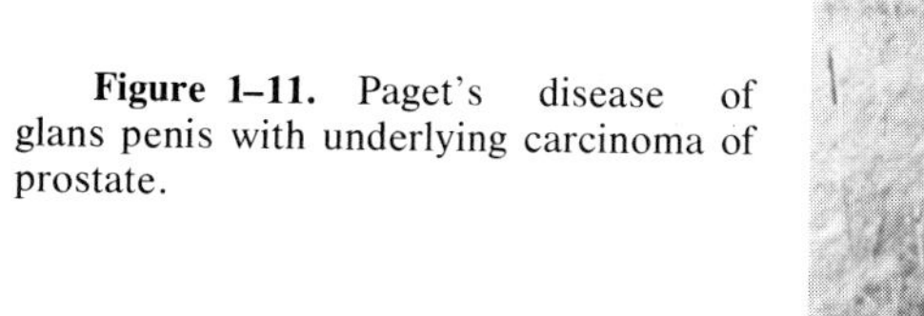

Figure 1–11. Paget's disease of glans penis with underlying carcinoma of prostate.

years.[21, 23-25] In two persons, adenocarcinomas of the apocrine glands and anal canal were diagnosed two and three years, respectively, after the clinical onset of Paget's disease.[26, 27] For practical purposes, then, it seems likely that the absence of detectable carcinoma at the time Paget's disease is diagnosed indicates an excellent prognosis for the patient. Prospective studies are needed to support or refute this notion.

The most common sites of metastases when they do occur are the regional inguinal and pelvic lymph nodes, liver, bone, lung, brain, bladder, prostate, and adrenals in that order, as reported by Helwig and Graham. Fourteen of 18 deaths in their series were directly attributable to the underlying or regional internal cancer. The median survival was 1.5 years, with a range of one month to eight years.[18]

In at least 50 per cent of patients, extramammary Paget's disease remains confined to the epidermis and its adnexa — apocrine, sebaceous, and eccrine sweat glands and the outer root sheath of the hair follicle — producing a histologic picture of carcinoma in situ. The apocrine gland and eccrine gland carcinomas that develop in patients are believed to arise by invasion of the dermis from the sites of carcinoma in situ.[18, 28]

The histogenesis of the Paget cell and the pathogenesis of extramammary Paget's disease ought to be less controversial in light of recent clinical observations and investigational studies. It is generally agreed that *mammary* Paget's is caused by the intraepidermal spread of malignant cells from an underlying ductal carcinoma of the breast which is present in virtually every instance. However, extramammary Paget's disease is probably associated with an underlying carcinoma in no more than 50 per cent of cases, and since some of the cancers have been of the urethra, cervix, and prostate, and even as distant as the breast, a concept has been proposed which states that a systemic carcinogenic stimulus simultaneously produces a *malignant transformation of keratinocytes into Paget cells, and the epidermal cells in adjacent structures and the cells in the regional organs such as the rectum and urethra into carcinomas in situ or carcinomas*.[18] The carcinomas in situ can eventually invade the dermis and metastasize. This concept proposes that the initial stimulus produces a multicentric effect, with carcinomas potentially arising from any of the altered structures, rather than there developing a malignant alteration in a single portion of the epidermis or regional tissues which is followed by migration of these neoplastic cells within or into the epidermis.[18]

There is considerable evidence against this multicentric hypothesis. First, the histology of Paget's disease, whether mammary or extramammary, indicates that cancer cells are living in symbiosis with keratinocytes and other epidermal cell populations. The hypothesis that the Paget cells have invaded the epidermis is supported by the findings in three unusual clinical cases, in addition to the general consensus about the origin of Paget cells in breast carcinoma. Greenwood and Minkowitz reported a patient who developed metastases to the skin 11 years after mastectomy for breast cancer.[29] The metastatic lesions were nodular and involved the chest and arm. Histologic examination of the nodules showed the pattern of Paget's disease in the epidermis. Carcinoma cells in the dermis were seen invading, but not destroying, the epidermis at multiple points and spreading intraepidermally from these entry sites. Pinkus and Mehregan described the remarkable case of a woman who developed an eccrine gland carcinoma on the foot which slowly spread to involve the leg, abdomen, and chest with multiple nodules over a two-year period.[30] Histologic studies showed tumor cells in lymphatic vessels in the skin, and at various points, where the lymphatics closely approached the epidermis, tumor cells were seen penetrating the epidermal layer and spreading out in an umbrella fashion to produce a histologic picture indistinguishable from Paget's disease. Dockerty and Pratt described a patient with transitional cell carcinoma of the bladder who developed in the skin of the anterior abdominal wall a metastatic lesion that had the histologic appearance of Paget's disease.[28] Secondly, it is hard to dismiss the conclusion that Paget's disease of the perianal area, in association with a rectal carcinoma or an anal canal carcinoma, is caused by intraepidermal spread of those cancers. Histochemical stains show the same reaction pattern in the Paget cells as in the goblet cells of the normal rectal mucosa and the cloacogenic zone of the anorectal junction.[31] Even the association of carcinoma of the prostate with Paget's phenomenon involving the glans penis or penile shaft, or carcinomas of the urethra and cervix with vulvar Paget's, can be explained by lymphatic spread of cancer cells to the epidermis with subsequent invasion and intraepidermal spread. The lymphatic vessels of the vagina anastomose with those of the cervix, vulva, and rectum. The lymphatics draining the female urethra connect with those of the vulva through the hypogastric lymph nodes. The lymphatic vessels of the cavernous urethra, glans penis, and penile skin all link up in the external iliac nodes with lymphatics which drain the posterior surface of the prostate gland. Therefore, the lymphatics of the perineal skin and organs are all interconnected and provide pathways for these various combinations of tumor spread even though the cancers may travel in retrograde fashion.[32]

What can one say about the histogenesis of the Paget cells in those instances where extramammary Paget's disease is confined to the skin and appendages in the absence of an associated cancer? The studies of Koss and Brockunier[20] and Belcher[24] employing electron microscopy and histochemistry indicate that Paget cells can have the characteristics of cells derived from eccrine sweat glands. However, Demopoulos, on the basis of electron microscopic studies of her case, found that the Paget cells resemble those derived from apocrine glands.[33] The evidence favors the view that this form of extramammary Paget's disease is a carcinoma in situ similar to Bowen's disease and that the malignant cells have arisen in the intra-epidermal ducts or upper parts of apocrine or eccrine sweat glands and spread intraepidermally — a concept proposed by Herman Pinkus long ago.[34]* The cause or nature of such a carcinogenic stimulus is as yet unknown. After an interval, in some patients, the carcinoma in situ may break through the basement membrane into the dermis to produce the focal apocrine gland cancer which is usually sought in the surgically excised specimens. This is the effect, not the cause, in this variety of extramammary Paget's disease. Dermal invasion and metastases, when

*An argument against this hypothesis is that no one has yet described an instance in which there has been apocrine gland involvement with spread only into the *adjacent* epidermis. However, the earliest histologic changes of Paget's disease would almost certainly not declare themselves clinically so that such lesions would not be biopsied. This point probably cannot be refuted or supported by current investigative methods.

they do occur, appear early rather than late in the course, as in Bowen's disease. The slowly expanding nature of the lesion may be related to ameboid spread of cells or expansion through mitoses or even a multicentric proliferation of cells in adnexal structures with clinical spread similar to that seen in multicentric superficial basal cell tumors.

Thus, the Paget phenomenon is a histologic syndrome that can be produced by different types of cells, provided that they are able to invade the epidermis and live there as symbionts. Such a view would divide extramammary Paget's disease into two groups: carcinoma in situ with possible future malignant degeneration (majority of cases) or intraepidermal spread of tumor cells from noncutaneous tumors (minority of cases).

The concept of a systemic carcinogenic stimulus acting upon eccrine or apocrine tissues is still reasonable. It could account for the 15 instances of extramammary Paget's disease associated with breast carcinoma,[19] as well as the induction of focal malignant change in the epidermal adnexa producing anogenital and axillary Paget's by intraepidermal migration. In one of our patients, a 56-year-old woman, both mammary and anogenital Paget's disease developed. First, mammary Paget's was diagnosed and the underlying carcinoma was treated by radical mastectomy. Two years later, an eczematous eruption appeared on her vulva. Biopsy of the skin revealed Paget's disease and an associated apocrine gland carcinoma was found in the surgical specimen after vulvectomy.

These reports teach us that all patients with extramammary Paget's disease should be examined for the possible presence of the various carcinomas noted above, including carcinoma of the breast, and that perhaps all patients with breast carcinoma should be examined for extramammary Paget's disease at the time of the initial diagnosis of breast cancer and at intervals during the management of that individual.

Extramammary Paget's disease may be difficult to distinguish from a melanoma on histologic examination. However, by staining for the presence of mucin in the abnormal clear cells in the epidermis, one can differentiate between Paget's disease and melanoma. The clear cells of melanomas do not stain for mucin.[18] This distinction is important because therapy and prognosis of the two diseases are different.

HUMORAL SYNDROMES FROM NONENDOCRINE TUMORS

One of the most interesting developments in oncology has been the observation that nonendocrine neoplasms can secrete substances that mimic endocrine disease and produce other distinctive syndromes. The two disorders most commonly recognized and studied have been the ectopic ACTH-producing syndrome and the carcinoid syndrome. The ectopic ACTH-producing syndrome (Cushing's syndrome with hyperpigmentation) is the one most commonly observed; approximately 120 cases have been reported.[35, 36] The typical clinical features are edema, proximal muscle weakness, mental confusion and paranoia, diabetes mellitus, hypertension, and intense hyperpigmentation. Treatment of the primary tumor can diminish or erase these features, but relapse develops when the cancer recurs. Most patients do not have the clinical appearance of Cushing's disease. Hyperpigmentation has been seen in 30 to 100 per cent of the patients reported in different series. The constant and significant laboratory findings have been the extreme degree of adrenocortical hyperactivity producing hypokalemic alkalosis, serum cortisol elevation, increased urinary excretion of 17-ketogenic steroids and 17-ketosteroids, and bilateral adrenal hyperplasia. Oat cell carcinoma is the most commonly associated tumor. Cancers of the pancreatic islet cells, thyroid, parotid, ovary, testes, colon, gallbladder, breast, and parathyroid glands, as well as thymoma-like and mediastinal tumors, neuroblastoma, pheochromocytoma, and malignant bronchial carcinoids, have also been associated with this syndrome.[37-39] In addition, benign bronchial carcinoids, intestinal carcinoids including those on the vermiform appendix, and medullary carcinoma of the thyroid have also been reported.[40, 41]

Excessive aldosterone secretion has been eliminated as the cause of the hypokalemic alkalosis and edema. The markedly elevated serum cortisol is responsible for most of the laboratory and clinical findings. In addition, peptides having ACTH and MSH (melanocyte-stimulating hormone) activity were identified by radioimmunoassay in the tumors and plasma of many of the patients.[42] On the basis of these studies, Abe et al. presented convincing data that beta-MSH, rather than ACTH or alpha-MSH, was the major factor responsible for the hyperpigmentation.[42] Recent studies, however, have shown that beta-MSH immunoreactivity is not related to beta-MSH but rather to a larger pituitary peptide beta-lipotropin, which contains within its sequence of 91 amino acids the 22 amino acid sequence of beta-MSH.[43-45] The peptide beta-MSH is an artifact produced in the mild extraction procedures through the degradation of beta-lipotropin. Beta-MSH immunoreactivity related to beta-lipotropin has been found in the plasma of patients with adrenal insufficiency, Nelson's syndrome, and Cushing's syndrome, as well as in the plasma and tumor tissue of individuals with the ectopic ACTH syndrome. Beta-MSH (amino acids 1 to 18) has been demonstrated as a minor component in tumor extracts, but it is not clear whether specific cleavage enzymes are present in these tumors or whether the degradation is merely the result of increased catabolic activity in actively growing neoplastic tissue.[46] The precise cause of the hyperpigmentation in this syndrome is not known at this time. The role played by beta-lipotropin or by any of its degradation products in the physiologic control of human pigmentation remains to be defined.

Most patients with Cushing's syndrome and hyperpigmentation associated with cancer die within several weeks after the diagnosis of adrenocortical hyperactivity has been made. Sometimes, when the tumors grow more slowly and possibly secrete less ACTH-like peptides, the patient survives for a longer period. In most instances, however, the diagnosis of adrenocortical hyperactivity in association with hyperpigmentation has been made shortly before the patient's death.

Profound proximal muscle weakness, or a myasthenia gravis–like syndrome, has been the striking clinical feature in some cases. Although in the past the muscle weakness has been ascribed to hypokalemia, it is likely that the muscular abnormalities represent polymyositis in association with the electrolyte and pigmentary disturbances.

An example of this syndrome was seen at the Yale-New Haven

Medical Center. A tumor not previously reported with this disorder was felt to be responsible.

The patient was a 74-year-old white woman who was admitted to the hospital because of intense hyperpigmentation, shortness of breath, and pain in the left hemithorax (Fig. 1–12). She had been seen three months earlier because of epigastric bloating. Her skin color was normal. A hiatus hernia and cholelithiasis were found. Her liver was enlarged three fingerbreadths below the right costal margin. During the succeeding three months, she developed generalized hyperpigmentation, peripheral edema, weakness, weight loss, muscle wasting, and glycosuria. On admission she had diabetes mellitus, increased urinary excretion of 17-ketosteroids and 17-ketogenic steroids, and hypokalemic alkalosis. Motor neuropathy was present. Biopsy of the liver did not reveal any abnormalities. At autopsy 10 weeks later, a primary anaplastic ductal carcinoma of the liver was found. In some areas the morphology of the tumor had a carcinoid pattern. Additional findings were bilateral cortical hyperplasia; acute and chronic pancreatitis with fat necrosis, which was ascribed to the high serum cortisol levels; and cytomegalic inclusion disease of the thyroid and lungs.

In the differential diagnosis of a patient with intense hyperpigmentation, the finding of hypokalemic alkalosis seems to point to malignant tumor.

Four cases of Cushing's syndrome, with and without hyperpigmentation, have been reported in which only adrenal hyperplasia was found and then surgically treated. Six months to three years later, a primary tumor became evident — a bronchial adenoma in three cases and a cancer of the pancreas with a carcinoid pattern in the fourth.[35, 40, 42] In one case the Cushing's syndrome cleared after adrenalectomy, but the patient developed hyperpigmentation postoperatively. Upon removal of the bronchial adenoma (carcinoid type), the pigmentation faded.[35]

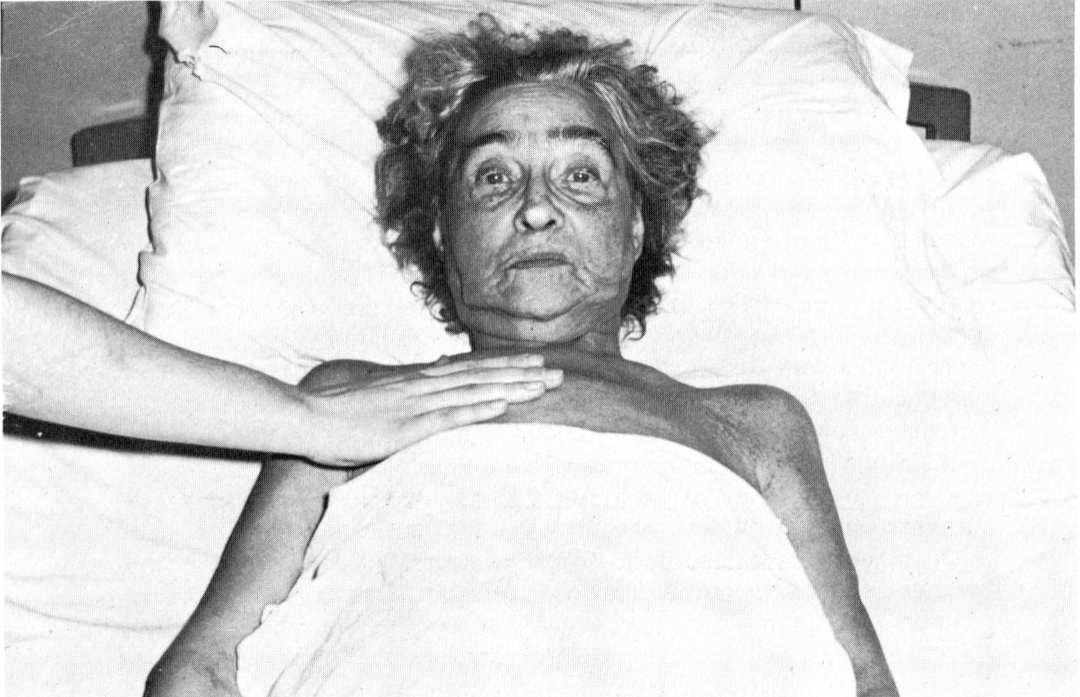

Figure 1–12. Hyperpigmentation and biochemical Cushing's syndrome produced by cancer of biliary tract.

There has been no evidence of insulin secretion in pancreatic islet cell tumors associated with Cushing's syndrome.

The tumors that have produced the ectopic ACTH syndrome have also secreted substances having the properties of antidiuretic hormone, parathormone, thyroid-stimulating hormone, growth hormone, glucagon, insulin, histamine, and serotonin.

Gonadotropin-like peptides are also secreted by these tumors and they can be associated with cutaneous markers. Fusco and Rosen described four patients with anaplastic bronchogenic carcinoma in whom gonadotropin activity could be demonstrated in the tumor and plasma.[47] Urinary gonadotropin and estrogen levels were also elevated. No evidence of a testicular tumor or of a burned-out choriocarcinoma was found in the testes of these four patients, nor was an extragenital trophoblastic neoplasm discovered at autopsy. Histologic examination of the pulmonary tumors revealed areas resembling choriocarcinoma, but the overall impression was that of a primary anaplastic carcinoma of the lung.

The striking clinical feature in Fusco and Rosen's patients was painful gynecomastia *in the absence of* hypertrophic osteoarthropathy. Gynecomastia has been reported with lung cancer many times, but in most instances, hypertrophic osteoarthropathy was also present; in only a few cases has there been evidence of increased urinary excretion of estrogen. Gynecomastia in association with elevated gonadotropin levels in the urine can also be seen with adrenocortical and undifferentiated retroperitoneal cancers, with tumors of the testes and extragonadal sites containing trophoblastic elements, and with some gastric and renal carcinomas. The most common tumors containing trophoblastic elements are choriocarcinoma, teratoma, and embryonal cell carcinoma. Three cases of precocious puberty have been reported in which hepatomas have exhibited gonadotropin activity.[48] Gonadotropins can also be produced by carcinomas of the colon, stomach, and pancreas.

Adults who develop gynecomastia, particularly if it is painful, should be evaluated carefully for the presence of nonendocrine, as well as endocrine, tumors even in the absence of elevated urinary gonadotropins. Gynecomastia can precede the clinical and radiographic recognition of lung cancer. Non-neoplastic causes of gynecomastia have to be considered in the differential diagnosis: treatment with hormones, digitalis, chlorpromazine, reserpine, or spirolactones. Gynecomastia can also be associated with chronic liver disease and malnutrition.

The second most studied example of these humoral syndromes is the carcinoid syndrome. This syndrome causes spectacular bright red cutaneous flushing, initially of the face, neck, and upper chest (Plate 2 *A*, *B*, *C*). The flush lasts from 10 to 30 minutes and tends to resolve centrally first, producing gyrate and serpiginous patterns. During repeated episodes, flushing may involve the entire trunk and extremities. Sensations of heat, edema, and stiffness may be present in the skin during flushing, and paresthesias may occur in the fingers. With successive attacks, the sclerae become injected, spots of cyanosis appear in the bright red flush, and eventually a bluish red flushing develops with each episode. After prolonged and repeated attacks, a permanent cyanotic flush of the face with telangiectasia develops, producing a plethoric appearance. The coarse telangiectasia resembles that of rosacea. The persistent edema and

PLATE 2

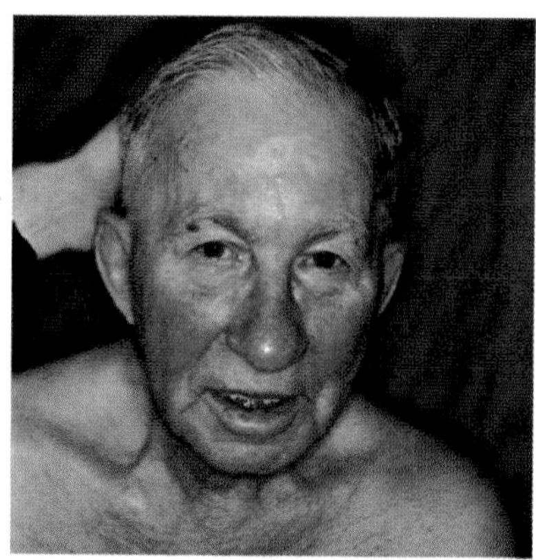

A, Carcinoid flush. Erythema on forehead has been pressed out by thumb in one place to demonstrate flush.

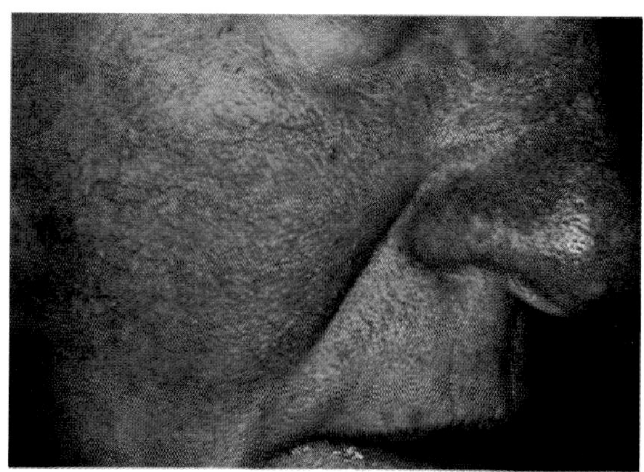

B, Close view of telangiectasia produced by recurrent carcinoid flushes.

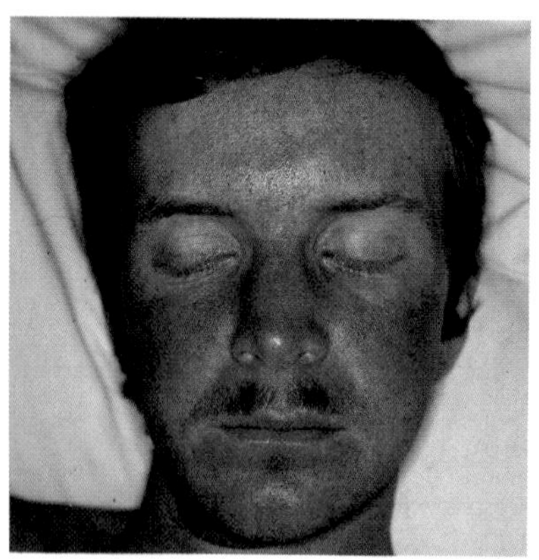

C, Carcinoid flush on cheeks and forehead.

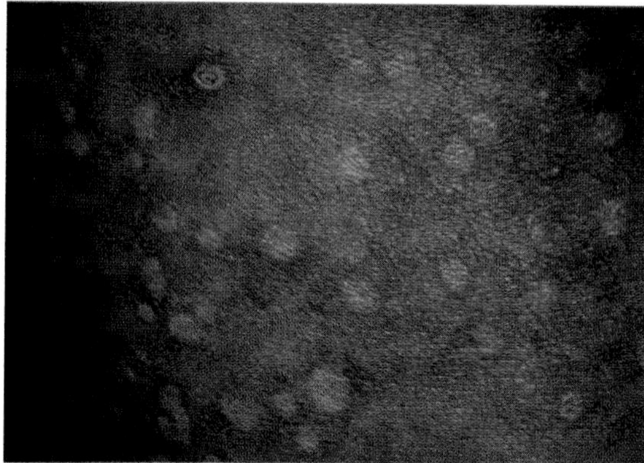

D, Close view of pityriasis rosea–like eruption in patient with carcinoma of stomach.

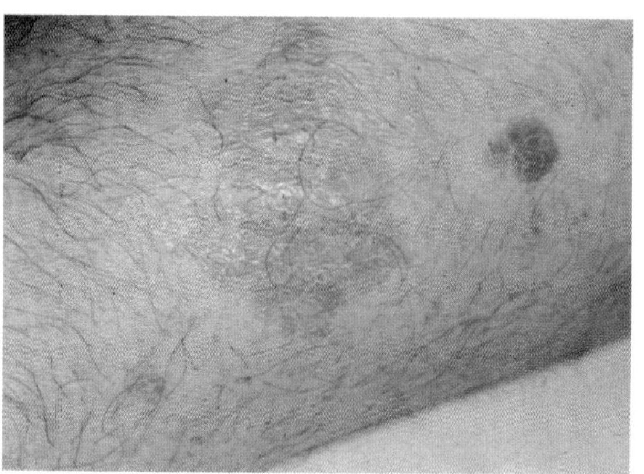

E, Bowen's disease produced by arsenism. Note similarity to eczema.

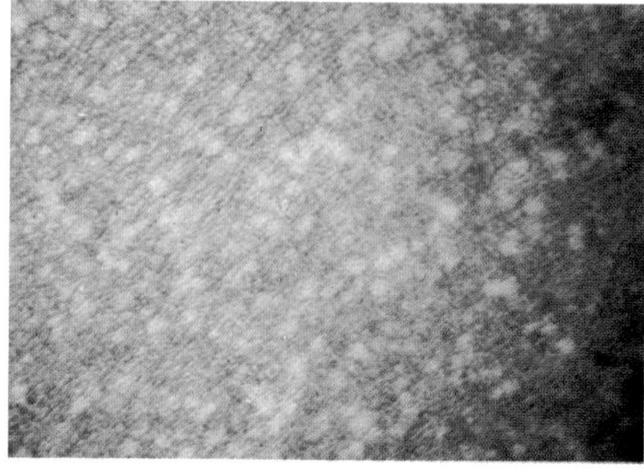

F, Arsenical hyperpigmentation. White spots are the areas of remaining normal skin pigmentation. (Courtesy of Dr. Thomas Kugelman.)

erythema can result in a leonine facies. Sjoerdsma described a patient with repeated episodes of intense purple flushing associated with facial edema, particularly of the eyelids. These episodes persisted for two weeks and subsided over a four- to five-day period. A pellagra-like picture has been reported in European patients with the carcinoid syndrome. Poor nutrition, consisting primarily of a tryptophane deficiency, has been given as the cause of the pellagra-like picture.[49, 50]

Associated with the cutaneous flushing are dyspnea, asthma, abdominal cramps with explosive watery diarrhea, and sometimes severe hypotension. Murmurs of pulmonary stenosis and tricuspid insufficiency, related to a thickening of the connective tissue of the right side of the heart, can develop.

Carcinoids represent 0.1 to 0.5 per cent of all tumors. Fifty per cent are found in the appendix; the rest are located in the small intestine. About 16 per cent of extra-appendiceal carcinoids metastasize to the liver or the lung. The carcinoid syndrome has been described primarily with intestinal carcinoid and hepatic metastases. However, the syndrome can be produced by bronchial adenomas of the carcinoid type with or without liver metastases.[51, 52]

The carcinoid syndrome associated with bronchial adenomas of the carcinoid variety is thought to be distinctive. Not only is the duration of flushing more prolonged — hours to days rather than the usual 10 to 30 minutes — but the individual may also exhibit marked anxiety, disorientation, fever, sweating, lacrimation, and salivation. These acute episodes respond dramatically to treatment with oral corticosteroids.[50]

Flushing in the carcinoid syndrome may be produced by palpation of liver metastases or abdominal tumor masses, alcohol ingestion, enemas, emotional stress, and sudden changes in body temperature. Cutaneous metastases from carcinoids are not common.

Serotonin (5-hydroxytryptamine) was initially considered to be the humoral agent responsible for the carcinoid syndrome. Serotonin could be extracted from the tumors, and its metabolite, 5-HIAA, was present in excess amounts in the urine of affected individuals. However, it has not been possible to demonstrate increased plasma or urine levels of serotonin and its metabolites in most patients during the spontaneous flush. Serotonin administered intravenously to carcinoid patients or to normal individuals does not consistently produce flushing. Reactions that are produced differ qualitatively from typical carcinoid flushes. The intravenous injection of epinephrine can produce typical carcinoid flushing without altering the hepatic venous blood level of serotonin in most carcinoid patients.

Current investigation implicates the vasoactive kinin peptides in the production of the carcinoid flush.[53] Epinephrine causes the release of kinins during flushing. The enzyme kallikrein, isolated from carcinoid tumors, converts kininogen, an alpha-2 globulin, into lysyl-bradykinin, which is then converted to bradykinin. These two peptides (a decapeptide and nonapeptide, respectively) are highly active compounds which can produce vasodilation, bronchoconstriction, and stimulation of smooth muscle. Synthetic bradykinin causes hypotension and carcinoid flushing when given to normal subjects and to patients with the carcinoid syndrome. Although the kinin system appears to be most important in the production of the carcinoid flush in the majority of patients, Roberts et al.

have recently proposed that histamine may be the principal vasodilator in the small subset of patients whose carcinoid syndrome is caused by metastatic gastric carcinoid. Persistently elevated urinary histamine is characteristic of this subgroup. These investigators were able to eliminate almost completely the attacks of carcinoid flushing in such a patient with the use of histamine H_1, and H_2 receptor antagonists.[55]

As more patients with the carcinoid syndrome were identified and studied, it became apparent that the clinical features of the syndrome varied considerably and that the disorder could be caused by two groups of neoplasms: intestinal carcinoids with hepatic metastases and extraintestinal carcinoids which arose in the bile ducts, pancreas, ovaries, and bronchi. It was also noted that various chemical substances in addition to serotonin were being produced by these tumors: histamine, catecholamines, kinins, and prostaglandins. For these two reasons, it became more appropriate to speak of the "carcinoid spectrum" rather than the "carcinoid syndrome" and to attempt to relate the various signs and symptoms being observed to the interactions of the various biologically active substances being released into the circulation at any one time from these tumors.[54]

The carcinoid spectrum has become more complex since that first conceptual revision because of the varied and mixed endocrine syndromes that have been produced by these tumors. For example, in one case, a carcinoid of the stomach with liver metastases produced bilateral adrenal hyperplasia, increased excretion of 17-ketosteroids and 17-hydroxysteroids, and the *clinical* features of Cushing's disease in addition to the carcinoid flush. The combination of these two syndromes has also been produced by a bronchial carcinoid and by an ovarian tumor of undetermined type.[37, 56] Hyperpigmentation of the skin, lips, and plantar and palmar creases was reported in a patient with the carcinoid flushing produced by a bronchial adenoma.[50] This was probably an instance of the tumor also producing ACTH- and MSH-like peptides, but this possibility was not considered.

As more such cases were reported it became clear that the carcinoid tumors could be associated with the carcinoid spectrum, the ectopic ACTH syndrome, a combination of the two disorders, or with other polypeptide hormone–secreting syndromes. This last group included carcinoid tumors secreting MSH-like peptides, glucagon, gastrin, vasoactive intestinal peptide (VIP), insulin, secretin, calcitonin, and antidiuretic hormone. An enormous variety of humoral syndromes both pure and in mixture were being reported in ever-increasing numbers. Individual carcinoid tumors were shown to be capable of producing more than one peptide or amine or a combination of both chemical species.[57]

It is frequently difficult to distinguish histologically between bronchial carcinoids, thymic carcinomas, and oat cell carcinomas when they are associated with the ectopic ACTH syndrome. Medullary carcinoma of the thyroid is histologically similar to oat cell carcinoma, carotid and aortic body tumors, carcinoids, and pancreatic islet cell tumors. Islet cell tumors of the pancreas and carcinoids in general are very difficult to distinguish histologically from each other, and the term "carcinoid–islet cell" tumor was coined by Weichert for this reason.[58] Histochemistry and electron microscopic studies have further strengthened the close relationship among these apparently diverse tumors. All of these tumors contain argentaffin granules in the cytoplasm and neurosecretory granules characteristic of argentaffin cells as defined by histochemistry and electron microscopy, respectively. The secretory granules are similar to those in cells of the juxtaglomerular apparatus and anterior pituitary that are known to secrete polypeptides.[58] All these observations, both clinical and laboratory, have suggested a common cellular origin for these seemingly different tumors.

A current unifying concept to explain the various ectopic humoral syndromes has as its cornerstone the APUD cell.[57, 59] The APUD cell has the following cytochemical properties: normal *A*mino content (5-hydroxytryptamine), high amine *P*recursor *U*ptake (DOPA, 5-hydroxytryptophan), and high content of amino acid *D*ecarboxylases.* In addition, these cells have been shown to be capable of secreting a variety of biologically active amines and polypeptide hormones discussed above, either singly or in combination.[57, 59] The APUD cells of the adult animal include the chromaffin cells of the adrenal medulla and paraganglia, the intestinal enterochromaffin system, the ganglia of the autonomic nervous system and chemoreceptor system, the corticotrophs and melanotrophs of the anterior pituitary, the cells in the hypothalamus producing posterior pituitary hormones, the thyroid C cells which secrete calcitonin, the beta, alpha, and D cells of the pancreas which are responsible for insulin, glucagon, and gastrin secretions, respectively, and the bronchial Kulchitsky cells. The technique of formaldehyde vapor–induced fluorescence is used to demonstrate intracellular amine stores in APUD cells, and immunochemical methods are used to demonstrate the presence of specific polypeptide hormones.[57]

The technique of formaldehyde vapor–induced fluorescence was used in embryologic studies to determine whether the precursors of the APUD cells could be found in the embryo, and such cells were identified in the neural crest. These neural crest cells were seen to migrate into the adrenal medulla, the ultimobranchial bodies which later were incorporated into the thyroid as C cells, the carotid bodies, and the foregut which gives rise to the stomach, duodenum, and pancreas. They were also seen to invade the bronchi and trachea which develop in the midst of the endocrine glands that develop from the foregut. The adenohypophysis is derived entirely from the neuroectoderm, predominantly from the ventral neural ridge. Part of the same neuroectoderm is incorporated into the developing hypothalamus.[60, 61]

However, the formaldehyde vapor–induced fluorescence technique shows only that neural crest cells have moved into the areas subsequently populated by adult APUD cells. This observation does not unequivocally establish that neural crest cells are the precursors of adult APUD cells; because the synthesis of polypeptide hormones probably does not begin until after the migrating neural crest cells have reached their destination. It has not been possible to apply both immunochemical and formaldehyde vapor–induced fluorescence techniques to study embryonic cells as one has been able to do with the adult APUD cell. The possibility exists that the fluorescent cells that migrate into an organ may not be those that later secrete specific polypeptides.

---

*High amine storage is a characteristic of these cells. Proliferating cells of many different types can take up the amino acid precursors of fluorogenic amines, but they are rapidly metabolized and not stored.[60]

The APUD cell concept implies that all cells of this series are derived from the definitive neural crest or from cells that arise earlier in the region of the ventral neural ridge or presumptive neural crest. Evidence in favor of this concept is twofold. Pearse, Polak, LeDouarin, and Le Lièvre established, by heterospecific grafting techniques in embryos in conjunction with anti-calcitonin immunofluorescence and formaldehyde vapor–induced fluorescence, that the thyroid C cells and the carotid body cells are derived from the neural crest.[62] Tischler et al. linked the APUD cells to a neural origin in a different way. He grew cells from a variety of tumors in culture and showed that he could produce action potentials in single cells by direct electrical stimulation and by iontophoretic application of acetylcholine which stimulates catecholamine secretion in vivo. The cells tested were from oat cell carcinomas, human medullary thyroid carcinomas, bronchial carcinoids, human neuroblastomas, and pituitary adenomas. Such action potentials have been observed in nerve and muscle but not in other cell types.[61]

Evidence against the common origin of APUD cells from the neural crest stems from studies related to the endocrine polypeptide APUD cells of the adult gastrointestinal tract and pancreas. Embryologic experiments employing heterospecific grafting techniques have failed to demonstrate neural crest cells localizing in gut epithelium. These same experiments showed that neural crest cells migrating into the developing foregut formed Auerbach and Meissner plexuses.[63] The origins of the gastrointestinal and pancreatic APUD cells remain to be determined.

Some medical writers have advocated using the word "apudoma" with a qualifying adjective for the secretory product rather than applying a histologic term to describe the tumors in these humoral syndromes, e.g., gastrin- and ACTH-secreting apudoma.[59] A functional rather than a morphologic diagnosis is sometimes more appropriate. The apudomas represent a series of tumors whose constituent cells may reproduce either the peptide-synthesizing or the amine-synthesizing properties, or both, of the cells of the APUD series. Neither the secreted amines nor any polypeptide hormone associated with these tumors is really "inappropriate" if it is accepted that the cells are totipotential with regard to amine and polypeptide synthesis because of their hypothesized common ancestry in the neural crest. The APUD cell concept has made the uniglandular and polyglandular neoplastic syndromes more understandable.

The main endocrine neoplasms or apudomas therefore include the following: corticotrophinoma (Cushing's syndrome), insulinoma, glucagonoma, gastrinoma (Zollinger-Ellison syndrome), calcitoninoma, enteroglucagonoma, VIPoma (watery diarrhea, hypokalemia, and achlorhydria — Verner-Morrison syndrome), secretinoma, pheochromocytoma, chemodectoma, carcinoid, bronchial adenoma, and oat cell tumor. Melanoma is a nonhumoral-secreting apudoma.

In addition to these single endocrine neoplasms there are a group of polyglandular endocrine neoplastic syndromes that become more understandable when thought of in terms of the APUD concept. Familial syndromes of multiple endocrine neoplasia (MEN) are known to occur in at least three separate clinical patterns. MEN type 1 (also known as multiple endocrine adenomatosis) is characterized by tumors of the pituitary gland, pancreatic islets, adrenal cortex, and parathyroid glands.[64] MEN type 2 is characterized by neoplasia of the C cells of the thyroid (medullary carcinoma), adrenal medulla (pheochromocytoma), and parathyroid glands (chief cell hyperplasia or adenoma).[65-67] MEN type 3 features medullary carcinoma of the thyroid and pheochromocytoma in association with a marfanoid habitus and multiple mucosal neuromas.[68, 69] Parathyroid hyperplasia is less frequent in type 3 than in types 1 and 2, and the mucocutaneous lesions and marfanoid habitus do not occur in MEN type 2. Sipple syndrome is an eponym frequently applied to MEN type 2. Multiple mucosal neuromas (MMN) syndrome is used by many authors to describe MEN type 3. In all 3 MEN syndromes, the disease is transmitted in a dominant autosomal fashion, although there are many sporadic cases of MEN type 3. The associated pheochromocytomas are usually bilateral in these syndromes. As of 1975, there were approximately 114 cases of MEN type 1, 105 cases of MEN type 2, and 41 cases of MEN type 3 reported in the literature.[68]

The parathyroid gland does not belong to the APUD series of cells. Therefore the frequent presence of parathyroid hyperplasia or adenoma needs to be explained in some other way. Pearse believed it was caused by direct stimulation by some as-yet-unidentified polypeptide product, or indirectly, as a response to the secretion of calcitonin produced by the medullary thyroid cancers (C cells).[59] Similarly, the adrenal cortical hyperplasia or adenoma is probably a secondary effect of trophic hormones from the other tumors associated with MEN type 1. However, patients with MEN type 2 have been reported with parathyroid hyperplasia in the presence of normal calcitonin levels.[67, 70] Patients with MEN type 3 have a very low incidence of parathyroid disease in spite of an almost uniform presence of medullary carcinoma of the thyroid, which is always associated with elevated calcitonin levels. These observations strongly suggest that the development of parathyroid hyperplasia or adenoma is not directly related to the medullary carcinoma of the thyroid in these syndromes.[68]

MEN type 2 or Sipple syndrome differs from MEN type 3 (MMN syndrome) in three important ways. In MEN type 2, the incidence of parathyroid hyperplasia or adenoma is at least 50 per cent, whereas in MEN type 3, only one of 41 patients had hyperparathyroidism. Gastrointestinal tract abnormalities were present in about one third of the 41 patients with MEN type 3 in the form of intestinal ganglioneuromatosis. This does not appear to be a feature of MEN type 2. The major distinction, of course, is the mucocutaneous lesions which occur only in MEN type 3. Although there are still investigators who lump MEN type 2 and MEN type 3 together, the current evidence strongly indicates that they should be kept separate.

The individual with the multiple mucosal neuromas syndrome is recognized by his characteristic facies (Fig. 1–13). The lips are thickened and slightly everted, with the upper lip being more affected than the lower. The surface of the lips may appear bumpy. The eyelids may also be thickened and slightly everted. The swelling and irregular surfaces of the lips and lids are produced by deep and superficial neuroma formation. The superficial neuromas are generally whitish to pink, one- to five-mm sessile papules that can be found on the lips, in the commissures, and on the tip or anterior half of the tongue (Fig. 1–14). Less frequently, they may be present on the buccal mucosa, gingivae, palate, and pharynx. Examina-

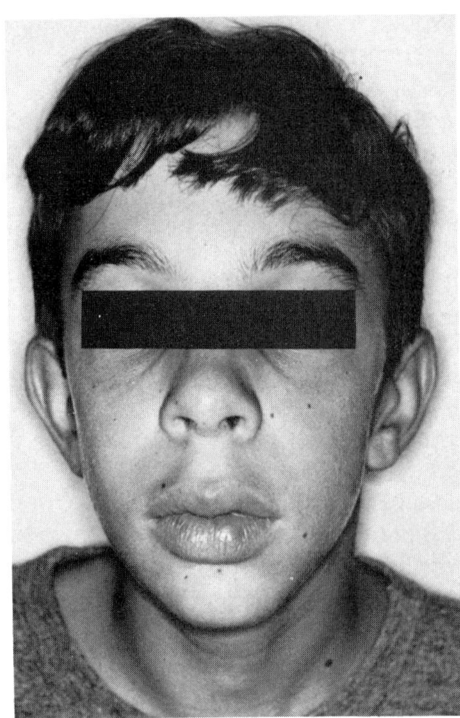

Figure 1–13. Multiple mucosal neuromas syndrome. Characteristic facies.

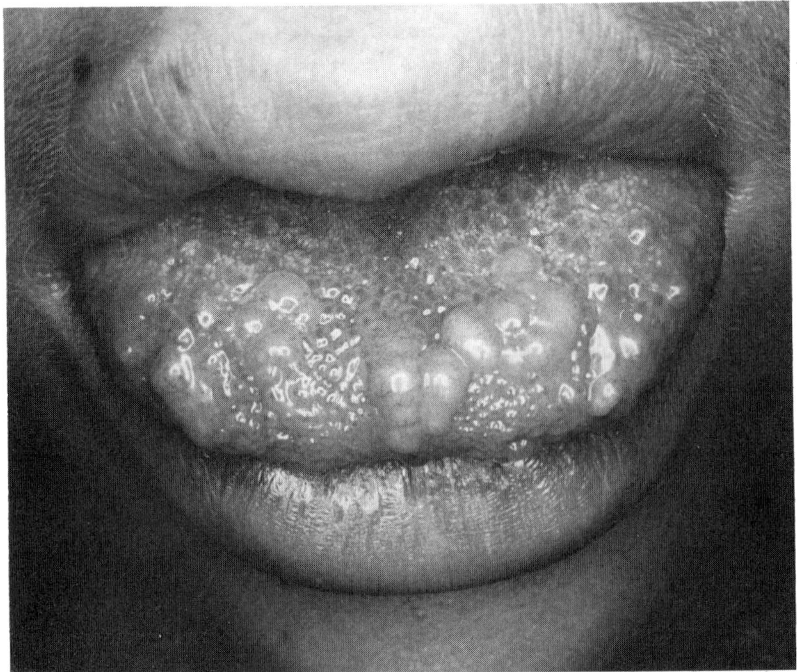

Figure 1–14. Multiple mucosal neuromas syndrome. Superficial neuromas on tongue.

tion of the eyes with a slit lamp may show easily detected thickened corneal nerves. Neuromas also develop on the conjunctivae and corneas.[68, 71] Associated prognathism is not frequent, but when it occurs, patients have been described as having an "acromegalic" facial appearance. The facies is otherwise so striking that unrelated individuals with this syndrome could be mistaken to be members of the same family.

Most of the patients have had a "marfanoid" habitus: slender body build with sparsity of body fat and poor development of body musculature. The extremities appear long and thin and sometimes there is muscular hypotonicity and increased laxity of joints. Some patients have had dorsal kyphosis, pectus excavatum, pes cavus, and a high arched palate. Ectopia lentis and aortic abnormalities are not present as in Marfan's syndrome, and homocystinuria has been excluded in the few patients in whom this was considered.[68]

Intestinal ganglioneuromatosis occurred in about one third and persistent diarrhea in one fourth of the patients in Khairi's series.[68] Some investigators believe that secretion of prostaglandins, serotonin, or calcitonin by the medullary carcinoma of the thyroid rather than neural abnormalities may be the most important factor in the pathogenesis of the diarrhea. Other gastrointestinal abnormalities associated with this syndrome have included diverticulosis, megacolon, and intestinal hypertrophy in 6 to 18 per cent of the patients about whom adequate information was available.[68]

An unusual abnormality in this syndrome is the absence of the axon flare when histamine is injected intradermally. Although there is no explanation for this, a generalized abnormality of neural structure or function is a reasonable speculation considering the extensive neuromatous hamartomas that are present in the skin and gastrointestinal tract.[71]

The main concern in both MEN type 2 and MEN type 3 is the development of medullary carcinoma of the thyroid. Since this tumor secretes calcitonin one can identify subjects at risk before metastases occur. Total thyroidectomy is indicated because the cancers are multifocal in origin.[69] Screening of family members for elevated plasma calcitonin levels is mandatory in the management of MEN type 2 disease. It is currently being performed at 6- to 12-month intervals.[72]

Gagel et al. have shown that the years of greatest risk for the development of medullary thyroid cancer in MEN type 2 is 8 to 18 years.[72] The same risk appears to hold true for MEN type 3. In Khairi's review, 24 of 38 patients had their thyroid cancer diagnosed between 8 and 18 years of age.[68] One patient was diagnosed at four years. However, six were diagnosed between 19 and 25 years of age and seven between 26 and 42 years. These data represent retrospective reviews of the literature. Prospective screening of these older individuals undoubtedly would have detected the cancers at an earlier age. According to Gorlin, only family members with the characteristic facies and mucosal lesions need to be studied for the development of the associated malignancies on the basis of currently available genealogic data.[73] In Khairi's review, over 90 per cent of individuals with MEN type 3 eventually developed thyroid cancer.

The distinctive facies of patients with MEN type 3 develops in the first few years of life, with the earliest changes having been observed in one patient at four weeks of age.[69] Thus, virtually every patient with

MEN type 3 should be able to be diagnosed early enough to detect medullary carcinoma of the thyroid before it metastasizes.

Pheochromocytomas developed in about 50 per cent of patients with MEN type 3 in Khairi's series. In two thirds of those affected, the pheochromocytomas were bilateral. These tumors have a higher prevalence in MEN type 2 where they are also bilateral in about 70 per cent of patients.[65] In both syndromes the pheochromocytomas are multifocal in the adrenal medulla. Extra-adrenal locations have occurred but are not common.[74]

Neurofibromatosis (von Recklinghausen's disease) is a member of the apudomas also. Multiple Schwann cell tumors develop in association with cafe-au-lait spots and sometimes with pheochromocytomas.

The glucagon-secreting alpha cell tumor of the pancreas is a recently described apudoma (glucagonoma syndrome). This disorder displays a spectacular and unique eruption. Wilkinson proposed the term *necrolytic migratory erythema* for this rash and it is an apt one.[75]

As a historical note, it is worth citing two cases reported by Stephen Rothman in 1925 and Becker, Kahn, and Rothman in 1942 that may have been the first examples of this syndrome reported in the literature.[76, 77] Rothman believed the skin was capable of destroying metastatic tumor cells and that inflammation and pruritus resulted from this defensive action. Metastases that eventually developed in pruritic inflammatory skin lesions were offered as evidence to support this theory. Rothman reported two cases with unusual inflammatory dermatoses which he believed were examples of this hypothesis.

In the first case[76] a markedly pruritic erythematous eruption which appeared on exposed areas and developed into an exfoliative dermatitis was seen in a patient who later died of gastric cancer. Ulcerations developed in areas of exfoliative dermatitis which quickly healed without therapy. Rothman believed that the spontaneous development and rapid healing of these ulcers suggested that they may have represented the defense mechanism of the skin against invading tumor cells. The rapid appearance and disappearance of the ulcerations may actually have been the superficial denudation seen in necrolytic migratory erythema. Although there was no pancreatic tumor found in this patient, the gastric cancer might have been a malignant carcinoid tumor arising in the stomach.

The other patient,[77] however, is clearly an example of the glucagonoma syndrome, now that the clinical features of this entity have been delineated.

This second patient developed an erythematous weeping vesicular eruption on the dorsa of the feet. This eruption slowly extended up the limbs and eventually involved the entire body at various times. Purpura and superficial denudation resembling a chemical burn were present. A biopsy of the skin showed nonspecific inflammation, and the patient eventually died with multiple venous thromboses. Autopsy revealed an islet cell tumor of the body and tail of the pancreas and thromboses of the inferior vena cava, left iliac, femoral, and common iliac veins.

In retrospect, a patient who was seen at the Yale-New Haven Hospital in 1957 was most likely also an example of this syndrome.

A 60-year-old white woman developed pulmonary tuberculosis in 1957. Shortly after she began therapy with PAS and INH, a weeping vesicular eruption appeared on the legs and slowly extended to her groin, abdomen, and chest. Urticarial plaques with fine scale and vesiculation were present over the chest. Oral corticosteroids suppressed the eruption, but it returned when the medication was discontinued. The differential diagnosis included contact dermatitis, nummular eczema, and seborrheic dermatitis with autoeczematization. Biopsies of the skin revealed nonspecific inflammation. A malabsorption syndrome with diarrhea, steatorrhea, and severe hypokalemia developed during the second year of her illness and was attributed to chronic pancreatitis. After an illness of two years, the patient died. Autopsy revealed an islet cell carcinoma of the body and tail of the pancreas with hepatic metastases.

In 1966, McGavran et al. reported the case of a woman with a bullous and eczematous eruption of the hands, feet, and legs which defied a specific diagnosis.[78] She was discovered to have a glucagon-containing alpha cell tumor of the pancreas in association with abnormally elevated serum levels of glucagon. Church and Crane recognized a similar case in 1967.[79] The validity and importance of the syndrome were established in 1971 when Wilkinson presented a case which had previously been diagnosed as pustular psoriasis with features of epidermal necrolysis. Church suggested an alternate diagnosis when he noted the similarity between this case and his own. Wilkinson's patient was surgically explored and found to have a carcinoma of the head of the pancreas with hepatic metastases.[80, 81] Approximately 22 cases have now been reported.[82, 83]

Characteristically, the eruption is widespread, with the severest areas of involvement being on the abdomen, groins, perineum, thighs, and buttocks (Plate 3*A*, *B*, *E*). The legs, feet, and hands can also be involved, and most patients have perioral lesions as well. The eruption waxes and wanes in intensity, but there can be intervals of complete remission lasting weeks or months. The eruption begins with patches of intense erythema that may be angular, annular, or highly irregular in outline. Flaccid vesicles and bullae develop over the surface, but their presence is sometimes difficult to appreciate because of their extensive superficiality. However, they break quickly, leaving denudation and crusts behind. The patches of erythema extend with flaccid vesicles, bullae, or simply a collarette of desquamating skin on the active margins (Plate 3*E*, and Fig. 1–15). The centers of the lesions heal, with hyperpigmentation sometimes being left behind. Circinate and polycyclic lesions frequently develop from the merging patches of erythema. In a few cases the rash has had the appearance of eczema craquelé (erythema with fine fissuring) Plate 3*C* and Fig. 1–16). Usually individual lesions run a course of 7 to 14 days, and typically one finds lesions in all stages of development in a patient. The perioral lesions are also characterized by patches of erythema with crusting or peripheral scaling. In a number of individuals, pressure, friction, or trauma has initiated or aggravated the eruption. In two patients, perforation of the ear lobes resulted from the clip of an earring and the rubber band of a hair net. The investigators wondered whether dermal fragility was a factor in this entity, because at the time the eruption was not present on the ears.[84]

Histologically, there is marked intercellular edema in the upper layers of the epidermis in association with swelling of the epidermal cells themselves. In some instances a hydropic degeneration of the superficial epidermal cells can be found (Figs. 1–17 and 1–18). This marked edema

PLATE 3

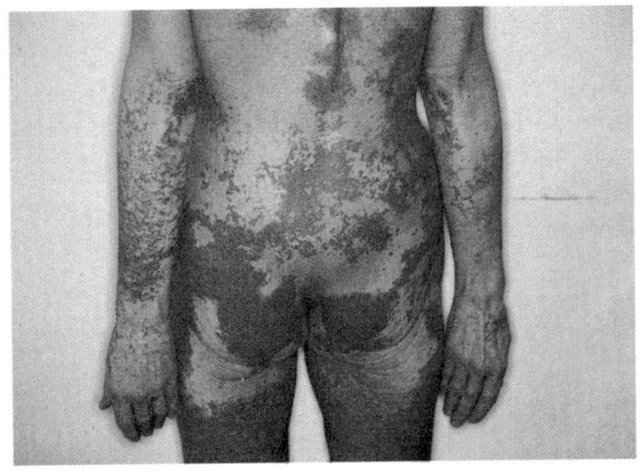

A, Glucagonoma. Migratory necrolytic erythema.

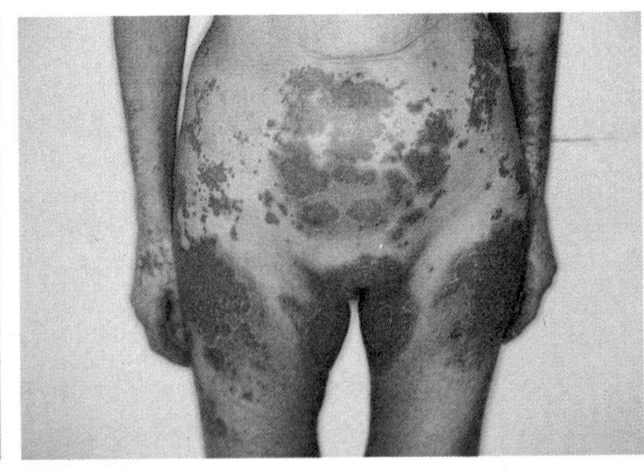

B, Glucagonoma. Migratory necrolytic erythema.

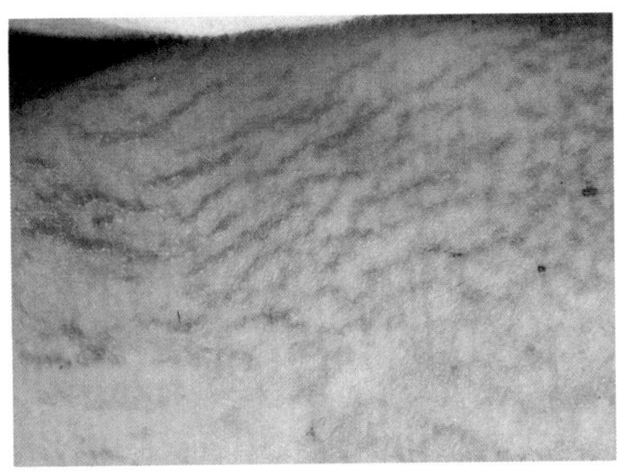

C, Glucagonoma. Eczema craquelé–type lesions.

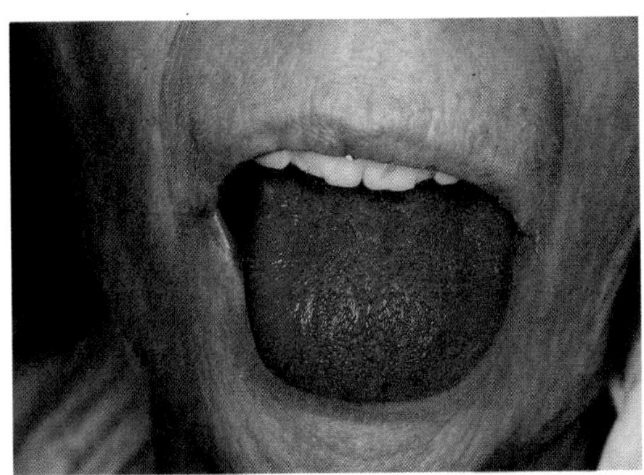

D, Glucagonoma. Beefy red tongue.

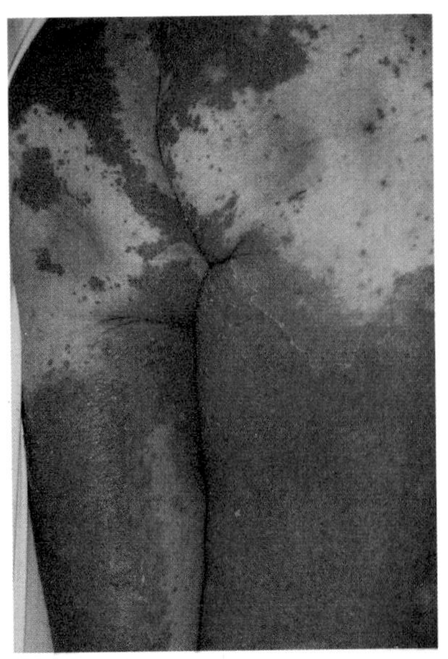

E, Glucagonoma. Migratory necrolytic erythema with peripheral collarette desquamation.

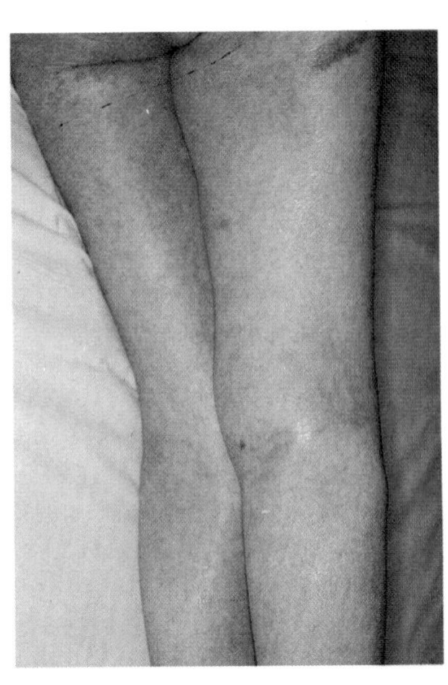

F, Glucagonoma. Necrolytic erythema resolving after diiodohydroxyquin.

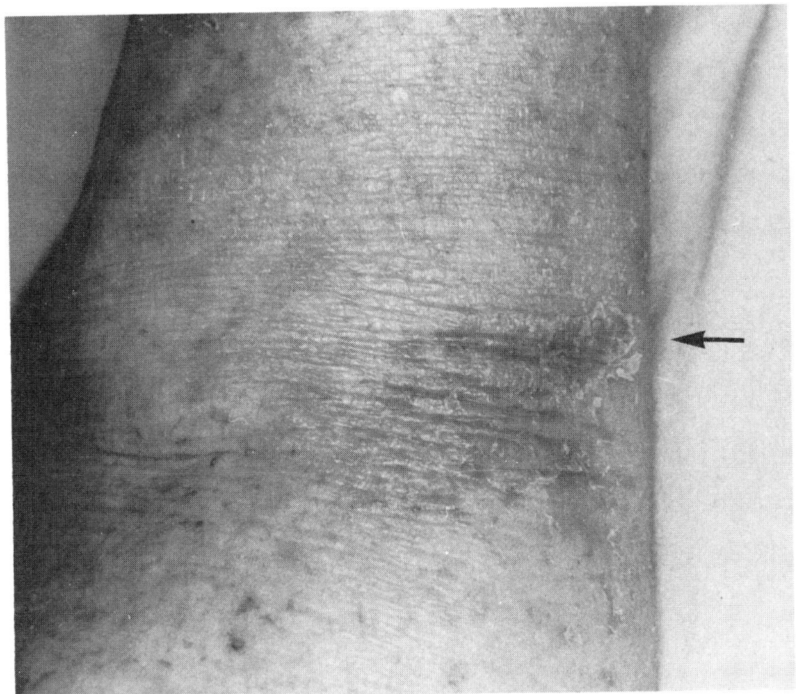

Figure 1-15. Glucagonoma syndrome. Erythema with collarette of desquamating skin (arrow).

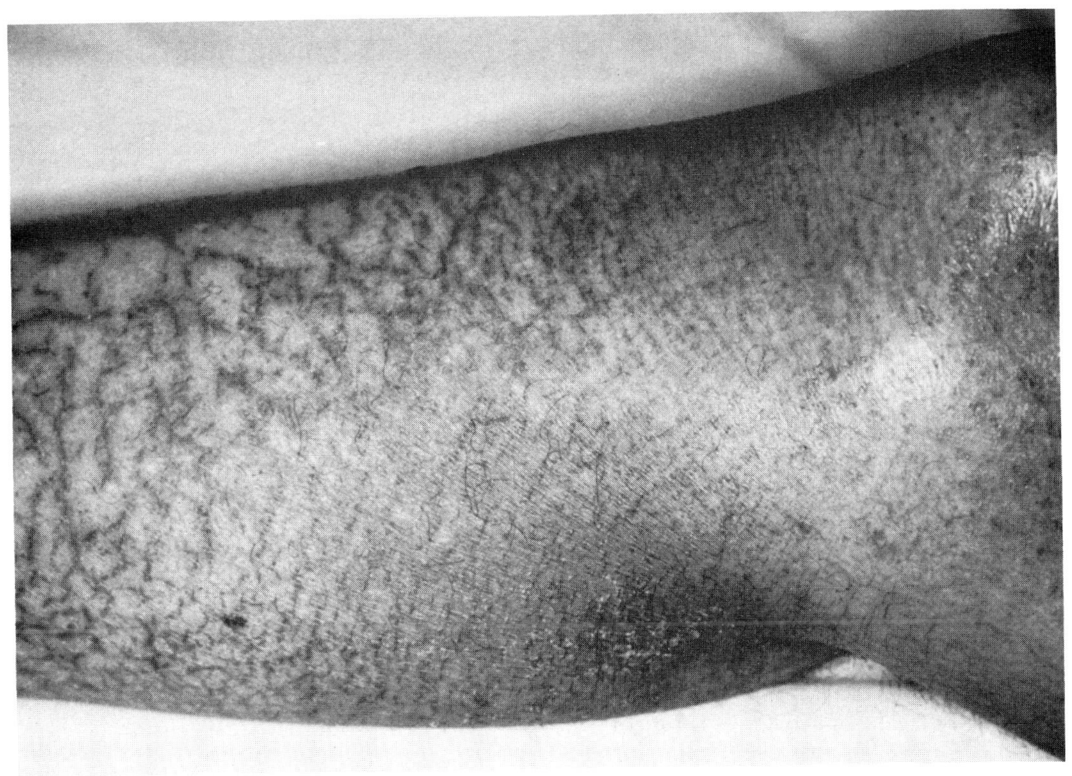

Figure 1-16. Eczema craquelé. Erythema with fine fissuring.

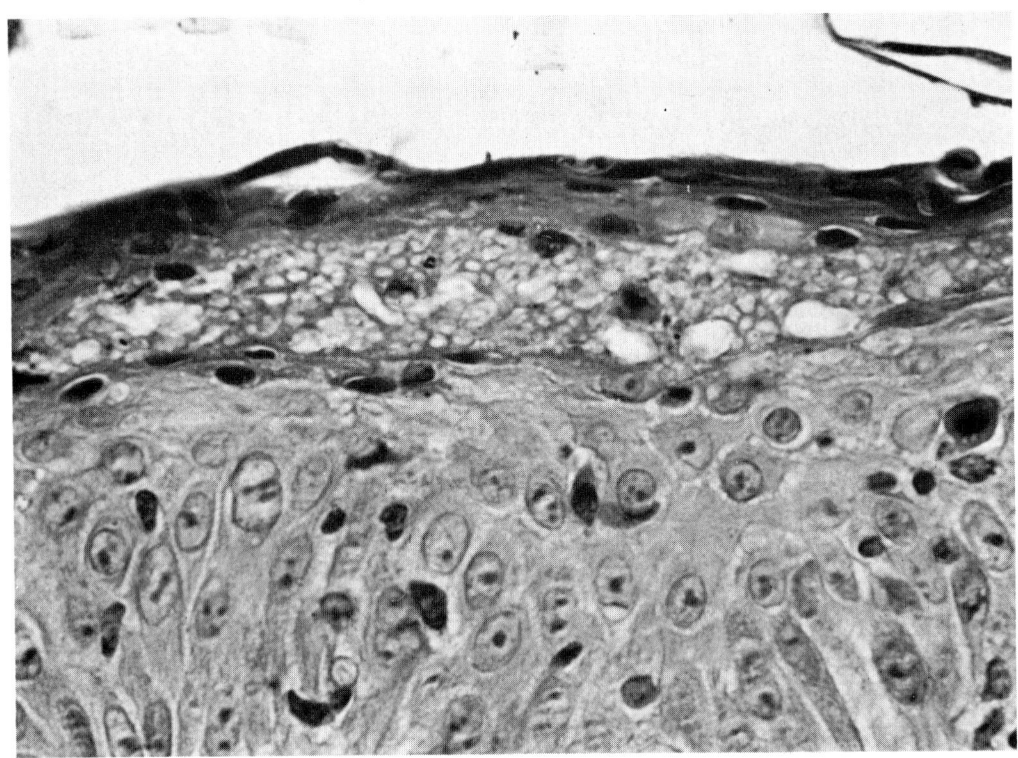

Figure 1-17. Glucagonoma syndrome. Marked intercellular edema in association with hydropic degeneration of epidermal cells.

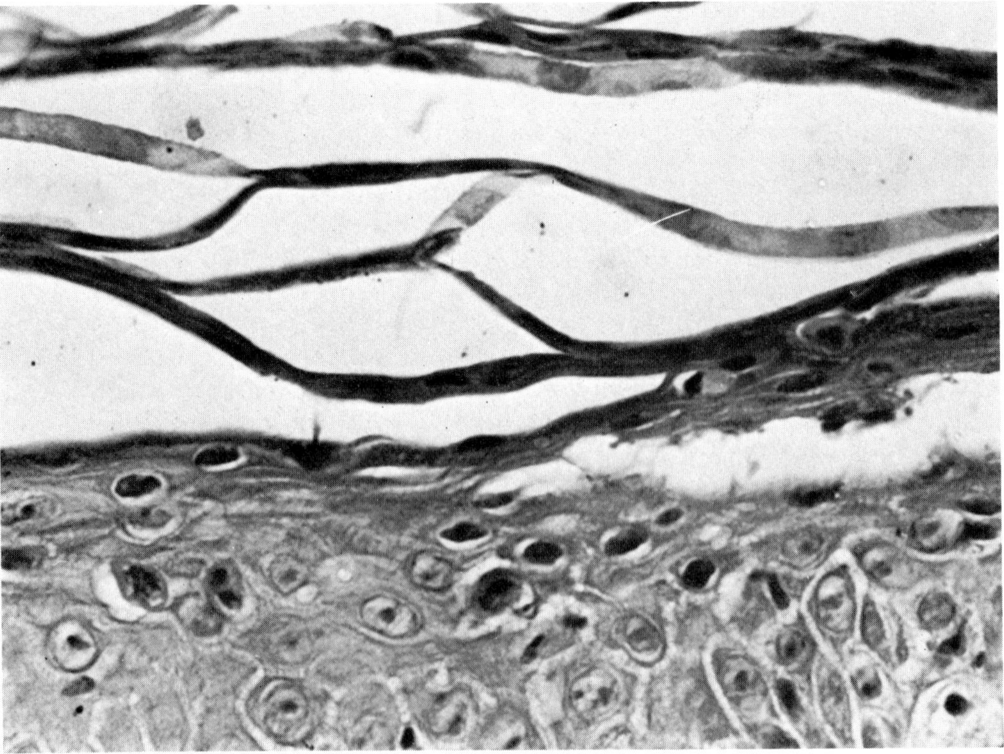

Figure 1–18. Glucagonoma syndrome. Edema and epidermal cell necrosis produce cleavage between epidermis and stratum corneum.

and epidermal cell death leads to cleavage between the epidermis and the stratum corneum, accounting for the development of flaccid vesicles and bullae and the collarette of scale. There is a minimal infiltrate of inflammatory cells in the dermis.[81, 85]

The eruption responds dramatically to oral diiodohydroxyquin, just as the rash of acrodermatitis enteropathica does (Plate 3*E, F*). However, unlike acrodermatitis enteropathica, which is produced by zinc deficiency, the serum zinc level in the glucagonoma syndrome is normal and the eruption does not respond to zinc therapy.[85]

Besides the distinctive cutaneous findings, patients with this syndrome have a glossitis (red, shiny, smooth tongue) (Plate 3*D*), angular cheilitis, normocytic normochromic anemia, weight loss, and low plasma amino acid levels. In most of the individuals, mild diabetes mellitus and diarrhea have also been present. In all of the patients thus far reported, an alpha cell tumor of the pancreas accompanied by markedly elevated serum glucagon levels has been found. In 62 per cent of the affected individuals the tumors have been metastatic to the liver, and in some there have been local metastases to the spine and adrenal glands. In a few patients, resection of the tumor has resulted in prompt resolution of the eruption, correction of the anemia, restoration of normal glucagon levels in the serum, and weight gain.[85] The alpha cell tumors in general are slowly progressive neoplasms and the courses in these patients have ranged from 4 months to 13 years.

Boden and Owen reported an instance of the glucagonoma syndrome in a 52-year-old man with MEN type 2.[86] The patient had both an islet cell tumor of the pancreas and a calcitonin-producing medullary carcinoma of the thyroid. The glucagonoma syndrome as a variant of MEN disorders is the exception rather than the rule.

The differential diagnosis of the eruption, because of its location and erosive qualities, includes acrodermatitis enteropathica, candidiasis, pemphigus foliaceus, and the annular lesions of pustular psoriasis of von Zumbusch. All of these entities can be easily distinguished from each other by biopsy and culture. The combination of features which superficially suggest toxic epidermal necrolysis and acrodermatitis enteropathica in the same patient should make one consider the glucagonoma syndrome.

Immunoreactive glucagon with a molecular weight of 3500 or 9000 daltons appears to be required for the development of the clinical glucagonoma syndrome. Molecular species of immunoreactive glucagon greater than 9000 daltons may not be fully active biologically.[86] Although the glucagonoma syndrome is associated with a marked elevation of glucagon in the serum, the hormone is probably not directly related to the pathogenesis of the eruption. The rash waxes and wanes in the presence of the tumor, and glucagon applied topically and injected intradermally does not produce any reaction.[84, 87] In two patients, described below, an identical cutaneous eruption both in its clinical and histologic appearance developed in the absence of elevated glucagon levels and pancreatic tumors. In one of the patients, removal of the pancreas was associated with prompt but not permanent disappearance of the eruption.

Mallinson et al. have suggested that glucagon-induced hypoaminoacidemia may be responsible for producing the skin lesions through deprivation so that epidermal proteins cannot be made.[82] Binnick et al.

point out that in acute kwashiorkor, caused by protein malnutrition, superficial bullae may occur and the skin appearance may resemble that of a burn.[85]

We have recently seen two additional examples of this syndrome and have been told of a third, all of which contribute additional information about this entity.

The first patient was a 50-year-old woman with classic Zollinger-Ellison syndrome (gastrin-producing islet cell tumor of the pancreas), whose disease ran a slowly deteriorating course over six years. During most of her illness she had recurring episodes of a widespread dermatitis that had the distribution characteristic of the glucagonoma rash and the appearance of eczema craquelé (Plate 3*C*, Fig. 1–15): patches of erythema with dryness and linear fissuring of the skin. Some areas showed patches of erythema with a collarette of desquamating skin. The eruption was present during the summer months and sometimes, but not always, responded to therapy with topical corticosteroids and lubrication. Several biopsies showed a nonspecific dermatitis. Serum zinc levels were normal. Serum glucagon levels were markedly elevated. This patient also had the typical changes of glossitis seen in this syndrome. At autopsy, there were widespread hepatic metastases from the islet cell tumor of the pancreas. No studies were performed on the tumor tissue, but we believe this case represents an instance of an islet cell tumor producing both gastrin and glucagon.

The second case is that of a 42-year-old woman with a 20-year history of anemia, weight loss, and watery diarrhea. In 1972, she was diagnosed as probably having celiac sprue on the basis of her symptoms, a small bowel biopsy which showed partial villous atrophy, and abnormally low levels of serum albumin, carotene, and potassium. She was placed on a gluten-free diet without any benefit. Prednisone therapy, oral potassium, vitamin supplementation, and a gluten-free diet resulted in the gradual correction of the anemia, level of serum albumin, abnormal lactose tolerance, and *d*-xylose excretion tests. A repeat small bowel biopsy was interpreted as normal. Her watery diarrhea continued, however. Approximately one year before she was seen at the Yale-New Haven Medical Center she had the following tests performed: pancreatic and superior mesenteric arteriograms and small bowel biopsy, which were normal; serum levels of insulin (fasting), 21 microunits per ml (normal 5–25); gastrin 209 pg/ml (normal <200); glucagon 475 pg/ml (normal 50–250); vasoactive intestinal peptide (VIP) 90 pg/ml (normal<50); no increase in excretion of stool fat. A secretin test revealed low bicarbonate and water output (exocrine hypofunction). Three months later, the assay for VIP revealed a high normal value of 50 pg/ml. Approximately six months before her eruption developed, repeat small bowel biopsies were performed before and after gluten challenge without change in symptoms or histology. In early 1977, approximately four months prior to the development of a generalized eruption the patient developed a hemorrhagic papule that evolved into a superficial ulceration on the left leg. It healed spontaneously within three to four weeks and no definitive diagnosis was made. Three months later she developed a generalized eruption on the right hip, perineum, trunk, legs, and arms. Initially it resembled a mild eczema craquelé but it evolved into many zones of bright erythema which displayed collarettes of desquamation as they extended (Plate 3*A*,*B*,*E*). There was intense burning associated with the eruption. A biopsy showed the characteristic histologic features of migratory necrolytic erythema (Figs. 1–17 and 1–18). She also had a red, smooth tongue.

She was reinvestigated for the presence of a pancreatic tumor by computerized axial tomography and arteriograms but none was found. Several determinations of serum glucagon levels were performed and showed normal levels (78–130 pg/ml). There was no evidence for hypercatabolism, and the secretory rate of glucagon was interpreted to be normal. The only abnormalities found were that somatostatin only partially suppressed glucagon secretion and an oral glucose tolerance test did not lower serum glucagon levels at all. Plasma amino acid levels were abnormally depressed to 25 to 50 per cent of normal values. Serum levels of zinc were normal. Treatment with diiodohydroxyquin produced a prompt and complete clearing of the eruption within one week (Plate 3*E,F*). The patient was explored to search for a pancreatic tumor but none was found. Two thirds of her pancreas was removed and after careful searching of the tissue, tumor was still not found. Surgery was followed by a stormy three-month postoperative course. Diarrhea and low body weight (86 lbs.) still persisted, but she felt stronger and had less diarrhea than before surgery.

Immediately postoperatively, there was a mild exacerbation of her eruption for two to three days, but it subsided without any specific treatment. The patient's skin remained normal without any therapy for an ensuing 11 months. At that point, a few patches of eczema and an eczema craquelé–like eruption developed over the feet and legs. However, it lacked the burning and painful sensations of the original rash. The lesions initially responded to topical steroids. Plasma amino acid levels determined at this time were abnormal and identical to those of one year previously. However, one month later the erythema became worse and a biopsy of the lesions showed the characteristic necrolytic changes at the junction of the epidermis and stratum corneum. Treatment was reinstituted with diiodohydroxyquin and the eruption was brought under control. During the next two years, the patient continued to have mild diarrhea and low body weight. She required continuous treatment with diiodohydroxyquin for control of her skin lesions, which were limited to her feet and lower legs. In the summer of 1980 she began to have difficulty maintaining her abnormally low body weight, resulting in hospitalization in October, 1980, for hyperalimentation. During this admission she developed gastrointestinal bleeding from a duodenal ulcer and died. Postmortem examination revealed no evidence of glucagonoma or other tumors.

In summary, this patient had a 20-year history of an illness thought to be celiac sprue, with suggestive evidence of pancreatic endocrine hyperfunction and exocrine hypofunction one year before developing the characteristic rash of the glucagonoma syndrome. No tumor was found at operation or in the surgical pathology specimen. Serum glucagon levels were normal at the time of surgery. The rash recurred one year later without any significant change in the patient's clinical picture.

This second case and a similar one were reported jointly by Dr. Stephen Katz and his colleagues and ourselves.[87a]

The patient was a 52-year-old woman who had the typical rash of the glucagonoma syndrome accompanied by weight loss and diarrhea. The stools were bulky and frothy. Stool fat was increased. Biopsy showed villous atrophy of the jejunum. Serum levels of zinc and glucagon were normal. No pancreatic tumor was found after thorough study. The bowel disorder improved on a gluten-free diet. A fall led to hospital admission where she developed pneumonia and died. Autopsy showed villous atrophy of the small bowel and focal chronic pancreatitis. No tumor was found.

Thivolet also reported a case of necrolytic migratory erythema without glucagonoma in a 38-year-old man with chronic pancreatitis.[87b] Plasma glucagon levels were not measured, but the histology of the skin lesions were characteristic. Following a cephalic duodenopancreatectomy, the rash disappeared. The length of follow-up was not given and no mention was made whether the eruption eventually reappeared, as it did in our patient 11 months after partial pancreatectomy. These three reports suggest that a normal level of plasma glucagon may be able to exclude pancreatic cancer in patients with this syndrome.

PROLIFERATIVE AND INFLAMMATORY DERMATOSES ASSOCIATED WITH INTERNAL CANCER

A number of dermatologic signs, symptoms, and disorders can be markers of internal cancer, although they are more commonly associated with non-neoplastic states. They have been considered at times to be manifestations of an internal cancer because of a temporal relation in the absence of other detectable causes and because, in a minority of cases, successful eradication of the cancer has resulted in a complete remission of the cutaneous disorder. A number of unusual skin reactions which cannot be classified among known dermatologic entities have also been reported in association with carcinomas. Individuals suffering from one of the following disorders should be examined for a carcinoma if the usual causes are not discovered or if the disorder is unusual in either its clinical appearance or its course.

Generalized pruritus or itching is an uncommon sign of cancer, but it frequently accompanies the lymphomatous diseases, especially Hodgkin's, lymphatic leukemia, and mycosis fungoides. Pruritus occurring with cancer is not as severe, generalized, or intolerable as it is with lymphomas. Cormia believes that the itching of carcinoma occurs primarily on the extremities and trunk and skips from site to site.[88] Hyperpigmentation, which may be diffuse or just accentuated in light-exposed areas, may develop in association with pruritus in individuals with cancer. Excoriated papules produced by a chronic itch-scratch cycle may be present as well. Unexplained pruritus, especially when generalized in an elderly individual, should prompt one to look for cancer or lymphoma. However, often one will find that xerosis (dry skin) associated with winter weather and excessive bathing is responsible for generalized pruritus in the elderly. Other possible etiologies to be excluded are eczema, drug reactions, chronic renal disease, and emotional problems.

Dermatomyositis, to be described in detail in Chapter 7, is associated with carcinoma, and occasionally with lymphoma and melanoma, in 15 to 50 per cent of adults over the age of 40. Carcinoma may involve almost any organ, but the lungs, gastrointestinal tract, and breast are most commonly affected. In children, dermatomyositis has not been associated with malignancy except for three instances which are described on page 313. In a recent review of the literature, Barnes was able to collect 258 cases of dermatomyositis. In 167, there was adequate documentation of the relationship between the diagnosis of dermatomyositis and the onset of cancer and vice versa. Table 1–1 is a summary of her findings.[89]

It is clear from these data that in the majority of patients with dermatomyositis preceding cancer, the discovery of the tumor occurs within the first year. The average is about six months. Likewise, in the majority of patients with cancer antedating dermatomyositis, the latter develops within the first year. The interval between the onset of dermatomyositis

Table 1–1. DERMATOMYOSITIS AND CANCER—TIME INTERVALS*

	Con-current	Within 1 Year	1–2 Years	2–3 Years	3–8 Years	Total No. Cases§
Interval between dermatomyositis and detection of cancer	17†	78 (79%)‡	9 (9%)	6 (6%)	6¶ (6%)	99
Interval between detection of cancer and onset of dermatomyositis		32 (62%)	10 (20%)	5 (10%)	4** (8%)	51

*From Barnes, B. E.: Dermatomyositis and malignancy. A review of the literature. Ann. Intern. Med., *84*:68, 1976.
†Seventeen cases showed concurrent development of cancer and dermatomyositis.
‡Percentage of total cases, exclusive of concurrent cases.
§Total number of cases exclusive of concurrent cases.
¶One individual developed cancer 8 years after the onset of dermatomyositis.
**Two individuals developed dermatomyositis 5 years after the detection of cancer.

and the discovery of cancer was as long as three to eight years in 6 per cent of the patients in Barnes' series. In one patient, the interval was eight years. In this particular case the woman was found to have a carcinoma of the uterus. Following a hysterectomy, the dermatomyositis went into remission and she was able to discontinue all steroid therapy.[90] In one of our patients, the interval between the onset of dermatomyositis and cancer proved to be six years. The neoplasm was discovered following a flu-like syndrome characterized by nausea, diffuse aches, and malaise, which did not resolve after several weeks. Hepatomegaly, an elevated alkaline phosphatase, hypercalcemia, and hypophosphatemia led to the diagnosis of an ectopic parathormone syndrome secondary to hepatic metastases from an APUD cell tumor, whose primary site was not found. These long intervals are best explained by a combination of slow-growing cancer and the development of lymphocyte-mediated striated muscle damage (see Chapter 7). Complete or partial removal of the malignancy may produce a remission of dermatomyositis. A relapse usually indicates either a recurrence of the tumor or metastatic spread.

It is obligatory to search for cancer in adults with dermatomyositis. At times painstaking scrutiny is required. In one of our cases the associated tumor was a transitional cell cancer in the anal area; the tumor had been considered to be a hemorrhoidal tag on two previous examinations. In another patient the tumor was a malignant calcium-encrusted polyp of the bladder. This patient had a known history of bladder gravel and renal stones, and it was during therapy for the urologic problem that the tumor was uncovered. Fulguration of the tumor induced a remission in this patient. In another individual, dermatomyositis appeared one and one-half years after radical mastectomy for breast cancer (Figs. 1–19 and 1–20). Intensive investigation failed to reveal either any signs of recurrence at the surgical site or evidence of metastases. Within three months, however, rapid growth of the tumor occurred in the surgical scar. Biopsy of the normal-appearing surgical scar three months earlier undoubtedly would have revealed cancer in this patient.

Dermatomyositis in adults arises either as a form of connective tissue disease or as a reaction to malignancy. I believe that the presence of Raynaud's phenomenon in the former distinguishes the connective tissue variety from that related to malignancy. In our series of 63 patients, 40

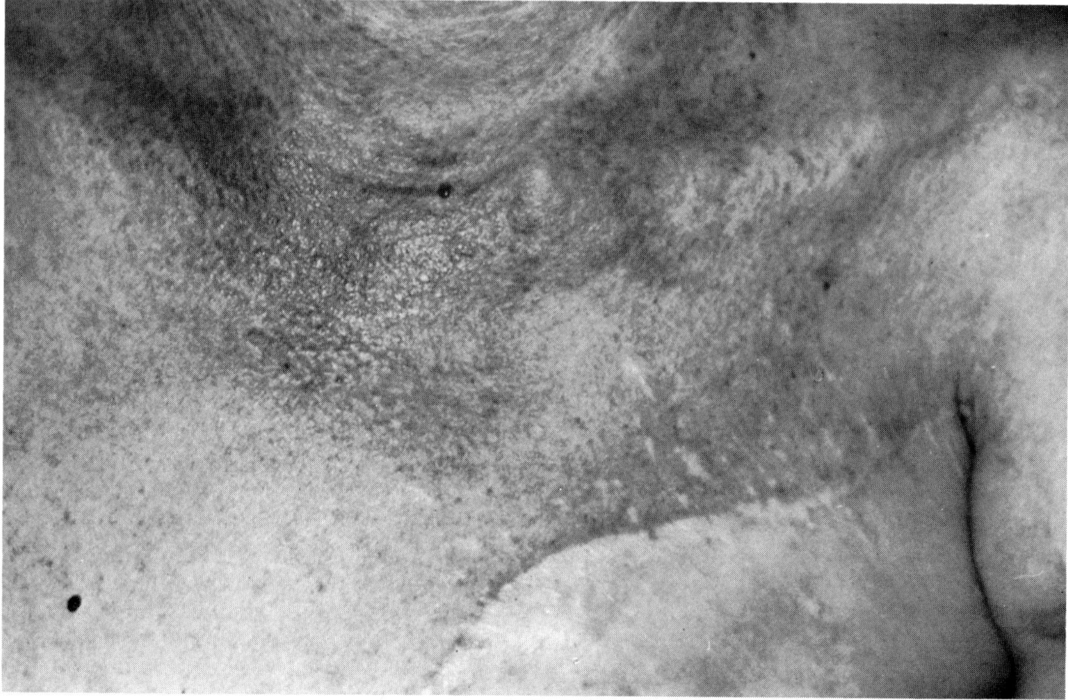

Figure 1–19. Dermatomyositis developed one and one-half years after radical mastectomy for breast cancer in this woman. Note that surgical scar appeared normal.

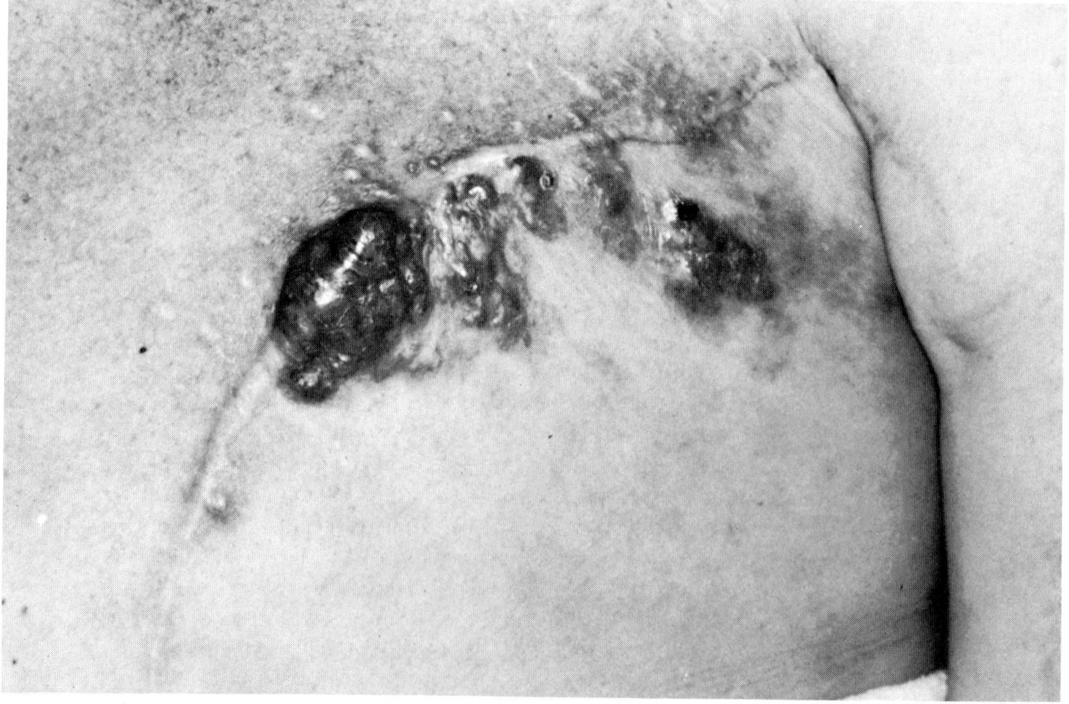

Figure 1-20. Recurrent breast cancer became visible three months after dermatomyositis began in patient shown in Figure 1–19.

were adults and 23 were children. Fifteen of 40 adults (37.5 per cent) over the age of 37 years had an associated malignancy. Raynaud's phenomenon occurred in 5 of 25 adults without cancer and in none of 15 with cancer — an increase of eight individuals in this latter category from the data reported in 1970. The presence of Raynaud's phenomenon in an adult with dermatomyositis may prove to be a way to exclude the presence of an underlying malignancy. In support of this hypothesis, Bohan et al. also found that none of their 13 patients with myositis and cancer had Raynaud's phenomenon. Their group consisted of eight patients with dermatomyositis and five patients with polymyositis.[91] Prospective studies should be able to confirm or deny the usefulness of this observation. Raynaud's phenomenon is usually not associated with childhood dermatomyositis.

A number of musculoskeletal disorders are associated with cancer: *clubbing, hypertrophic osteoarthropathy, pachydermoperiostosis, polyarthritis simulating rheumatoid arthritis, tenosynovitis, and fibrositis*.[92]

Clubbing of the fingers and toes is a well-known manifestation of bronchogenic carcinoma, mesothelioma, and metastatic cancer to the thorax (from the colon, larynx, breast, and ovary); it occurs in 5 to 12 per cent of cases.[93] Metastatic melanoma to the lung has also been reported to be associated with hypertrophic osteoarthropathy. Clubbing may develop insidiously or abruptly and be painless or painful. Hypertrophic osteoarthropathy is the term used for clubbing that is accompanied by subperiosteal new bone formation along the shafts of the tibia, radius, and phalanges. The ankles, knees, wrists, and hands can be painful. With more extensive involvement, new bone formation may occur beneath the periosteum of the iliac crests, ribs, clavicles, and vertebral column. Tenderness to palpation over these areas can be elicited. Aching or burning paresthesias may affect the fingertips. Deep boring and burning pain in the legs may be major complaints. Joint swelling, synovitis, and periarticular swelling can occur with osteoarthropathy. Hyperhidrosis and palmar erythema may be present in addition to the joint pain — a picture simulating early rheumatoid arthritis.

In some patients cutaneous thickening of the forearms and legs produces cylindrical limbs; hyperkeratosis of the palms and soles occurs, and the hand may be shaped like a spade (Figs. 1–21 and 1–22). The facial features may become coarse; a deepening of the facial furrows simulates acromegaly (Fig. 1–23). Pachydermoperiostosis is the term applied to hypertrophic osteoarthropathy with acromegaloid features. Usually it occurs as a familial genetic disorder unassociated with malignant disease, but lung cancer can produce an identical phenocopy.

Thus far there have been no cases of hypertrophic osteoarthropathy associated with a completely extrathoracic malignant tumor. Excision of the intrathoracic tumor, denervation of the lung root, or section of the vagus nerve at the lung root can induce remission of the pain and joint swelling of hypertrophic osteoarthropathy within a few hours after surgery.

Although clubbing and pachydermoperiostosis are associated chiefly with carcinomas, they may also be the presenting signs of Hodgkin's disease. Clubbing is commonly seen with diffuse intestinal lymphoma (alpha heavy chain disease, Mediterranean lymphoma).

Polyarthritis may occur in the absence of osteoarthropathy and

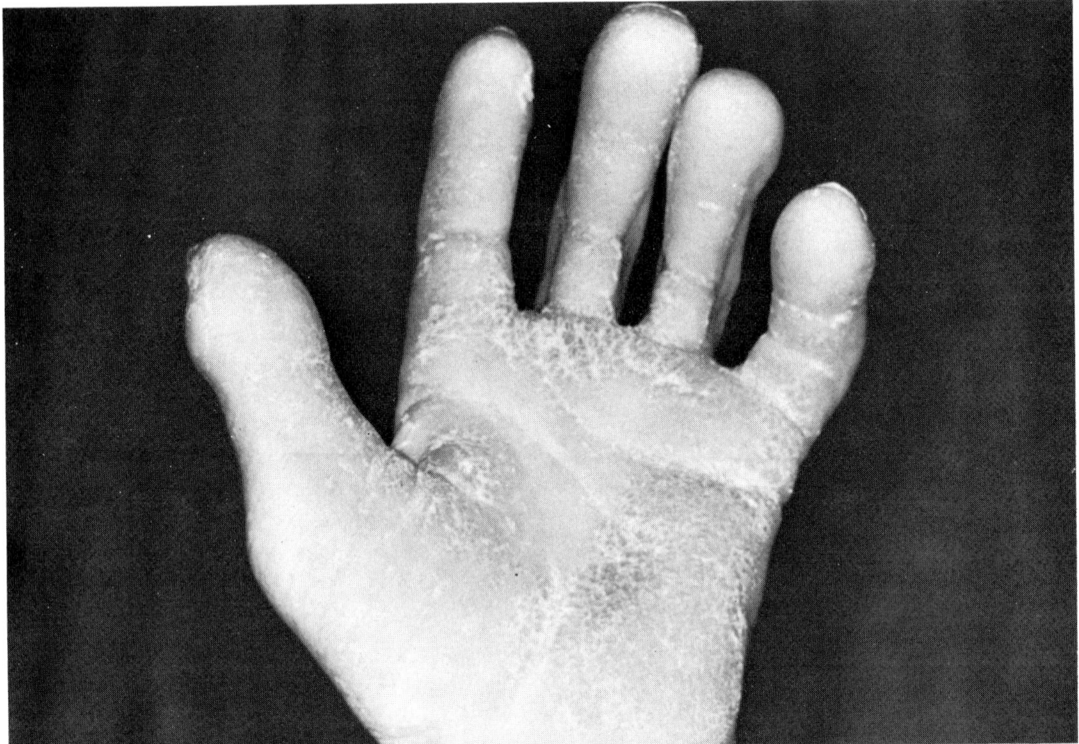

Figure 1-21. Hyperkeratosis of palm, clubbing, and spade-like hand in man with familial osteoarthropathy.

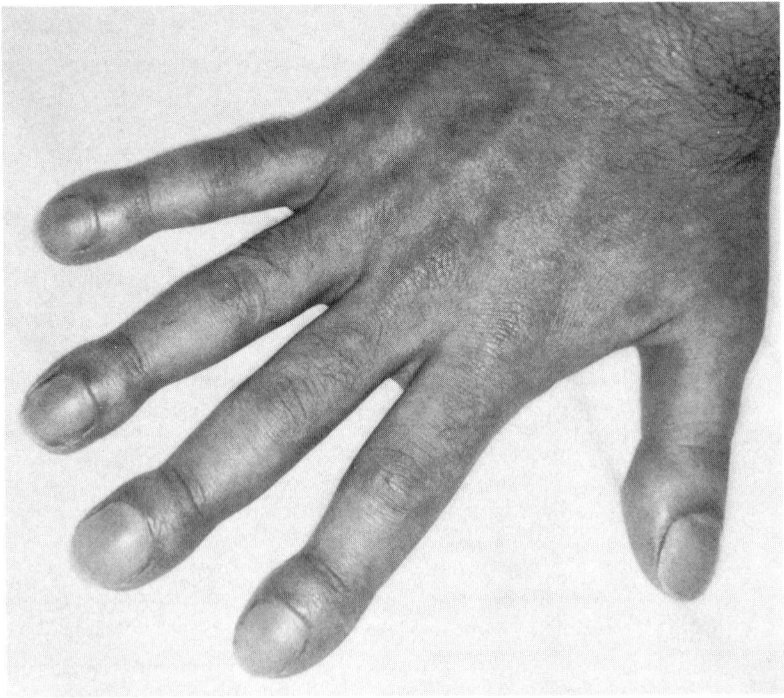

Figure 1–22. Hypertrophic osteoarthropathy with clubbing.

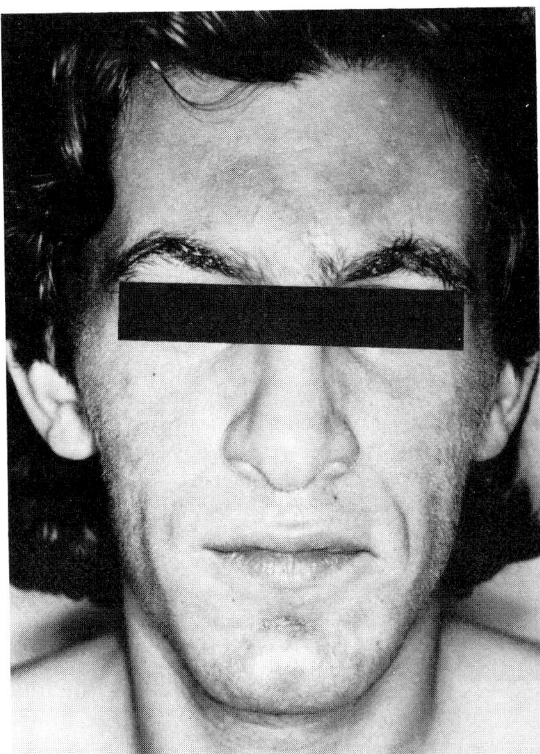

Figure 1–23. Hypertrophic osteoarthropathy with coarse facial features.

clubbing in patients with carcinoma; this situation often mimics rheumatoid arthritis. Mackenzie and Scherbel described 18 cases of rheumatoid arthritis–like disease in association with cancer.[94] In 10 cases the arthritis began abruptly and asymmetrically with relative sparing of the wrists and small joints of the hands. The knees, ankles, and metatarsals were more commonly involved. Rheumatoid nodules were absent, family history for rheumatoid disease was negative, and a positive rheumatoid factor was detected in only one patient. The carcinomas found in these 18 patients were located in the prostate in eight individuals, in the breast in three, and in the bladder in two. Tumors of the bronchus, colon, cervix, liver, and kidney occurred in the rest. The average age of the patients was 64 years, and the arthritis preceded the discovery of cancer by 10 months in 11 of the patients.

Acute monoarthritis, tenosynovitis, and fibrositis syndromes have also been reported in association with cancer, and there may be a mixed picture of musculoskeletal disorders in these patients. As in dermatomyositis, the musculoskeletal disorders remit with successful treatment of the neoplasms and then recur, but not invariably, with a recurrence of the cancer.

Polyarthritis of the small joints of the hands, feet, and elbows, in association with tender subcutaneous nodules resembling Weber-Christian disease, together with fever and eosinophilia, constitute a unique syndrome of pancreatic disease.[95, 96] Although most cases are produced by a functioning acinar cell cancer of the pancreas, identical signs and symptoms occur in acute and chronic pancreatitis.[97] The subcutaneous nodules produced by fat necrosis are often tender and fluctuant with varying shades of erythema. Central necrosis with leakage of oily material can occur. The lesions may be multiple and located anywhere on the body. Markedly elevated serum lipase and amylase are present. Although fat necrosis may occur anywhere, the skin, omentum, and perirenal and pelvic fat are primarily affected. Tumor cells are not found in the areas of fat necrosis, and it seems highly probable that the circulating increased levels of lipase, amylase, possibly trypsin, and other unidentified factors from the pancreas are responsible for this unique syndrome. The arthritis is caused partly by fat necrosis in the periarticular tissue. The tumor is assumed to be a functioning neoplasm because of the presence of zymogen granules.[98, 99] Differentiation from Weber-Christian disease (febrile nonsuppurative panniculitis) is made by the presence of polyarthritis and histologic examination of the areas of fat necrosis (see Chapter 14).

Superficial thrombophlebitis and deep venous thromboses are common medical and surgical problems and are related usually to trauma, debility, prolonged immobilization, and infection. However, *migratory superficial thrombophlebitis* and multiple deep venous thromboses that cannot be readily explained by ordinary causes are likely to be manifestations of cancer (Fig. 1–24). Armand Trousseau drew attention to the clinical association between thrombophlebitis and neoplasia in 1862.[100] Sproul, in 1938, emphasized two points based upon 4000 consecutive autopsies: venous thromboses and carcinomas of the body and tail of the pancreas were often associated, and thromboses developed in the absence of significant inflammation of the vessel wall and in the absence of mural invasion by tumor cells.[101] Sack et al. pointed out, on the basis of their review of the literature, that approximately 77 per cent of the underlying cancers arose in the pancreas, lung, stomach, prostate, or hematopoietic system. Approximately 13 per cent were accounted for by carcinomas of the colon, ovary, gallbladder, and biliary tract.[102] The study of Miller et al. is representative of the many investigations carried out on the hemostatic and coagulation mechanisms in patients with disseminated malignancy.[103] The most common pattern found was a short bleeding time; decrease in both silicone coagulation and partial thromboplastin times; increased tolerance to heparin; marked elevation of plasma levels of Factors I, II, V, VII, IX, and XI; acceleration of the thromboplastin generation; and an increase in platelet number. These types of observations have been the basis for the concept of the *hypercoagulable state* to explain the increased tendency for thrombosis in malignancies.

However, a *defibrination syndrome*, characterized by easy bruising, widespread purpura, and bleeding from multiple sites may also be a feature of malignancy. The most probable mechanism is contact of circulating blood with clot-promoting substances derived from the neoplastic cells or with the cells themselves, which leads to hypofibrinogenemia, reduced levels of Factors V and VIII, decreased levels of platelets, and impaired platelet plug formation.[104, 105] The fibrinolytic system is activated, so that local deposits of fibrin are lysed with resultant accumulation of fibrinogen-fibrin degradation products in the circulation. The causes of altered blood coagulability in patients with malignant disease are complex and not yet completely understood.

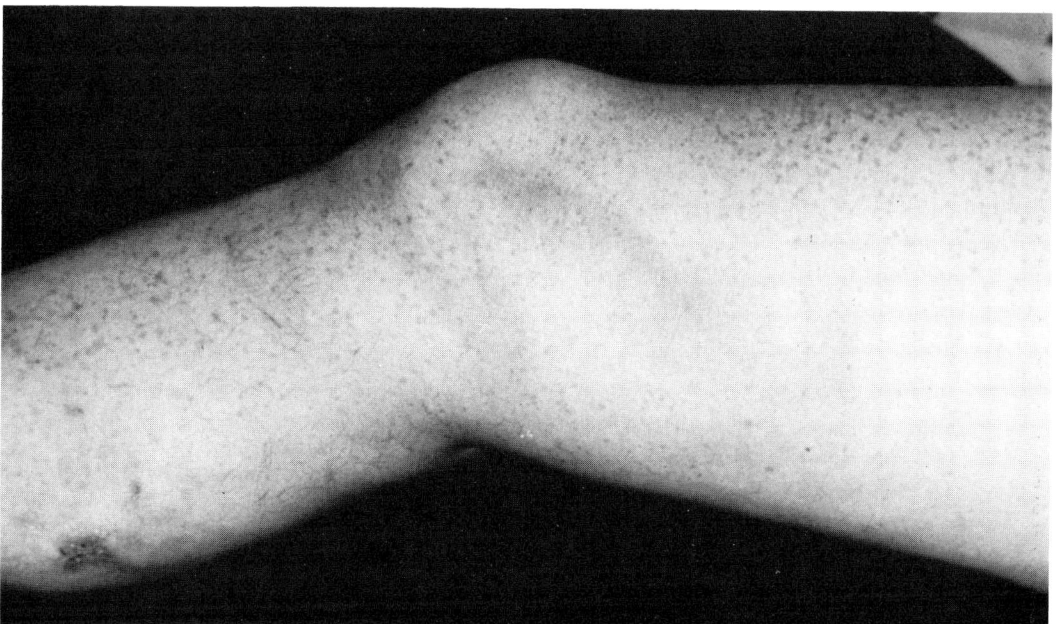

Figure 1–24. Superficial thrombophlebitis. Mildly erythematous linear cord along medial aspect of knee.

The presumed pathophysiologic basis for the *hypercoagulable state* and the *defibrination syndrome* is the initiation and sustaining of disseminated intravascular coagulation by activation of thrombin, with resultant coagulation of fibrinogen and subsequent fibrinolysis with its attendant phenomena. Trousseau's syndrome represents one pole of the spectrum of disseminated intravascular coagulation (DIC), and the defibrination syndrome the other pole.

Thromboses and hemorrhage may be occurring in the patient at the same time. The term *purpura fulminans* is currently used to describe this mixed phenomenon and is no longer restricted to the syndrome following viral and bacterial infections in children. Activation of the coagulation mechanism may have many causes, such as release of tissue factor into the circulation, which occurs in obstetrical accidents or severe trauma, or activation by bacterial endotoxin. The latter plays a significant role in the pathogenesis of the cutaneous lesions in acute meningococcemia. The coagulopathy syndromes associated with obstetrical, traumatic, and infectious catastrophes represent *acute* DIC, and are usually more fulminant, but short lived.

Migratory thrombophlebitis and deep venous thromboses develop in the neck, chest, abdominal wall, pelvis, and limbs. Several areas may be involved simultaneously or sequentially. The veins are palpable as tender cords. Often the episodes of phlebitis last only a few days and correlate with the absent or mild inflammation of the vessel wall seen on histologic examination. Pulmonary embolism and infarction may occur but are not common.

The phlebitis can be severe enough to produce massive edema and redness (phlegmasia cerulea dolens).

Migratory phlebitis can precede the detection of cancer by as long as six months. In general, the cancers associated with chronic DIC have been inoperable. Although most cancers are accompanied by thrombotic episodes rather than hemorrhagic phenomena, carcinoma of the prostate and acute leukemia are associated more with the latter than the former. The derangements in coagulation are frequently corrected or improved by successful therapy of the underlying malignancy.[102]

In their analysis of 182 patients with chronic DIC, Sack et al. found that 50 per cent had migratory phlebitis, 60 per cent had at least one episode of thrombophlebitis, 40 per cent had hemorrhagic complications, 25 per cent suffered from arterial embolization, and 7 per cent had the triad of thrombophlebitis, hemorrhage, and arterial emboli, often sequentially.[102] The arterial emboli were composed of fibrin which arose in almost all cases from nonbacterial thrombotic endocarditis involving the aortic and mitral valves and rarely the tricuspid. The common sites of embolization were the cerebrum, myocardium, retina, mesentery, and kidney.

The fibrin degradation products can behave as a cryoprotein (cryofibrinogen) as well as an anticoagulant.[102] The cryofibrinogen may be responsible for the localization of hemorrhagic gangrenous changes on the digits, ears, and nose in some patients (see p. 817).

Hawley and associates described six patients who developed digital gangrene in association with malignancy.[106] The neoplastic disorders included carcinomas of the maxillary sinus, kidney, ovary, colon, and uterus. One patient had Hodgkin's disease. Digital gangrene in association with the thrombotic phase of DIC also occurs in nonmalignant disease. I have observed this phenomenon in two patients with ulcerative colitis (see p. 596).

The dermatologic gamut of *blistering disease* can be seen with cancer.[107] Pruritic, grouped vesicles, either over extensor surfaces or widely distributed, simulate dermatitis herpetiformis. Choriocarcinoma and malignant tumors of the ovary, uterus, prostate, bladder, rectum, and breast have been reported with dermatitis herpetiformis-like disease. In three cases, the eruption disappeared after removal of choriocarcinoma and cancers of the uterus and ovary.[108-110]

An eruption, simulating pemphigus vulgaris, which consists of large bullae on normal skin and sometimes on the mucous membranes is called pemphigoid. Although pemphigoid is of unknown etiology, it has been associated with melanoma and carcinoma of the stomach and lung. It usually occurs idiopathically in elderly people. It is differentiated from pemphigus vulgaris, which is not associated with cancer, by the histopathology: the bullae are subepidermal, and acantholysis does not occur. In two cases of pemphigoid associated with gastric and lung cancers, ocular mucosal erosions resulted in adhesions that resembled ocular pemphigus.[111]

Erythema multiforme is also seen with cancer. In addition, deep x-ray therapy for malignancy can produce an erythema multiforme reaction that is thought to be an allergic response to necrotic tumor tissue. Scarlatiniform, urticarial, and eczematous eruptions with fever also appear after deep x-ray therapy for cancer.[112, 113]

All of these blistering eruptions can arise with lymphomas and leukemias. Blistering diseases are not rare in general medical practice and usually they are *not* accompanied by cancer. However, the relationship of pemphigoid to malignancy remains controversial. Two recent publications have stressed that the association between pemphigoid and cancer is not statistically significant,[114, 115] while a third one supports this link.[116] However, there is no question that bullous eruptions can be associated with and parallel the course of malignant disease. It would be medically sound judgment to consider the possibility of an underlying neoplasm in a patient if the bullous disorder has an atypical appearance or course, or if it occurs in an elderly patient. A carefully performed history and physical examination, coupled with a hemogram, urinalysis, chest x-ray, and examination of the stool for occult blood would be an efficient and effective way to uncover malignancies in most patients. The following case histories illustrate this striking skin marker:

A 70-year old debilitated white woman with diabetes mellitus had suffered from recurrent bullous pemphigoid for one year before admission to the Yale-New Haven Hospital. A gastric carcinoma was discovered and successfully resected; a complete remission of the pemphigoid resulted (Fig. 1–25).

A 35-year-old white man had had recurrent erythema multiforme of unknown etiology for five and one half years. A carcinoma of the sigmoid was found and successfully resected. Neither the erythema multiforme nor the cancer recurred after 10 years of follow-up.

A 65-year-old white man developed an epidermoid cancer of his maxillary sinus. One week after the start of deep x-ray therapy he developed a generalized erythema multiforme reaction with marked erythema and edema at the radiation port.

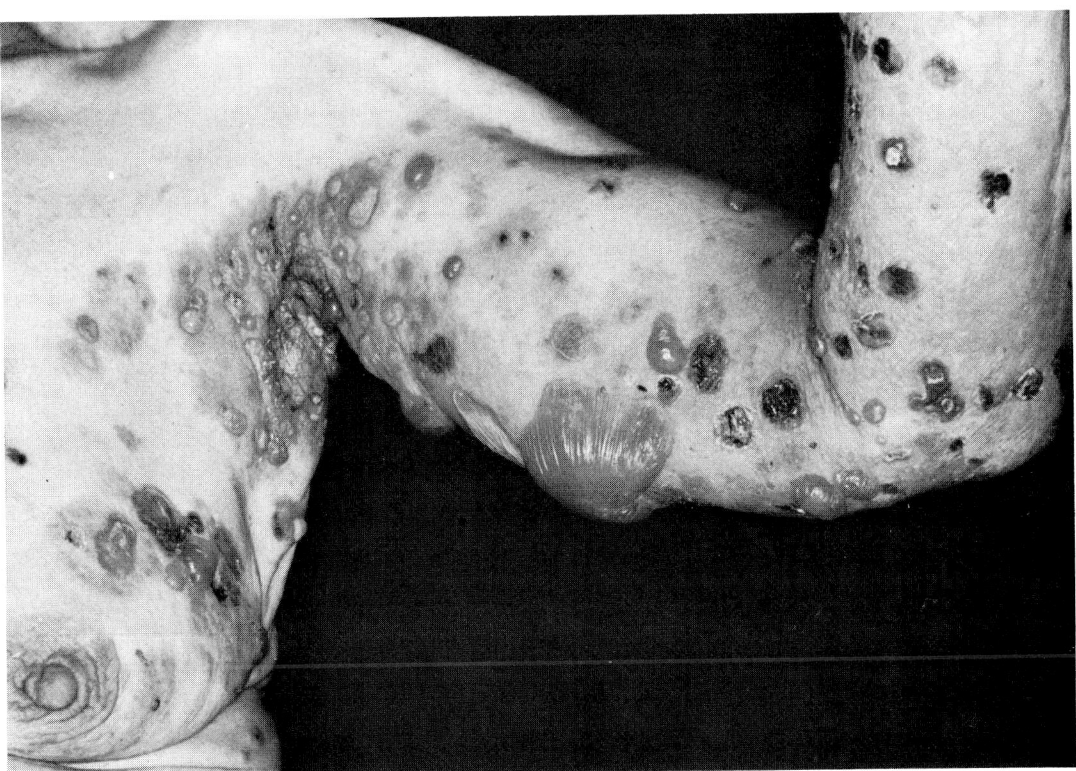

Figure 1–25. Pemphigoid in patient with gastric cancer. Eruption disappeared and did not recur following surgical removal of the tumor.

Urticaria is very uncommon as a manifestation of neoplasia, but it has been described together with choriocarcinoma and cancer of the rectum. In both instances, successful removal of the tumors prompted disappearance of the urticaria.[117]

A spectacular sign of cancer is erythema gyratum repens, which looks like the grain of wood. Multiple wavy erythematous urticarial bands with a peripheral fine scale slowly migrate over the skin surface (Fig. 1–26). Gammel first described this entity, and since then 20 additional cases have been reported.[118, 119] There have been seven cancers of the lung, two of the breast, two of the stomach, one each of the bladder, prostate, cervix, hypopharynx, tongue, and uterus, and one case of multiple myeloma. In two patients metastatic carcinomas, primary sites unknown, were found. In most instances where the malignancy had not disseminated too widely, there was dramatic to moderate improvement of the eruption following therapy for the neoplasm. In the report by Leavell et al. the patient initially developed urticaria, which was then followed by erythema annulare centrifugum, a simple form of the more complex disorder, erythema gyratum repens.[120] The cancer was discovered when the gyrate erythema appeared. In the patient described by Skolnick and Mainman, the initial lesions were also those of erythema annulare centrifugum, which progressed to erythema gyratum repens.[119] At this point, the tumor became symptomatic and was discovered. In most of the patients the eruption developed between five months before to seven months after the cancer was detected. In five instances, the intervals varied from nine to 21 months before to 16 to 20 months after the tumor was diagnosed.

Shelley and Hurley described the case of a 26-year-old white woman with benign virginal hypertrophy of the breasts who developed a similar gyrate erythema. Their studies showed that the eruption was a hypersensitivity reaction to her cystic breast tissue.[121] At the time, she also had serological evidence, but none of the clinical manifestations, of systemic lupus erythematosus. A follow-up of this interesting case disclosed that the gyrate erythema almost completely disappeared after bilateral mastectomy. However she continued to have weakly positive serological evidence of lupus erythematosus (elevated gamma globulins, LE cell tests, and false positive serology) for the next 12 years. Her sister developed severe lupus erythematosus complicated by nephritis and died.[122] About 6 years post-mastectomy the patient developed verrucae vulgares in generalized fashion over the legs. Review of the surgical specimens revealed hematoxylin bodies in the breast tissues.

Barber et al. reported erythema gyratum repens in a 63-year-old man with a cavitary pulmonary lesion on the upper lobe. He was thought to have a bronchogenic carcinoma, but after resection tuberculosis was diagnosed. Careful sectioning of the lung tissue showed no evidence of malignancy.[123]

With the exception of these two cases, all instances of erythema gyratum repens have been associated with malignancy. Shelley has suggested that the figurate erythemas (erythema perstans) be classified into three groups: erythema annulare centrifugum, erythema chronicum migrans, and erythema gyratum repens.[124] These three forms have different morphologies and are easily distinguished from one another (see Chap. 9). Erythema annulare centrifugum is only rarely associated with

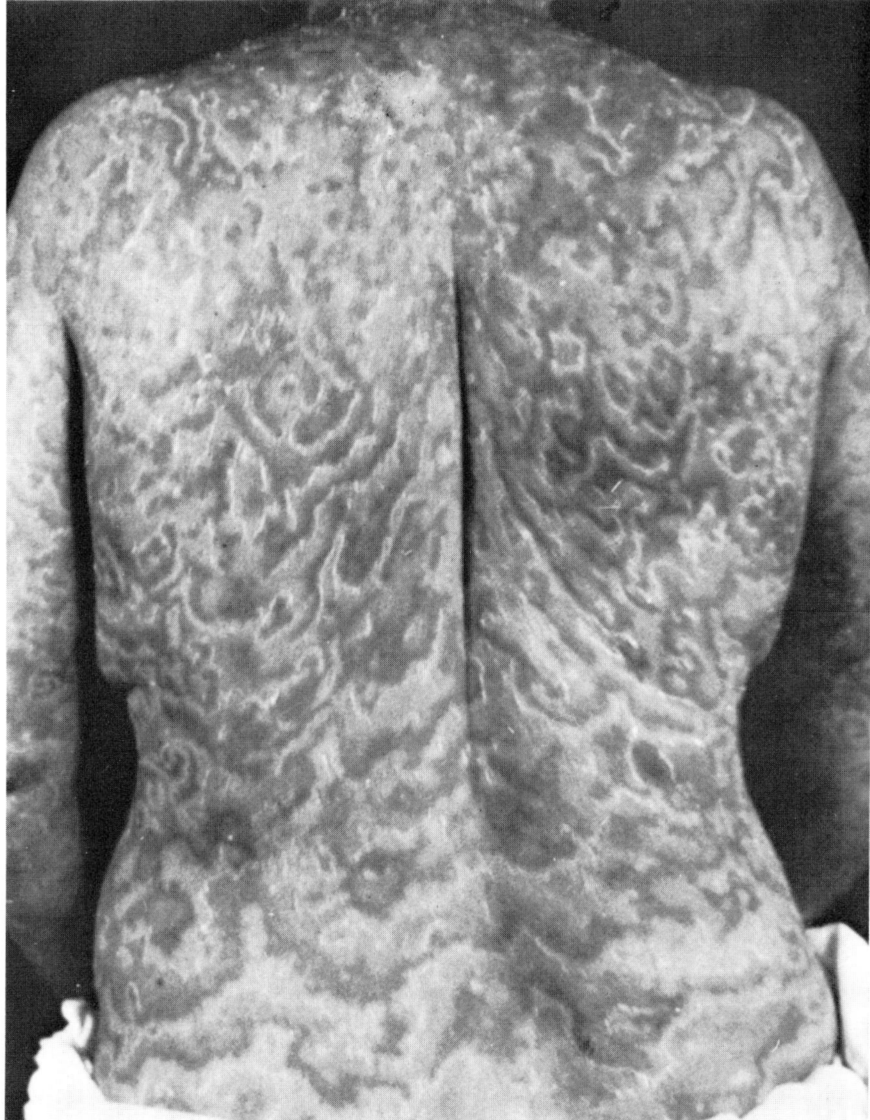

Figure 1–26. Erythema gyratum repens in patient reported by Gammel. (From Gammel, J. A.: Erythema gyratum repens. Arch. Dermatol., *66*:494, 1952. Courtesy of Drs. Helen Curth and Thomas Fitzpatrick.)

malignancy but has been associated with a variety of causative factors: cheese fungi, chloroquine therapy, autoimmune disease, mycotic infections, and candidiasis. Erythema chronicum migrans follows a tick bite and erythema gyratum repens thus far has been almost always associated with cancer.

We recently had the opportunity to observe the association between erythema annulare centrifugum and a benign ovarian tumor — a cystadenoma. The patient was a 45-year-old woman who had had erythema annulare centrifugum in a chronic and recurrent fashion over the thighs, perineum, and trunk for 10 years (Figs. 1–27 and 1–28). Two years before admission to the hospital, she noted a slowly increasing girth to her abdomen. At laporatomy the surgeon found an enormous benign ovarian tumor which proved to be a cystadenoma on histologic examination.

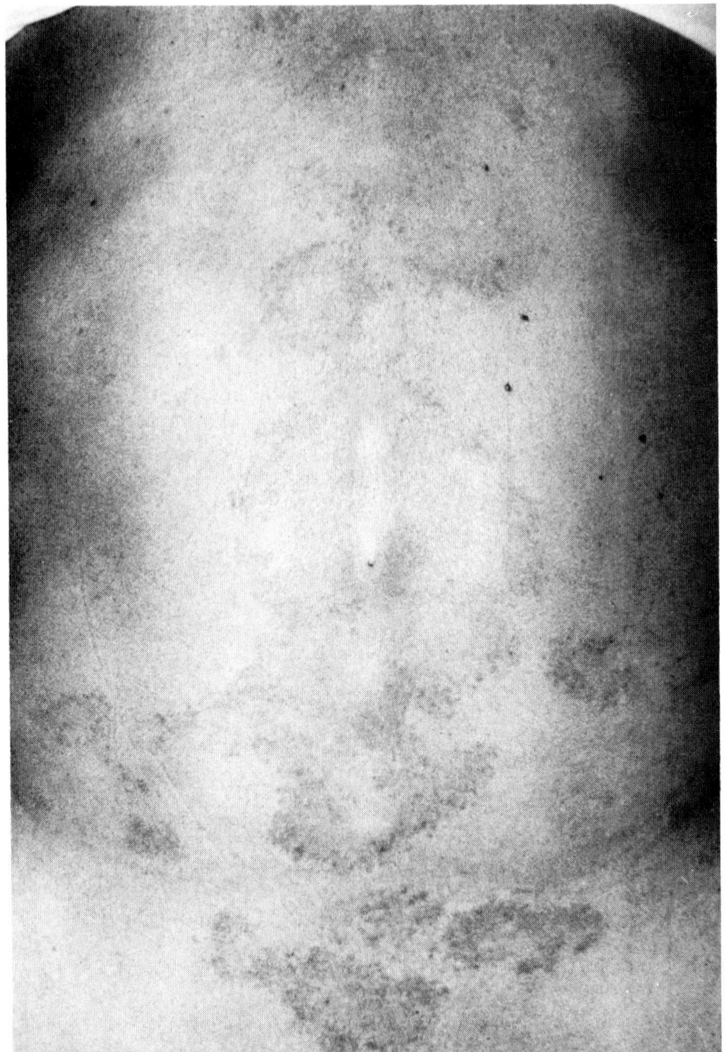

Figure 1–27. Erythema annulare centrifugum associated with ovarian tumor.

Within one week after removal, the generalized erythema annulare centrifugum disappeared and did not recur during two years of further observations. Ikada et al. reported an identical case from Japan in which the erythema annulare centrifugum was also generalized and pruritic and disappeared within ten days after removal of an ovarian cystadenoma.[125]

Hyperkeratosis of the palms and soles, also known as tylosis or keratoderma, is a dominantly transmitted genodermatosis which usually develops within the first few months of life. The marked thickening of the stratum corneum can be spotty or diffuse, producing a wartlike or callous appearance (Figs. 1–29 and 1–30). In some families the tylosis develops late in childhood. The thickening of the palms and soles may be accompanied by painful fissures and hyperhidrosis. In addition to being a disease *sui generis*, keratoderma can also be a feature of acanthosis nigricans, pachydermoperiostosis, psoriasis, and a number of disorders of keratinization.

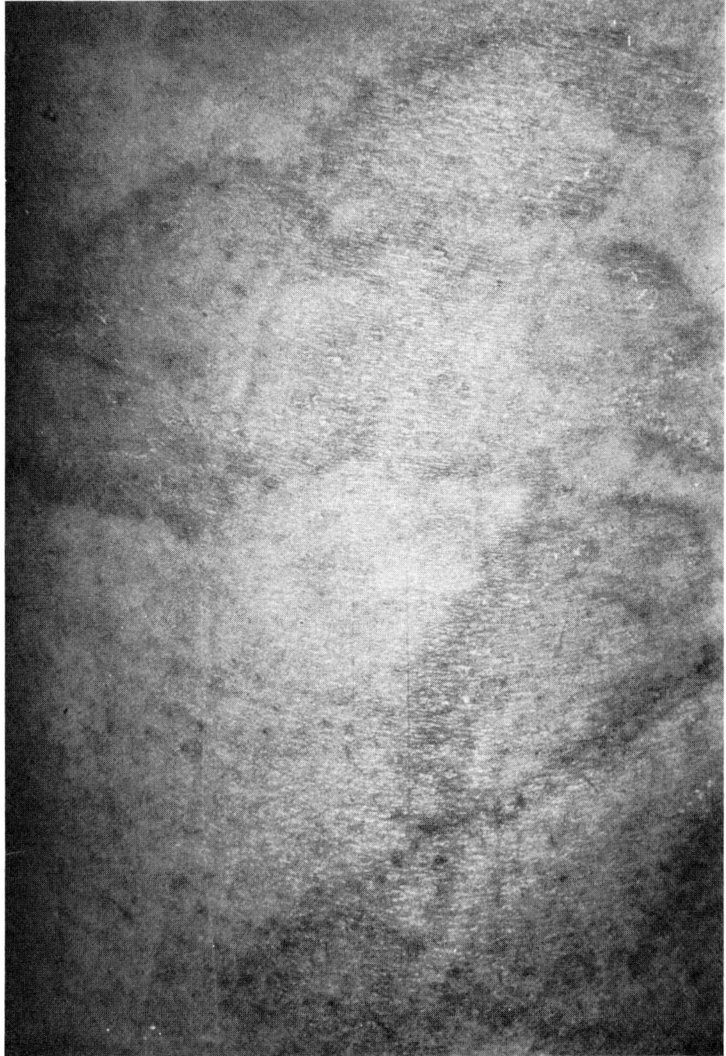

Figure 1–28. Close-up of erythema annulare centrifugum in Figure 1–27. Central clearing with slightly scaly erythematous border.

Tylosis can be a marker of systemic disease. Howel-Evans et al. reported the association of tylosis and esophageal cancer in two English families from Liverpool.[126] When the individual was about 10 years of age, the keratoderma appeared on the palms and soles, although some members had only plantar involvement. At the time of the original report, 14 of 48 persons with tylosis had developed esophageal cancer in the fourth and fifth decades. None of the 87 nontylotic individuals had developed cancer. In two persons the keratoderma underwent temporary remission during convalescence from esophagogastrectomy. A follow-up report of these families in 1963 revealed that an additional 2 of 11 tylotics past the age of 35 had developed esophageal cancer.[127] Further review of the family in 1969 indicated that the trend of tylotics to develop esophageal cancer was continuing.[128] Keratotic changes have not been found in the esophagus as precursors of the malignancy. The tylosis occurring in

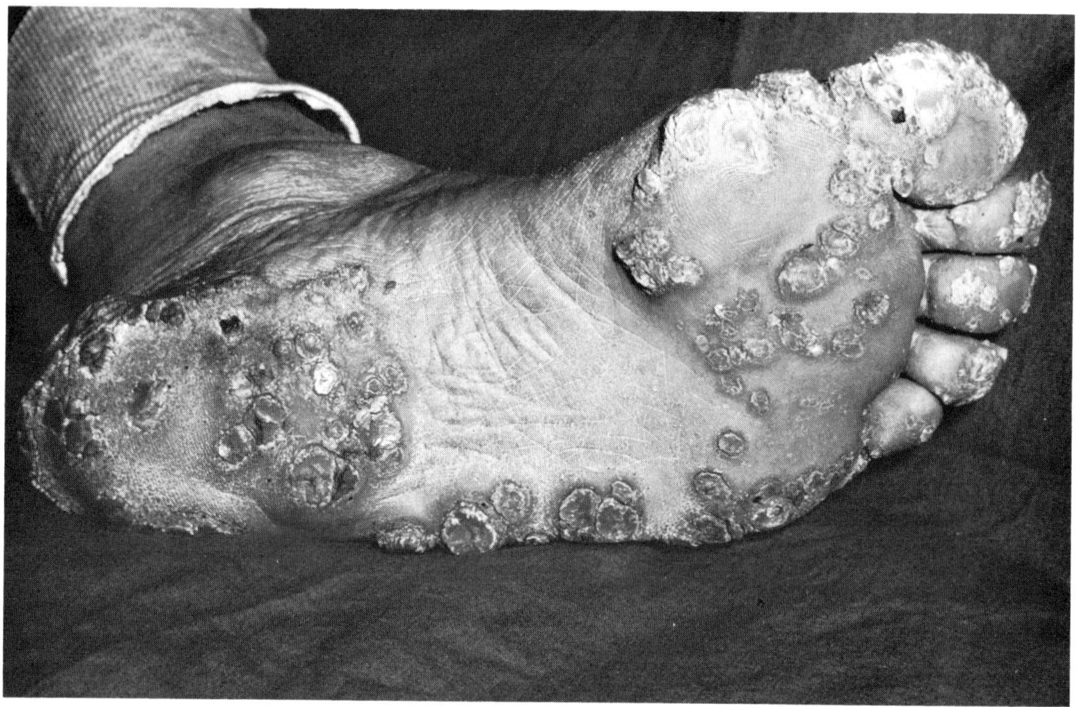

Figure 1–29. Plantar hyperkeratosis displaying a warty appearance.

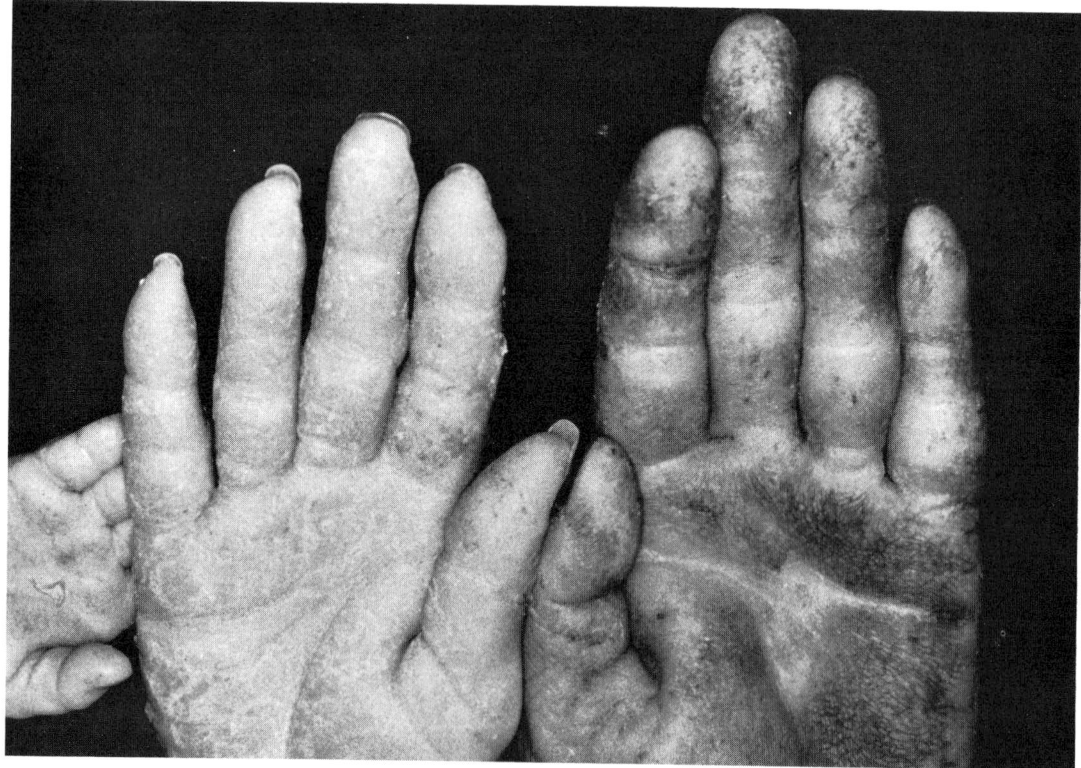

Figure 1–30. Palmar hyperkeratosis in three members of one family. The keratoderma is diffuse.

these families differs from the benign dermatologic disorder only in its later onset. The two families are thought to be related, but definite evidence on this point is lacking. Everall, in a personal communication to Howel-Evans, reported that he had seen tylosis associated with lung cancer, but details were not given.

Although these two kindreds are the only ones reported with this unique syndrome, tylosis has been described with another esophageal disease in a physician, his mother, and his son.[129] These individuals had a short esophagus, the stomach being pulled up into the thorax. Stricture of the esophagus was symptomatic and present from birth in the father and son. Esophageal cancer developed in the physician, probably secondary to the stricture and reflux esophagitis. In the son, the esophageal stricture was resected and replaced by a loop of jejunum as a prophylactic measure. According to her history and symptoms, the physician's mother most likely had the same esophageal abnormalities.

Parnell and Johnson reported the histories of five patients, two of whom they personally examined and three of whom they discovered by review of medical records, who had keratoderma of palms and/or soles in association with cancer.[130] Four had esophageal carcinomas and one had widespread metastases of a cancer that probably arose in the lung. In only one patient were they certain that the keratoderma was of recent onset. The duration of the tylosis in the other patients was unknown. Although such observations provide only circumstantial evidence, it would be worthwhile to look for an underlying carcinoma of the esophagus or lung in adults who develop tylosis unassociated with a benign dermatosis.

Bizarre and unclassifiable dermatoses should suggest the possibility of occult malignancy, as in the following instance:

A 51-year-old black man was admitted to Yale-New Haven Hospital in September, 1964, for treatment of "psoriasis." He stated that at the ages of 13 and 25, he was covered by an acute generalized eruption which resolved after three weeks following three injections of unknown medication. He was told that he had had "psoriasis." Fourteen months before admission to this hospital, many oval and circular lesions with a fine peripheral white scale developed on his trunk. They measured 3 centimeters in diameter and were slightly hypopigmented. They did not look like psoriasis clinically, and a biopsy of one lesion showed a nonspecific perivascular lymphocytic infiltrate in the dermis. A hematocrit of 35 per cent and occult blood in the feces on admission led to the discovery of an antral gastric cancer. Gastrectomy was successfully performed, and a single regional node was positive for cancer. Within two weeks after surgery, the skin lesions began to fade; they were completely gone in three months. During the following 21 months, the patient remained in good health and was free of skin lesions. He then suddenly became ill, developed ascites, and died within 12 weeks because of metastatic carcinoma to the liver. The skin lesions did not recur. His dermatosis, which can best be described as a pityriasis rosea–like eruption, is illustrated in Figures 1–31 and 1–32 and in Plate 2*D*.

Behan, in 1965, reported a patient who seems to be similar to ours, although no illustrations of the lesions were included in his paper:[131]

The patient was a 53-year-old white man admitted to the hospital because of weight loss and vomiting for one month. He also had had a skin rash for one month which covered his forearms, legs, and buttocks. The eruption, simulating pityriasis

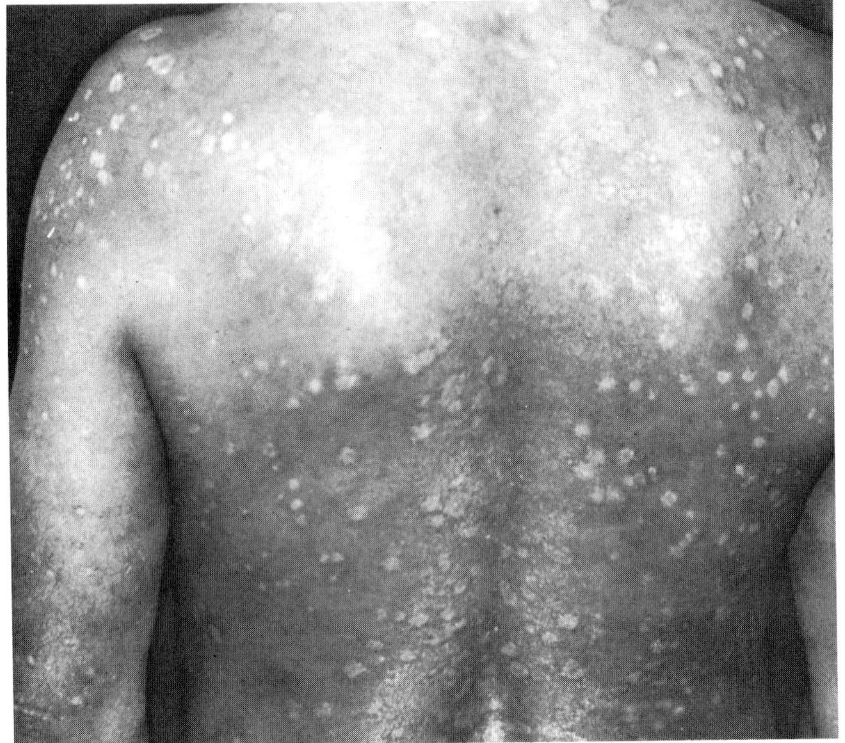

Figure 1–31. Pityriasis rosea–like eruption in patient with gastric cancer.

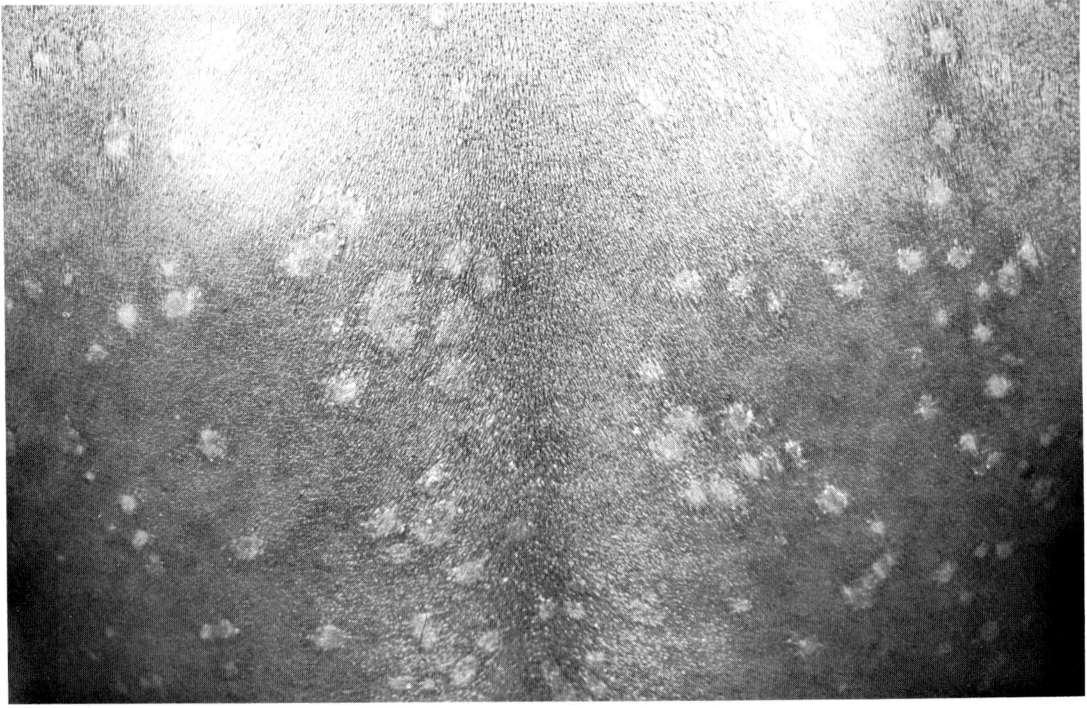

Figure 1–32. Closer view of lesions shown in Figure 1–31. The eruption is composed of hypopigmented slightly scaling macules.

rosea, consisted of oval macules and small red plaques, with marginal scaling. A bronchogenic carcinoma was detected and the patient died three weeks later. Autopsy revealed bronchogenic carcinoma with metastases to the liver, adrenal glands, and brain. The histopathology of the skin lesions was not described in this brief report.

We have seen two other examples of "psoriasis" associated with carcinoma:

The first patient was a 48-year-old white man who denied any previous skin disease. In October, 1966, he developed an erythematous dry scaling eruption in the finger webs and on the dorsa of his hands. This eruption rapidly became generalized but spared the face and knees (Figs. 1–33 to 1–36). The areas most heavily involved were the elbows, popliteal spaces, trunk, scalp, and plantar surfaces. Over the next five months he developed pruritus and anorexia, and he lost 15 pounds. He was referred to the Yale-New Haven Hospital in March, 1967, for treatment of "psoriasis." On physical examination the scaling in his scalp, the hyperkeratosis on his soles, and most of the remaining cutaneous lesions had the appearance of psoriatic plaques. In a few areas there were poorly demarcated patches of dry scaling erythema that were more characteristic of xerosis than of psoriasis.

Biopsy of a typical "psoriatic" plaque showed a nonspecific dermatitis and nothing to suggest psoriasis. A chest x-ray revealed a mediastinal mass. The patient's dermatosis responded well to Goeckerman treatment with coal tar and ultraviolet light, but he refused any further investigation of the thoracic lesion and left the hospital.

After discharge, his dermatosis promptly recurred, and his general symptoms progressed. Four weeks later he was readmitted to the hospital for further study. The dermatosis was present on the scalp, elbows, thighs, and soles. The lesions on

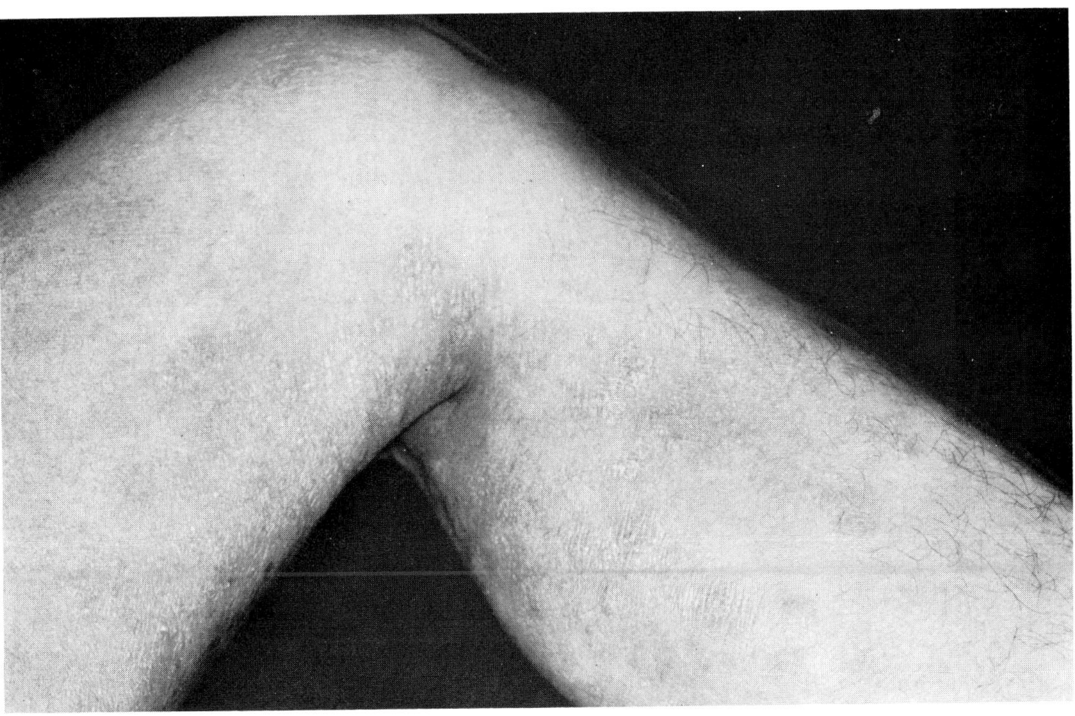

Figure 1–33. Psoriasiform eruption in patient with lung cancer.

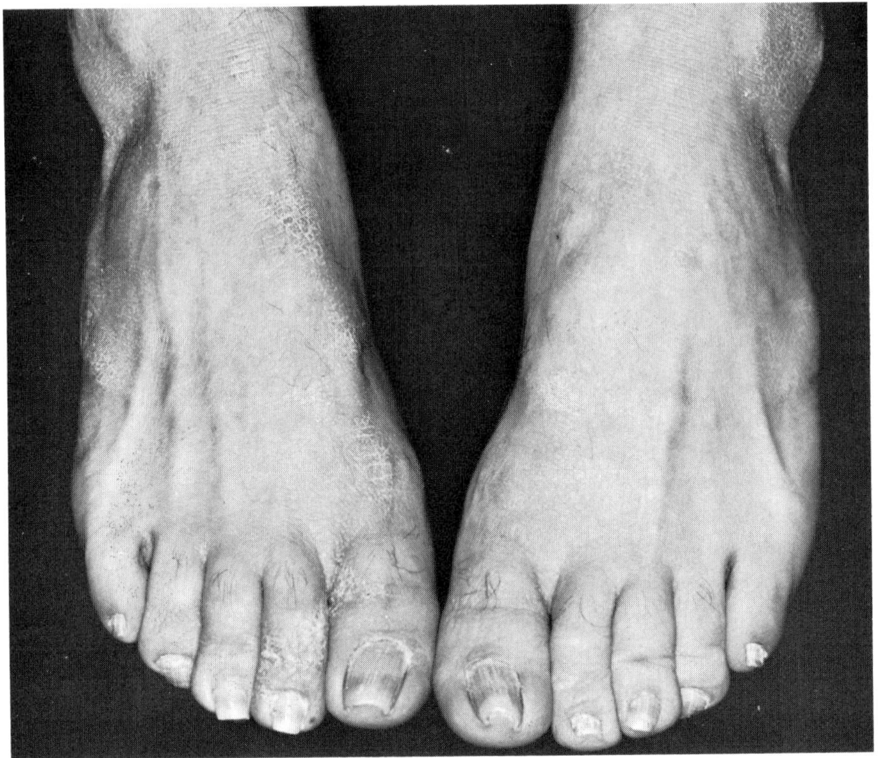

Figure 1–34. Psoriasiform eruption in patient shown in Figure 1–33.

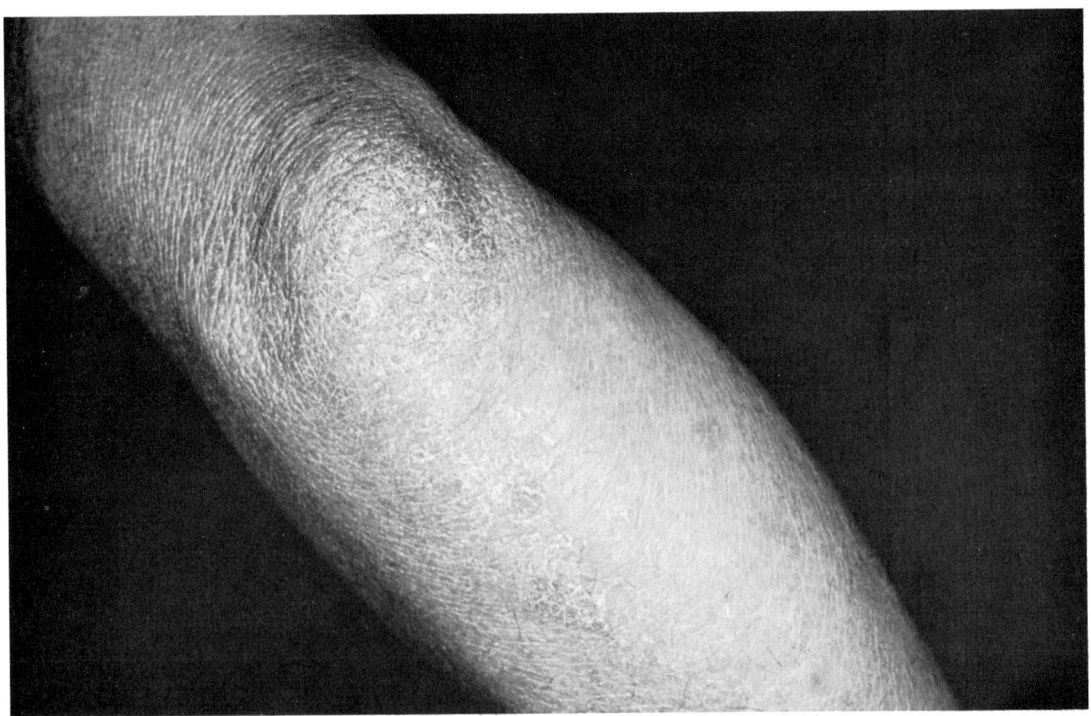

Figure 1–35. Involvement of skin over elbow in patient shown in Figure 1–33.

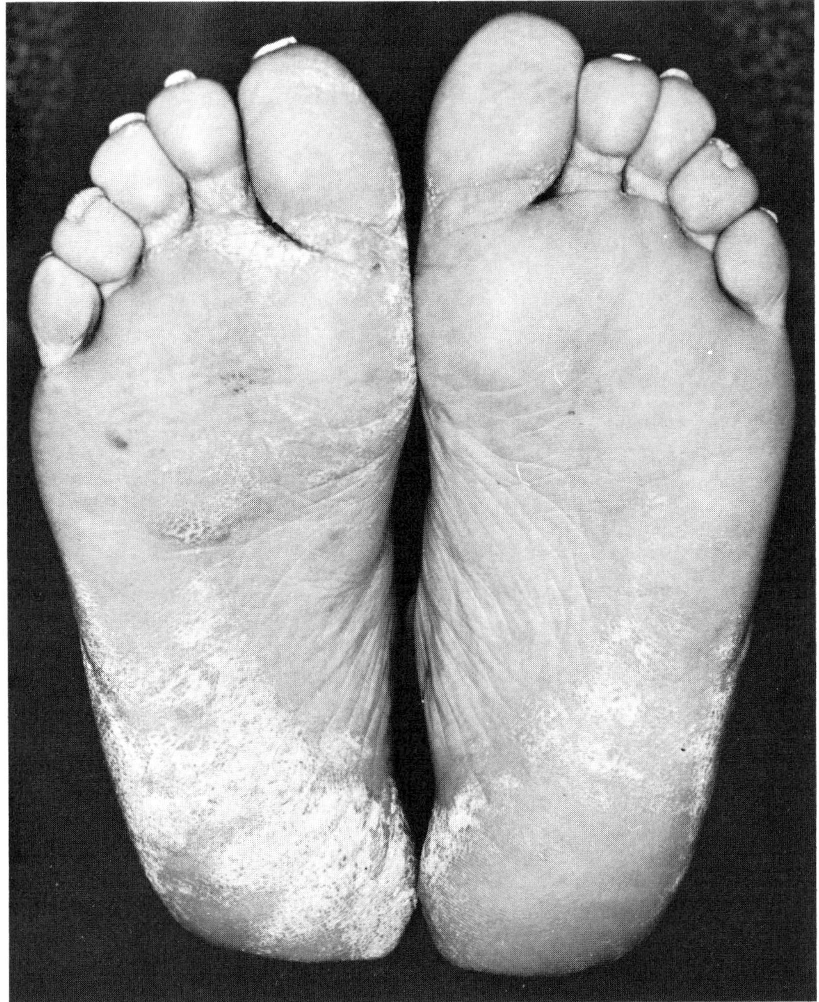

Figure 1–36. Psoriasis-like lesions on feet of patient in Figure 1–33.

the scalp, soles, and parts of the thighs again resembled psoriasis, but those on the elbows and other areas looked more like xerosis or dermatitis. The mediastinal tumor was proved to be an undifferentiated epidermoid cancer probably arising from the lung. He was treated with deep x-ray therapy, but he steadily deteriorated and subsequently died two months later.

The second patient was a 61-year-old man who developed subacute eczematous lesions on the nose, face, and ears and a psoriasiform eruption on the knees, backs of the hands, and toes (Figs. 1–37 to 1–41). The fingernails were longitudinally ridged; some were brittle and crumbling at the distal margins. The skin on the palmar surfaces of the fingers was thick and had a honeycomb appearance. Biopsy of a "psoriatic" lesion revealed a nonspecific dermatitis; no histologic features of psoriasis were found.

Coincident with the appearance of the psoriasiform dermatosis, the patient was noted to have a 5 centimeter, firm, freely movable lymph node on the left of his neck. Further studies revealed that the node contained anaplastic epidermoid cancer that was metastatic from a small primary focus in the base of the tongue. Radiography of the chest revealed a mass in the left upper lobe which, by means of percutaneous needle biopsy, was shown to be an anaplastic epidermoid carcinoma.

The tongue and node were treated with radon seed implants and iridium ribbons, and the lesion in the lung was treated with deep x-ray therapy.

The three foci of cancer disappeared within four months after therapy had been initiated. The skin lesions also vanished. The fingernails returned toward normal, but they remained slightly ridged. The patient remained in good health without detectable cancer for about eight months. At this time a metastasis appeared in his left pectoral muscle, and a radiograph of the chest revealed a new mass in the left lower lobe. Carcinomatosis slowly developed, and he died eight months later with metastases in the liver, lung, kidneys, and bones. His skin lesions did not recur.

Autopsy disclosed that there was no recurrence of tumor in either the tongue or the lymph node. The histology of the epidermoid carcinoma had changed from an anaplastic to a well-differentiated state.

This second patient with "psoriasis," although unique in our experience, was first described by Bazex in 1965. The disease is well known in France as acrokératose paranéoplastique (Bazex's syndrome).[131a, 132] I am indebted to Dr. J. Thivolet for bringing this extraordinary syndrome to my attention. A total of 17 other patients have thus far been described and the details of this disorder have been published by Namour.[133] Individuals with this syndrome have had eczematous and psoriasiform lesions on the ears, nose, cheeks, hands, feet, and knees as illustrated in Figures 1–37 to 1–41. The elbows, lower legs, scalp, and neck have been involved in a few patients. There may be a violaceous color to the lesions and the scale may be adherent, so that sometimes the eruption may resemble that of cutaneous lupus erythematosus. There is hyperkeratosis of the palms and soles and nail dystrophy. All the patients with this syndrome resemble

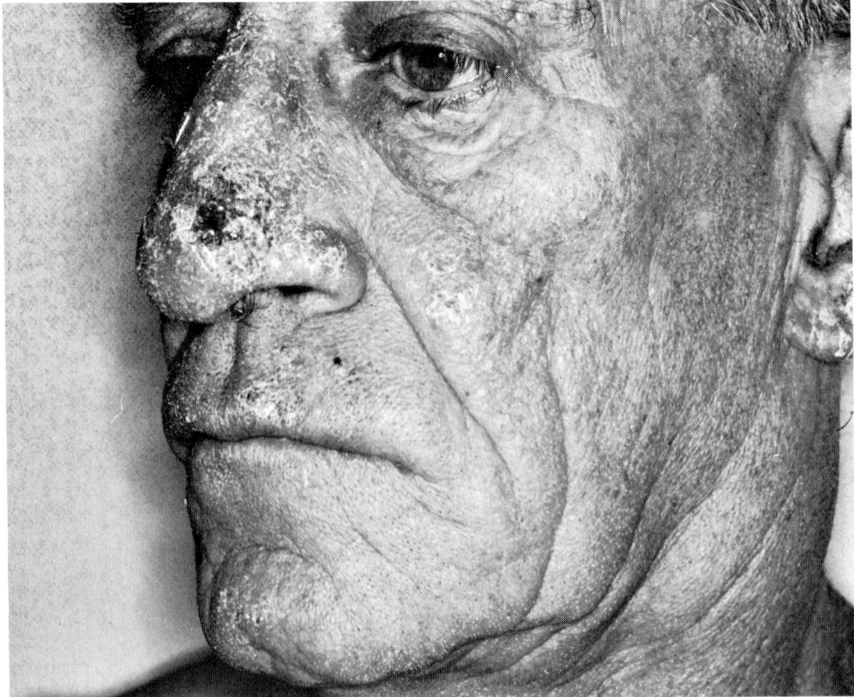

Figure 1–37. Bazex's syndrome. Psoriasiform and eczematous eruptions in patient with cancer of the tongue.

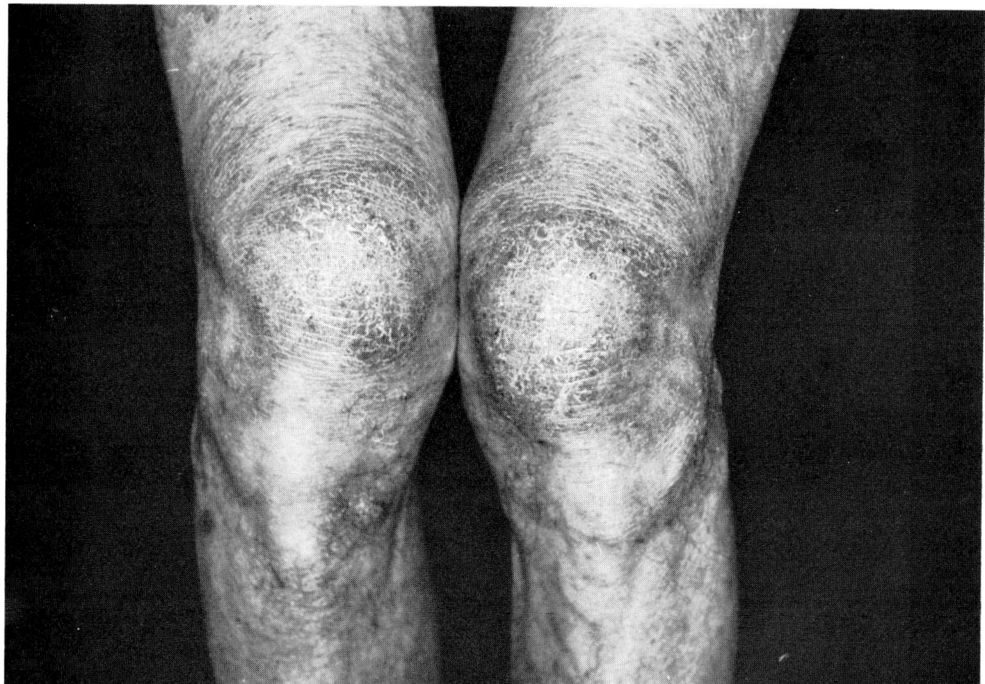

Figure 1–38. Bazex's syndrome. Psoriasiform lesions on knees of patient shown in Figure 1–37.

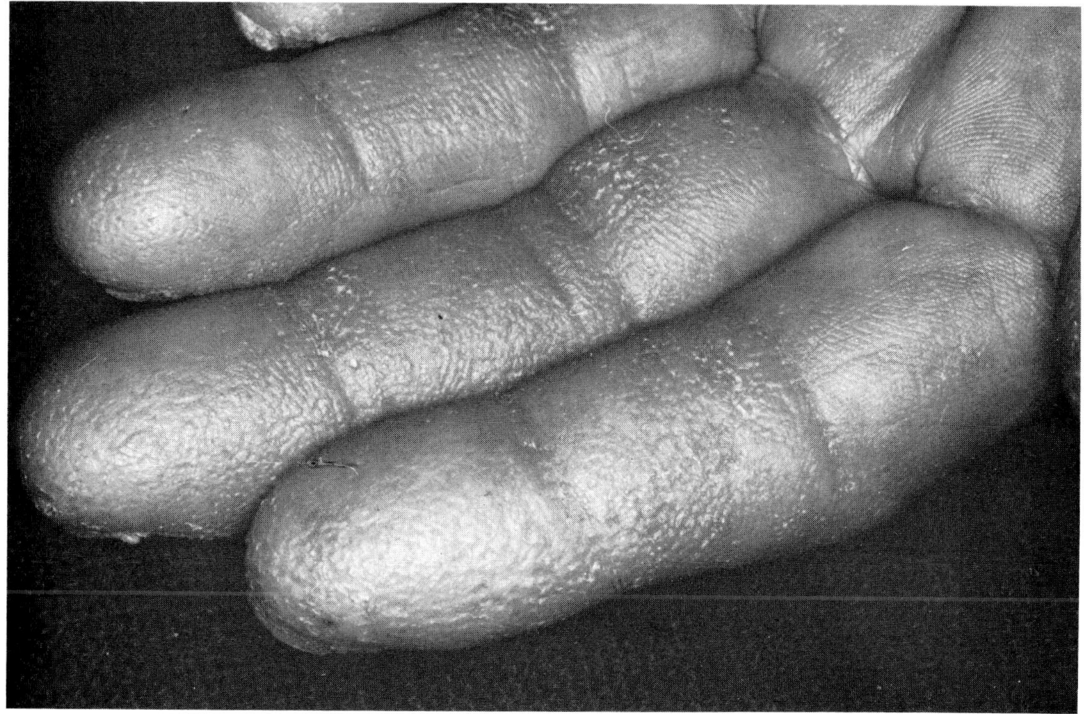

Figure 1–39. Bazex's syndrome. Hyperkeratosis of fingers and palms producing honeycomb appearance in patient shown in Figure 1–37.

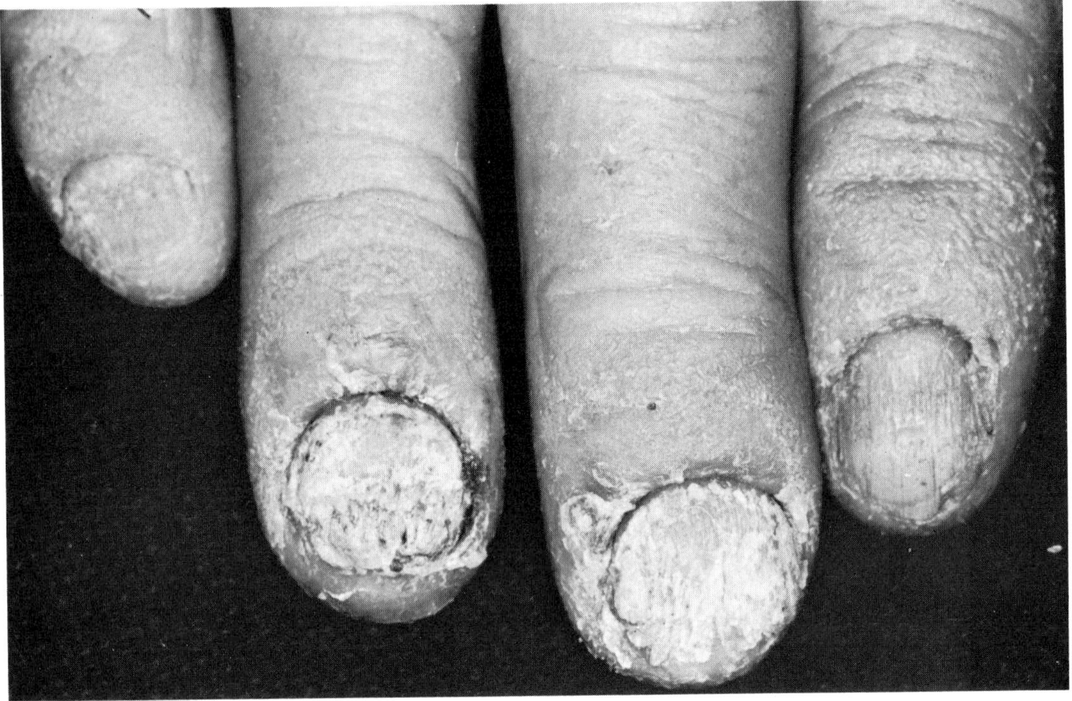

Figure 1–40. Bazex's syndrome. Ridged and brittle nails of patient shown in Figure 1–37.

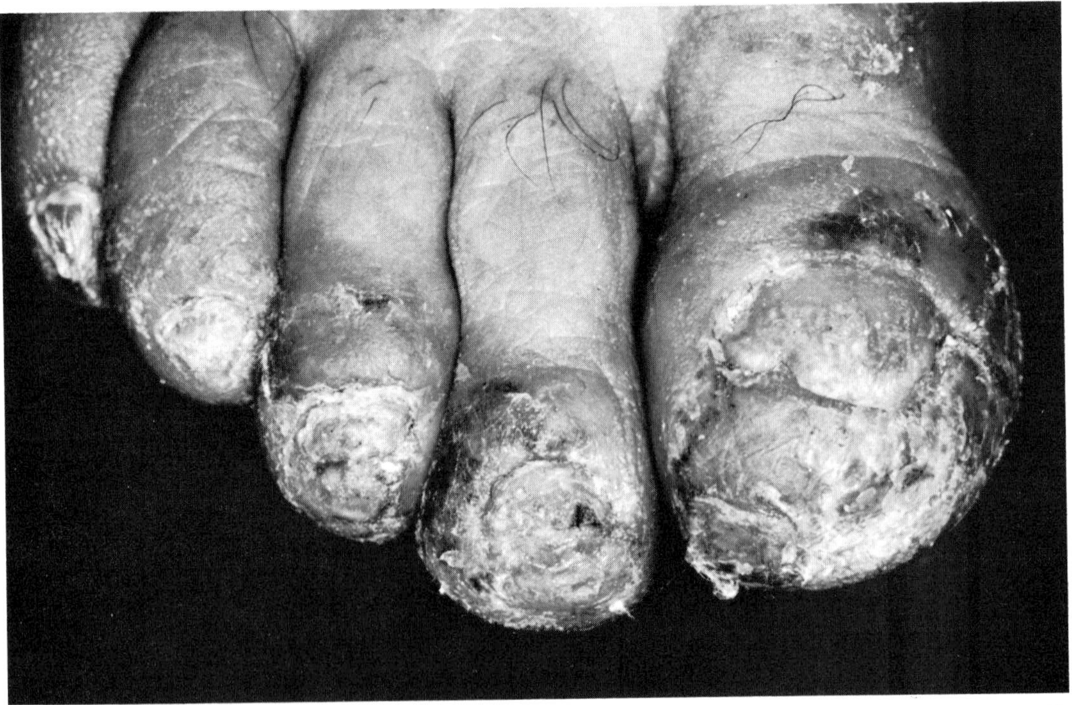

Figure 1–41. Bazex's syndrome. Psoriasiform changes of toes and nails of patient shown in Figure 1–37. The eruption also resembles that seen in Reiter's syndrome.

one another and the drawing in Figure 1–42 may be a helpful way in which to remember this disorder. This paraneoplastic syndrome is specific for carcinomas of the upper respiratory and digestive tracts. The 17 patients have had carcinomas of the tonsil, pyriform sinus, tongue, larynx, pharynx, soft palate, and esophagus, and in one patient the cancer arose in an area adjacent to the larynx and esophagus. In another patient, there were metastases to submaxillary nodes from an undetermined primary site. Two patients were said to have carcinomas of the lung, but the exact type and localization within the lungs were not stated. Successful treatment of the underlying cancer was followed by resolution of the dermatitis in several cases. This entity which seems to be a specific sign of cancer in the upper airway and upper digestive tract belongs in the same category of signficant skin signs as do dermatomyositis, erythema gyratum repens, and acanthosis nigricans.

Exfoliative dermatitis is a relatively frequent manifestation of lymphomas, leukemias, and mycosis fungoides, but it is extremely uncommon as a marker of solid cancers. However, it can occur with carcinoma, which the following situations demonstrate. Schweigl described a woman with a carcinoma of the cervix and exfoliative dermatitis; the exfoliative dermatitis disappeared after the tumor was surgically removed.[134] Graham, Nicolis, and Helwig have reported exfoliative dermatitis in association with carcinomas of the stomach, liver, prostate, lung, and thyroid.[135, 136] Gougerot and Ruppe reported exfoliative dermatitis and keratoderma of the palms and soles; both disorders were secondary to a cancer of the tongue.[137] In their report, they also described the case of a 38-year-old woman who had the acute onset of generalized eczema that proved unresponsive to therapy. She was subsequently found to have a carcinoma of the rectovaginal septum. McGaw and McGovern published three instances of exfoliative dermatitis and cancer of the lung in which

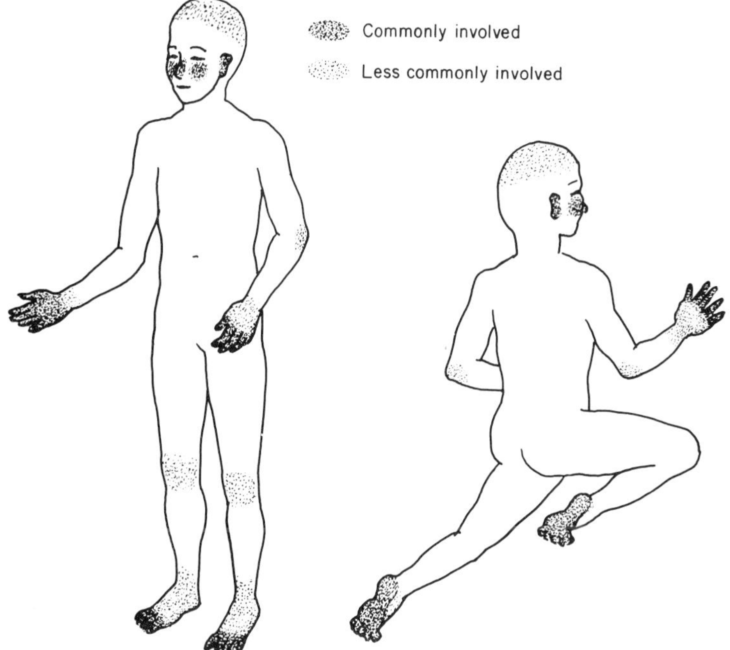

Figure 1–42. Bazex's syndrome. Distribution of cutaneous lesions.

the skin lesions preceded the detection of the malignancy by 5, 8, and 13 months. In one patient, successful surgical removal of the cancer was followed by the disappearance of the exfoliative dermatitis.[138]

Ichthyosis appearing *de novo* in adults is another relatively specific sign of lymphoma. However, it has been reported with multiple myeloma three times and with individual cases of oat cell cancer of the lung and mammary cancer.[139, 140] It may be more common than is realized, because Flint et al. have reported four more cases with this manifestation. Two of the patients had carcinomas of the lung, one had a mammary cancer, and one had a carcinoma of the cervix.[141]

Acquired ichthyosis should not be confused with asteatotic eczema (xerosis), which is common in older individuals, particularly in the winter months when the temperature is cold and the humidity is low. In its extreme form, the dryness and fine scaling of xerosis may be accompanied by erythema and red superficial fissures producing the picture of eczema craquelé (Fig. 1–16). Histologic examination will differentiate eczema or dermatitis from ichthyosis and exclude sarcoidosis, which can sometimes produce an ichthyotic picture on the legs (Fig. 10–12). Hypothyroidism also needs to be excluded because of its capability of producing an ichthyotic eruption (Fig. 13–14).

Acquired growth of lanugo hair (acquired hypertrichosis lanuginosa) appears to be another marker of cancer (Fig. 1–43). In this syndrome, an excessive growth of lanugo hair covers almost the entire face (cheeks, nose, ears, and eyelids), neck, trunk, and eventually the extremities. The hair is soft, silky, long, and unpigmented. In at least three patients there was excessive growth of terminal hairs on the scalp and eyebrows as

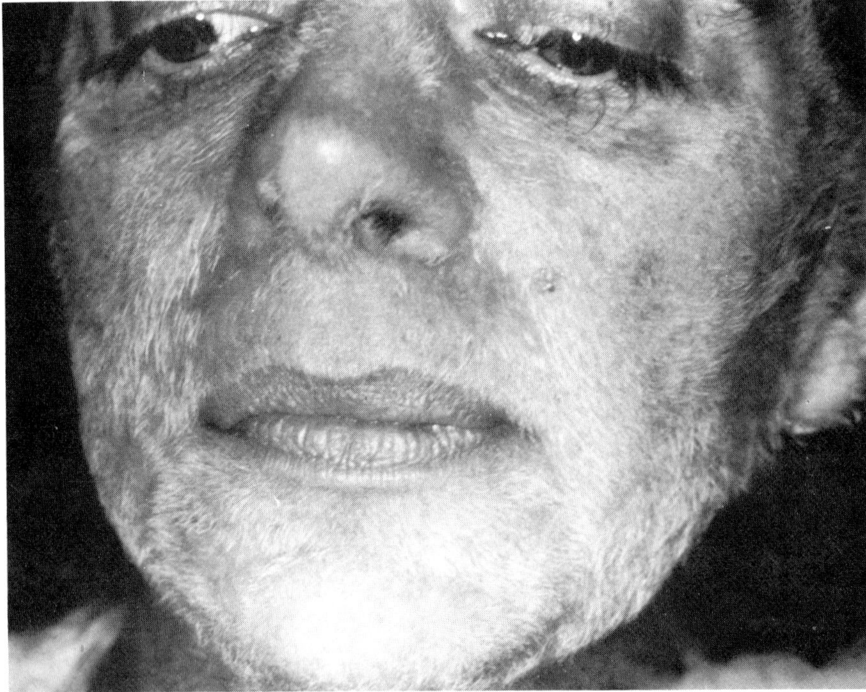

Figure 1–43. Acquired hypertrichosis lanuginosa. (From Schorr, W.: Acquired hypertrichosis lanuginosa and malignancy. Arch. Dermatol., *106*:84, 1972.)

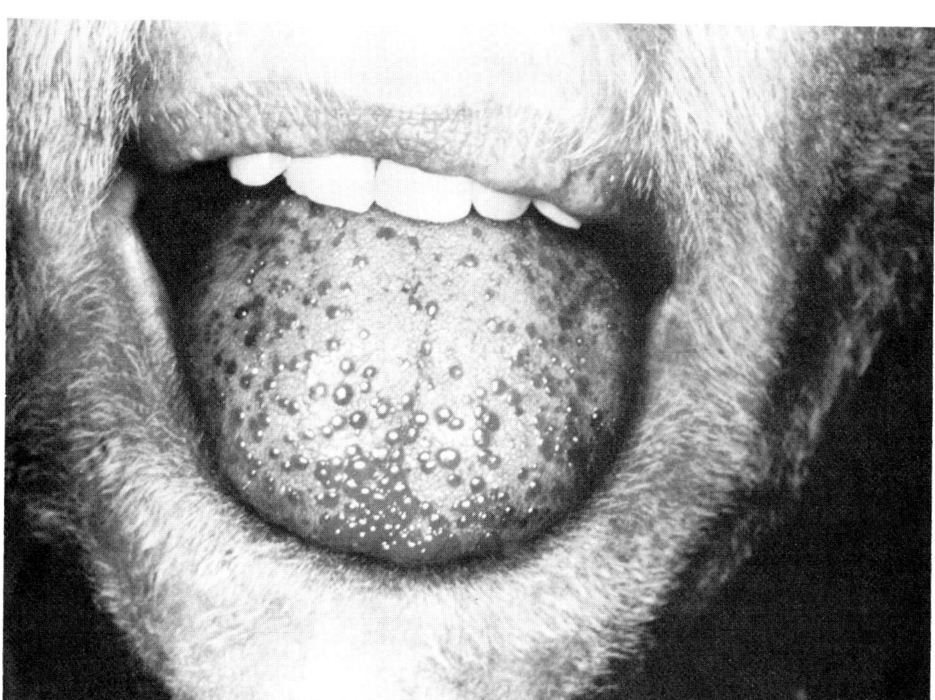

Figure 1–44. Acquired hypertrichosis lanuginosa. Associated red swollen papules on anterior tongue. (From Schorr, W.: Acquired hypertrichosis lanuginosa and malignancy. Arch. Dermatol., *106*:84, 1972.)

well.[142, 143] Congenital examples of this condition, which occurs more frequently than the acquired type, have been associated with dental abnormalities, deformities of the ears, and mental retardation. The acquired type is not accompanied by such abnormalities. Fretzin reported a patient who had this condition in association with an anaplastic carcinoma of the lung.[144] He coined the term "malignant down" for this disorder. At least 16 cases have been described and carcinomas have been found in 13 persons. A pancreatic islet cell tumor was probably present in the fourteenth individual.[145-148] The two persons in whom cancers were not discovered had not been followed long enough to exclude the later development of a neoplasm. In most patients, the cancer was present at the time the lanugo hair growth occurred. In two patients the lanugo hair growth developed two months and four months after the cancer was detected. In a third patient the lanugo hair growth developed four years and four months after a carcinoma of the colon was resected and a presumed metastasis or recurrence developed in the left iliac fossa.[149, 150] In two cases the hair growth preceded the recognition of the cancer by intervals of one and two years.[146, 147] The cancers in these patients have included those of the lung, bladder, gallbladder, rectum, colon, uterus, and breast. One patient had a histiocytic lymphoma[147] and another probably had the Zollinger-Ellison syndrome with a pancreatic islet cell tumor. Treatment of the malignancy was associated with disappearance of the lanugo hair in only one patient,[148] but the hair stopped growing in several other instances. A painful glossitis or disturbance of taste has been present in half of the patients. In a few, the tongue has been described as having red swollen papules or red swollen fungiform papillae on the anterior half of the tongue (Fig. 1–44). Furrowing and cleft formation of the lingual surface have also been described in association with these papules. No endocrine abnormalities or other factors have been uncovered in any of the patients to explain the growth of the lanugo hair.[147, 148]

Acanthosis nigricans is probably the most well-known cutaneous marker of internal malignancy. However, it occurs in a variety of situations unrelated to neoplasia: as a congenital or familial lesion; in association with puberty, endocrine disease, and excessive weight gain: and with a number of congenital anomalies. Juvenile, benign, and pseudoacanthosis nigricans, which are the terms applied to this dermatosis when it is not accompanied by cancer, will be discussed more fully later.

The clinical and histologic features of acanthosis nigricans are identical in all the disorders with which it is associated. Acanthosis nigricans chiefly affects the flexures: neck, axillae, groin, and antecubital spaces (Figs. 1–45 to 1–48). With extensive involvement, lesions can be found on the areolae, around the umbilicus, and in the perineal area. The lips and buccal mucosa may also be affected. McKissic described a patient with metastatic adenocarcinoma, primary site unknown, in whom extensive papillomatous changes of acanthosis nigricans developed on the gums, buccal mucosa, tongue, palate, and lips. In addition, there were papillary masses, presumed to be part of the same process, demonstrated by x-ray in the lower pharynx and esophagus.[151] Hyperkeratosis of the palms and of the skin over the elbows, knees, and interphalangeal joints can occur as well.

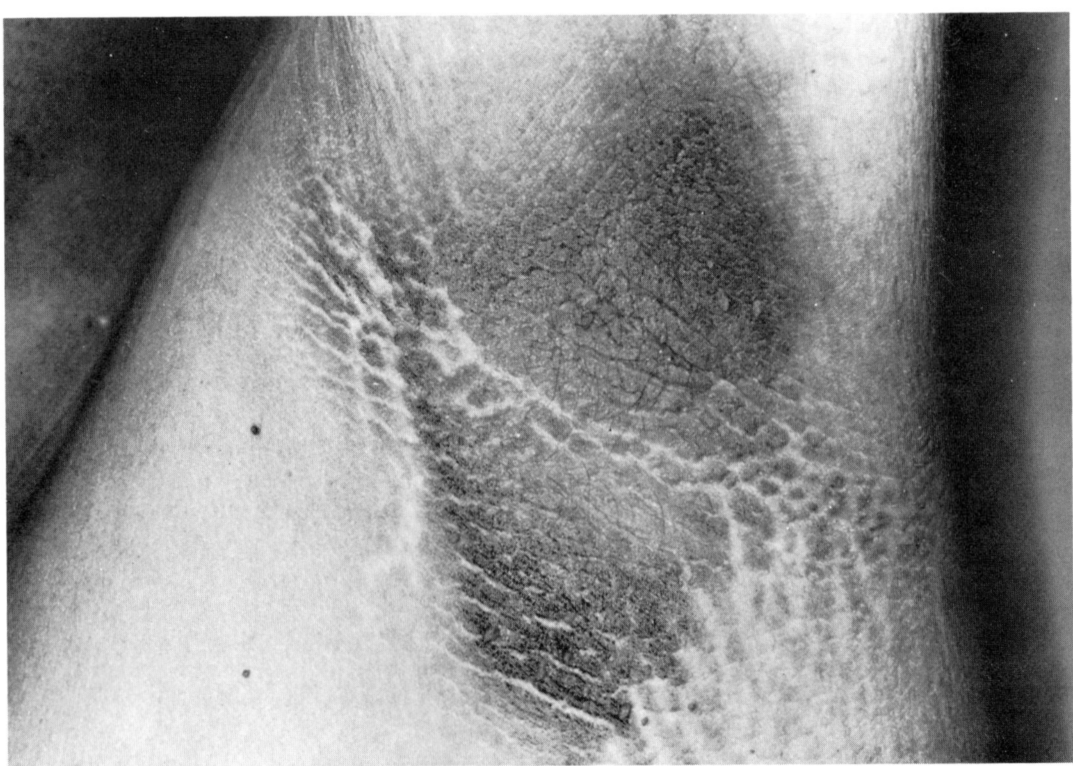

Figure 1–45. Acanthosis nigricans in axilla.

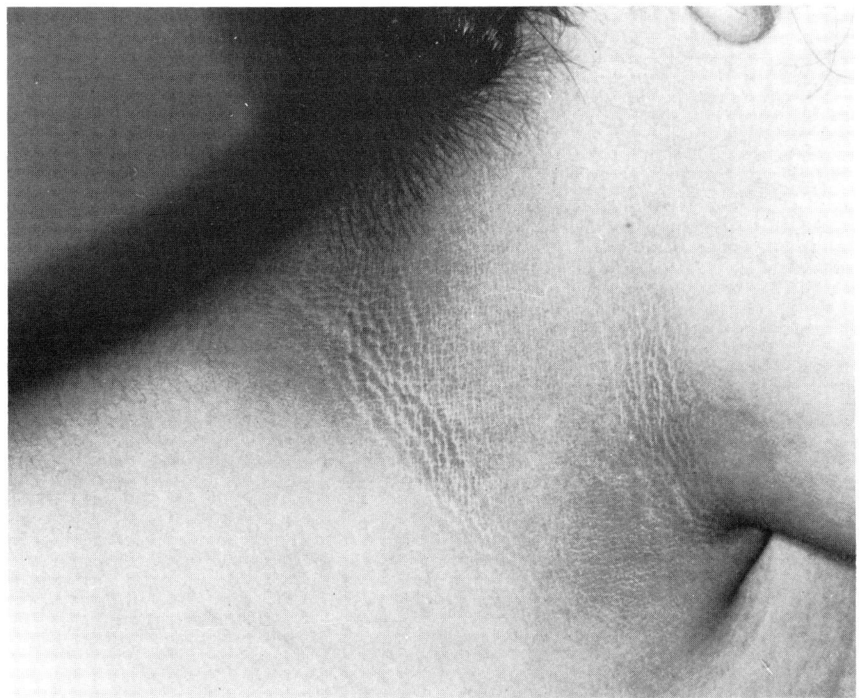

Figure 1–46. Acanthosis nigricans on neck.

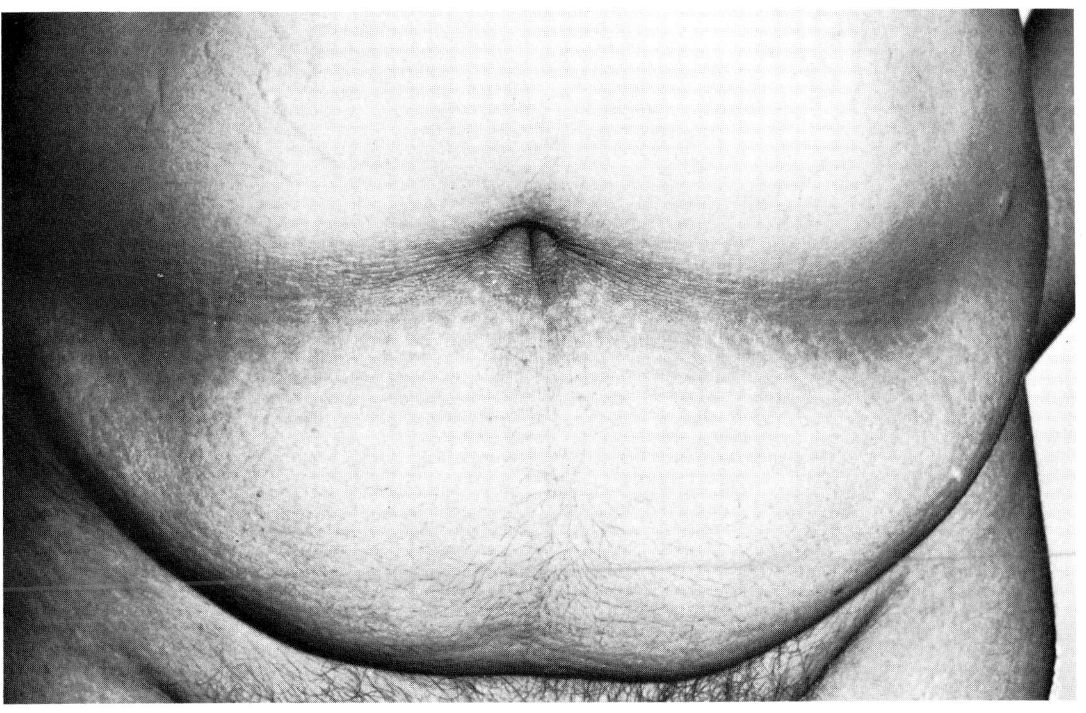

Figure 1–47. Acanthosis nigricans on abdominal wall.

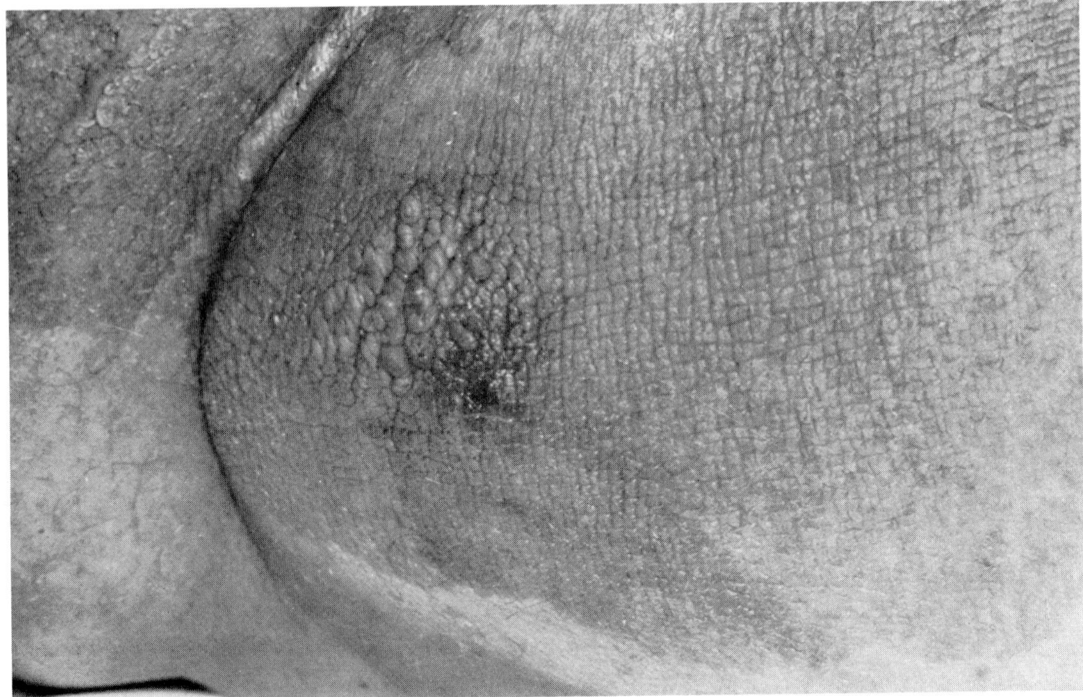

Figure 1–48. Acanthosis nigricans on inner thigh. Papillomatosis has developed in the center of lesion.

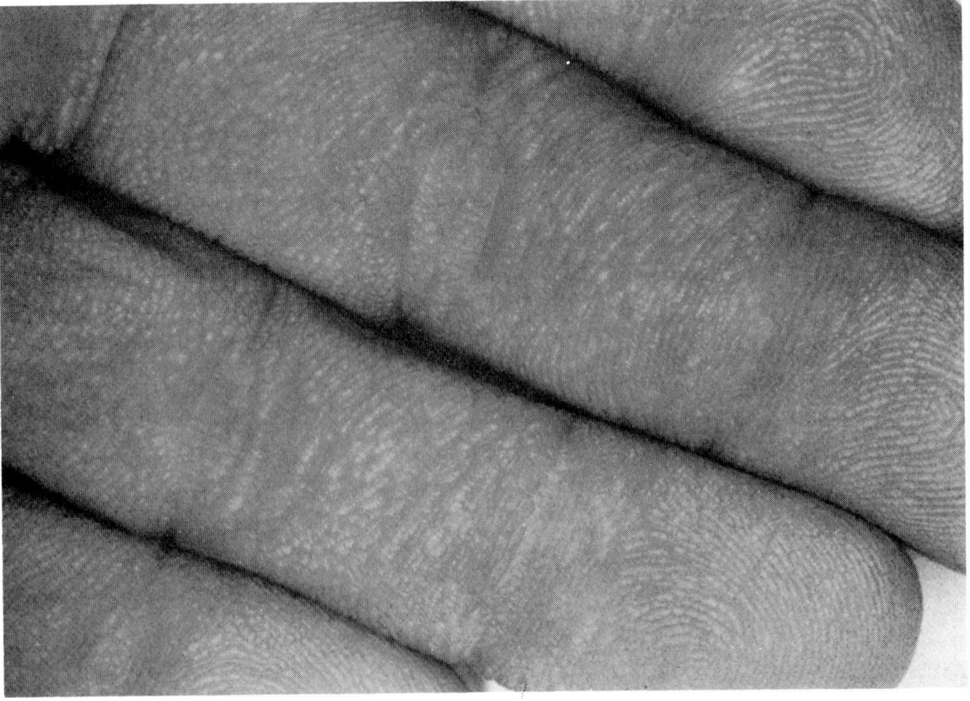

Figure 1-49. Keratoderma in association with carcinoma of stomach.

In acanthosis nigricans, the skin is thrown up into folds. Microscopically, it has a papillomatous appearance. Hyperpigmentation varying from brown to black is associated with this hyperplastic change. In its mildest form, acanthosis nigricans looks like exaggerated skin lines and is often thought by patients and their families to be dirty skin. As the dermatosis becomes more severe, a verrucose, velvety, and at times shaggy appearance develops, and gross papillomas can be found. When acanthosis nigricans is associated with cancer, it may spread as the neoplasm disseminates and may regress temporarily when the malignancy is resected. Möller et al. reported the case of a 64-year-old man with widespread acanthosis nigricans involving the hands, shoulders, face, lips, tongue, and oral mucosa as well as the axillae and groins. Following removal of hilar and mediastinal lymph nodes containing metastatic squamous cell carcinoma from an unknown site, the acanthosis nigricans completely disappeared. The patient was free of relapse from both the tumor and the acanthosis nigricans during three years of observation.[152] It has not been established how frequently acanthosis nigricans resolves

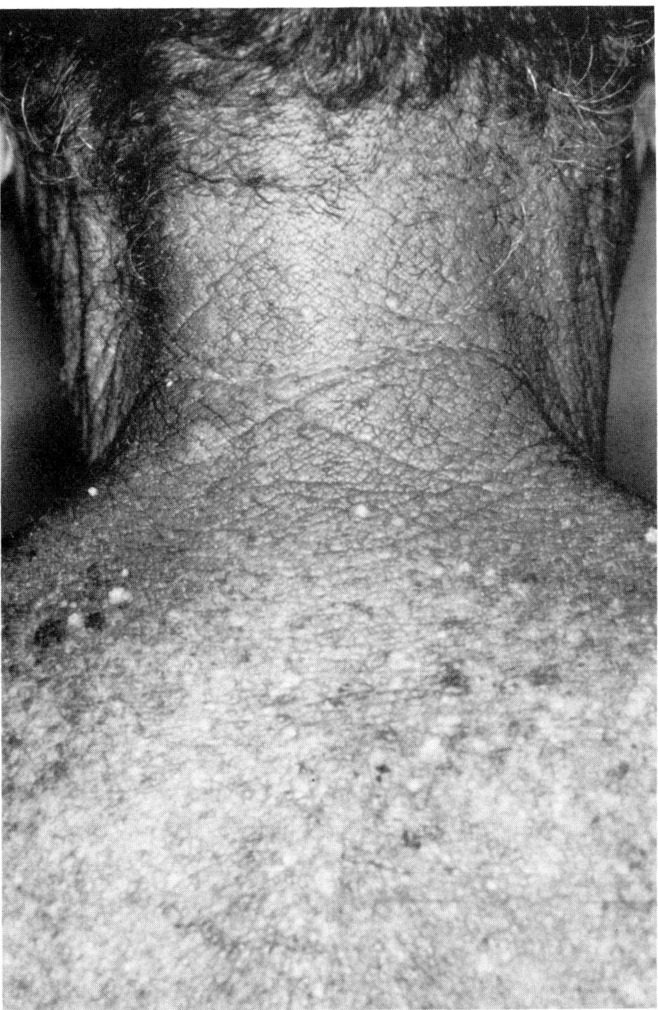

Figure 1–50. Acanthosis nigricans and diffuse hyperpigmentation in patient illustrated in Figure 1–49.

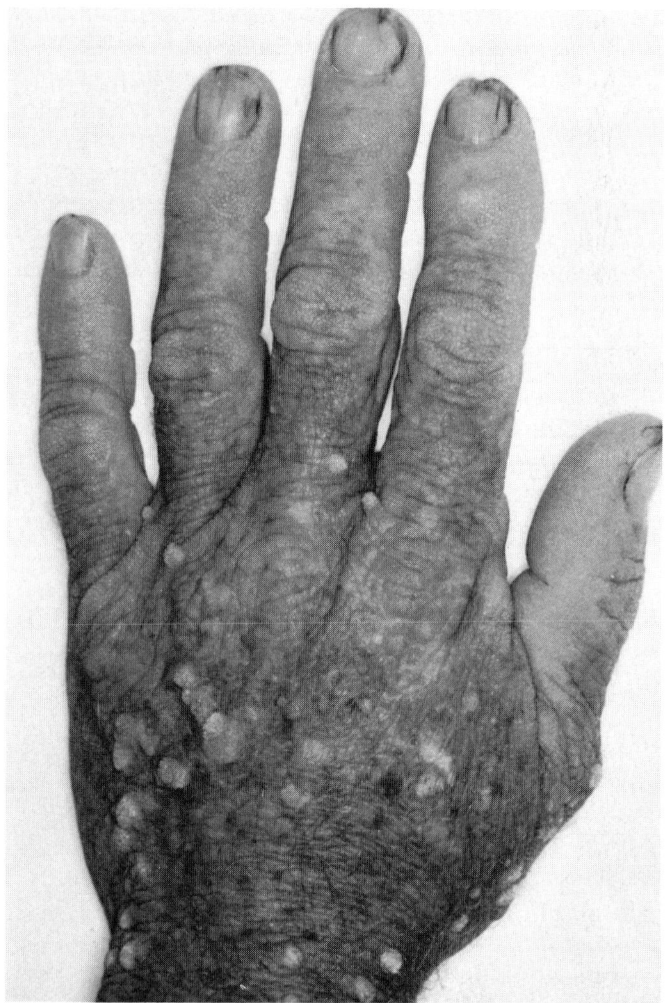

Figure 1–51. Disseminated common warts in patient shown in Figure 1–49.

after its associated disorders (cancer, obesity, or endocrine disease) have been successfully treated.

Figures 1–49 to 1–51 illustrate a patient with acanthosis nigricans secondary to carcinoma of the stomach. In addition to diffuse hyperpigmentation and hyperkeratosis of the palms, he had disseminated common warts as well. The immunodepression sometimes associated with advanced cancer may have been a factor in allowing the warts to become generalized in this patient. The spread of warts is not unusual in patients on immunosuppressive therapy (Fig. 1–52).

The terms *benign* and *malignant* acanthosis nigricans refer to the associated disorders and not to the dermatosis, which never undergoes malignant change.

Acanthosis nigricans associated with cancer is a disease of adults, the youngest patient reported being a 17-year-old white girl. In 80 to 90 per 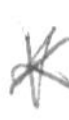 cent of all instances, the cancer is abdominal; in 60 per cent, the cancer arises in the stomach. Other associated carcinomas have included those of the uterus, liver, esophagus, pancreas, prostate, ovary, kidney, colon, and rectum. Almost all cancers accompanying this dermatosis have been adenocarcinomas. However, there have also been reported instances of

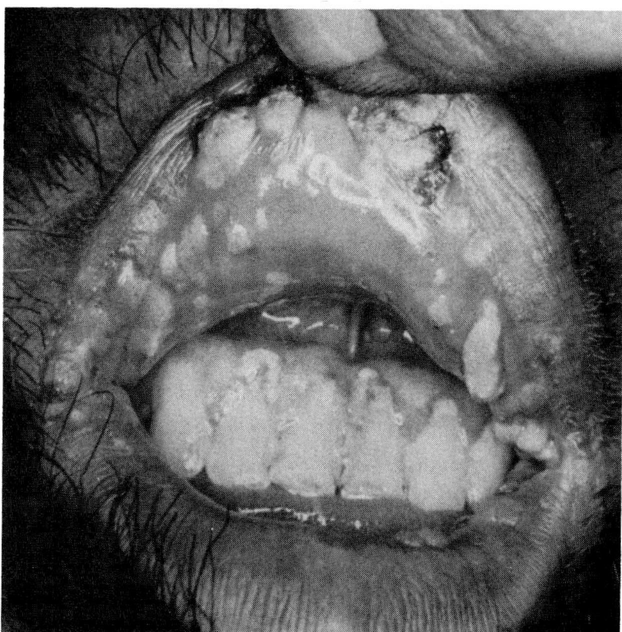

Figure 1–52. Common warts on lips of immunosuppressed patient with renal transplant.

anaplastic carcinoma of the lung and stomach, squamous cell carcinoma of the cervix and lung, choriocarcinoma, lymphosarcoma, reticulum cell sarcoma, and Hodgkin's disease in association with acanthosis nigricans.[153-155]

In 60 per cent of approximately 140 cases tabulated by Curth, the dermatosis and cancer appeared at the same time.[156] In 17 per cent (25 cases), the dermatosis preceded the detection of the malignancy. In 11 of these 25 cases, the dermatosis preceded the cancer by 5 to 18 years, and in the remainder of the cases, the dermatosis preceded the cancer by one to three years; the acanthosis nigricans may have been related to other causes in these 11 cases, and the cancers may have been coincidental. In 22 per cent (31 cases), the acanthosis nigricans appeared up to two years after the tumor was detected and was usually associated with metastases.

The tumors associated with acanthosis nigricans are highly malignant, and the average survival after the cancer is discovered or resected is 12 months. The mechanism by which the tumor produces these hyperplastic changes in the skin is not known, but it is reasonable to believe that the neoplasm may be secreting an as-yet-unidentified peptide that directly stimulates the skin to become hyperplastic.[157] In support of this hypothesis, Hage and Hage described a patient with acanthosis nigricans in whom many tumor cells of the associated gastric carcinoma had histochemical and ultrastructural features resembling those of the enterochromaffin cells of the APUD series.[158] In addition, this patient also had generalized common warts similar to those in our patient shown in Figures 1–49 to 1–51.

Curth has pointed out an interesting feature of patients with both *benign* and *malignant* acanthosis nigricans: there is an apparently high incidence of cancer, predominantly gastric carcinoma, in family members. These relatives, however, do not have acanthosis nigricans.

These observations need to be pursued further. Familial *malignant* acanthosis nigricans has not been reported.[159]

In dogs, especially Swedish dachshunds, acanthosis nigricans occurs as a benign and familial trait.[159] Two dogs with acanthosis nigricans and cancer have been studied, but the association in these animals is very uncommon.[160]

How is acanthosis nigricans in an adult evaluated? In the majority of cases, one will find a fat individual who has been obese since childhood and who probably has had acanthosis nigricans since that time. A minority of adults with obesity and acanthosis nigricans may have an endocrine abnormality such as Cushing's disease. Special concern must be given to *nonobese* adults who develop acanthosis nigricans, for they are the ones in whom a malignancy is almost always present.

The differential diagnosis of acanthosis nigricans includes primarily erythrasma and Addison's disease. In erythrasma, produced by *Corynebacteria,* one finds hyperpigmentation and fine scaling, without verrucous change, in the axillae and groin. This chronic superficial cutaneous infection responds rapidly to oral or topical antibiotics. In Addison's disease, which can also be associated with axillary hyperpigmentation, the cutaneous surface remains normal.

Sneddon reported two patients in whom cancer of the stomach was associated with a sudden increase in the number and size of their seborrheic keratoses.[161] Although they did not have acanthosis nigricans, he thought that the increase in the size and number of the keratoses might represent a variant of acanthosis nigricans. Sneddon referred to similar observations by Gougerot and Duperrat[162] and Josserand et al.[163] A review of these papers reveals different, but none the less interesting, observations.

Gougerot and Duperrat reported the case of a 64-year-old French woman who for one year had had a pruritic weeping eczematous dermatitis involving the pubic and perineal areas, thighs, and ankles. Verrucous papules and plaques were present on the hands, fingers, dorsal interphalangeal joints, and elbows. Most of the verrucous lesions occurred as small patches on the palmar and dorsal aspects of the hands and fingers and clinically resembled common warts (verrucae vulgares) or a patchy keratoderma. However, on the radial aspect of the right hypothenar eminence, the verrucous papules were arranged in a longitudinal band that resembled a linear epidermal nevus or a Koebner reaction involving warts. Over each elbow was a large plaque made up of linear bands oriented along the axis of the arms. The bands composing the plaques were made up of verrucous papules. The clinical appearance of the plaques on the elbow resembled acanthosis nigricans, epidermal nevi, or confluent verrucae vulgares. Histological examination of this lesion was most consistent with either acanthosis nigricans or an epidermal nevus. Seborrheic keratosis and verruca vulgaris were excluded. The patient died suddenly and at autopsy she was found to have a carcinoma of the head of the pancreas. The description of weeping eczematous dermatitis in the perineal area and on the thighs in association with a carcinoma of the pancreas makes it very likely that this patient had the *glucagonoma* syndrome. I interpret the accompanying verrucous lesions to have represented acanthosis nigricans, which has a hyperkeratotic appearance in nonintertriginous areas.

Josserand et al. described a 32-year-old woman with a breast carcinoma that produced marked edema and gave a peau d'orange appearance to the overlying skin. She developed many common warts (verrucae vulgares) in this area. Over a period of six months, the edema secondary to the cancer spontaneously disappeared and so did the warts.

Gougerot and Duperrat also refer to a book entitled *Warts, Papillomas and Cancer* by two Hungarian physicians, Balo and Korpassy, who believe that adults with many seborrheic keratoses have three times as many visceral cancers as those adults that do not have seborrheic keratoses. This skin manifestation has been called the sign of Leser-Trélat in recognition of two surgeons — one French, Ulysse Trélat (1828–1890) and the other German, Edmund Leser (1853–1916) — who espoused this hypothesis.[164] Although the sign of Leser-Trélat is a controversial one, primarily because of its rarity, the sudden appearance and rapid increase in size and number of seborrheic keratoses over a period of three to six months should arouse suspicion of an internal malignancy. Liddell et al. published a well-documented report of three patients in whom the sudden and rapid development of seborrheic keratoses was associated with adenocarcinomas of the large bowel.[165] In one of the patients, the seborrheic keratoses virtually disappeared following treatment of the primary tumor with radiotherapy, but they recurred when the tumor began to extend six months later. Sneddon's two cases are also examples of this sign.[161] Approximately 10 documented instances of this syndrome have been described and are listed in the article by Liddell et al.[165] The case reports of Josserand et al. and Gougerot and Duperrat described in detail above are not examples of this syndrome, although they are always included in reviews of this sign.

The carcinomas in documented cases of the Leser-Trélat syndrome have included those of the stomach, ovary, uterus, colon, and one of unspecified site and type. Dantzig reported a patient with Sézary's syndrome in whom "warty" and numerous velvety and papillary papules 2 to 6 mm in diameter were present over the back, shoulders, and chest.[166] No biopsies were performed on these lesions, so it is not clear whether they represented seborrheic keratoses or the localized areas of epidermal hyperplasia ("acanthomas") which develop in areas of erythroderma caused by eczema, psoriasis, or the application of tar.[167] The "acanthomas" do not have the histological features of seborrheic keratoses. They also differ from them in being smaller, lacking the "stuck-on" appearance, being only slightly elevated and not nearly as pigmented, and tending to disappear spontaneously within a few months.

SYNDROMES INDICATIVE OF SYSTEMIC OR ORGAN-RELATED CARCINOGENESIS

In 1959 Graham and Helwig made a remarkable observation: Bowen's disease of the skin (epidermoid carcinoma *in situ*) was associated with the eventual development of internal cancer.[135] In their series of 35 patients who had Bowen's disease and who had died, 20 were discovered to have carcinomas of the hypopharynx, larynx, lung, esophagus, breast, ovary, stomach, kidney, urinary bladder, or prostate. Both epidermoid and adenocarcinomas were found. Four patients developed a reticuloendothelial disease: lymphosarcoma, chronic myelogenous leukemia, or chronic lymphatic leukemia. In four others, squamous cell carcinoma of the skin, which in two instances arose from Bowen's disease, and malignant melanoma were present. In six patients the internal malignancy was found only at autopsy. In seven patients no internal neoplasm was found, but four of these seven persons had actinic keratoses, basal cell tumors, or a sweat gland neoplasm. Thus, 80 per cent of their patients had an associated malignancy, and in only one case did the Bowen's disease appear after the cancer had been detected. At the time of their report, in 23 of over 100 living patients with Bowen's disease, primary cancers of the lips, the cornea, the conjuctivae, the urethra, the thyroid, and the organs mentioned previously had developed. A follicular lymphoma occurred in one patient. The average latent period between the onset of Bowen's disease and the detection of a neoplasm was eight and one half years. The average latent periods for the development of malignancy in different organs are summarized in Table 1–2.

A family history of cancer was elicited in 48 per cent of 77 families. The cancer involved all three germ layers, and the sites, in order of frequency, were the skin, respiratory tract, gastrointestinal system, genitourinary organs, reticuloendothelial system, endocrine system, breast, and eye. These data were updated in 1961 to include 155 patients, both living and dead, 48 per cent of whom had associated premalignant and malignant lesions.[168] It seems likely that the association of Bowen's disease of the skin with internal and cutaneous cancer is a manifestation of a systemic carcinogenic process.

These data have been confirmed and extended by Peterka et al. and by Sneddon and Russell, who pointed out that Bowen's disease on covered parts of the body is even more significant than it is on exposed areas, with regard to the development of internal cancer. Actinic keratoses may exhibit Bowenoid changes and be confused with true Bowen's disease. In Peterka's series, 33 per cent of the patients with Bowen's disease had an internal cancer, and in Sneddon's and Russell's series the incidence was 50 per cent.[161, 169] In Peterka's cases, only 5 per cent of patients with lesions in areas of actinic exposure had internal cancer; in Russell's series the incidence was 4.4 per cent. Epstein, Hugo, and Conway confirmed the association between cutaneous Bowen's disease and malignancy but did not differentiate between covered and uncovered areas.[170, 171]

Andersen et al. studied the Danish population to determine whether this association could be confirmed. They found six cancers where only

Table 1–2. LATENT PERIODS FOR DEVELOPMENT OF MALIGNANCY

Organ	Average Latent Period (in years)
Reticuloendothelial system	1.3
Genitourinary tract	4.5
Respiratory tract	8.4
Endocrine organs	12
Gastrointestinal tract	13
Skin	14.2

2.78 were expected in their group of 31 patients with Bowen's disease, but the observed number of cancers was not judged to be statistically significant.[172]

Bowen's disease of the skin is epidermoid carcinoma *in situ.* In 5 per cent of the patients, it becomes invasive; in one third of such patients in Graham and Helwig's series, there were metastases to internal organs.

Clinically, the lesions of Bowen's disease usually are circumscribed, oval to arciform, and have varying degrees of induration. In the mildest form, the lesion is erythematous and flat with scaling that resembles eczema or psoriasis (Fig. 1–53; Plate 2*E*). The lesion can also be nodular with heavy scaling and crusting. Pigmentation may be intense or absent. Ulceration usually denotes local invasion and malignant change.

The appearance of an asymptomatic eczematous or psoriasiform lesion which has been slowly expanding for months or years should be suspect. Multicentric superficial basal cell tumors are often confused with Bowen's disease. They can be distinguished clinically by the presence of a thin elevated pearly border. The histologic differentiation presents no difficulties.

From the available data, a general rule can be formulated: a person with Bowen's disease on a covered part of the body — trunk, legs, or arms — has one chance in two or three of developing an internal cancer in five to ten years. The latent period, which varies from one to 14 years, depends upon the organ system affected.

The histology of the palmar keratoses that develop in chronic arsenical intoxication may show disorder in orientation of epidermal cells resembling those of actinic keratoses. When squamous cell carcinoma

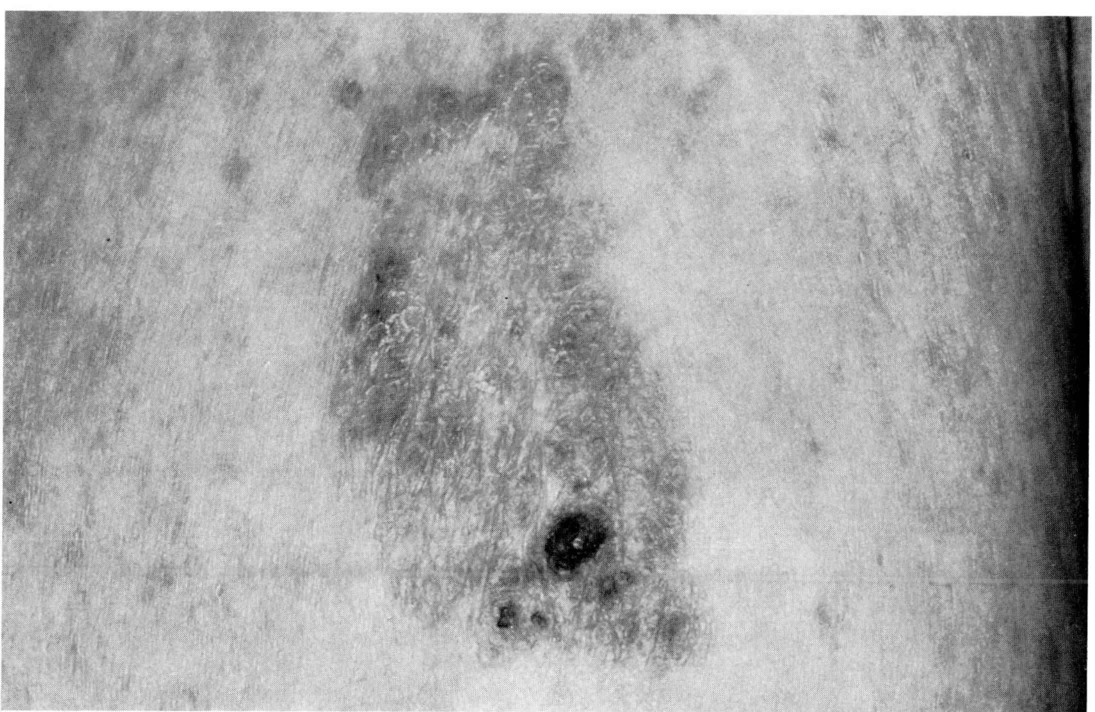

Figure 1–53. Bowen's disease on breast. Dark oval spot is biopsy site.

arises from arsenical keratoses, vacuolization of epidermal cells resembling those in Bowen's disease can be found as well.[173] Since chronic arsenical intoxication can produce cutaneous Bowen's disease and internal malignancies, Graham and Helwig looked for and found increased amounts of arsenic in Bowen's lesions.[174] Other investigators have not confirmed this finding, but different analytical methods were used in these various studies.[175, 176] The role of arsenic in the etiology of Bowen's disease remains highly controversial.

It is easy for individuals to develop chronic arsenical intoxication because the routes of entry are many, some being obvious and some subtle. Arsenic can be ingested as a medication in the form of potassium arsenite ($KAsO_2$) in Fowler's solution. Inorganic arsenic was combined with potassium iodide in cough medications for the symptomatic treatment of asthma. Although arsenic is rarely used in the current practice of medicine, it still finds its way into unorthodox medications from time to time. Tay reported an epidemic of arsenic poisoning caused by a particular group of Chinese herbal medicines used in Singapore from 1972 to 1973.[177] Lead arsenate is an ingredient of food additives and of insecticides and herbicides used in agriculture. Until the early 1950's, it was used to spray tobacco crops, so that American cigarettes became contaminated with arsenic. The arsenic content of cigarettes rose from 12.6 μg per cigarette in 1932 to 42 μg in 1951.[178] Recognition of this problem resulted in a decrease in the arsenic content to 7.7 μg per cigarette by 1968.[179] Arsenic is also used in electroplating, is important in the manufacture of dyes — Schweinfurth green and Scheele's green — and is combined with sulfur for sheep dip. Miners are exposed to arsenic via inhalation during the processing and smelting of copper and other ores. The increased incidence of lung cancer among copper smelters in Montana is attributed to arsenical intoxication based upon the increased arsenic content in the foliage near the smelters. In ores, arsenic exists as the trioxide (synonyms: white arsenic, arsenous anhydride, arsenous acid). In many parts of the world, arsenic is present in the well water used for drinking.[180]

A new use for arsenic has recently been introduced. In the forestry industry, cacodylic acid (dimethylarsenic acid) and MSMA (monosodium acid methanearsenate) are being injected into trees as silvicides in order to thin out forests so that properly spaced tree crops can be planted and harvested for economic purposes.[181] In spite of protective clothing, gloves, and masks, foresters engaged in this process are absorbing significant quantities of arsenic. In addition, the cacodylic acid and MSMA are microbially transformed into arsine gas which persists for up to three weeks in the forest after the initial spraying is carried out.[181, 182] Although cacodylic acid and MSMA are classified as organic arsenicals, they behave like inorganic arsenic because they are converted in the body to arsenous acid (As_2O_3).[183] Whether the chronic exposure to cacodylic acid, MSMA, and arsine gas will produce the same chronic toxic effects in man as do the other forms of arsenic remains to be determined.

Inorganic, not organic, arsenic is responsible for the cutaneous and systemic changes to be described. In organic arsenicals, the arsenic is covalently bonded to a benzene ring, which prevents its being converted to an inorganic arsenic compound. Because arsenic has been shown to be carcinogenic only for human beings, an experimental animal model is not available for study. Exposure to arsenic for a time as short as six months or as long as 30 years causes identical changes in man.

Arsenical toxicity produces hyperpigmentation, palmar and plantar keratoses, Bowen's disease of the skin, multicentric superficial basal cell tumors, and internal cancers. Pigmentation and keratoses develop from three to four years after exposure to arsenic. Although all features noted above are not always present in an individual case, either the pigmentation or the keratoses are necessary to make a diagnosis of arsenism. However, multiple patches of either Bowen's disease or multicentric basal cell tumors in the absence of pigmentation or keratoses should alert one to the possibility of arsenical intoxication.

The hyperpigmentation appears primarily on the trunk but can also be seen in the axillae, on the areolae, in the perineal area, and on pressure sites. A mottled or reticulated brown to gray pigmentation interspersed with oval areas of normal appearing skin develops (Plate 2*F*). The oval areas of normal skin have been called "dew drops" and have been misinterpreted as depigmentation.

Hyperkeratotic yellowish papules, discrete or coalescent, are typically present on the palms and soles but may also occur over the dorsa of the hands. Malignant transformation of these papules into epidermoid carcinoma with widespread metastases can take place. The exact incidence is not known, but it is probably low. Arsenical keratoses do not have central depressions and are distinct from the keratotic papules described by Dobson (see p. 99).

Typical lesions of Bowen's disease develop especially on covered parts of the body. In Sanderson's experience, the production of multiple superficial basal cell tumors occurs in the absence of hyperpigmentation and keratoses.[184]

Arsenical keratoses are illustrated in Figures 1–54 to 1–57. This patient had received Fowler's solution as a nerve tonic 20 years previously. One of her palmar keratoses degenerated into an epidermoid carcinoma which metastasized to her median nerve and axillary nodes and necessitated forelimb amputation.

The patient illustrated in Figure 1–58 has hundreds of superficial multicentric basal cell tumors on the trunk. She had been given Fowler's solution for therapy of acne vulgaris 10 years previously. She did not have arsenical keratoses or pigmentation, in keeping with Sanderson's observations, nor did she exhibit stigmata of the basal cell nevus syndrome (see p. 83).

On the southwest coast of Taiwan there is an area in which the artesian wells are highly contaminated with arsenic.[185] Approximately 160,000 people drink from these wells. Similar situations have been described in Reichenstein, Silesia, and in Cordoba, Argentina. In Taiwan, in contrast to other areas of the world where arsenic is present in the drinking water, no mucous membrane or internal cancers have been found, but cutaneous malignancies have developed: epidermoid carcinoma, basal cell tumors, and Bowen's disease.

The prevalence of arsenical intoxication was determined in six villages. More than 3000 people, 80 per cent of the population, were examined. The average incidence was 36 per cent, but because there was a progressive increase with age, 84 per cent of the population over 50 years old had keratoses and typical hyperpigmentation. The incidence of

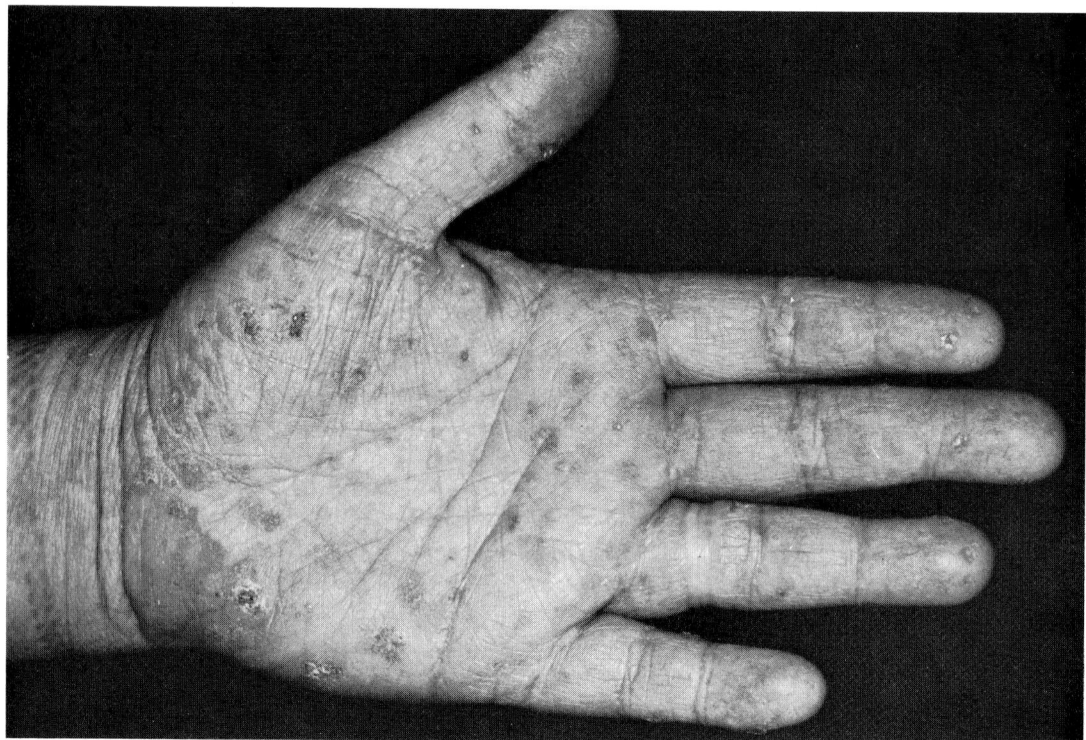

Figure 1–54. Arsenical keratoses.

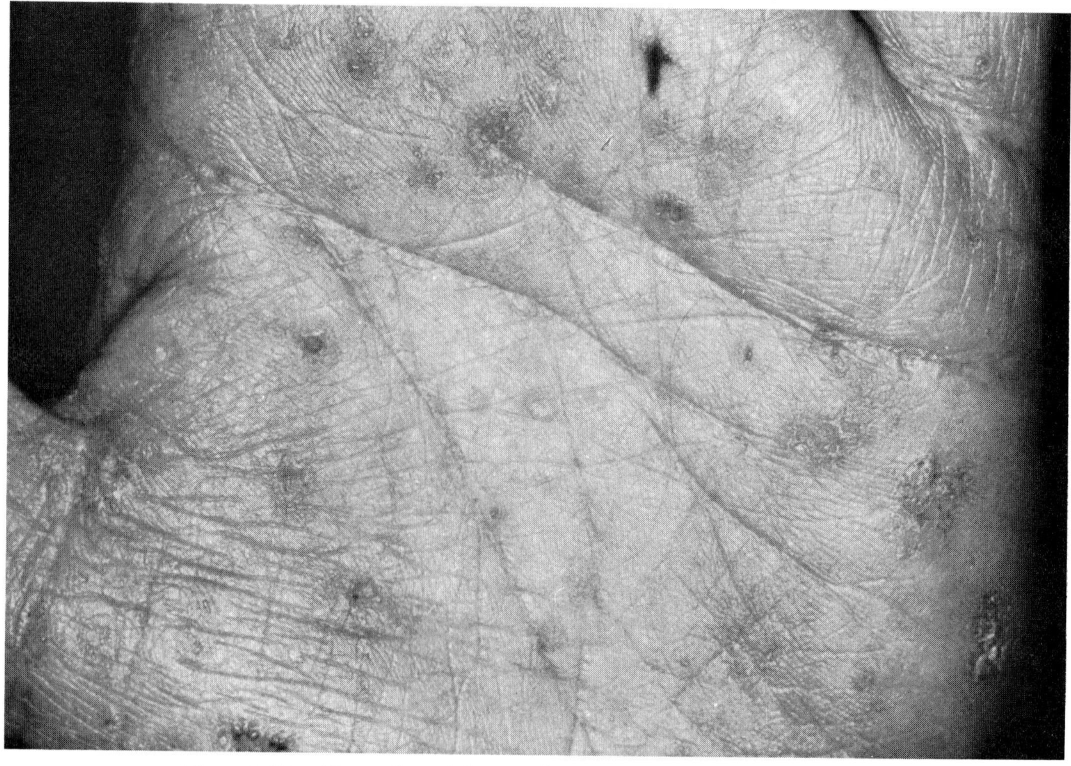

Figure 1–55. Closer view of the arsenical keratoses shown in Figure 1–54.

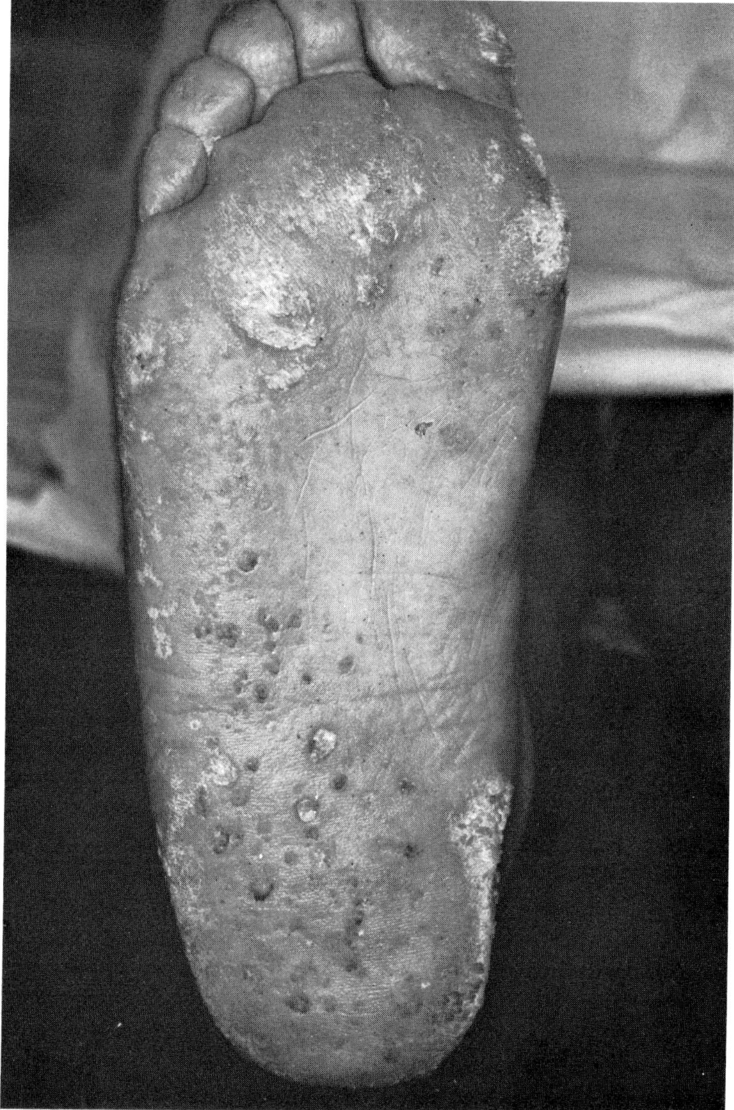

Figure 1-56. Arsenical keratoses on feet. Same patient as in Figure 1–54.

skin cancer in persons more than 50 years old was 6.8 per cent. These people also developed a peripheral vascular disorder called "blackfoot" disease; it is related to arsenical intoxication and resembles Buerger's disease.

The latent period for the development of the signs of arsenical intoxication on Taiwan varied from person to person and village to village. However, hyperpigmentation was observed in children seven to eight years old, and skin cancer was seen in a 24-year-old woman.

Ninety-four people moved from this endemic focus on Taiwan to another region where the well water was free of arsenic. Follow-up revealed that at least five years of exposure to arsenic was necessary for the development of pigmentation, 15 years for keratoses, and 20 years for skin cancer. Twenty-five per cent of the people showed no signs of arsenism. However, these data are different from those reported in other

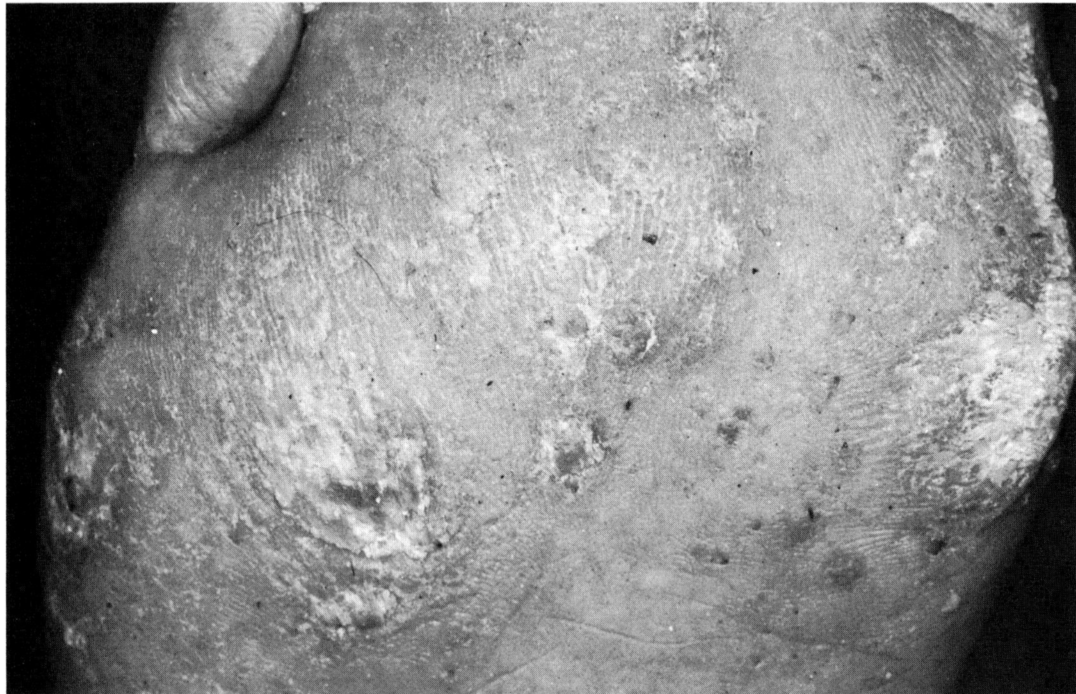

Figure 1–57. Closer view of the arsenical keratoses shown in Figure 1–56. Although these keratoses resemble warts, the *characteristic features* of verrucae (discrete borders and multiple capillaries) would not be found when the keratoses are pared down with a scalpel blade.

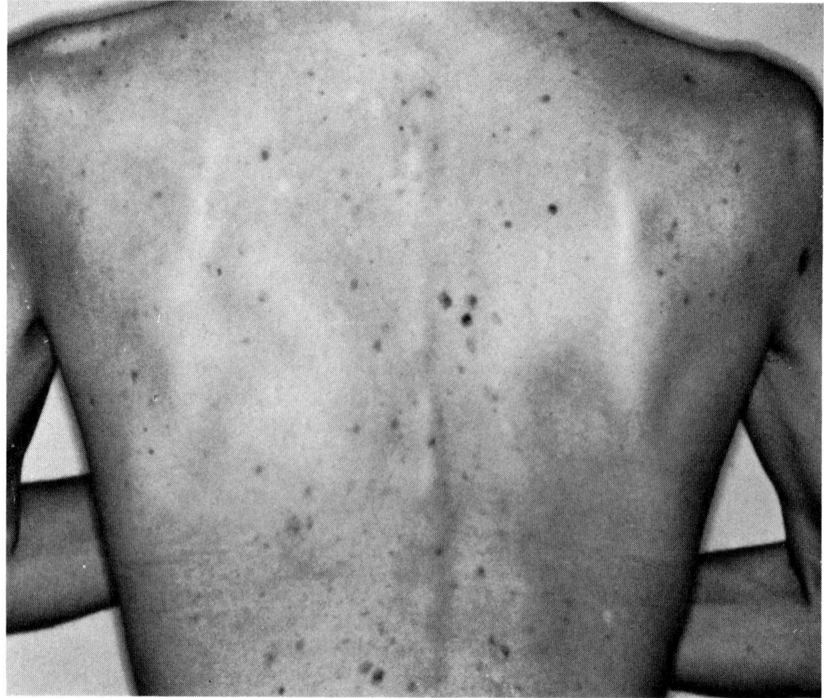

Figure 1–58. Multiple superficial basal cell tumors in woman who was given Fowler's solution 10 years before.

regions of the world. Yen has published a more current and complete account of chronic arsenism in this endemic focus on Taiwan.[186]

Roth described the plight of the Moselle vineyard workers who used arsenical sprays and drank a house wine made from the contaminated grapes.[187] He found 10 instances of bronchogenic cancer and three hepatic malignancies (hemangiosarcomas) in 24 autopsies on these vineyard workers. One individual had a carcinoma of the bile duct in addition to the lung cancer. In six patients with typical cutaneous signs of arsenism, death resulted from carcinoma of the lung. Most instances of internal cancer secondary to arsenism have the skin markers of arsenical intoxication.

Sommers and McManus studied 27 individuals with arsenism and found 10 cases of internal malignancy. The organs involved were the tonsil, esophagus, lung, pancreas, breast, colon, and those of the genitourinary tract; in addition, a chest wall sarcoma was found.[188] Russell studied 331 individuals with basal cell tumors. In 11 patients there was a history of arsenic ingestion. Five of these eleven persons, but only seven of the remaining 320 individuals, developed lung cancer.[189]

A study at Dow Chemical Company, where an inorganic arsenic insecticide product was being manufactured from 1919 to 1956, showed that workers developed cancer of the respiratory tract 2 to 3.5 times more often than expected because of presumed exposure to the manufacture and packaging of the product which contained lead arsenate, calcium arsenate, copper acetoarsenite, and magnesium arsenate.[190] There was also an increase in lymphomas — 6 observed versus 2.8 expected — that was considered statistically significant. The lymphomas were diagnosed as lymphoblastoma, reticulum cell sarcoma, and Hodgkin's disease. However, there was no evidence that the employees as a group had a shorter life span than would be expected. In 1973, the National Institute of Occupational Safety and Health estimated that 1.5 million American workers were potentially exposed to inorganic arsenic.[190]

Although the mechanism of arsenical carcinogenesis in man is unknown, the profound effects of inorganic arsenic on cellular metabolism and replication provide some clues toward its eventual understanding. Arsenic inhibits the enzymes responsible for oxidative phosphorylation because of its reactivity with sulfhydryl groups. Arsenic added to cultures of lymphocytes will suppress cell division and produce increased numbers of chromosomal breaks and sister chromatid exchanges.[191] Burgdorf et al. have demonstrated that there is an increased rate of sister chromatid exchange in lymphocytes of individuals with skin cancers related to previous arsenic ingestion.[192] These workers have not yet studied patients with arsenic ingestion who do not have skin cancer or other signs of arsenical toxicity. Arsenism and Bowen's disease behave similarly: cancer of varied types develops in all organs. The skin is most frequently involved, followed by the squamous epithelium of the mouth and esophagus, the metaplastic squamous epithelium of the respiratory tract, and the epithelium of the kidney, ureter, and urinary bladder.

A discussion of Bowen's disease, multicentric basal cell tumors, internal cancer, and arsenism is not complete without some general remarks about skin carcinogenesis. The differential diagnosis of these entities includes the common types of skin cancers which arise in the following precancerous situations: the susceptible individual, the prema-

PLATE 4

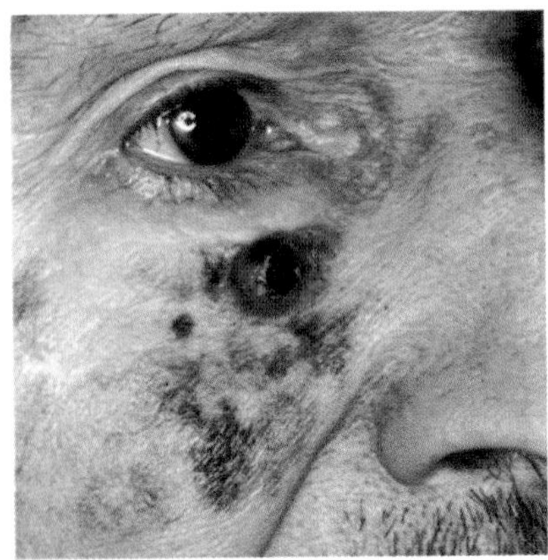

A, Melanotic freckle with developing melanoma. (Courtesy of Dr. Donald Shedd.)

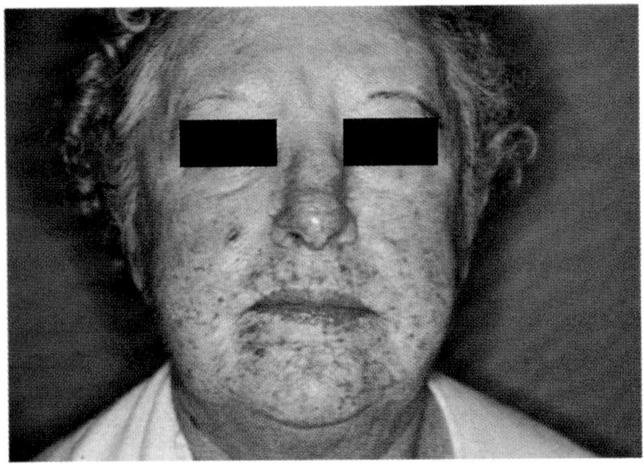

B, Radiodermatitis of face produced by x-ray therapy for hirsutism.

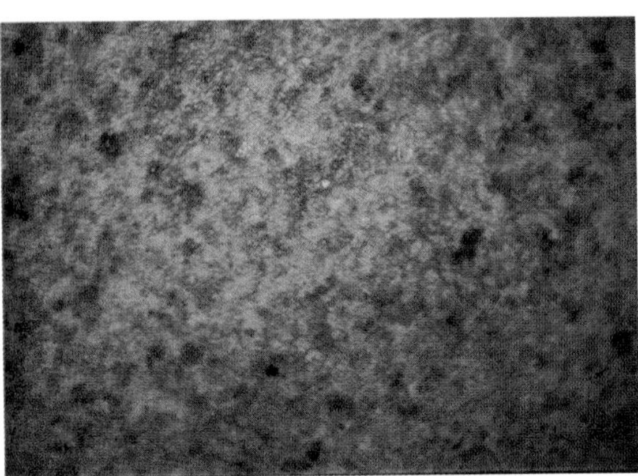

C, Close view of the skin in xeroderma pigmentosum. Radiodermatitis is mimicked.

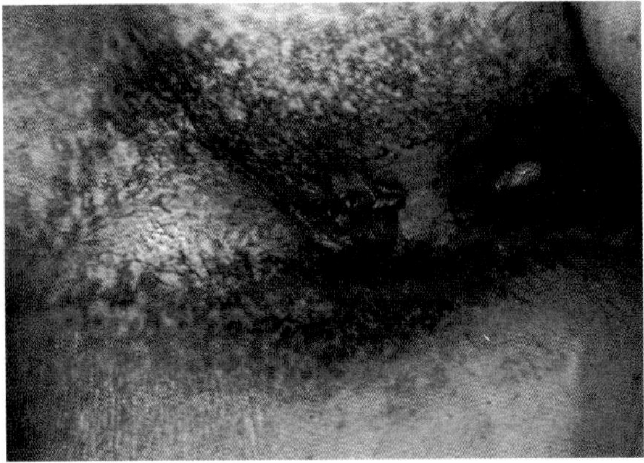

D, Reticulated hyperpigmentation in the perineal area of a woman with familial polyposis (Courtesy of Dr. Sherwin Nuland.)

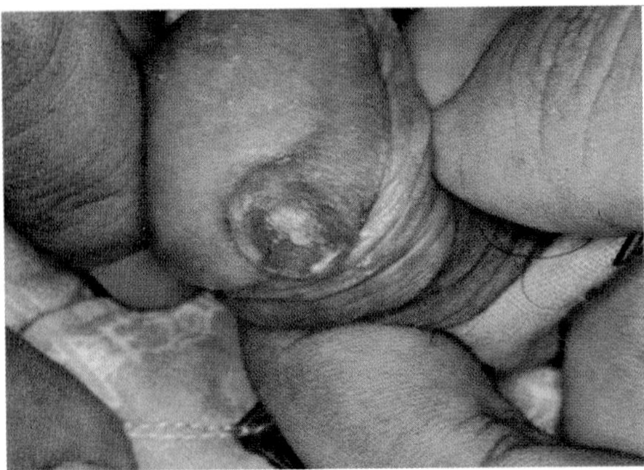

E, Reticulum cell sarcoma involving the glans penis.

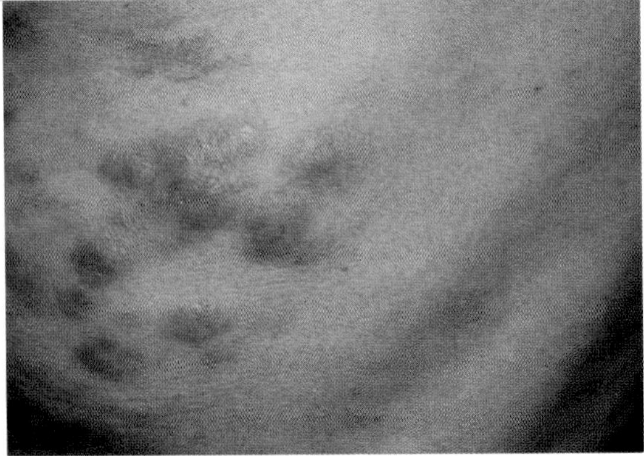

F, Close view of specific cutaneous lesions in Hodgkin's disease. Note characteristic erythematous-violaceous color of the lymphomatous diseases.

lignant dermatosis, and the severely scarred skin. Awareness of these precancerous situations is important because they may be responsible for the induction of metastatic disease in the viscera. In addition, the presence of multiple skin cancers can be a marker for non-neoplastic systemic diseases.

Actinically damaged skin in blue-eyed individuals of fair complexion is predisposed to the development of basal cell tumors, squamous cell tumors, and even malignant melanoma. Incidence of these skin cancers can be correlated with the amount and intensity of sun exposure. Those persons living in latitudes close to the equator are particularly vulnerable to these malignant transformations. The increased amount of melanin pigment protects the Negro skin against the deleterious effects of ultraviolet radiation. Albinos lack this protective pigmentation.

Lentigo maligna (melanotic freckle of Hutchinson) often appears on actinically damaged areas but can also occur on covered portions of the body. This premalignant lesion gives rise to malignant melanoma which behaves differently from the usual type of melanoma arising *de novo* or from a junctional nevus (Plate 4*A*). The melanoma arising from a melanotic freckle is usually only locally invasive and rarely metastasizes widely. Local surgical excision often controls the tumor.[193, 194]

Epidermoid carcinomas that arise in actinically damaged skin—almost always from an actinic keratosis — behave in a benign fashion. They grow very slowly, are only locally invasive, and *almost never* metastasize. This behavior is in contrast to that of aggressive epidermoid carcinomas which arise from other types of premalignant conditions: arsenical keratoses, Bowen's disease on a covered portion of the body, exposure to pitch and tar, scars, radiodermatitis, and the skin of patients with xeroderma pigmentosum. Epidermoid carcinomas arising from skin normally protected from sun exposure (rare), lip, penis, vulva, and anus, however, are usually highly invasive and run a considerable risk of metastasis.[195]

Squamous cell carcinoma can develop in cutaneous scars that result from third degree burns, lupus vulgaris, lupus erythematosus, dystrophic epidermolysis bullosa,[196, 197] from the edges of chronic draining osteomyelitic sinuses and from chronic ulcerations, especially those on the legs.

Skin cancers of the scrotum and other areas can be produced by pitch, tar, creosote oil, mineral oil, and paraffin oil. The reader is referred to excellent discussions of these topics by Huepner and Henry.[198, 199] There are at least 250,000 workers exposed to these carcinogenic hazards in the United States. A recent survey by Wahlberg disclosed that in Sweden there were 34 cases of squamous cell carcinoma of the scrotum diagnosed from 1958 to 1970. Thirty-nine per cent were of occupational origin — exposure to machine oils. The causes of the rest were not determined. In England from 1939 to 1948, there were 34 cases uncovered. Twenty-five of the 34 were related to exposure to oil or pitch. In Manchester, England, from 1963 to 1968, 103 cases were found. Where information was available in 89 individuals, there was a clear relation to occupation in 84. The problems of the chimney sweeps are still with us.[200]

Radiodermatitis, primarily of the hands and face, is another premalignant dermatosis. It is seen most commonly in medical personnel and in certain groups of women (Fig. 1–59). Basal cell tumors and squamous cell carcinomas may arise. The poor calibration of x-ray machines, a lack of proper shielding, and an incomplete knowledge of the harmful effects of radiation in the early days of radiotherapy were responsible for the many cases of radiodermatitis on the hands of medical and dental personnel. Many women were treated for hirsutism and acne vulgaris during this same period, 1910 to 1930. We are currently seeing the late radiation effects in these two groups of people (Plate 4*B*). Radiodermatitis is characterized by atrophy, coarse telangiectasia, and mottled hyper- and hypopigmentation (Fig. 1–60). Tumors arise as ulcerations or as ulcerated papules within the area of radiodermatitis.

Xeroderma pigmentosum is a recessively inherited disorder in which there is an incredibly rapid development of aging and neoplastic change in the skin in response to sunlight. Investigators employing high energy monochromators have studied the cutaneous reactivity of these patients to narrow wave bands throughout the ultraviolet and visible light spectrum.[201, 202] Most patients with xeroderma pigmentosum have reacted abnormally to wave lengths of ultraviolet light between 290 and 320 nm, by forming a papular, and rarely a vesicular lesion, in association with the induced erythema. The erythema develops much later than expected after the irradiation and also persists for a longer period of time. In most patients the minimal erythema dose has been normal, but at least one patient had a significantly lower minimal erythema dose than normal.[201] Two patients have reacted like normal individuals to this test procedure.[202] These abnormal reactions to irradiation with ultraviolet light occur both in the abnormal skin of the patient with xeroderma pigmentosum as well as in the clinically normal skin of very young patients who

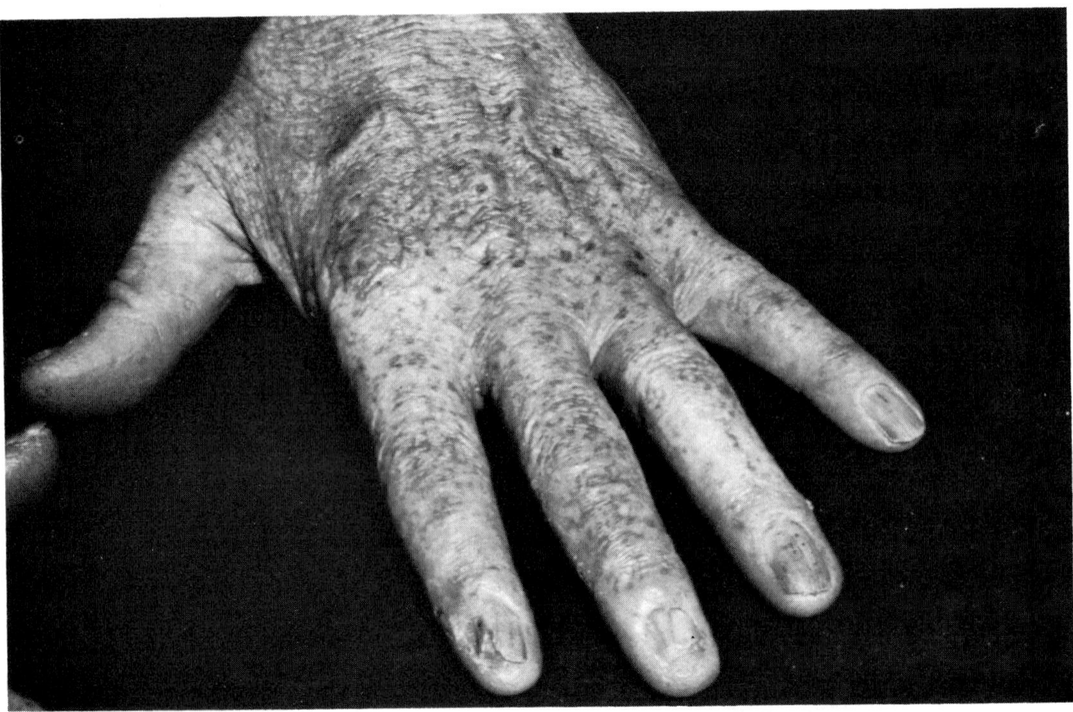

Figure 1–59. Radiodermatitis with nail dystrophy in dental technician.

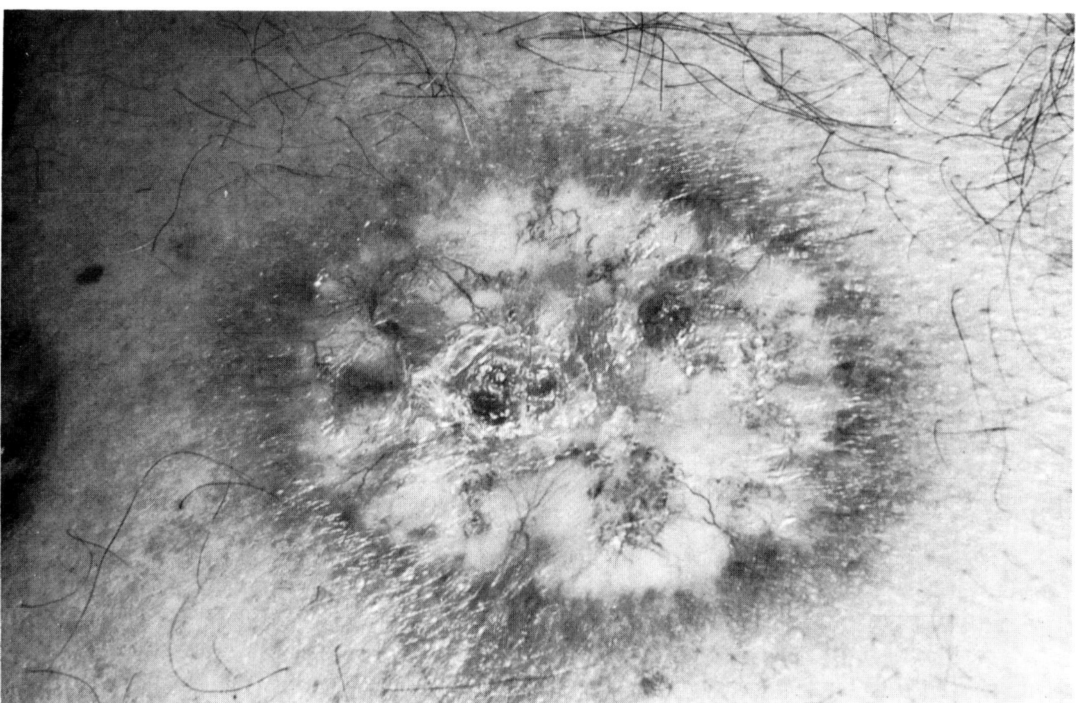

Figure 1-60. Radiodermatitis following x-ray treatment of skin cancer. Note characteristic telangiectasia, atrophy, and dyspigmentation.

have not yet developed the typical pigmentation and telangiectatic changes.[202]

Children with this disorder develop erythema, freckling, and increased pigmentation after their initial exposures to sunlight (Fig. 1–61; Plate 4*C*). Dryness, scaling, and atrophy of the skin with fine telangiectasia soon follow. By two or three years of age many youngsters have senile skin and tumors: basal cell tumors, squamous cell epitheliomas, hemangiomas, keratoacanthomas, and malignant melanomas. Photophobia, keratitis, and ectropions are common and are responsible for corneal opacities and loss of vision. Epidermoid carcinoma and malignant melanoma have arisen in the cornea and limbus.[203, 204] The clinical appearance of xeroderma pigmentosum resembles chronic radiodermatitis. The skin of the axillae and buttocks, which is protected from sunlight, remains relatively normal. The severity of the disease varies and cannot be correlated with sex, age of onset, blood groups, or the number of affected siblings in a family. In the more severely affected individuals, metastatic disease from skin tumors can cause death. Although xeroderma pigmentosum occurs almost exclusively in Caucasians, it has been reported in deeply pigmented blacks.[205] The greatest number of reports come from Egypt and the Near East where consanguinity is common.

In various studies, 25 to 80 per cent of children with xeroderma pigmentosum exhibited one or more developmental or neurological disorders (deSanctis-Cacchione syndrome): microcephaly, mental deficiency, spastic paralysis, deafness, ataxia, choreoathetosis, dwarfism, delay in bony maturation, and gonadal underdevelopment. Histological studies of patients with involvement of the central nervous system show a

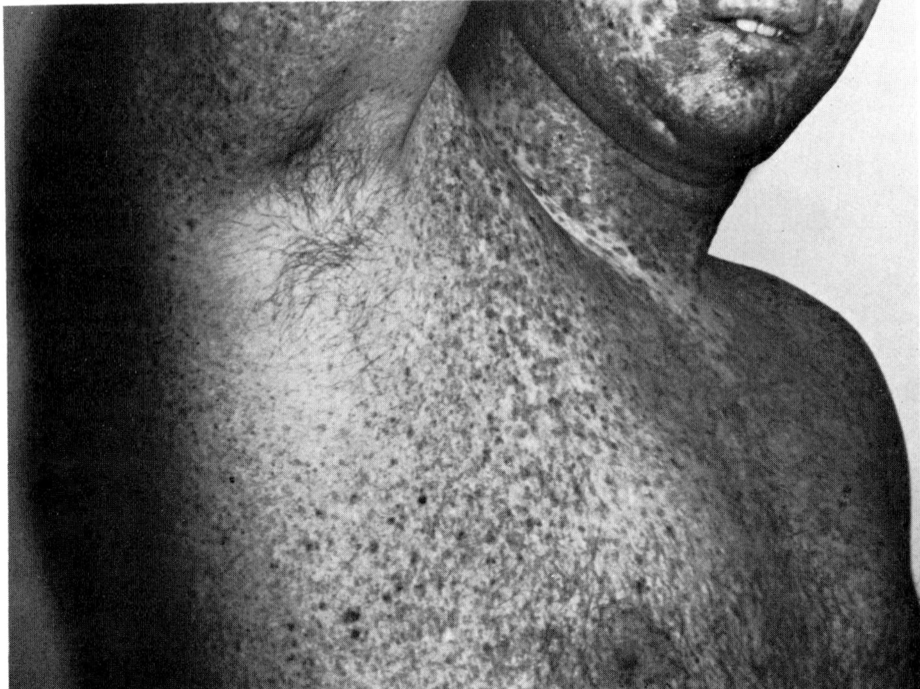

Figure 1–61. Xeroderma pigmentosum. Axillary skin is normal because it has not been exposed to sunlight.

neuronal loss or deficiency that lacks distinctive features.[206] The terms *common* and *neurological* have been introduced to distinguish these two major forms of xeroderma pigmentosum (see below). In Reed's series of four patients, chromosomal studies were normal, and no abnormalities were found in porphyrin excretion.[207] In a series of 24 patients, El-Hefnawi and co-workers found elevated serum copper, aminoaciduria, and low urinary excretion of 17-ketosteroids and 17-hydroxysteroids.[208-210] In a more recent study, xeroderma pigmentosum was shown to be linked to blood group O.[211]

Cleaver made an important discovery in 1968. He demonstrated that cultures of fibroblasts from the skin of patients with xeroderma pigmentosum are unable to repair ultraviolet-damaged DNA.[212] Epstein and his colleagues subsequently demonstrated the same defect *in vivo* in ultraviolet-irradiated epidermis of patients with xeroderma pigmentosum.[213] Since then, cultured fibroblasts from different patients have been shown to vary in their ability to perform excision repair of ultraviolet-damaged DNA.[214] Some cultures are unable to excise dimers to any measurable extent, while others can function at 90 per cent of normal levels. Cells from patients with the *common* and the *neurological* forms of the syndrome behave qualitatively similarly. The fibroblastic cultures from affected siblings show similar levels of repair, indicating that this function is inherited as a genetic trait. On the basis of hybridization experiments that combine cells from different patients with xeroderma pigmentosum, investigators have established that there are five complementation groups in this disorder — A, B, C, D, and E. Groups A, B, and D have one or more neurological abnormalities associated with them, but there is no specific neurological syndrome associated with any group. Each group is characterized by exhibiting the same level of DNA repair. Groups C and E are associated with the *common* form of the disease. In all of these groups, the fibroblasts share an additional common feature: irradiation with ultraviolet light results in poor cell survival.

A group of patients with classic xeroderma pigmentosum has been identified whose fibroblasts show normal levels of DNA repair and normal cell survival following ultraviolet irradiation. These individuals have been called xeroderma pigmentosum variants (XP variants). Their cells have been shown to be defective in postreplication repair. The XP variants form a set outside the five complementation groups. In the photosensitivity studies performed by Ramsay and Giannelli, one of the patients who did not show an abnormal reaction to ultraviolet light also exhibited normal levels of DNA repair in fibroblastic cultures.[202] Further studies are necessary to indicate whether all XP variants show a normal cutaneous reaction to ultraviolet light.

Xeroderma pigmentosum can now be diagnosed prenatally by testing amniotic cells for their ability to perform excision repair of damaged DNA. Postnatally, tests for excision repair of DNA in skin fibroblasts, coupled with observation of cutaneous reactivity to ultraviolet light, will enable one to diagnose the disease in an infant before the development of the diagnostic skin lesions. Only the XP variants, the minority of patients with this disorder, will not be detected by these techniques.[202]

It is currently believed that a close correlation exists between the mutagenic and carcinogenic activity of many chemical agents.[215] Cleaver and Bootsma propose that damaged DNA that is repaired defectively may result in mutagenesis and that the mutation of some critical region of the genome may be an important step in carcinogenesis. They also believe that both the excision repair system and the postreplication repair system are important in preventing radiation-induced carcinogenesis because of the clinical identity between the XP variants and the *common* and *neurological* forms of the disease.[214]

Locally aggressive squamous cell carcinoma is also a feature of epidermodysplasia verruciformis. This entity was described by Lewandowsky and Lutz in 1922 and initially was believed to represent the widespread development of small, flat-topped epidermal nevi.[216] Because of its frequently observed familial nature, it was thought to be a recessively transmitted genodermatosis, although there were some reported cases compatible with a dominant transmission. Histological examination of the papules revealed histologic changes characteristic of flat warts (verruca plana), but the fact that squamous cell carcinomas and Bowen's disease frequently arose among the lesions made it seem likely that the lesions were actually premalignant epidermal nevi. (Basal cell tumors may rarely arise in these sites.)

However, it has finally been established by auto- and heteroinoculation experiments[217-219] and by the demonstration of viral particles and viral antigen within the lesions by electron microscopy and immunofluorescent methods, respectively, that epidermodysplasia verruciformis represents widespread and persistent dissemination of flat warts.[220-222] The viral agent is a papova virus, related to human wart virus. Equally clear is the observation that the histological features of wart and early squamous cell carcinoma may be present in the same lesion, and in such situations, viral particles are still present but in fewer numbers.[220, 223, 224] However, in the developed lesions of Bowen's disease and squamous cell carcinoma, the viral particles or viral antigens can no longer be detected.[220, 221] This phenomenon is similar to that associated with the Shope viral papillomas in rabbits in which virus can be recovered from the benign papillomas, but not from the transformed malignant tumors.[225, 226]

Thus far, the squamous cell carcinomas in this entity have been only locally invasive, and metastases have not been reported. In almost every case, the carcinomas have developed in sun-exposed areas. An instance of microscopic malignant degeneration within a non–sun-exposed verrucous lesion has been reported.[224] It is currently assumed, but by no means rigorously proven, on the basis of lesions which contain virus and show histologic evidence of both wart and malignant change, that the verruca plana lesions are being transformed into malignancies.[223, 224]

Epidermodysplasia verruciformis typically begins in early childhood with the development of flat-topped papules, a few millimeters in diameter, which vary in colors from pink and flesh to gray or brown. The papules increase in number and become confluent, producing large plaques. Fine wrinkling and scaling may be present over the surface (Figs. 1–62 and 1–63).

The sites of predilection for the plaques and papules are the face, neck, back of the hands and wrists, dorsa of the feet and extremities. The trunk may be involved in cases in which there is widespread dissemination of the lesions. In some individuals, as in our patient, the disseminated papules and plaques can simulate a reticulated erythema or tinea versicolor. Only on close inspection does the true nature of this "erythema" become apparent (Fig. 1–63). From among the papules and plaques, large verrucous crusted and ulcerating tumors arise — mainly on the face, neck, and hands (Figs. 1–64 and 1–65). Malignant degeneration develops in the second and third decades. At the present time, therapy with x-ray, excision, electrodesiccation and curettage, and topical 5-fluorouracil would seem to be indicated because of the locally invasive behavior of these tumors.

The competency of the immune system has begun to be studied in these patients, and future studies will tell us whether or not immunodeficiency plays a role in the pathogenesis of the disease. In our patient, a 29-year-old man whose eruption began at the age of three years, the only abnormalities were borderline low levels of IgM and IgA in the serum. Cell-mediated immunity as evaluated by skin tests to microbial antigens, response of circulating lymphocytes to stimulation by phytohemagglutinin and Candida antigens, mixed lymphocyte culture, and quantitation of circulating B and T cells were all normal. Our patients also had unexplained eosinophilia, lymphadenopathy, and splenomegaly. Because of mild hypersplenism, a splenectomy was performed, but no evidence of lymphoma or other pathology was discovered on histologic examination.

Prawer et al. reported a case in which there was a 75 per cent depression of lymphocyte response to phytohemagglutinin, conconavalin-A, and streptokinase-streptodornase. The mixed lymphocyte culture test and quantitation of circulating B and T cells were normal. The patient was anergic to intracutaneous testing with microbial antigens and epicutaneous testing with 34 standard contact allergens.[227] Ultraviolet-induced DNA repair synthesis was impaired by 40 per cent in a patient studied by

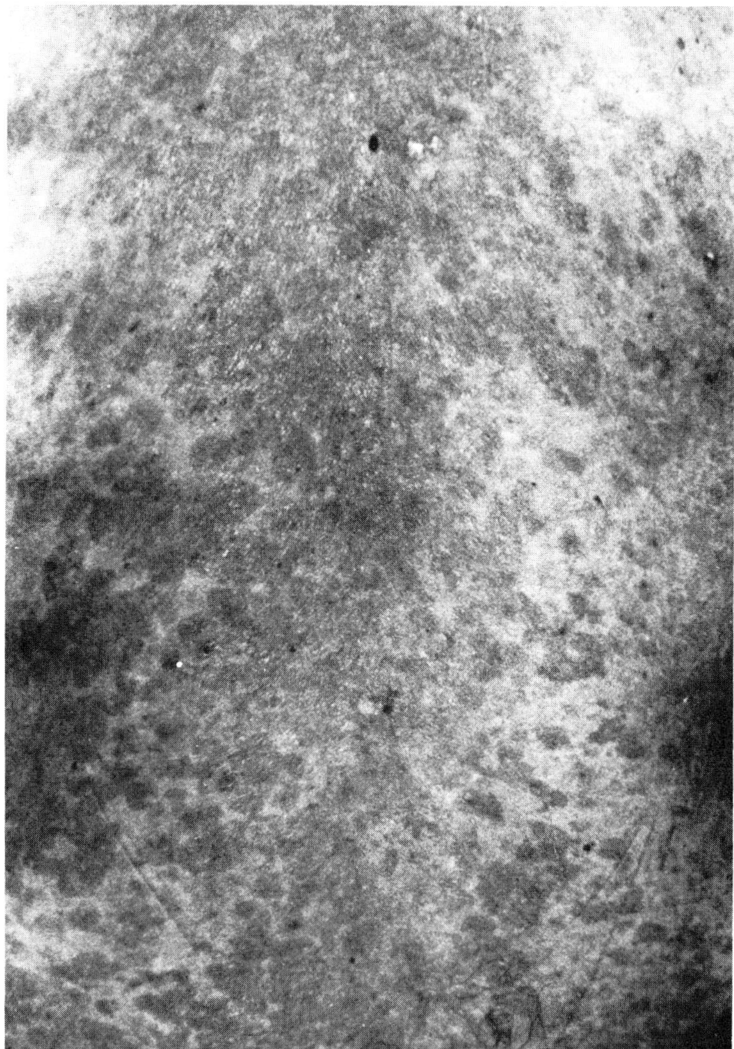

Figure 1–62. Epidermodysplasia verruciformis. Disseminated plaques and papules on back simulate a reticulated erythema or tinea versicolor.

Hammat et al., but cell-mediated immunity as evaluated by intracutaneous testing with PPD, Candida, and mumps antigens and induction of sensitivity to DNCB were normal.[228] We are at the beginning of our understanding of this unusual syndrome. Is the widespread viral infection responsible for the varying degrees of immunodepression or is there an inherited or acquired immunodeficiency responsible for the widespread viral infection with its subsequent and presumptive oncogenic properties?

The etiology of most cases of basal cell tumors is attributed to chronic actinic damage in a susceptible person: a fair complexioned, blue-eyed individual who works outdoors and who is usually of Anglo-Saxon background. A person in his twenties or thirties may be affected if he has been living in a sunny semitropical or tropical climate.

Basal cell tumors can develop on a genetic basis without chronic sun exposure. The basal cell nevus syndrome was first delineated in 1959, and since then over 100 cases have been reported.[229, 230] This genodermatosis which is transmitted in a dominant fashion includes three definite stigmata and is associated with multiple other abnormalities.

The basal cell tumors, which comprise the first stigma, encompass all clinical varieties including the multicentric superficial type. They may develop as early as six years of age and number in the hundreds. The tumors can behave as ordinary basal cell tumors with ulceration and deep tissue invasion. Fortunately, this process is not seen during childhood.

The development of multiple dentigerous cysts, either unilocular or multilocular and more frequent in the mandible than in the maxilla, is the second feature of this syndrome (Fig. 1–66). The cysts continue to develop during the patient's life.

Pits on the palms and soles and occasionally on the lateral aspects of the digits and dorsa of the hands and feet constitute the third stigma of this syndrome. The pits are 1 to 4 millimeters, and when large, they tend to be slightly erythematous. They look like linear slits or irregularly punched

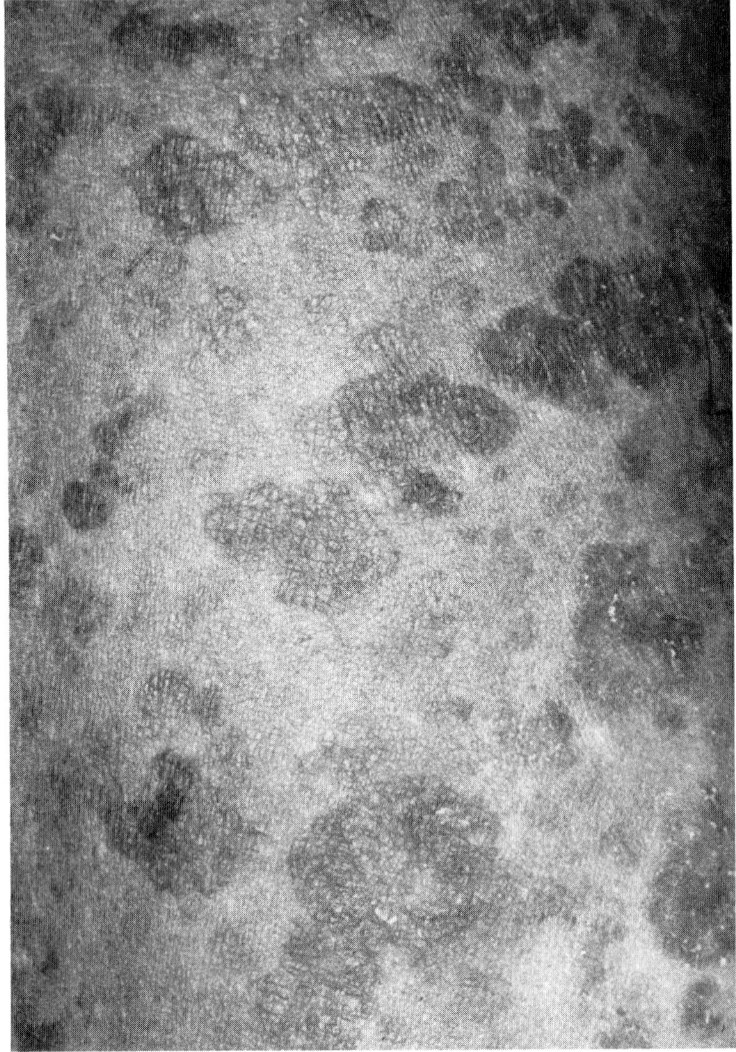

Figure 1–63. Epidermodysplasia verruciformis. Closer view demonstrates resemblance of papules and plaques to tinea versicolor.

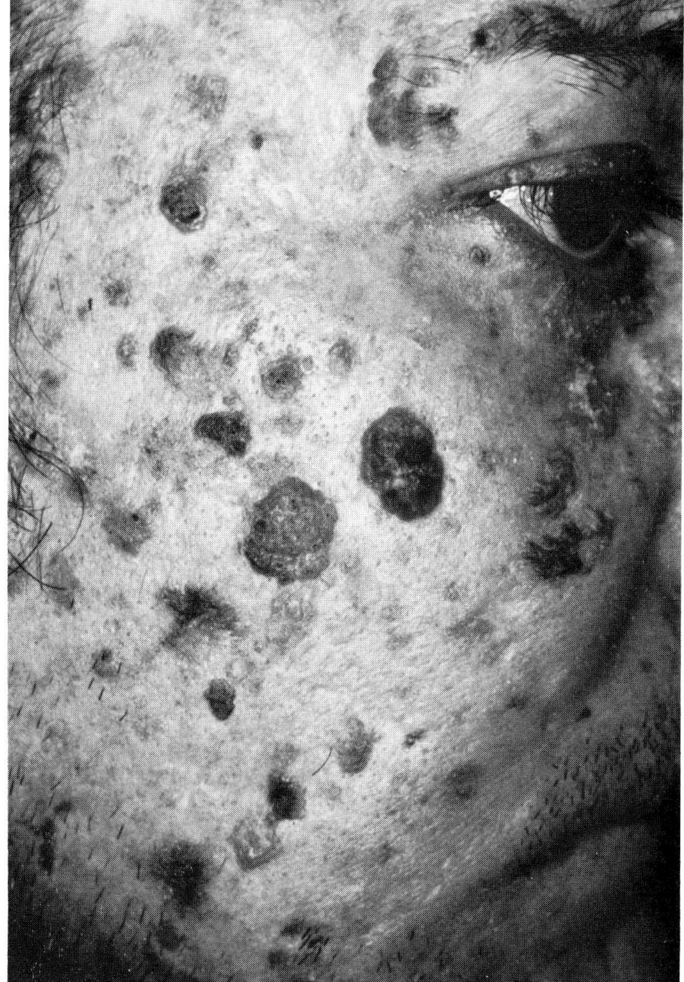

Figure 1–64. Epidermodysplasia verruciformis. Verrucous tumors.

out ice pick punctures (Figs. 1–67 and 1–68). They are asymptomatic. Histologically the epidermis is normal, but there is an absence of the keratin layer which corresponds to the pit. The development of a basal cell tumor in the base of the pit is a rare accompaniment of this syndrome.[231-233]

An individual with multiple basal cell tumors that appear early in life or with dentigerous cysts or pitted palms probably exhibits the basal cell nevus syndrome. Other anomalies associated with this disorder are listed in Table 1–3.

Clendenning and co-workers noted that five of their female patients with this syndrome had shortening of the fourth metacarpal. Three women had ovarian fibromas with calcification, and a fourth patient was strongly suspected of having an ovarian fibroma. One had the clinical features of pseudohypoparathyroidism and was subsequently shown to be hyporesponsive to parathormone. Four other patients were also shown to be hyporesponsive to parathormone even though they did not have the clinical features of pseudohypoparathyroidism. The genetic abnormality in the basal cell nevus syndrome may also produce a defect in renal tubular reabsorption of phosphate.[234]

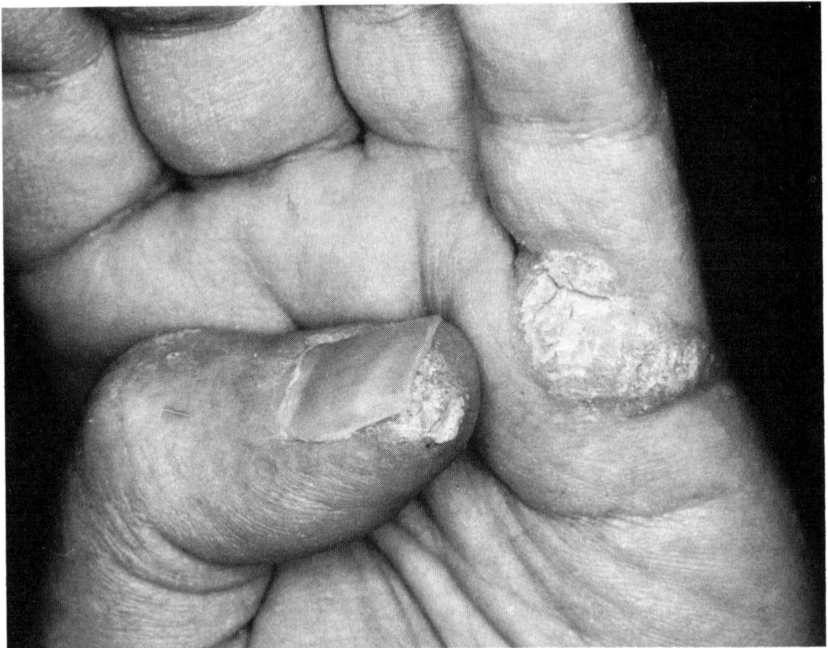

Figure 1–65. Epidermodysplasia verruciformis. Verrucous tumors.

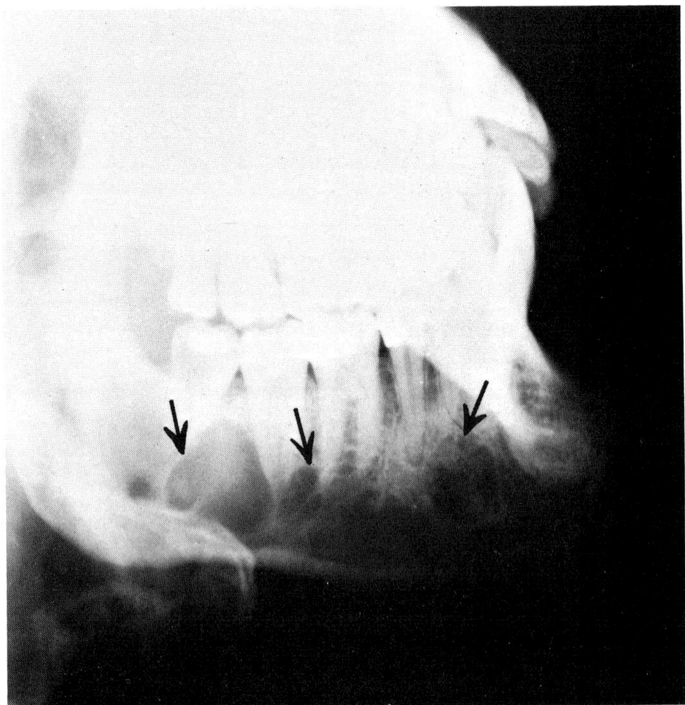

Figure 1–66. Radiograph of jaw. Multiloculated cysts (arrows) associated with roots of second and third lower molars and first bicuspid in patient with basal cell nevus syndrome. (From Katz, J., Savin, R. S., and Spiro, H. M.: Basal cell nevus syndrome and inflammatory disease of the bowel. Am. J. Med., *44*:483, 1968.)

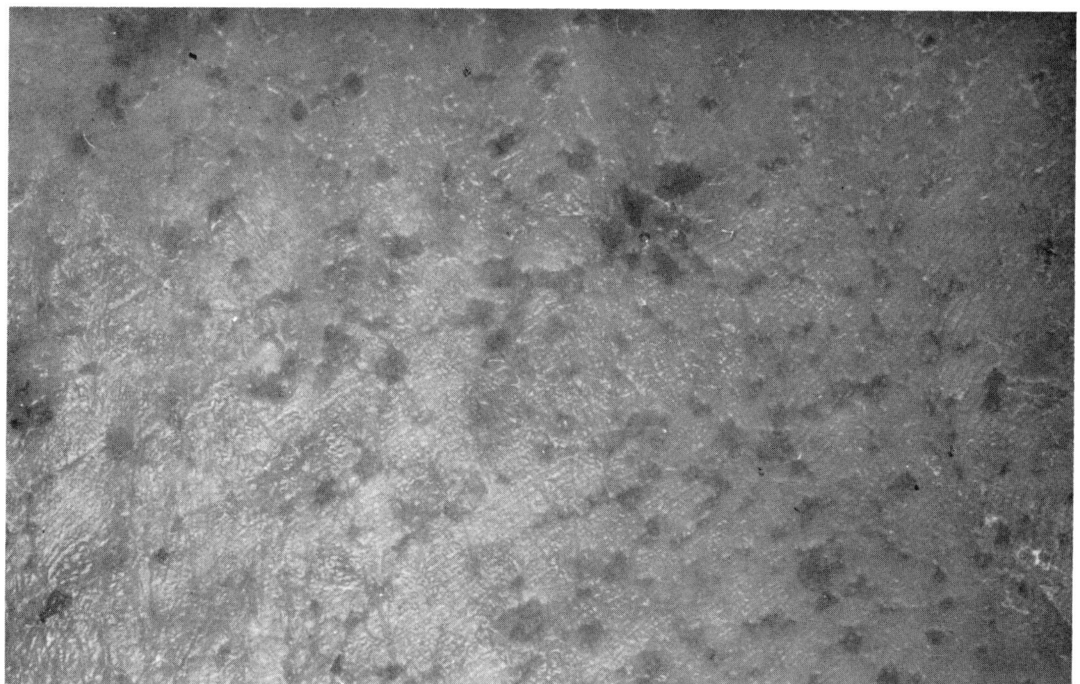

Figure 1-67. Basal cell nevus syndrome. Broad pits on sole.

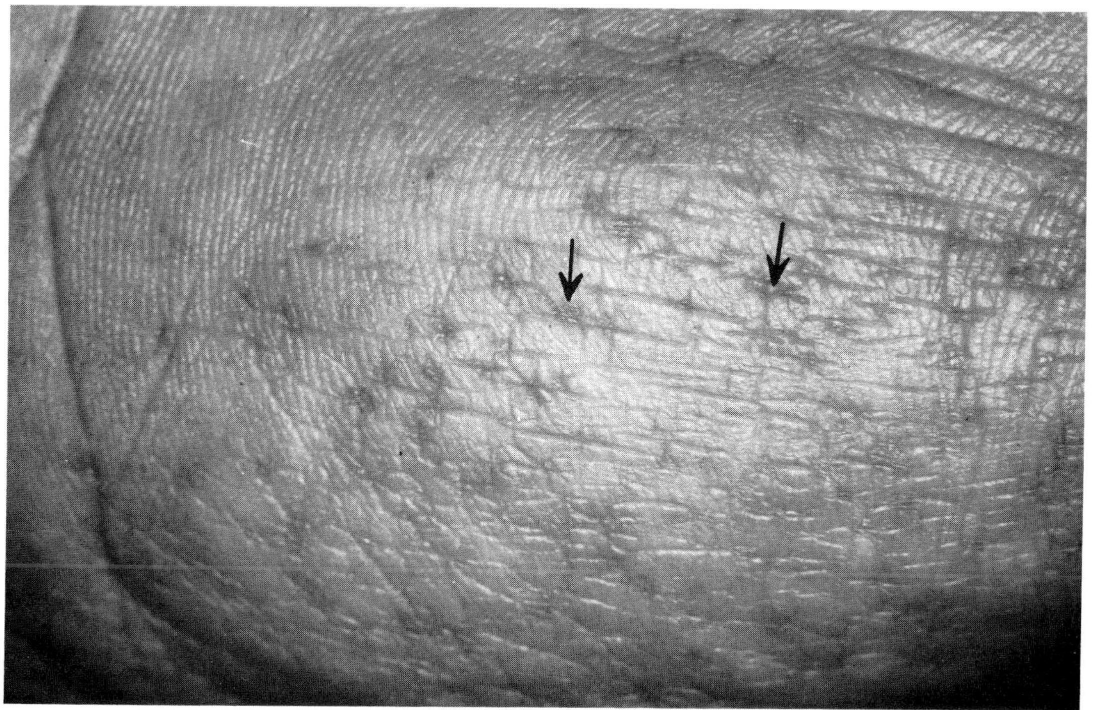

Figure 1–68. Basal cell nevus syndrome. Slit-like pits (arrows) on palm.

Table 1–3. Anomalies Associated with Basal Cell Nevus Syndrome

Hypertelorism
Broad nasal root
Parietal and frontal bossing
Strabismus
Bifid, fused, or splayed ribs
Scoliosis
Kyphosis
Spina bifida occulta
Brachymetacarpalism
Calcification of falx cerebri, tentorium cerebelli, and basal ganglia
Bridging of sella turcica
Agenesis of corpus callosum

The basal cell nevus syndrome and inflammatory disease of the bowel (regional ileitis and ulcerative colitis) were associated in a large kindred that was studied at the Yale-New Haven Hospital (Fig. 1–69).[235] Three generations were available for study. All of the adults, except for one having inflammatory disease of the bowel, had either the stigmata of the basal cell nevus syndrome or the ability to transmit the gene for this syndrome to their offspring. The children of the woman who seemed to be an exception were in their teens and early twenties and may yet develop skin or dental lesions. The concurrence of these two diseases is unique in this family; it may be coincidental, but the association should be looked for in future studies. The same may be said for the following observation.

Schwartz described an additional gastrointestinal disorder not previously reported with this syndrome.[236] The patient was a 54-year-old man who complained of dyspepsia, the evaluation of which led to the discovery of several hamartomatous polyps in the prepyloric and antral regions of the stomach and a jejunal mesenteric cyst. A barium enema study showed no colonic polyps.

Epithelioma adenoides cysticum (Brooke's tumors) must be differentiated from the basal cell nevus syndrome.[237] In this dominantly transmitted genodermatosis, cutaneous adnexal tumors differentiating toward hair follicles develop on the face, in the nasolabial folds, and occasionally on the scalp, neck, and trunk. They appear in early childhood or at puberty. They rarely transform into basal cell tumors even though both arise from

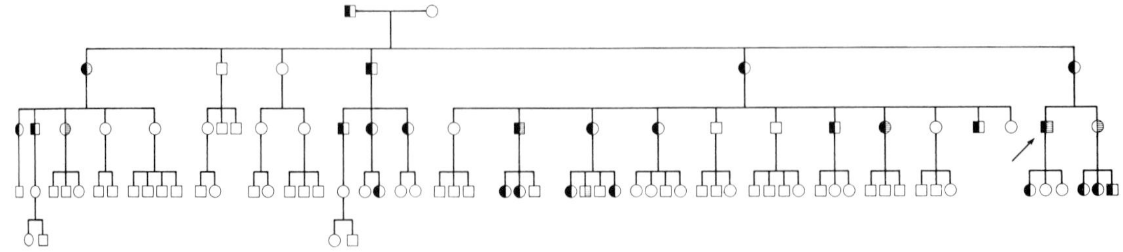

Figure 1–69. Family pedigree. Members with basal cell tumors, odontogenic cysts, or pitted palms are considered to have basal cell nevus syndrome. Propositus indicated by arrow. (From Katz, J., Savin, R. S., and Spiro, H. M.: Basal cell nevus syndrome and inflammatory disease of the bowel. Am. J. Med., *44*:483, 1968.)

common primary epithelial germ cells. Brooke's tumors are not associated with other systemic abnormalities.

Acrodermatitis chronica atrophicans is very rare and is seen almost exclusively in people of European origin.[238] Initially the skin is edematous and red, but soon it becomes atrophic, wrinkled, and blue. The subcutaneous veins can easily be seen and are sometimes mistaken for varicosities. This dermatosis can be unilateral or bilateral; its etiology is not known. Both epidermoid carcinomas and sarcomas have been reported to arise from the atrophic skin after a number of years.[239-241]

An example of this disorder was seen at the Yale-New Haven Hospital in 1959:

A 70-year-old German woman was referred to the medical center because of acute dermatomyositis. For at least 10 years she had had unilateral acrodermatitis chronica atrophicans of the left leg, the thigh, and the buttock, where the acrodermatitis extended to the anus. Intensive studies were carried out to uncover a neoplasm underlying her dermatomyositis. At first none was found. After several rectal examinations, a presumed thrombosed hemorrhoid proved to be a transitional cell carcinoma which had developed in the area of acrodermatitis adjacent to the anus. The tumor was successfully resected, but the patient died postoperatively. Permission for autopsy was refused. It seems likely that the dermatomyositis was secondary to the transitional cell carcinoma, which in turn may have been related to the acrodermatitis chronica atrophicans.

Three varieties of polyposis of the bowel are considered in any discussion of premalignant lesions: Gardner's syndrome, Peutz-Jeghers syndrome, and familial polyposis. They will be briefly considered here and discussed more fully in Chapter 12.

Gardner's syndrome is characterized by cutaneous osteomas, fibromas, and multiple large disfiguring sebaceous cysts, in association with polyps of the small and large bowel. Malignant transformation of the polyps is frequent.

In Peutz-Jeghers syndrome, freckle-like lesions on the lips, nose, buccal mucosa, fingertips, and under the nails are present in association with polyps of the small intestine, stomach, and colon. Polyps may also develop in the esophagus, mouth, nostrils, maxillary sinus, and nasopharynx.[242] Originally the gastrointestinal polyps were thought to be premalignant, but the current consensus is that the polyps are hamartomas whose histology has been confused with malignancy. Development of cancer is relatively uncommon, and the diagnosis of Peutz-Jeghers syndrome does not engender the same anxiety as do the diagnoses of Gardner's syndrome and familial polyposis.

However, there have been case reports of 24 patients with Peutz-Jeghers syndrome who have developed gastrointestinal cancer.[243-252] The cancers have arisen in the ileum in two, jejunum in three, small intestine, not further specified, in one, stomach in three, duodenum in seven, and colon in eight. Dormandy, in his classic review of Peutz-Jeghers syndrome, mentioned that four of his 21 patients died from carcinoma arising in a rectal or colonic polyp.[253] Achord and Proctor reported a 13-year-old black girl with typical pigmentation and multiple gastric, duodenal, and jejunal polyps. A gastric polyp became malignant, and hepatic metastases soon followed.[254] In another patient, there was only serosal invasion from two adenocarcinomas arising in ileal polyps.[245] In these various reports, the mucosa of the stomach, duodenum, and less commonly the ileum is often described as showing micropolyposis when gross polyps are not present. The gastrointestinal cancers in this syndrome have arisen from areas of micropolyposis, individual polyps, and normal appearing mucosa in the stomach, duodenum, colon, and small bowel. In some instances, however, where the cancer is large, it has been impossible to determine whether it arose from a polyp or the mucosa. While everyone agrees that the small bowel polyps are hamartomas, there is controversy over the nature of the large bowel polyps: whether they be hamartomas, adenomas, or a mixture of both existing side by side.[255, 256]

According to Dozois et al., 326 cases of Peutz-Jeghers syndrome had been reported in the literature as of 1969.[255] Twenty of them had developed gastrointestinal cancer, suggesting that approximately 6 per cent of patients with Peutz-Jeghers syndrome are at risk for this neoplastic complication.

Two of our own patients illustrate this point:

A 60-year-old white woman had been admitted to the Yale-New Haven Hospital on several occasions over a 30-year period for recurrent gastrointestinal bleeding of unknown etiology. On her first admission, a duodenal ulcer was thought to be present, but this finding could not be confirmed during subsequent hospitalizations. When she was 60 years old, she was admitted again for gastrointestinal bleeding. At this time, typical Peutz-Jeghers pigmentation was found on the lips and buccal mucosa, and jejunal polyps were demonstrated radiographically. A review of the x-ray studies performed 14 years earlier revealed that the polyps had been present at that time. Persistent bleeding required surgical intervention. The jejunal polyp showed malignant transformation to a leiomyosarcoma, and metastases were found in the liver. The patient died two years later. Permission for autopsy was denied.

An 81-year-old Italian woman was admitted to the Yale-New Haven Hospital because of epigastric pain which had been radiating to the back for the past six weeks. Physical examination revealed typical Peutz-Jeghers pigmentation of the lips and buccal mucosa; this pigmentation had been present for 40 years (Fig. 1–70). Her five siblings had the same pigmentation, but they were not investigated further. She stated that her maternal grandmother, but not her mother, had had similar spots. A more detailed family history could not be obtained. The patient had a carcinoma of the pancreas. At autopsy no polyps were found. This patient probably represents an instance of the Peutz-Jeghers syndrome with a coincidental pancreatic cancer. Pigmentation without polyps, and vice versa, can occur as a limited form of the disease.[257]

Peutz-Jeghers pigmentation has also been reported in a patient with generalized hemangiomatosis of the small bowel.[258]

Christian and associates described a four and one half-year-old white girl with Peutz-Jeghers syndrome and precocious puberty that was produced by a benign functioning granulosa theca cell tumor of the ovary.[259] Polyposis of the stomach and small intestine was present. Two patients in Dormandy's series also had granulosa cell tumors. A case of Peutz-Jeghers syndrome with a Brenner tumor and a dysgerminoma has been reported as well. Ovarian tumors are another feature of the Peutz-Jeghers syndrome. To date there have been 19 patients with 21 ovarian tumors. Their ages ranged from 4½ to 60 years at the time the ovarian neoplasm was diagnosed, and more importantly 12 of the 19 were

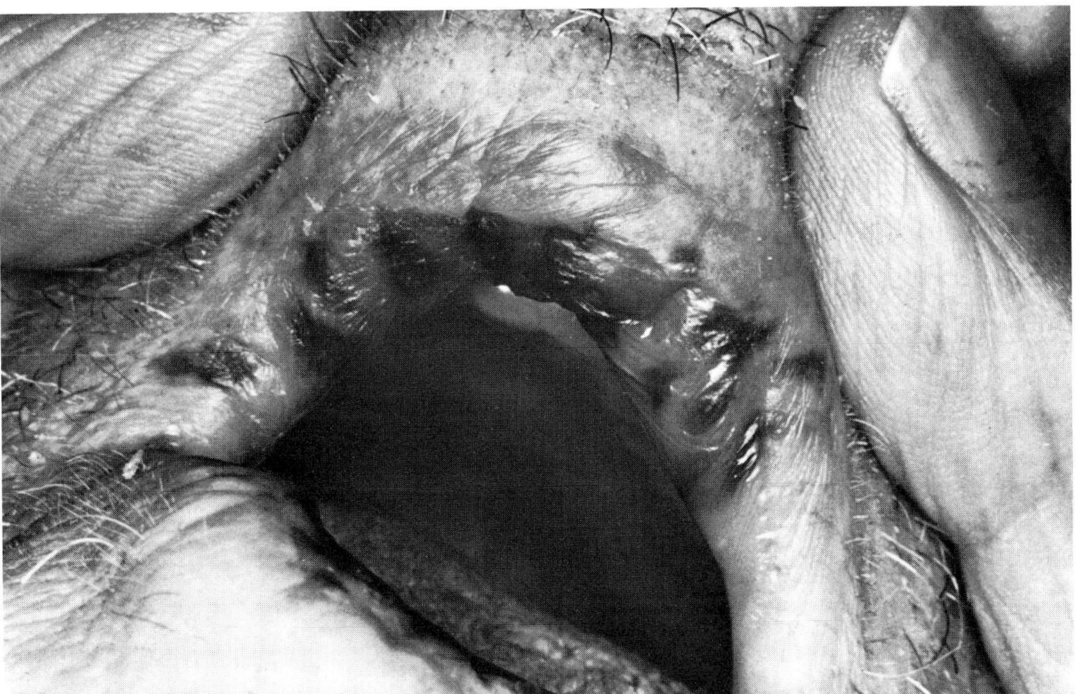

Figure 1–70. Pigmentation of lips in Peutz-Jeghers syndrome. This patient also had carcinoma of the pancreas.

less than 23 years old. Six of these women had "sex cord tumors with annular tubules." (Only 13 such tumors have been reported in the world's literature.) Five women had cystadenomas, a common epithelial tumor. Dysgerminoma, simple cyst, lipoid cell tumor, carcinosarcoma, Sertoli tumor, and one tumor with an indeterminate diagnosis occurred in the other eight patients.[260, 261] Therefore, careful pelvic examinations should be done in women and children with Peutz-Jeghers syndrome; three of the above 19 were children less than 15 years old, and one was 4½ years old.

There seems to be no doubt that there is a small but definite increased risk of intestinal cancer in patients with Peutz-Jeghers syndrome, arising chiefly from the duodenum and colon. Since the individual polyps in this syndrome can grow quickly or even spontaneously disappear, the therapy and management of each patient becomes highly individualized.

Familial polyposis of the large bowel has not been thought to be associated with skin markers. However, Dr. Sherwin Nuland called our attention to an unusual cutaneous lesion associated with familial polyposis in one of his patients. This instance will be described briefly, since it may prove to be a useful marker in identifying this disorder:

A 49-year-old white woman was admitted to Yale-New Haven Hospital in 1964 for treatment of a herniated vertebral disc. On physical examination she was found to have a polypoid rectal mass. A barium enema revealed polyposis of the colon. Surgery revealed two carcinomas in the bowel as well as peritoneal implants and metastases to the ovaries. A double barrel colostomy was constructed after the colonic neoplasms were resected. The patient died 18 months later. Polyposis of the colon was found in her 13-year-old daughter but not in her son. Neither child had abnormal pigmentation. The patient had two types of skin lesions. A reticu-

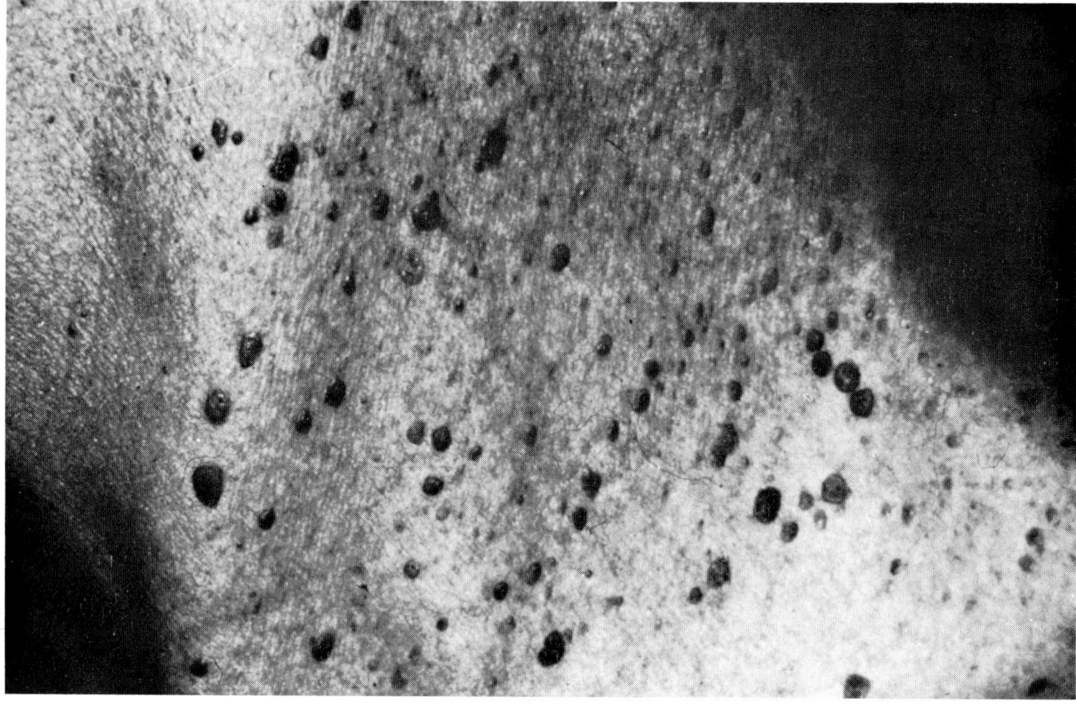

Figure 1–71. Widespread seborrheic keratoses in patient with familial polyposis. (Courtesy of Dr. Sherwin Nuland.)

lated hyperpigmentation, which the patient had never noticed, was present over the perineum and extended onto the inner thighs (Plate 4*D*). Over the neck, the V of the chest, and in the antecubital spaces were hundreds of seborrheic keratoses (Fig. 1–71). The unusual pigmentation in the perineum may prove to be related to the polyposis, as is the pigmentation in Peutz-Jeghers disease. The significance of the seborrheic keratoses in this situation is unclear.

Torre's syndrome is a recently recognized entity in which multiple carcinomas, primarily of the gastrointestinal tract, are associated with *multiple sebaceous gland neoplasms* (not cysts).[262-264] The sebaceous gland tumors are found chiefly on the trunk, and less often on the face, and include adenomas, carcinomas, and less frequently basal cell tumors with sebaceous differentiation. Clinically they present as yellowish or violaceous nodules that may have an ulcerated surface. These tumors tend to remain localized in the skin without any significantly aggressive local growth.

Thus far, 12 patients have been described, and in 11, the carcinomas have been in the colon. The twelfth patient had a carcinoma of the endometrium. The carcinomas have preceded the sebaceous gland tumors by intervals of up to ten years. In addition to carcinoma of the colon, many of the patients have had multiple cancers involving other areas of the gastrointestinal tract as well as other systems developing over an interval of years. The neoplasms have included cancers of the ampulla of Vater, duodenum, stomach, larynx, ovary, and genitourinary tract and endometrium. None of these patients has had polyposis of the colon. In five of the 12 patients, there was a strong family history of cancer.

In only one or two patients did the multiple sebaceous gland tumors precede the development of the visceral cancer and in that instance, the interval was 11 years.[263]

The visceral cancers appear to be low grade malignancies because the reported survival times in virtually all the patients have been between 5 and 21 years. The value of this skin sign is not as an early warning system for the first cancer, but rather as an alert to anticipate the possible development of additional neoplasms.

Cowden's disease, multiple hamartoma syndrome, is another recently appreciated syndrome linking benign mucocutaneous lesions with the later development of internal cancer. Twenty-nine patients have been described — 18 women and 11 men. The mucocutaneous lesions occur in a distinctive combination and seem to herald the eventual development of tumors and cancers involving the thyroid, breast, and gastrointestinal tract. The disease appears to be inherited in an autosomal dominant fashion.[265-271]

A variety of cutaneous lesion are found.

Lichenoid Papules. These are flat-topped papules which range from less than 1 mm to 4 mm. They are flesh colored and not scaly. In many, one can see a central pore or depression filled with a keratotic plug. The lesions may remain discrete or become confluent, producing a larger lesion with a cobblestone surface. These lesions are found most commonly on the pinnae, and surrounding skin, on the sides of the neck, and over the central part of the face with a tendency to cluster around the eyes, nose, and mouth and over the glabella. These lesions are *not* found on the trunk or elsewhere on the body (Figs. 1–72 to 1–75). In some individuals, papillomatous and

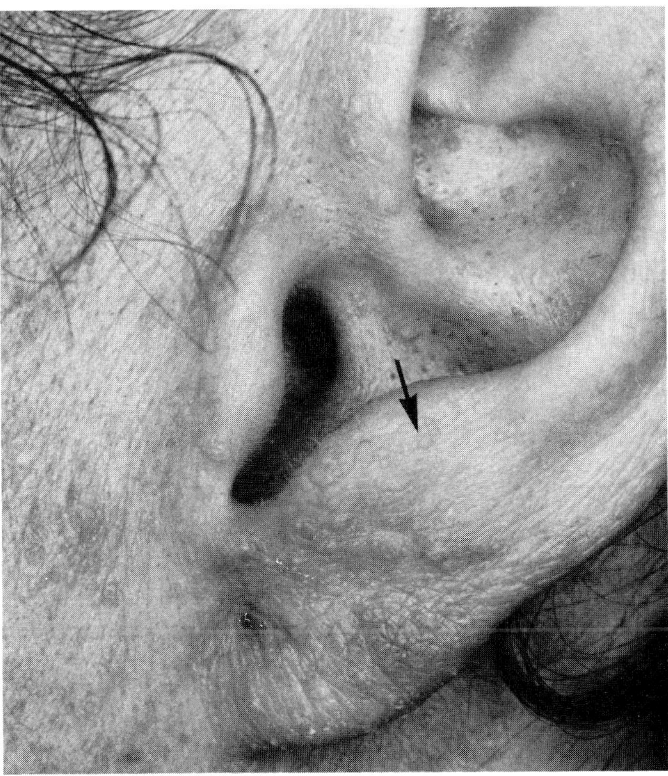

Figure 1–72. Cowden's disease. Lichenoid papules on ear lobes (arrow).

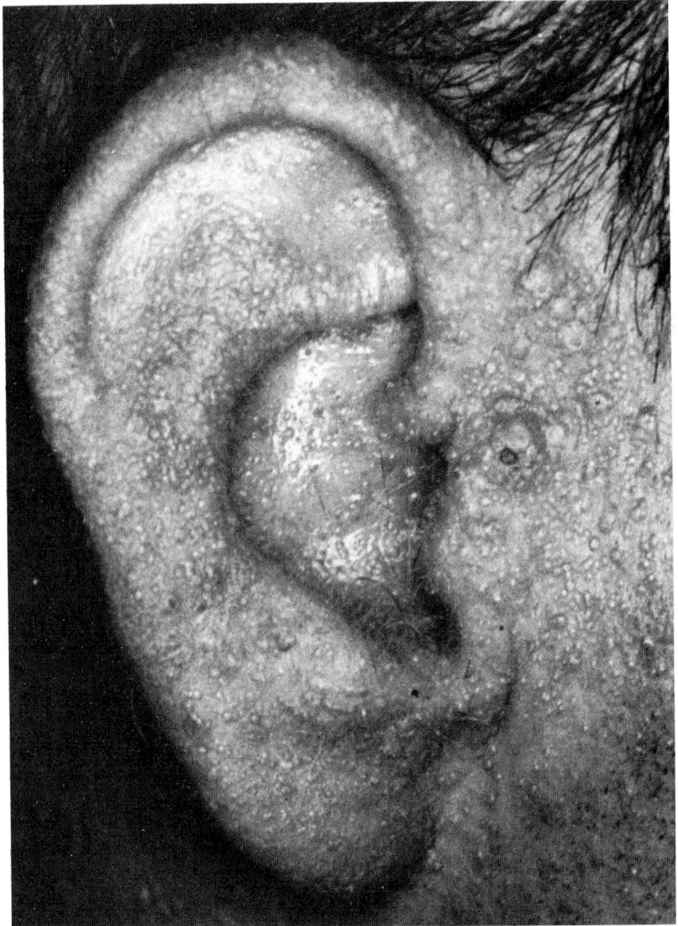

Figure 1–73. Cowden's disease. Lichenoid papules. (From Weary, P.: Multiple hamartoma syndrome (Cowden's disease). Arch. Dermatol., *106*:682, 1970.)

filiform wartlike lesions are found around the eyes, ears, nose, and mouth. They probably represent a larger proliferating version of the lichenoid lesions.

Flat Wartlike Papules. Hyperkeratotic, flat-topped papules, resembling verruca plana or the lesions of acrokeratosis verruciformis, are found on the dorsa of the hands and wrists *but not* on the dorsa of the feet.

Keratosis Punctata. Hyperkeratotic papules with central delling or umbilication are present on the soles and sides of the feet and on the palms and digits (Fig. 1–76). They are identical in appearance to the punctate keratoses, illustrated in Fig. 1–80, which had been described by Dobson et al. as a possible sign of internal cancer.[272]

Multiple *lipomas* and *cavernous hemangiomas* have been present in almost half of the cases and are probably part of the Cowden syndrome.

The mucosal lesions consist of papules scattered over the gingivae (Fig. 1–77) and to a lesser extent over the palate. They vary in size from 1 to 3 mm and tend to coalesce, producing a faint cobblestone appearance. They tend to be whiter than the surrounding mucosa. These lesions may also become papillomatous and verrucoid and may be found on the buccal, oropharyngeal, and faucial mucosae. In one patient, lesions were also present in the esophagus, stomach, and duodenal bulb.[270] In some patients they have extended down into the laryngeal area, interfering with speech and requiring periodic removal. The tongue may be studded with hundreds of papules producing a pebbly appearance (Fig. 1–78). The vermillion border of the lips and the commissures of the lips may be similarly affected (Fig. 1–79).

There is disagreement about the histological interpretation of the cutaneous lichenoid lesions. Brownstein et al. claim them to be trichilemmomas[273] and Ackerman[274] believes them to be old verrucae in which the virus can no longer be found by electron microscopy. Their papillomatous counterparts which show irregular acanthosis and hyperkeratosis of the epidermis with masses of squamous cells containing squamous eddies beneath, are probably the same type of lesion. The acrokeratotic papules on the backs of the hands and wrist show only acanthosis and hyperkeratosis of the epidermis and are not viral warts. The mucosal lesions show the

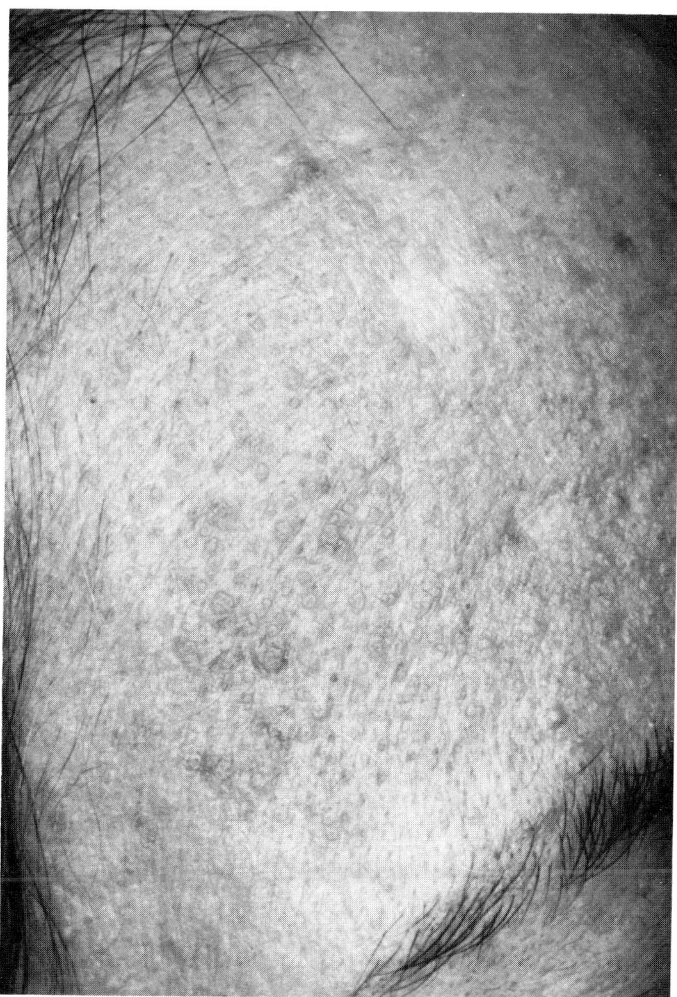

Figure 1–74. Cowden's disease. Lichenoid papules on forehead.

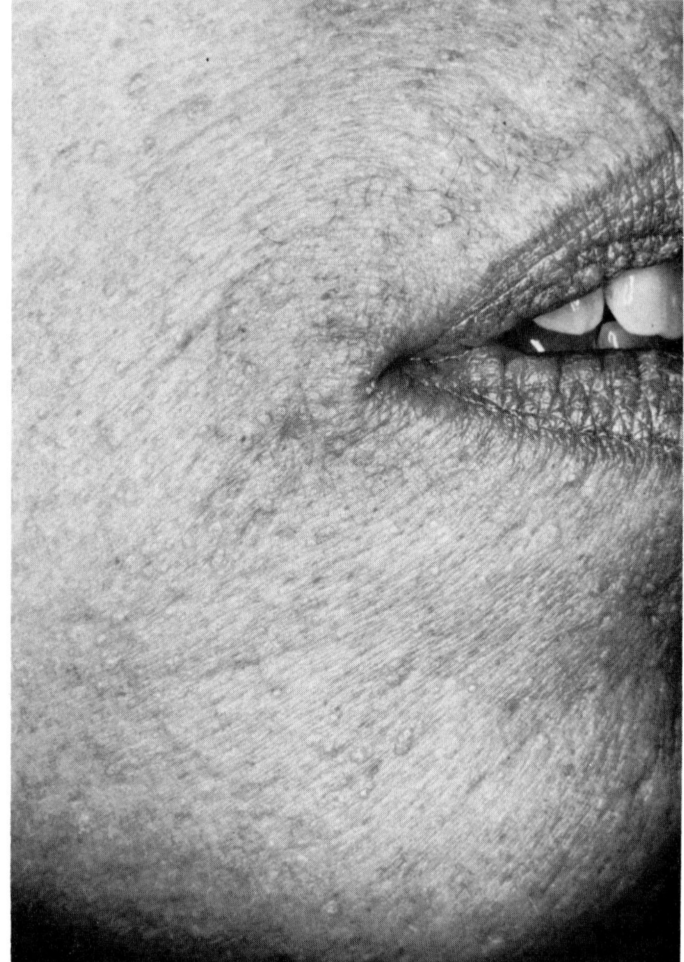

Figure 1–75. Cowden's disease. Lichenoid papules around mouth.

histologic features of either nonspecific papillomas or fibromatous nodules.[266]

Although all patients exhibit mucocutaneous lesions there is some degree of variability in the expression of each type of lesion. The lesions can appear as early as childhood and as late as the third and fourth decades.

Almost all of the women have had fibrocystic disease of the breasts and thus far, eight of 18 have developed carcinomas of the breast. Three women each had female relatives with carcinomas of the breast and two of the latter had Cowden's syndrome by description. Thyroid tumors occurred in 75 per cent of the patients and have included adenomas, goiters, thyroiditis, and carcinomas (three of 29). Gastrointestinal polyposis had been found in 33 per cent of the patients and on biopsy they have been shown to be inflammatory or adenomatous polyps, and pedunculated and sessile ganglioneuromas. In one case, the polyps were diagnosed histologically as fibrous polyps. In five patients, pectus excavatum and an adenoid facies with beaked nose were present. These two features may also prove to be part of the syndrome.

A variety of syndromes bear a superficial resemblance to Cowden's

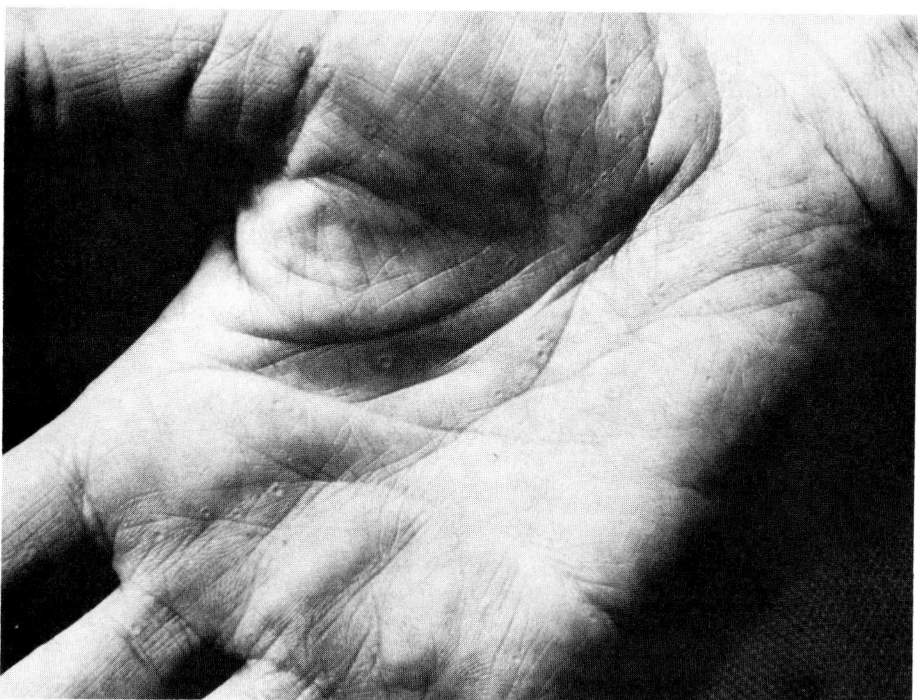

Figure 1–76. Cowden's disease. Umbilicated papules on palm. (From Burnett, J. W., Goldner, R., and Calton, G. J.: Cowden disease. Report of two additional cases. Br. J. Dermatol., *93*:329, 1975.)

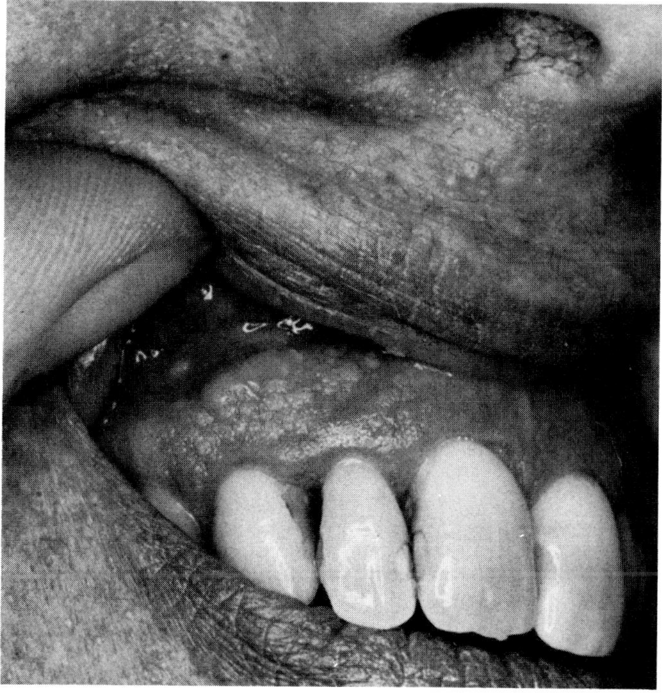

Figure 1–77. Cowden's disease. Papules producing cobblestone appearance on gums.

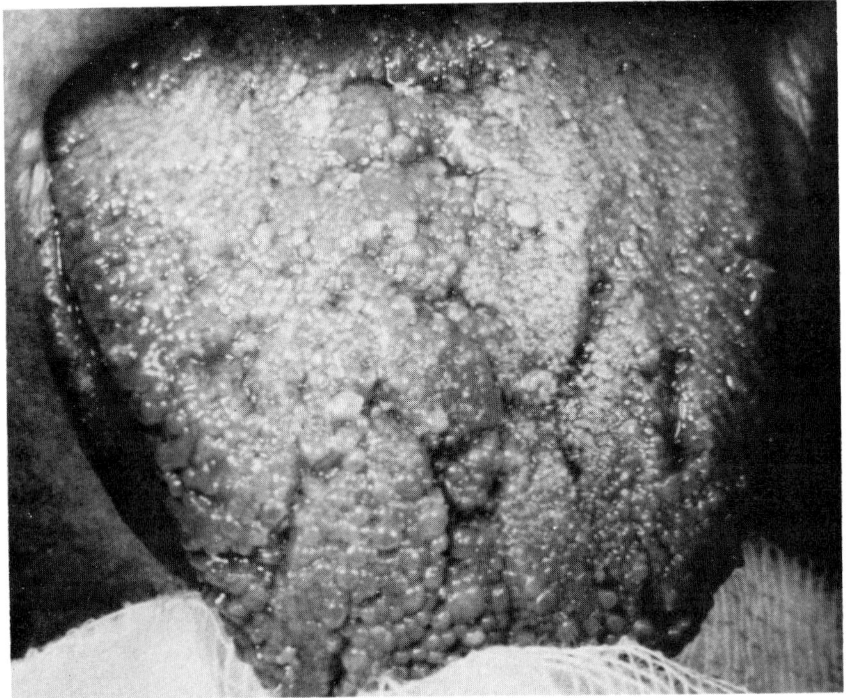

Figure 1–78. Cowden's disease. Papules on tongue produce a pebbly appearance. (From Weary, P., Gorlin, R. J., Gentry, W. C., Jr., et al.: Multiple hamartoma syndrome (Cowden's disease). Arch. Dermatol., *106*:682, 1972.)

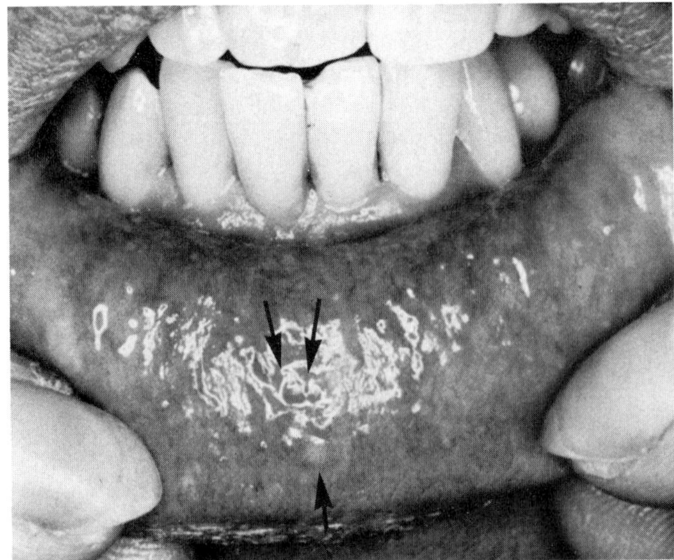

Figure 1–79. Cowden's disease. Papules on vermilion border of lip (arrows.)

disease: multiple mucosal neuromas syndrome, Darier's disease, and lipoid proteinosis. Biopsy of a cutaneous lesion will easily distinguish one from the other.

The observation that the facial lesions may be trichilemmomas is of diagnostic importance. Undoubtedly, patients will be encountered with milder forms of the disease, and the diagnosis of multiple trichilemmomas as opposed to a solitary lesion should alert the physician that he may be dealing with Cowden's disease. Also, the combination of papillary mucocutaneous lesions, warty papules on the dorsa of the hands, and umbilicated papules on the palms and soles is a distinctive triad. This morphologic combination should alert physicians to the presence of this syndrome, regardless of whether the facial lesions are trichilemmomas or warts. Gastrointestinal polyps, unusually large lipomas and cavernous hemangiomas, or thyroid tumors alone or in combination with these cutaneous lesions should raise the possibility of Cowden's disease in the evaluation of the patient.

The multiple hamartoma syndrome appears to be a very important marker for identifying the eventual development of thyroid disease and breast carcinoma arising in the setting of fibrocystic disease.

The astute clinician is always looking for a skin marker to detect internal disease. In 1965, Dobson and co-workers reported the association of palmar hyperkeratotic papules with a variety of cancers, including melanoma and lymphoma. Thirty-two per cent of the tumor group and 7 per cent of a control group exhibited these lesions.[272] Bean et al. were unable to confirm this association.[275] Dobson described the lesions as punctate pearly yellow, or flesh-colored translucent hyperkeratotic papules sur-

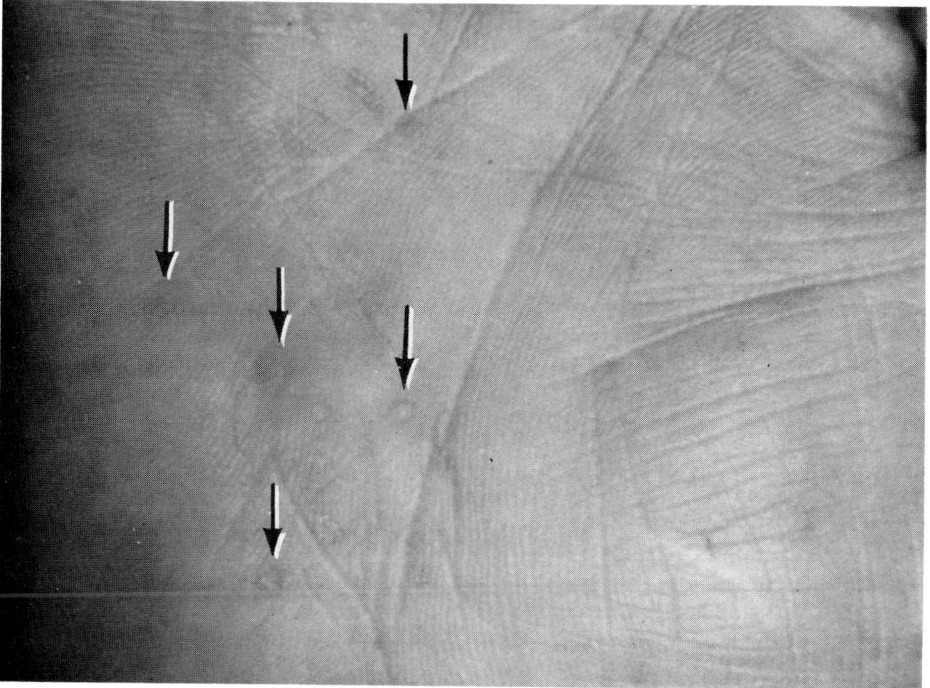

Figure 1–80. Crater-like punctate keratoses (arrows) on palm.

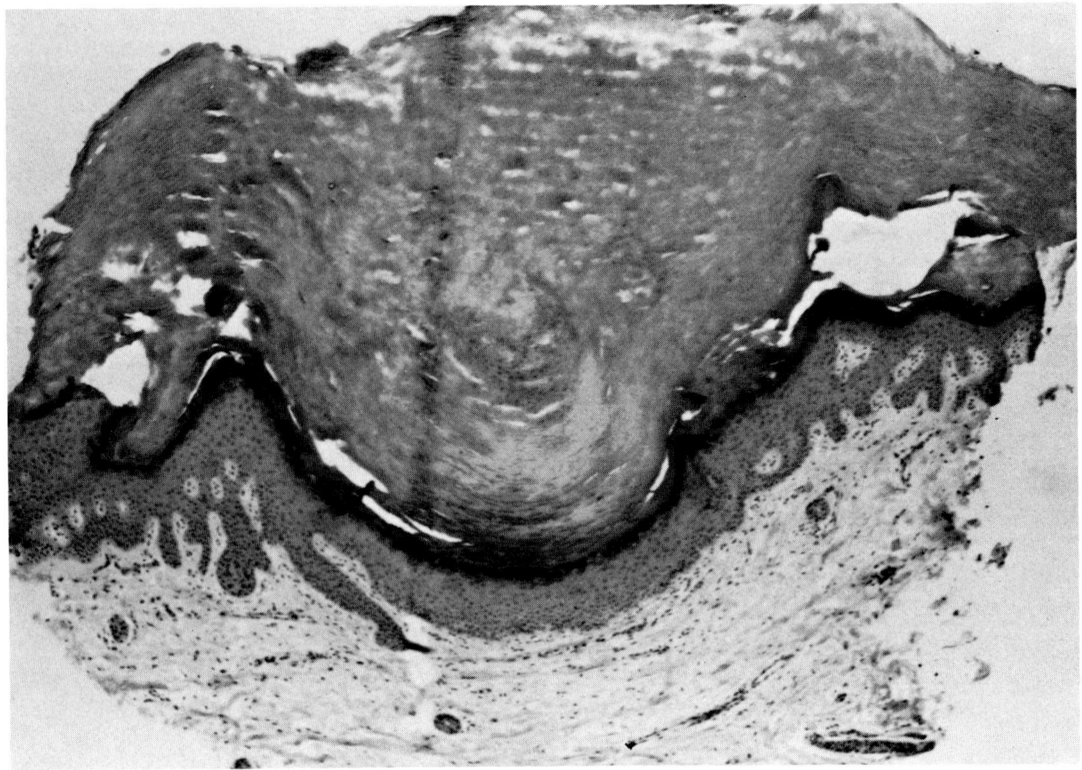

Figure 1–81. Photomicrograph of punctate keratosis. Epidermal cells have a normal cytologic appearance. Hematoxylin and eosin. 40.

rounded by a collarette of scale. Histologically, many of the epidermal cells showed pyknotic nuclei and prominent vacuolization, thereby resembling the changes in arsenical keratoses. The lesions tended to be localized on the thenar and hypothenar eminences and varied in size from one to several millimeters.

My experience leads me to a different interpretation of these lesions. They appear to be papules with central depressions, or they may be merely pitted areas in the palm with a thin elevated border forming a structure similar to that of a volcanic crater (Fig. 1–80). In our histological material, one sees cup-shaped depressions in the epidermis filled with keratin (Fig. 1–81). Vacuolization of cells is not seen. I believe that these lesions represent punctate keratoses (keratosis punctata), and in no way resemble those lesions associated with arsenic.[276] Our observations were confirmed by the later studies of Woodside and Dobson.[277] The relationship between punctate keratoses and cancer was reexamined by Stolman et al., who were also unable to confirm this relationship.[278] However, it is important to be able to recognize punctate keratoses for two reasons: they appear to be one of the significant lesions in Cowden's disease and they should not be mistaken for arsenical keratoses or the palmar pits of the basal cell nevus syndrome.

REFERENCES

1. Gates, O.: Cutaneous metastases of malignant disease. Am. J. Cancer *30*:718, 1937.
2. Mehregan, A. H.: Metastatic carcinoma to the skin. Dermatologica, *123*:311, 1961.
3. Willis, R. A.: The Spread of Tumors in the Human Body. Butterworth and Co., London, 1952.
4. Brownstein, M. H., and Helwig, E. B.: Spread of tumors to the skin. Arch. Dermatol., *107*:80, 1973.
5. Ginzburg, E., Catz, B., Nelson, C. L., Kozikowski, B. M., and Chesne, E. L.: Hyperthyroidism secondary to metastatic functioning thyroid carcinoma. Ann. Intern. Med., *58*:684, 1963.
6. Wheelock, M. C., Frable, W. J., and Urnes, P. D.: Bizarre metastases from malignant neoplasms. Am. J. Clin. Pathol., *37*:475, 1962.
7. Markser, L. S., Stoops, C. W., and Kanter, J.: Metastatic transitional cell carcinoma of the penis simulating a chancre. Arch. Dermatol. *59*:50, 1949.
8. Brownstein, M. H., and Helwig, E. B.: Patterns of cutaneous metastases. Arch. Dermatol., *105*:862, 1972.
9. Montgomery, H., and Kierland, R. R.: Metastases of carcinoma to the scalp. Arch. Surg., *40*:672, 1940.
10. Cohen, I., Levy, E., and Schreiber, H.: Alopecia neoplastica due to breast cancer. Arch. Dermatol., *84*:490, 1961.
11. Stewart, F. W., and Treves, N.: Lymphosarcoma in post-mastectomy lymphedema. Report of 96 cases of elephantiasis chirurgica. Cancer, *1*:64, 1948.
12. Gray, C. F., Jr., Gonzales-Licea, A., Hartmann, W. H., and Woods, A. C.: Angiosarcoma in lymphedema. An unusual case of Stewart-Treves syndrome. Bull. Hopkins Hosp., *119*:117, 1966.
13. Fitzpatrick, T. B., Montgomery, H., and Lerner, A. B.: Pathogenesis of generalized dermal pigmentation secondary to malignant melanoma and melanuria. J. Invest. Dermatol., *22*:163, 1954.
14. Konrad, K., and Wolff, K.: Pathogenesis of diffuse melanosis secondary to malignant melanoma. Br. J. Dermatol., *91*:635, 1974.
15. Fenster, L. F., and Klatskin, G.: Manifestations of metastatic tumors of the liver. Am. J. Med., *31*:238, 1961.
16. Kawatsu, T., and Miki, Y.: Triple extramammary Paget's disease. Arch. Dermatol., *104*:316, 1971.
17. Cawley, L. P.: Extramammary Paget's disease. Am. J. Clin. Pathol., *27*:559, 1966.
18. Helwig, E. B., and Graham, J. H.: Anogenital (extramammary) Paget's disease. Cancer, *16*:387, 1963.
19. Friedrich, E. G., Jr., Wilkinson, E. J., Steingraeber, P. H., and Lewis, J. D.: Paget's disease of the vulva and carcinoma of the breast. Obstet. Gynecol., *46*:130, 1975.
20. Koss, L. G., and Brockunier, A., Jr.: Ultrastructural aspects of Paget's disease of the vulva. Arch. Pathol., *87*:592, 1969.
21. Tchang, F., Okagaki, T., and Richard, R. M.: Adenocarcinoma of Bartholin's gland associated with Paget's disease of vulvar area. Cancer, *31*:221, 1973.
22. Murrell, T. W., Jr., and McMullen, F. H.: Extramammary Paget's disease. A report of two cases. Arch. Dermatol., *85*:600, 1962.
23. Becker, S. W., Brennan, B., and Weichselbaum, P. K.: Genital Paget's disease. Arch. Dermatol., *82*:857, 1960.
24. Belcher, R. W.: Extramammary Paget's disease. Enzyme, histochemical and electron microscopic study. Arch. Pathol., *94*:59, 1972.
25. Fenn, M. E., Moreley, G. W., and Abell, M. R.: Paget's disease of the vulva. Obstet. Gynecol., *38*:660, 1971.
26. Holleran, W. M., and Schmutzer, K. J.: Paget's disease of the groin. J.A.M.A., *193*:193, 1965.
27. Yoell, J. H., and Price, W. G.: Paget's disease of the perineal skin with associated adenocarcinoma. Arch. Dermatol., *82*:986, 1960.
28. Dockerty, M. P., and Pratt, J. H.: Extramammary Paget's disease. A report of four cases in which certain features of histogenesis were exhibited. Cancer, *5*:1161, 1952.
29. Greenwood, S. M., and Minkowitz, S.: Paget's disease in metastatic breast carcinoma. Arch. Dermatol., *104*:312, 1971.
30. Pinkus, H., and Mehregan, A. H.: Epidermotropic eccrine carcinoma. A case combining features of eccrine poroma and Paget's dermatosis. Arch. Dermatol., *88*:165, 1963.
31. Fisher, E. R., and Beyer, F., Jr.: Differentiation of neoplastic lesions characterized by large vacuolated intradermal (Pagetoid) cells. Arch. Pathol., *67*:140, 1959.
32. Gray, H.: Anatomy of the Human Body, 25th ed. Edited by Charles Mayo Goss. Lea and Febiger, Philadelphia, 1948, pp. 715–726.
33. Demopoulos, R. I.: Fine structure of the extramammary Paget's cell. Cancer, *27*:1202, 1971.
34. Pinkus, H.: Discussion of paper. *In* Becker, S. W., Brennan, B., and Weichselbaum, P. K.: Genital Paget's disease. Arch. Dermatol., *82*:863, 1960.
35. O'Riordan, J. L. H., Blanshard, G. P., Moxham, A., and Nabarro, J. D. N.: Corticotrophin-secreting carcinomas. Q. J. Med., *35*:137, 1966.
36. Friedman, M., Marshall-Jones, P., and Ross, E. J.: Cushing's syndrome: Adrenocortical hyperactivity secondary to neoplasms arising outside the pituitary-adrenal system. Q. J. Med., *35*:193, 1966.
37. Davis, R. B., and Kennedy, B. J.: Carcinoid

associated with adrenal hyperplasia. Arch. Intern. Med., *109*:192, 1962.
38. Escovitz, W. E., and Reingold, I. M.: Functioning malignant bronchial carcinoid with Cushing's syndrome and recurrent sinus arrest. Ann. Intern. Med., *54*:1248, 1961.
39. Liddle, G. W., Island, D. P., Ney, R. L., Nicholson, W. E., and Shimizu, N.: Nonpituitary neoplasms and Cushing's syndrome. Arch. Intern. Med., *111*:471, 1963.
40. Cohen, R. B., Toll, G. D., and Castleman, B.: Bronchial adenomas in Cushing's syndrome: their relation to thymomas and oat cell carcinomas associated with hyperadrenocorticism. Cancer, *13*:812, 1960.
41. Johnston, W. H., and Waisman, J.: Carcinoid tumor of the vermiform appendix with Cushing's syndrome. Cancer, *27*: 681, 1971.
42. Abe, K., Nicholson, W. E., Liddle, G. W., Island, D. P., and Orth, D. N.: Radioimmunoassay of β-MSH in human plasma and tissues. J. Clin. Invest., *46*:1609, 1967.
43. Bloomfield, G. A., Scott, A. P., Lowry, P. J., Gilkes, J. J. H., and Rees, L. H.: A reappraisal of human β-MSH. Nature, *252*:492, 1974.
44. Gilkes, J. J. H., Bloomfield, G. A., Scott, A. P., Lowry, P. J., Ratcliffe, J. G., Landon, J., and Rees, L. H.: Development and validation of a radioimmunoassay for peptides related to β-melanocyte-stimulating hormone in human plasma: The lipotropins. J. Clin. Endocrinol. Metab., *40*:450, 1975.
45. Hirata, Y., Matsukura, S., Imura, H., Nakamura, M., and Tanaka, A.: Size heterogenity of β-MSH in ectopic ACTH-producing tumors: Presence of β-LPH-like peptide. J. Clin. Endocrinol. Metab., *42*:33, 1976.
46. Brown, J. D., and Doe, R. P.: Pituitary pigmentary hormones. Relationship of melanocyte-stimulating hormone to lipotropic hormone. J.A.M.A., *240*:1273, 1978.
47. Fusco, R. D., and Rosen, F. D.: Gonadotropin producing carcinomas of the lung. N. Engl. J. Med., *275*:507, 1966.
48. Case records of the Massachusetts General Hospital (Case 46451). N. Engl. J. Med., *263*:965, 1960.
49. Kierland, R. R., Sauer, W. G., and Dearing, W. H.: The cutaneous manifestations of the functioning carcinoid. Arch. Dermatol., *77*:86, 1958.
50. Melmon, K. L., Sjoerdsma, A., and Mason, D. T.: Distinctive clinical and therapeutic aspects of syndrome associated with bronchial carcinoid tumor. Am. J. Med., *39*:568, 1965.
51. Steele, C. W.: Malignant carcinoid. Ann. Intern. Med., *110*:763, 1962.
52. Hyman, G. A., and Wells, J.: Bronchial carcinoid with osteoblastic metastases. Arch. Intern. Med., *114*:541, 1964.
53. Mason, D. T., and Melmon, K. L. M.: New understanding of the mechanism of the carcinoid flush. Ann. Intern. Med., *65*:1334, 1966.
54. Melmon, K. L.: Kinins — one of the many mediators of the carcinoid spectrum. Gastroenterology, *55*:545, 1968.
55. Roberts, L. J., II, Marney, S. R., Jr., and Oates, J. A.: Blockade of the flush associated with metastatic gastric carcinoid by combined histamine H_1, and H_2 receptor antagonists. Evidence for an important role of H_2 receptors in human vasculature. N. Engl. J. Med., *300*:236, 1979.
56. Brown, H., and Lane, M.: Cushing's and malignant carcinoid syndromes from ovarian neoplasm. Arch. Intern. Med., *115*:490, 1964.
57. Pearse, A. G., Polak, J. M., and Heath, C. M.: Polypeptide hormone production by "carcinoid" apudomas and their relevant cytochemistry. Virchows Arch. [Cell. Pathol.], *16*:95, 1974.
58. Weichert, R. F.: The neural ectodermal origin of the peptide-secreting endocrine glands. Am. J. Med., *49*:232, 1970.
59. Pearse, A. G. E.: The APUD cell concept and its implications in pathology. Pathol. Annu., *9*:27, 1974.
60. Pearse, A. G. E., and Polak, J. M.: Neural crest origin of the endocrine polypeptide (APUD) cells of the gastrointestinal tract and pancreas. Gut, *12*:783, 1971.
61. Tischler, A. S., Dichter, M. A., Biales, B., and Greene, L. A.: Neuroendocrine neoplasms and their cells of origin. N. Engl. J. Med., *296*:919, 1977.
62. Polak, J. M., Pearse, A. G. E., LeLièvre, C., Fontaine, J., and LeDouarin, N. M.: Immunocytochemical confirmation of the neural crest origin of avian calcitonin-producing cells. Histochemistry, *40*:209, 1974.
63. Fontaine, J., and LeDouarin, N. M.: Analysis of endoderm formation in the avian blastoderm by use of quail-chick chimaeras. The problem of the neuroectodermal origin of the cells of the APUD series. J. Embryol. Exp. Morphol., *41*:209, 1977.
64. Ballard, H. S., Frame, B., and Hartsock, R. J.: Familial multiple endocrine adenoma–peptic ulcer complex. Medicine, *43*:481, 1964.
65. Steiner, A. L., Goodman, A. D., and Powers, S. R.: Study of a kindred with phaeochromocytoma, medullary thyroid carcinoma, hyperparathyrodism and Cushing's disease: multiple endocrine neoplasia, type 2. Medicine, *47*:371, 1968.
66. Catalona, W. J., Engelman, K., Ketcham, A. S., and Hammond, W. G.: Familial medullary thyroid carcinoma, phaeochromocytoma, and parathyroid adenoma (Sipple's syndrome). Study of a kindred. Cancer, *28*:1245, 1971.
67. Keiser, H. R., Beaven, M. A., Doppman, J., Wells, S., Jr., and Buja, L. M.: Sipple's syndrome: medullary thyroid carcinoma, phaeochromocytoma, and parathyroid

disease. Studies in a large family. Ann. Intern. Med., *78*:561, 1973.
68. Khairi, M. R. A., Dexter, R. N., Burzynski, N. J., and Johnston, C. C.: Mucosal neuroma, phaeochromocytoma and medullary thyroid carcinoma: multiple endocrine neoplasia type 3. Medicine, *54*:89, 1975.
69. Brown, R. S., Colle, E., and Tashjian, A. H., Jr.: The syndrome of multiple mucosal neuromas and medullary thyroid carcinoma in childhood. Importance of recognition of the phenotype for the early detection of malignancy. J. Pediatrics, *86*:77, 1975.
70. Melvin, K. E. W., Miller, H. H., and Tashjian, A. H.: Early diagnosis of medullary carcinoma of the thyroid gland by means of calcitonin assay. N. Engl. J. Med., *285*:1115, 1971.
71. Baum, J. L., and Adler, M. E.: Phaeochromocytoma, medullary thyroid cancer, multiple mucosal neuroma. Arch. Ophthalmol., *87*:574, 1972.
72. Gagel, R. F., Melvin, K. E. W., Tashjian, A. H., Jr., Miller, H. H., Feldman, Z. T., Wolfe, H. J., DeLellis, R. A., Cervi-Skinner, S., and Reichlin, S.: Natural history of the familial medullary thyroid carcinoma–pheochromocytoma syndrome and the identification of preneoplastic stages by screening studies: a five year report. Trans. Assoc. Am. Physicians, *88*:177, 1975.
73. Gorlin, R.: Cited in reference 69, p. 81.
74. Marks, A. D., and Channick, B. J.: Extra-adrenal pheochromocytoma and medullary thyroid carcinoma with pheochromocytoma. Arch. Intern. Med., *134*:1106, 1974.
75. Wilkinson, D. S.: Necrolytic migratory erythema with pancreatic carcinoma. Proc. R. Soc. Med., *64*:25, 1971.
76. Rothman, S.: Über Hauterscheinungen bei bösartigen Geschwülsten innerer Organe. Arch Dermat. Syph., *149*:99, 1925.
77. Becker, S. W., Kahn, D., and Rothman, S.: Cutaneous manifestations of internal malignant tumors. Arch. Dermatol., *45*:1069, 1942.
78. McGavran, M. H., Unger, R. H., Recant, L., Polk, H. C., Kilo, C., and Levin, M. E.: A glucagon-secreting alpha-cell carcinoma of the pancreas. N. Engl. J. Med., *274*:1408, 1966.
79. Church, R. E., and Crane, W. A. J.: A cutaneous syndrome associated with islet cell carcinoma of the pancreas. Br. J. Dermatol., *79*:284, 1967.
80. Wilkinson, D. S.: Necrolytic migratory erythema with pancreatic carcinoma. Proc. R. Soc. Med., *64*:1197, 1971.
81. Wilkinson, D. S.: Necrolytic migratory erythema with carcinoma of the pancreas. Trans. St. Johns Hosp. Dermatol. Soc., *59*:244, 1973.
82. Mallinson, C. N., Bloom, S. R., Warin, A. P., Salmon, P. R., and Cox, B. A.: Glucagonoma syndrome. Lancet, *2*:1, 1974.
83. Swenson, K. H., Amon, R. B., and Hanifin, J. M.: The glucagonoma syndrome. A distinctive marker of systemic disease. Arch. Dermatol., *114*:224, 1978.
84. Warin, A. P.: Necrolytic migratory erythema with carcinoma of pancreas. Proc. R. Soc. Med., *67*:2, 1974.
85. Binnick, A. N., Spencer, S. K., Dennison, W. L., Jr., and Horton, E. S.: Glucagonoma syndrome. Report of two cases and literature review. Arch. Dermatol., *113*:749, 1977.
86. Boden, G., and Owen, O. E.: Familial hyperglucagonemia — an autosomal dominant disorder. N. Engl. J. Med., *296*:534, 1977.
87. Sweet, R. D.: A dermatosis specifically associated with a tumor of pancreatic alpha cells. Br. J. Dermatol., *90*:301, 1974.
87a. Goodenberger, D. M., Lawley, T. J., Strober, W., Wyatt, L., Sangree, M. H., Jr., Sherwin, R., Rosenbaum, H., Braverman, I. M., and Katz, S. I.: Necrolytic migratory erythema without glucagonoma. Report of two cases. Arch. Dermatol., *115*:1429, 1979.
87b. Thivolet, J.: Necrolytic migratory erythema without glucagonoma. Arch. Dermatol., *117*:4, 1981.
88. Cormia, F. E.: Pruritus, an uncommon but important symptom of systemic carcinoma. Arch. Dermatol., *92*:36, 1965.
89. Barnes, B. E.: Dermatomyositis and malignancy. A review of the literature. Ann. Intern. Med., *84*:68, 1976.
90. Bluefarb, S. M., Walk, S., and Gigli, L.: Dermatomyositis (remission following surgery for carcinoma of the uterus). Arch. Dermatol., *83*:168, 1961.
91. Bohan, A., Peter, J. B., Bowman, R. L., and Pearson, C. M.: A computer-assisted analysis of 153 patients with polymyositis and dermatomyositis. Medicine, *56*:255, 1977.
92. Mills, J. A.: Connective tissue disease associated with malignant neoplastic disease. J. Chronic Dis., *16*:797, 1963.
93. Knowles, J. H., and Smith, L. H., Jr.: Extrapulmonary manifestations of bronchogenic carcinoma. N. Engl. J. Med., *262*:505, 1960.
94. Mackenzie, A. H., and Scherbel, A. L.: Connective tissue syndromes associated with cancer. Geriatrics, *18*:745, 1963.
95. Osborne, R. R.: Functioning acinous cell carcinoma of the pancreas accompanied with widespread focal fat necrosis. Arch. Intern. Med., *85*:933, 1950.
96. Burns, W. A., Matthews, M. J., Hamosh, M., Weide, G. V., Blum, R., and Johnson, F. B.: Lipase-secreting acinar cell carcinoma of the pancreas with polyarthropathy. A light and electron microscopic, histochemical, and biochemical study. Cancer, *33*:1002, 1974.
97. Szymanski, F. J., and Bluefarb, S. M.: Nodular fat necrosis and pancreatic diseases. Arch. Dermatol., *83*:224, 1961.
98. Wuketich, S., and Pavlik, F.: Syndrome of metastasizing lipase forming pancreatic adenoma: differential diagnosis of Pfeifer-Weber-Christian disease. Arch. Klin. Exp. Dermatol., *216*:412, 1963.

99. Schmid, M.: Über das Syndrom des sekretorischaktiven metastierenden exokrinen Pankreas-adenomas. Z. Klin. Med., *154*:439, 1957.
100. Trousseau, A.: Phlegmasia alba dolens. Clinique medicale de l'Hotel-Dieu de Paris. The New Sydenham Society, *3L*:94, 1865.
101. Sproul, E. E.: Carcinoma and venous thrombosis: the frequency of association of carcinoma in the body or tail of the pancreas with multiple venous thrombosis. Am. J. Cancer, *34*:566, 1938.
102. Sack, G. H., Jr., Levin, J., and Bell, W. R.: Trousseau's syndrome and other manifestations of chronic disseminated coagulopathy in patients with neoplasms: clinical, pathophysiologic and therapeutic features. Medicine, *56*:1, 1977.
103. Miller, S. P., Sanchez-Avalos, J., Stefanski, T., and Zuckerman, L.: Coagulation disorder in cancer. I. Clinical and laboratory studies. Cancer, *20*:1452, 1967.
104. Merskey, C.: Pathogenesis and treatment of altered blood coagulability in patients with malignant tumors. N.Y. Acad. Sci., *230*:289, 1974.
105. Goodnight, S. H., Jr.: Bleeding and intravascular clotting in malignancy: A review. N.Y. Acad. Sci., *230*:271, 1974.
106. Hawley, P. R., Johnston, A. W., and Rankin, J. T.: Association between digital ischaemia and malignant disease. Br.. Med. J., *3*:208, 1967.
107. Skog, E.: Cutaneous manifestations associated with internal malignant tumors with particular reference to vesicular and bullous lesions. Acta Dermatovener., *44*:114, 1964.
108. Elliott, J. A.: Bullous dermatoses of toxic origin: report of a case involving an association with choriocarcinoma. Arch. Dermatol., *37*:219, 1938.
109. Davis, H.: On two cases of exudative erythema associated with malignant disease of the uterus. Br. J. Dermatol., *34*:12, 1922.
110. Tobias, N.: Dermatitis herpetiformis associated with visceral malignancy. Urol. Cutan. Rev., *55*:352, 1951.
111. Marks, J. M.: Pemphigoid with malignant melanoma. Proc. R. Soc. Med., *54*:225, 1961.
112. Arnold, H. L., Jr.: Erythema multiforme following high voltage roentgen therapy. Arch. Dermatol., *60*:143, 1949.
113. Loewe, L., and Camiel, M. R.: Exanthem complicating neoplastic disease. Am. J. Roentgenol., *43*:587, 1940.
114. Stone, S. P., and Schroeter, A. L.: Bullous pemphigoid and associated malignant neoplasms. Arch. Dermatol., *111*:991, 1975.
115. Ahmed, A. R., Chu, T. M., and Provost, T. T.: Bullous pemphigoid. Clinical and serologic evaluation for associated malignant neoplasms. Arch. Dermatol., *113*:969, 1977.
116. Chorzelski, T. P., Jablonska, S., Maciejowska, E., Beuntner, E. H., and Wronkowski, L.: Coexistence of malignancies with bullous pemphigoid. Arch. Dermatol., *114*:964, 1978.
117. Urbach, E.: Endogenous allergy. Arch. Dermatol., *45*:697, 1942.
118. Gammel, J. A.: Erythema gyratum repens. Arch. Dermatol., *66*:494, 1952.
119. Skolnick, M., and Mainman, E. R.: Erythema gyratum repens with metastatic adenocarcinoma. Arch. Dermatol., *111*:227, 1975.
120. Leavell, U. W., Winternitz, W. W., and Black, J. H.: Erythema gyratum repens and undifferentiated carcinoma. Arch. Dermatol., *95*:69, 1967.
121. Shelley, W. B., and Hurley, H. J.: Unusual autoimmune syndrome: erythema annulare centrifugum, generalized pigmentation and breast hypertrophy. Arch. Dermatol., *81*:889, 1960.
122. Shelley, W. B.: An unusual autoimmune syndrome. A followup with reference to breast hypertrophy, SLE and verrucae. Acta Dermatovener., *52*:33, 1972.
123. Barber, P. V., Doyle, L., Vickers, D. M., and Hubbard, H.: Erythema gyratum repens with pulmonary tuberculosis. Br. J. Dermatol., *98*:465, 1978.
124. Shelley, W. B.: Erythema annulare centrifugum. A case due to hypersensitivity to blue cheese Penicillium. Arch. Dermatol., *90*:54, 1964.
125. Ikada, J., Kishimoto, S., Kagami, K., and Nakano, Y.: Erythema annulare centrifugum with ovarian cystadenoma. Arch. Dermatol., *111*:1537, 1975.
126. Howel-Evans, W., McConnell, R. B., Clarke, C. A., and Sheppard, P. M.: Carcinoma of the esophagus with keratosis palmaris et plantaris (tylosis). Q. J. Med., *27*:413, 1958.
127. McConnell, R. B.: The Genetics of Gastrointestinal Disorders. Oxford University Press, London, 1966, p. 40.
128. Harper, P. S., Harper, R. M. J., and Howell-Evans, A. W.: Carcinoma of the oesophagus with tylosis. Q. J. Med., *39*:317, 1970.
129. Shine, I., and Allison, P. R.: Carcinoma of the esophagus with tylosis (keratosis palmaris et plantaris). Lancet, *1*:950, 1966.
130. Parnell, D. D., and Johnson, S. A. M.: Tylosis palmaris et plantaris. Its occurrence with internal malignancy. Arch. Dermatol., *100*:7, 1969.
131. Behan, P. O.: Internal malignancy associated with a dermatologic condition. Br. J. Clin. Pract., *19*:305, 1965.
131a. Bazex, A., Salvador, R., Dupre, A., and Christol, B.: Syndrome paranéoplasique à type d'hyperkératose des extrémités. Guérison aprés le traitement de l'épithélioma larynge. Bull. Soc. Fr. Derm. et Syph. *72*:182, 1965.
132. Bazex, A., Dupre, A., Christol, B., Cantala, P., and Geerts, J. M.: Acrokératose paranéoplasique. Bull. Soc. Fr. Dermatol. Syph., *76*:537, 1969.
133. Namour, M. N.: Acrokératose Paranéoplasique ou Syndrome de Bazex. Imprimerie Toulouse, Régionale, 1971.

134. Schweigl, R. L.: Erythrodermie und Uteruskarzinom. Zbi. Gynaek., *57*:94, 1933.
135. Graham, J. H., and Helwig, E. B.: Bowen's disease and its relationship to systemic cancer. Arch. Dermatol., *80*:133, 1959.
136. Nicolis, G. D., and Helwig, E. B.: Exfoliative dermatitis. A clinicopathologic study of 135 cases. Arch. Dermatol., *108*:788, 1973.
137. Gougerot, H., and Ruppe: Dermatose erythemato-squameuse avec hyperkératose palmo-plantarie, porectasies digitales et cancer de la langue latent. Paris Méd., *43*:234, 1922.
138. McGaw, B., and McGovern, V. J.: Exfoliative dermatitis associated with carcinoma of the lung. Aust. J. Dermatol., *3*:115, 1956.
139. Van Dijk, E.: Ichythyosiform atrophy of the skin associated with internal malignant disease. Dermatologica, *127*:413, 1963.
140. Reiches, A. J.: Acquired ichthyosis: report of a case associated with breast cancer. Urol. Cutan. Rev., *54*:160, 1950.
141. Flint, G. L., Flam, M., and Soter, N. A.: Acquired ichthyosis. A sign of nonlymphoproliferative malignant disorders. Arch. Dermatol., *111*:1446, 1975.
142. Herzberg, J. J., Potjan, K., and Gebauer, D.: Hypertrichose lanugineuse acquise. Ann. Dermatol. Syph. (Paris), *96*:129, 1969.
143. van der Lugt, L., and deWit, C. D.: Hypertrichosis lanuginosa acquisita. Dermatologica, *146*:46, 1973.
144. Fretzin, D. F.: Malignant down. Arch. Dermatol., *95*:294, 1967.
145. Hensley, G. T., and Glynn, K. P.: Hypertrichosis lanuginosa as a sign of internal malignancy. Cancer, *24*:1051, 1969.
146. Wadskov, S., Bro-Jørgensen, A., and Sondergaard, J.: Acquired hypertrichosis lanuginosa. Arch. Dermatol., *112*:1442, 1976.
147. Samson, M. K., Buroker, T. R., Henderson, M. D., Baker, L. H., and Vaitkevicius, V. K.: Acquired hypertrichosis lanuginosa. Report of two new cases and a review of literature. Cancer, *36*:1519, 1975.
148. Kaiser, I. W., Perry, G., and Yoonessi, M.: Acquired hypertrichosis lanuginosa associated with endometrial malignancy. Obstet. Gynecol., *47*:479, 1976.
149. Lyell, A., and Whittle, C. H.: Hypertrichosis lanuginosa, acquired type. Br. J. Dermatol., *63*:411, 1951.
150. Hegedus, S. I., and Schorr, W. F.: Acquired hypertrichosis lanuginosa and malignancy. Arch. Dermatol., *106*:84, 1972.
151. McKissic, E. D.: Malignant acanthosis nigricans and anesthesia. Anesthesiology, *42*:357, 1975.
152. Möller, H., Eriksson, S., Holen, O., and Waldenström, J. G.: Complete reversibility of paraneoplastic acanthosis nigricans after operation. Acta Med. Scand., *203*:245, 1978.
153. Curth, H. O.: Cancer associated with acanthosis nigricans. Arch. Surg., *47*:517, 1943.
154. Curth, H. O., Hilberg, A. W., and Machacek, G. F.: The site and histology of cancer associated with malignant acanthosis nigricans. Cancer, *15*:364, 1962.
155. Ackerman, A. B., and Lantis, L. R.: Acanthosis nigricans associated with Hodgkin's disease. Arch. Dermatol., *95*:202, 1967.
156. Curth, H. O.: Dermatoses and malignant internal tumors. Arch. Dermatol., *71*:95, 1955.
157. Lerner, A. B.: On the cause of acanthosis nigricans. N. Engl. J. Med., *281*:106, 1969.
158. Hage, E., and Hage, J.: Malignant acanthosis nigricans — a paraendocrine syndrome? Acta Dermatovener., *57*:169, 1977.
159. Curth, H. O., and Aschner, B. M.: Genetic studies on acanthosis nigricans. Arch. Dermatol., *79*:55, 1959.
160. Curth, H. O., and Slanetz, C. A.: Acanthosis nigricans and cancer of the liver in a dog. Am. J. Cancer, *37*:216, 1939.
161. Sneddon, I. B.: The skin markers of malignancy. Br. Med. J., *2*:405, 1963.
162. Gougerot, H., and Duperrat, B.: Dermatose verruqueuse "Monitrice" d'un cancer viscéral. Ann. Dermatol. Syph., *2*:193, 1942.
163. Josserand, A., Dargent, M., and Mayer, M.: Evolution et involution simultanées de carcinose du sein et de verruses de la region mammaire. Presse Med., *56*:674, 1948.
164. Ronchese, F.: Keratoses, cancer and the sign of Leser-Trélat. Cancer, *18*:1003, 1965.
165. Liddell, K., White, J. E., and Caldwell, I. W.: Seborrhoeic keratoses and carcinoma of large bowel. Br. J. Dermatol., *92*:449, 1975.
166. Dantzig, P. I.: Sign of Leser-Trélat. Arch. Dermatol., *108*:700, 1973.
167. Williams, M. G.: Acanthomata appearing after eczema. Br. J. Dermatol., *68*:268, 1956.
168. Graham, J. H., and Helwig, E. B.: Bowen's disease and its relationship to systemic cancer. Arch. Dermatol. *83*:738, 1961.
169. Peterka, E. S., Lynch, F. W., and Goltz, R. W.: An association between Bowen's disease and internal cancer. Arch. Dermatol., *84*:623, 1961.
170. Epstein, E.: Association of Bowen's disease with visceral cancer. Arch. Dermatol., *82*:349, 1960.
171. Hugo, N. E., and Conway, H.: Bowen's disease: its malignant potential and relationship to systemic cancer. Plast. Reconstr. Surg., *39*:109, 1967.
172. Andersen, S. La C., Nielsen, A., and Reymann, F.: Relationship between Bowen disease and internal malignant tumors. Arch. Dermatol., *108*:367, 1973.
173. Lever, W. F.: Histopathology of the Skin, 4th ed., Lippincott, Philadelphia, 1967, p. 261.
174. Graham, J. H., Mazzanti, G. R., and Helwig, E. B.: Chemistry of Bowen's disease: relationships to arsenic. J. Invest. Dermatol., *37*:317, 1961.

175. Domonkos, A. N.: Neutron activation analyses of arsenic in normal skin, keratoses and epitheliomas. Arch. Dermatol., *80*:672, 1959.
176. Fergusson, A. G., Dewar, W. A., and Smith, H.: Arsenic values in various skin diseases. (Estimation by activation analyses). Arch. Dermatol., *81*:931, 1960.
177. Tay, C. H.: Cutaneous manifestations of arsenic poisoning due to certain Chinese herbal medicine. Australasian J. Dermatol., *15*:121, 1974.
178. Satterlee, H. S.: The problem of arsenic in American cigarette tobacco. N. Engl. J. Med., *254*:1149, 1956.
179. Lee, B. K., and Murphy, G.: Determination of arsenic content of American cigarettes by neutron activation analyses. Cancer, *23*:1315, 1969.
180. Currie, A. N.: The role of arsenic in carcinogenesis. Br. Med. Bull., *4*:402, 1947.
181. Wagner, S. L., and Weswig, P.: Arsenic in blood and urine of forest workers. Arch. Environ. Health, *28*:77, 1974.
182. Bollen, W. B., Norris, L. A., and Stowers, K. L.: Effect of cacodylic acid and MSMA on microbes in forest floor soil. Weed Science, *22*:557, 1974.
183. Goodman, L. A., and Gilman, A.: The Pharmacological Basis of Therapeutics, 5th ed. Macmillan, New York, 1975, pp. 924–927.
184. Sanderson, K. V.: Arsenic and skin cancer. Trans. St. John Hosp. Dermatol. Soc., *49*:115, 1963.
185. Yeh, S.: Relative incidence of skin cancer in Chinese in Taiwan: with special reference to arsenical cancer. (Conference on Biology of Cutaneous Cancer.) Nat. Cancer Inst. Monogr., *10*:81, 1963.
186. Yeh, S.: Skin cancer in chronic arsenicism. Hum. Pathol., *4*:469, 1973.
187. Roth, F.: Über die chronische Arsenvergiftung der Moselwinzer unter besonderer Berücksichtigung des Arsenkrebses. Z. Krebsforsch., *61*:287, 1956.
188. Sommers, S. C., and McManus, R. G.: Multiple arsenical cancers of skin and intestinal organs. Cancer, *61*:347, 1953.
189. Data of Russell cited by Sanderson, K. V., Trans. St. John Hosp. Dermatol. Soc., *49*:115, 1963.
190. Ott, M. G., Holder, B. B., and Gordon, H. L.: Respiratory cancer and occupational exposure to arsenicals. Arch. Environ. Health, *29*:250, 1974.
191. Oppenheim, J. J., and Fishbein, W. N.: Induction of chromosome breaks in cultured normal human leukocytes by potassium arsenite, hydroxyurea, and related compounds. Cancer Res., *25*:980, 1965.
192. Burgdorf, W., Kurvink, K., and Cervenka, J.: Elevated sister chromatid exchange rate in lymphocytes of subjects treated with arsenic. Hum. Genet., *36*:69, 1977.
193. Costello, M. J., Fisher, S. B., and DeFeo, C. P.: Melanotic freckle. Arch. Dermatol., *80*:753, 1959.
194. Davis, J., Pack, G. T., and Higgins, G. K.: Melanotic freckle of Hutchinson. Am. J. Surg., *113*:457, 1967.
195. Stoll, H. L., Jr.: Squamous cell carcinoma. *In* Fitzpatrick, T. B., et al.: Dermatology in General Medicine. McGraw Hill Book Co., New York, 1971, p. 407.
196. Wechsler, H. L., Krugh, F. J., Domonkos, A. N., Scheen, S. R., and Davidson, C. L., Jr.: Polydysplastic epidermolysis bullosa and development of epidermal neoplasms. Arch. Dermatol., *102*:374, 1970.
197. Reed, W. B., College, J., Jr., Frances, J. O., Zachariae, H., Mohs, F., Sher, M. A., and Sneddon, I. B.: Epidermolysis bullosa dystrophica with epidermal neoplasms. Arch. Dermatol., *110*:894, 1974.
198. Huepner, W. C.: Recent developments in environmental cancer. Arch. Pathol., *58*:360, 475, 645, 1954.
199. Henry, S. A.: Occupational cutaneous cancer attributable to certain chemicals in industry. Br. Med. Bull., *4*:389, 1947.
200. Wahlberg, J. E.: Occupational and non-occupational scrotal cancer in Sweden 1958–1970. Acta Dermatovener, *54*:471, 1974.
201. Cripps, D. J., Ramsay, C. A., and Ruch, D. M.: Xeroderma pigmentosum: abnormal monochromatic action spectrum and autoradiographic studies. J. Invest. Dermatol., *56*:281, 1971.
202. Ramsay, C. A., and Giannelli, F.: The erythema action spectrum and deoxyribonucleic acid repair synthesis in xeroderma pigmentosum. Br. J. Dermatol., *92*:49, 1975.
203. Hadida, E., Marill, F-G., and Sayag, J.: Xeroderma pigmentosum: 48 personal cases. Ann. Dermatol. Syph., *90*:467, 1963.
204. El-Hefnawi, H., El-Nabawi, M., and Rasheed, A.: Xeroderma pigmentosum. I. A clinical study of 12 Egyptian cases. Br. J. Dermatol., *74*:201, 1962.
205. King, H., and Hamilton, C. M.: Xeroderma pigmentosum in a Negress. Arch. Dermatol., *42*:570, 1940.
206. Robbins, J. H., Kraemer, K. H., Lutzner, M. A., Festoff, B. W., and Coon, H. G.: Xeroderma pigmentosum: an inherited disease with sun sensitivity, multiple cutaneous neoplasms, and abnormal DNA repair. Ann. Intern. Med., *80*:221, 1974.
207. Reed, W. B., May, S. B., and Nickel, W. R.: Xeroderma pigmentosum with neurological complications. Arch. Dermatol., *91*:224, 1965.
208. El-Hefnawi, H., El-Nabawi, M., and El-Hawary, M. F. S.: Xeroderma pigmentosum. III. Studies of serum cooper and blood glutathione. Br. J. Dermatol., *74*:218, 1962.
209. El-Hefnawi, H., and El-Hawary, M. F. S.: Chromatographic studies of amino acids in sera and urine of patients with xeroderma pigmentosum and their normal relatives. Br. J. Dermatol., *75*:235, 1963.
210. El-Hefnawi, H., El-Hawary, M. F. S., El-Komy, H. M., and Rasheed, A.: Xeroder-

ma pigmentosum. V. Studies of 17-ketosteroids and total 17-hydroxycorticosteroids. Br. J. Dermatol., *77*:484, 1963.
211. El-Hefnawi, H., and Smith, S. M.: Xeroderma pigmentosum. A brief report on its genetic linkage with ABO blood groups in the United Arab Republic. Br. J. Dermatol., *77*:35, 1965.
212. Cleaver, J. E.: Defective repair replication of DNA in xeroderma pigmentosum. Nature, *218*:652, 1968.
213. Epstein, J. H., Fukuyama, K., Epstein, W. L., and Reed, W. B.: An in vivo study of a defect in DNA synthesis in xeroderma pigmentosum. J. Clin. Invest., *48*:23a, 1969.
214. Cleaver, J. E., and Bootsma, D.: Xeroderma pigmentosum: biochemical and genetic characteristics. Annu. Rev. Genet., *9*:19, 1975.
215. Ames, B. M.: The detection of chemical mutagens with enteric bacteria. *In* Hollander, A. (ed.): Chemical Mutagens: Princples and Methods for Their Detection. Plenum Press, New York, 1971, p. 267.
216. Lewandowsky, F., and Lutz, W.: Ein Fall einer bisher nicht beschriebenen Hauterkrankung (Epidermodysplasia verruciformis). Arch. Derm. Syph., *141*:193, 1922.
217. Lutz, W.: A propos de l'epidermodysplasie verruciforme. Dermatologica, *92*:30, 1946.
218. Jablonska, S., and Formas, I.: Weitere positive Ergebnisse mit Auto- und Heteroinokulation bei Epidermodysplasia verruciformis Lewandowsky-Lutz. Dermatologica, *118*:86, 1959.
219. Jablonska, S., Fajanska, L., and Formas, I.: On the viral etiology of epidermodysplasia verruciformis. Dermatologica, *132*:369, 1966.
220. Yabe, Y., and Sadakane, H.: The virus of epidermodysplasia verruciformis: electron microscopic and fluorescent antibody studies. J. Invest. Dermatol., *65*:324, 1975.
221. Aaronson, D. M., and Lutzner, M. A.: Epidermodysplasia verruciformis and epidermoid carcinoma. Electron microscopic observations. J.A.M.A., *201*:149, 1967.
222. Ruiter, M., and Van Mullem, P. J.: Demonstration by electron microscopy of an intranuclear virus in epidermodysplasia verruciformis. J. Invest. Dermatol., *47*:247, 1966.
223. Ruiter, M., and Van Mullem, P. J.: Behavior of virus in malignant degeneration of skin lesions in epidermodysplasia verruciformis. J. Invest. Dermatol., *54*:324, 1970.
224. Yabe, Y., Yasui, M., Yoshino, N., Fujiwara, T., Ohkuma, N., and Nohara, N.: Epidermodysplasia verruciformis: viral particles in early malignant lesions. J. Invest. Dermatol., *71*:225, 1978.
225. Rous, P., and Beard, J. W.: Carcinomatous changes in virus induced papillomas of the skin of the rabbit. Proc. Soc. Exp. Biol. Med., *32*:578, 1935.
226. Kidd, J. G., and Rous, P.: Cancers derived from the virus papillomas of wild rabbits under natural conditions. J. Exp. Med., *71*:469, 1940.
227. Prawer, S. E., Pass, F., Vance, J. C., Greenberg, L. J., Yunis, E. J., and Zelickson, A. S.: Depressed immune function in epidermodysplasia verruciformis. Arch. Dermatol., *113*:495, 1977.
228. Hammar, H., Hammar, L., Lambert, B., and Ringborg, U.: A case report including EM and DNA repair investigations in a dermatosis associated with multiple skin cancers: Epidermodysplasia verruciformis. Acta Med. Scand., *200*:441, 1976.
229. Howell, J. B., Anderson, D. E., and McClendon, J. L.: The basal cell nevus syndrome. J.A.M.A., *190*:274, 1964.
230. Anderson, D. E., Taylor, W. B., Falls, H. F., and Davidson, R. T.: The nevoid basal cell carcinoma syndrome. Am. J. Hum. Genet., *19*:12, 1967.
231. Holubar, K., Matras, H., and Samlik, A. V.: Multiple palmar basal cell epitheliomas in basal cell nevus syndrome. Arch. Dermatol., *101*:679, 1970.
232. Howell, J. B., and Mehregan, A. H.: Pursuit of the pits in the nevoid basal cell carcinoma syndrome. Arch. Dermatol., *102*:586, 1970.
233. Taylor, W. B., and Wilkins, J. W., Jr.: Nevoid basal cell carcinoma of the palm. Arch. Dermatol., *102*:654, 1970.
234. Clendenning, W. E., Block, J. B., and Radde, I. C.: Basal cell nevus syndrome. Arch. Dermatol., *90*:38, 1964.
235. Katz, J., Savin, R. S., and Spiro, H. M.: Basal cell nevus syndrome and inflammatory disease of the bowel. Am. J. Med., *44*:483, 1968.
236. Schwartz, R. A.: Basal-cell-nevus syndrome and gastrointestinal polyposis. N. Engl. J. Med., *299*:49, 1978.
237. Gray, H. R., and Helwig, E. B.: Epithelioma adenoides cysticum and solitary trichoepithelioma. Arch. Dermatol., *87*:102, 1963.
238. Hopf, H. Ch.: Acrodermatitis Chronica Atrophicans (Herxheimer) and Nervensystem. Springer-Verlag, Berlin, 1966.
239. Striltzer, C.: Acrodermatitis chronica atrophicans. Arch. Dermatol., *81*:280, 1960.
240. Dougherty, J. W.: Squamous cell epithelioma in acrodermatitis chronica atrophicans treated with skin grafting. Arch. Dermatol., *77*:349, 1958.
241. Lewis, G. A., and Sachs, W.: Anaplastic epithelioma in patient with acrodermatitis chronica atrophicans. Arch. Dermatol., *63*:790, 1951.
242. Jancu, J.: Peutz-Jeghers syndrome. Involvement of the gastrointestinal and upper respiratory tracts. Am. J. Gastroenterol., *56*:545, 1971.
243. Reid, J. D.: Intestinal carcinoma in the Peutz-Jeghers syndrome. J.A.M.A., *229*:833, 1974.
244. Bailey, D.: Polyposis of gastrointestinal tract: the Peutz syndrome. Br. Med. J., *2*:433, 1957.

245. Beinfeld, M. S., and Chargus, G. W.: Peutz-Jeghers syndrome. Report of a case of small intestinal polyposis and carcinoma associated with melanin pigmentation of the lips and buccal mucosa. Gastroenterology, *35*:534, 1959.
246. Kyle, J.: Peutz-Jeghers syndrome. Scot. Med. J., *6*:361, 1961.
247. Morson, B. C.: Precancerous lesions of upper gastrointestinal tract. J.A.M.A., *179*:311, 1962.
248. de la Pava, S., Cabrera, A., and Studenski, E. R.: Peutz-Jeghers syndrome with jejunal carcinoma. N.Y. State J. Med., *62*:97, 1962.
249. Humphries, A. L., Shepherd, M. H., and Peters, H. J.: Peutz-Jeghers syndrome with colonic adenocarcinoma and ovarian tumors. J.A.M.A., *197*:138, 1966.
250. Shibata, H. R., and Phillips, N. J.: Peutz-Jeghers syndrome with jejunal and colonic adenocarcinomas. Can. Med. Assoc. J., *103*:285, 1970.
251. Dodds, W. J., Schulte, W. J., Hensley, G. T., and Hogan, W. J.: Peutz-Jeghers syndrome and gastrointestinal malignancy. Am. J. Roentgenol., *115*:374, 1972.
252. Papaioannon, A., and Critselis, A.: Malignant changes in the Peutz-Jeghers syndrome. N. Engl. J. Med., *289*:694, 1973.
253. Dormandy, T. L.: Gastrointestinal polyposis with mucocutaneous pigmentation (Peutz-Jeghers syndrome). N. Engl. J. Med., *256*:1093, 1141, 1186, 1957.
254. Achord, J. L., and Proctor, H. D.: Malignant degeneration and metastases in Peutz-Jeghers syndrome. Arch. Intern. Med., *111*:498, 1963.
255. Dozois, R. R., Judd, E. S., Dahlin, D. C., and Bartholomew, L. G.: The Peutz-Jeghers syndrome. Is there a predisposition to the development of intestinal cancer? Arch. Surg., *98*:509, 1969.
256. Altemeier, W. A.: in discussion of ref. 255, p. 517.
257. Farmer, R. G., Hawk, W. A., and Turnbull, R. B., Jr.: The spectrum of the Peutz-Jeghers syndrome. Am. J. Dig. Dis., *8*:953, 1963.
258. Bandler, M.: Hemangiomas of small intestine associated with mucocutaneous pigmentation. Gastroenterology, *38*:641, 1960.
259. Christian, C. D., McLoughlin, T. G., Cathcart, E. R., and Eisenberg, M. M.: Peutz-Jeghers syndrome associated with functioning ovarian tumor. J.A.M.A., *190*:157, 1964.
260. Scully, R. E.: Sex cord tumor with annular tubules. A distinctive ovarian tumor of the Peutz-Jeghers syndrome. Cancer, *25*:1107, 1970.
261. Dozois, R. R., Dahlin, D. C., and Bartholomew, L. G.: Ovarian tumors associated with the Peutz-Jeghers syndrome. *In* Ariel, I. M. (ed.): Progress in Clinical Cancer. Grune and Stratton, New York, 1973, p. 187.
262. Torre, D.: Multiple sebaceous tumors. Arch. Dermatol., *98*:549, 1968.
263. Sciallis, G. F., and Winkelmann, R. K.: Multiple sebaceous adenomas and gastrointestinal carcionoma. Arch. Dermatol., *110*:913, 1974.
264. Leonard, D. D., and Deaton, W. R., Jr.: Multiple sebaceous gland tumors and visceral carcinomas. Arch. Dermatol., *110*:917, 1974.
265. Lloyd, K. M., and Dennis, M.: Cowden's disease. A possible new symptom complex with multiple system involvement. Ann. Intern. Med., *58*:136, 1963.
266. Weary, P. E., Gorlin, R. J., Gentry, W. C., Jr., Comer, J. E., and Greer, K. E.: Multiple hamartoma syndrome (Cowden's disease). Arch. Dermatol., *106*:682, 1970.
267. Gentry, W. C., Jr., Eskritt, N. E., and Gorlin, R. J.: Multiple hamartoma syndrome (Cowden disease). Arch. Dermatol., *109*:521, 1974.
268. Burnett, J. W., Goldner, R., and Calton, G. J.: Cowden disease. Report of two additional cases. Br. J. Dermatol., *93*:329, 1975.
269. Siegel, J. M.: Cowden disease: Report of a case with malignant melanoma. Cutis, *16*:255, 1975.
270. Nuss, D. D., Aeling, J. L., Clemons, D. E., and Weber, W. N.: Multiple hamartoma syndrome (Cowden's disease). Arch. Dermatol., *114*:743, 1978.
271. Wade, T. R., and Kopf, A. W.: Cowden's disease: a case report and review of the literature. J. Dermatol. Surg. Oncol., *4*:459, 1978.
272. Dobson, R. L., Young, M. R., and Pinto, J. S.: Palmar keratoses and cancer. Arch. Dermatol., *92*:553, 1965.
273. Brownstein, M. H., Mehregan, A. H., and Bikowski, J. B.: Trichilemmomas in Cowden's disease. J.A.M.A., *238*:26, 1977.
274. Ackerman, A. B.: Trichilemmoma. Arch. Dermatol., *114*:286, 1978.
275. Bean, S. F., Foxley, E. G., and Fusaro, R. M.: Palmar keratoses and internal malignancy. A negative study. Arch. Dermatol., *97*:528, 1968.
276. Ross, J. B.: Keratosis punctata. Br. J. Dermatol., *75*:478, 1963.
277. Woodside, J. R., and Dobson, R. L.: Histopathology of palmar keratoses associated with cancer. Arch. Dermatol., *98*:648, 1968.
278. Stolman, L. P., Kopf, A. W., and Garfinkel, L.: Are palmar keratoses a sign of internal malignancy? Arch. Dermatol., *101*:52, 1970.

2

Lymphomas and Allied Disorders

The skin markers of Hodgkin's disease and non-Hodgkin's lymphomas, and their allied disorders — mycosis fungoides and Kaposi's hemorrhagic sarcoma — are discussed in this chapter. The leukemias are dealt with in Chapter 3.

The malignant lymphomas have undergone considerable reevaluation and reclassification in the past decade. Formerly, lymphomas were classified into three major groups — lymphosarcoma, reticulum cell sarcoma, and Hodgkin's disease. In 1966, Rappaport proposed a classification of the non-Hodgkin's lymphomas based upon their histological growth patterns and cytologic features observed in affected lypmph nodes.[1] This classification has proved to be useful for prognostic and descriptive purposes. The malignant lymphomas were divided into nodular (follicular) and diffuse types and each category was further subdivided on the basis of whether the cells were well differentiated or poorly differentiated lymphocytes, histiocytes, or a mixture of lymphocytes and histiocytes. *Reticulum cell sarcoma* was renamed histiocytic lymphoma, but subsequently it was demonstrated by other workers that the reticulum cells actually were transformed lymphocytes and not macrophages.[2,3] True histiocytic lymphomas do occur but are very uncommon. Nevertheless, for purposes of discussion in this chapter the non-Hodgkin's lymphomas will be referred to as histiocytic and lymphocytic lymphomas.*

More recently, Lukes and Collins proposed a classification of non-Hodgkin's lymphomas based upon the morphological and immunocytochemical properties observed in the B and T lymphocytic cell systems of current immunology. They proposed that the non-Hodgkin's lymphomas were B cell tumors arising from cells of the follicular centers of the lymph node.[3,4] The lymphomas were divided basically into nodular and diffuse types, depending upon the infiltrative pattern in the lymph node, and further subdivided on the basis of the predominant cell population — small cleaved, large cleaved, small noncleaved, or large noncleaved. Lukes and Collins postulated that the small lymphocytes in the node have cleaved nuclei and as they become transformed following antigenic stimulation, they initially enlarge, retain their cleaved nuclei, and begin to develop pyroninophilia within the cytoplasm. As enlargement continues,

*However, the terms *lymphosarcoma* and *reticulum cell sarcoma* will be used when reference is made to papers published before the Rappaport classification came into general use.

the nuclear cleavage disappears, the nucleus becomes oval or round and develops two nucleoli, and the cytoplasm becomes more extensive and more pyroninophilic. At their maximum size, the cells are four times as large as the original small lymphocyte and are referred to as immunoblasts. They eventually serve as the precursors of plasma cells. The complete proposed classification is a combination of morphology and function based upon the B and T lymphocytic cell systems (Table 2–1). The eventual establishment of a definitive classification will depend upon future correlations between morphological and functional studies utilizing fresh nonfixed lymphomatous tissue that can be examined for the presence of surface membrane and histochemical markers characteristic of lymphocytes and histiocytes. The criteria for distinguishing between B and T cells and monocytes (histiocytes) on the basis of membrane markers are only in the early stages of development. The assumption that these criteria derived from studies on normal lymphoid cells and monocytes are also applicable for identifying and characterizing the tumor cells of the lymphoreticular system remains to be proved.[5] Currently, the classifications of Rappaport and Lukes and Collins are both important and useful for the diagnosis and management of the malignant lymphomas. The reader is referred to the papers of these authors for a more detailed account of their proposals.[1, 3, 5]

Lukes and Collins have also introduced into clinical medicine the concept of cellular immune proliferations with the immunoblast — defined as a transformed lymphocyte — as the significant replicating cell. Both B and T cell types are included in this concept, although it is not currently possible to distinguish between them morphologically. They have defined three types of immunoblastic proliferations: (a) immunoblastic reaction that occurs in the interfollicular tissue of lymph nodes in

Table 2–1. CLASSIFICATION OF LYMPHOMAS (LUKES AND COLLINS)*

U cell (undefined cell) type
T cell types
  Mycosis fungoides including Sézary syndrome
  Convoluted lymphocyte (acute lymphocytic leukemia with mediastinal mass)
  ?Hodgkin's disease
  ?Immunoblastic sarcoma of T cells
B cell types
  Small lymphocyte (chronic lymphatic leukemia)
  Plasmacytoid lymphocyte

Follicular center cell types (FCC)
(follicular, diffuse, follicular and diffuse, and sclerotic)
  small cleaved
  large cleaved
  small noncleaved
  large noncleaved

  Immunoblastic sarcoma of B cells
Histiocytic type
Unclassifiable

*The outlined area represents the majority of non-Hodgkin's lymphomas encountered in medical practice. (From Lukes, R. J., and Collins, R. D.: New approaches to the classification of the lymphomata. Br. J. Cancer, *31* (Suppl. II): 1, 1975.)

immune reactions, in severe forms of infectious mononucleosis, and in postvaccination lymphadenitis; (b) immunoblastic lymphadenopathy — a non-neoplastic appearing proliferation of immunoblastic and plasma cells which obliterates lymph node architecture and is associated with a characteristic clinical picture; and (c) immunoblastic sarcoma — a monomorphous malignant counterpart of immunoblastic lymphadenopathy. The latter two entities will be discussed later in this chapter.

The lymphomas previously classified under the term *reticulum cell sarcoma* (histiocytic lymphoma) have either the morphologic features of large noncleaved follicular center cells, often with a component of cleaved cells, or the histology of immunoblastic sarcoma, wherein the cells exhibit plasmacytoid features.

The natural history and histopathology of the non-Hodgkin's lymphomas — histiocytic lymphoma (reticulum cell sarcoma) and lymphocytic lymphoma — establish these disorders as malignancies of lymphoreticular tissues. However, a consensus on the nosology of Hodgkin's disease is lacking. Some investigators object to the inclusion of Hodgkin's disease with the lymphomas because the clinical features often resemble an infectious disease with a spontaneously remitting course and because the histopathology shows an atypical granulomatous reaction with atypical histiocytes.[6] The two major non-Hodgkin's lymphomas are sometimes called monomorphous lymphomas, since histologic examination of the cutaneous and visceral lesions reveals a tumor infiltrate consisting of uniformly malignant-appearing cells. Hodgkin's disease has been termed a polymorphous lymphoma because the infiltrate in the skin and viscera is composed of a mixture of inflammatory and "neoplastic" cells. Neutrophils, lymphocytes, plasma cells, eosinophils, histiocytes, and fibroblasts make up the bulk of the lesion in an inflammatory granulomatous reaction. Atypical histiocytes, including the pathognomonic Sternberg-Reed cell, are dispersed within this inflammatory phase. Sternberg-Reed cells can be either rare or plentiful in the lesions of Hodgkin's disease.

Another important difference exists between the polymorphous and monomorphous lymphomas. Abnormalities of delayed hypersensitivity are characteristic of Hodgkin's disease, whereas immunologic reactivity is unimpaired in the non-Hodgkin's lymphomas until the late states of the diseases.[7, 8]

Many clinicians equate mycosis fungoides with lymphoma. However, impressive evidence has accumulated which indicates that mycosis fungoides is a unique lymphoreticular disease of the skin. It behaves in many ways like Hodgkin's disease and not like the monomorphous lymphomas. In mycosis fungoides, a polymorphous inflammatory reaction with abnormal appearing mononuclear cells is the distinctive histopathologic finding. The abnormal cell was considered to be a histiocyte, but current evidence indicates that it has the membrane markers of a T lymphocyte. (However, the abnormal mononuclear cells do not resemble Sternberg-Reed cells, and an experienced pathologist would not confuse the histologic picture of Hodgkin's disease with mycosis fungoides.) The course of mycosis fungoides is long and punctuated by spontaneous remissions. The cutaneous manifestations are manifold.

Kaposi's hemorrhagic sarcoma is discussed in this section because it coexists with the monomorphous lymphomas, Hodgkin's disease, and mycosis fungoides more often than mere chance permits.

LYMPHOMAS

Cutaneous manifestations occur at some time in approximately 50 per cent of patients with lymphomas.[9] As with carcinoma, both specific and nonspecific lesions are found. Specific lesions, composed of the characteristic malignant cells, are seen most frequently with histiocytic lymphoma and lymphocytic lymphoma. Morphologically, the specific skin lesions are identical in both Hodgkin's disease and the non-Hodgkin's lymphomas. The nonspecific lesions, such as exfoliative dermatitis, bullous eruptions, pruritus, and ichthyosis, are associated more often with the polymorphous disorder, Hodgkin's disease. Likewise, there are many nonspecific dermatoses which characterize the early or premycotic phase of mycosis fungoides.

The specific lesions consist of papules, nodules, and tumors located at all levels of the skin, from the superficial dermis to the subcutaneous layer. The lesions vary from a few millimeters to several centimeters and typically are pink, violaceous, or plum-colored; sometimes they are reddish-brown (Plate 5*A*, *B*, *C*). Ulceration can occur but is not common. However, the involved lymph nodes can become necrotic, produce sinus tracts, and result in ulceration of the overlying skin. The specific nodules and tumors are often distributed in a generalized fashion, but they can also cluster, assume circinate and arciform configurations, and even coalesce into large plaques, thereby mimicking the lesions of mycosis fungoides (see p. 114). These specific lesions can appear anywhere on the body surface and in the oral cavity. It is not unusual to find tumors involving the scalp, conjunctivae, or genitalia (Figs. 2–1 and 2–2; Plate 4*E*). The nodules and tumors are firm but not stony-hard like the metastatic nodules of carcinoma. The tonsils, palate, tongue, and nasopharynx may show nodules and ulcerations.

Lymphoctyic lymphoma and histiocytic lymphoma can begin with skin lesions and remain localized to the skin for months or years before visceral involvement becomes evident, although this is not a common occurrence.[10] Long et al. reviewed the clinical and histopathologic findings in 25 cases of malignant lymphoma of the skin, other than mycosis fungoides.[11] All of the patients had skin lesions as the primary manifestation of the disorder, and none had histopathologic evidence of extracutaneous involvement at the time of skin biopsy. (However, eight individuals had either peripheral, retroperitoneal, or mediastinal adenopathy or pleural effusion as clinical evidence of systemic involvement.) Fifteen of 25 patients had lesions on the head or neck, seven had lesions on the extremities, and three on the trunk. Nodules were present in 21 individuals and red plaques in four. The lesions were single in 21 individuals. Ulcerated nodules were present in only three patients. Twenty-two of the patients developed extracutaneous lymphoma six months to five years (mean duration 21 months) after the diagnosis of lymphoma was made by biopsy of a cutaneous nodule. Sixteen of the 25 patients died from disseminated lymphoma. Lymphocytic lymphoma was diagnosed in 22, and histiocytic lymphoma in three individuals. Three patients were still alive and well without recurrent disease for one, six, and eight years following therapy. No cases of Hodgkin's disease were encountered in their series.

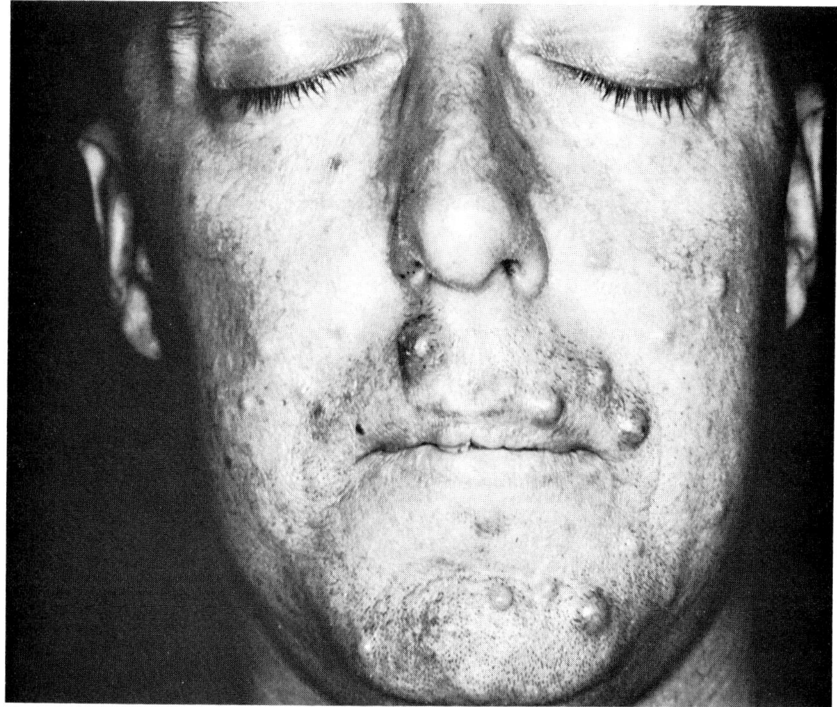

Figure 2–1. Reticulum cell sarcoma.

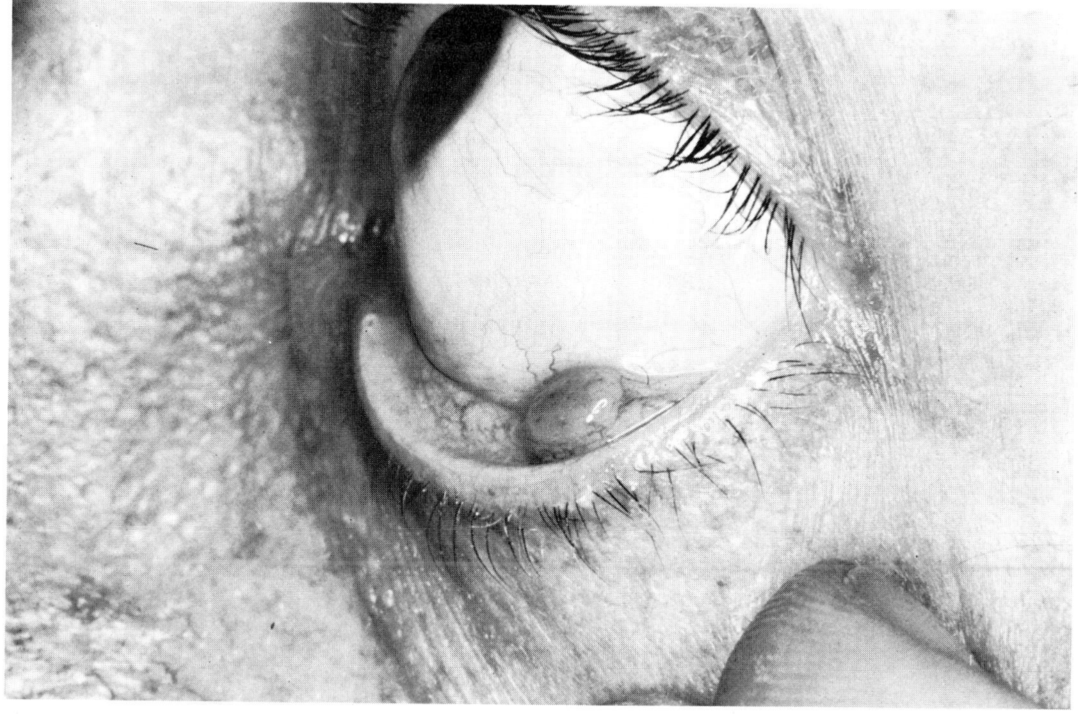

Figure 2–2. Reticulum cell sarcoma. Conjunctival tumor.

Specific cutaneous lesions have been noted to be the initial sign of Hodgkin's disease and may be localized to the skin without detectable visceral involvement, or with only localized nodal involvement, for up to six years. However, they usually appear during the course of the illness, primarily as a late manifestation.[12, 13] Beninghoff et al. have suggested that the pathogenesis of the skin involvement in Hodgkin's disease is related to neoplastic cells being carried to the skin in a retrograde flow of lymph secondary to regional lymph node obstruction. Hence, the mechanism would be a passive one, rather than an active cutaneous invasion or proliferation *de novo* in skin.[13]

The patient shown in Figure 2–3 and in Plate 4*F* developed specific nodules and plaques in her chest wall and breast three years after the onset of Hodgkin's disease. Figures 2–4 and 2–5 show an erythematous plaque with nodule formation on the leg of a patient with Hodgkin's disease. The lesion arose during the course of the illness and clinically simulated a lesion of mycosis fungoides. Ulcerated plaques and nodules were present at the onset of Hodgkin's disease in the patient shown in Plate 6*A*, *B*. Ulceration is not a common feature of the specific lesions in monomorphous lymphomas and Hodgkin's disease, but is common in the lesions of mycosis fungoides.

Mikulicz's syndrome is seen more frequently with the monomorphous lymphomas than with Hodgkin's disease. The symmetrical swelling of the lacrimal, orbital, and salivary glands is produced by neoplastic cellular infiltration.

The presence of lymphomatous disease should always be considered

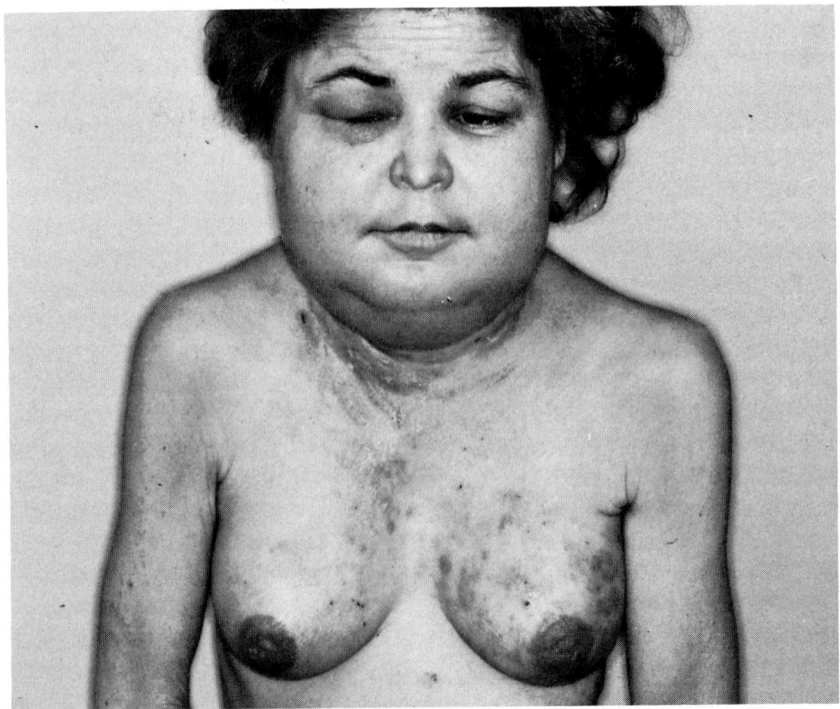

Figure 2–3. Hodgkin's disease. These nodules on the breasts showed the diagnostic histopathology of Hodgkin's disease. The nodules are shown in closer detail in Plate 4*F*.

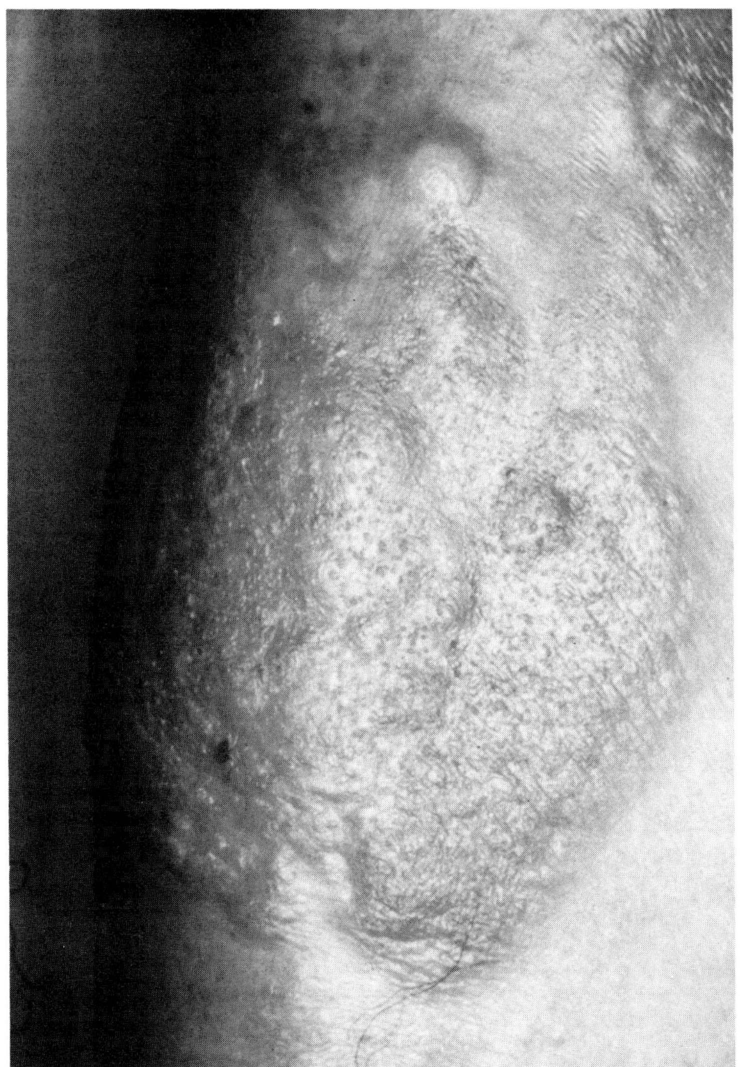

Figure 2–4. Hodgkin's disease. Erythematous plaque with nodule formation simulating mycosis fungoides.

PLATE 5

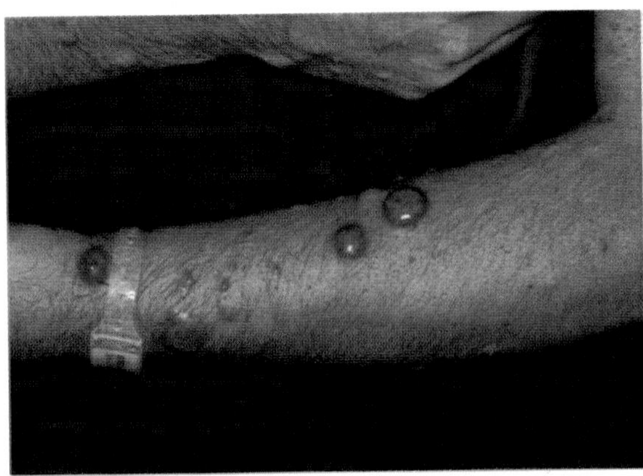

A, Reticulum cell sarcoma. Both deep and superficial tumors are present.

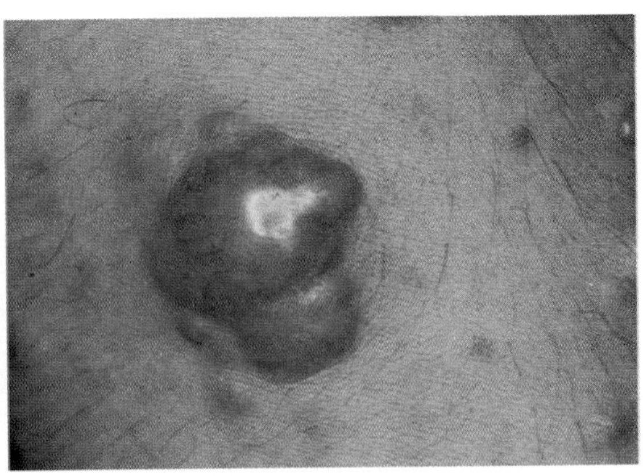

B, Close view of tumors in reticulum cell sarcoma. Note characteristic erythematous-violaceous color.

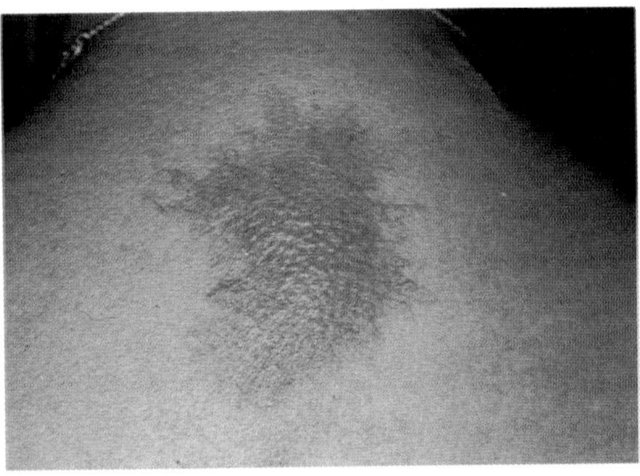

C, Close view of tumor in reticulum cell sarcoma. Note erythematous-violaceous color and prominent dilated blood vessels.

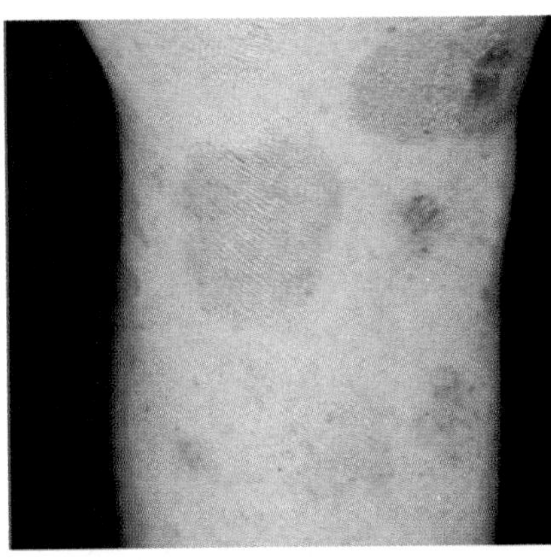

D, Mycosis fungoides. These eczematous patches showed the diagnostic histopathology of mycosis fungoides.

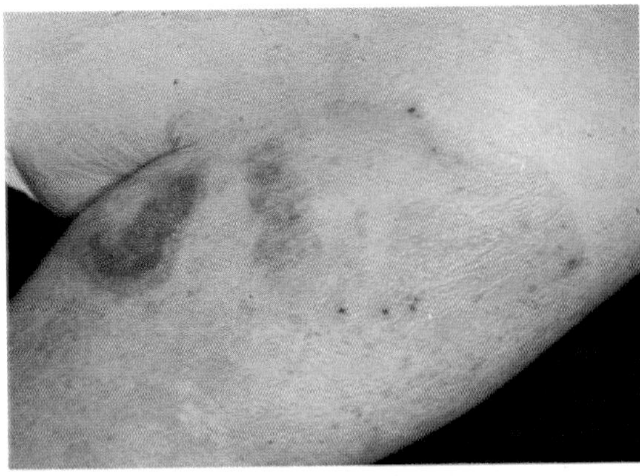

E, Mycosis fungoides. Arciform lesion with superficial ulceration adjacent to an eczematous patch of mycosis fungoides.

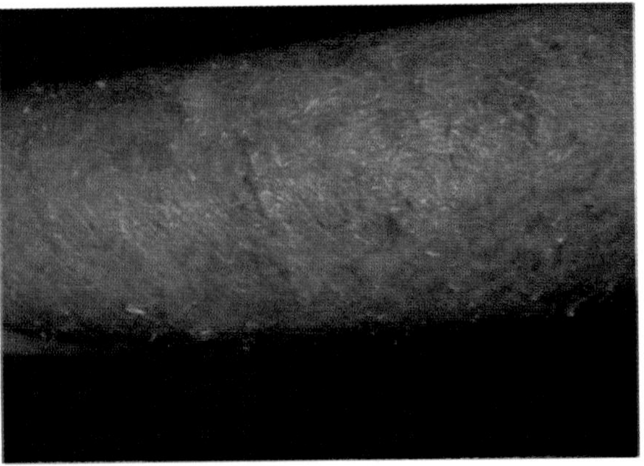

F, Mycosis fungoides. Weeping eczematous lesions which showed diagnostic histopathology.

PLATE 6

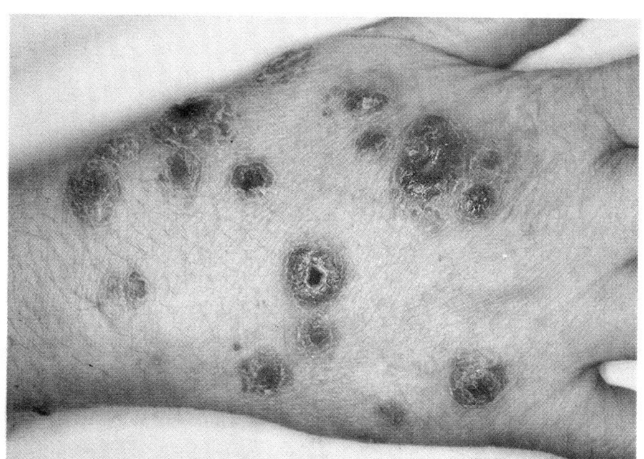

A, Hodgkin's disease. Erythematous ulcerating nodules.

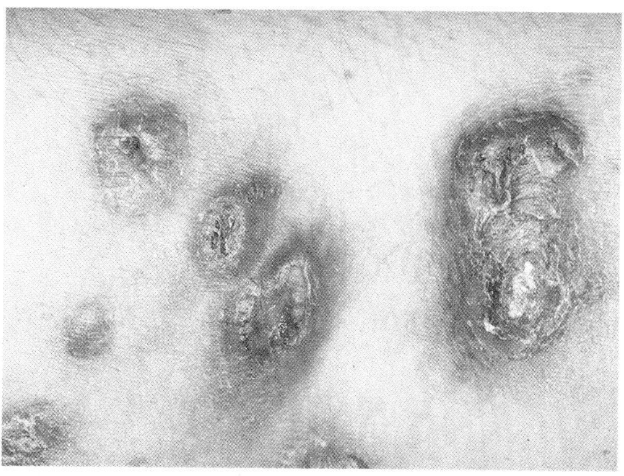

B, Hodgkin's disease. Close-up of ulcerating nodules shown in *A*.

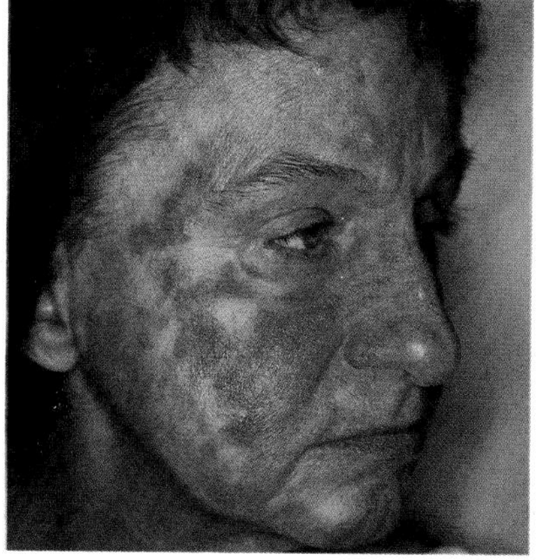

C, Hodgkin's disease. Violaceous plaques and eczematous patches as expressions of a graft-versus-host reaction.

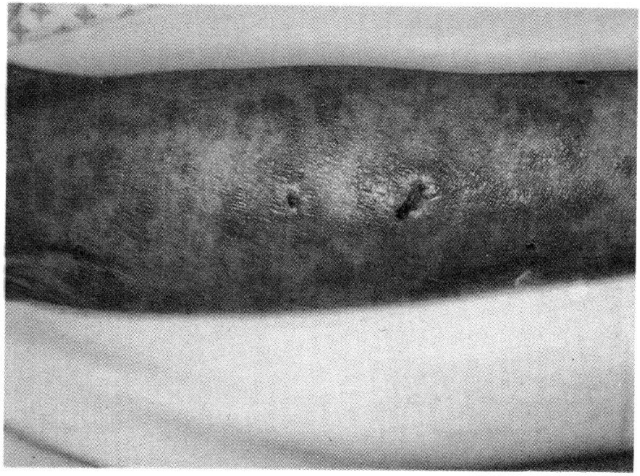

D, Hodgkin's disease. Graft-versus-host reaction in patient shown in *C*.

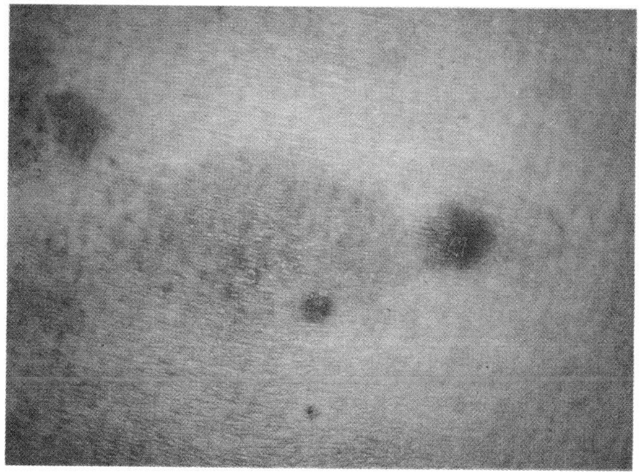

E, Parapsoriasis en plaques with nodule formation. Close-up of lesion shown in Figure 2–23.

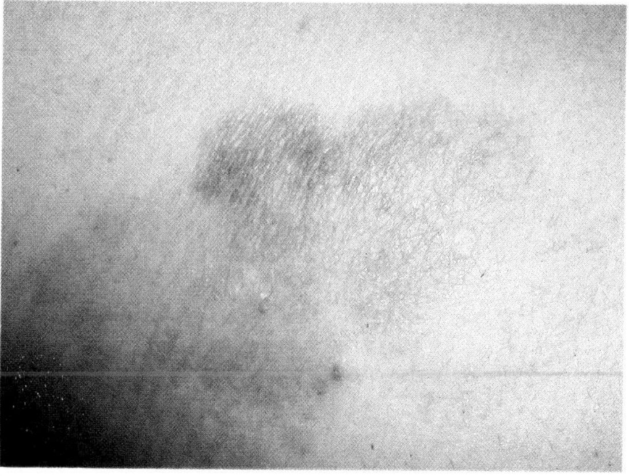

F, Parapsoriasis en plaques as manifestation of mycosis fungoides. Close-up of lesion shown in Figure 2–24.

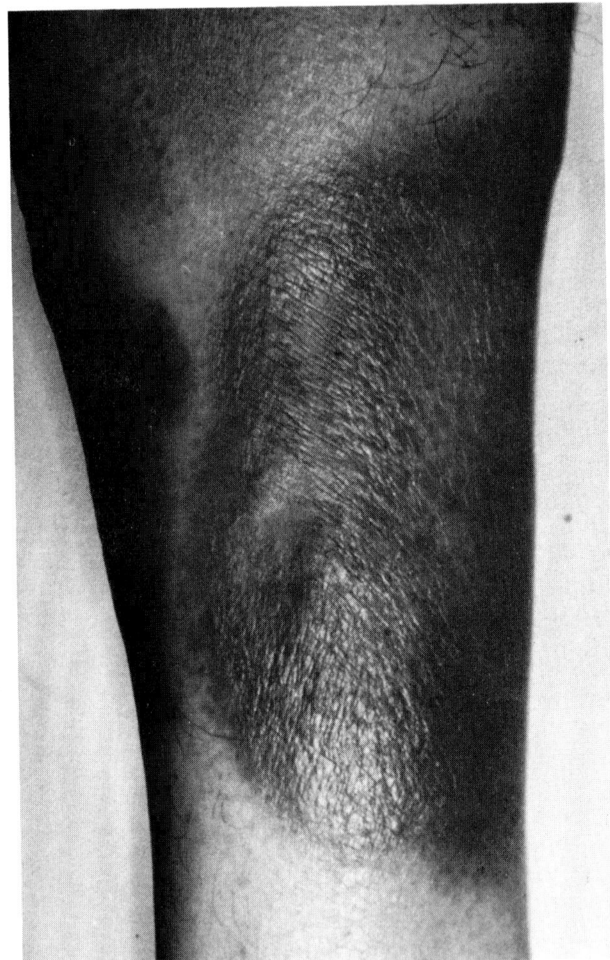

Figure 2–5. Hodgkin's disease. Erythematous plaque simulating mycosis fungoides.

when one finds pink, purplish, or reddish-brown papules, nodules, or tumors in the skin. The differential diagnosis of such lesions chiefly includes sarcoidosis, lupus erythematosus, leukemia cutis, lymphocytoma cutis, granuloma faciale, and insect bite reactions. Sometimes the history and physical findings will resolve a perplexing case, but usually histologic examination of the lesion is necessary to establish the correct diagnosis.

The most fascinating aspects of the skin markers in lymphomatous disease are the nonspecific dermatoses and symptoms. These features are associated much more frequently with Hodgkin's disease than with the monomorphous lymphomas. The pathogenesis of these nonspecific markers is not understood, but their frequent association with the polymorphous disorders — Hodgkin's disease and mycosis fungoides — is consistent with the hypothesis that these two illnesses begin as reactive disorders that eventually develop a neoplastic behavior rather than developing as malignant processes *de novo*.

Generalized pruritus may be the only manifestation of Hodgkin's disease for years before other evidence of the illness becomes apparent. This symptom is found much less frequently with monomorphous lymphomas and carcinoma. Excoriations can be widespread in the absence of any other identifiable lesion (Fig. 2–6).

However, nonspecific cutaneous lesions in association with pruritus have been described under the designation of "prurigo-like papules."[14] These lesions are said to be erythematous edematous papules which appear in crops and are surmounted by a minute vesicle. Scratching, which removes the tops of these lesions, leaves denuded areas. Healing produces hyperpigmented scars. Some clinicians believe that these lesions represent a nonspecific cutaneous reaction associated with pruritus and are related to the same factors producing the itch, while others believe that these lesions are produced by rubbing and scratching. When associated with polycythemia vera, this identical cutaneous reaction pattern has been called "acne urticata."[15, 16] Kaposi originally described and named acne urticata, but none of his patients had polycythemia vera.

The histopathology of acne urticata is identical to that seen with erythema mulitforme.[15, 16] I believe that *prurigo-like papules* and *acne urticata* are identical disorders and are a morphological variant of either erythema multiforme or bullous pemphigoid, both of which are seen with lymphoma and carcinoma.

Fuller described a patient who developed erythema nodosum two months before, and erythema multiforme one month before, the diagnosis of Hodgkin's disease was established. This protocol strongly suggests that these hypersensitivity phenomena were related to the Hodgkin's disease.[17]

Exfoliative dermatitis can also be the sole stigma of malignant lymphoma for years before disease is diagnosed in the lymph nodes or the viscera. In Nicolis and Helwig's series, five of eight patients with Hodgkin's disease were affected by episodes of exfoliative dermatitis for four to 16 years before the disease appeared in the lymph nodes. In two patients, the dermatitis developed after the disease was diagnosed and in one, both appeared simultaneously.[18] Exfoliative dermatitis is associated

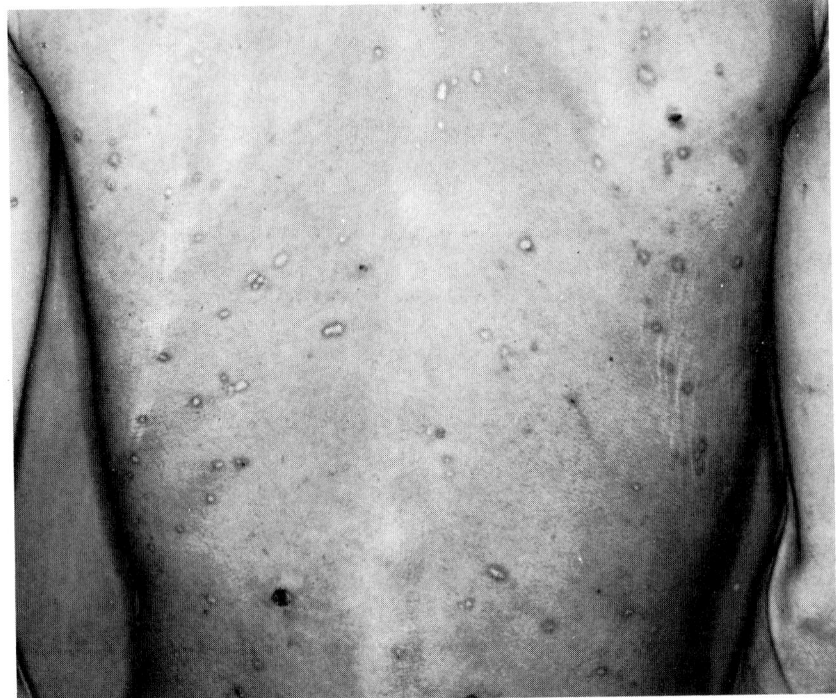

Figure 2–6. Hodgkin's disease. Excoriations resulting from generalized pruritus.

primarily with Hodgkin's disease and develops only infrequently with the monomorphous lymphomas. In this recent review of 135 cases of exfoliative dermatitis by Nicolis and Helwig, there were eight cases of Hodgkin's disease and two of histiocytic lymphoma. In addition there were four cases of visceral carcinomas — liver, lung, thyroid, and prostate — discovered at atuopsy.[18] Exfoliative dermatitis can also be an expression of mycosis fungoides.

Exfoliative dermatitis often begins as a patchy erythroderma that becomes generalized and eventually associated with marked scaling. The hair may fall, the nails can become dystrophic and be shed, and hyperkeratosis of the palms and soles may develop. Pruritus is almost always associated with the exfoliative state. The affected individual complains of being cold and chilly; these sensations are caused by a heat loss from the tremendously increased blood flow in the vasodilated skin. It is usually possible to make the histologic diagnosis of a specific lymphoma by biopsy of the exfoliative dermatitis.[18-20]

The usual cause of exfoliative dermatitis, however, is either a drug reaction or a preexisting dermatosis which has become generalized. Psoriasis, seborrheic dermatitis, stasis, and contact dermatitis are the dermatoses most frequently found to be the cause of exfoliative dermatitis. Often no associated disease will be uncovered. In various series, the percentages of patients with exfoliative dermatitis and lymphomatous diseases such as Hodgkin's disease, mycosis fungoides, monomorphous lymphomas, and leukemias have ranged from 8 to 25 per cent.[18-21] Drug reactions accounted for 11 to 40 per cent and preexisting skin disease for 26 to 31 per cent. In 12 to 50 per cent of cases, no cause could be determined.

Although exfoliative dermatitis and erythroderma have been reported to be manifestations of chronic lymphatic leukemia, Edelson et al. have questioned the validity of this association.[22] In their experience, they discovered that such patients actually had the Sézary syndrome — the leukemic phase of mycosis fungoides — which had been misdiagnosed as chronic lymphatic leukemia. Our patient shown in Plate 11*C* is an example of such an error. On reviewing her skin biopsies, course, and laboratory data, it is clear that she had had the Sézary syndrome and not chronic lymphatic leukemia. This observation is clinically and therapeutically important and needs to be evaluated further. The purported association between exfoliative dermatitis and chronic lymphatic leukemia may prove to be rare or nonexistent.

Unfortunately, the presence or absence of enlarged lymph nodes is not helpful in differentiating benign from lymphomatous erythroderma because lymphadenopathy develops in virtually all cases of long-standing exfoliative dermatitis. Histologic examination of these nodes reveals reticuloendothelial hyperplasia with melanin and fat-laden histiocytes. The terms *lipomelanotic reticulosis* and *dermatopathic lymphadenopathy* have been applied to these histologic changes, which should not be misinterpreted as indicative of a malignant lymphoma.[23]

Acquired ichthyosis is almost unique to the lymphomatous diseases and is seen more commonly with Hodgkin's disease than with the monomorphous lymphomas. Adults do not develop acquired ichthyosis except in association with lymphomas, drugs which inhibit cholesterol synthesis (triparanol and occasionally nicotinic acid), and a rare case of carcinoma. The ichthyosis varies from generalized dry skin to a picture indistinguishable from the oridinary genetically determined ichthyosis vulgaris with its fish-like scales accentuated on extensor surfaces (Fig. 2–7). Hyperkeratosis of the palms and soles may be an additional feature. Ichthyosis can be the only manifestation of Hodgkin's disease for months or years, or it can develop during the course of the disease. The ichthyosis can disappear when the lymphoma enters a remission.[24, 25] Although ichthyosis is a characteristic feature of Hodgkin's disease, it is not seen with mycosis fungoides.

The pathogenesis of the ichthyosis is not understood. Glazebrook and Tomaszewski have postulated that a vitamin A deficiency produced by lymphomatous involvement of the liver was the important factor in two instances, but this theory requires confirmation.[26]

The following two histories illustrate some variations of this unique eruption:

A 22-year-old white man developed generalized dryness of his skin two years after the diagnosis of Hodgkin's disease had been made. Over the knees, elbows, and knuckles, the skin was especially dry and hyperkeratotic, resembling the changes often seen with acanthosis nigricans (Fig. 2–8 to 2–10).

A 12-year-old white boy developed dryness and roughening of the skin over the extensor surfaces of the major joints, shins, and upper back at a time when he felt completely well. The cutaneous eruption, illustrated in Figure 2–11, can best be described as lichen spinulosus, an exaggerated keratosis pilaris. Six months later he developed cervical lymphadenopathy, and a diagnosis of Hodgkin's disease was made.

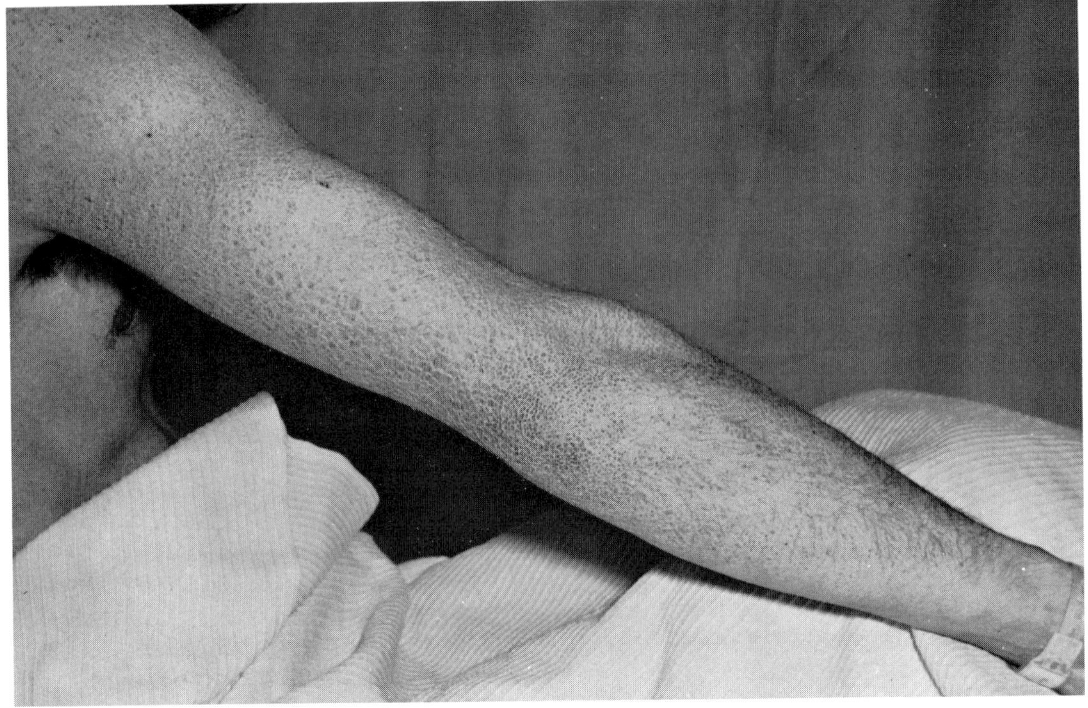

Figure 2–7. Ichthyosis vulgaris. Extensor surfaces are dry and scaly.

A nonspecific eczema can appear during the course of the disease, as illustrated in Figure 2–12. In this particular case, pityriasis rosea was simulated. In another patient referred by Dr. Haskell Rosenbaum, discrete psoriasiform and eczematous patches were present on the face, trunk, and extremities for two years before the diagnosis of nodular sclerosing Hodgkin's disease was made by biopsy of an enlarged submandibular lymph node. The cutaneous lesions were pruritic, and on histologic examination they showed features compatible with parapsoriasis en plaques, an eruption characteristic of the premycotic phase of mycosis fungoides. Only the liver, spleen, and celiac lymph nodes proved to be involved by Hodgkin's disease. The disease went into remission and the rash disappeared after five months of chemotherapy. However, two months after low dose radiation of the involved areas had been started, a few erythematous macules and papules appeared on the forearms, legs, and right cheek. Biopsies showed epidermal edema (spongiosis) and a nonspecific perivascular infiltrate. The rash persisted in this mild form for the next six months before suddenly becoming more extensive and severe. The patient developed violaceous plaques and extensive eczematous patches over her body (Fig. 2–13; Plate 6*C,D*). Some of the areas spontaneously developed superficial erosions which healed with crusting. Biopsies showed vacuolization of the basal cell layer with mild exocytosis of mononuclear cells compatible with a graft-versus-host reaction. Reexamination of the patient failed to reveal recurrence of the Hodgkin's disease. The rash became even more severe and bullae followed by denudation of large areas of skin developed. Multiple biopsies revealed focal thinning of the epidermis, individual necrotic epidermal cells, and

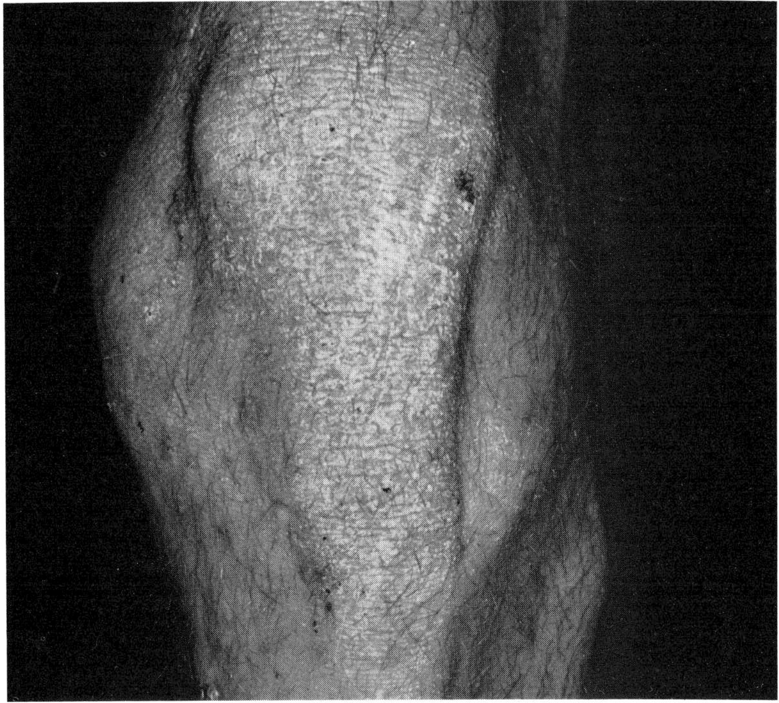

Figure 2–8. Hodgkin's disease. Dryness and scaling are present over the knees.

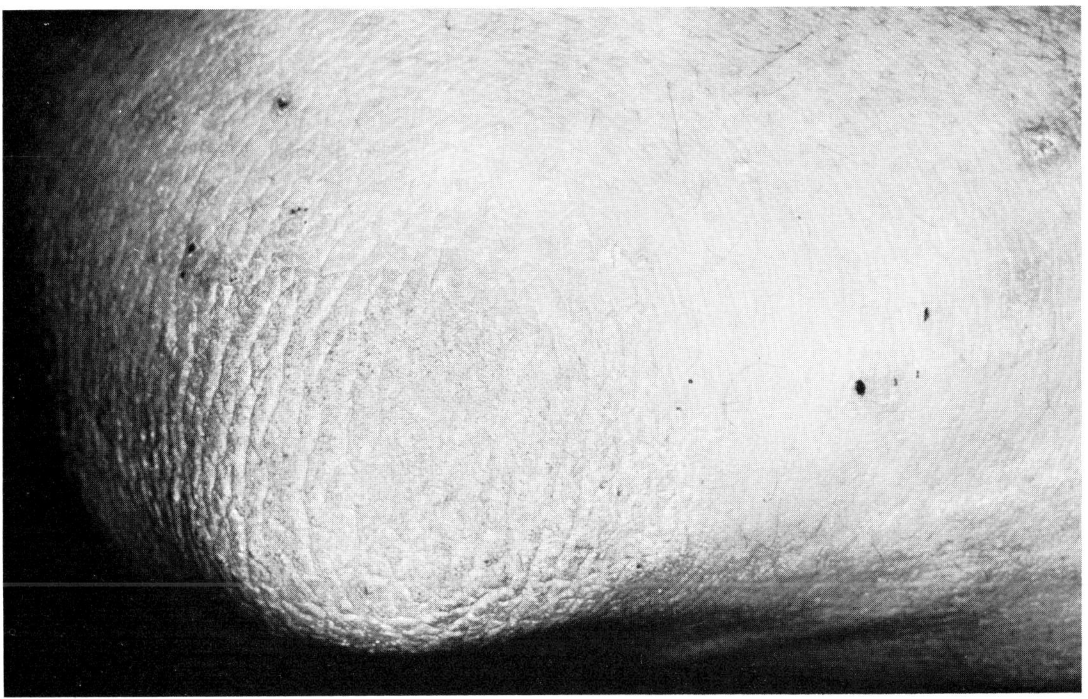

Figure 2–9. Hodgkin's disease. The skin over the elbows is dry, scaly, and thickened in this patient.

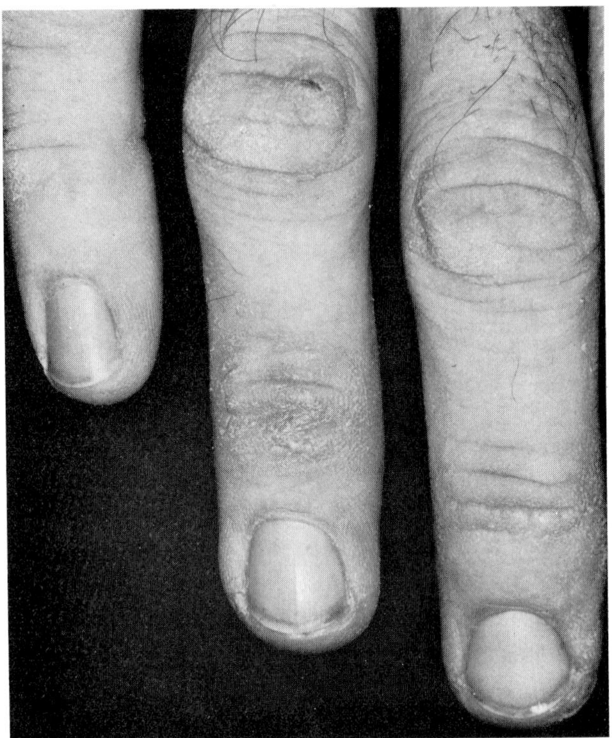

Figure 2–10. Hodgkin's disease. Same patient as in Figure 2–9. The skin over the knuckles is dry, thickened, and scaly. These changes over the elbows and knuckles resemble those of acanthosis nigricans.

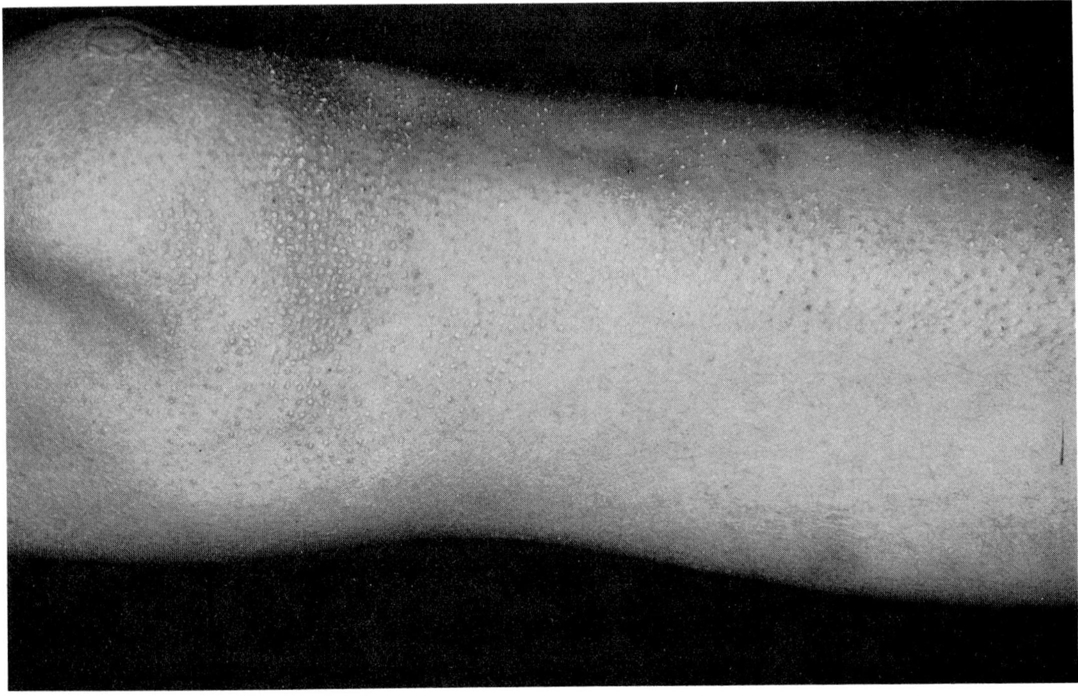

Figure 2–11. Hodgkin's disease. A lichen spinulosus–like eruption preceded the clinical appearance of this lymphoma by several months.

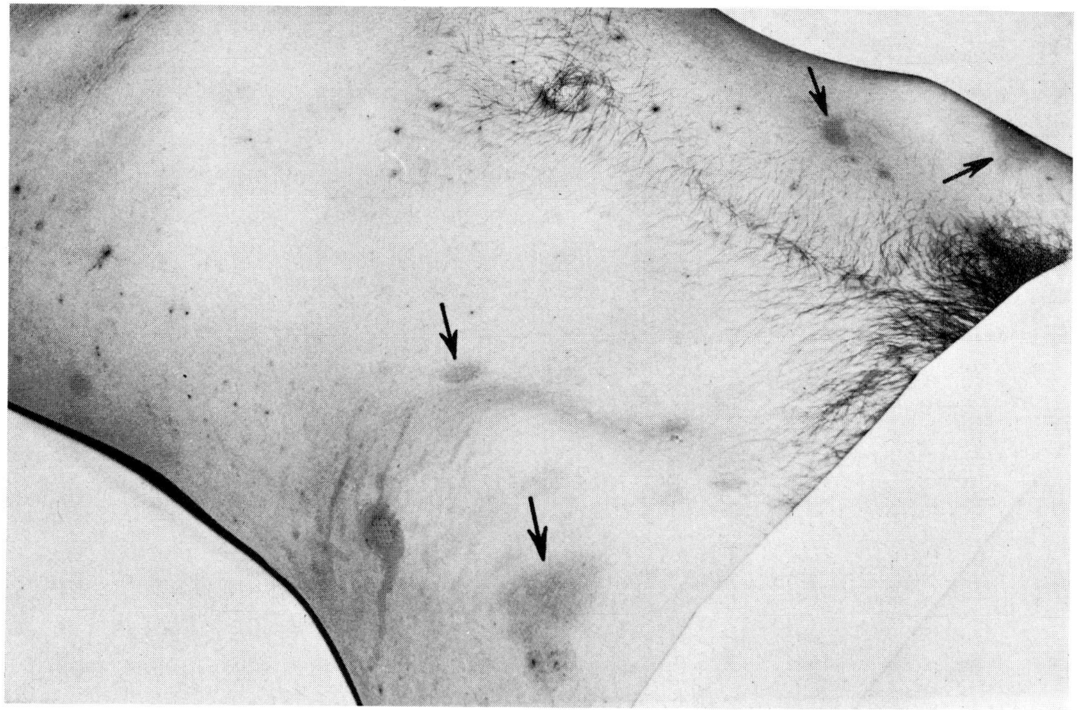

Figure 2–12. Hodgkin's disease. Nonspecific eczematous eruption (arrows).

vacuolization of the basal cell layer compatible with a graft-versus-host reaction. Restudy for a second time failed to reveal recurrence of Hodgkin's disease. The patient developed staphylococcal septicemia which led to her death. Permission for an autopsy was not granted. The psoriasiform and eczematous rash that evolved into a bullous ulcerating eruption probably represented a graft-versus-host reaction that was somehow initiated by the underlying Hodgkin's disease. It continued autonomously after the disease went into apparent remission and was responsible for the patient's death.

Hyperpigmentation develops in 10 to 30 per cent of patients with Hodgkin's disease and much less frequently in those with monomorphous lymphomas.[27] The hyperpigmentation may be either generalized or confined to the flexural areas as it is in adrenal insufficiency, or it may develop in a patchy fashion as does a postinflammatory reaction to scratching. The pathogenesis of the increased pigmentation is not understood.

Other nonspecific manifestations include pallor and purpura that are related to hematopoietic disturbances (Fig. 2–14). Cutaneous bacterial infections are common because of the increased susceptibility of the host. Jaundice can result from lymphomatous infiltration of the liver and from biliary obstruction by locally enlarged nodes. Urticaria can be a reflection of activity as well as the first sign of lymphomatous disease.[28]

Enlarged lymph nodes can produce lymphatic and venous obstruction resulting in edema, especially of the genitalia and legs. In the case of Hodgkin's disease, illustrated in Figure 2–3, cervical lymphadenopathy

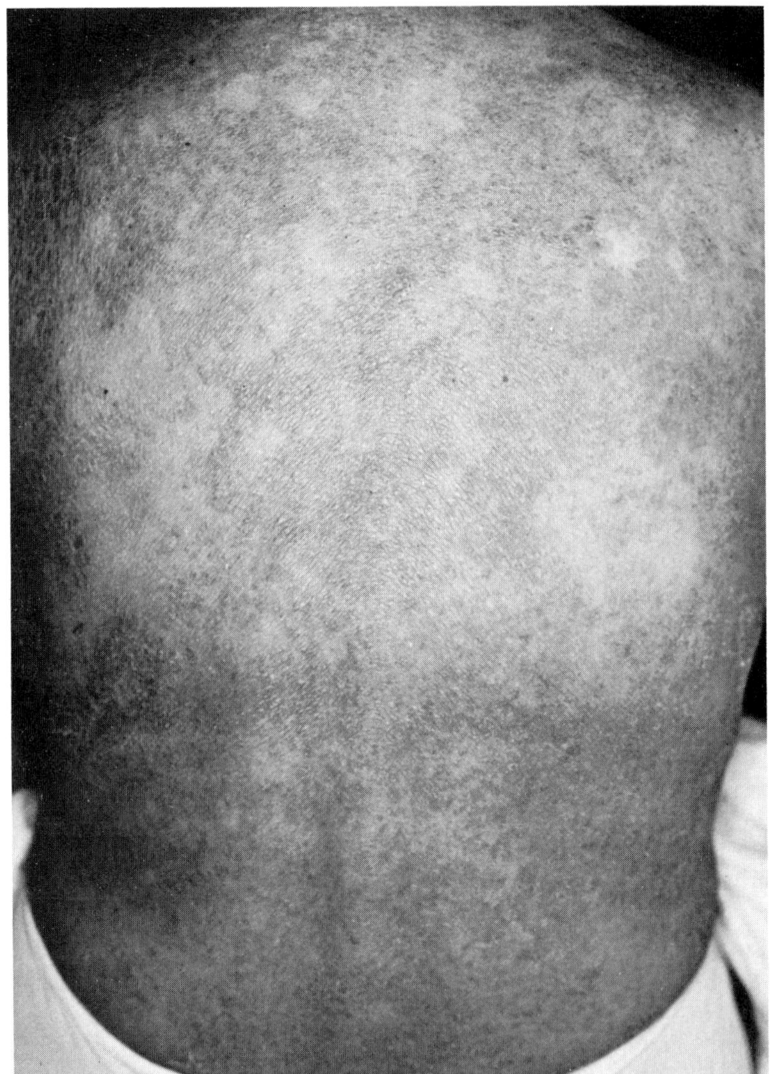

Figure 2–13. Hodgkin's disease. Graft-versus-host reaction.

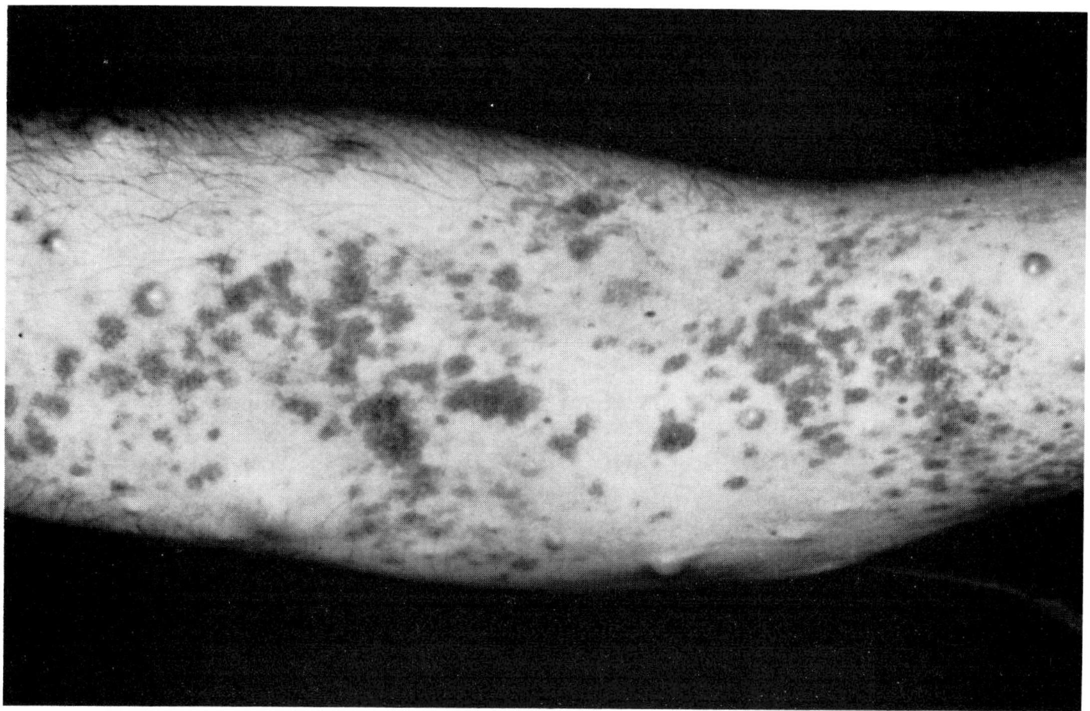

Figure 2–14. Reticulum cell sarcoma. Purpura secondary to thrombocytopenia. Tumor nodules are visible.

and postradiation fibrosis were responsible for the facial lymphedema. Treatment with nitrogen mustard greatly reduced the facial swelling.

Hypertrophic pulmonary osteoarthropathy is an uncommon complication of Hodgkin's disease. About 14 instances have been reported. This syndrome was usually present at the time the disease was diagnosed, and in all the cases in which data were available, a mediastinal mass was present. Atkinson et al. reported a patient in whom there was complete resolution of the hypertrophic osteoarthropathy following successful chemotherapy.[29] This syndrome in a young person suspected of having a malignancy should alert one to the possibility of Hodgkin's disease.

Skin lesions that exhibit the histologic features of granulomatous angiitis and atypical "reticulum" cells and which occur in association with a systemic illness can be a manifestation of malignant lymphoma. In three cases, ulcerated nodular and arciform cutaneous lesions were associated with fever and a clinical illness that suggested either lymphoma or an angiitis syndrome.[30-32] Histologic examination of the skin lesions disclosed a granulomatous angiitis with necrosis and atypical "reticulum" cells. At autopsy, the following diagnoses were made in the three cases: malignant lymphoma of mixed cell type, reticulum cell sarcoma, and histiocytic leukemia. Christianson and Fine have made similar observations.[33]

Pseudolymphoma

The term pseudolymphoma has been applied to a number of entities which have a benign course in spite of clinical and histologic findings that strongly suggest malignant lymphoma. Allied to these disorders are a newly emerging group of syndromes which, in some instances, do pursue a fatal course but still cannot be classified strictly as malignant lymphoma because of normal cellular histology.

Lymphocytoma cutis can be confused clinically and histologically with lymphoma. The synonyms for this entity include Spiegler-Fendt sarcoid, lymphadenosis benigna cutis, miliary lymphocytoma, and cutaneous lymphoplasia. The clinical appearances of the skin lesions range from a solitary plaque or nodule to several regionally localized lesions. They are indistinguishable from the specific lesions of lymphoma both in color and in morphology. The face (malar area, tip of nose, ear lobes), scrotum, areolae of the breasts, and the forearms are the sites of predilection.

Histologic examination reveals a proliferation of mature non-neoplastic appearing lymphoid and reticulum cells in the dermis which occur either diffusely or in nodules. When nodular, follicles with germinal centers are simulated. Sometimes the lymphoreticular cells are admixed with other mature cells and produce a polymorphous infiltration; at other times an associated proliferation of capillaries produces a granulomatous picture. Successive biopsies may reveal one or more of these histologic models, thereby indicating that these are fluid patterns.

Follicular patterns also can be found in the malignant lymphomas, but the presence of the characteristic malignant lymphoreticular cell in the germinal centers differentiates the lymphomas from the benign lymphoplasias.

Lymphocytoma cutis can occur in a disseminated form. The long-term observations of Bäfverstedt indicate that the disseminated variety of the disease is both benign and identical to the localized form.[34, 35]

The follicular pattern of lymphocytoma cutis is similar to that found in Brill-Symmers disease (giant follicular lymphoma of the lymph nodes), but there is no evidence that they are related.

Mach and Wilgram wish to change the name *lymphocytoma cutis* to *cutaneous lymphoplasia* because there is no evidence that this is a neoplastic disease. None of their 115 cases developed into a lymphoma.[36] The localized disorder in some patients appears to be a reactive proliferation of lymphoreticular cells to at least two known stimuli: insect bites and mechanical trauma. Their proposal for a change in nomenclature has merit.

The histologic features of cutaneous lymphoplasia are not always unequivocally benign. As is illustrated in the following, each case must be studied carefully to eliminate a possible malignant lymphoma.

The lesions of a 74-year-old Italian woman with cutaneous lymphoplasia are shown in Figure 2–15. The clinical appearance of the lesions was characteristic of lymphomatous disease. A biopsy revealed a diffuse lymphoreticular proliferation with many atypical histiocytes, and a diagnosis of malignant lymphoma, possibly Hodgkin's disease, was made. Extensive laboratory tests did not uncover any systemic involvement. The patient refused superficial radiotherapy for the lesions and did not return to the clinic until two years later. Many of the lesions had spontaneously disappeared and a few new ones had formed (Fig. 2–16). Rebiopsy showed that the lymphoreticular proliferation had a more benign appearance and that a follicular pattern was now present. The entire area was excised and histologic examination showed many follicles with benign-appearing cells. Three years after the excision, the patient was in excellent health and free of lesions.

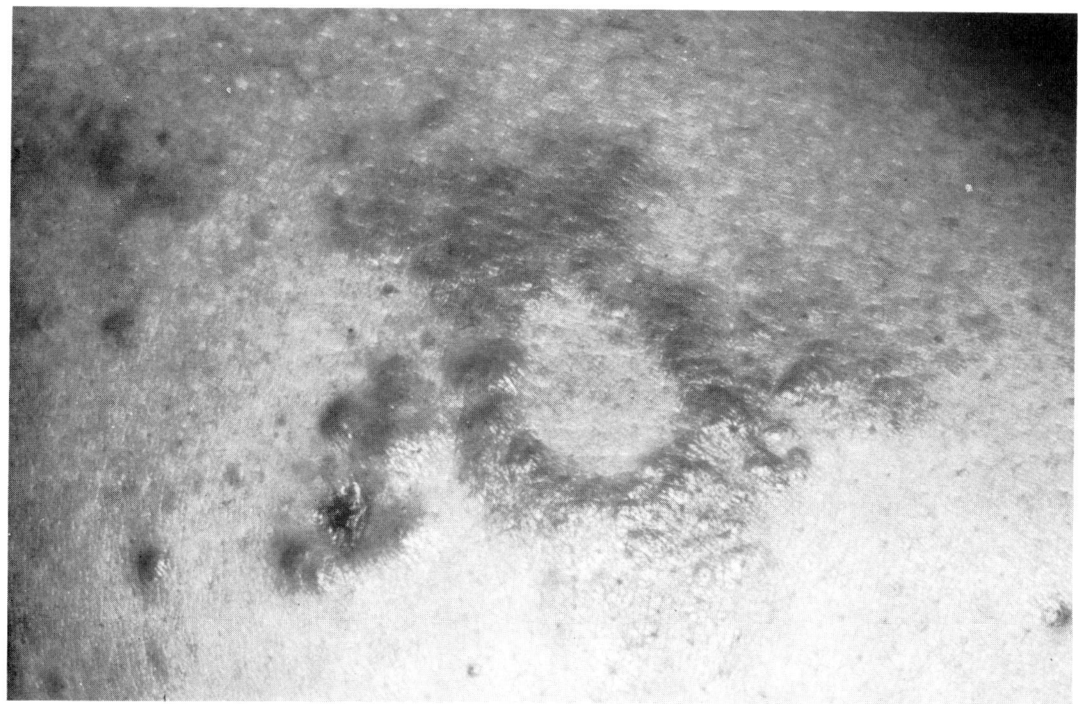

Figure 2–15. Lymphocytoma cutis.

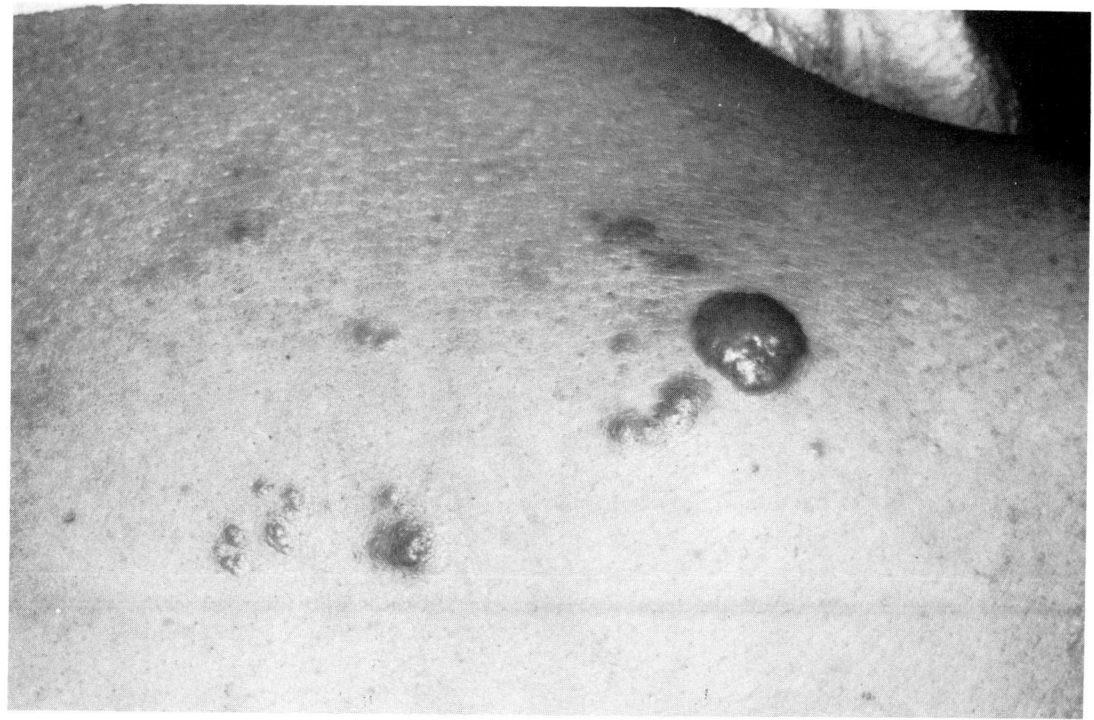

Figure 2–16. Lymphocytoma cutis. Same patient shown in Figure 2–15 two years later. Most of the nodules disappeared without treatment.

Lymphomatoid papulosis is an uncommon entity in which the cutaneous lesions display a neoplastic-like histology in the face of a benign chronic clinical course.[37-38] Individuals with this disorder develop crops of erythematous to reddish-brown papules which undergo central necrosis and eventual spontaneous healing with scar formation (Figs. 2–17 to 2–22). The individual lesions persist for two to four weeks before resolving, and the papules arise in crops over the trunk and extremities for periods ranging from weeks to months. The disorder can persist for as long as 30 years. The lesions are usually asymptomatic except when they first erupt, when they may itch or be painful. Clinically, the eruption most closely resembles that of Mucha-Habermann disease (see p. 444), and investigators believe that it is a variant of that disease. Histologic examination of a papule shows a bandlike lymphocytic infiltrate below the epidermis and epidermal edema or necrosis associated with migration of mononuclear cells from the dermis into the epidermis, sometimes producing an intraepidermal collection of mononuclear cells resembling a Pautrier microabscess. Endothelial cell swelling and intense perivascular accumulations of mononuclear cells simulate a necrotizing vasculitis, but fibrinoid changes are absent. Atypical mononuclear cells resembling neoplastic "reticulum" cells are present in varying numbers, and because of these cells the biopsy material is frequently interpreted as representing possible malignant lymphoma. These atypical cells have been shown to have the surface markers of T lymphocytes.[39]

At least 68 patients with lymphomatoid papulosis have been cited in the literature since 1965.[37-40] In three individuals, malignant lymphomas (undifferentiated lymphoma, anaplastic sarcoma, and pleomorphic reticulum cell sarcoma) developed 8, 18, and 40 years, respectively, after a typical course of lymphomatoid papulosis. However, complete clinical and autopsy data were available only in the last instance. In two of three additional cases,[39, 40] the lesions of lymphomatoid papulosis and mycosis fungoides coexisted, while in the third case, erythroderma and lymphomatoid papulosis were present together. Mycosis fungoides can produce lesions mimicking lymphomatoid papulosis, both in morphology and histology. Nevertheless it does appear that lymphomatoid papulosis in almost all instances has pursued a benign, although protracted course, in spite of its malignant-appearing histology. Both lymphomatoid papulosis and lymphocytoma cutis require careful observation of the patients with periodic biopsies for proper evaluation and management.

Anticonvulsant therapy with Mesantoin, Dilantin, Tridione, and other related compounds can produce fever and lymphadenopathy that mimic lymphoma both clinically and histologically.[41] At least one patient with this syndrome has been treated with chemotherapy for a lymphoma before the relevance of anticonvulsant medication to her illness was appreciated.[42] The syndrome has almost always been reversible after the medication was discontinued. However, Hyman and Sommers reported seven patients who developed either lymphosarcoma or Hodgkin's disease after having been treated for epilepsy with anticonvulsants for 2 to 19 years.[43] Since then, five additional examples of Dilantin-associated lymphomas have been reported.[44-46] In addition, one patient with Mikulicz's disease converted to lymphocytic lymphoma during therapy with Dilantin.[47] In six of the seven patients reported by Hyman and Sommers, the initial lymph node biopsies were interpreted as true lymphoma and not

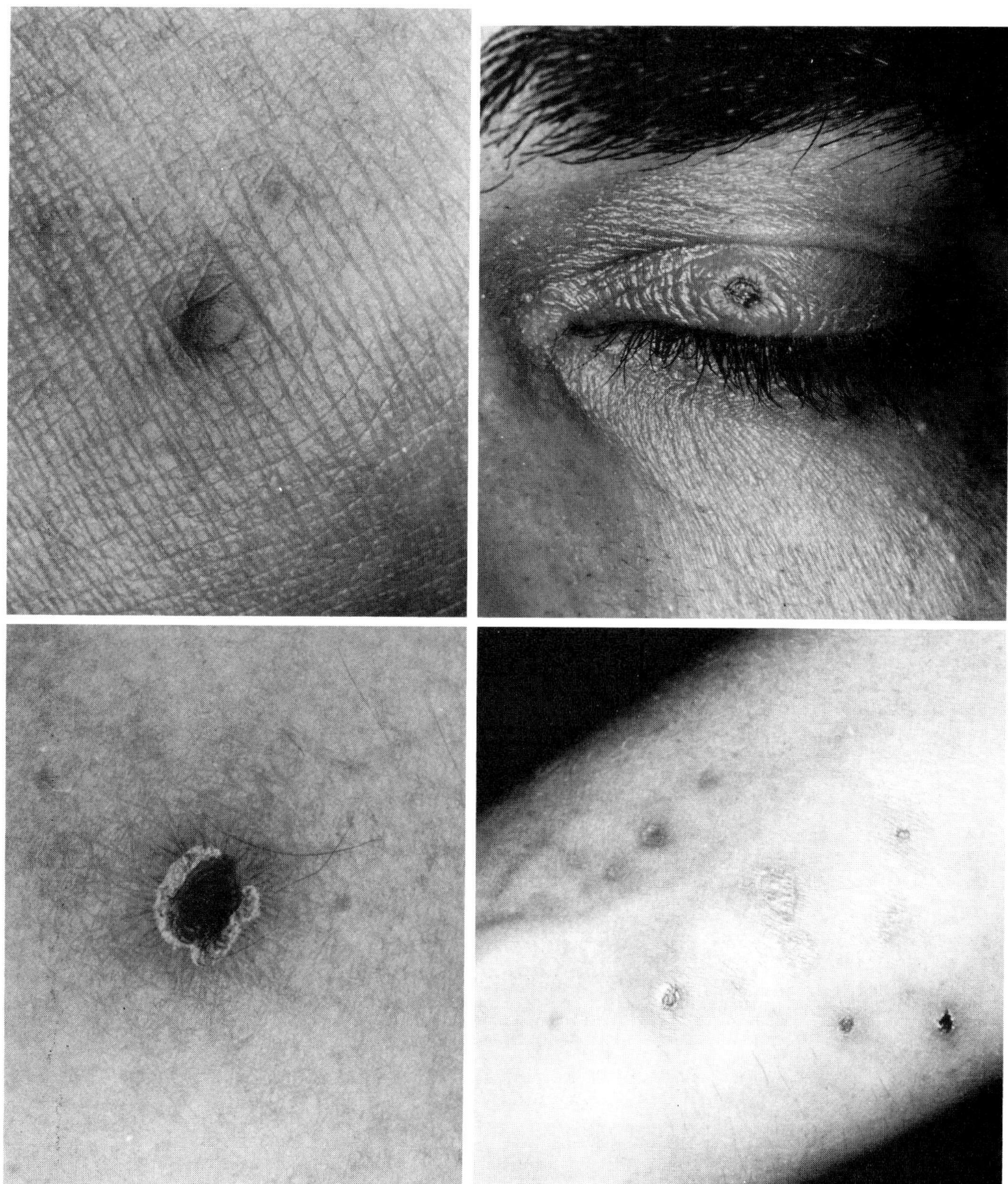

Figure 2–17. Top left. Lymphomatoid papulosis. Course of individual lesion shown in Figures 2–17 to 2–20. Initial lesion is a papule.

Figure 2–18. Top right. Lymphomatoid papulosis. Papule undergoing umbilication because of necrosis.

Figure 2–19. Bottom left. Lymphomatoid papulosis. Papule is necrotic with overlying crust.

Figure 2–20. Bottom right. Lymphomatoid papulosis. End stage of the papule is a punched-out depressed scar.

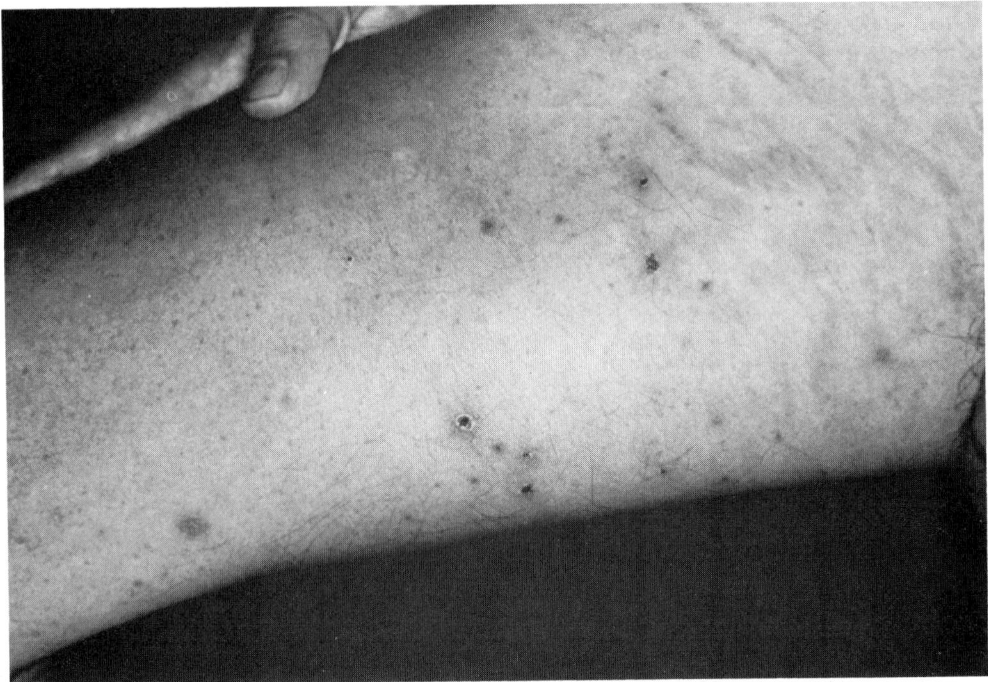

Figure 2–21. Lymphomatoid papulosis. Distribution of lesions.

pseudolymphoma. In one patient, the first node biopsy was interpreted by some pathologists as atypical hyperplasia and by others as lymphosarcoma. A second biopsy two years later showed definite lymphosarcoma.

These observations raise two questions: Is the atypical hyperplasia of lymph nodes (pseudolymphoma) that is sometimes observed during anticonvulsant therapy a precancerous state, and can Dilantin and related compounds act as carcinogens? Currently, this general problem can be viewed in a different way. The newly described entity of immunoblastic lymphadenopathy has been reported following Dilantin therapy.[48, 49] Lukes and Tindle have noted that in their experience there was a morphological similarity between immunoblastic lymphadenopathy and the abnormal lymph nodes associated with anticonvulsant therapy.[49] They believe that these patients are likely to be abnormal reactors to Dilantin, which "switches on" an abnormal immune system to a progressive proliferation manifesting itself as immunoblastic lymphadenopathy rather than Hodgkin's disease or a non-Hodgkin's lymphoma. Since anticonvulsants have been shown to depress cellular immunity,[50, 51] the "switch on" theoretically could be related to a decrease in the suppressor T cell compartment, which might allow for abnormal B cell proliferation. Alternatively, a depression in cellular immunity might manifest itself as a decrease in immunosurveillance, resulting in an increased risk for lymphoreticular malignancies in these patients.

Immunoblastic lymphadenopathy, also known as angioimmunoblastic lymphadenopathy with dysproteinemia,[52] is being increasingly recognized as a clinical and pathologic entity that may have been confused with Hodgkin's disease in the past. Over 70 cases have thus far been reported since its initial description in 1973.[49, 52, 53] In most instances, this disorder

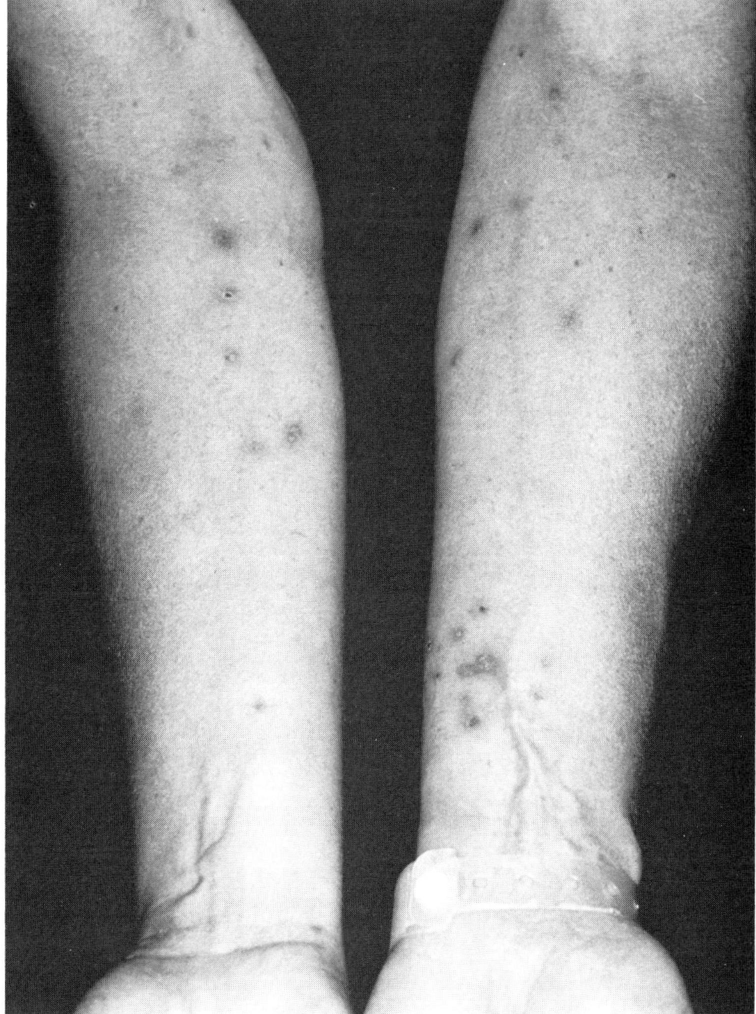

Figure 2–22. Lymphomatoid papulosis. Distribution of lesions.

appears to result from chronic antigenic stimulation induced by drugs and, in one case, by injections of liver extract.[54] Clinically, individuals have generalized lymphadenopathy, fever, weight loss, and polyclonal hyperglobulinemia. Hemolytic anemia with an occasionally positive Coombs' test was present in less than half of the cases in the series of Lukes and Tindle.[49] A pruritic generalized maculopapular eruption is present in about 40 per cent of patients.[49] In two patients, there were in addition to the rash, subcutaneous nodules on the face and trunk[52] and plaques and nodules on the posterior surfaces of the thighs resembling those of mycosis fungoides.[55] Petechiae and purpura have been manifestations in a few patients.

The histology of the lymph nodes presents a unique picture: a non-neoplastic-appearing proliferation of immunoblasts (transformed lymphocytes), plasmacytoid immunoblasts, and plasma cells; a proliferation of small vessels in an arborizing pattern; and the deposition of unidentified amorphous acidophilic material in the interstitial tissues. All of these features combine to obliterate the nodal architecture. The same histologic features are present in the skin lesions, although the arborization of the vessels is not developed to the same degree.[52, 55] In addition to these features, histiocytes and eosinophils are present in variable degrees which produce a mixed histologic picture resembling Hodgkin's disease — the disorder most often confused with this condition. Sometimes the immunoblasts resemble Sternberg-Reed cells. The history of preceding drug exposure, hyperglobulinemia, and hemolytic anemia is unusual in Hodgkin's disease and will serve to distinguish the otherwise similar clinical picture from Hodgkin's disease. Systemic involvement occurs in this disorder, and the histologic triad can be found in the bone marrow, spleen, lung, and *skin.* Lukes and Tindle observed three cases of monomorphous proliferation of immunoblasts arising in patients with immunoblastic lymphadenopathy which they call immunoblastic sarcoma and which has a rapidly progressive and fatal course.[3, 4, 49]

Although immunoblastic lymphadenopathy can resolve spontaneously, 18 of 28 cases in Lukes and Tindle's series ended fatally after a median survival of 15 months. The majority of cases occur in the sixth and seventh decades, but the disease has been described in persons between 25 and 30 years old. The natural history of the disease remains to be characterized because most cases have been diagnosed retrospectively after being treated as a neoplastic process. Although definitive studies for detection of surface membrane markers have yet to be done, it appears likely that immunoblastic lymphadenopathy does represent an abnormal hyperimmune disorder of the B cell system. The moderate to marked proliferation of immunoblasts, plasmacytoid immunoblasts, and plasma cells, in association with a constant hyperglobulinemia, supports this hypothesis. Although immunoblastic lymphadenopathy displays a benign cellular histology, it often behaves as a malignant disease and also has the potential for transformation into a histologically malignant lymphoma which Lukes and Tindle call immunoblastic sarcoma. Yataganas et al. reported the case of a 33-year-old man with angioimmunoblastic lymphadenopathy that terminated as Hodgkin's disease.[56]

Immunoblastic sarcoma is a monomorphous proliferation of immunoblasts that involves lymph nodes either focally or completely. A *monoclonal* gammopathy may be associated with it, and the course is rapidly progressive and fatal over two to three months.[3, 4, 49] Lukes and Tindle have observed immunoblastic sarcoma arising in patients with systemic lupus erythematosus, rheumatoid arthritis, and Sjögren's syndrome, and in elderly individuals without any obvious immunological disorders. They also believe, on the basis of their personal experiences, that the lymphomas developing in patients on immunosuppressive therapy, in those with alpha chain disease, and in those with congenital immune defects, exhibit the features of immunoblastic sarcoma rather than those of "reticulum cell" sarcoma as commonly reported.[3, 49] They propose that immunoblastic sarcoma may develop in abnormal, damaged, or senescent immune systems following chronic antigenic stimulation. Thus far, the immunoblastic sarcomas have had the *morphological* features suggestive of the B cell type. However, Lukes and Collins were able to document a T cell variety of immunoblastic sarcoma by functional studies in one of their cases.[3]

Hossfeld et al. found chromosome abnormalities in lymph node–derived cells of two individuals with angioimmunoblastic lymphadenopathy.[57] Long-term studies are necessary to determine whether or not all patients with immunoblastic lymphadenopathy have chromosome abnormalities and whether those with such abnormalities are more likely to develop immunoblastic sarcoma or other malignant lymphomas.

Virtually all the information one has about immunoblastic lymphadenopathy has been gleaned retrospectively. Prospective studies are needed to delineate the spectrum of clinical features associated with the disorder. Wechsler and Stavrides have recently published such a case.[58] This patient was a 53-year-old woman with cervical and axillary adenopathy that showed the classic histological features of this entity. However, she did not have fever, weight loss, hemolytic anemia, or hypergammaglobulinemia. Instead, she had abnormally depressed serum levels of IgG, increased levels of serum IgM, and a mixed cryoglobulinemia exhibiting rheumatoid factor activity. The last abnormality was associated with leukocytoclastic angiitis of the lower extremities. She also showed depression of cellular immunity by her poor response to microbial, fungal, and viral skin tests and epicutaneous testing to DNCB. Blastogenic transformation of her lymphocytes by phytohemagglutinin was abnormally low. She died after a course of approximately 21 months with ulcers of the legs caused by the angiitis, thrombocytopenia of unknown cause, and septicemia caused by *Escherichia coli* and *Streptococcus faecalis*. At autopsy there was also evidence of generalized cytomegalic virus inclusion disease. Mixed cryoglobulinemia, a manifestation of circulating immune complexes, was also present in the case reported by Schultz and Yunis.[54] In that individual, repeated injections of liver extract were believed to be the antigenic stimulation for the development of the immunoblastic lymphadenopathy.

MYCOSIS FUNGOIDES

Mycosis fungoides has been one of the most confusing and bewildering diseases in medicine. However, in the past decade there have been significant advances in our understanding of this disorder. This progress is of more than academic and therapeutic interest because the eventual discovery of its etiology and pathogenesis may prove to be important for lymphoreticular malignancies and hyperplasias in general. A brief account of the historical development of mycosis fungoides will explain the reasons for some of the confusion surrounding this disease.

Alibert described this disorder in 1806 and called it *pian fungoides* because he believed it was a form of yaws with large necrotic tumors. Alibert later changed the name to *mycosis fungoides* because the tumors resembled mushrooms. (He could not have meant to imply that this disease was a fungal infection, since human mycotic diseases had not yet been discovered.) Bazin, one of Alibert's students, recognized that there were three phases of mycosis fungoides and described them in 1876. In 1885 Vidal and Brocq introduced the term *mycosis fungoides à tumeurs d'emblée* to delineate disorders having mushroom-like tumors that appeared in the absence of the first two phases of the disease. In 1891 Hallopeau applied the term *mycosis fungoides* to diseases in which exfoliative dermatitis was the prime feature. Affected persons were called *l'homme rouge*.[59]

PLATE 7

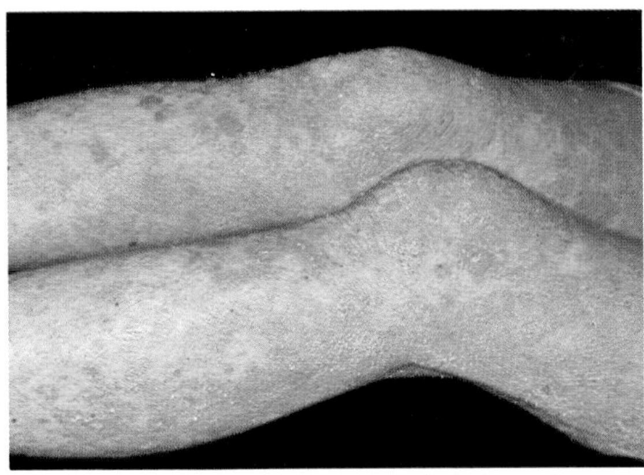

A, Mycosis fungoides. Lesions mimic those of psoriasis.

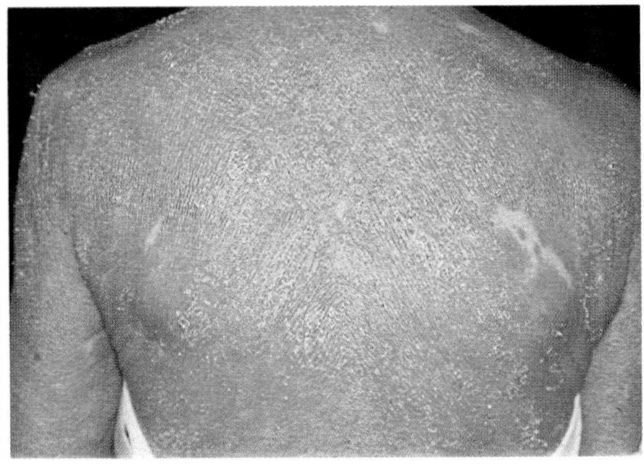

B, Mycosis fungoides. Eruption simulates psoriasis in the exfoliative phase. A few islands of normal skin still remain.

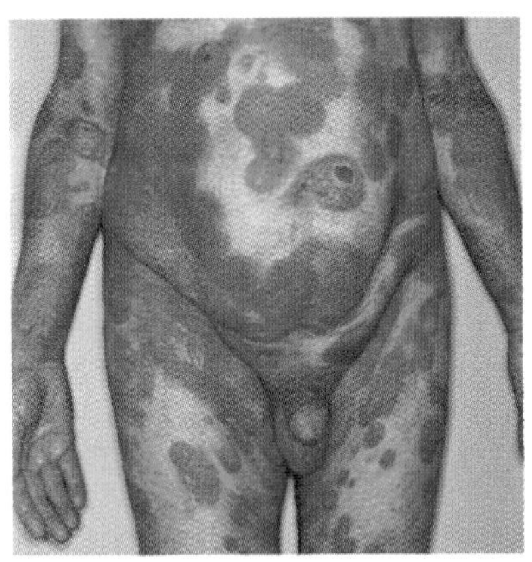

C, Mycosis fungoides. Plaques and tumors.

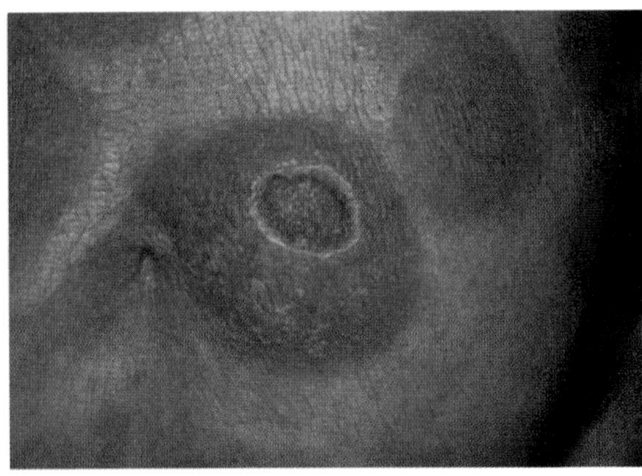

D, Mycosis fungoides. Close view of necrotic tumor.

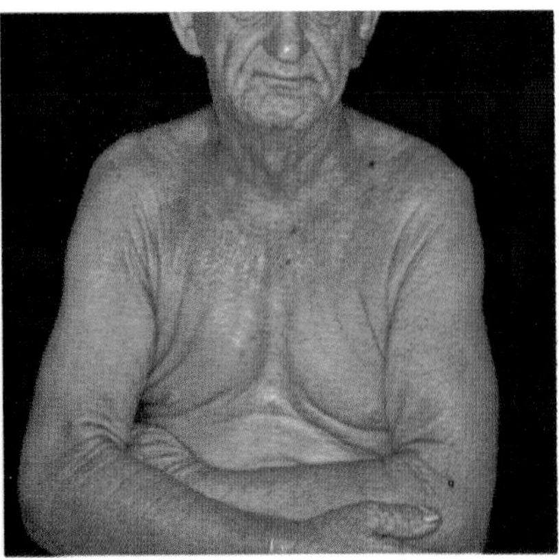

E, Mycosis fungoides. Exfoliative dermatitis with marked edema of skin. This patient had Sézary syndrome.

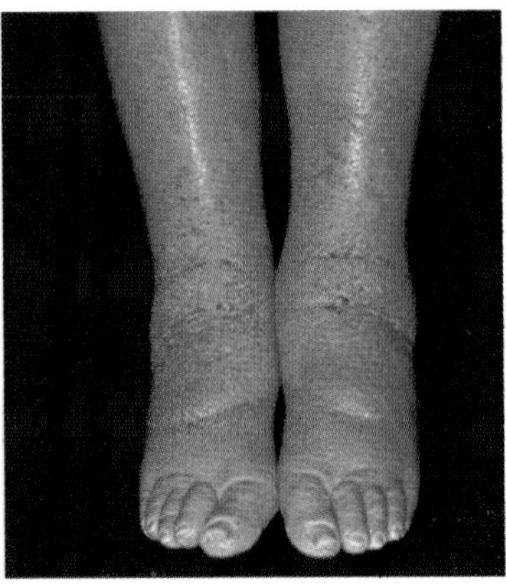

F, Mycosis fungoides. Same patient as in *E*. Marked edema of legs accompanied exfoliative dermatitis.

PLATE 8

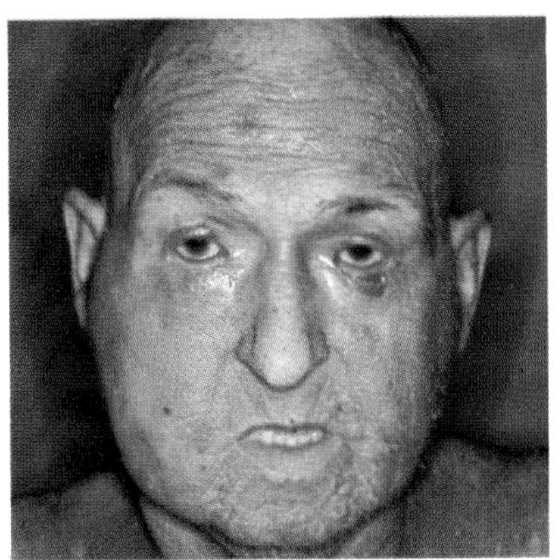

A, Mycosis fungoides. Diffuse infiltration of skin. Note ulcerations under left eye.

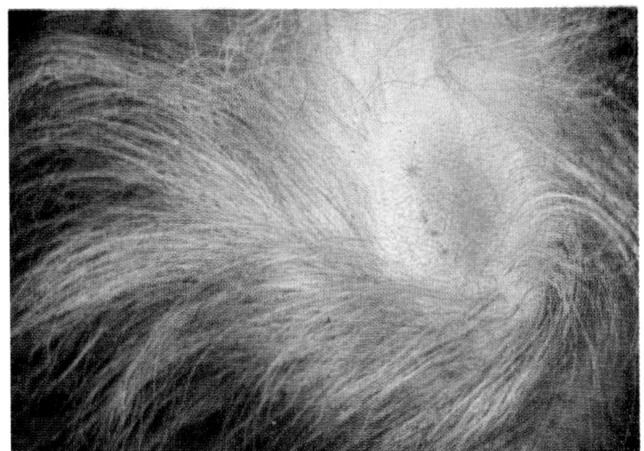

B, Mycosis fungoides. Alopecia associated with tumor of mycosis fungoides.

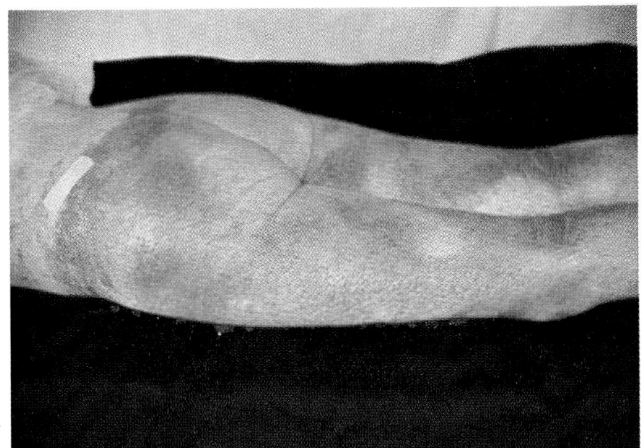

C, Mycosis fungoides. Poikilodermatous form. This distribution and presence of islands of normal skin are characteristic.

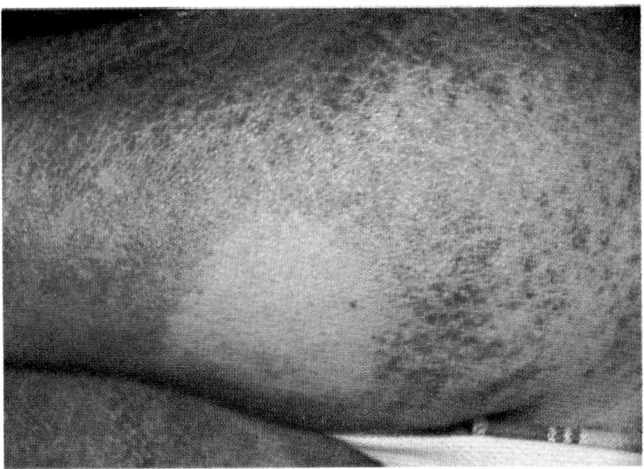

D, Mycosis fungoides. Close view of poikilodermatous form of mycosis fungoides.

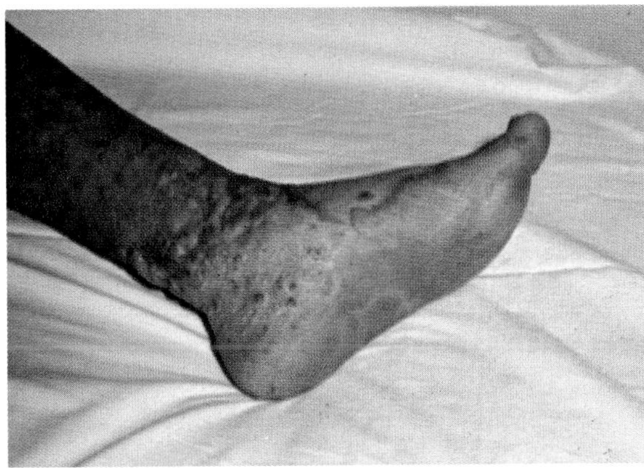

E, Kaposi's sarcoma. Characteristic plaques on sole. Typical nodules on ankle and leg.

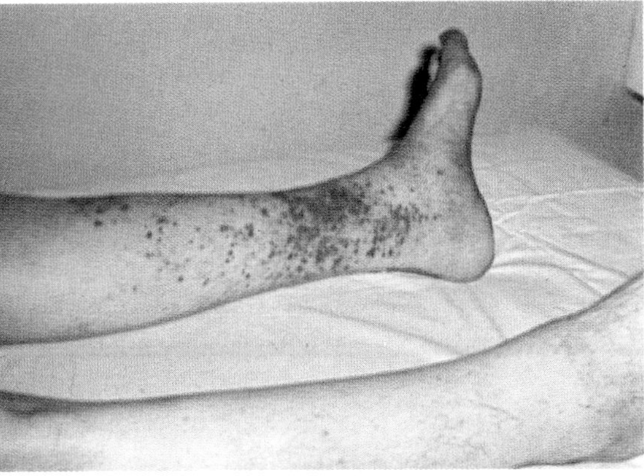

F, Kaposi's sarcoma. Characteristic nodules on leg.

Since then, most cases of lymphoma with tumors have been called mycosis fungoides and vice versa: Mycosis fungoides as defined by Alibert and Bazin has been considered by many to be the cutaneous expression of malignant lymphoma.[60-62]

The natural history and histopathology of mycosis fungoides are strikingly different from those of the monomorphous lymphomas and are analogous to those of Hodgkin's disease.[63-66]

There are three phases of mycosis fungoides: the premycotic (erythematous, eczematous) stage, the plaque (mycotic) stage, and the tumor stage. The premycotic phase can persist from a few months to more than 40 years. A variety of dermatoses, usually associated with intense pruritus, is the prime feature, or pruritus may be the sole manifestation in this stage. The dermatoses resemble banal eruptions: psoriasis, seborrheic dermatitis, and eczema. But the morphology of the lesions, their clinical course, and their response to conventional therapy are often somewhat atypical. The dermatoses can remit spontaneously only to reappear later. On occasion the premycotic eruptions are exact duplicates of banal dermatologic disorders, and the correct diagnosis is made after biopsy or in retrospect. Histologic examination of a premycotic lesion usually discloses only chronic nonspecific inflammation in the dermis. However, there may be histologic features that make one suspicious of mycosis fungoides even though the cellular elements appear benign and mature: The infiltrate may be present as a band below the epidermis; the inflammatory cells may be polymorphic; and the overlying epidermis may be slightly thickened. In some patients, sequential biopsies over the course of months or years will display progressive histologic changes that become diagnostic of mycosis fungoides. In the plaque and tumor stages, the diagnostic histologic abnormalities are always present.

In the plaque stage, the premycotic lesions become infiltrated, and pruritus continues. Indurated plaques can also arise from previously uninvolved skin. These lesions assume horseshoe, arciform, and other bizarre shapes, and their color varies from shades of red to reddish-brown and purple. The entire integument may be infiltrated and produce a thickened red hide with or without scaling (exfoliative dermatitis and erythroderma). A few islands of normal skin may remain for a time before universal erythroderma is complete (Plate 7*B*). Alopecia is seen in hairy areas involved by plaques or diffuse infiltration (Plate 8*B*).

In the final stages, tumors develop from preexisting plaques, erythroderma, or previously uninvolved skin. The size of the tumors varies from a few centimeters to as many as 10, and their colors are the same as those seen in the plaques.

The tumors characteristically undergo necrosis, but they also can spontaneously disappear as the lesions in the premycotic and plaque stages sometimes do. The intensity of the pruritus often diminishes with the onset of the tumor stage.

Necrosis is not limited to tumors. Plaques may become necrotic, and the ulceration may extend to involve large areas of the body (see Fig. 2–36). Ulcers can also develop on a background of generalized erythroderma and exfoliative dermatitis produced by cellular infiltration (see Fig. 2–37). In spite of extensive cutaneous involvement with tumors and plaques, the individual usually does not appear acutely ill.

One does observe this three-stage sequence in most instances of mycosis fungoides, and often lesions from the three phases are present at the same time. In other patients, only the plaque and tumor stages appear. Regional or generalized lymphadenopathy may develop at any stage in this disease, and it is a sign that should be carefully looked for in the management of patients because its presence generally indicates a prognostic change for the worse.

The d'emblée form of mycosis fungoides is usually a manifestation of a malignant lymphoma. This view, championed by Bluefarb,[63] has been supported by the observations of Reed and Cummings[67] and by our own data. However, mycosis fungoides can begin with tumors. In the series of 144 patients from the National Institutes of Health studied and reported over the years by Block et al.[65] and Epstein et al.,[68] ten patients presented with tumors. Allen reported similar examples.[69]

In our experience, exfoliative dermatitis and erythroderma are not unusual manifestations of mycosis fungoides. In ten of 144 patients in Epstein's series, mycosis fungoides began as an exfoliative erythroderma.[68] The skin can become markedly edematous and thickened, producing *l'homme rouge* with leonine facies and ectropion. This markedly edematous phase of the disease responds dramatically to oral steroid therapy. Two of our patients lost several pounds when the skin returned to normal. The reason for the marked fluid retention was not determined; these patients did not have cardiac or renal disease. Mycosis fungoides manifesting itself as erythroderma without circulating abnormal mononuclear cells is a legitimate manifestation of the disease. Erythroderma in mycosis fungoides does not always signify the presence of the Sézary syndrome (p. 158).

In one of our patients, an interesting series of dermatologic disorders developed:

> A 60-year-old white man developed alopecia totalis which was followed by an exfoliative dermatitis two years later. Repeated biopsies of the skin showed only nonspecific dermal inflammation. When the erythroderma was effectively treated by oral corticosteroids, his hair regrew. Six years after the onset of the alopecia totalis, typical plaques of mycosis fungoides, histologically verified, arose from his generalized erythroderma.

This case is similar to others collected and reported by Bluefarb.[70]

Mycosis fungoides is often suspected because of atypical dermatoses in the premycotic stage. However, there is a distinctive and easily recognized premycotic dermatosis which is a harbinger of the disease. Clinically, one sees large flat reddish-brown patches composed of fine telangiectasia, stippled pigmentation, fine wrinkling, and scaling on the lower abdomen, flanks, buttocks, and thighs (Plates 6 *E, F;* 8 *C, D;* Figs. 2–23 and 2–24). In addition to these sites of predilection, the lesions can also develop on the arms and chest. Pruritus may be present. The histologic features only rarely suggest the presence of mycosis fungoides. This dermatosis can be present for as long as 35 years before the plaques and tumors of mycosis fungoides develop.[71]

Some have called this dermatosis *poikiloderma vasculare atrophicans,* and others, *parapsoriasis en plaques.* This semantic confusion is responsible for the interminable discussions among dermatologists as to whether or not parapsoriasis en plaques is a premycotic lesion. (Ordinary guttate parapsoriasis is a benign disorder unrelated to the dermatosis under discussion [Figs. 2–25 and 2–26].)

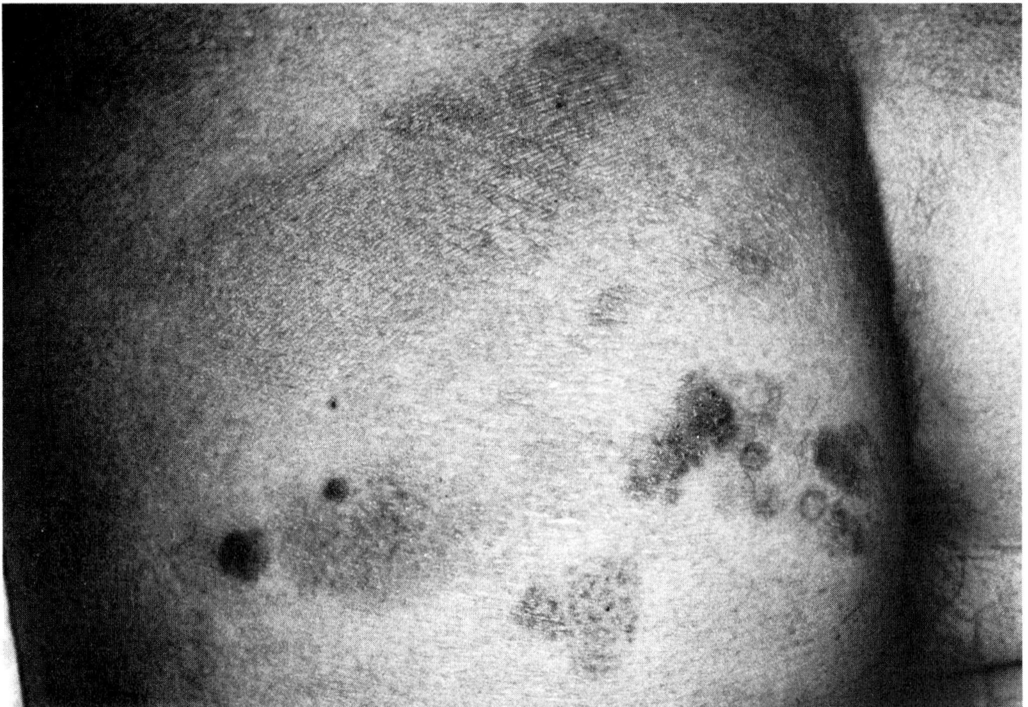

Figure 2–23. Parapsoriasis en plaques with poikilodermatous features which has developed nodules histologically diagnostic of mycosis fungoides. See Plate 6*E* for close-up.

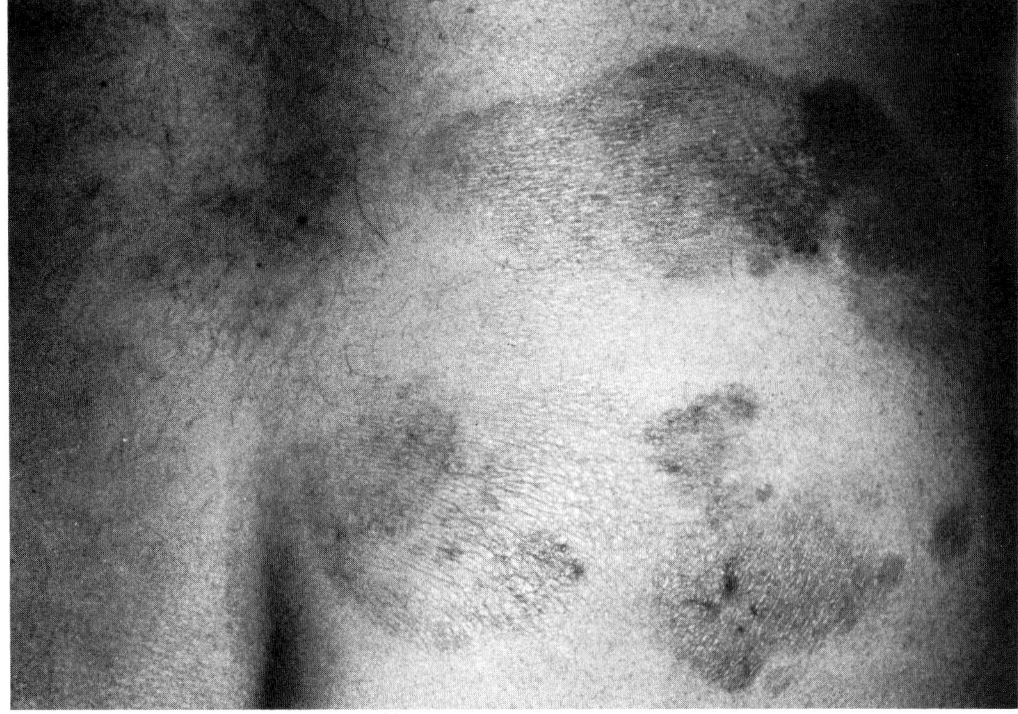

Figure 2–24. Parapsoriasis en plaques which showed histologic changes of mycosis fungoides. See Plate 6*F* for close-up.

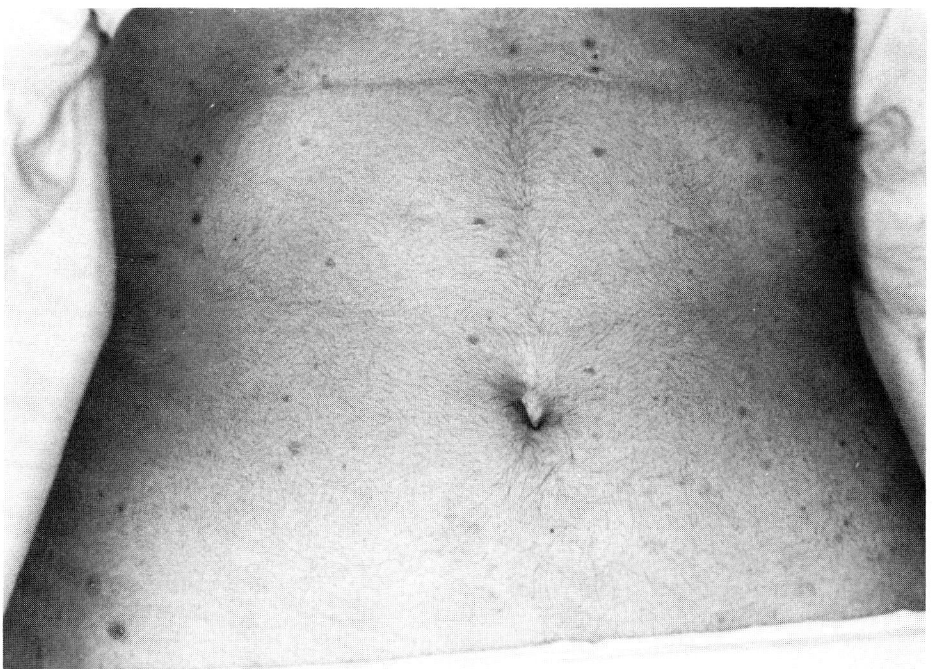

Figure 2–25. Guttate parapsoriasis. Oval papulosquamous lesions that remain benign.

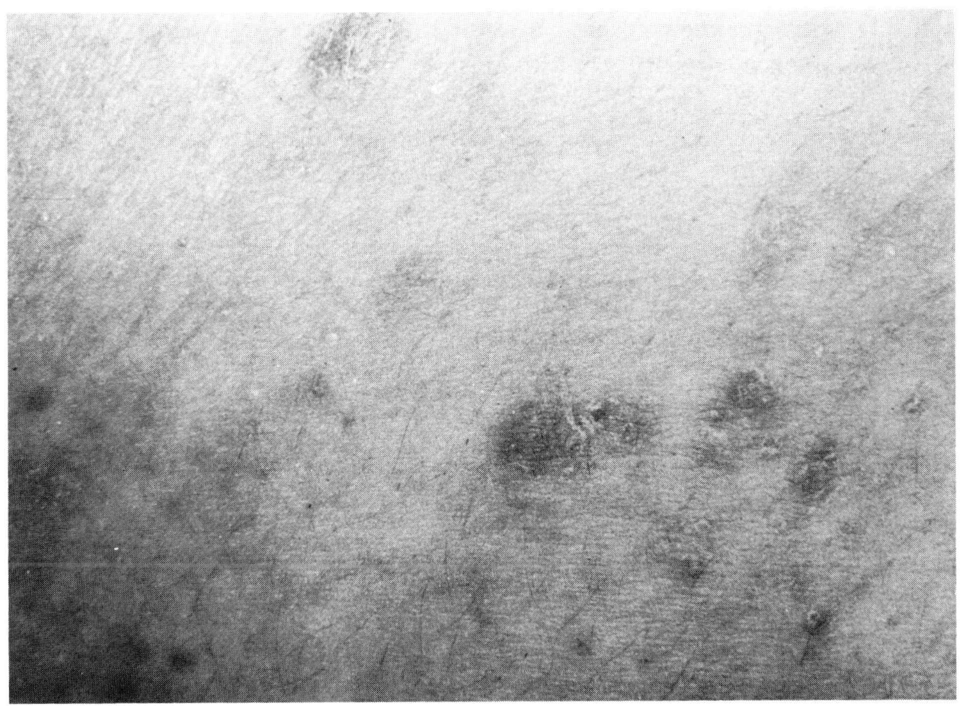

Figure 2–26. Guttate parapsoriasis. Close-up of papulosquamous lesions in Figure 2–25.

Samman calls this lesion *poikiloderma*. He reported a series in which 12 of 25 patients with this dermatosis developed mycosis fungoides. Most of the patients developed mycosis fungoides 6 to 10 years after the poikiloderma appeared, but in some individuals this transition was not observed until 30 years later.

Samman restricts the term *parapsoriasis en plaques* to lesions having a faint erythema sometimes accompanied by a yellowish cast, a fine scale, and slightly wrinkled surface. On the trunk and limbs, the lesions are usually small, round, oval or finger-like in shape (Fig. 2–27). On the buttocks and thighs where they occur more commonly, parapsoriasis en plaques is usually present in large patches.

In his original series,[71] only one of 59 persons with this type of lesion developed mycosis fungoides. The appearance of poikilodermatous changes in the benign form of parapsoriasis en plaques is an ominous sign. In a later paper, Samman reported that in a few patients with this presumed benign dermatosis, poikiloderma was observed to develop two to three years after the eruption appeared.[72] Similarly in a few instances, the first biopsy of the *benign* form of parapsoriasis en plaques showed histologic features suggesting pre–mycosis fungoides. Therefore periodic biopsies of parapsoriasis en plaques (Samman) and careful long-term observations are necessary not only for the proper management of this dermatosis but also for learning more about the natural history of this presumed benign dermatosis.[72]

Fleischmajer et al. reported that 7 of 13 cases of parapsoriasis en plaques eventually terminated in mycosis fungoides.[73] However, the morphologic descriptions of the dermatoses were those of poikiloderma and not parapsoriasis as defined by Samman. Irrespective of nomenclature, the "poikilodermatous-parapsoriasis" lesion is a highly distinctive and easily recognized premycotic lesion.

A variant of the "poikilodermatous-parapsoriasis" lesion is called parapsoriasis variegata or parapsoriasis lichenoides. Initially, it develops as a netlike pattern of minimally elevated red papules, which evolve into spots of fine wrinkling with telangiectases and pigmentation. It then has the appearance of poikiloderma vasculare atrophicans in a reticulated pattern, as well as the same significance.

We have seen several unusual manifestations of mycosis fungoides in our series of 59 patients. Three women developed petechiae in their eczematous and poikilodermatous lesions whenever their disease flared. Reactions to medications, thrombocytopenia, and angiitis were excluded as causes for bleeding. Three men developed several 1- to 2-cm oval lesions of parapsoriasis en plaques (Samman) in a necklace distribution around the neck and upper chest (Fig. 2–28). The histologic features of these lesions were those of a dense band of mature lymphohistiocytic cells in the upper dermis that suggested pre–mycosis fungoides. These patients developed plaques and nodules clinically and histologically characteristic of mycosis fungoides in other areas 12 months, 18 months, and five years later.

A 73-year-old white man had had intermittent oozing from the right ear canal for 30 years; this eventually resulted in an occluded canal and a chronically swollen pinna. When he was first seen in 1962, he had many eczematous patches over the scalp, body, and neck in addition to the swollen canal and pinna. A diagnosis of chronic external otitis with an autosensitization reaction was made. Over the next

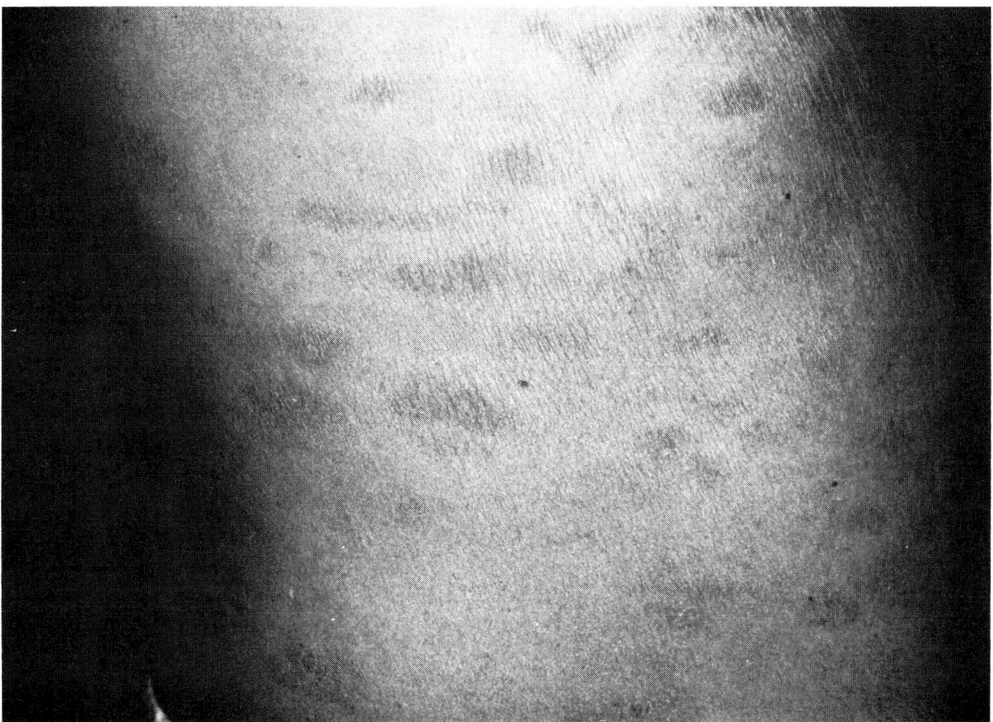

Figure 2–27. Parapsoriasis en plaques (Samman). Faint erythema with a fine scale and a slightly wrinkled surface.

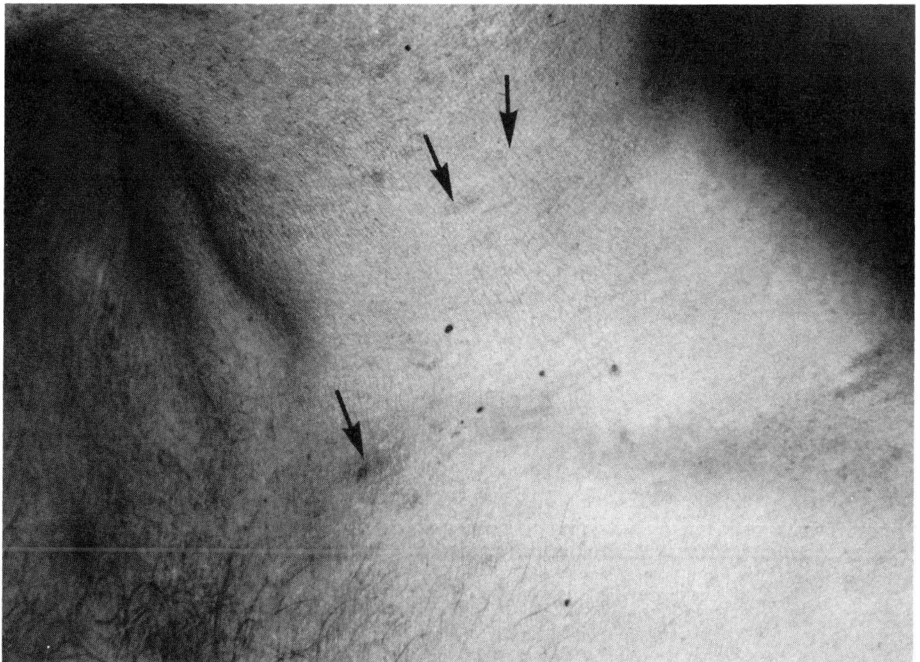

Figure 2–28. Parapsoriasis en plaques (Samman) in a necklace distribution around the neck and upper chest (arrows). Mycosis fungoides developed 12 months later.

six months his eczematous dermatitis evolved into a generalized erythroderma which proved on histologic examination to be mycosis fungoides. He was treated successfully with electron-beam radiation. The erythroderma cleared and his swollen right pinna returned to normal size.

A 66-year-old white woman had had severe generalized pruritus with moderate hyperpigmentation for one year. Several axillary nodes were enlarged bilaterally. Histologic examination of the skin and an axillary node revealed the classic changes of mycosis fungoides. Following electron beam therapy, the pruritus persisted for an additional six months before disappearing. At follow-up 5½ years later, the patient was free of pruritus and skin lesions and there was no detectable lymphadenopathy. Follow-up by telephone 8½ years later disclosed that the patient was still free of symptoms and that her skin lesions had not recurred.

Other rare manifestations of this disease include bullae, pustules, alopecia mucinosa, and involvement of the tonsils, tongue, and palate.[74, 77] Price et al. described a 60-year-old man with mycetoma-like lesions on one foot for 24 years. Several circumscribed, hyperkeratotic plaques with a verrucous surface extended from the dorsum of the toes and plantar and dorsal surfaces of the foot to just above the malleoli. In some lesions, ulcers and fissures exuding a bloody purulent exudate were present. Areas of relatively normal appearing skin (slightly erythematous and edematous) separated the plaques. The patient had no other significant lesions, nor palpable lymphadenopathy.[78]

A rare variant of mycosis fungoides is Woringer-Kolopp disease, in which the epidermal invasion by tumor cells is massive and not focal as in the formation of Pautrier microabscesses. On the basis of this histologic picture, names such as epidermotropic reticulosis and Pagetoid reticulosis have been proposed. Electron microscopic studies have demonstrated that these cells have the serpentine and grooved nuclear features characteristic of mycosis fungoides.[79] In some patients, the lesions have been described as well-defined, polycyclic, red scaling patches which enlarge slowly or not at all; while in others, the lesions have spread rapidly, producing necrosis in their centers. In one patient, the lesion had the clinical appearance of parapsoriasis variegata.[79] The rapid enlargement of such lesions paralleled the fatal course of the illness in these patients.[80] Some authors do not consider the patients with the slowly enlarging plaques to have a variant of mycosis fungoides because the cutaneous lesions have been present for 6 to 16 years without evidence of organ involvement.[81]

Alopecia mucinosa (follicular mucinosis) has recently been shown to be a feature of mycosis fungoides and, rarely, malignant lymphoma.[82] Three morphologic forms exist: a flat rough patch of follicular papules, a scaly plaque of follicular papules, and a boggy erythematous infiltrated area (Figs. 2–29 to 2–31). Lesions develop on the face, neck, scalp, trunk, and extremities and are associated with hair loss. Histologically, one finds an accumulation of acid mucopolysaccharide in the outer root sheath of the hair follicles and in the secretory epithelium of associated sebaceous glands. An inflammatory infiltrate surrounds the affected follicles.

Ninety-two cases have been reported in the literature since Pinkus described this entity in 1957.[83, 84] Sixty-four have occurred in individuals under 40 years of age. The course has been benign with spontaneous remission occurring a few months to a year after onset. However, in 28

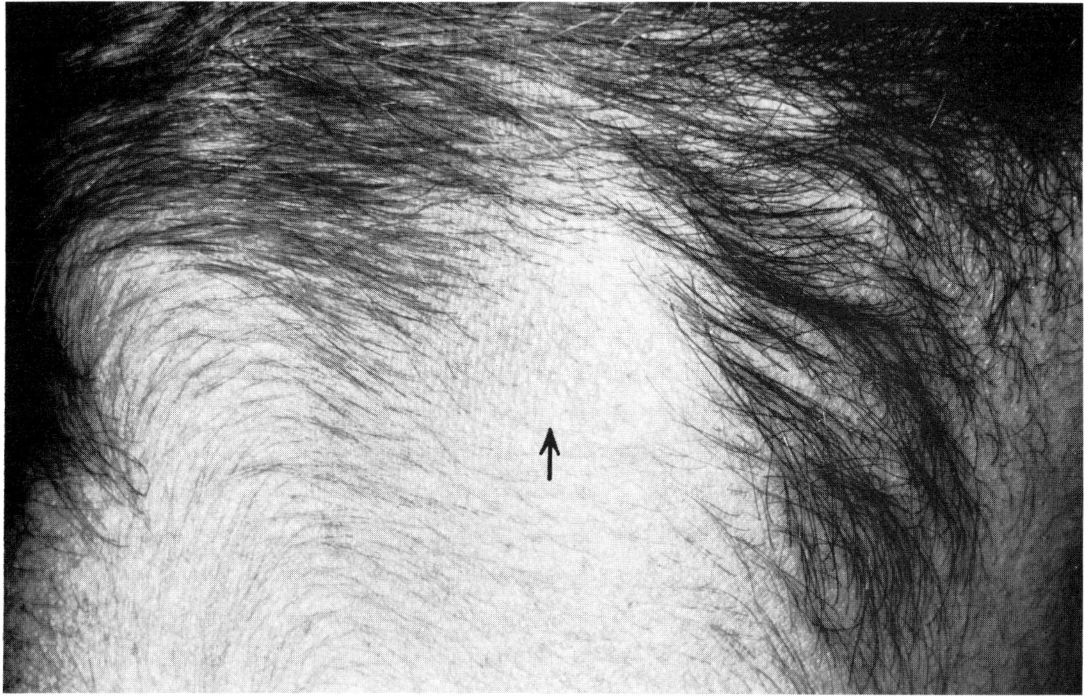

Figure 2–29. Alopecia mucinosa (benign variety). Hair loss associated with perifollicular papules (arrow).

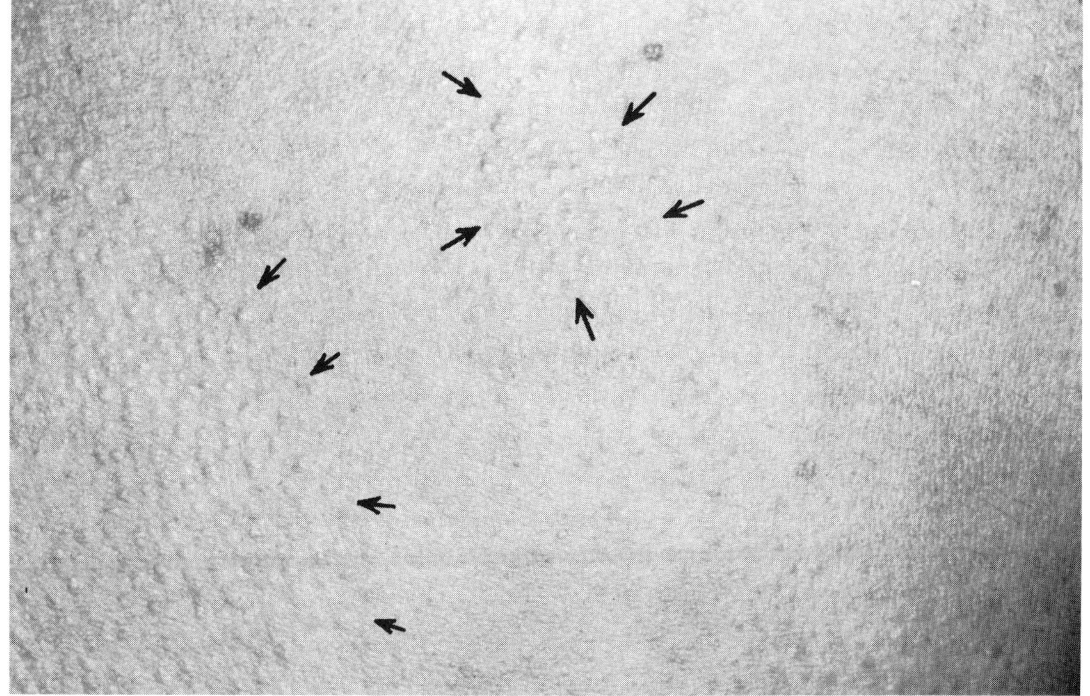

Figure 2–30. Alopecia mucinosa (benign variety). Clusters of perifollicular papules (arrows).

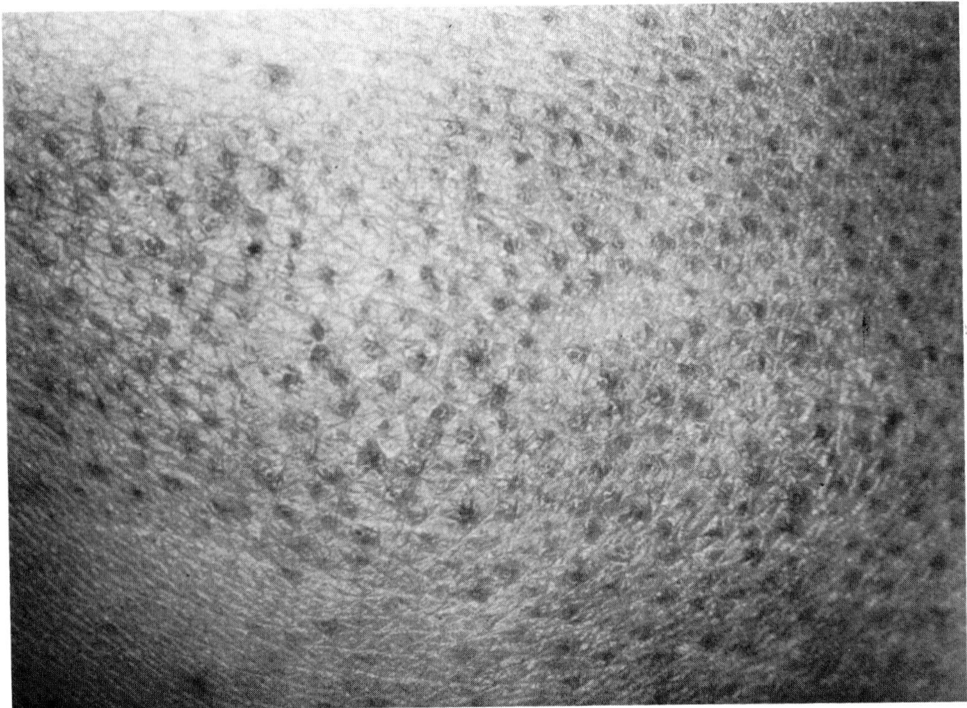

Figure 2–31. Alopecia mucinosa indistinguishable from the benign variety, as a manifestation of mycosis fungoides. Biopsy showed the histologic findings of mycosis fungoides.

persons over the age of 40, the duration of the disorder ranged from one to 14 years. In six cases the histologic abnormalities of follicular mucinosis were present in lesions of known cases of mycosis fungoides and lymphoma; but in four other cases, alopecia mucinosa began as an idiopathic disorder which evolved into either mycosis fungoides or reticulum cell sarcoma. These recent observations point up the malignant potential of this uneventful and curious dermatosis in individuals past the age of 40.

Pyoderma vegetans (dermatitis vegetans, pyodermite végétante Hallopeau) is a rare disorder that represents a reaction pattern of skin. Although there are probably multiple but as-yet-undetermined causes underlying this entity, the most commonly identified associated condition is ulcerative colitis.[85] The lesions begin as small pustules or groups of vesicopustules that tend to coalesce into boggy erythematous plaques. These lesions often spread, producing a center composed of crusts and granulation tissue behind the slowly expanding pustular border. Although pyoderma vegetans has a predilection for the flexures, it may appear anywhere. Histologic examination reveals epidermal hyperplasia with spongiotic edema and focal to diffuse accumulations of eosinophils and neutrophils within the epidermis. Within the dermis there is diffuse infiltration with neutrophils, eosinophils, and mononuclear cells, sometimes accompanied by foci of necrosis.

One of our patients with mycosis fungoides developed lesions that clinically and histologically mimicked this condition. The patient was a 50-year-old man who sought medical attention because of several 1- to 3-cm oval parapsoriasis en plaques lesions which appeared around his neck,

PLATE 9

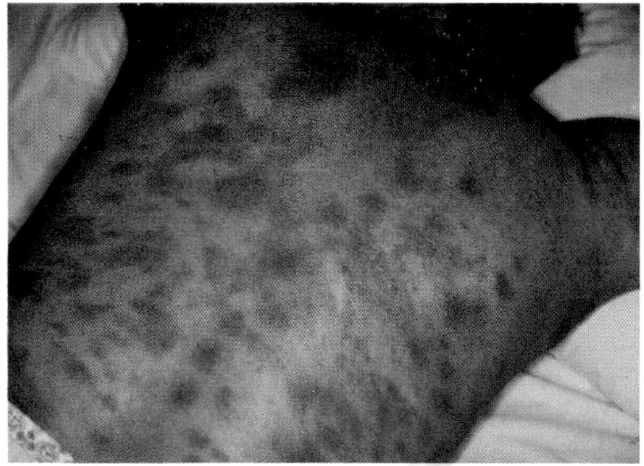

A, Mycosis fungoides. Patches and plaques show histologic features of pyoderma vegetans. Same patient in *A* through *E*.

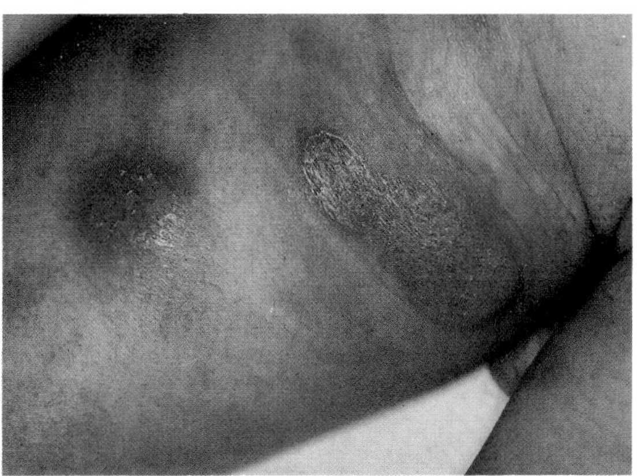

B, Mycosis fungoides. Lesions of pyoderma vegetans.

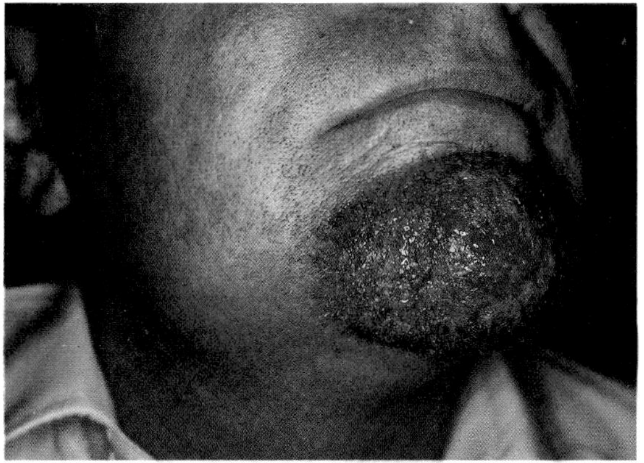

C, Mycosis fungoides. Pyoderma vegetans on chin.

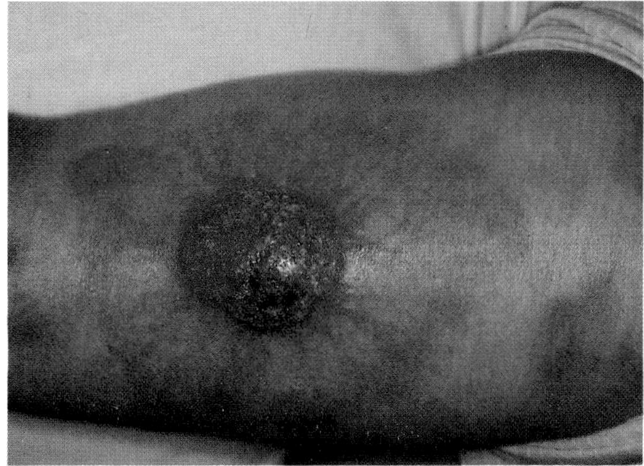

D, Mycosis fungoides. Pyoderma vegetans with wide red halo. Superficial pustules and erosions on surface of tumors.

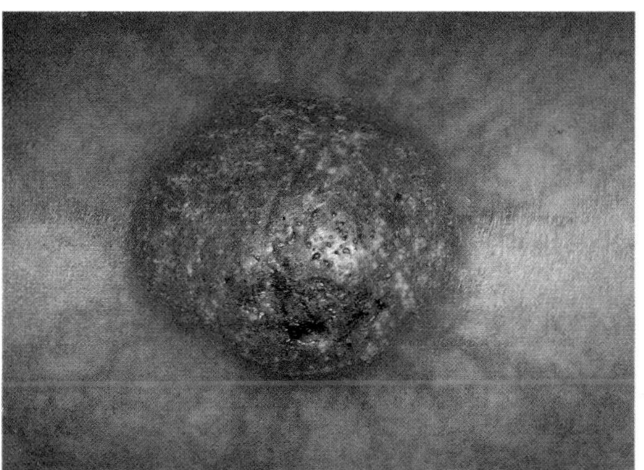

E, Mycosis fungoides. Close-up of lesion shown in *D*.

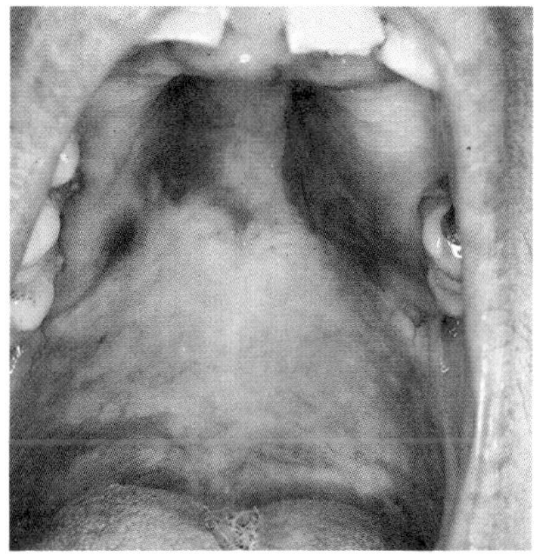

F, Kaposi's hemorrhagic sarcoma. Tumors of Kaposi's disease on hard palate.

upper chest, and face. A small 5-mm nodule was present on the upper left eyelid and was the only one which showed the histologic features of mycosis fungoides. One year after successful treatment with high-energy electrons, he gradually developed an extensive eruption of 3- to 5-cm oval scaly patches resembling those of pityriasis rosea and parapsoriasis en plaques on the trunk and extremities. Histologic examination of these lesions revealed a mild nonspecific inflammatory reaction without cellular atypia, characteristic of pityriasis rosea or chronic guttate parapsoriasis. After about five months, boggy red plaques with superficial pustules that constantly exuded purulent material arose from these banal-appearing lesions. No bacterial, fungal, or mycobacterial organisms could be identified in or isolated from biopsies of these boggy pustular plaques. Multiple histologic examinations revealed the characteristic features of dermatitis vegetans, and no atypical cells of mycosis fungoides could be found by light and electron microscopy. Except for the pain and swelling associated with the development of these lesions, the patient had no signs or symptoms of a systemic illness. Plate 9 *A, B, C, D, E,* illustrate the spectrum of lesions which were present. Some of the lesions had wide zones of erythema surrounding the boggy plaque, and other lesions were merely reddish brown flat macules. The latter lesions also showed the histologic features of dermatitis vegetans. Although some of the lesions responded to local x-ray irradiation, and a few disappeared spontaneously, new lesions kept developing. A variety of cancer chemotherapeutic agents and dapsone were used, but none was helpful. The only effective therapy proved to be daily intramuscular injections of 20 to 40 units of ACTH gel which completely suppressed the lesions within 12 to 24 hours. High doses of oral prednisone (60 to 100 mg) were ineffective. When the ACTH was discontinued, the lesions reappeared within 24 hours. He was treated with 20 to 40 units of ACTH and 10 mg of prednisone daily for 1½ years. Multiple biopsies of the lesions of dermatitis vegetans, which would reappear whenever the ACTH dose was lowered, failed to reveal histological evidence of mycosis fungoides. The patient eventually died from staphylococcal sepsis and infection with *Candida albicans* in the blood and lungs. At autopsy, there was a histologic infiltrate of mycosis fungoides in the fat and deep dermis underlying one of the suppressed lesions of dermatitis vegetans. Mycosis fungoides was also found in a solitary 1-cm nodule on the trunk which had not been observed during the terminal illness. The lymph nodes were normal. There was no evidence of mycosis fungoides in the viscera.

The adrenal glands were not found at autopsy and were assumed to be completely atrophic. Unfortunately the pituitary gland was not available for study. These findings support the thesis that ACTH is able to exert an anti-inflammatory effect through a nonadrenal pathway.

The eruption of dermatitis vegetans in this patient is believed to have represented an exaggerated hypersensitivity response by the patient to his mycosis fungoides.

The variety of lesions found in mycosis fungoides are illustrated in Figures 2–29 to 2–39 and in Plates 5*D, E, F;* 6*E, F;* 7; 8*A, B, C, D;* and 9*A, B, C, D, E.*

Although mycosis fungoides is basically a disorder of the lymphoreticular system of the skin, visceral and lymph node involvement can be found in 20 to 80 per cent of the autopsies performed on patients with

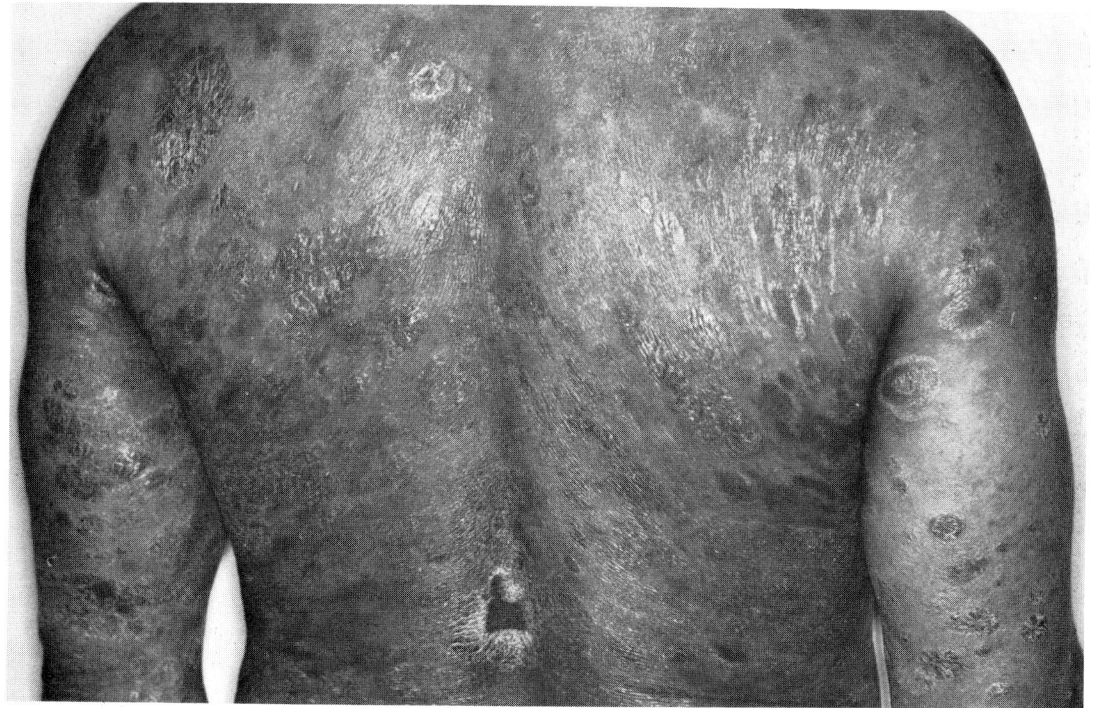

Figure 2–32. Mycosis fungoides. Plaques and eczematous lesions.

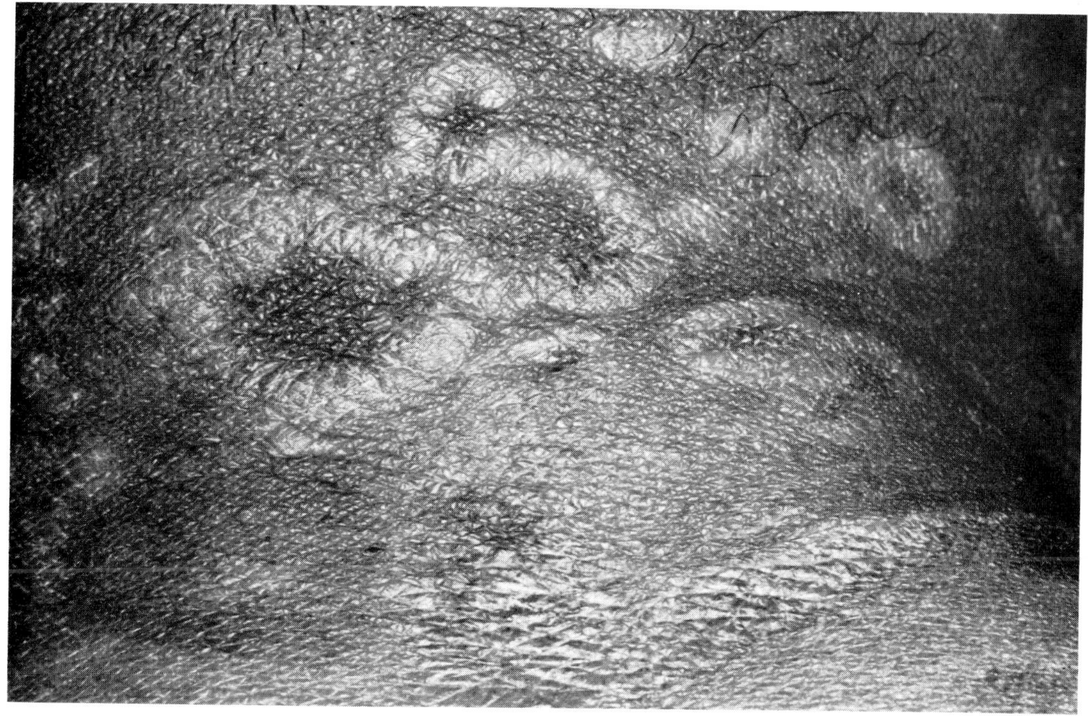

Figure 2–33. Mycosis fungoides. Same patient shown in Figure 2–32. Circinate plaques on neck.

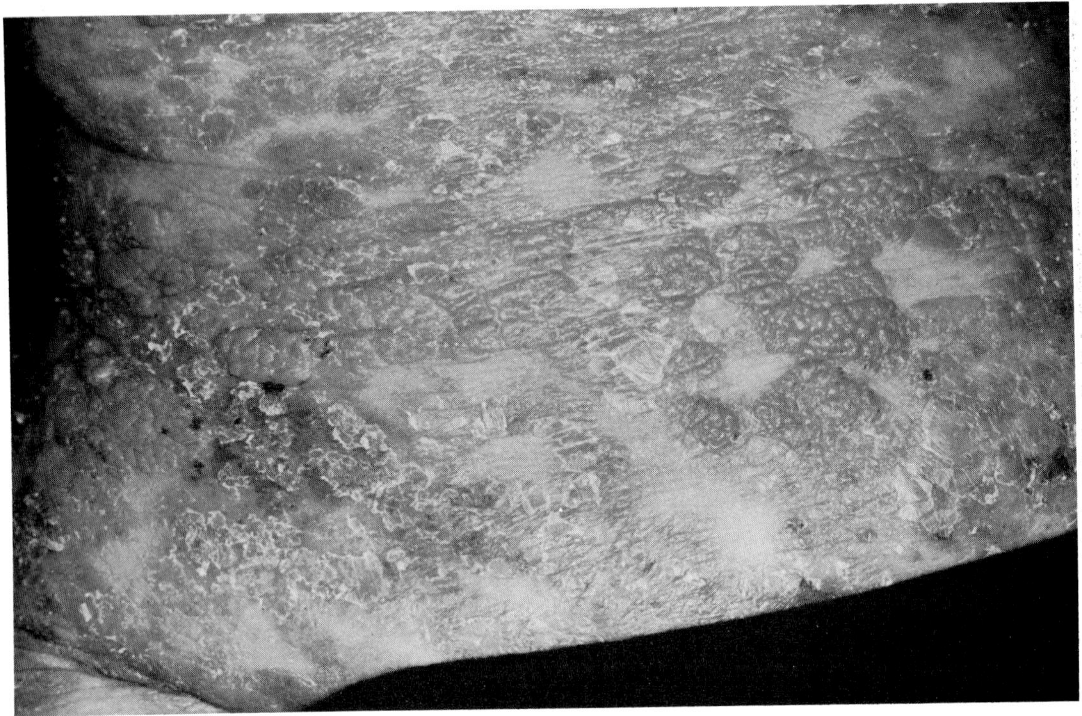

Figure 2–34. Mycosis fungoides. Many plaques have a pebbly surface.

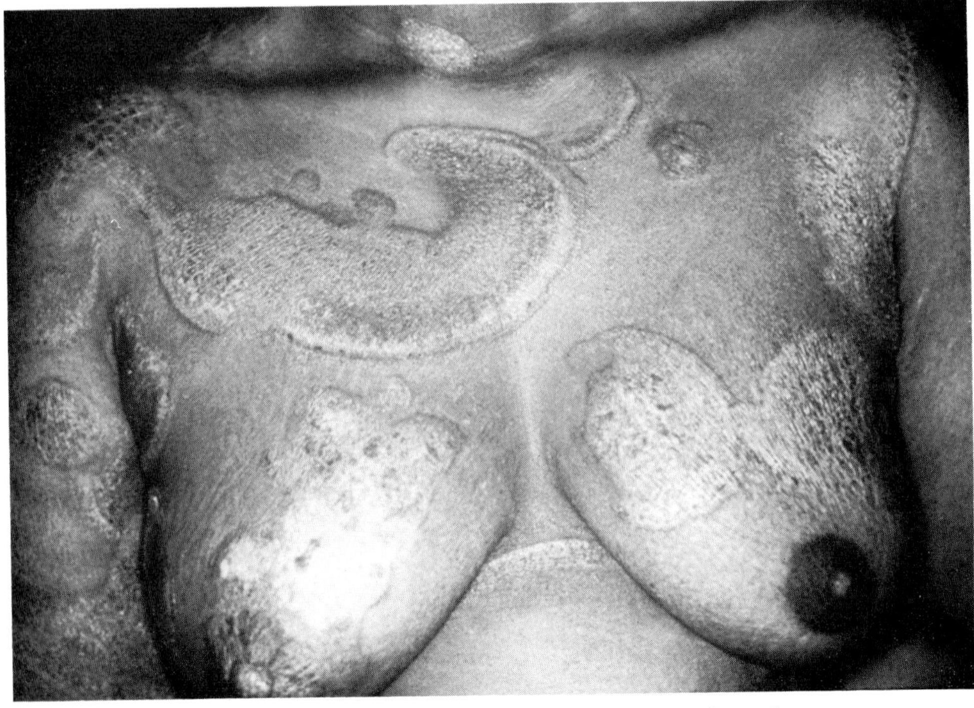

Figure 2–35. Mycosis fungoides. Plaque stage. Note semilunar shape.

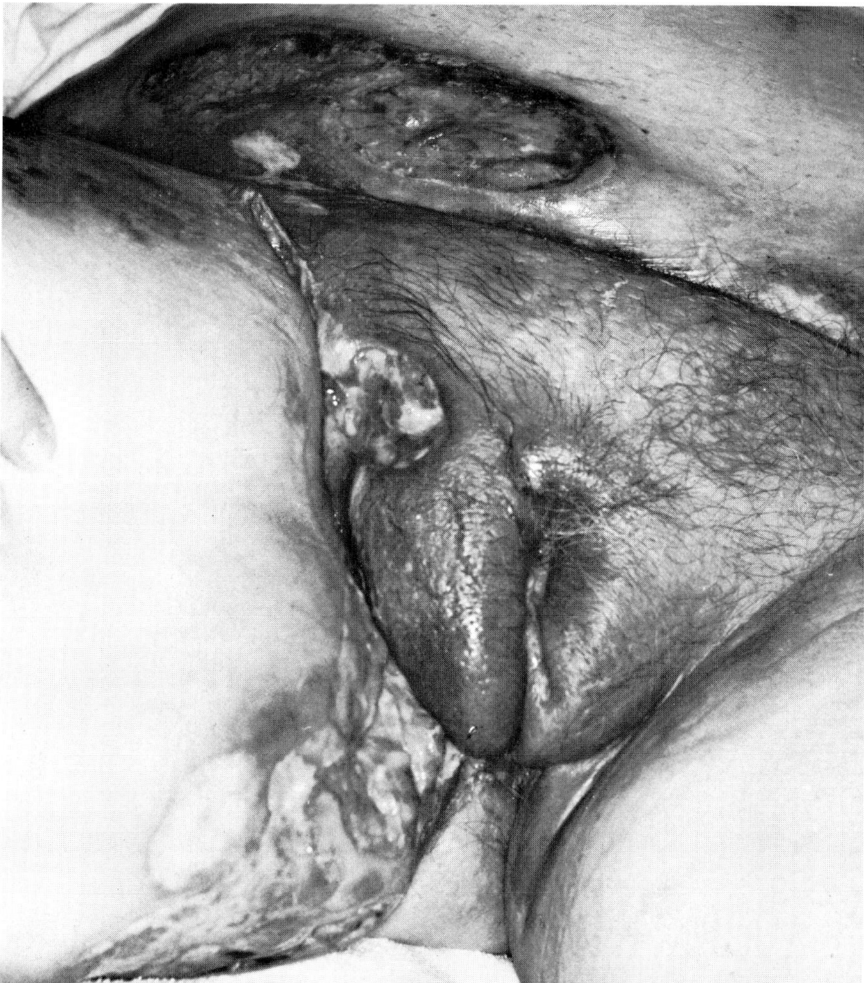

Figure 2–36. Mycosis fungoides. Extensive ulceration in plaques.

mycosis fungoides. In our series of 59 patients, 17 have come to autopsy and nine have had visceral involvement. The cellular infiltration is identical to that seen in the skin and will be described more fully later.

Functional impairment of internal organs is unusual in mycosis fungoides because visceral tumor formation is uncommon. However, there are reports of dysfunctions involving the central nervous system, heart, kidneys, lungs, gastrointestinal tract, and corneas.[86-92] Figure 2–40 is a radiograph of the pulmonary lesions of mycosis fungoides in one of our patients.

Fever is a very unusual manifestation of mycosis fungoides when infection is absent.[93] One of our patients consistently developed temperatures of 101 to 103°F. whenever her disease flared, and another, in association with widespread necrotic tumors and plaques, developed a hectic fever course for the last three weeks of her life. Septicemia was never established in this patient either during her life or at postmortem examination, nor did her fever and toxic state respond to antibiotic therapy. Although infection, often arising in necrotic skin, is the most common cause of death in mycosis fungoides, it is not always possible to

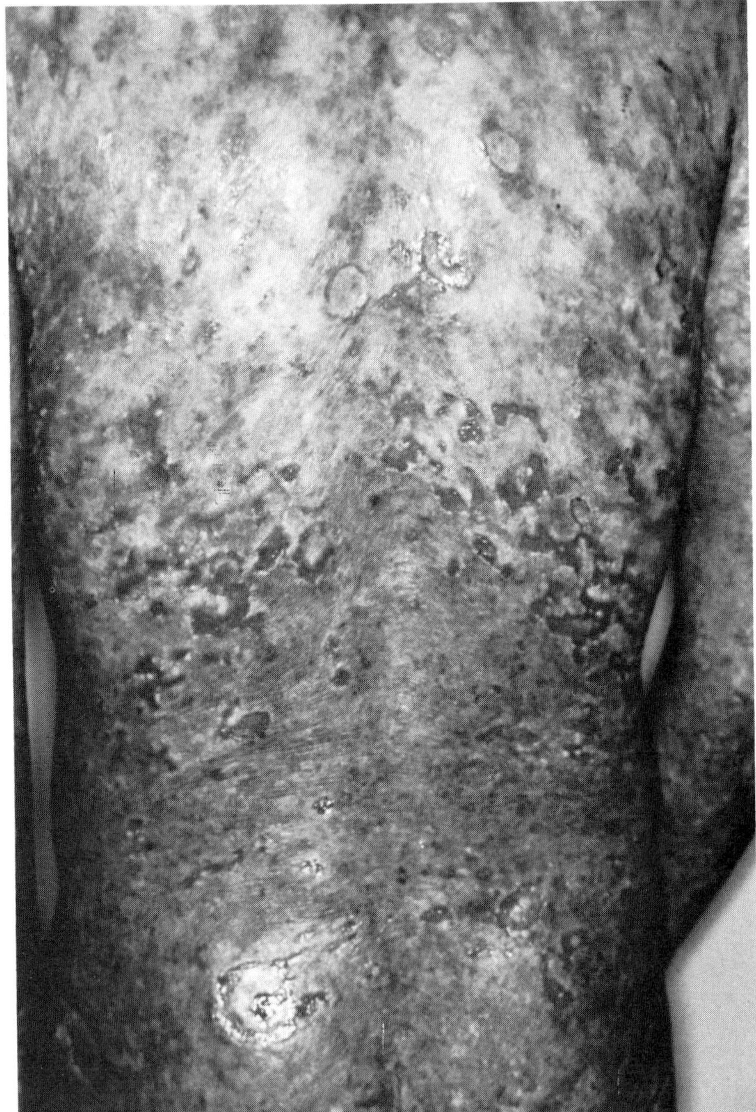

Figure 2–37. Mycosis fungoides. Generalized ulcerations produced by diffuse infiltration of skin with mycosis fungoides.

determine the exact cause of death. In the latter of the two patients just mentioned, the toxemia, fever, and progressive deterioration could have been produced by unidentified factors from the widespread necrosis in the skin. At autopsy, only the skin and superficial lymph nodes were involved by mycosis fungoides; the internal organs and deep nodes were unaffected.

Mycosis fungoides is more common in men and the sex ratio varies from 2:1 to 1.3:1 in different series.[59, 66, 68, 94] Most cases are diagnosed in the fifth and sixth decades, but individuals can develop this disease in their teens. The duration of the illness, measured from its earliest phase, varies from one to more than 48 years. In some instances the disease is fulminant, and death occurs in less than one year. In other cases there can be a mild and protracted course for several decades. The average duration

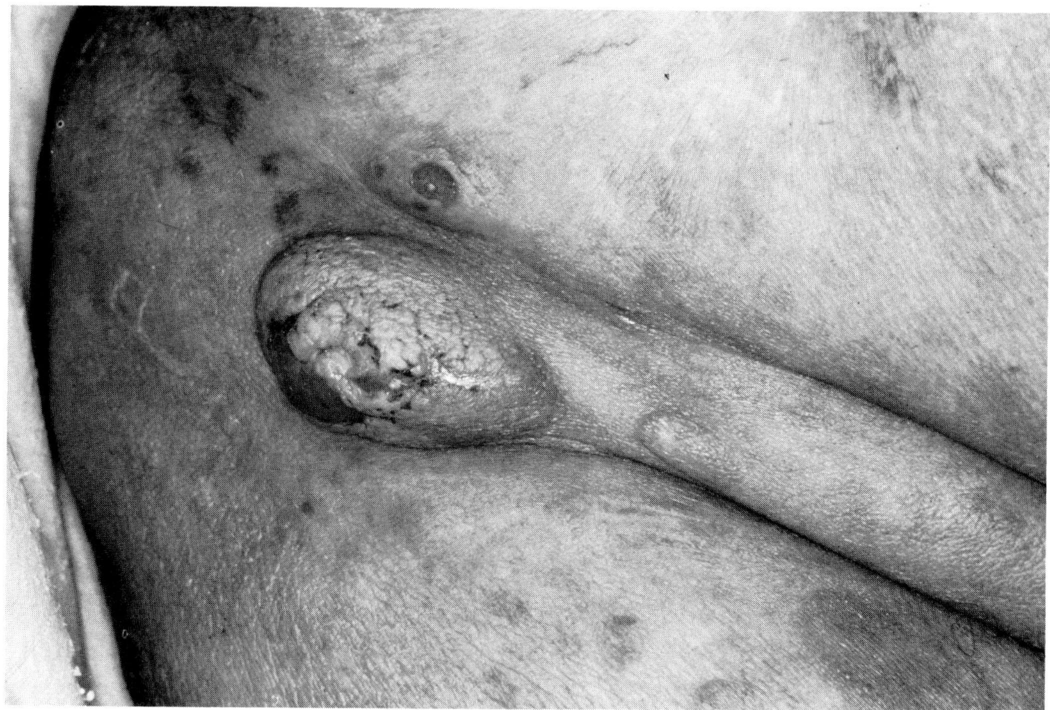

Figure 2–38. Mycosis fungoides. Plaques, ulcerated plaques, and tumors.

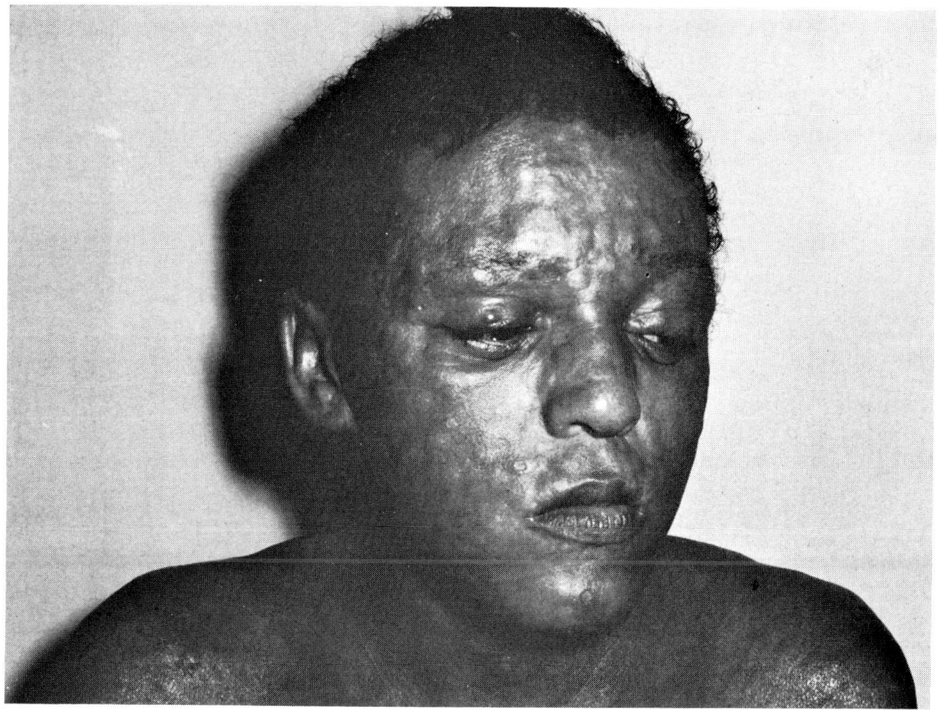

Figure 2–39. Mycosis fungoides. Tumors producing early stage of leonine facies.

of the disease is 8 to 12 years, but following the appearance of tumors, the survival time is less than three years.

The recent analysis by Epstein et al. of 144 patients from the National Institutes of Health provides us with more precise information about prognosis.[68] The development of lymphadenopathy, tumors, or cutaneous ulceration during the course of the disease indicates that the median survival time from the point at which diagnosis has been made by skin biopsy is approximately four years (0.1 to 48.3 years, average six years). Table 2–2 summarizes these important indicators as determined by analysis of the graphs in their paper. Their data emphasize the following points. No patient died of mycosis fungoides without first developing one of these three major prognostic signs. Irrespective of the order in which these signs developed, the appearance of the third was associated with a median survival time of one year. Of 35 patients who were initially seen at the National Institutes of Health and who did not have tumors, ulcers, or palpably enlarged lymph nodes, 80 per cent died or eventually developed one of these signs of progressive disease by the time of their report. The type of therapy initially administered to these patients did not affect survival, nor was the response or lack of response to any therapy associated with a longer survival. In addition, no prediction regarding survival could be made on the basis of the patient's sex, race, duration of lesions before biopsy diagnosis, age at onset of lesions, or type of lesion

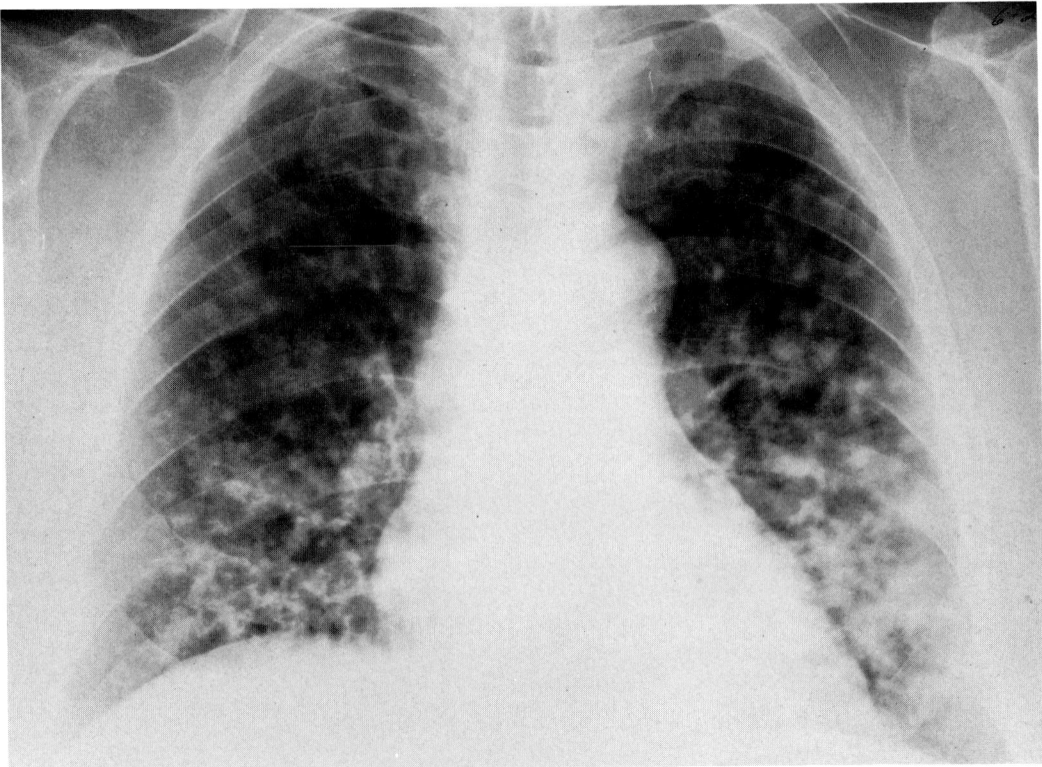

Figure 2–40. Mycosis fungoides. Radiograph of chest showing pulmonary involvement by mycosis fungoides in one of our patients.

Table 2–2. MYCOSIS FUNGOIDES—SURVIVAL STATISTICS*

Prognostic Indicator	Survival Time for 50% of Patients	Survival Time for 30% of Patients
After initial diagnostic biopsy	4 yr	9 yr
Older than 60 years when diagnosed	3.5 yr	–†
Younger than 51 years when diagnosed	6.5 yr	–
Signs at time of diagnostic biopsy:		
Absence of nodes, tumors and ulcers	5 yr	–
Presence of only one sign	4 yr	–
Presence of two or three signs	2.5 yr	–
Appearance at any time in course of disease:		
Tumors or palpable nodes	2.5 yr	5 yr
Development of third sign	1 yr	2.5 yr
After lymph node biopsy:		
Diagnosis of dermatopathic node	34 months	–
Diagnosis of mycosis fungoides node	18 months	–
Clinically recognized hepatomegaly or splenomegaly	3 months	–

*From Epstein, E. H., Jr., Levin, D. L., Croft, J. D., Jr., and Lutzner, M. A.: Mycosis fungoides. Survival, prognostic features, response to therapy, and autopsy findings. Medicine, *51*:61, 1972.

†(—) indicates information not available.

noted at the onset of disease. Dr. Steven Cohen analyzed the data in our 59 patients in an identical fashion and found identical survival curves.[94] Our series is composed almost completely of previously untreated patients who came from the New Haven area or State of Connecticut and were either diagnosed at Yale or referred here shortly after diagnosis elsewhere. Most of these individuals have been closely followed since the earliest manifestations of their illness, whether in the premycotic or mycotic stages. Our study confirms the findings of Epstein et al., whose series was made up predominantly of patients with more extensive disease who had been referred to the National Institutes of Health for consultation after the onset of skin lesions (average 7.3 years) and after biopsy diagnosis (average 1.2 years). The series from Stanford University reported by Fuks et al. also demonstrated similar time courses for these prognostic factors.[95]

It is important to take note of those patients with mycosis fungoides whose disease runs a benign and mild course in the absence of any significant therapy, because they may represent a subset of individuals who eventually undergo spontaneous remissions or are able to control their disease through as-yet-undetermined mechanisms related to host resistance. If one does not recognize the existence of such patients, one may claim therapeutic success where no such claim is warranted. Epstein et al. noted that three of 35 individuals in their series had not developed any of the three prognostic signs of progressive disease and were in apparent remission from 3.4 to 5.5 years after biopsy diagnosis. The three had entered remissions either spontaneously or following what was considered to be "mild" treatment. There were no clinical or histological features at the time of biopsy diagnosis which distinguished these three patients from those who did not achieve unmaintained remissions. Review of the original skin in these patients confirmed the diagnosis of mycosis fungoides. A fourth patient was initially placed in this group also, but on reviewing the original biopsy a definite diagnosis could not be made histologically. It is likely that the 66-year-old woman cited on page 144 entered a spontaneous remission because of the long interval of six months between the completion of electron beam therapy and the disappearance of her signs and symptoms. In the Stanford series 14 of 132 patients treated by electron beam therapy have had disease-free intervals of three to 14 years.[95] However, one should maintain an open and objective viewpoint about therapeutic responses in this disease, because although our current therapies have made patients symptom-free for longer periods than formerly, there is no unequivocal evidence that they have increased survival time.

Patients with mycosis fungoides who have primarily the poikiloderma-parapsoriasis lesions have not been studied as a subset with regard to their prognosis. One does not know whether their survival times differ from those individuals who have eczema, plaques, and tumors, once the histologic changes of mycosis fungoides appear in their poikilodermatous lesions. The poikiloderma-parapsoriasis lesions represent a stage of pre–mycosis fungoides, which can persist for as long as 35 years.

The histopathology of mycosis fungoides is distinctive. In the premycotic stage, a banal inflammatory infiltrate of lymphocytes and histiocytes, present perivascularly in the mid-dermis and the upper dermis, conforms to a histologic diagnosis of a chronic nonspecific dermatitis.

In the plaque stage, the histologic features become pathognomonic of the disease. The infiltrate is heavier; it consists of mature lymphocytes, histiocytes, plasma cells, eosinophils, and polymorphonuclear leukocytes; and it forms a dense band in the upper dermis. This layer of polymorphous cells presses against the epidermis and obliterates the narrow zone of normal collagen (grenz zone) which ordinarily separates the epidermis from dermal inflammatory and infiltrative processes. Within the polymorphous infiltrate, one finds a spectrum of atypical lymphoid cells with irregularly shaped nuclei that frequently exhibit deep folds. These atypical lymphoid cells correspond cytologically most closely to what had been called the differentiated histiocytic cell of reticulum cell sarcoma. Some of the cells were indistinguishable from the reticulum cells of "reticulum cell" sarcoma. However, current studies, to be discussed later, have indicated that the abnormal cells belong to the lymphocytic rather than the histiocytic system of cells. In addition to this predominant atypical lymphoid population, a miniority of so-called *mycosis cells* can be found. They differ from the majority of the abnormal cells by having a nucleus that is more irregularly shaped and indented and more deeply stained. The size of the nucleus is usually larger than in other atypical cells, but some mycosis cells may have small nuclei. The atypical lymphoid cells may also form multinucleated cells. The mycosis cells are not pathognomonic of the disease as Sternberg-Reed cells are for Hodgkin's disease. Small foci of these abnormal lymphoid cells are usually present within the epidermis (Pautrier's microabscesses). The epidermis is thickened in response to the dermal infiltrate.

In the tumor phase, the polymorphous band no longer confines itself to the upper dermis but invades the entire dermis and the subcutaneous layer. The atypical lymphoid cells increase in number and sometimes produce a monomorphous collection of cells. In most cases, however, the mass of atypical cells continues to be associated with mature lymphocytes, eosinophils, histiocytes, plasma cells, and polymorphonuclear leukocytes. In those instances when the histologic appearance of a tumor is truly monomorphous, one can sometimes find the characteristic polymorphous infiltrate in an adjacent field.[96] An extensive plasma cell infiltration can also be a histologic feature of mycosis fungoides.[69] The atypical lymphoid cells in mycosis fungoides are not as malignant-appearing as are the cells of histiocytic lymphoma, lymphocytic lymphoma, or the Sternberg-Reed cells of Hodgkin's disease.

The histopathology of mycosis fungoides differs from that of the monomorphous lymphomas and Hodgkin's disease in the following ways. (1) The dermal and subcutaneous tumor masses of malignant lymphoma result in pressure atrophy rather than in acanthosis of the epidermis. (2) A grenz zone is almost always present between the epidermis and the dermal infiltrate of lymphoma. (3) A band of infiltrate confined to the upper dermis is not seen with lymphomas. (4) The *mycosis cells* are distinct from the Sternberg-Reed cells. (5) Gross tumors in visceral organs are characteristic of lymphoma but are uncommon in mycosis fungoides. When visceral involvement occurs, the cellular infiltrate is polymorphous, as it is in the skin.

The clinical and histopathologic features of mycosis fungoides are clearly distinct from those of the monomorphous lymphomas and Hodgkin's disease. Although there has been controversy in the past over whether mycosis fungoides was a clinical and pathologic entity[60, 62] and whether it eventually terminated in lymphocytic or histiocytic lymphoma or Hodgkin's disease,[66] this is no longer at issue. The earlier studies of Rappaport[97] and Allen,[69] which showed this transition to be rare, have been amplified and corroborated by more recent ones.[98, 99] The confusion had stemmed from the inclusion of cases of malignant lymphoma in series dealing with mycosis fungoides and from the misinterpretation of the reactive alterations in the lymph nodes and viscera as representing lymphoma. The large series reported by Block et al.,[65] included in the series of Epstein et al.,[68] is an example of the problem that was encountered in the interpretation of involved lymph nodes and viscera in mycosis fungoides. These workers had stated:

> Once visceral metastases have occurred, histopathologic examination of these metastases shows morphologic changes that can be identified as malignant lymphoma, but often cannot be classified further. However, the cutaneous histopathology characteristically remains unchanged and permits the diagnosis of mycosis fungoides.

In Block's series there obviously was a preponderance of atypical lymphoreticular cells in the viscera and nodes, but the criteria for a definitive diagnosis of reticulum cell sarcoma, lymphosarcoma, or Hodgkin's disease were lacking. Rappaport and Thomas recently reviewed the tissue sections from the series of Block et al. and found the histologic changes in the viscera to be those of mycosis fungoides rather than of lymphoma.[98]

Reed and Cummings also settled the question about the histologic identity of mycosis fungoides.[67] They reviewed the tissues of 72 patients who had been diagnosed clinically as having either mycosis fungoides, exfoliative dermatitis, or lymphoma cutis. The tissue sections were studied without knowledge of the clinical findings. They were able to divide the specimens into four histologic groups: 47 showed chronic nonspecific dermatitis, 11 had changes which they called hyperplastic reticulosis and malignant reticulosis *in situ*, and 14 had reticulum cell sarcoma. On clinicopathologic correlation, all of the patients with a tissue diagnosis of hyperplastic reticulosis and malignant reticulosis in situ (identical to the histopathology of mycosis fungoides just described) had either the Alibert-Bazin (three-stage sequence) or the erythrodermic form of mycosis fungoides.

Reed and Cummings also described four cases of lymphoma of several years' duration presenting with erythroderma and nonspecific cutaneous changes, thereby reemphasizing the point that occasionally lymphoma can have a long course and can clinically mimic mycosis fungoides but that a biopsy will establish the correct diagnosis.

Reed and Cummings further reported that only one of 11 cases of mycosis fungoides evolved into a reticulum cell sarcoma.[67] In our series, none of the 17 cases examined at autopsy had been found to have a lymphoma. Now that the histologic criteria for diagnosing mycosis fungoides in skin and viscera are fairly well established and accepted, future prospective studies will be able to determine whether mycosis fungoides evolves into malignant lymphoma. The current evidence indicates that this phenomenon must be exceedingly rare if it does occur.

If mycosis fungoides were the cutaneous manifestation of a lymphoma, one should expect to find clinical and histological evidence of mycosis fungoides after the diagnosis of lymphoma has been made, but this has never been observed. There no longer can be any question that mycosis fungoides is a clinical and histologic entity.

Sézary Syndrome

Although the Sézary syndrome was believed at first to be an independent entity, the available evidence now indicates that, with infrequent exceptions, it is merely one of the many manifestations of mycosis fungoides. In a rare instance there may be an underlying monomorphous lymphoma.[100]

The classic description of Sézary syndrome consists of generalized pruritus, exfoliative dermatitis with edema and thickening of the skin, ectropion, leonine facies, alopecia, dystrophic nails, keratoderma of the palms and soles, and lymphadenopathy associated with leukocytosis and abnormal mononuclear cells. In some cases, however, there is simply patchy to universal erythema over the body with redness, fissuring, and mild thickening of the palms and soles. Alopecia and leonine facies may be absent and ectropion minimal. It is not unusual in my experience to see the erythema wax and wane during the course of the day as well as over the course of weeks, without any detectable change in the histological pattern of cutaneous involvement. The cutaneous features of the Sézary syndrome form a spectrum which is indistinguishable from that seen in the erythrodermic form of mycosis fungoides. The published histopathologic descriptions of the erythroderma are those of mycosis fungoides.[101–105] Leukocytosis or circulating abnormal mononuclear cells or both have been found in as many as 20 per cent of patients with mycosis fungoides, the majority of whom did not have erythroderma.[65, 66, 105] In blood smears, the Sézary cell appears as a mononuclear cell with a grooved nucleus and cytoplasmic vacuoles which often can be stained by periodic acid–Schiff reagent.[102, 105, 107] Glycogen is responsible for the staining in some, but not in all, of the vacuoles. Sézary cells exist as small and large cell variants, with the smaller cell measuring about 8 μm and the larger one, 15 to 20 μm in diameter.[108]

The immediate source of the circulating abnormal cells is thought to be the skin, since they cannot be demonstrated in abnormal amounts in bone marrow; moreover, they have been observed to disappear when the skin lesions resolve.[109] In one of our patients, shown in Plate 7*E* and *F*, leukocytosis and abnormal cells disappeared after the skin was treated successfully with electron-beam therapy.

Lutzner compared the ultrastructure of the abnormal cells in the skin, lymph nodes, and peripheral blood of patients with the Sézary syndrome and mycosis fungoides and found that the cells were similar. This is another bit of evidence supporting the identity of the Sézary syndrome and mycosis fungoides.[110]

The case history of Walter B. Cannon, the famous American physiologist, also is pertinent.[109] Dr. Cannon had mycosis fungoides for 14 years. Eight years before he died, he entered the erythrodermic phase (l'homme rouge), which was accompanied by a leukocytosis of 32,000 with 80 per cent circulating atypical lymphocytes. This "leukemic" phase, as it was called then, subsided after four years coincident with

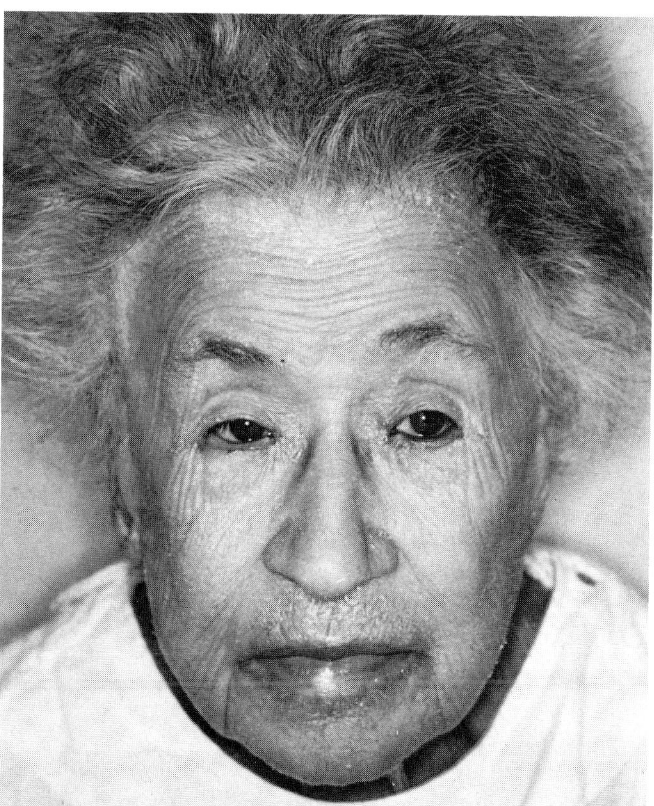

Figure 2–41. Sézary syndrome. Erythroderma with ectropion formation.

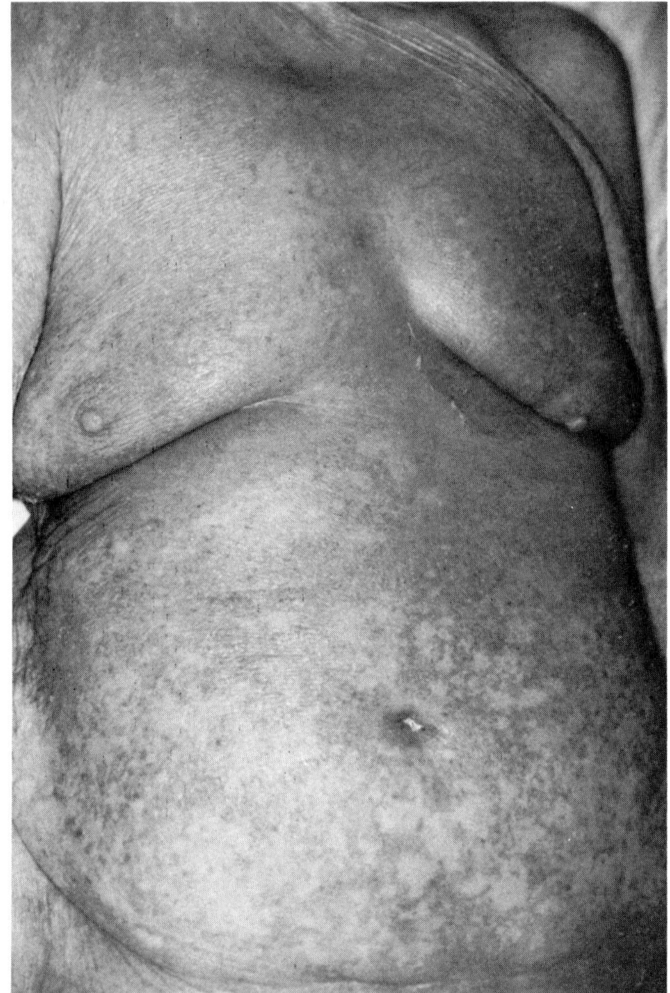

Figure 2–42. Sézary syndrome. Erythroderma of trunk. Same patient as in Figure 2–41.

spontaneous regression of the erythroderma. Dr. Cannon died four years later of bronchopneumonia. Courses similar to those of Dr. Cannon's have now been observed by Lutzner et al.[108] and ourselves. Figures 2–41 to 2–43 illustrate the appearance of one of our patients with mycosis fungoides that presented as a typical Sézary syndrome which was kept under control with prednisone and chlorambucil for three years, only to relapse with plaques and tumors one year before she died of progressive disease. The evidence to date indicates that the Sézary syndrome is the leukemic phase of mycosis fungoides.

RECENT ADVANCES

Major insights into the nature of mycosis fungoides have occurred since 1968. As discussed earlier, Rappaport and Thomas[98] reviewed the autopsy material from 45 patients with mycosis fungoides and demonstrated unequivocally that mycosis fungoides does not evolve into a malignant lymphoma but is a disease *sui generis* during its entire course.

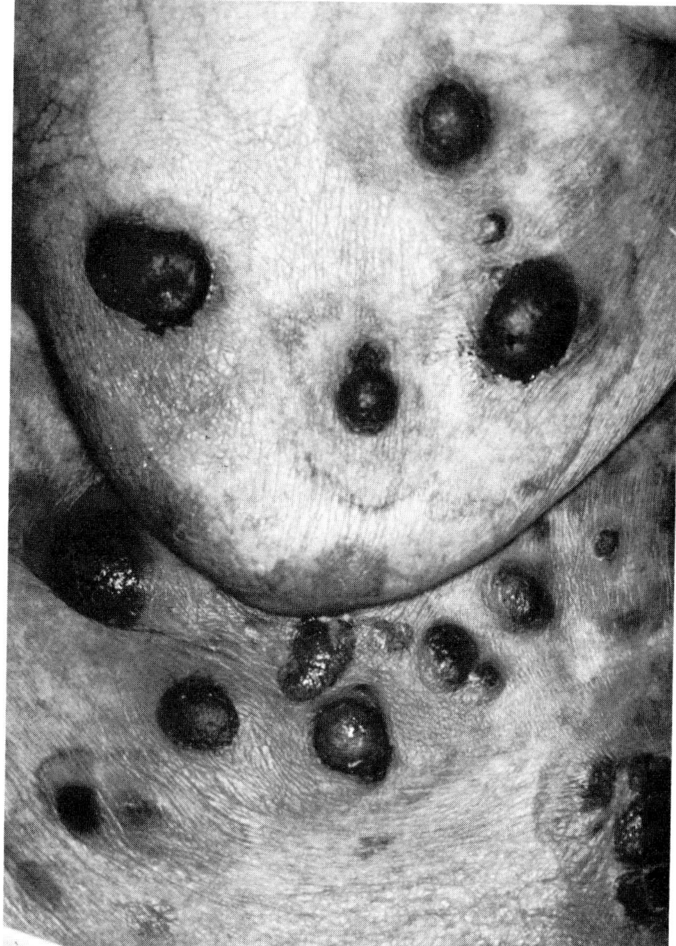

Figure 2–43. Sézary syndrome. Same patient as in Figures 2–41 and 2–42. Erythroderma disappeared and was replaced by plaques and tumors one year before she died.

Microscopic involvement of internal viscera with the same polymorphous infiltrate as occurs in the skin was found in the majority of autopsied cases, but gross tumor nodules were rare. They also showed that the disease initially is confined to the skin and that involvement of regional lymph nodes was associated with internal organ involvement in the majority of cases. The skin appears to be the main barrier to the disease and not the regional lymph nodes. Rappaport and co-workers also showed that so-called "dermatopathic" lymph nodes in mycosis fungoides are associated with visceral involvement. Epstein et al. had demonstrated that lymphadenopathy in mycosis fungoides, whether "dermatopathic" or histologically diagnostic of mycosis fungoides, had a similar poor prognosis.[68]

Lutzner and Jordan showed that the Sézary cell had a deeply convoluted and cerebriform-appearing nucleus which appeared serpentine in electron microscopic sections.[110] Subsequently, identical-appearing cells were found in the lymph nodes in Sézary's syndrome and in the skin lesions of mycosis fungoides. The "mycosis" cell with its irregular nucleus had the same ultrastructural features as the Sézary cell.[111] Because of this unique ultrastructure, the Sézary cell and "mycosis" cell were believed to be diagnostic of mycosis fungoides. However, similar-appearing individual cells were subsequently found in benign conditions such as lichen planus, psoriasis, lupus erythematosus, vasculitis, and actinic keratosis.[111, 112] Yeckley et al. demonstrated that normal human lymphocytes transformed by pokeweed mitogen and phytohemagglutinin develop cerebriform nuclei resembling Sézary cells.[113] Nevertheless, Rappaport and his co-workers showed that although individual Sézary-like cells may not be diagnostic of mycosis fungoides, their presence in sheets and clusters within tissues does make them diagnostic.[98, 114]

The Sézary cell as well as the cells present in the skin lesions of mycosis fungoides form rosettes with sheep red blood cells.[22, 115, 116] Because they also lack the surface cell markers of B cells, they have been placed in the class of T lymphocytes. They are not histiocytes because they are nonadhesive and nonphagocytic.[116] Broder et al. demonstrated that circulating Sézary cells can function as helper T cells. Suppressor T cell function could not be elicited.[117] Although the Sézary cell appears to be lymphocytic, it contains a prominent network of cytoplasmic filaments 7.5 to 8 nm in diameter which are not found in normal lymphocytes but have been seen in peritoneal macrophages, other neoplastic cells, and occasional thoracic duct lymphocytes.[116] Sézary cells cannot be distinguished morphologically from those of chronic lymphatic leukemia by scanning electron microscopic techniques.[118]

The Sézary cell and the similar appearing cells in the skin lesions of mycosis fungoides have been assumed by most workers to be the malignant cells in this disease on the basis of the following criteria: they are present in the skin lesions and viscera; they have abnormal numbers of chromosomes and abnormal karyotypes including marker chromosomes;[119-122] and in individual patients, the same abnormal karyotype has been found in skin lesions, lymph nodes, peripheral blood, spleen, and bone marrow for periods up to 18 months,[119] supporting the concept that a single clone of cells, arising in an as-yet-undetermined site, has spread to involve all of the affected organs.

On the basis of the above studies, it is highly probable but not rigorously proven that the chromosomal abnormalities observed are those of the Sézary and "mycosis" cells. It is also likely, but not proven, that these cells are the malignant elements in this disease. Although similar appearing cells can be found in benign inflammatory disorders and in mitogen-stimulated lymphocyte cultures, such cells have not been studied for their chromosomal characteristics or DNA content as have the cells in mycosis fungoides, so that one does not know how closely they are related to the Sézary and "mycosis" cells.

Exploiting the abnormality of chromosomal numbers in "mycosis" cells, Van Vloten et al. measured the distribution of DNA content in cell imprints from cutaneous lesions of mycosis fungoides, suspected pre–mycosis fungoides lesions such as erythroderma and parapsoriasis en plaques, and benign lesions such as psoriasis, lichen planus, and dermatitis.[123] Employing the technique of Feulgen-DNA cytophotometry, they were able to differentiate mycosis fungoides from benign skin lesions and to predict the eventual appearance of mycosis fungoides within a year in six of eight patients with suspected premycotic lesions. The cells in the other seven patients of this group had a normal distribution curve of DNA content, and these individuals were still well at the time of the report two and one-half years after the measurements were made.

The histogenesis and site of origin of the Sézary and mycosis cells have not been determined. However, the cells home to the dermis and exhibit tropism for the epidermis. Edelson et al. demonstrated there was a flux between the skin and peripheral blood in patients with the Sézary syndrome. By employing leukapheresis, they were able to cause cutaneous tumors to disappear by lowering the level of circulating leukocytes that were composed predominantly of Sézary cells.[124] Discontinuation of the leukapheresis was followed by the reappearance of erythroderma which once again improved after a second leukapheresis. In one of their patients, there was a spontaneous fluctuation in circulating Sézary cells. Whenever the number of cells increased, the skin lesions improved, and when they decreased the skin lesions recurred.[39] It has been established that the bone marrow is not the site of replication of these cells.

Levels of B and T cells in the peripheral blood of patients with Sézary syndrome and mycosis fungoides have been measured in several series.[39, 116, 125, 126] Although determinations have not been performed serially in individual patients, the results from these studies indicate that the levels of B and T cells are normal in the early stages of the disease, but both elements may be depressed in the advanced phase with a concomitant increase in the level of null cells (lymphocytes without markers for either B or T cells). Skin tests for recall antigens, induction of contact sensitivity to dinitrochlorobenzene (DNCB), and humoral antibody formation are usually normal early in the disease,[124] but in the late stages there may be impairment of cell-mediated hypersensitivity. In one patient with mycosis fungoides, the level of circulating T cells returned to normal following successful treatment.[126] Phytohemagglutinin stimulation of blood lymphocytes appears to yield a normal response in the early stages of mycosis fungoides, but may show inhibition in the tumor stage of the disease.[127] Although the serum levels of immunoglobulins G, M, and A have generally been normal, IgE has been found to be markedly elevated in some, but not in all series of patients with mycosis fungoides.[128-130]

The mixed lymphocyte reaction may be impaired in the Sézary syndrome and mycosis fungoides. It appears to be caused by an intrinsic but as yet unidentified defect in the lymphocytes of these patients.[39] In addition, patients with Sézary syndrome have been shown to contain a migration inhibitory factor (MIF)-like substance in their sera. Paradoxically, the peripheral lymphocytes in most of these patients fail to liberate MIF *in vitro* after appropriate stimulation.[131] However, the MIF-like material produced erythema and induration when injected intradermally into guinea pigs. Yoshida et al. speculated that the same MIF-like material was responsible for producing the erythroderma in Sézary's syndrome.[131]

What is the nature of mycosis fungoides? There are two hypotheses which seem equally probable to me. There is certainly a progressive proliferation of cutaneous lymphoreticular tissue in association with a polymorphous mature cell infiltrate. The polymorphous infiltrate could represent host defense against a low-grade neoplasm of lymphoreticular tissue represented by the atypical lymphoid cells. In the premycotic phase, the defense reaction is so effective that these abnormal cells cannot be found by light microscopy, and the disease cannot be diagnosed histologically. In the plaque and tumor stages, the cells become more numerous and obvious as host resistance begins to wane.

In most patients, host resistance eventually breaks down and the abnormal lymphoid cells proliferate to form tumors which had been previously erroneously diagnosed as some form of malignant lymphoma in 10 to 30 per cent of cases.[66] This is a current popular view, and because of the tumor formation, mycosis fungoides is considered as a special type of lymphoma of the skin.

Dr. Stephen Rothman believed that the pruritus associated with the first two stages of the disease was a symptom of host defense and that its diminution in the third stage correlated with the ability of the abnormal cells to proliferate and form tumors.

A second hypothesis for the pathogenesis of mycosis fungoides includes a two-stage process. The polymorphous cellular proliferation could represent one aspect of the immune response against unknown stimuli, infectious or otherwise. At first, chronic antigenic stimulation produces a benign proliferation of lymphoid cells. Later, these chronically stimulated cells appear atypical and eventually become malignant, proliferating freely in the skin to produce tumors. If the stimulation were active for a sufficient length of time, the lymphoreticular tissues of the internal organs might also react to produce visceral mycosis fungoides. However, an alternate possibility, based upon recent morphological and cytogenetic studies is more likely: there is lymphatic and hematogenous spread of the atypical cells from the skin to the regional and internal lymph nodes and viscera to account for the generalized involvement observed in the late stages of the disease.[120]

Experimental evidence supports the concept of a benign proliferation of lymphoreticular tissue undergoing neoplastic change. Metcalf produced reticulum cell sarcoma and plasma cell tumors in mice by repeatedly injecting them with bovine serum albumin or *Salmonella adelaide* vaccine.[132] Schwartz and Beldotti demonstrated that when mice were subjected to a graft-versus-host reaction, the spleen cells of the host underwent neoplastic transformation and produced a transplantable tumor with histologic changes that resembled reticulum cell sarcoma or Hodgkin's disease.[133] Walford made similar observations.[134] The continuous or repetitive exposure of lymphoid tissue to antigens could result in a sustained cellular proliferative response which would culminate in neoplasia. Fialkow has called this process *immunologic oncogenesis*.[135] Schwartz and colleagues have postulated that the immunostimulation may have activated latent oncogenic viruses that transformed the lymphoid cells into malignant elements.[136]

Recent clinical observations provide additional support to the concept of immunologic oncogenesis: the delineation of diseases such as immunoblastic lymphadenopathy, pseudolymphoma syndrome caused by Dilantin, and the lymphomatous diseases appearing in immunosuppressed renal transplant patients; the finding of elevated serum levels of IgE in the absence of other immunoglobulin increases in mycosis fungoides; and the observation that Sézary cells are related to T lymphocytes and can function as T helper cells *in vitro,* enabling B cells from hypogammaglobulinemic patients to produce immunoglobulins.

Schuppli also has proposed recently that mycosis fungoides is a disease related to chronic antigenic stimulation. Many of his patients developed marked contact sensitivity to nickel, chromium, paraphenylenediamine, and other allergens.[137] Tan et al. have viewed mycosis fungoides as being a disease of antigen persistence because of elevated serum levels of IgE, absence of immune depression, and the presence of autoantibodies to gastric parietal cells, thyroid tissue, and smooth muscle and antinuclear antibodies in 14 of 23 patients.[128] Dr. Steven Cohen in our department found that in our series of 59 patients, employment in manufacturing or construction industries was attended by a significant risk factor for developing mycosis fungoides (relative risk = 4.3, p value = 0.02).[94] Occupations included machinists, construction workers, foundry operators, hatters, and industrial electricians. Dr. Mark Greene of the National Cancer Institute independently discovered that the manufacturing and petrochemical industries were the most frequent occupations in his survey of 211 patients with mycosis fungoides. Twenty-nine per cent of these individuals were engaged in work situations in which they were exposed to petroleum products and metals.[138] An additional hazard to machinists has been uncovered by Fan et al., who found extremely high levels of the carcinogen N-nitrosodiethanolamine in several brands of synthetic cutting fluids to which such workers may be exposed.[139] The frequent finding of eczematous eruptions as premycotic lesions is consistent with the concept of chronic antigenic stimulation as an underlying mechanism in mycosis fungoides. Rowden and Lewis have related this concept to the recent developments in the biology of the Langerhans cell.[140]

Epidermotropism of the atypical lymphoid cells in mycosis fungoides is a striking feature of the disease. Rowden and Lewis have proposed that the Langerhans cell system may play an important role in this phenomenon and in the pathogenesis of mycosis fungoides.[140] The Langerhans cells constitute a dendritic cell population within the epidermis and are easily identified with the electron microscope by their cytoplasmic "racquet"-shaped granules. Silverberg et al. have shown that these cells can pick up and transport cutaneously applied antigen to the regional lymph nodes.[141, 142] In guinea pigs passively sensitized to DNCB, a challenge application of this chemical on the skin is followed by the detection of Langerhans cells within dermal lymphatics and the apposition of mononuclear cells resembling lymphocytes to Langerhans cells in the dermis. In man and guinea pigs actively sensitized against contact allergens, Langerhans cells and similar appearing mononuclear cells are found in apposition within the epidermis. In addition one may observe signs of damage to the Langerhans cells. The Langerhans cell has been shown to carry Ia (immune response–associated) antigens on its surface, as well as receptors for Fc and C3.[143-146] These three surface markers are characteristic of macrophages. The Langerhans cells may perform functions similar to those of the monocyte-macrophage system, both by initiating the immune response to external antigens and by facilitating an enhanced reaction in the secondary response. The Langerhans cells may represent the most peripheral outpost of the afferent limb of the immune system.

Rowden and Lewis noted that the atypical lymphoid cells in mycosis fungoides were frequently in close association with epidermal Langerhans cells, many of which showed ultrastructural changes suggestive of cytotoxic damage.[140] They proposed that mycosis fungoides may develop after chronic exposure to a variety of contact allergens. The Langerhans cell would trap the antigen, transport it to the regional lymph nodes where they would initiate the primary immune response, and induce the formation of specifically sensitized lymphocytes. These transformed cells would then home to sites of initial antigen fixation in the epidermis. Their accumulation in the epidermis would produce the Pautrier microabscess where through direct contact or secretion of lymphokines they could produce various degrees of specific and nonspecific damage to Langerhans cells and surrounding keratinocytes. The persistence of antigen for the presumedly necessary chronic stimulation of the immune system might be the result of chronic environmental exposure or from failure of the Langerhans cell in certain individuals to rid itself of the antigens on its surface, or both.

It is humbling to note that the hypothesis about mycosis fungoides proposed by the eminent physicians who prepared the case report of Dr. Walter B. Cannon in 1955 (p. 159) is identical to the current leading proposal:

> On the basis of this material [clinical features and autopsy findings] it seems a legitimate speculation that mycosis fungoides should not be considered a neoplasm but a reaction (to agents unknown) which like other known premalignant processes leads to development of neoplastic properties in responsive cells.

A pathogenesis for Hodgkin's disease can be similarly postulated. The immunologic defect in Hodgkin's disease selectively affects cell-mediated immunity, thereby placing the disease in the broad category of T cell lymphomas. Order and Hellman suggested that in Hodgkin's disease, some T cells undergo alteration of their cell surface antigens following a viral infection.[147] Normal immunocompetent T cells within the same lymphoid organ react against the antigenically altered cells and T cell depletion follows. A chronic immune reaction similar to graft-versus-host disease leads to the appearance of neoplastic "reticulum" cells. Tumor-associated antigens are present in Hodgkin's disease. The fever and night sweats, weight loss, and pruritus had been proposed as possibly being caused by a tumor-versus-host reaction as far back as 1959 by Kaplan and Smithers.[148] Mycosis fungoides and Hodgkin's disease could have a similar pathogenetic mechanism — chronic antigenic stimulation — but of different etiologies, with the disorders developing along different tracks. In mycosis fungoides the cutaneous lymphoreticular system is primarily affected, whereas in Hodgkin's disease the lymph nodes and the visceral lymphoreticular system are involved, with resultant immunologic aberrations.

The premycotic dermatoses that evolve into the plaque and tumor stages are nonspecific reactions to unknown stimuli, and there is no evidence that the banal dermatoses of, for instance, psoriasis and eczema evolve into mycosis fungoides.

The evidence is clear that mycosis fungoides is a unique clinical and histologic entity. It is also clear that Sézary's syndrome and mycosis fungoides represent variant clinical manifestations of the same underlying disease. Because these terms still engender confusion among physicians, it would be better to use the designation "cutaneous T cell lymphoma with or without leukemic phase" as proposed by Schein et al.[149] as we continue to study and understand this disorder.

KAPOSI'S HEMORRHAGIC SARCOMA

Kaposi's hemorrhagic sarcoma is a disorder of lymphoreticular and endothelial cell proliferation. It may be a reactive rather than a neoplastic disorder; if neoplastic, it is low grade and does not behave as a sarcoma.[150, 151] This disease exhibits distinct skin markers that are rarely confused with any other entity.

No discussion of this disorder would be complete without allusion to the proper pronunciation of the name of this physician who has contributed so much to medicine. Most people pronounce the name as Kă-pō′-sē. However, the accent, as in all Hungarian words, is on the first syllable. The correct pronunciation is Kô′-pô-shē.[152]

Kaposi's sarcoma occurs primarily in North America, central Europe, Italy, and in Equatorial and South Africa. Men are affected ten times as frequently as women. The peak incidence occurs in the fifth and sixth decades in Western countries and in the third and fourth decades in Africa. Infants and children have developed Kaposi's sarcoma. The average duration of this disease is 10 years, although it may cause death within three years or persist for as long as 50 years. Older people with this disorder often die from an intercurrent illness. In the Congo, Kaposi's sarcoma accounts for 9 per cent of all cancers compared with 0.06 per cent in Chicago.[153]

This disease is important because multicentric visceral involvement is the cause of death in many cases. The feet and legs are usually the initial sites, but the lesions can also first appear on the genitalia, hands, pinnae, and even the tip of the nose. In rare cases visceral involvement can develop one to two years before cutaneous lesions appear. The lesions multiply during the course of the disease, but spontaneous resolution does occur. There is no correlation between the extent of visceral and cutaneous involvement.

Kaposi's sarcoma begins as dark blue or purplish macules, papules, or nodules; a red-brown component may also be present, and sometimes the lesions may be red-brown initially and later develop a bluish hue as vascular proliferation becomes rapid. Early lesions can present as sharply demarcated macules on the dorsal, lateral, or plantar surfaces of the feet and toes (Plates 8 *E, F* and 10 *A, B, C*). At first glance they may be mistaken for a bruise or an area of cyanosis, but the sharp borders of the macules are the clue to the correct diagnosis.

Single or multiple discrete smooth nodules can be the initial lesions, or macules may become infiltrated plaques from which nodules can arise. Several plaques may coalesce to involve an entire extremity, or a single plaque may slowly expand peripherally.

Purpura may be the initial lesion and may be followed by nodules and plaques in that area weeks later. In rare cases, large plaques may resolve spontaneously, leaving atrophy, telangiectasia, and hyperpigmentation. The differential diagnosis of the macules, plaques, and nodules includes pyogenic granuloma, hemangioma, and glomus tumor.

The skin of the leg characteristically becomes thick and bound down in areas of involvement; lymphedema is common. The normal contours of the leg from mid-tibia to ankle are replaced by straight lines (Plate 10 *B*). In some instances, marked pitting edema or lymphedema of the legs may be present for months or years before cutaneous lesions appear; this sequence is presumably a result of early and microscopic lymphatic obstruction by the disease process. Elephantiasis or a verrucose, ichthyotic picture can develop around the feet, ankles, and lower legs as a consequence of multiple lesions and chronic edema. Ulceration is not common, but when it occurs it is related to trauma rather than to spontaneous necrosis.

The most common extracutaneous site of Kaposi's sarcoma is the gastrointestinal tract. The characteristic bluish nodules can be found on the tongue, palate, pharynx, esophagus, and in the remainder of the gut (Plate 9 *F*). The major complication in this disease is gastrointestinal bleeding. The patient shown in Figures 12–2 and 12–3 and in Plate 10 *C* had melena for two years before cutaneous lesions developed. Lymphocytic lymphoma appeared in this patient four years after the onset of Kaposi's disease. Novis et al. reported a unique presentation of Kaposi's sarcoma in a 14-year-old boy from South Africa — diarrhea and protein-losing enteropathy secondary to involvement of the gastrointestinal tract from the stomach to the rectum.[154]

The respiratory tract (larynx, lungs, and pleura) is the next most frequently involved area, but bleeding from these sites is uncommon. Almost every organ has been involved by Kaposi's sarcoma: liver, lymph nodes, spleen, pancreas, kidneys, adrenals, testes, myocardium, and infrequently, the central and peripheral nervous systems. Although the involvement of the tissues in these organs is usually microscopic and not clinically important, three recent case reports have described instances of significant involvement of the heart,[155] brain,[156] and lymph nodes.[157] The frequency of clinically detectable visceral lesions can be as high as 20 percent.[151] Cox et al. reported a case in which Kaposi's sarcoma was localized to the glans penis and coronal sulcus.[158]

Feuerman and Potruch-Eisenkraft noted in their series of 38 patients that there was a good prognosis and less of a tendency for extracutaneous involvement in those individuals in whom Kaposi's sarcoma initially appeared on the legs and feet. There was a tendency to dissemination and a fatal outcome in those whose initial lesions appeared on the hands, forearms, thighs, breast, and ears. Five of 32 in the former group died of their disease, compared with four of six in the latter group.[159]

Geographic and racial factors play important roles in the epidemiology of Kaposi's sarcoma. The vast majority of reported cases are from central and eastern Europe, Italy, the United States of America, and Equatorial and South Africa. The largest number of cases in the world occurs in Africa among the Bantus. Although Kaposi's sarcoma is seen in many other parts of the world, such as Scandinavia, South America, Japan, and France, the number of these cases is a minority.

Dörffel believed that the distribution of Kaposi's sarcoma followed a geographic rather than a racial pattern because the majority of the patients were from Russia, Poland, or northern Italy.[160] The 258 cases he collected from the literature included 111 Italians, 45 Russian and Polish

PLATE 10

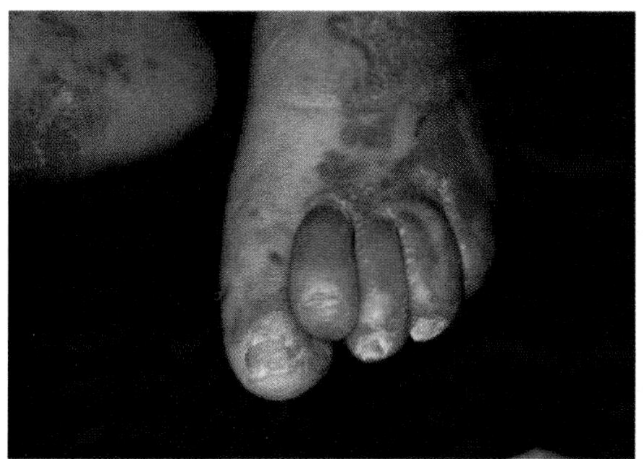

A, Kaposi's sarcoma. Involvement of the toes is another characteristic feature of this disease.

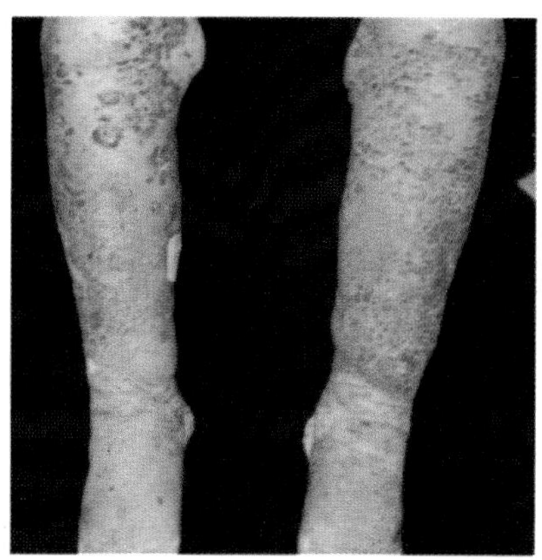

B, Kaposi's sarcoma.

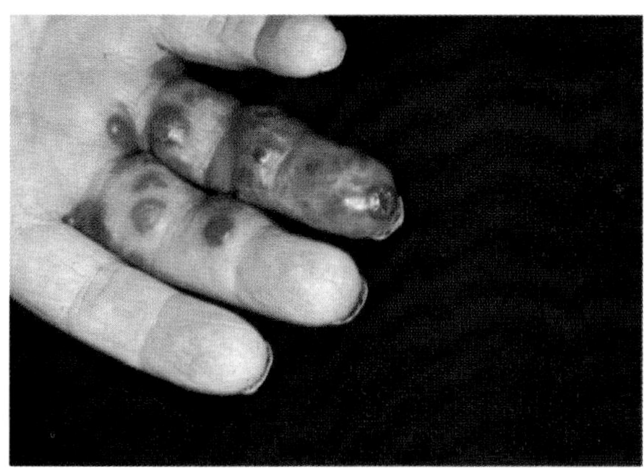

C, Kaposi's sarcoma. Involvement of fingers.

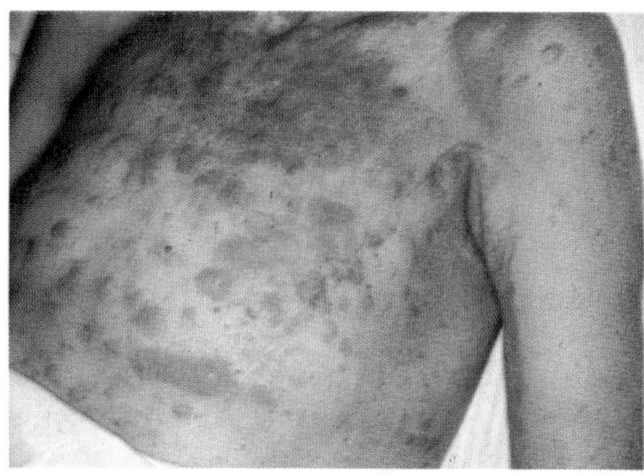

D, Chronic granulocytic leukemia. Cutaneous infiltrates.

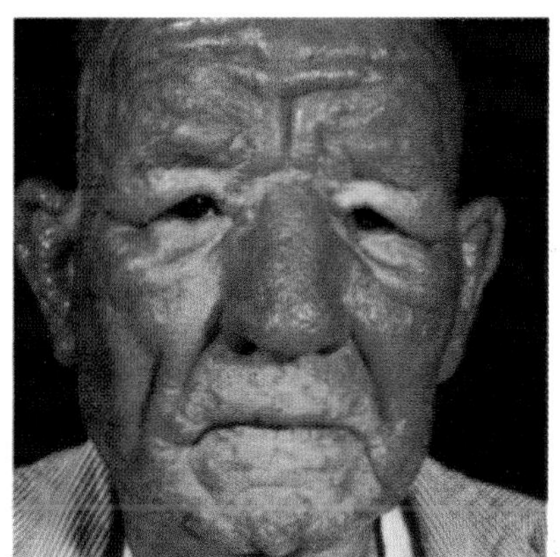

E, Chronic lymphocytic leukemia. Leonine facies produced by diffuse leukemic infiltration.

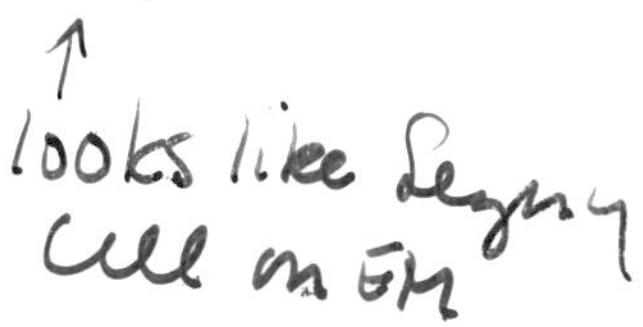

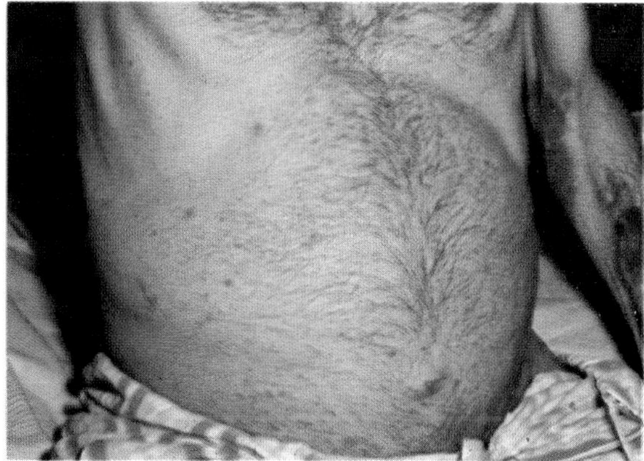

F, Chronic granulocytic leukemia. The cutaneous infiltrates are 3 to 7 mm. in diameter and are scattered over the abdominal wall. Note the characteristic red-purple color.

Jews, 70 Russian and Polish gentiles, 12 Austrians, 7 Hungarians, 5 Germans, and 8 Americans. However, these same data would also allow other conclusions. The Jews constituted 10 per cent of the population in the Polish-Russian borderlands where Kaposi's sarcoma was prevalent. Therefore, Kaposi's sarcoma occurred six times more frequently among the Jews than among the non-Jewish population in these areas. If the environmental and geographic factors are important, one still must explain the reasons for the increased incidence among the Jews.

Furthermore, the geographic distribution of Dörffel's cases is not as significant as it might seem because most Jews outside of the United States lived in Russia and Poland before 1939. The distribution of Kaposi's sarcoma correlates with the population centers of the Italians and Jews rather than with the geographic locations of Poland, Russia, and Italy. Ronchese recently pointed out that the oft-quoted statement to the effect that northern Italians are predisposed to this disease is erroneous because southern Italians make up the bulk of patients with Kaposi's sarcoma.[161]

Other evidence can be cited to support the idea of racial proclivity to Kaposi's sarcoma among Italians and Jews. Rothman noted that the emancipated Jews in western Austria and Hungary were affected as often as their co-religionists living under extreme social restrictions in Poland and Russia; these observations suggest that ethnic rather than environmental factors were more important.[153] In the United States, the majority of cases of Kaposi's sarcoma have occurred in Jewish and Italian immigrants. More than 80 per cent of the patients seen by Wise and McCarthy and Pack in New York City were Jewish and Italian immigrants.[162, 163]

In 1959, Cox and Helwig reviewed 50 cases of Kaposi's sarcoma submitted to the Armed Forces Institute of Pathology by the Veterans Administration and Armed Services.[164] Among them were 11 American blacks, 8 Americans of Italian descent, and 31 other native Americans. None was known to be Jewish. The major reasons for the absence of known Jewish patients in their series is as follows. The bulk of Jewish emigration from eastern Europe took place between 1900 and 1920. The majority of the adult immigrants were too old, and their children were too young, for service in the United States forces in World War I. Although their children were old enough to serve in the Second World War, the majority of them were not yet old enough to develop Kaposi's sarcoma.

The question of racial predisposition to Kaposi's sarcoma among Jews and Italians can be settled in the next 20 to 30 years by studying the incidence of the disease in Americans of Italian and Jewish descent who are now approaching the age at which Kaposi's sarcoma develops. Cox and Helwig reported eight cases of Kaposi's sarcoma in Americans of Italian descent.[164]

As of 1969 we had seen 24 examples of this disease in our clinics. Twenty patients were Italian or Jewish, and the other four were Puerto Rican, American of French-Canadian descent, Norwegian, and Polish. Of the 13 Italians, four were born in Connecticut; of the seven Jews, two were born in the United States of Russian parents. The rest were emigrants from either Italy or eastern Europe. One of our 24 patients was a Norwegian woman. From 1970 to 1978, an additional seven patients have been seen. Four were Jewish men born in the United States but whose parents were born in Russia, two were Italian men born in this country, and one was an Italian man born in Italy.

These preliminary statistics of Italian and Jewish Americans from our series and from that of Cox and Helwig support the theory of racial predisposition.

The racial and environmental aspects could be further evaluated by comparing the incidence of the disease among Sephardic Jews — the inhabitants of North Africa, Spain, Portugal, and Turkey — with the eastern European, or Ashkenazic, Jews. Although significant statistics are not yet available, Degos et al. reported 28 patients with Kaposi's sarcoma; 15 came from North Africa, and 5 of them were Jewish.[165] Sagher noted 14 instances in Israel from 1956 to 1965. Two patients were of Sephardic origin, and 12 were of Ashkenazic origin.[166] Feuerman and Potruch-Eisenkraft reported additional data on 38 patients seen between 1960 and 1970 in Israel. There were 30 men and 8 women, 26 of whom had been born in Eastern and Central Europe. The rest originated in North Africa and Middle Eastern countries.[159]

In Africa, Kaposi's sarcoma is seen most frequently in the Congo. In Transvaal, South Africa, the Bantus are affected 10 times more frequently than the Caucasians; the Coloureds and Indians living beside the Bantus do not seem to be affected. Although the Bantus are predisposed to this disease, there is a striking difference in prevalence among the Bantus from country to country. A geographical difference is superimposed upon a racial proclivity.

The prevalence of Kaposi's sarcoma is low among the West African blacks, from whom the black American derives his origin.

In 1966, Williams and Williams had noted a correlation between the distribution of Kaposi's sarcoma and free-flowing streams harboring the Simulium black fly, the vector of onchocerciasis. Although there was no direct relationship between onchocerciasis and Kaposi's sarcoma, the possibility existed that the Simulium fly might be involved in the etiology of the disease by acting as a vector for an infectious agent.[167] However, this hypothesis has been negated by subsequent field studies which found areas with a high prevalence of Kaposi's sarcoma in the absence of Simulium flies, and an area relatively free of Kaposi's disease that was endemic for the black flies.[168]

All the evidence supports a greater likelihood of Kaposi's sarcoma developing in Italians, Jews, and Bantus than in other ethnic groups. Environmental factors, perhaps a viral infection, acting upon a genetically susceptible host may prove to be important in Kaposi's disease. The association between Kaposi's sarcoma and cytomegalic virus, one strain of which has oncogenic potential, is currently being investigated.[169]

Kaposi's sarcoma in the United States and Europe differs from the African disorder in a few ways. In Africa the peak incidence is in the 30 to 50 year age group, whereas primarily the 50 to 70 year group is affected in the Western world; moreover, the disease frequently develops in Bantu children. Lymphadenopathy with minimal cutaneous involvement is the most common expression of the disorder in African youngsters, and in adults the ulceration of cutaneous lesions and bony involvement is common.[170]

The African disease can be divided into three basic types: *Nodular disease.* Subcutaneous nodules develop on the limbs. The disease progresses by an irregular appearance of new nodules and regression of old ones. The prognosis is good and the majority of patients become free of disease following chemotherapy. *Locally aggressive disease.* Tumors arise *de novo* or from preexisting nodules. The tumor tends to ulcerate and erode local structures, extending often to the deep fascia and bone. The prognosis is poorer than with nodular disease, but the patients may survive for many years with their lesions reasonably well controlled by chemotherapy, although relapse is common. *Generalized disease.* Widespread tumors are present. In children, the lymph nodes are predominantly affected, with minimal cutaneous or visceral involvement. In young adults, there are widespread lesions in the nodes, viscera, and skin. Untreated, this form of the disease can run a fatal course within three years, and sometimes more rapidly within weeks.[171, 172]

Templeton and Bhana found that the ability to develop a contact sensitivity to DNCB in a patient could be correlated with prognosis. In general, virtually everyone with nodular disease, but only 50 per cent of those with locally aggressive disease could be sensitized to DNCB. No patient with the generalized form was able to be sensitized. In two patients with locally aggressive disease who were successfully treated, the initial negative reaction to challenge with DNCB became positive after the tumor was eradicated. Six of nine patients with locally aggressive disease and negative contact sensitivity to DNCB died, whereas only two of seven patients with positive contact sensitivity to DNCB did so. The finding of nonreactivity to DNCB was generally associated with visceral lesions or a locally aggressive superficial tumor. This appears to be a useful way to gauge prognosis in the African disease and perhaps could be applied to the Western European form of the disease. Dobozy et al. have reported mild depression of humoral and cell-mediated immunity in several European cases.[173]

The association of lymphoma and leukemia with Kaposi's sarcoma occurs in 10 per cent of the patients in the West but is rare in Africans.[168, 174] Curiously, in neither Europe nor Africa can a high rate of leukemia or lymphoma be correlated with an increased prevalence of Kaposi's sarcoma. Kaposi's sarcoma presumably requires specific conditions for its development and is not simply induced by stimuli capable of producing leukemia and lymphoma. A number of observations have implicated immunodepression or defects in immunologic surveillance in the initiation of the disease. Kaposi's sarcoma has arisen in several patients with renal transplants who were being maintained on immunosuppressive therapy. The tumors disappeared after discontinuing the immunosuppressive agents.[175] In Uganda, Kaposi's disease is more common in the western part of the country. However the majority of children with the lymphadenopathic form of the disease as well as all the young adults with generalized disease came from the eastern part of Uganda. It has been postulated that the severe forms of the disease develop in individuals who are suffering or have suffered from malaria, which is known to induce a period of immunologic unresponsiveness.[176]

Although immunological mechanisms are most likely operative in Kaposi's disease, other factors may be important as well. Rothman suggested that a metabolic defect secondary to faulty tissue respiration might be important in the pathogenesis of Kaposi's sarcoma because the disease first appears in areas with precarious circulatory mechanisms such as the extremities, fingers, toes, tip of the nose, and pinnae of the ears.[153]

The lymphomatous diseases can precede or follow the onset of Kaposi's sarcoma. Cases have been recorded in which a single lymph node showed the histologic features of Hodgkin's disease and Kaposi's sarcoma side by side.[177] Kaposi's sarcoma occurs in 6 to 10 per cent of the cases of leukemia and lymphoma that develop a second neoplastic disorder. No particular type of leukemia is associated with Kaposi's sarcoma, but among the lymphomas, follicular lymphoma and Hodgkin's disease are seen four times more often than lymphosarcoma and reticulum cell sarcoma. The combination of Kaposi's sarcoma with mycosis fungoides and with multiple myeloma has also been reported.[178] Our patient illustrated in Plate 11 *C* developed Kaposi's sarcoma after she had had the Sézary syndrome for several years.

Other associations with Kaposi's sarcoma have been dermatomyositis in one patient[179] and acquired ichthyosis in three others.[180]

The histopathology of Kaposi's sarcoma is characterized by proliferating capillaries intermixed with masses of spindle cells and fibroblasts. Clefts lacking an endothelial lining but filled with red blood cells within the whorls of spindle cells are a diagnostic histologic feature. The vascular proliferation is responsible for the color, the rapid growth, and the occasional spontaneous resolution of lesions by thromboses, but the origin of the spindle cell is believed to be the key to the classification and nature of this disease.

Schwann cells and reticuloendothelial cells have both been proposed as the origin of the spindle cell,[181-183] but the accumulated and current evidence supports the endothelial cell or the undifferentiated vasoformative cell of the vascular adventitia as the cellular sources of Kaposi's sarcoma.[184]

Moertel and Hagedorn believe that Kaposi's sarcoma is a malignant disease of the reticuloendothelial system.[185] However, cytologic features of malignancy are missing in the lesions, and frank sarcomatous degeneration has been reported in 3 per cent of the cases in two series and in 30 per cent of the cases in a third series.[151, 164, 165] When a sarcoma does develop, it may be only locally invasive, or it may metastasize widely. Kaposi's sarcoma is most likely a multifocal proliferative and reactive process rather than a malignant disorder with disseminated metastases. The cutaneous and visceral lesions histologically exhibit all stages of development. A primary focus which progressively enlarges is lacking, and instead, widely disseminated lesions appear in crops.[151]

REFERENCES

1. Rappaport, H.: Tumors of the hematopoietic system. *In* Atlas of Tumor Pathology, section III, fasc. 8. Washington, D.C., Armed Forces Institute of Pathology, 1966.
2. Stein, H., Lennert, K., and Parwaresch, M. R.: Malignant lymphomas of B cell type. Lancet, *2*:855, 1972.
3. Lukes, R. J., and Collins, R. D.: New approaches to the classification of the lymphomata. Br. J. Cancer, *31*(Suppl. II):1, 1975.
4. Lukes, R. J., and Collins, R. D.: Immunologic characterization of human malignant lymphomas. Cancer, *34*:1488, 1974.
5. Whiteside, T. L., and Rowlands, D. T., Jr.: T-cell and B-cell identification in the diagnosis of lymphoproliferative disease. A review. Am. J. Pathol., *88*:754, 1977.
6. Aisenberg, A. C.: Hodgkin's disease — prognosis, treatment and etiologic and immunologic considerations. N. Engl. J. Med., *270*:508, 617, 1964.
7. Lapes, M., Rosenzweig, M., Barbieri, B.,

Joseph, R. R., and Smalley, R. V.: Cellular and humoral immunity in non-Hodgkin's lymphoma. Correlation of immunodeficiencies with clinicopathologic factors. Am. J. Clin. Pathol., *67*:347, 1977.
8. Kaplan, H. S.: Hodgkin's disease and other human malignant lymphomas: advances and prospects. G.H.A. Clowes Memorial Lecture. Cancer Res., *36*:3863, 1976.
9. Epstein, E., and MacEachern, K.: Dermatologic manifestations of the lymphoblastoma-leukemia group. Arch. Intern. Med., *60*:867, 1937.
10. Kim, R., Winkelmann, R. K., and Dockerty, M.: Reticulum cell sarcoma of the skin. Cancer, *16*:646, 1963.
11. Long, J. C., Mihm, M. C., and Qazi, R.: Malignant lymphoma of the skin. A clinicopathologic study of lymphoma other than mycosis fungoides diagnosed by skin biopsy. Cancer, *38*:1282, 1976.
12. Van der Meiren, L.: Three cases of Hodgkin's disease with predominantly cutaneous localization. Br. J. Dermatol., *60*:181, 1948.
13. Benninghoff, D. L., Medina, A., Alexander, L. L., and Camiel, M. R.: The mode of spread of Hodgkin's disease to the skin. Cancer, *26*:1135, 1970.
14. Bluefarb, S. M.: Cutaneous Manifestations of the Malignant Lymphomas. Charles C Thomas, Springfield, 1959, p. 251.
15. Baxter, D. L., and Lockwood, J. H.: Acne urticata polycythemica. Report of a case. Arch. Dermatol., *78*:325, 1958.
16. Weidman, F. D., and Klauder, J. V.: Acne urticata polycythemica. Arch. Dermatol. Syph., *39*:645, 1938.
17. Fuller, C. J.: Hodgkin's disease with erythema nodosum. Br. Med. J., *2*:1172, 1934.
18. Nicolis, G. D., and Helwig, E. B.: Exfoliative dermatitis. A clinicopathologic study of 135 cases. Arch. Dermatol., *108*:788, 1973.
19. Montgomery, H.: Exfoliative dermatitis and malignant erythroderma: the value and limitations of histopathologic studies. Arch. Dermatol. Syph., *27*:253, 1933.
20. Abrahams, I., McCarthy, J. T., and Sanders, S. L.: 101 cases of exfoliative dermatitis. Arch. Dermatol., *87*:96, 1963.
21. Wilson, H. T. H.: Exfoliative dermatitis. Its etiology and prognosis. Arch. Dermatol., *69*:577, 1954.
22. Edelson, R. L., Kirkpatrick, C. H., Shevach, E. M., Schein, P. S., Smith, W. W., Green, I., and Lutzner, M.: Preferential cutaneous infiltration by neoplastic thymus-derived lymphocytes. Morphologic and functional studies. Ann. Intern. Med., *80*:685, 1974.
23. Schnyder, V. W., and Schirren, C. G.: So-called "lipomelanotic reticulosis" of Pautrier-Woringer. Arch. Dermatol., *70*:155, 1954.
24. Ronchese, F.: Ichthyosiform atrophy of the skin in Hodgkin's disease. Arch. Dermatol. Syph., *47*:778, 1943.
25. Sneddon, I. B.: Acquired ichthyosis in Hodgkin's disease. Br. Med. J., *1*:763, 1955.
26. Glazebrook, A. J., and Tomaszewski, W.: Ichthyosiform changes of skin associated with internal diseases. Arch. Dermatol. Syph., *55*:28, 1947.
27. Bluefarb, S. M.: *op. cit.*, p. 256.
28. Bluefarb, S. M.: *Ibid.*, p. 266.
29. Atkinson, M. K., McElwain, T. J., Peckhem, M. J., and Thomas, P. R. M.: Hypertrophic pulmonary osteoarthropathy in Hodgkin's disease. Reversal with chemotherapy. Cancer, *38*:1729, 1976.
30. Case records of the Massachusetts General Hospital (case 13-1966). N. Engl. J. Med., *274*:620, 1966.
31. New England Dermatological Society Seminar on Cutaneous Pathology. Case 6. May 15, 1966, Boston, Mass.
32. Baler, G. R.: Personal communication.
33. Christianson, H. B., and Fine, R. M.: Vasculitis with or without panniculitis in leukemia, lymphoma and multiple myeloma. Southern Med. J., *60*:567, 1967.
34. Bäfverstedt, B.: Über Lymphadenosis benigna cutis. Acta Derm. Venereol., *24* (Suppl. 11), 1943.
35. Bäfverstedt, B.: Lymphadenosis benigna cutis (LABC), its nature, course and prognosis. Acta Derm. Venereol., *40*:10, 1960.
36. Mach, K. W., and Wilgram, G. F.: Characteristic histopathology of cutaneous lymphoplasia (lymphocytoma). Arch. Dermatol., *94*:26, 1966.
37. Macaulay, W. L.: Lymphomatoid papulosis. Arch. Dermatol., *97*:23, 1968.
38. Brehmer-Andersson, E.: Mycosis fungoides and its relation to Sézary's syndrome, lymphomatoid papulosis, and primary cutaneous Hodgkin's disease. A clinical, histopathologic and cytologic study of fourteen cases and a critical review of the literature. Acta Derm. Venereol., *56* (Suppl. 75), 1976.
39. Lutzner, M. A., Edelson, R., Schein, P., Green, I., Kirkpatrick, C., and Ahmed, A.: Cutaneous T-cell lymphomas: the Sézary syndrome, mycosis fungoides and related disorders. Ann. Intern. Med., *83*:534, 1975.
40. Thomsen, K., and Schmidt, H.: Lymphomatoid papulosis. Arch. Dermatol., *113*:232, 1977.
41. Salzstein, S. L., and Ackerman, L. V.: Lymphadenopathy induced by anticonvulsant drugs and mimicking clinically and pathologically malignant lymphoma. Cancer, *12*:164, 1959.
42. Rosenfeld, S., Swillen, A. I., Shenoy, Y. M. V., and Morrison, A. N.: Syndrome simulating lymphosarcoma induced by diphenylhydantoin sodium. J.A.M.A., *176*:491, 1961.
43. Hyman, G. A., and Sommers, S. C.: The development of Hodgkin's disease and lymphoma during anticonvulsant therapy. Blood, *28*:416, 1966.
44. Rausing, A., and Trell, E.: Malignant lym-

phogranulomatosis and anticonvulsant therapy. Acta Med. Scand., *189*:131, 1971.
45. Tashima, C. K., and De los Santos, R.: Lymphoma and anticonvulsive therapy. J.A.M.A., *228*:286, 1974.
46. Bichel, J.: Hydantoin derivatives and malignancies of the haemopoietic system. Acta Med. Scand., *198*:327, 1975.
47. Lapes, M., Antoinades, K., Gartner, W., Jr., and Vivacqua, R.: Conversion of a benign lymphoepithelial salivary gland lesion to lymphocytic lymphoma during Dilantin therapy. Correlation with Dilantin-induced lymphocyte transformation in vitro. Cancer, *38*:1318, 1976.
48. Lapes, M. J., Vivacqua, R. J., and Antoniades, K.: Immunoblastic lymphadenopathy associated with phenytoin (diphenylhydantoin). Lancet, *1*:198, 1976.
49. Lukes, R. J., and Tindle, B. H.: Immunoblastic lymphadenopathy. A hyperimmune entity resembling Hodgkin's disease. N. Engl. J. Med., *292*:1, 1975.
50. Masi, M., Paolucci, P., Perocco, P., and Franchesi, C.: Immunosuppression by phenytoin. Lancet, *1*:860, 1976.
51. Massimo, L., Pasino, M., Rosanoa-Vadala, C., Tonini, G. P., DeNegri, M., and Saccomani, L.: Immunological side-effects of anticonvulsants. Lancet, *1*:860, 1976.
52. Frizzera, G., Moran, E. M., and Rappaport, H.: Angio-immunoblastic lymphadenopathy with dysproteinemia. Lancet, *1*:1070, 1974.
53. Moore, S. B., Harrison, E. G., Jr., and Weiland, L. H.: Angioimmunoblastic lymphadenopathy. Mayo Clin. Proc., *51*:273, 1976.
54. Schultz, D. R., and Yunis, A. A.: Immunoblastic lymphadenopathy with mixed cryoglobulinemia. A detailed case study. N. Engl. J. Med., *292*:8, 1975.
55. Matloff, R. B., and Neiman, R. S.: Angioimmunoblastic lymphadenopathy. A generalized lymphoproliferative disorder with cutaneous manifestations. Arch. Dermatol., *114*:92, 1978.
56. Yataganas, X., Papadimitriou, C., Pangalis, G., Loukopoulos, D., Fessas, P., and Papacharalampous, N.: Angioimmunoblastic lymphadenopathy terminating as Hodgkin's disease. Cancer, *39*:2183, 1977.
57. Hossfeld, D. K., Hoffken, K., Schmidt, C. G., and Diedrichs, H.: Chromosome abnormalities in angioimmunoblastic lymphadenopathy. Lancet, *1*:198, 1976.
58. Wechsler, H. L., and Stavrides, A.: Immunoblastic lymphadenopathy with purpura and cryoglobulinemia. Arch. Dermatol., *113*:636, 1977.
59. Bluefarb, S. M.: *op. cit.*, p. 7.
60. Symmers, D.: Mycosis fungoides as a clinical and pathologic nonexistent. Arch. Dermatol. Syph., *25*:1, 1932.
61. Gates, O.: Cutaneous tumors in leukemia and lymphoma. Arch. Dermatol. Syph., *37*:1015, 1938.
62. Cawley, E. P., Curtis, A. C., and Leach, J. E. K.: Is mycosis fungoides a reticuloendothelial neoplastic entity? Arch. Dermatol. Syph., *64*:255, 1951.
63. Bluefarb, S. M.: Is mycosis fungoides an entity? Arch. Dermatol., *71*:293, 1955.
64. Farber, E. M., Schneiderman, H. M., and Llerena, G. J.: Natural history of mycosis fungoides. Calif. Med., *87*:225, 1957.
65. Block, J. B., Edgcomb, J., Eisen, A., and Van Scott, E. J.: Mycosis fungoides. Natural history and aspects of its relationship to other malignant lymphomas. Am. J. Med., *34*:228, 1963.
66. Cyr, C. P., Geokas, M. C., and Worsley, G. H.: Mycosis fungoides. Arch. Dermatol., *94*:558, 1966.
67. Reed, R. J., and Cummings, C. E.: Malignant reticulosis and related conditions of the skin. A reconsideration of mycosis fungoides. Cancer, *19*:1231, 1966.
68. Epstein, E. H., Jr., Levin, D. L., Croft, J. D., Jr., and Lutzner, M. A.: Mycosis fungoides. Survival, prognostic features, response to therapy, and autopsy findings. Medicine, *51*:61, 1972.
69. Allen, A. C.: The Skin. A Clinicopathologic Treatise. 2nd ed. Grune & Stratton, New York, 1967, p. 1120.
70. Bluefarb, S. M.: Cutaneous Manifestations of the Malignant Lymphomas. p. 99.
71. Samman, P. D.: Survey of reticulosis and premycotic eruptions. A preliminary report. Br. J. Dermatol., *76*:1, 1964.
72. Samman, P. D.: The natural history of parapsoriasis en plaque (chronic superficial dermatitis) and prereticulotic poikiloderma. Br. J. Dermatol., *87*:405, 1972.
73. Fleischmajer, R., Pascher, F., and Sims, C. F.: Parapsoriasis en plaques and mycosis fungoides. Dermatologica, *131*:149, 1965.
74. Roenigk, H. H., Jr., and Castrovinci, A. J.: Mycosis fungoides bullosa. Arch. Dermatol., *104*:402, 1971.
75. Bluefarb, S. M., Lazar, P., Dunlap, F., and Lewis, R.: Mycosis fungoides with bullous lesions. Arch. Dermatol., *81*:282, 1960.
76. Ackerman, A. B., Miller, R. C., and Shapiro, L. C.: Pustular mycosis fungoides. Arch. Dermatol., *93*:221, 1966.
77. Bluefarb, S. M.: Cutaneous Manifestations of the Malignant Lymphomas. p. 129.
78. Price, N. M., Fuks, Z. Y., and Hoffman, T. E.: Hyperkeratotic and verrucous features of mycosis fungoides. Arch. Dermatol., *113*:57, 1977.
79. Haneke, E., Tulusan, A. H., and Weidner, F.: Histological features of "Pagetoid reticulosis" (Woringer-Kolopp) in premycosis fungoides. Arch. Dermatol. Res., *258*:265, 1977.
80. Degreef, H., Holovoet, C., Van Vloten, W. A., Desmet, V., and De Wolf-Peeters, C.: Woringer-Kolopp disease. An epidermotropic variant of mycosis fungoides. Cancer, *38*:2154, 1976.
81. Medencia, M., and Lorincz, A. L.: Pagetoid reticulosis (Woringer-Kolopp Disease). Arch. Dermatol., *114*:262, 1978.

82. Kim, R., and Winkelmann, R. K.: Follicular mucinosis (alopecia mucinosa). Arch. Dermatol., *85*:490, 1962.
83. Pinkus, H.: Alopecia mucinosa. Arch. Dermatol., *76*:419, 1957.
84. Plotnick, H., and Abbrecht, M.: Alopecia mucinosa and lymphoma. Report of two cases and review of literature. Arch. Dermatol., *92*:137, 1965.
85. Brunsting, L. A., and Underwood, L. J.: Pyoderma vegetans in association with chronic ulcerative colitis. Arch. Dermatol. Syph., *60*:161, 1949.
86. Weber, M. B., and McGavran, M. H.: Mycosis fungoides involving the brain. Arch. Neurol., *16*:645, 1967.
87. Bluefarb, S. M.: Cutaneous Manifestations of the Malignant Lymphomas. p. 120.
88. Kitchen, C. K.: Mycosis fungoides keratitis. Presentation of a case. Am. J. Ophthalmol., *55*:758, 1963.
89. Lundberg, W. B., Cadman, E. C., and Skeel, R. T.: Leptomeningeal mycosis fungoides. Cancer, *38*:2149, 1976.
90. Keltner, J. L., Fritsch, E., Cykiert, R. C., and Albert, D. M.: Mycosis fungoides. Intraocular and central nervous system involvement. Arch. Ophthalmol., *95*:645, 1977.
91. Cohen, M. I., Widerlite, L. W., Schechter, G. P., Jaffe, E., Fischmann, A. B., Schein, P. S., and Macdonald, J. S.: Gastrointestinal involvement in the Sézary syndrome. Gastroenterology, *73*:145, 1977.
92. Chang, A. H., and Ng, A. B. P.: The cellular manifestations of mycosis fungoides in cerebrospinal fluid. A case report. Acta Cytol., *19*:148, 1975.
93. Post, C. F., and Lincoln, C. S.: Mycosis fungoides. Report of two unusual cases with autopsy findings. J. Invest. Dermatol., *10*:135, 1948.
94. Cohen, S. R., Stenn, K. S., Braverman, I. M., and Beck, G. J.: Mycosis fungoides: a retrospective study with observations on occupation as a new prognostic factor (abstract). J. Invest. Dermatol., *70*:221, 1978.
95. Fuks, Z. Y., Bagshaw, M. A., and Farber, E. M.: Prognostic signs and the management of the mycosis fungoides. Cancer, *32*:1385, 1973.
96. Montgomery, H.: Dermatopathology. Harper & Row, New York, 1967, pp. 1207, 1212, fig. 37–4.
97. Rappaport, H.: Tumors of the hematopoietic system. *In* Atlas of Tumor Pathology, section III, fasc. 8. Washington, D.C., Armed Forces Institute of Pathology. 1966, p. 345.
98. Rappaport, H., and Thomas, L. B.: Mycosis fungoides: the pathology of extracutaneous involvement. Cancer, *34*:1198, 1974.
99. Long, J. C., and Mihm, M. C.: Mycosis fungoides with extracutaneous dissemination: a distinct clinciopathologic entity. Cancer, *34*:1745, 1974.
100. Winkelmann, R. K.: Clinical studies of T-cell erythroderma in the Sézary syndrome. Mayo Clin. Proc., *49*:519, 1974.
101. Fleischmajer, R., and Eisenberg, S.: Sézary's reticulosis. Its relationship with neoplasias of the lymphoreticular system. Arch. Dermatol., *89*:9, 1964.
102. Taswell, H. F., and Winkelmann, R. K.: Sézary syndrome — a malignant reticulemic erythroderma. J.A.M.A., *177*:465, 1961.
103. Alderson, W. E., Barrow, G. I., and Turner, R. L.: Sézary's syndrome. Br. Med. J., *1*:256, 1955.
104. Main, R. A., Goodhall, H. B., and Swanson, W. C.: Sézary's syndrome. Br. J. Dermatol., *71*:335, 1959.
105. Clendenning, W. E., Brecher, G., and Van Scott, E. J.: Mycosis fungoides. Relationship to malignant cutaneous reticulosis and the Sézary syndrome. Arch. Dermatol., *89*:785, 1964.
106. Brody, J. I., Cypress, E., Kimball, S. G., and McKenzie, D.: The Sézary syndrome. Arch. Intern. Med., *110*:205, 1962.
107. Tedeschi, L. G., and Lansiger, D. T.: Sézary syndrome. A malignant leukemic reticuloendotheliosis. Arch. Dermatol., *92*:257, 1965.
108. Lutzner, M., Edelson, R., Schein, P., Green, I., Kirkpatrick, C., and Ahmed, A.: Cutaneous T-cell lymphomas: The Sézary syndrome, mycosis fungoides, and related disorders. Ann. Intern. Med., *83*:534, 1975.
109. Aub, J. C., Wolbach, S. B., Kennedy, B. J., and Bailey, G. T.: Mycosis fungoides followed for 14 years; The case of Dr. W. B. Cannon. Arch. Pathol., *60*:535, 1955.
110. Lutzner, M. A., and Jordan, H. W.: The ultrastructure of an abnormal cell in Sézary's syndrome. Blood, *31*:719, 1968.
111. Lutzner, M. A., Hobbs, J. W., and Horvath, P.: Ultrastructure of abnormal cells in Sézary syndrome, mycosis fungoides and parapsoriasis en plaque. Arch. Dermatol., *103*:375, 1971.
112. Flaxman, B. A., Zelazny, G., and Van Scott, E. J.: Non-specificity of characteristic cells in mycosis fungoides. Arch. Dermatol., *104*:141, 1971.
113. Yeckley, J. A., Weston, W. L., Thorne, E. G., and Krueger, G. G.: Production of Sézary like cells from normal human lymphocytes. Arch. Dermatol., *111*:29, 1975.
114. Rosas-Uribe, A., Variakojis, D., Molnar, Z., and Rappaport, H.: Mycosis fungoides: an ultrastructural study. Cancer, *34*:634, 1974.
115. Brouet, J-C., Flandrin, G., and Seligmann, M.: Indications of the thymus derived nature of proliferating cells in six patients with Sézary's syndrome. N. Engl. J. Med., *289*:341, 1973.
116. Zucker-Franklin, D., Melton, J. W., III, and Quagliata, A.: Ultrastructural, immunologic, and functional studies on

Sézary cells: a neoplastic variant of thymus-derived (T) lymphocytes. Proc. Nat. Acad. Sci., *71*:1877, 1974.

117. Broder, S., Edelson, R. L., Lutzner, M. A., Nelson, D. L., MacDermott, R. P., Durm, M. E., Goldman, C. K., Meade, B. D., and Waldmann, T. A.: The Sézary syndrome. A malignant proliferation of helper T-cells. J. Clin. Invest., *58*:1297, 1976.
118. Polliack, A., Djaldetti, M., Reyes, F., Biberfeld, P., Daniel, M. T., and Flandrin, G. F.: Surface features of Sézary cells: A scan electron microscopy study of 5 cases. Scand. J. Haematol., *18*:207, 1977.
119. Lutzner, M. A., Emerit, I., Durepaire, R., Flandrin, G., Grupper, C., and Prunieras, M.: Cytogenetic, cytophotometric and ultrastructural study of large cerebriform cells of the Sezary syndrome and description of the small cell variant. J. Nat. Cancer. Inst., *50*:1145, 1973.
120. Erkman-Balis, B., and Rappaport, H.: Cytogenetic studies in mycosis fungoides. Cancer, *34*:626, 1974.
121. Prunieras, M.: DNA content and cytogenetics of the Sézary cell. Mayo Clin. Proc., *49*:548, 1974.
122. Dewald, G., Spurbeck, J. L., and Vitek, H.: Chromosomes in a patient with the Sézary syndrome. Mayo Clin. Proc., *49*:553, 1974.
123. Van Vloten, W. A., Van Duijn, P., and Schaberg, A.: Cytodiagnostic use of Feulgen-DNA measurements in cell imprints from the skin of patients with mycosis fungoides. Br. J. Dermatol., *91*:365, 1974.
124. Edelson, R., Fackton, M., Andres, A., Lutzner, M. A., and Schein, P.: Successful management of the Sézary syndrome. Mobilization and removal of extravascular neoplastic T cells by leukapheresis. N. Engl. J. Med., *291*:293, 1974.
125. Flandrin, G., and Brouet, J-C.: The Sézary cell: cytologic, cytochemical, and immunologic studies. Mayo Clin. Proc., *49*:575, 1974.
126. Nordquist, B. C., and Kinney, J. P.: T and B cells and cell mediated immunity in mycosis fungoides. Cancer, *37*:714, 1976.
127. Langner, A., Glinski, W., Pawinska, M., and Obalek, S.: Lymphocyte transformation in mycosis fungoides. Arch. Derm. Forsch., *251*:249, 1975.
128. Tan, R. S-H., Butterworth, C. M., McLaughlin, H., Malka, S., and Samman, P. D.: Mycosis fungoides: a disease of antigen persistence. Br. J. Dermatol., *91*:607, 1974.
129. Mackie, R., Sless, F. R., Cochran, R., and DeSousa, M.: Lymphocyte abnormalities in mycosis fungoides. Br. J. Dermatol., *94*:173, 1976.
130. Cooperrider, P. A., and Roenigk, H. H., Jr.: Selective immunological evaluation of mycosis fungoides. Arch. Dermatol., *114*:207, 1978.
131. Yoshida, T., Edelson, R., Cohen, S., and Green, I.: Migration inhibitory activity in serum and cell supernatants in patients with Sezary syndrome. J. Immunol., *114*:915, 1975.
132. Metcalf, D.: Reticular tumors in mice subjected to prolonged antigenic stimulation. Br. J. Cancer, *15*:769, 1961.
133. Schwartz, R. S., and Beldotti, L.: Malignant lymphomas following allogeneic disease: transition from an immunological to neoplastic disorder. Science, *149*:1511, 1965.
134. Walford, R. L.: Increased incidence of lymphoma after injection of mice with cells differing at weak histocompatability loci. Science, *152*:78, 1966.
135. Fialkow, P. J.: "Immunologic" oncogenesis. Blood, *30*:388, 1967.
136. Melief, C. J. M., Datta, S., Louie, S., and Schwartz, R. S.: Immunologic activation of murine leukemia viruses. Cancer, *34*:1481, 1974.
137. Schupplli, R.: Is mycosis fungoides an "immunoma"? Dermatologica, *153*:1, 1976.
138. Greene, M. H., Dalager, N. A., Lamberg, S. I., Argyropoulos, C. E., and Fraumeni, J. F., Jr.: Mycosis fungoides: epidemiologic observations. Cancer Treat. Rep., *63*:597, 1979.
139. Fan, T. Y., Morrison, J., Rounbehler, D. P., Ross, R., Fine, D. H., and Miles, W.: N-nitrosodiethanolamine in synthetic cutting fluids: a part-per-hundred impurity. Science, *196*:70, 1977.
140. Rowden, G., and Lewis, M. G.: Langerhans cells: involvement in the pathogenesis of mycosis fungoides. Br. J. Dermatol., *95*:665, 1976.
141. Silberberg, I., Baer, R., and Rosenthal, S. A.: The role of Langerhans cells in allergic contact hypersensitivity. A review of findings in man and guinea pigs. J. Invest. Dermatol., *66*:210, 1976.
142. Silberberg-Sinakin, I., Thorbecke, G. J., Baer, R. L., Rosenthal, S. A., and Berezowski, V.: Antigen bearing Langerhans cells in dermal lymphatics and in lymph nodes. Cell Immunol., *25*:137, 1976.
143. Rowden, G., Lewis, M. G., and Sullivan, A. K.: Ia antigen expression on human epidermal Langerhans cells. Nature, *268*:247, 1977.
144. Klareskog, L., Tjernlund, V. M., Forsum, U., and Peterson, P. A.: Epidermal Langerhans cells express Ia antigens. Nature, 268:248, 1977.
145. Stingl, G., Wolff-Schreiner, E. C., Pichler, W. J., Gschnait, F., and Knapp, W.: Epidermal Langerhans cells bear Fc and C3 receptors. Nature, *268*:245, 1977.
146. Stingl, G., Katz, S. I., Shevach, E. M., Rosenthal, A. S., and Green, I.: Analogous functions of macrophages and Langerhans cells in the initiation of the immune response. J. Invest. Dermatol., *71*:59, 1978.
147. Order, S. E., and Hellman, S.: Pathogenesis of Hodgkin's disease. Lancet, *1*:571, 1972.

148. Kaplan, H. S., and Smithers, D. W.: Autoimmunity in man and homologous disease in mice in relation to the malignant lymphomas. Lancet, *2*:1, 1959.
149. Schein, P. S., Macdonald, J. S., and Edelson, R.: Cutaneous T-cell lymphoma. Cancer, *38*:1859, 1976.
150. Bluefarb, S. M.: Kaposi's sarcoma. Charles C Thomas, Springfield, 1957.
151. Reynolds, W. A., Winklemann, R. K., and Soule, E. H.: Kaposi's sarcoma: a clinicopathologic study with particular reference to its relationship to the reticuloendothelial system. Medicine (Balt.), *44*:419, 1965.
152. Rothman, S.: Some remarks on Moricz Kaposi and on the history of Kaposi's sarcoma. Acta Un. Int. Cancer, *18*:321, 1962.
153. Rothman, S.: Remarks on sex, age and racial distribution of Kaposi's sarcoma and possible pathogenic factors. *Ibid.*, p. 326.
154. Novis, B. H., King, H., and Bank, S.: Kaposi's sarcoma presenting with diarrhea and protein-losing enteropathy. Gastroenterology, *67*:996, 1974.
155. Levison, D. A., and Semple, P. D'a: Primary cardiac Kaposi's /sarcoma. Thorax, *31*:595, 1976.
156. Rwomushana, R. J. W., Bailey, I. C., and Kyalwazi, S. K.: Kaposi's sarcoma of the brain. A case report with necropsy findings. Cancer, *36*:1127, 1975.
157. Ramos, C. V., Taylor, H. B., Hernandez, B. A., and Tucker, E. F.: Primary Kaposi's sarcoma of lymph nodes. Am. J. Clin. Pathol., *66*:998, 1976.
158. Cox, J. W., Halprin, K., and Ackerman, A. B.: Kaposi's sarcoma localized to the penis. Arch. Dermatol., *102*:461, 1970.
159. Feurerman, E. J., and Potruch-Eisenkraft, S.: Kaposi's sarcoma. A follow-up of 38 patients. Dermatologica, *146*:115, 1973.
160. Dörffel, J.: Histogenesis of multiple idiopathic hemorrhagic sarcoma of Kaposi. Arch. Dermatol. Syph., *26*:608, 1932.
161. Ronchese, F.: Kaposi's sarcoma and northern Italy. A 68 year old error continues to be repeated. Arch. Dermatol., *93*:148, 1966.
162. Wise, F.: Idiopathic hemorrhagic multiple sarcoma of the skin (Kaposi) with special reference to early diagnosis. M. Rec., *88*:513, 1915.
163. McCarthy, W. D., and Pack, G. T.: Malignant blood vessel tumors. A report of 56 cases of angiosarcoma and Kaposi's sarcoma. Surg. Gynecol. Obstet., *91*:465, 1950.
164. Cox, F. H., and Helwig, E. B.: Kaposi's sarcoma. Cancer, *12*:289, 1959.
165. Degos, R., Touraine, R., Civatte, J., Belaich, S., and Franck, D.: Maladie de Kaposi (à propos de 28 cas). Ann. Dermatol. Syph., *91*:113, 1964.
166. Sagher, F., Personal communication.
167. Williams, E. H., and Williams, P. H.: A note on an apparent similarity in distribution of onchocerciasis, femoral hernia and Kaposi's sarcoma in the West Nile District of Uganda. E. Afr. Med. J., *43*:208, 1966.
168. Taylor, J. F., Smith, P. G., Bull, D., and Pike, M. C.: Kaposi's sarcoma in Uganda: geographic and ethnic distribution. Br. J. Cancer, *26*:483, 1972.
169. Glaser, R., Geder, L., St. Jeor, S., Michelson-Fiske, S., and Haguenau, F.: Partial characterization of a herpes-type virus (K9V) derived from Kaposi's sarcoma. J. Nat. Cancer Inst., *59*:55, 1977.
170. Oettle, A. G.: Geographical and racial differences in the frequency of Kaposi's sarcoma as evidence of environmental or genetic causes. Acta Un. Int. Cancr., *18*:330, 1962.
171. Taylor, J. F., Templeton, A. C., Vogel, C. I., Ziegler, J., and Kyalwazi, S. K.: Kaposi's sarcoma in Uganda — a clinical pathological study. Int. J. Cancer, *22*:122, 1971.
172. Templeton, A. C., and Bhana, D.: Prognosis in Kaposi's sarcoma. J. Natl. Cancer Inst., *55*:1301, 1975.
173. Dobozy, A., Husz, S., Hunyadi, J., Berko, G., and Simon, N.: Immune deficiencies and Kaposi's sarcoma. Lancet, *2*:625, 1973.
174. Lothe, F., and Murray, J. F.: Kaposi's sarcoma: autopsy findings in the African. Acta Un. Int. Cancr., *18*:429, 1962.
175. Hardy, M. A., Goldfarb, P., Levine, S., Dattner, A., Muggia, F. M., Levitt, S., and Weinstein, E.: De novo Kaposi's sarcoma in renal transplantation. Case report and brief review. Cancer, *38*:144, 1976.
176. Templeton, A. C.: Kaposi's sarcoma. *In* Templeton, A. C.: Tumors in a Tropical Country. A Survey of Uganda. Springer-Verlag, New York, 1973, p. 268.
177. Uys, C. J., and Bennett, M. B.: Kaposi's sarcoma: a neoplasm of reticular origin. S. Afr. J. Lab. Clin. Med., *5*:39, 1959.
178. Ettinger, D. S., Humphrey, R. L., and Skinner, M. D.: Kaposi's sarcoma associated with multiple myeloma. Johns Hopkins Med. J., *137*:88, 1975.
179. Dantzig, P. I.: Kaposi sarcoma and polymyositis. Arch. Dermatol., *110*:605, 1974.
180. Krakowski, A., Brenner, S., and Covo, J.: Acquired ichthyosis in Kaposi sarcoma. Arch. Dermatol., *111*:1213, 1975.
181. Levan, N. E., Korn, C. S., Booker, J., and Rounds, D. E.: Tissue culture of Kaposi's sarcoma. Arch. Dermatol., *106*:37, 1972.
182. Becker, B. J.: The histogenesis of Kaposi's sarcoma. Acta Int. U. Canc., *18*:477, 1962.
183. Dayan, A. D., and Lewis, P. D.: Origin of Kaposi's sarcoma from the reticuloendothelial system. Nature, *213*:889, 1967.
184. Gokel, J. M., Kurzl, R., and Hubner, G.: Fine structure and origin of Kaposi's sarcoma. Pathol. Eur., *11*:45, 1976.
185. Moertel, C. G., and Hagedorn, A. B.: Leukemia or lymphoma and coexisting primary malignant lesions. A review of the literature and a study of 120 cases. Blood, *12*:788, 1957.

3

Leukemia and Allied Disorders

The basic skin markers of leukemia and polycythemia vera will be discussed in this chapter. Photographs of our own patients illustrate the characteristic lesions. For a detailed review of the literature on leukemia cutis, the reader is referred to Bluefarb's excellent monograph.[1] The relation of herpes zoster to lymphoma, leukemia, and carcinoma will also be considered.

LEUKEMIA

Leukemias and lymphomas are alike in two ways: the morphology of the specific cutaneous lesions is identical, and similar types of specific and nonspecific eruptions arise during the course of both diseases. Specific cutaneous lesions are found in 10 to 50 per cent of patients with monocytic leukemia and in 6 to 20 per cent of those with lymphocytic and granulocytic leukemias.[2-6] Although the skin markers in the various leukemias closely resemble one another in appearance, each type of leukemia tends to have its own distinctive distribution of specific lesions: in acute and chronic lymphocytic leukemia, primarily the face and the extremities are involved; in granulocytic leukemia, the trunk is affected; and in monocytic leukemia, the entire skin surface is involved. Acute monocytic leukemia tends to have more florid oral and cutaneous lesions than the other two types.

Although involvement of the mouth is the striking feature of acute leukemia, especially the monocytic variety, oral lesions can also develop in chronic leukemia. The specific leukemic infiltrates often produce hyperplasia of the gums, which at times cover the teeth completely. The red friable gingivae may bleed spontaneously or after mild trauma. If the gums and buccal mucosa ulcerate, the picture simulates Vincent's infection. Oral lesions are less severe and less common in children with monocytic leukemia than in adults.

The specific lesions of leukemia are morphologically identical to those of malignant lymphomas: the macules, papules, and tumors range in color from pink and red-brown to purple (Plate 10*D*). The solid masses are firm but not stony-hard. The tumors of monocytic leukemia tend to be large and purplish and are often referred to as "plum-colored." In several patients with monocytic leukemia, the eruption of diagnostic purplish macules and papules on the trunk resembled roseola or secondary syphilis.[7] Histologically specific cutaneous infiltrates are seen most often in chronic lymphatic and granulocytic leukemias and in the acute monocytic variety. Specific nodules, intact or ulcerated, can also arise on the buccal mucosa, palate, and tonsils, but such oral lesions are found more commonly in patients with lymphocytic lymphoma than in persons with leukemia.

When thrombocytopenia occurs, purpura often develops in the specific cutaneous nodules. Leukemia cutis can form plaques and arciform lesions, thereby simulating mycosis fungoides, and diffuse and massive infiltration can produce a leonine facies, especially in chronic lymphocytic leukemia (Plate 10*E*). The ulceration of cutaneous lesions is seen most frequently in monocytic leukemia. Leukemic infiltration of the subcutaneous fat can produce flesh-colored or erythematous nodules simulating erythema nodosum (see p. 482).[8, 9]

Unusual pictures are caused by the peculiar deposition of leukemic infiltrates: genital ulceration simulates venereal disease; periarticular subcutaneous nodules mimic juxta-articular nodes; facial involvement resembles rosacea or lupus erythematosus; the infiltration of male and female erectile tissue produces priapism; and perineal lymphatic obstruction gives rise to the appearance of esthiomene.[10, 11] Leukemia cutis can be diagnosed by biopsy, but the cell type cannot always be identified with certainty. As in lymphoma cutis, examination of touch preparations from the freshly cut surface of a cutaneous biopsy is the best way to identify the abnormal cell type.

Chloroma (granulocytic sarcoma) is a green tumor that is the sole pathognomonic lesion of leukemia. It can arise at the same time as acute granulocytic leukemia or it may precede this disease by as long as one year.[12] Chloroma is seen primarily in children and young adults under the age of 18 and results from the infiltration of immature granulocytic cells chiefly within the periosteum of the orbital and cranial bones. The sinuses, sternum, vertebrae, pelvis, and long bones can also be involved. Proptosis and tumors of the scalp occur when the orbit and cranium are severely affected. The chloromas can expand subdurally and epidurally and compress the brain, cranial nerves, and spinal cord. One of our patients with acute granulocytic leukemia had green-colored intradermal nodules on the trunk as a manifestation of leukemia cutis. Chloroma was named for its green color, which fades within one to three hours after the cut tumor is exposed to air. The green pigment is an enzyme, myeloperoxidase (verdoperoxidase), which can be regenerated temporarily by exposure to hydrogen peroxide.[13]

Sweet's syndrome — acute febrile neutrophilic dermatosis — is characterized by multiple warm, painful, discrete red plaques or papules that usually arise in crops on the face, neck, upper chest, arms, and legs (see p. 753). High fever, leukocytosis, and neutrophilia frequently accompany these cutaneous lesions, and the affected individual appears and feels ill. Although most reported cases have followed an infectious illness, seven of 66 patients had acute myelogenous leukemia and two, acute blastic leukemia.[14-16]

Many authors in the past have cited instances of individuals with lymphocytic leukemia whose disease seemed to have arisen in the skin or subcutaneous tissues. They had specific cutaneous lesions that were present for months before the hematologic abnormalities appeared and that sometimes behaved independently of the peripheral blood findings.[17] Currently, one would interpret these cases as representing well-differentiated lymphocytic lymphoma (small lymphocytic, B-cell type lymphoma) that has subsequently involved the bone marrow or has passed from the tissue phase into the hematologic phase. Some authors believe that lymphocytic lymphoma may develop in either direction.[18, 19]

Leukemic infiltrates may arise in scars from recent surgery, trauma, burns, herpes zoster, and herpes simplex. They are also found at the sites of intramuscular injections. Plate 12*A* illustrates this principle. This patient with acute myeloblastic leukemia and thrombocytopenia developed a painful hemorrhagic nodule on her breast either spontaneously or following minor trauma. A biopsy revealed both extensive red blood cell extravasation and a moderate leukemic infiltrate.

Nonspecific cutaneous manifestations of leukemia include the pallor of anemia, purpura and bleeding from the mucous membranes secondary to thrombocytopenia, and the general wasting of malignant disease. Pruritus and herpes zoster are seen more frequently with chronic lymphocytic leukemia than with the two other types. Prurigo-like papules, erythema multiforme, bullous pemphigoid, hyperpigmentation, and nonspecific eczematous eruptions have also been observed with leukemia, but they are more frequently associated with the malignant lymphomas. Acquired ichthyosis and keratoderma of the palms and soles have not been reported in leukemia. Because of decreased host resistance, pyoderma is common in acute leukemia.

Typical and unusual eruptions observed in our own patients with leukemia are illustrated in the following photographs. Figures 3–1 and 3–2 show gingival hyperplasia and widespread purpuric nodules in patients with acute and subacute monocytic leukemia, respectively. The characteristic specific lesions of the leukemias — red-purple nodules of varying size — are distributed over the trunk of a patient with chronic granulocytic leukemia (Plate 10*F*). Over the ankles and dorsa of the feet, this same patient had a purplish confluent eruption composed of discrete papules, which on casual examination might have been confused with a stasis dermatitis (Plate 11*A*). Biopsy of these lesions showed a specific cellular infiltrate.

The patient in Plate 11*B* had subacute lymphoblastic leukemia. Hyperpigmented spots together with nodules and plaques are scattered over the entire skin. Histologic examination revealed that hyperpigmentation was confined to those areas of lymphoblastic infiltrate. The intervening normal skin showed a few leukemic cells or none at all. The infiltrating leukemic cells may have stimulated the overlying melanocytes to produce more pigment.

Although erythroderma and exfoliative dermatitis have been considered to be features of chronic lymphatic leukemia, Edelson et al. have questioned the validity of these associations on the basis of their recent observations (see p. 121). It is likely that most, if not all, of the cases diagnosed as chronic lymphatic leukemia with erythroderma actually represent patients with the Sézary syndrome. The case reports summarized by Bluefarb[20] are compatible with the Sézary syndrome. Prospective studies will clarify this point. In the patient shown in Plate 11*C*, the erythroderma had been attributed to chronic lymphatic leukemia. After reviewing her course and skin biopsies, it was clear that she had the Sézary syndrome. The biopsies showed an upper dermal, bandlike

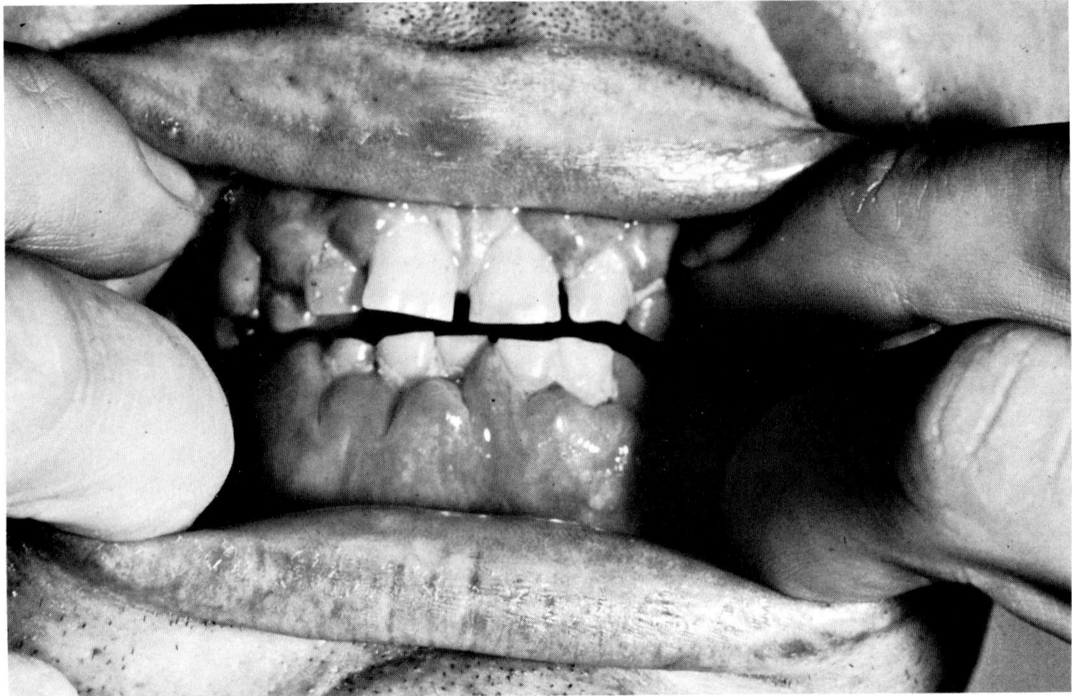

Figure 3–1. Monocytic leukemia. Gingival hypertrophy produced by leukemic infiltrates. (From Evans, T. S., and Lomardo, R.: The skin and mucous membrane manifestations of monocytic leukemia. Conn. Med., *23*:644, 1959.)

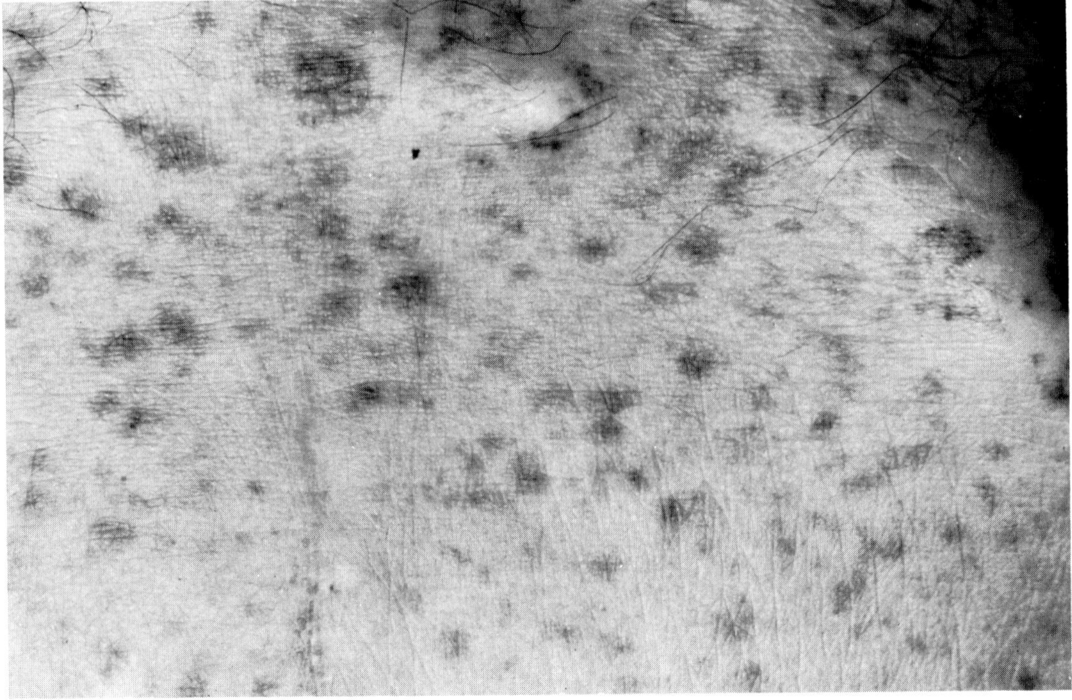

Figure 3–2. Monocytic leukemia. Purpura present in cutaneous infiltrates.

infiltrate composed of lymphoid cells with grooved nuclei. Two years before her death, she developed Kaposi's sarcoma superimposed on the erythroderma, which had been treated continuously by corticosteroids and chlorambucil for several years.

A specific tumor mass of chronic lymphatic leukemia is shown in Plate 11D. Hemorrhage and necrosis are present in the center of the tumor, which is indistinguishable from those seen in the malignant lymphomas.

An unusual lesion in a child with acute lymphoblastic leukemia is illustrated in Figure 3–3. Many erythematous and purpuric papules exhibiting a central necrotic spot were present on the extremities. Biopsy revealed an acute angiitis in the upper dermis and marked perivascular cuffing by lymphoblasts in the lower dermis. Angiitis in leukemia, lymphoma, and plasma cell dyscrasias is being recognized more frequently and is usually associated with monoclonal or mixed cryoglobulins, which can produce immune complex disease.[21]

Plate 11*E* and *F* shows a patient with diffuse, polycyclic, reddish-brown, and minimally infiltrated patches over the trunk and shoulders. The lesions simulated most closely a fungal infection caused by *Trichophyton rubrum*. However, biopsy demonstrated the characteristic lesion of chronic granulocytic leukemia. Specific leukemic infiltrates often involve the subcutis and produce flesh-colored or pink nodules as illustrated in Figure 3–4. Such lesions are seen best in profile. In this particular patient an acute granulocytic leukemia arose during the course of myeloid metaplasia. The lesions were stony-hard — a most unusual finding in leukemia and lymphoma cutis.

The patient shown in Figure 3–5 and in Plate 13*A* developed a pruritic red-brown mildly eczematous eruption on her legs as a nonspecific

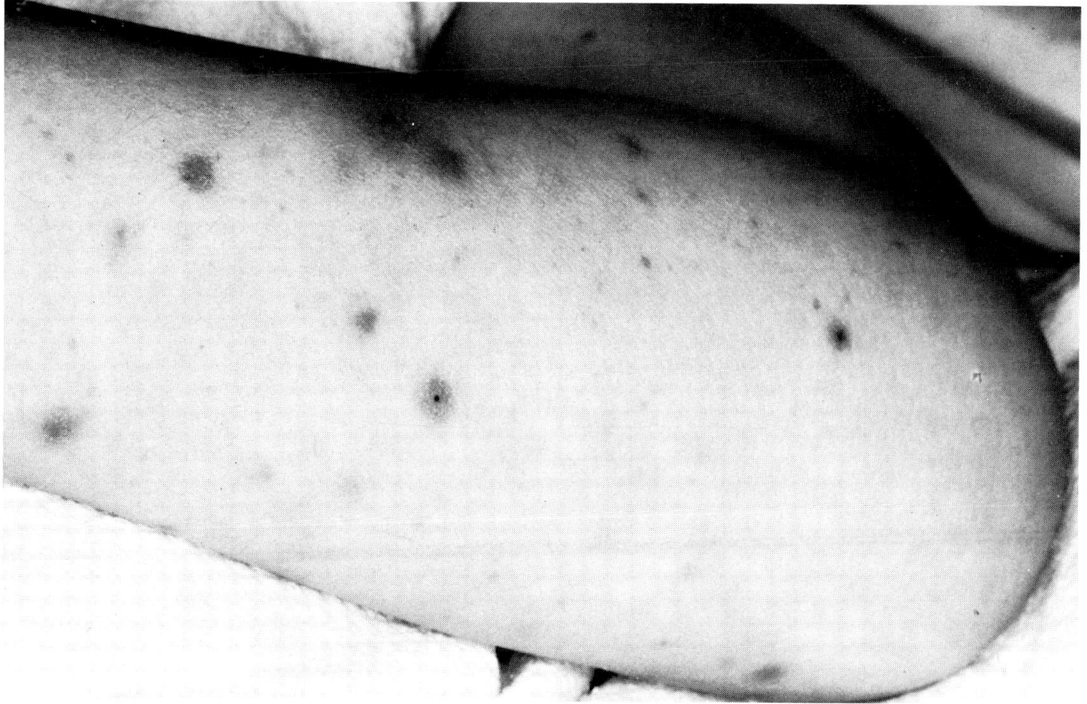

Figure 3–3. Acute lymphoblastic leukemia. Purpuric spots showed necrotizing angiitis as well as leukemic infiltrates.

PLATE 11

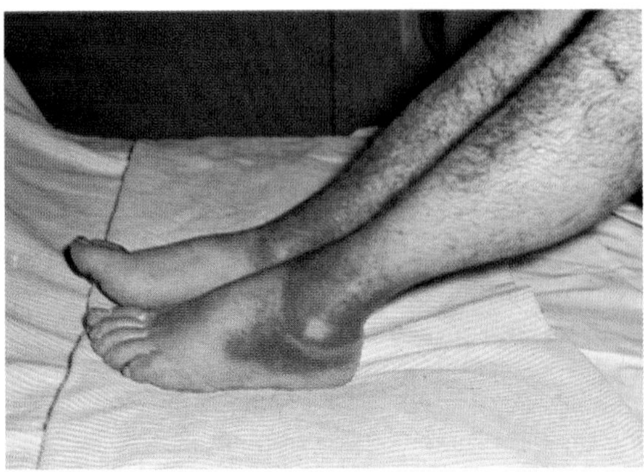

A, Chronic granulocytic leukemia. Infiltrates mimic stasis dermatitis.

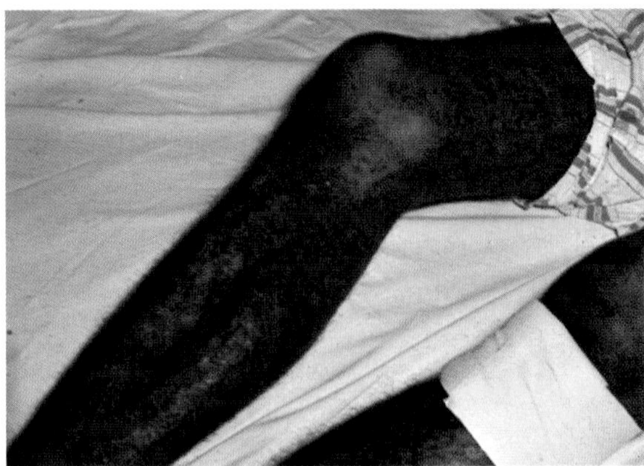

B, Subacute lymphoblastic leukemia. Hyperpigmentation confined to sites of cutaneous infiltration.

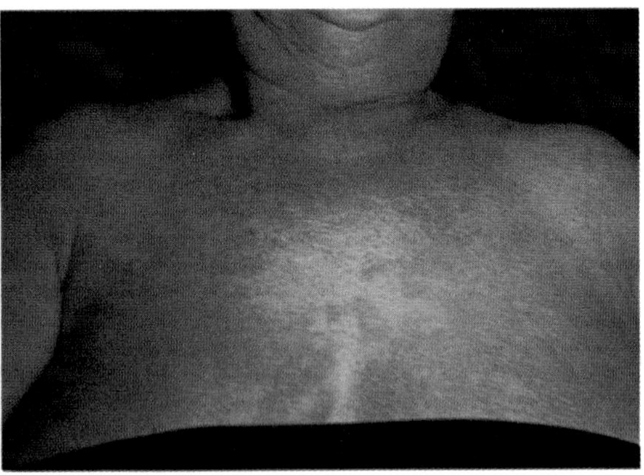

C, Chronic lymphocytic leukemia. Diffuse infiltration produced an erythroderma.

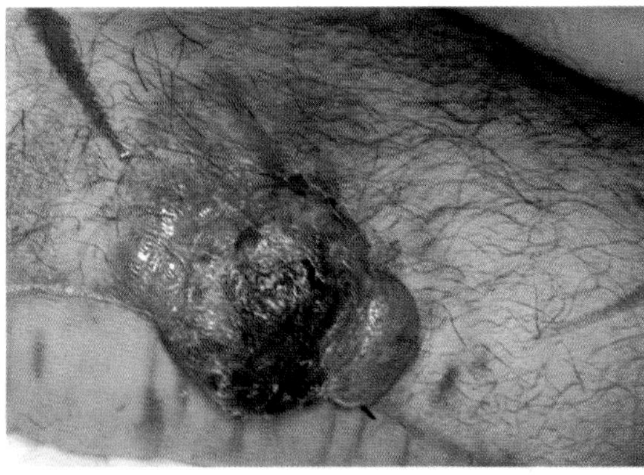

D, Chronic lymphocytic leukemia. Localized tumor.

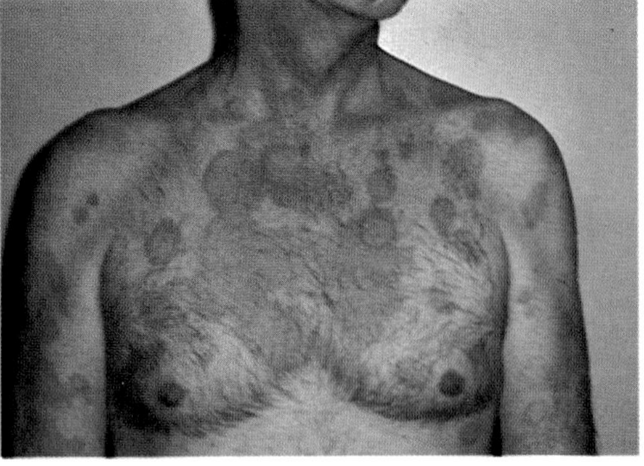

E, Chronic granulocytic leukemia. Infiltrates mimic a tinea infection.

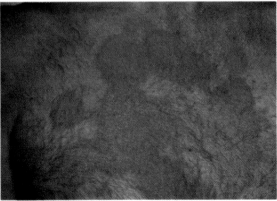

F, Chronic granulocytic leukemia. Close view of lesions in *E*.

PLATE 12

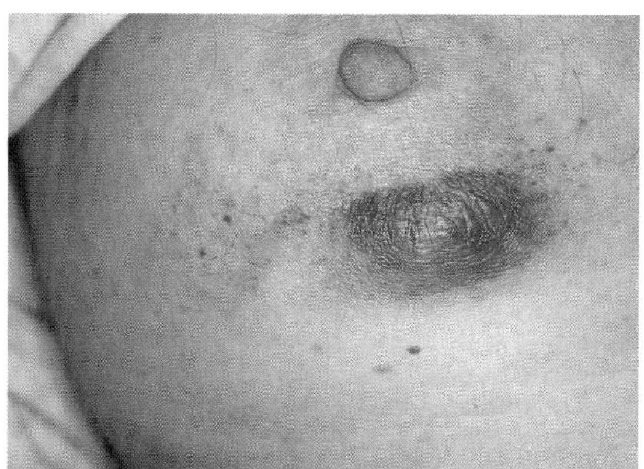

A, Acute myeloblastic leukemia. Nodule showed both red cell extravasation and leukemic infiltrate. Produced by trauma in patient with thrombocytopenia.

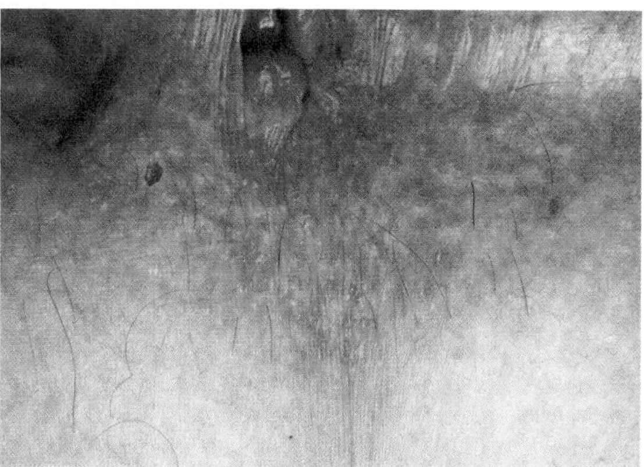

B, Histiocytosis X. Perianal lesion mimicking extramammary Paget's disease.

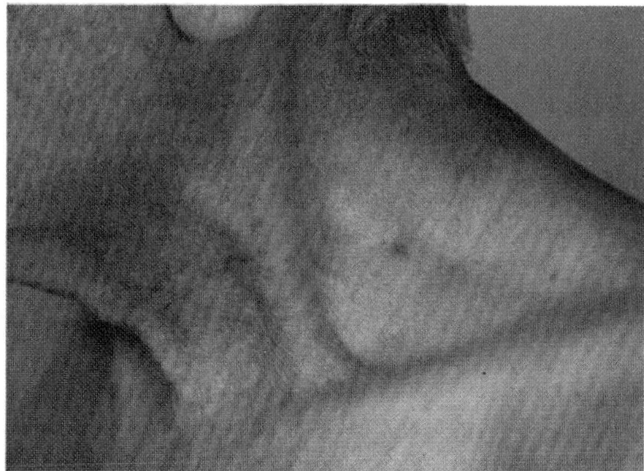

C, Normolipemic plane xanthoma in patient with plasmacytosis in bone marrow. Marrow findings not yet diagnostic of multiple myeloma.

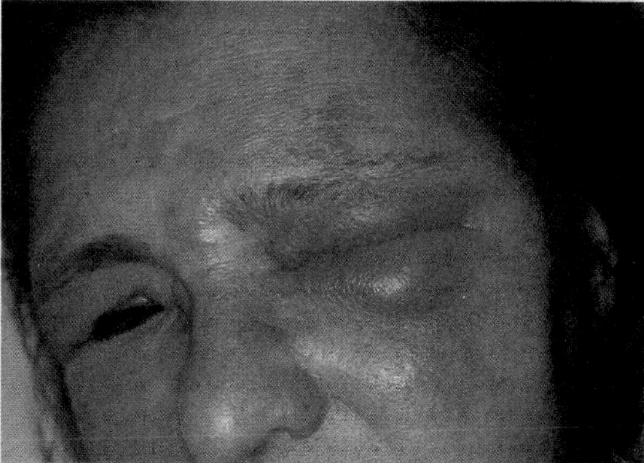

D, One of several recurrent episodes of erysipelas in a woman with idiopathic acquired agammaglobulinemia.

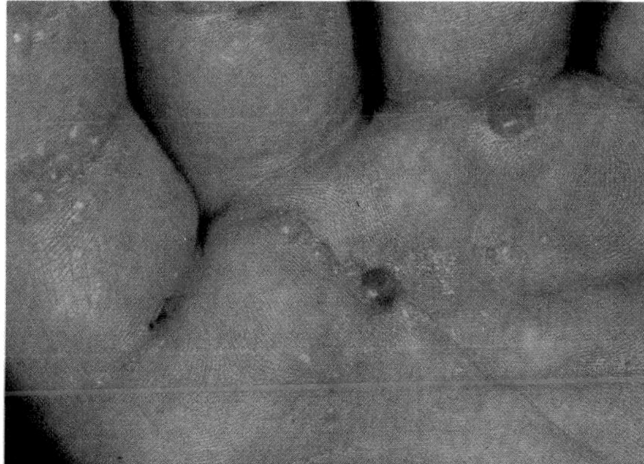

E, Generalized amyloidosis secondary to myeloma. Amyloid nodules on palm, one of which has become purpuric after trauma.

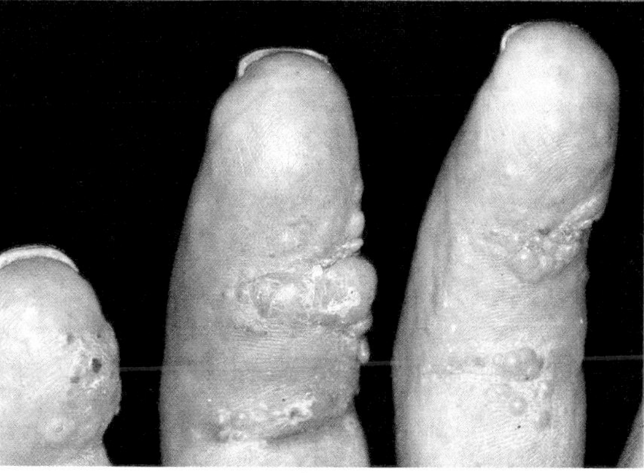

F, Generalized amyloidosis secondary to myeloma. Nodules on fingers. Same patient as in *E*.

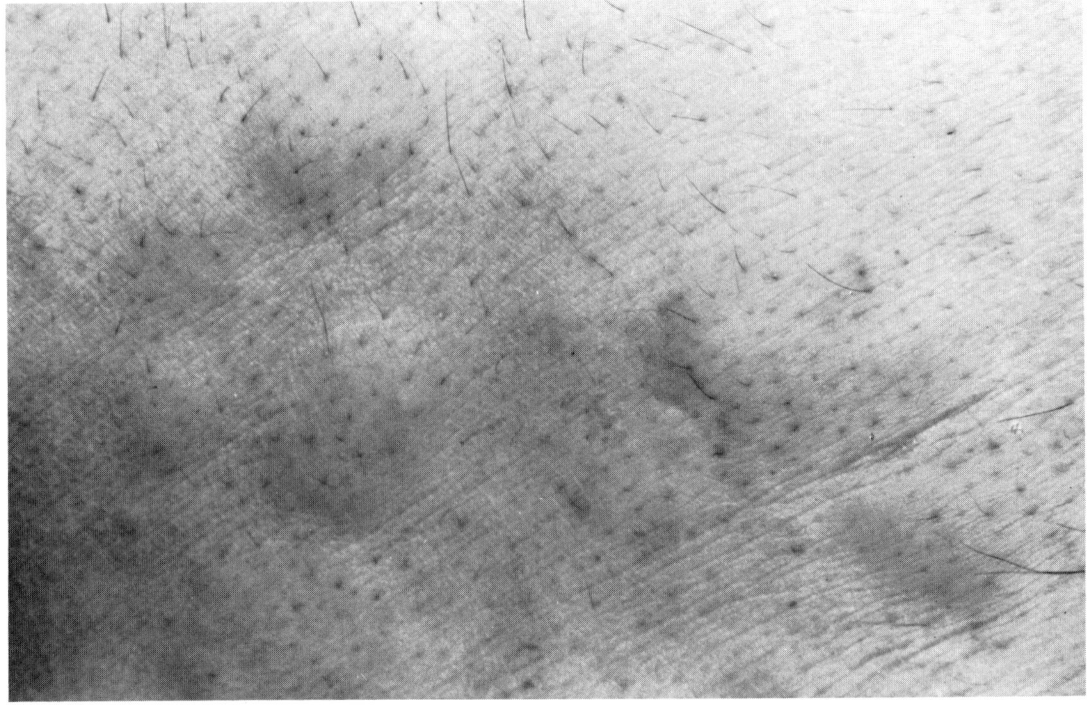

Figure 3–4. Acute granulocytic leukemia. Subcutaneous leukemic infiltrates.

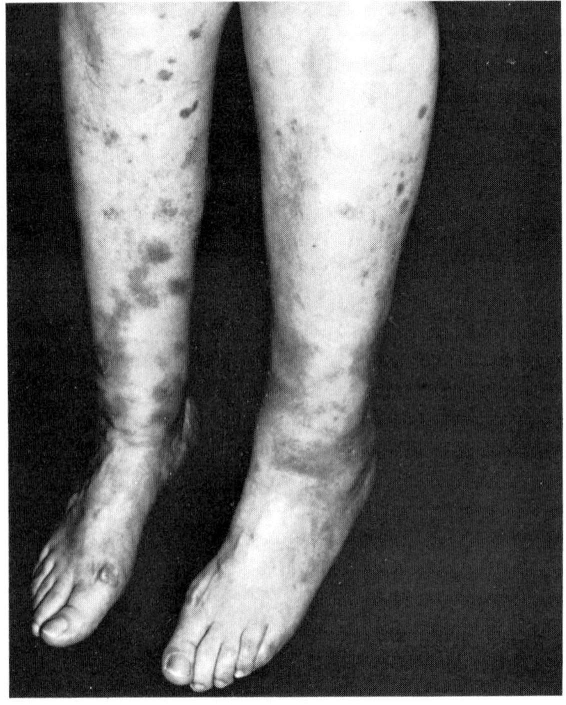

Figure 3–5. Chronic granulocytic leukemia. Nonspecific eczematous eruption. Same patient shown in Plate 13*A*.

manifestation of chronic granulocytic leukemia. Histologic examination revealed a chronic inflammatory reaction. At first glance the diagnosis seemed to be stasis dermatitis, but the character and distribution of the lesions, the lack of venous insufficiency, and the histopathology excluded that diagnosis.

Although there are many variations in the specific lesions of the leukemias, one feature is common to all: the erythematous red-brown or purplish color. A papule, nodule, or tumor with these colors should alert one to the possibility of lymphoma or leukemia. Sarcoidosis, lupus erythematous, and occasionally histiocytosis must also be considered.

HERPES ZOSTER AND MALIGNANCY

The increased incidence of herpes zoster in patients with lymphoma and leukemia, especially Hodgkin's disease and chronic lymphocytic leukemia, has been recognized for many years (Fig. 3–6). Zoster and carcinoma, primarily mammary cancer, have also been linked. Hope-Simpson proposed a hypothesis based in part upon his meticulous study of 192 patients with zoster to explain these associations. From 1947 to 1962, he saw virtually every case of zoster in his practice of 3500 people in a rural community in England.[22] In his series, the annual incidence of zoster was three to four cases per 1000 individuals. The disease did not follow a seasonal pattern, nor was there an increased incidence during four epidemics of varicella. None of his patients with zoster transmitted the virus to another individual. Furthermore, the disease did not appear in any adult who had been exposed to children with chickenpox. Adults with

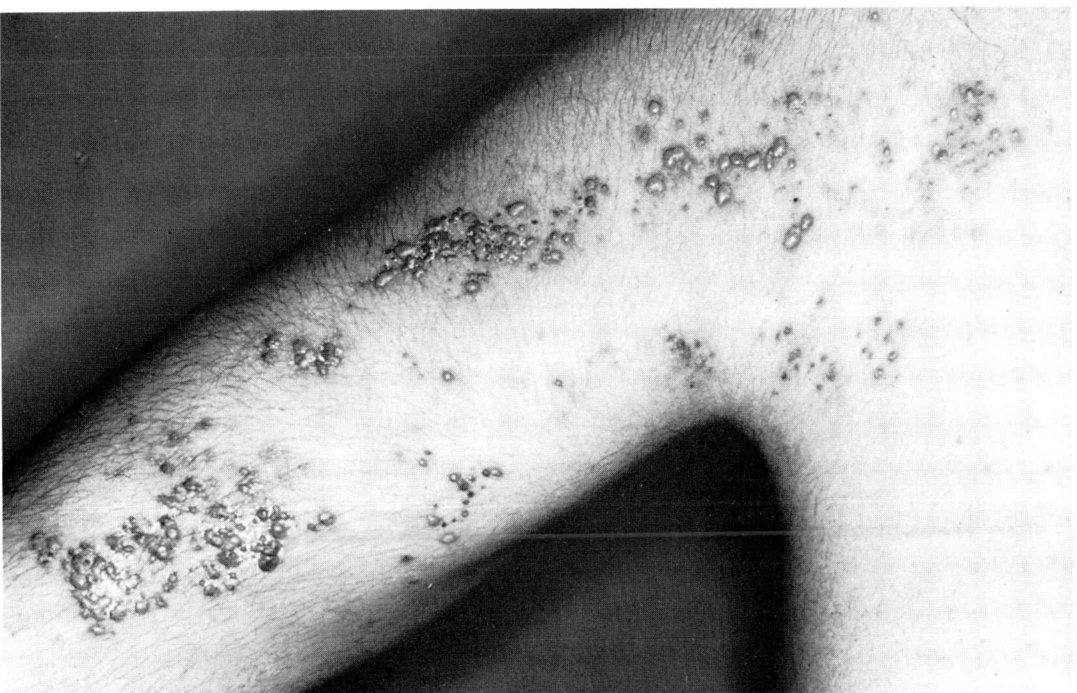

Figure 3–6. Herpes zoster.

zoster are infectious and can therefore transmit the virus to susceptible children and produce chickenpox. Although zoster has been reported in adults exposed either to other adults with zoster or to children with varicella, these examples are probably exceptions to the usual course of events in zoster.

During an episode of varicella, the virus invades the neurons in the dorsal root ganglia and becomes latent and noninfectious. Hope-Simpson postulated that since the zoster-varicella virus is an obligate parasite for man, it would be eliminated from humans within a single generation if it were not able to leave the host and infect a susceptible person. Thus the development of zoster in the adult permits the virus to complete its life cycle by infecting a susceptible child.

The zoster virus could be reactivated and become infectious in two ways: cellular death might reactivate the virus and liberate infectious particles, or a latent virus in a viable neuron could be induced to replicate and become infectious through the action of infiltrating cells in the ganglion. Clinical disease would develop when the number of viral particles was in excess of the neutralizing capacity of the available antibodies. This ratio could be critical. If neutralizing antibodies were in excess, the infectious particles could act as an immunizing booster. Brunell et al. found that individuals previously exposed to varicella and then intimately reexposed to patients with chickenpox or zoster developed an increase in the level of serum antibodies against this virus. Thus, reinfection can be an immunizing booster without producing clinical disease. Hope-Simpson's hypothesis and the observation of Brunell et al. probably represent the natural course of zoster in normal individuals.[23]

However, in terminal monomorphous lymphomas, Hodgkin's disease and chronic lymphatic leukemia, the increased frequency of zoster may be related to depression of cellular immunity in association with viral activation by a variety of mechanisms that are still speculative.[25] Neuronal death with viral replication could result from trauma to the spinal cord, from neoplasms impinging upon or infiltrating the dorsal roots, spinal cord, and nerves, or from gliosis and vascular insufficiency produced in the nervous tissue by deep x-irradiation. Sabin and Koch demonstrated that a latent virus could be activated without the death of the host cells, by the exposure of that virus to certain other cells.[24] It is possible that the leukemic cells, which are known to infiltrate the dorsal ganglia, can induce the latent zoster virus to become infectious. Another major factor that seems to be responsible for the increased prevalence of zoster in Hodgkin's and non-Hodgkin's lymphomas is splenectomy combined with extended-field radiation therapy and chemotherapy.[26, 27] In one series, the zoster tended to become generalized,[26] while in another, dissemination did not occur.[27]

In most cases of zoster associated with carcinoma (usually mammary), the patient had been treated with deep x-ray and the spinal cord was situated within the radiation port. The development of zoster three to six months after the administration of x-ray therapy correlates with the interval necessary for both the production of gliosis and the vascular insufficiency in nervous tissue that results in the death of neurons.[28]

Disseminated zoster often appears in association with neoplasms. Five to eight days after the initial zonal outbreak, zoster vesicles can erupt over the entire body without any relation to dermatomes. The vesicles may be umbilicated or look like varicella. Dissemination usually lasts from two days to two weeks. Stevens and Merigan have shown that the kinetics of interferon appearance in the vesicle fluid correlate most closely with the course of the zoster.[29] Cessation of dissemination follows the development of peak levels of interferon in the vesicles. Those in whom the zoster remained localized had an early and sharp rise in vesicular interferon levels, whereas in those in whom dissemination developed, the rise in interferon levels began later and was slower. However, both groups reached comparable peak levels of interferon in the vesicle fluid. Dissemination stopped 48 hours after peak levels were reached, regardless of its time of onset after its first appearance of zoster, or the length of time it remained generalized. Humoral antibodies were relatively unimportant in preventing dissemination, because in some patients complement-fixing antibodies to zoster virus were detected before the development of the generalized spread, and in others, antibodies did not appear until after the dissemination had ended. The relation between local interferon production and the humoral and cellular immune systems is not fully understood.

The initial zonal eruption and the disseminated vesicles can be hemorrhagic and destructive. Herpes zoster tends to produce severe necrosis in patients with malignancies as well as in those with chronic illnesses such as diabetes mellitus. Although widespread dissemination occurs primarily in persons with an underlying serious disorder, it can also develop in a healthy individual. It is not uncommon to see several vesicles resembling chickenpox outside the dermatome distribution in a

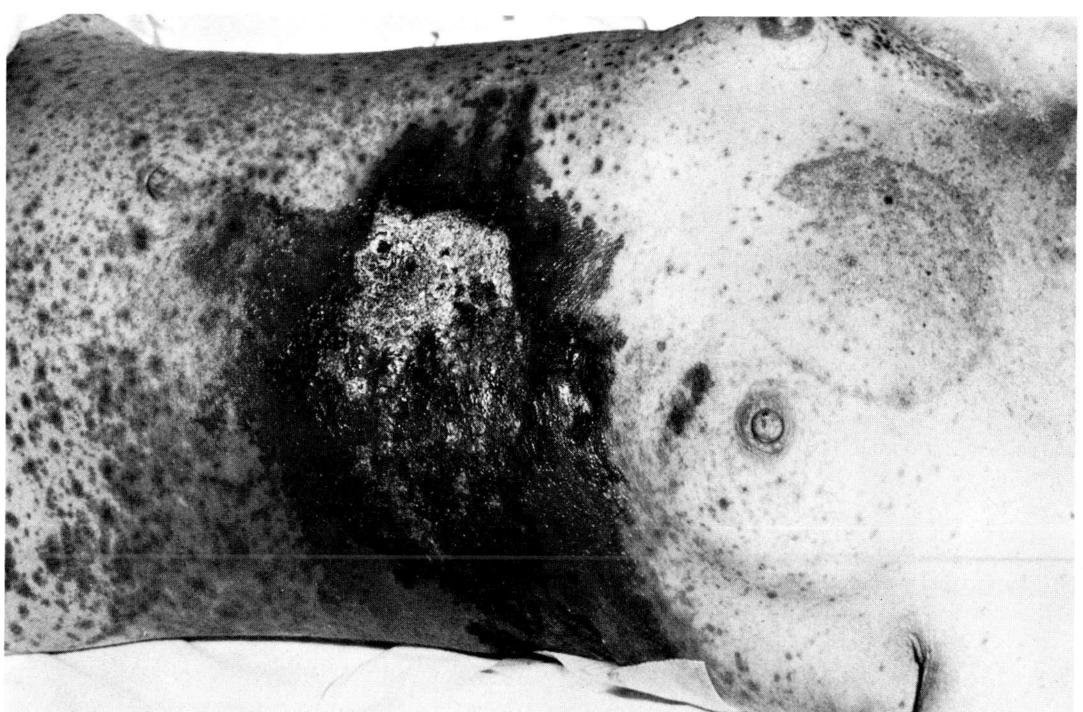

Figure 3–7. Herpes zoster and disseminated herpes simplex in patient with Hodgkin's disease.

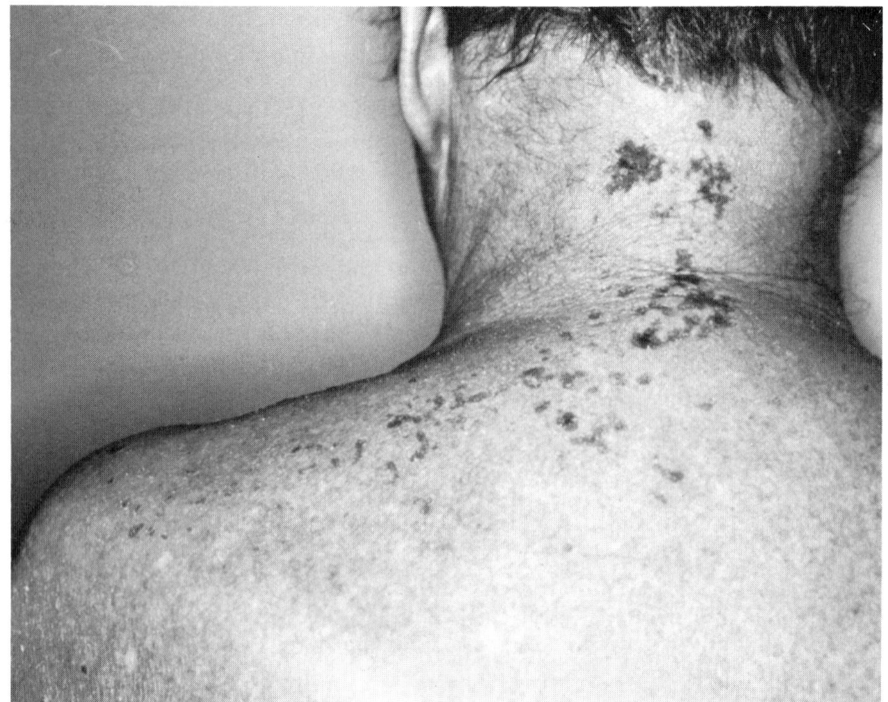

Figure 3–8. Herpes zoster in patient with mycosis fungoides. Sequence of events leading to dissemination shown in Figures 3–8 to 3–11. Initial eruption of zoster.

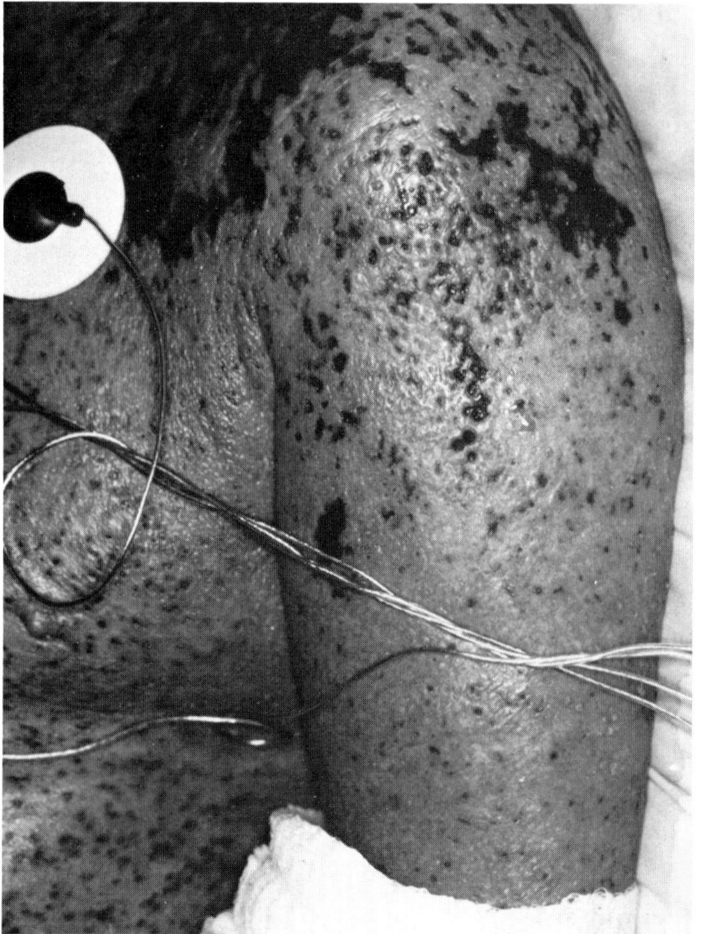

Figure 3–9. Initial eruption of zoster has become hemorrhagic and ulcerative.

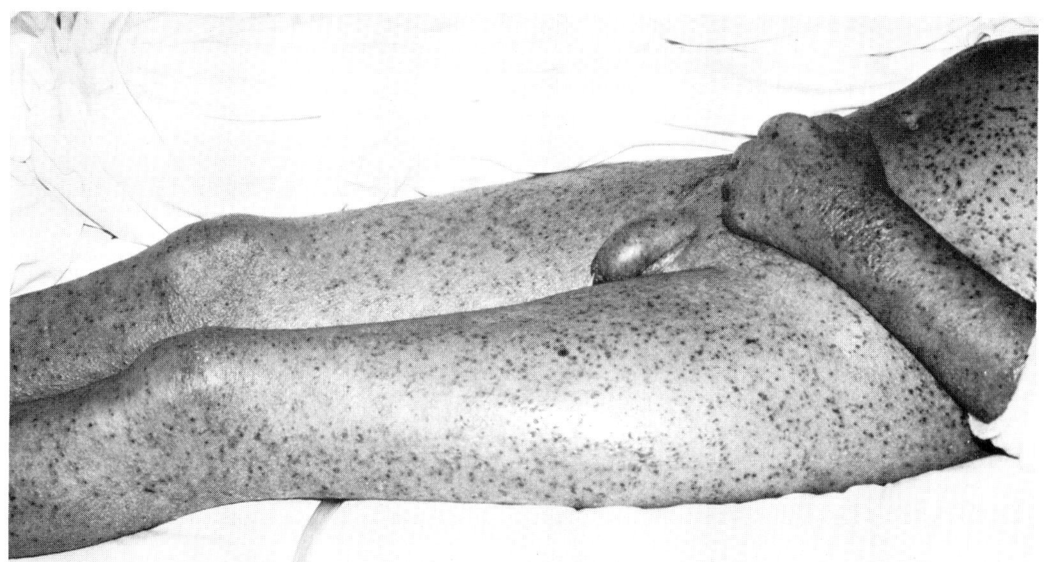

Figure 3–10. Zoster has become generalized, producing confluent umbilicated vesicles over the entire body surface.

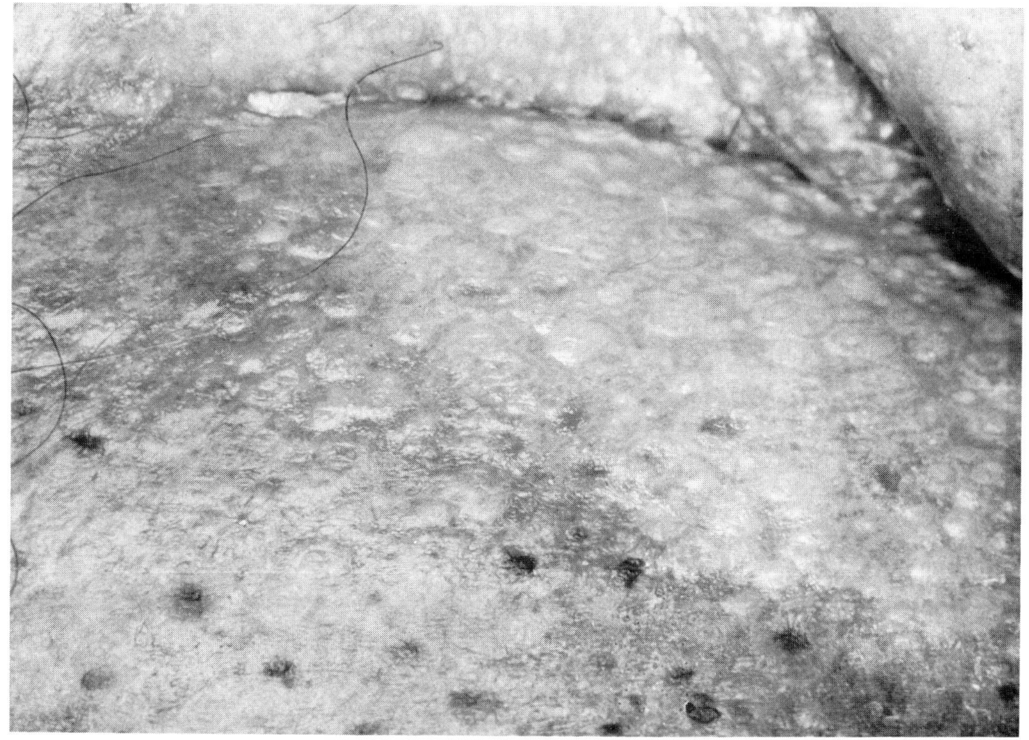

Figure 3–11. Close-up of the confluent umbilicated vesicles of generalized zoster in the patient shown in this sequence.

healthy person with zoster. Viremia is responsible for this phenomenon.

Herpes zoster usually develops during the course of lymphomatous disease and rarely is the presenting sign. Only patients having destructive lesions or an unusually prolonged course should be investigated for underlying disease.

In one of our patients with Hodgkin's disease and zoster, an unusual course occurred (Fig. 3–7). The zonal eruption arose on the left flank. One week later a scattered vesicular eruption appeared and continued to spread for 53 days. Herpes simplex was cultured from the generalized lesions. It is likely that this patient had both herpes zoster and a disseminated herpes simplex infection. In another patient with mycosis fungoides on chemotherapy, culture-proven dissemination by zoster produced confluent umbilicated vesicles over the entire skin surface (Figs. 3–8 and 3–11).

In the past, persons with lymphoma or chronic lymphatic leukemia who were vaccinated were liable to develop a progressive vaccinial reaction. In progressive vaccinia, the primary vaccination site does not heal because of continued viral replication and a resultant progressive infection of the surrounding skin. Vaccinial lesions develop in uninoculated areas because of viremia; visceral organs may also be infected. This complication of vaccination is associated with an absence of delayed hypersensitivity to inactivated vaccinia virus. Since smallpox now appears to have been eradicated from the world, there is no longer any medical indication for vaccination. Progressive vaccinia should never again occur in clinical medicine.

MYELOPROLIFERATIVE DISORDERS

The myeloproliferative disorders comprise a group of conditions characterized by an uncontrolled proliferation of one or more bone marrow elements. The entities include polycythemia vera, myelofibrosis (myelosclerosis) with or without extramedullary hematopoiesis, primary thrombocytosis (hemorrhagic thrombocythemia), and chronic granulocytic leukemia.[31] It is common to see transformations from the less malignant to the more malignant disorders in this group but not the reverse. For example, the initial picture of polycythemia vera is that of hyperplasia of red and white blood cells and platelet precursors within a very hypercellular marrow. As the illness progresses, there may be a tendency for the development of fibrosis in the marrow with an accompanying sequela of extramedullary hematopoiesis. Later, pancytopenia secondary to marrow failure may develop, accompanied by massive hepato- and splenomegaly. Approximately 10 per cent of such patients develop granulocytic leukemia. The designation *myeloproliferative diseases* is also employed as a concept by which one can view a group of disorders that have the common features of marrow element proliferation, marrow fibrosis, and splenic involvement without requiring a transformation from one entity to another. These disorders also have a number of abnormal laboratory findings and clinical features in common, which makes it useful to consider them as a group. However, one specific abnormality, the Philadelphia chromosome, is present only in chronic granulocytic leukemia and not in any of the other disorders.

In polycythemia vera, all three components of the bone marrow — erythrocytes, leukocytes, and platelets — proliferate. A marked increase in blood volume accompanies the persistent erythrocytosis and produces vascular engorgement of the viscera and skin. At autopsy, dark blood flows freely from cut parenchymatous organs.[32]

Individuals with polycythemia typically appear plethoric and have a ruddy complexion secondary to an overdistended cutaneous vasculature. This deep red color occurs primarily on the face, neck, and distal extremities. The veins of the sclerae and retinae may be dark and distended. Because numerous telangiectatic vessels are superimposed upon the facial erythema, the misdiagnosis of rosacea has been made in many patients. The oral musocal vessels are also dilated, and a deep red-blue color can be seen in the pharynx, tonsils, and tongue. Vascular engorgement may be severe enough to cause enlargement of the tongue.

Not all patients with polycythemia vera are deeply erythematous, and the intensity of color can vary from day to day. In patients successfully treated by venesection or other means, erythema may persist in spite of a normal hematocrit.

Petechiae and ecchymoses are frequently produced in the skin by relatively mild injury. Dental extractions are often followed by severe bleeding; epistaxis is not uncommon; and intramuscular injections cause hematomas. The other myeloproliferative disorders exhibit similar bleeding problems. In primary thrombocytosis, there is the additional problem of gastrointestinal hemorrhage. In all of the myeloproliferative diseases, one can demonstrate one or more of the following: poor clot retraction, abnormalities in platelet adhesiveness or defective platelet aggregation in response to adrenalin, ADP, collagen, and thrombin. Mild disseminated intravascular coagulation can be demonstrated in some patients.[33] Not all patients show the same hematologic abnormalities. There is no clear correlation between any specific abnormality of platelet, coagulation, or fibrinolytic function and clinical bleeding in a given patient. However, it has been suggested that platelet dysfunction and coagulation abnormalities in the same patient may act synergistically to precipitate bleeding. Figure 3–12 illustrates extensive purpura following minor trauma in a patient with polycythemia vera.

Acne urticata has been considered a specific sign of polycythemia vera, but it also occurs in the lymphomatous diseases as well as in healthy people (see previous discussion, p. 119).

Twenty to 50 per cent of patients with polycythemia vera develop severe pruritus or cutaneous sensations of burning following a hot shower.[34, 35] These paresthesias may persist for 15 to 30 minutes and be so severe that the patient refuses to bathe again. Pruritus after bathing is not unusual in individuals with eczema and ichthyosis, but the severity and duration of itching is minimal compared to that seen in patients with polycythemia vera. Gilbert et al. have correlated the pruritus with elevated levels of histamine found in the blood and urine. The production of histamine appeared to be localized to the basophils and other granulocytes.[36] Gilbert et al. also found that patients with an elevated level of histamine in any of the myeloproliferative disorders were five times as likely to have pruritus as those individuals with normal levels of histamine. The pruritus in polycythemia vera is sometimes relieved by reduction of the red cell mass. Chanarin and Szur reported that oral

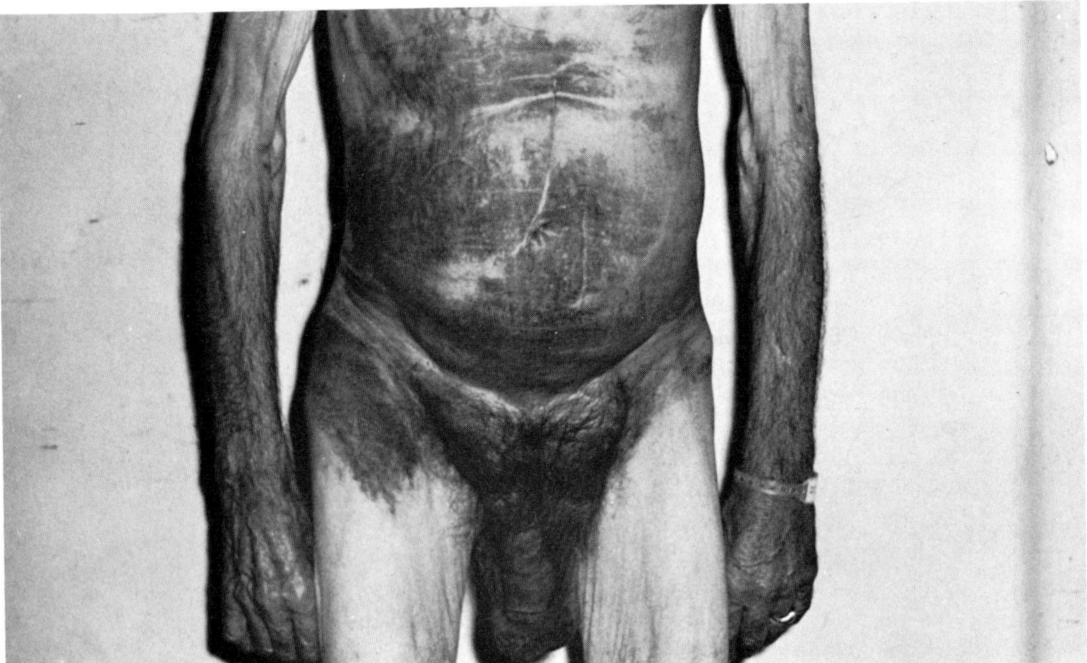

Figure 3–12. Polycythemia vera. Extensive cutaneous purpura in a patient with polycythemia vera following the removal of a mustard plaster.

cholestyramine was successful in alleviating pruritus in four patients with polycythemia vera,[37] and Easton and Galbraith found that cimetidine, a histamine H_2 receptor antagonist, was strikingly effective in one patient.[38] The latter observation is especially interesting, since pruritus is thought to be histamine H_1 receptor mediated.

Erythromelalgia (erythermalgia) is a peculiar vascular response seen most frequently in patients with polycythemia vera and the other myeloproliferative disorders.[39-41] It may precede the appearance of polycythemia by as much as three to 14 years.[40] Sensations of heat and pain accompany erythematous swelling of the legs. The pain is variously described as burning, stinging, sharp, or stabbing. The lower extremities are usually affected, although sometimes the hands or fingers may be involved. The entire leg or simply the feet, soles, or toes may show this peculiar vascular reaction. Although an attack is usually bilateral, unilateral episodes occur. Erythromelalgia may persist for minutes to hours or even for two to three days. Increased environmental temperature, walking, standing, exercising, and, in some susceptible individuals, the wearing of gloves or shoes may set off erythromelalgia. Elevation of the extremities and cooling alleviate the symptoms. Aspirin is often an effective remedy. If the polycythemia is successfully treated, the erythromelalgia may disappear.

Polycythemia vera and primary thrombocytosis are complicated by venous and arterial thromboses in 30 to 50 per cent of cases.[42, 43] Increased blood viscosity secondary to an enlarged red cell mass, elevated numbers of platelets, and occasional spontaneous platelet aggregation[44] are believed to be responsible for the vascular complications. In one series, the most frequently involved vessels in decreasing order were the cerebral, peripheral, coronary, and retinal.[42] Usually the episodes of ischemia are recurrent and transient before permanent loss of function develops. Disturbances in vision, aphasia, transient hemiparesis, and facial weakness are common signs and symptoms. Involvement of peripheral arteries produces gangrene of fingers and toes. Sometimes only single digits may be affected. Superficial and deep thrombophlebitis, livedo reticularis, leg ulcers, and cold sensitivity producing chilblain-like lesions are also common findings in this group of disorders.[45] Both arterial and venous thromboses can occur in the same patient. A picture simulating thromboangiitis obliterans can be produced. In a few patients with ischemia of the toes, the cause was shown to be not local thromboses, but emboli from a mural thrombus in the proximal femoral or popliteal arteries. In this series of 200 patients with polycythemia vera,[42] cerebrovascular occlusion occurred four times more often than coronary artery disease, and ischemic changes of the fingers and toes developed before the warning symptoms of claudication, the reverse of the findings in atherosclerosis. Although ischemia and gangrenous changes of the digits are most frequently seen in patients with atherosclerosis, diabetes mellitus, and scleroderma, one should consider the possibility of polycythemia vera and idiopathic thrombocytosis when digital ischemia and gangrene develop without prior warning. Although these vascular complications often occur during the course of untreated disease, they have been the presenting features of the illness.

In the differential diagnosis of polycythemia, the absence of clubbing helps to distinguish polycythemia vera from the secondary polycythemia of pulmonary and cardiac disease. In addition, there exists a group of patients with red faces in whom the hematocrit and levels of hemoglobin are elevated, thereby simulating polycythemia vera. This group is composed of hypertensive individuals who are being treated with diuretics.[46] These patients have a normal red cell mass with a decreased plasma volume which has spuriously raised the hematocrit to mimic polycythemia vera. "Stress" polycythemia and "relative" polycythemia are terms that have been used to describe similar syndromes in the past.

REFERENCES

1. Bluefarb, S. M.: Leukemia Cutis. Charles C Thomas, Springfield, Ill., 1960.
2. Fairburn, E. A., and Burgen, A. S. V.: The skin lesions of monocytic leukemia. Br. J. Cancer, *1*:352, 1947.
3. Doan, C. A., and Wiseman, B. K.: Monocyte, monocytosis and monocytic leukosis — a clinical and pathologic study. Ann. Intern. Med., *8*:383, 1934.
4. Osgood, E. E.: Monocytic-leukemia: report of six cases and review of one hundred twenty-seven cases. Arch. Intern. Med., *59*:931, 1937.
5. Epstein, E., and MacEachern, K.: Dermatologic manifestations of the lymphoblastoma-leukemia group. Arch. Intern. Med., *60*:867, 1937.
6. Freeman, H. E., and Koletsky, S.: Cutaneous lesions in monocytic leukemia. Report of two cases with pathologic study. Arch. Dermatol. Syph., *40*:218, 1939.
7. Mercer, S. T.: The dermatosis of monocytic leukemia. Arch. Dermatol. Syph., *31*:615, 1935.
8. Lynch, F. W.: Cutaneous lesions associated with monocytic leukemia and reticuloendotheliosis. Arch. Dermatol. Syph., *34*:775, 1936.
9. Gaté, J., and Cuilleret, P.: A propos des manifestations cutanées des leucémies. Bull. Soc. Franc. Dermatol. Syph., *44*:1213, 1937.
10. Bluefarb, S. M., and Webster, J. R.: Leukemia cutis simulating venereal disease. Quart. Bull. Northwestern Univ. Med. School, *27*:18, 1953.

11. Yaffee, H. S.: Esthiomene secondary to chronic lymphatic leukemia. Arch. Dermatol., *85*:408, 1962.
12. Rappaport, H.: Tumors of the hematopoietic system: *In* Atlas of Tumor Pathology. section III, fasc. 8, Armed Forces Institute of Pathology, Washington, 1966, p. 241.
13. Agner, K.: Verdoperoxidase. A ferment isolated from leucocytes. Acta Physiol. Scand., *2* (Suppl. 8):1, 1941.
14. Klock, J. C., and Oken, R. L.: Febrile neutrophilic dermatosis in acute myelogenous leukemia. Cancer, *37*:922, 1976.
15. Raimer, S. S., and Duncan, W. C.: Febrile neutrophilic dermatosis in acute myelogenous leukemia. Arch. Dermatol., *114*:413, 1978.
16. Pipard, C., and Delannoy, A.: Syndrome de Sweet et leucémie myéloide aigue. Ann. Dermatol. Venereol., *104*:160, 1977.
17. Bluefarb, S. M.: Leukemia Cutis. Charles C Thomas, Springfield, Ill., 1960, pp. 48–58.
18. Discussion II: Roundtable discussion of histopathologic classification. Cancer Treat. Rep., *61*:1037, 1977.
19. Lukes, R. J., and Collins, R. D.: New approaches to the classification of the lymphomata. Br. J. Cancer, *31* (Suppl. II):1, 1975.
20. Bluefarb, S. M.: Leukemia Cutis. Charles C Thomas, Springfield, Ill., 1960, pp. 246–262.
21. Brouet, J.-C., Clauvel, J.-P., Danon, F., Klein, M., and Seligmann, M.: Biologic and clinical significance of cryoglobulins. A report of 86 cases. Am. J. Med., *57*:775, 1974.
22. Hope-Simpson, R. E.: The nature of herpes zoster: a long term study and a new hypothesis. Proc. R. Soc. Med., *58*:9, 1965.
23. Brunell, P. A., Gershon, A. A., Uduman, S. A., and Steinberg, S.: Varicella-zoster immunoglobulins during varicella, latency, and zoster. J. Infect. Dis., *132*:49, 1975.
24. Sabin, A. B., and Koch, M. A.: Behavior of non-infectious SV40 viral genome in hamster tumor cells: induction of synthesis of infectious virus. Proc. Natl. Acad. Sci. USA, *50*:407, 1963.
25. Ruckdeschel, J. C., Schimpff, S. C., Smyth, A. C., and Mardiney, M. R., Jr.: Herpes zoster and impaired cell-associated immunity to the varicella-zoster virus in patients with Hodgkin's disease. Am. J. Med., *62*:77, 1977.
26. Monfardini, S., Bajetta, E., Arnold, C. A., Kenda, R., and Bonadonna, G.: Herpes zoster-varicella infection in malignant lymphomas. Influence of splenectomy and intensive treatment. Eur. J. Cancer, *11*:51, 1975.
27. Goffinet, D. R., Glatstein, E., and Kaplan, H. S.: Herpes zoster infections in lymphoma patients. Natl. Cancer Inst. Monogr., *36*:463, 1973.
28. Ellis, F., and Stoll, B. A.: Herpes zoster after irradiation. Br. Med. J., *2*:1323, 1949.
29. Stevens, D. A., and Mergian, T. C.: Herpes zoster: recent studies. Natl. Cancer Inst. Monogr., *36*:465, 1973.
30. Feldman, S., Chaudary, S., Ossi, M., and Epp, E.: A viremic phase for herpes zoster in children with cancer. J. Pediatr., *91*:597, 1977.
31. Laszlo, J., and Huang, A. T.: Diagnosis and management of myeloproliferative disorders. Current problems in Cancer, *11*:1, 1977.
32. Rappaport, H.: *Op. Cit.,* p. 303.
33. Stathakis, N. E., Papayannis, A. G., Arapakis, G., and Gardikas, C.: Haemostatic defects in polycythemia vera. Blut, *29*:77, 1974.
34. Brumpt, L. C.: Le prurit des polyglobuliques. Presse Med., *60*:1397, 1952.
35. Bluefarb, S. M.: Cutaneous manifestations of polycythemia vera. Quart. Bull. Northwestern Univ. Med. School, *29*:8, 1955.
36. Gilbert, H. S., Warner, R. R. P., and Wasserman, L. R.: A study of histamine in myeloproliferative disease. Blood, *28*:795, 1966.
37. Chanarin, I., and Szur, L.: Relief of intractable pruritus in polycythemia rubra vera with cholestyramine. Br. J. Haematol., *29*:669, 1975.
38. Easton, P., and Galbraith, P. R.: Cimetidine treatment of pruritus in polycythemia vera. N. Engl. J. Med., *299*:1134, 1978.
39. Babb, R. R., Alarcon-Segovia, D., and Fairbairn, J. F., II: Erythermalgia: review of 51 cases. Circulation, *29*:136, 1964.
40. Alarcon-Segovia, D., Babb, R. R., Fairbairn, J. F., II, and Hagedorn, A. B.: Erythermalgia: a clue to the early diagnosis of myeloproliferative disorders. Arch. Intern. Med., *117*:511, 1966.
41. Fitzgerald, G., McCarthy, D., and O'Connell, L. G.: Burning feet. Br. Med. J., *1*:1149, 1976.
42. Barabas, A. P., Offen, D. N., and Meinhard, E. A.: The arterial complications of polycythemia vera. Br. J. Surg., *60*:183, 1973.
43. Gillespie, G.: Peripheral gangrene as the presentation of myeloproliferative disorders. Br. J. Surg., *60*:377, 1973.
44. Barbui, T., Battista, R., and Dini, E.: Spontaneous platelet aggregation in myeloproliferative disorders. A preliminary study. Acta Haematol., *50*:25, 1973.
45. Clarke, J., and Wells, G. C.: Livedo reticularis with thrombocythaemia in association with polycythemia rubra vera. Br. J. Dermatol., *95* (Suppl. 14):63, 1976.
46. Davies, S. W., Glynne-Jones, E., and Lewis, E. P. J.: Red face and reduced plasma volume. J. Clin. Pathol., *27*:109, 1974.

4

Histiocytosis X

Histiocytosis X includes three clinical entities: Letterer-Siwe disease, Hand-Schüller-Christian disease, and eosinophilic granuloma of bone.[1,2] Eosinophilic granuloma should not be confused with granuloma faciale, which is an entirely different disorder (see p. 292). The pathologic basis of histiocytosis X is the disseminated, progressive, and invasive proliferation of atypical but well-differentiated histiocytes. Although the disorder is included among the neoplastic diseases, this point of malignancy has not been definitely established. The three syndromes are believed to be variations of a single pathologic process: Letterer-Siwe disease represents the acute phase, whereas Hand-Schüller-Christian disease and eosinophilic granuloma of bone represent the chronic phase.

Letterer-Siwe disease rarely arises in adults; it is almost exclusively limited to children two months to three years old. Hand-Schüller-Christian disease usually develops in children between two and seven years old but can occur in younger children and in adults. Eosinophilic granuloma characteristically develops in older children and young adults, but occasionally it appears in children as young as three years.

Three histologic patterns involving histiocytes are found in histiocytosis X: a proliferative reaction composed almost exclusively of histiocytes; a granulomatous picture characterized by histiocytes and eosinophils primarily, with an admixture of neutrophils, lymphocytes, and plasma cells; and a xanthomatous pattern in which there are many foam cells accompanied by histiocytes, eosinophils, and lymphocytes. Giant cells, usually of the foreign body type but also of the Touton variety, are present. Each pattern tends to accompany a clinical type: proliferative, with Letterer-Siwe disease; granulomatous, with eosinophilic granuloma; and xanthomatous, with Hand-Schüller-Christian disease. Although each of the three entities presents a reasonably discrete clinical picture, overlapping of symptoms and cutaneous signs accompanied by their respective histologic patterns commonly occurs.[3] Histiocytosis X can be recognized easily if the character and distribution of the cutaneous lesions are kept in mind. The diagnosis can be established by biopsy of the skin.

The lesions of histiocytosis X show a predilection for seborrheic areas: the scalp, hairline, retroauricular region, axillae, and inguinal folds. The eruption may be either localized to these sites or disseminated. Even when lesions are generalized, the eruption is accentuated in the seborrheic zones.

Skin markers occur in virtually all patients with Letterer-Siwe disease but in only 30 to 50 per cent of those with Hand-Schüller-Christian disease. The frequency of cutaneous involvement in eosinophilic granuloma is not known exactly, but it is low. The skin lesions of histiocytosis X can undergo spontaneous regression.

LETTERER-SIWE DISEASE

Letterer-Siwe disease is an acute fulminant disease characterized by fever, anemia, thrombocytopenia, and histiocytic proliferation in the liver, spleen, lung, bone, and lymph nodes.[4, 5] The typical eruption resembles seborrheic dermatitis: a scaly erythema on the scalp; along the hairline; behind the ears; and in the axillary, inguinal, and perineal areas (Figs. 4–1 to 4–3; Plate 13*B,C*). However, on close inspection one will notice yellow-brown and red-brown papules 1 to 3 mm. in diameter at the periphery of the eruption. Coalescence of the papules produces the characteristic flat, scaly, erythematous, and sometimes weeping eruption behind the ears, in the groin, and on the scalp. Papular and infiltrated lesions never occur in seborrheic dermatitis. Frequently ulcers evolve from the confluent papules behind the ears and in the inguinal folds (Fig. 4–2). When thrombocytopenia is present, the dermatosis generally is purpuric.

The yellow-brown and red-brown papules, the basic lesions in this disease, do not always become confluent. They can remain discrete when either generalized or confined predominantly to seborrheic areas.

Involvement of the epithelium in the external auditory canal produces the picture of acute or chronic external otitis and may be a presenting feature of Letterer-Siwe disease. Ulceration of the buccal

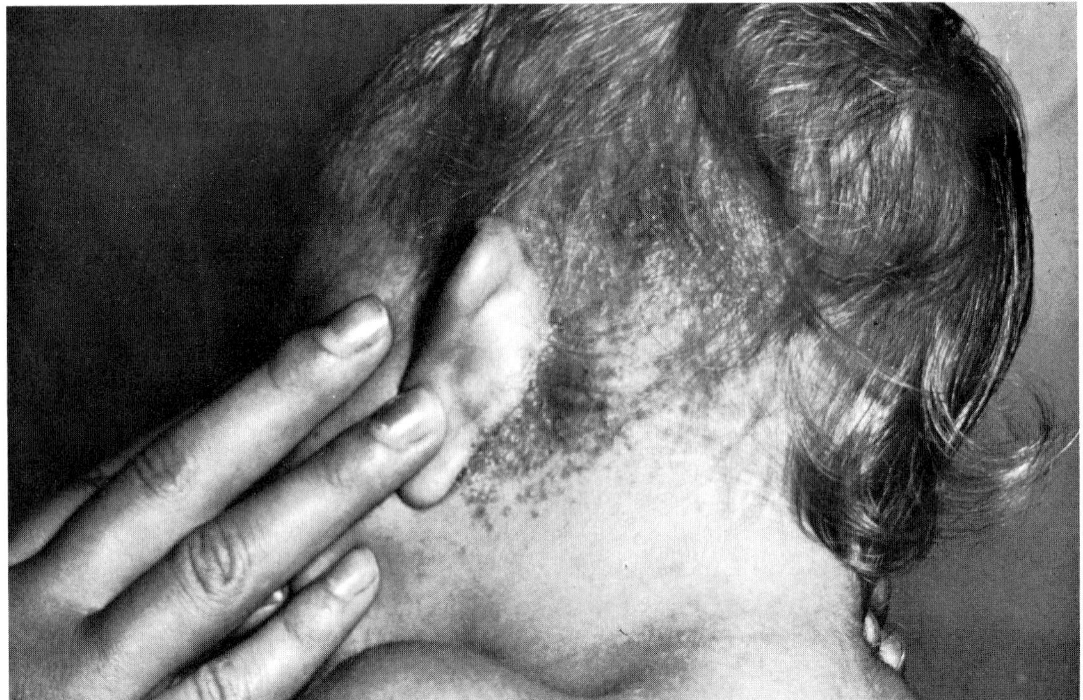

Figure 4–1. Letterer-Siwe disease. Characteristic seborrheic-like eruption is composed of discrete papules.

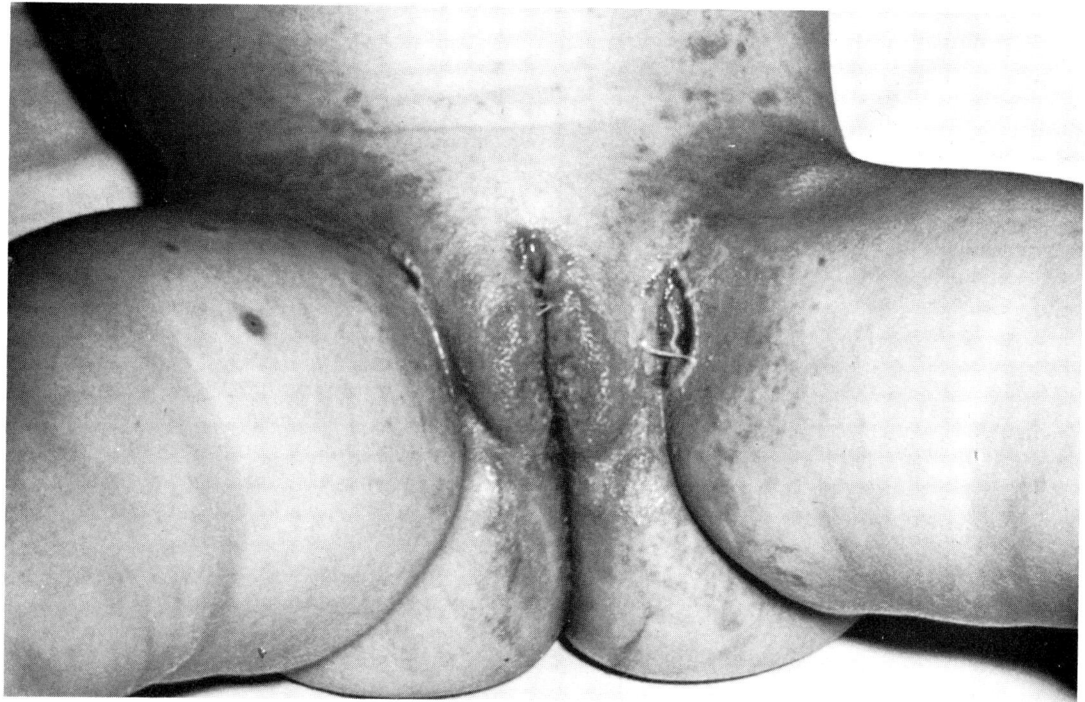

Figure 4–2. Letterer-Siwe disease. Ulceration and papules in an area often affected by seborrheic dermatitis.

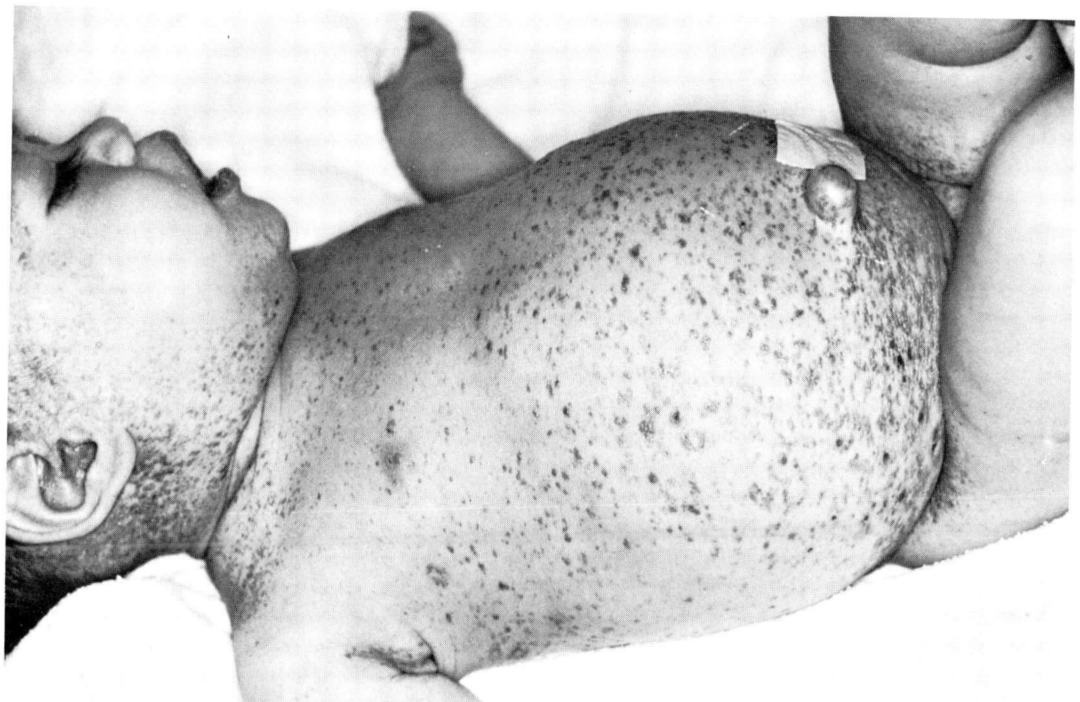

Figure 4–3. Letterer-Siwe disease. Hemorrhagic papules.

PLATE 13

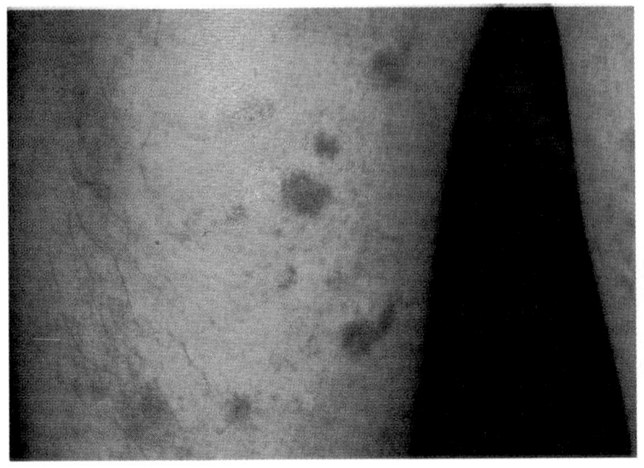

A, Chronic granulocytic leukemia. Nonspecific eczematous eruption both clinically and histologically. Same patient as in Figure 3–5.

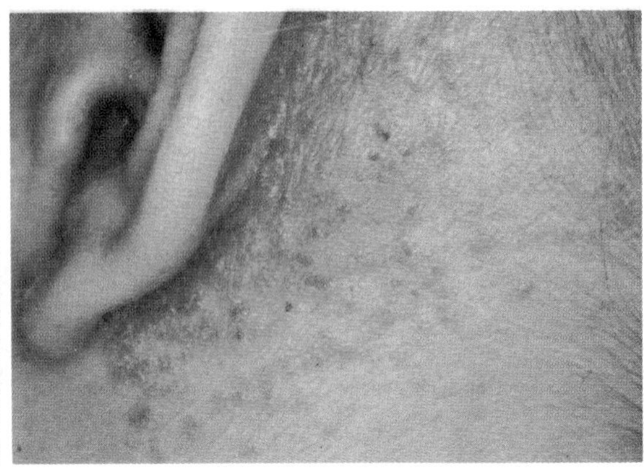

B, Letterer-Siwe disease. Seborrheic dermatitis-like eruption. Note the infiltrative papules, a feature never found in seborrheic dermatitis.

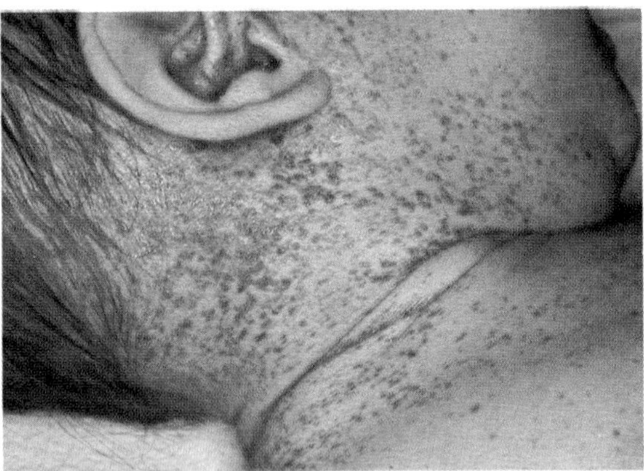

C, Letterer-Siwe disease. Hemorrhage papular eruption. The lesions in both *B* and *C* show the diagnostic histopathology of this entity.

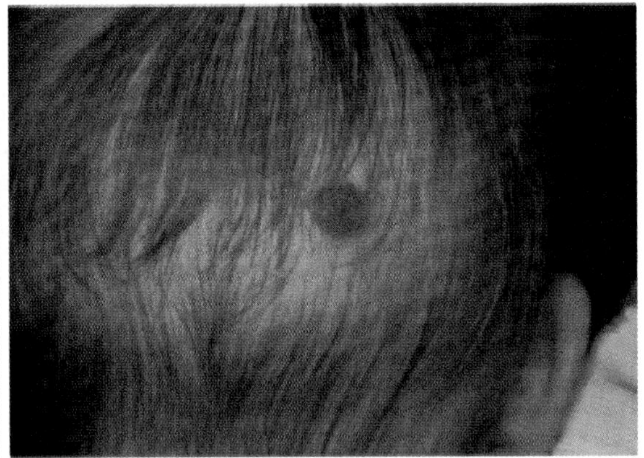

D, Nevoxanthoendothelioma on scalp.

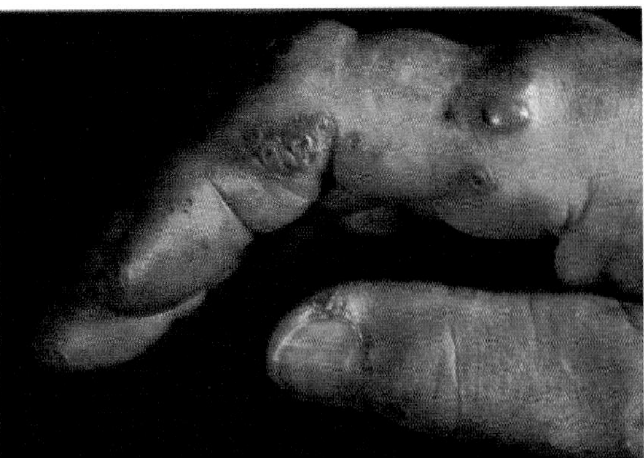

E, Reticulohistiocytoma. Red-brown papules on fingers that have a flexion deformity.

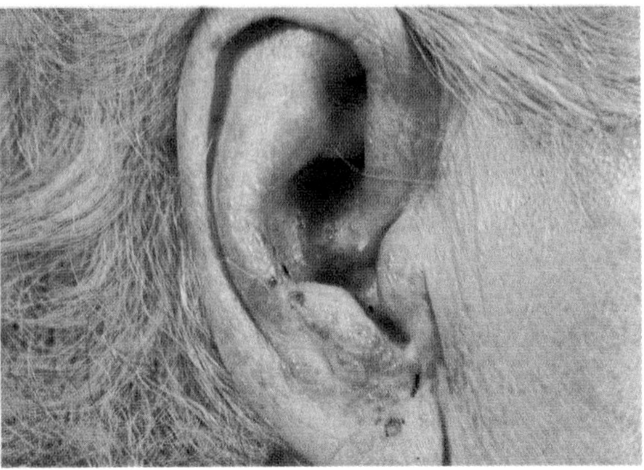

F, Reticulohistiocytoma. Grouped papules on pinna. (Plates *E* and *F* are from Arch. Dermatol, *89*:640, 1964. Courtesy of Dr. Milton Orkin.)

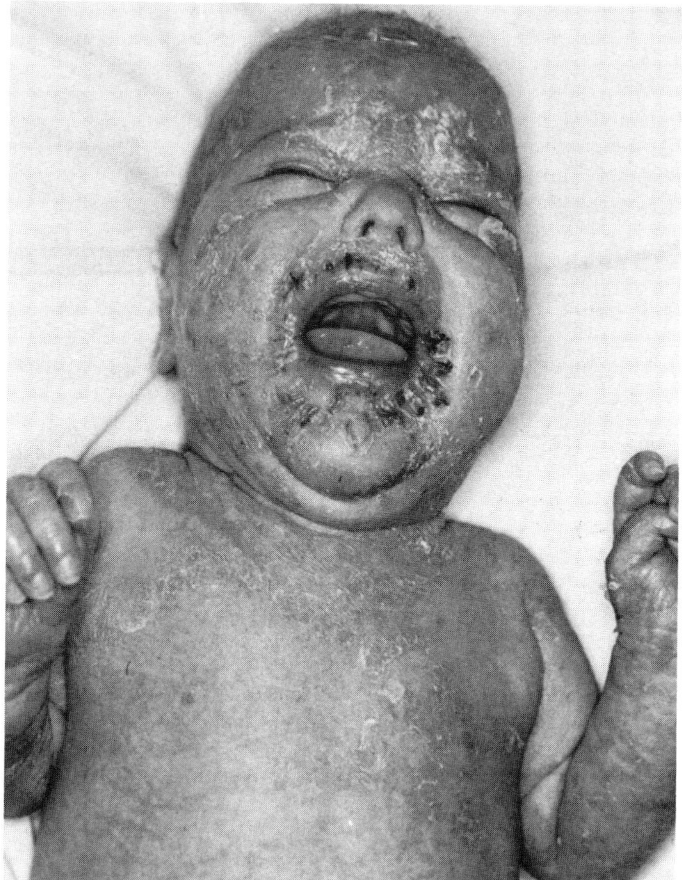

Figure 4–4. Letterer-Siwe disease simulating generalized seborrheic dermatitis.

mucosa and gums, secondary to histiocytic proliferation, is also an important sign.

A hemorrhagic seborrheic dermatitis-like eruption or a chronic ulceration of the perineum in a child less than three years old should immediately suggest a possible diagnosis of Letterer-Siwe disease. Figure 4–4 illustrates one of our patients with an eruption indistinguishable both histologically and clinically from seborrheic dermatitis. She was thought to have Leiner's disease, but a lymph node biopsy revealed the characteristic changes of Letterer-Siwe disease.

Although Letterer-Siwe disease is usually fatal, spontaneous remissions occur. Sometimes the illness evolves into a more chronic phase of histiocytosis X such as Hand-Schüller-Christian disease.

HAND-SCHÜLLER-CHRISTIAN DISEASE

The typical patient with this variant of histiocytosis X shows osteolytic defects of the calvarium and long bones, diabetes insipidus, and exophthalmos.[5, 6] Although bone lesions are invariably present, diabetes insipidus occurs in 50 per cent, and exophthalmos in only 10 per cent of the cases of Hand-Schüller-Christian disease. The cutaneous lesions seen in 30 to 50 per cent of the patients are identical to those in Letterer-Siwe disease except that in Hand-Schüller-Christian disease, purpura is not common.

Bony involvement is the basis for a number of clinical signs and symptoms. The histiocytic tumor formation responsible for the osteolytic lesions may extend into the overlying subcutaneous fat and produce deep cutaneous nodules. In addition to the characteristic hypertrophy and necrosis of the gums caused by local histiocytic proliferation, the mandible is also frequently involved, causing the teeth to become loose and fall out. Chronic otitis media commonly follows histiocytic proliferation in the mastoid and can be a presenting sign of Hand-Schüller-Christian disease.

As in the Letterer-Siwe variant, small tumors which may ulcerate occur on the oral mucous membranes. Hyperpigmentation occurs infrequently in this disorder and is a nonspecific sign. The lungs are affected in approximately 30 per cent of the patients, whereas the liver, spleen, and lymph nodes are implicated much less often. The development of anemia frequently indicates a transition to the acute Letterer-Siwe phase.

Endocrine dysfunction, manifesting as diabetes insipidus and growth retardation, is present in about 50 per cent of patients with this chronic form of histiocytosis X.[7,8] The finding of histiocytic infiltration of the hypothalamus in the absence of anterior pituitary involvement makes it likely that a derangement of hormonal releasing and inhibitory factors is responsible for the endocrine disorders.[7,9] Histiocytic infiltration of the posterior pituitary does occur, but it is rare.[9-12] The deficiency of antidiuretic hormone may be partial or complete. Elevated levels of prolactin can be found in the blood because the normal tonic inhibition of this hormone by the hypothalamus is no longer completely effective.[7] The growth retardation in these children is caused by deficiency of growth hormone and not by the debilitating effects of the disease. These patients respond to replacement therapy with growth hormone no differently than children who are deficient for other reasons.[13] Panhypopituitarism is rare in Hand-Schüller-Christian disease.[7]

Although diabetes insipidus is often associated with histiocytic involvement of the hypothalamus and, rarely, of the posterior pituitary, there have been at least four patients in whom histiocytic proliferation in the hypothalamus and pituitary has not been found.[9-11] Although the periosteum of the sella turcica is frequently infiltrated by histiocytes, there is no evidence that it is responsible for producing endocrine dysfunction by compression or any other mechanism. Involvement of the sella has occurred both with and without diabetes insipidus, and the healing of the periosteal lesion has not been accompanied by disappearance of the diabetes insipidus.[5,9]

The prognosis in histiocytosis X is related to the age of onset and the number of organs involved. Children less than two years old have a poorer prognosis than those who are older. The prognosis also becomes poorer when more than five organs are affected. Diabetes insipidus is not a bad prognostic sign.[14]

EOSINOPHILIC GRANULOMA OF BONE

Skin lesions of eosinophilic granuloma are uncommon.[2, 5] When present, they can be identical to those seen in Letterer-Siwe and Hand-Schüller-Christian disease, or they may consist of a few isolated papules and nodules in the perineal and retroauricular areas (Fig. 4–5). Often these lesions ulcerate.

As in the other two variants of histiocytosis X, the lungs and the oral mucosa, including the palate and gums, can be affected.

The long bones are involved more frequently than the vertebrae and calvarium. Fever, leukocytosis, and pain can be present, but usually the bony disease is asymptomatic. In the adult, eosinophilic granuloma of bone is often a benign, chronic, and stationary disease, but in a youngster it is usually a harbinger of Hand-Schüller-Christian or Letterer-Siwe disease.

Etiology

Lichtenstein considered the term *histiocytosis X* to be "a useful broad designation [under which] the recognized types of clinical involvement can be grouped and still be differentiated so that useful distinctions having a bearing on treatment and prognosis are maintained."[1] At least two groups, Lieberman et al.[9] and Vogel and Vogel,[15] have objected to considering these three entities a nosological unit and prefer to subclassify "idiopathic histiocytosis" into two groups, a benign variety — unifo-

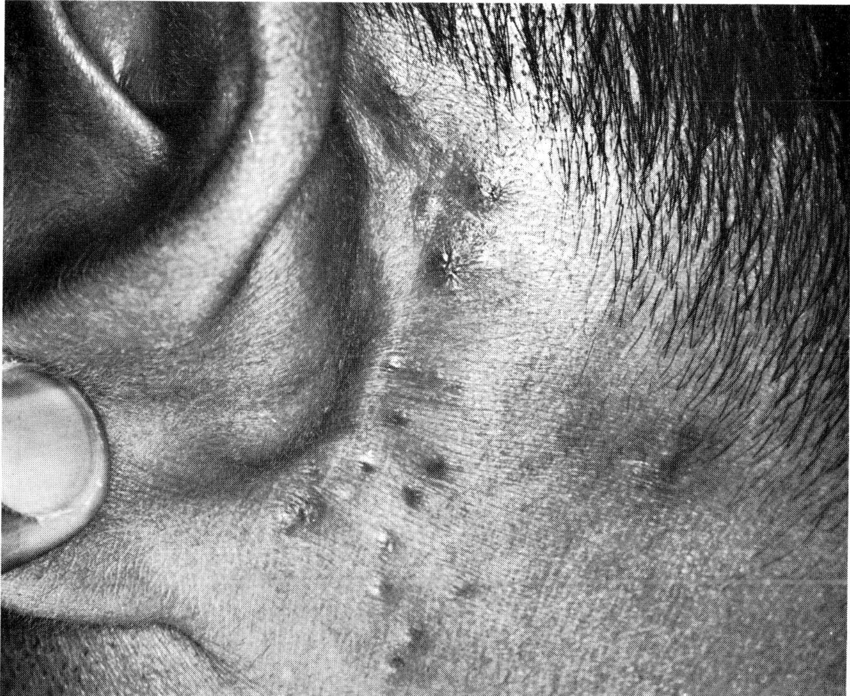

Figure 4–5. Eosinophilic granuloma of bone. Papules in retroauricular zone showed diagnostic histopathology of histiocytosis X. This patient also had similar lesions in inguinal area.

cal and multifocal eosinophilic granuloma — and a malignant variety — Letterer-Siwe disease. They felt that the term *Hand-Schüller-Christian syndrome* represented an entity with too great a variability in its clinical expression to be useful and that it was not a pathologic entity. Lieberman et al. did not believe that there was any purpose in using the term "Hand-Schüller-Christian disease" as a synonym for multifocal eosinophilic granuloma. They also believed that *Letterer-Siwe disease* was a clinical term that had been used to characterize various malignant histiocytic lymphomas and, occasionally, infectious processes. Their arguments, based upon interpretation of clinical syndromes and pathologic tissue, are less cogent today. In 1965 and subsequently, Basset and colleagues have described cytoplasmic inclusions, shaped like "tennis raquets" in the histiocytic cells of all three clinical syndromes encompassed by the term *histiocytosis X,* and these observations have been amply confirmed by others.[16, 17] These granules are basically identical in morphology, size, and three-dimensional configuration to those found in the Langerhans cells,[17, 18] a dendritic cell population found chiefly in normal epidermis. Langerhans cells have also been seen occasionally both in normal dermis and in normal human esophageal mucosa.[19, 20] Only minor differences exist. In histiocytosis X, the granules occasionally are observed to branch and form an interconnected network in the cytoplasm; the granules are attached to the cell membrane more often than in epidermal Langerhans cells; and the granules are sometimes found within the nuclei of cells in histiocytosis X, a phenomenon thought to be caused by trapping during abnormal mitoses.[18] The presence of the Langerhans granules has become virtually diagnostic of histiocytosis X because they are not found in any other disease in such large numbers. Although a few Langerhans granules have been found in pathologic human lung — one case of desquamative interstitial pneumonia, four cases of interstitial alveolar fibrosis, and one case of bronchoalveolar carcinoma — they have not been found in pulmonary sarcoidosis, hypersensitivity pneumonitis, or normal human lung.[21] A characteristic of the lesions in histiocytosis X is the predilection for skin and mucous membrane involvement, and the distribution of histiocytic cells in a bandlike, sometimes polymorphous infiltrate in the upper dermis with invasion of the epidermis. The latter feature is analogous to the histopathology of mycosis fungoides. The recent finding that the Langerhans cell is a histiocyte with probable participation as a macrophage in the immune system makes it reasonable to consider that the cells of histiocytosis X might have an analogous function (see p. 165). The distinctive granules may be a marker for certain types of histiocytes without requiring that they all originate from the same cell of origin. Basset et al. have demonstrated in tissue culture that the histiocytic X cells phagocytize opsonized red cells, adhere to glass, and contain certain lysosomal enzymes.[21] A search for complement and immunoglobulin receptors on these cells has not yet been reported. Histiocytosis X could arise in the skin and mucous membranes and become disseminated in a manner similar to that in mycosis fungoides. The acute and chronic forms of the disease would be determined by the immunologic status of the host. The occasional spontaneous remissions in Letterer-Siwe disease, as well as the benign nature of eosinophilic granuloma, indicate that these disorders are more likely to be reactive processes than neoplastic ones.

Three patients illustrate the spectrum of histiocytosis X.

A 44-year-old white woman had developed diabetes insipidus, lytic lesions of the right femur and left tibia, and an intensely pruritic perianal rash five years earlier. The perianal lesion was an infiltrated plaque with an uneven surface that produced a reticulated pattern of red-pink and hypopigmentation and was clinically indistinguishable from extramammary Paget's disease (Fig. 4–6; Plate 12*B*). Biopsy of the perianal lesion showed the proliferative histologic pattern of histiocytosis X. The vulvar mucosa eventually became involved, producing identical-appearing lesions. Deficiencies in ACTH and growth hormone secretion were found following insulin-induced hypoglycemia, and the serum level of prolactin was elevated. Thyroid function was normal. The perineal lesions were treated three times with radiation therapy because of short-lived remissions of several months.

Feuerman and Sandbank described a man with a 25-year history of cutaneous histiocytosis X without any systemic involvement.[22] The lesions were distributed on the face, neck, retro-auricular areas, back, axillae, and inguinal regions and over the sacrum. The eruption was composed of pink to reddish-brown papules, pinhead to 3 mm in size. Some had small central ulcerations or crusts. Langerhans granules were demonstrated by electron microscopy. The lesions disappeared following x-ray therapy on three occasions, but they always recurred.

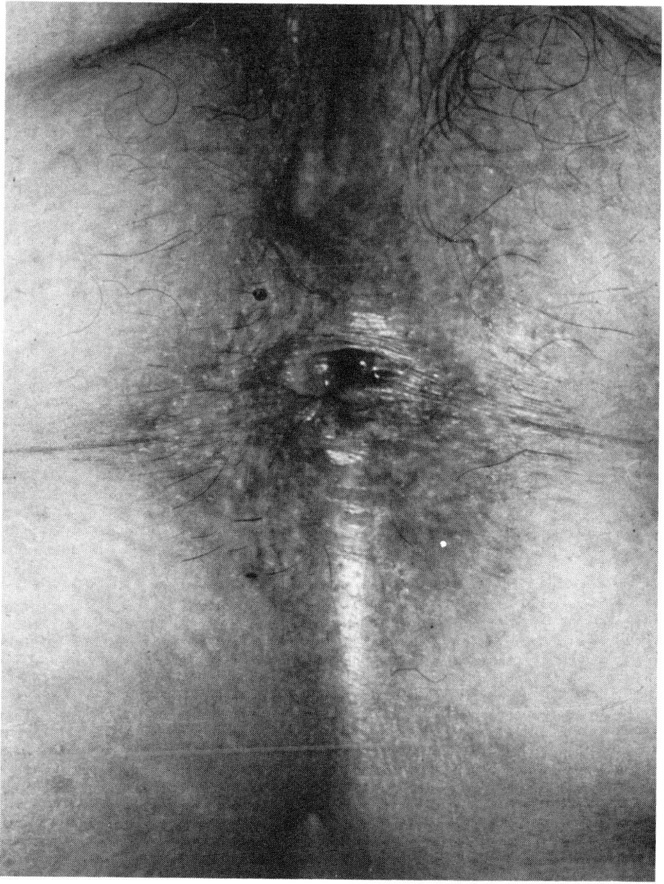

Figure 4–6. Histiocytosis X of the perianal skin simulating extramammary Paget's disease. See Plate 12*B* for close-up.

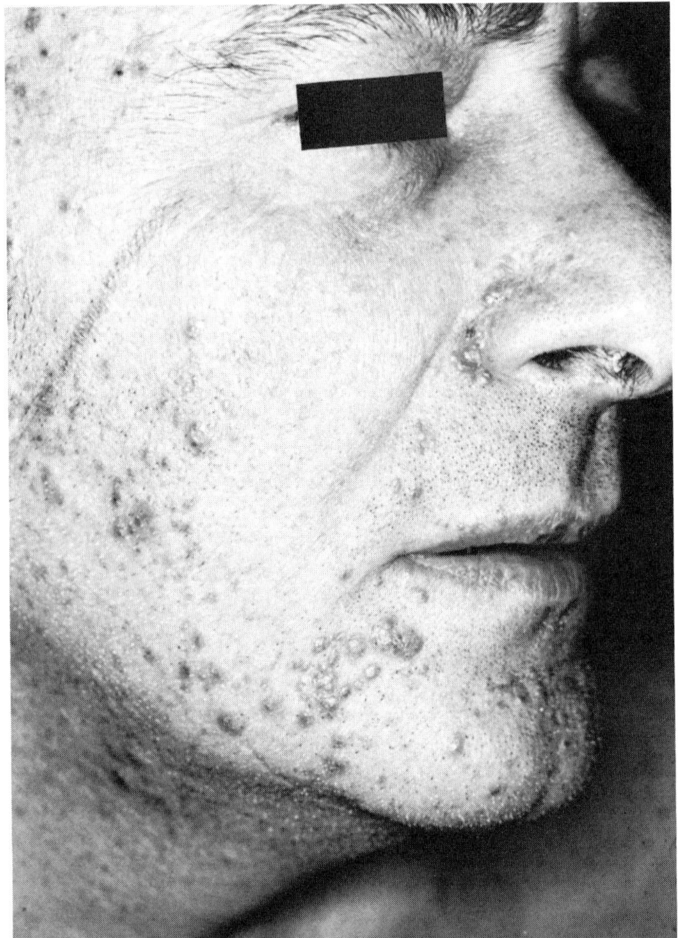

Figure 4–7. Histiocytosis X. Reddish-brown papules in an acneiform distribution. (Courtesy of Dr. Joseph McGuire.)

Figure 4–7 illustrates a patient who had histiocytosis X for 22 years. At age 32, this patient developed diabetes insipidus. At age 38, he began to develop red-brown papules on the face and scalp which eventually spread to the lower back and legs. At age 53, the skin lesions and a lymph node were biopsied for the first time and the histologic features of eosinophilic granuloma were found. Purulent drainage from both ear canals, believed to be caused by granulomatous involvement of the skin of the ear canal, was also present. Although a bone scan showed increased uptake in the posterior aspect of several ribs, both knees and maxillae, no lytic lesions were found on x-ray studies. However, one year later, at age 54, lytic lesions were discovered in the left humerus, and generalized lymphadenopathy developed. The skin lesions and enlarged lymph nodes promptly resolved following chemotherapy.

RELATED DISORDERS

Benign histiocytic proliferation with secondary uptake of lipid is also the characteristic feature of xanthoma dissemination, juvenile xanthogranuloma, multicentric reticulohistiocytosis, and lipogranulomatosis disseminata. They form a spectrum of diseases with histiocytosis X and are usually classified among the lipid storage diseases. The serum lipids are normal in all of these disorders, which are usually designated as the normolipemic xanthomatoses. Cerebrotendinous xanthomatosis, a newly described entity, and lipoid proteinosis (hyalinosis cutis et mucosae), which has been traditionally placed in the group of normolipemic xanthomas, will also be discussed in this section.

Xanthoma Disseminatum

Xanthoma disseminatum is not common; only about 50 cases have been reported in the literature.[23] In 60 per cent of the patients the disease began before the age of 25 years, and in 30 per cent it began before the age of 15. Xanthoma disseminatum is characterized by red-brown or red-yellow papules and nodules concentrated in the axillae, the antecubital and popliteal fossae, and the intertriginous areas. These papules and nodules characteristically coalesce to form furrowed plaques. Xanthomatous deposits have been observed in the tongue, gums, tonsils, uvula, buccal mucosa, epiglottis, larynx, trachea, and bronchi in 40 per cent of the cases; frequently they have produced dysphagia and dyspnea, and in five instances they have necessitated a tracheostomy.

Xanthomas can involve the floor of the third ventricle and the infundibulum, thus producing diabetes insipidus; this sequence has been noted in 40 per cent of the case reports.

In spite of similarities, xanthoma disseminatum probably is not a forme fruste of Hand-Schüller-Christian disease. The significant differences between the two entities can be summarized as follows: (1) the histopathology of xanthoma disseminatum is that of a xanthoma with normal histiocytes; (2) exophthalmos, bone lesions, and the characteristic distribution pattern of cutaneous lesions in histiocytosis X are not found in xanthoma disseminatum; (3) involvement of the upper respiratory tract is not a feature of histiocytosis X; (4) xanthoma disseminatum is a benign self-limited disorder with a good prognosis as opposed to the usually progressive course and poor outlook of Hand-Schüller-Christian disease; and (5) the diabetes insipidus of xanthoma disseminatum is mild and usually remits spontaneously.

Thannhauser believed that xanthoma disseminatum was a forme fruste of Hand-Schüller-Christian disease and subsequently referred to all the cutaneous lesions of histiocytosis X as xanthoma disseminatum.[24] However, the concurrence of Hand-Schüller-Christian disease and xanthoma disseminatum as previously defined is extremely rare and has been reported only once.[25] Xanthomas secondary to hypercholesterolemia are rare in Hand-Schüller-Christian disease and have been reported only three times.[26-29] In each case the patient also had biliary cirrhosis with secondary hypercholesterolemia. The inclusion of the three patients with xanthomas secondary to hypercholesterolemia in the early reports of Hand-Schüller-Christian disease, in addition to an overemphasis on, and a misdiagnosis of, xanthoma disseminatum in histiocytosis X, has confused the relationship between true xanthomas and histiocytosis X in the medical literature.[30]

Another instance of this confusion can be cited. Thannhauser described an unusual cutaneous lesion in one of his patients with Hand-Schüller-Christian disease.[31] The entire scalp was covered with an infiltrated yellow-brown plaque. The eyelids were similarly involved. These lesions were believed to be xanthoma planum and xanthelasma. Unfortunately they were not examined by biopsy, since the color and distribution favored the specific lesions of histiocytosis X more than those of true xanthomas.

Juvenile Xanthogranuloma

Juvenile xanthogranuloma, or nevoxanthoendothelioma, is a benign proliferation of histiocytes with secondary lipidization that appears shortly after birth and is only rarely associated with visceral involvement.[32] The eruption may be composed of solitary or multiple papules and nodules which are yellow-brown or red-brown and vary in size from a few millimeters to several centimeters. The scalp and extensor surfaces of the extremities are the sites of predilection (Plate 13*D*).

Xanthogranuloma usually involutes spontaneously, but it can persist for more than 20 years.[33] Histologically, the lesions are composed of mature histiocytes, foam cells, multinucleated giant cells, and polymorphonuclear leukocytes, but the picture can vary greatly. Nevertheless, an experienced pathologist would not confuse xanthogranuloma with histiocytosis X or true xanthomas. There is no compelling evidence to indicate that xanthogranuloma and histiocytosis X are closely related.

Systemic involvement in xanthogranuloma is rare. When it does occur, lesions arise in the iris and ciliary body of the eye and produce hemorrhage in the anterior chamber and secondary glaucoma.[34, 35] Bilateral ocular involvement is uncommon but does occur.[36] In a few cases the testes, vulva, lung, liver, and tongue have also been involved in xanthogranuloma.[37, 38] In those patients with pulmonary involvement, the granulomatous lesions eventually regressed spontaneously. In one infant lesions of xanthogranuloma were also present on the pericardial surface of the heart, which caused a hemopericardium that compressed the left lung and produced repiratory distress.[39] Several reports have linked xanthogranuloma with neurofibromatosis.[40] Further observations in this regard should be made. Juvenile xanthogranuloma is not limited to children, however. Eighteen adults, aged 24 to 80, have been reported to have xanthogranuloma, but without ocular involvement.[41, 42] Three adults with biopsy-proven ocular xanthogranuloma in the absence of skin lesions have also been reported.[43]

Multicentric Reticulohistiocytosis

Multicentric reticulohistiocytosis is also characterized by histiocytic proliferation with secondary lipidization in the presence of normal serum lipids.[44] Synonyms for this entity include generalized giant cell histiocytomatosis, reticulohistiocytoma of skin, multicentric reticulohistiocytosis of skin and synovia, reticulohistiocytic granuloma, and lipoid dermatoarthritis. The salient features are mucocutaneous lesions, severe arthritis, and a distinctive histopathology. Approximately 40 cases have been reported, and in about three quarters of these the patients have been women. The age of onset may range from 11 to 70 years, but the average age is about 43 years.[45-47]

In 25 per cent of the patients, the arthritis and skin lesions appear simultaneously. The skin lesions can precede the arthritis by one year, but it is more common for the lesions to develop about three years after the arthritis has begun.

The primary cutaneous lesion is a firm papule or nodule ranging in color from that of the skin to yellow, red, or brown. The sites of predilection are the fingers, backs of the hands, pinnae, face, and scalp (Plate 13*E,F*). The papules characteristically involve the paronychial zones and the extensor and lateral surfaces of the fingers around the joints. Dystrophic nails are often present.[48] Papules may also arise on the forehead, eyelids, and nose, and in some patients a leonine facies can develop. The trunk may show lesions, and the papules can coalesce to form plaques over the sacrum, coccyx, and perineum. Deep subcutaneous nodules may develop over the elbows and knees and simulate the nodules of rheumatic fever, rheumatoid arthritis, and even the juxta-articular nodes of syphilis.

Individual lesions can be pruritic. The mucous membranes of the lips, tongue, gums, pharynx, larynx, and the sclerae are affected. One quarter of the patients have xanthelasma. Soft cystic swellings resembling ganglia may develop over the extensor and flexor surfaces of the wrists in some patients.

The distinctive histologic picture is that of a dense dermal infiltrate with round and oval giant cells that are usually PAS-positive and sudanophilic.[44, 49] The giant cells can contain as many as 20 nuclei. Mitoses are not found. In early lesions the dense dermal infiltrate is composed of histiocytes, eosinophils, and lymphocytes, with few or no giant cells. The PAS-positive material is believed to be a mucoprotein or a glycoprotein and the sudanophilic material, a varying mixture of triglycerides, free cholesterol, cholesterol esters, and phospholipids that are secondarily phagocytized by the proliferating histiocytes.[47] The lipid components may vary from case to case. In some, there may be no lipid; in some, a mixture of lipids; and in others, only a simple glycolipid.[47]

A symmetric seronegative polyarthritis that mimics rheumatoid arthritis develops in almost every patient. Any joint, including the vertebral and temporomandibular, may be affected, but the terminal interphalangeal is the one most commonly involved. The earlier the disease begins, the more severe the eventual arthritis tends to become. In 20 per cent of the cases, arthritis mutilans (opera glass hand), indistinguishable from that seen in rheumatoid arthritis and psoriasis, eventually develops. The fingers are short and stubby. Radiographs show not only extensive osteoporosis and resorption but also partial dissolution and telescopic subluxation of the joints of the fingers and wrists.[46]

Weight loss, chills, and fever occur in 15 to 30 per cent of the patients with this disease. X-ray studies have demonstrated pulmonary infiltration in 20 per cent of the women with this disorder, but the nature of the histopathology underlying these radiographic shadows is not known.[44]

One of the characteristics of this illness is the tendency for the cutaneous lesions to regress, even though the arthritis may become progressively worse. Orkin et al. reviewed the published cases and found that the eruption cleared in 25 per cent, improved in 25 per cent, and in the rest of the cases either remained the same with fluctuations or steadily progressed.[44] The arthritis was progressive in half and stationary in half.

In three patients the arthritis disappeared or improved. In the majority of cases the disease became inactive after about eight years, but the patients were left with crippling arthritis.

Autopsy studies were performed on three patients who had died eleven months, three years, and four years after the onset of disease. In the first case, death was due to metastatic adenocarcinoma of the lung, but in the other two instances, death followed clinical deterioration attributed to the disease. In all three autopsies the distinctive histopathologic changes were found in the pharynx, larynx, bronchial lymph nodes, skeletal muscles, synovia, bone, and endocardium.[44] Five additional patients have had carcinomas of the colon, breast, bronchus, cervix, and of an unknown primary site. This association requires further study to determine its significance.[45]

Orkin and associates performed comprehensive immunologic studies on their patients in an effort to uncover evidence of immunologic deficiency, but no abnormalities were found.

Approximately 55 cases of reticulohistiocytoma without arthritis have been reported. In the majority of the patients, only a solitary lesion was present, in eight there were as many as four lesions, and in one patient there were 150 lesions. Whether these cases represent a forme fruste is not known.[50, 51]

Urbach et al. reported an instance of a 74-year-old woman with a 30-year history of multiple lesions in the absence of arthritis. However, this patient did have cystic ganglia–like lesions which were shown by histologic examination to exhibit the features of reticulohistiocytosis, not ganglia.[52]

Farber's Disease

Farber's disease, or disseminated lipogranulomatosis, is a rare and fatal lipid storage disease of infants.[53, 55] At least 17 cases have now been reported.[56] Almost all the children have died before two years of age, but in three the disease pursued a milder course. Two children were still alive at six years of age and one had died at 16 years.[57-59] Farber et al. had originally believed that this new entity was related to the other granulomatous histiocytic proliferative disorders in which secondary lipid storage developed.[53]

Within a few months of life, the affected infant develops tender and swollen joints and has a hoarse, weak cry. Gross mental and motor retardation becomes evident in most cases as the infant grows. Nodular and diffuse erythematous or yellowish-red swellings develop around the wrists, interphalangeal joints, elbows, knees, and toes (Figs. 4–8 to 4–10). Flexion contractures eventually occur. The lumbar spine, occiput, infraorbital ridges, sacrum, and heels are also the sites of nodular swellings; this process is analogous to the formation of rheumatoid nodules in an area of chronic pressure and trauma. The epiglottis, vocal cords, and laryngeal joints are involved, resulting in dysphonia, laryngeal stridor, hoarse cry, and noisy respirations. It appears as if the major pathology is concentrated in joints and tissues subjected to vigorous mechanical stress and trauma, which may explain why the heart valves and chordae tendineae are also affected in some patients.

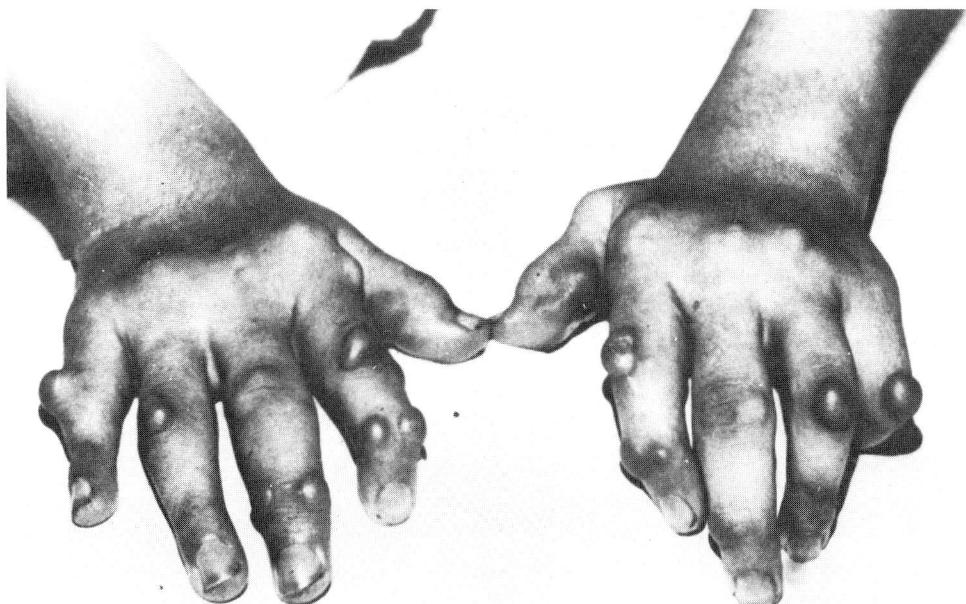

Figure 4–8. Disseminated lipogranulomatosis (Farber's disease). Nodules around interphalangeal joints. (Courtesy of Dr. Hugo Moser.)

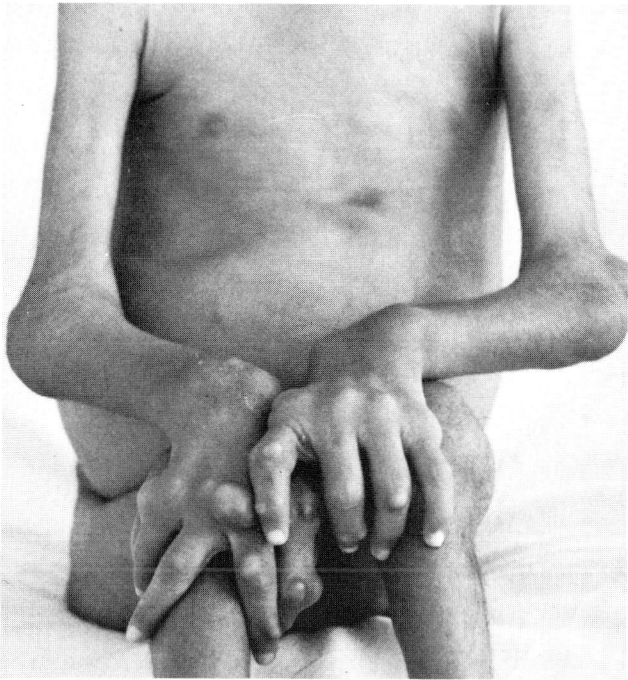

Figure 4–9. Disseminated lipogranulomatosis (Farber's disease). Nodules around elbows, wrists, and interphalangeal joints. Muscle wasting and growth retardation are also present. (Courtesy of Dr. G. Amirhakimi.)

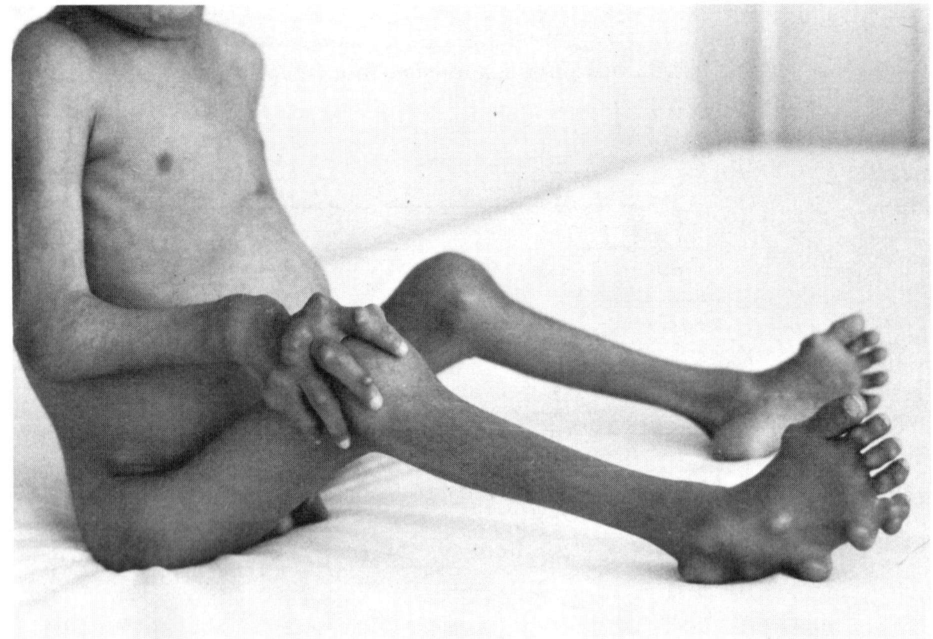

Figure 4–10. Disseminated lipogranulomatosis (Farber's disease). Nodules on knees, ankles, and feet. (Courtesy of Dr. G. Amirhakimi.)

The periarticular granulomatous inflammation responsible for the major signs of the disease frequently extends into adjacent ligaments, synovial tissue, and articular cartilage to produce destruction of joints. The periarticular granulomas can undergo calcification. The ears become diffusely thickened and enlarged if the child lies on them for prolonged periods.

The lipid storage material has also been found in lymph nodes, thymus, gastrointestinal tract, kidney, spleen, lung, pericardium, and peritoneum.[53-55, 60] Death has resulted from complications related to the respiratory tract, nervous system, and cachexia.

There is a dichotomy in histopathologic findings between those of the skin, joints, and viscera and those of the central nervous system. In the skin and periarticular tissues, one observes a proliferation of histiocytic and inflammatory cells that form granulomas. Foam cells are prominent and the lesions eventually undergo fibrosis. In early granulomas, the foam cells are distended with material that stains strongly with periodic acid–Schiff reagent and weakly with lipid stains. As the lesions evolve, the reaction with PAS weakens and the sundanophilia increases. Eventually the foam cells degenerate and release the storage material into the interstitial space. This substance was originally thought to be a nonsulfonated abnormal acid mucopolysaccharide or a glycolipid. The reticuloendothelial system is only minimally affected in this disorder.

In the nervous system, on the other hand, the pathologic finding is distention of neuronal cytoplasm with PAS-positive material in the absence of granulomatous inflammation. The anterior horn cells and large nerve cells of the medulla, pons, and cerebellum have been most frequently involved, and those of the cerebral cortex least affected. The autonomic and visceral ganglia have also been involved. The white matter has shown focal myelin degeneration and gliosis of variable severity.[60]

Recent investigations have established that this disease belongs to the sphingolipidoses rather than the histiocytic group of disorders. The cutaneous and visceral lesions contain 10 to 60 times more free ceramide and the affected nervous system tissue, two to five times more than normal.[60] The abnormality in this disease is a genetically determined deficiency of lysosomal acid ceramidase which catalyzes the hydrolysis of ceramide to sphingosine and fatty acid.[61] The diagnosis should be able to be made prenatally by measuring the levels of ceramides in cultured fibroblasts.[56] The disease is recessively transmitted.

Electron microscopic studies have demonstrated rectilinear and curvilinear structures in the cytoplasm of histiocytes in the granulomatous inflammation found in cutaneous nodules and periarticular tissues.[60] It appears that ceramide containing nonhydroxylated fatty acids is responsible for producing the granulomas and the curvilinear profiles. If one overloads cultures of fibroblasts from patients with ceramide containing nonhydroxylated fatty acids, the typical curvilinear inclusions are produced. Ceramide containing hydroxylated fatty acids will not produce these changes.[60] Moser et al. had shown earlier that ceramide containing nonhydroxylated fatty acids, isolated from the liver of a patient with Farber's disease, produced granulomatous inflammation when injected subcutaneously into rat skin, but ceramide containing hydroxylated fatty acids did not.[59] In general, curvilinear inclusions have not been found in cerebellum, liver, and kidney, an observation which correlates with the almost constant presence of ceramide containing hydroxylated fatty acids in these sites. Uncommonly, ceramide in visceral lesions has been shown to contain nonhydroxylated fatty acids.[58, 59] The difference in ceramide composition relating to the fatty acids may indicate a local synthesis of the latter.[60]

There may be two manifestations of the disease: a common severe variant and a rarer milder form, which differ on the basis of whether there is a significant accumulation of ceramide within the nervous system.[57, 59]

Cerebrotendinous Xanthomatosis

Cerebrotendinous xanthomatosis is a rare familial disorder that superficially resembles Type II lipoproteinemia (familial hypercholesterolemic xanthomatosis). Twenty patients with this syndrome have now been reported.[62-66] The disorder is inherited as a Mendelian recessive trait.

Cholestanol and cholesterol are deposited in all tissues of the body, but their accumulation as xanthomas in the tendons, brain, and lungs produces the major clinical manifestations of this illness. Deposition begins in childhood and produces xanthomas in the Achilles tendons, which are the hallmark of the disease. The xanthomas usually develop in the proximal part of the Achilles tendon in contrast to the distal portion, which is the favored site of xanthoma formation in familial hypercholesterolemia. The xanthomas also can develop in the tendons of the patella, biceps, triceps, and quadriceps, as well as in the long extensor tendons of the fingers. At least two patients have developed xanthomas within the skin (tuberous xanthomas). Cataracts develop in a majority of patients and a progressive dementia may develop. Cerebellar ataxia and pseudobulbar paralysis, which gradually worsens and often contributes to the patient's death, are the main neurological deficits that characteristically develop in adult life. Sterol deposition in the lungs produces infiltrates detectable by x-ray or abnormalities in pulmonary function tests. Symptomatic atherosclerosis with acute myocardial infarction has been a feature in three patients.

Serum cholestanol levels are markedly elevated in this disorder. Serum levels of cholesterol are normal or low. Within the body tissues, however, the levels of cholesterol may be as much as four times normal while the levels of cholestanol may be from 10 to 900 times normal. Cholesterol occurs in much greater amounts than cholestanol in normal human tissues. The serum level of cholestanol can be diagnostic in a patient with xanthomas and cataracts who has not yet developed any of the neurological signs and symptoms.

The biosynthesis of cholesterol and cholestanol is greatly increased, but the formation of bile acids is markedly decreased. The increased synthesis has been ascribed in part to the lack of negative feedback regulation by bile acids on several hepatic microsomal enzymes. The decreased production of bile acids from cholesterol has been attributed to a deficiency of an enzyme that catalyzes the degradation of the side chain of cholesterol. However, these biochemical findings do not explain the reasons for the low serum levels of cholesterol, the accumulation of cholestanol and cholesterol in the brain and other tissues, or the development of the clinical symptoms.[67-69]

Lipoid Proteinosis

Lipoid proteinosis (hyalinosis cutis et mucosae, Urbach-Wiethe's disease) is traditionally included with the lipid storage diseases, even though it does not exhibit any of the histologic features of these disorders.[70-72] Microscopic examination of the cutaneous lesions reveals a hyaline and homogeneous-appearing material deposited diffusely through the dermis as well as in the mantles around vessels, sebaceous and sweat glands, and nerves. The material accumulates in the absence of foam cells, necrosis, inflammation, or granuloma formation. This substance is believed to be a glycoprotein loosely associated with lipids. Cholesterol, neutral fat, and a trace of phospholipid have been identified in the lipid fraction.[73, 74]

Lipoid proteinosis is inherited as an autosomal recessive trait. The abnormal glycoprotein is deposited in skin and mucosae in the absence of serum lipid abnormalities. In a typical case the skin is yellow-white, resembling old ivory. Individual lesions consist of discrete or confluent papules and are found most frequently on the face, eyelids, neck, and hands. On the lid margins, the papules resemble a string of beads (Fig. 4–11). Multiple confluent papules produce verrucose plaques on the elbows, knees, hands, and feet. Alopecia results when the scalp is affected, and plaques simulating morphea (localized scleroderma) have also been described.

The lips may be everted and their surfaces studded with tiny yellow nodules. The papules may produce radiating fissures at the corners of the

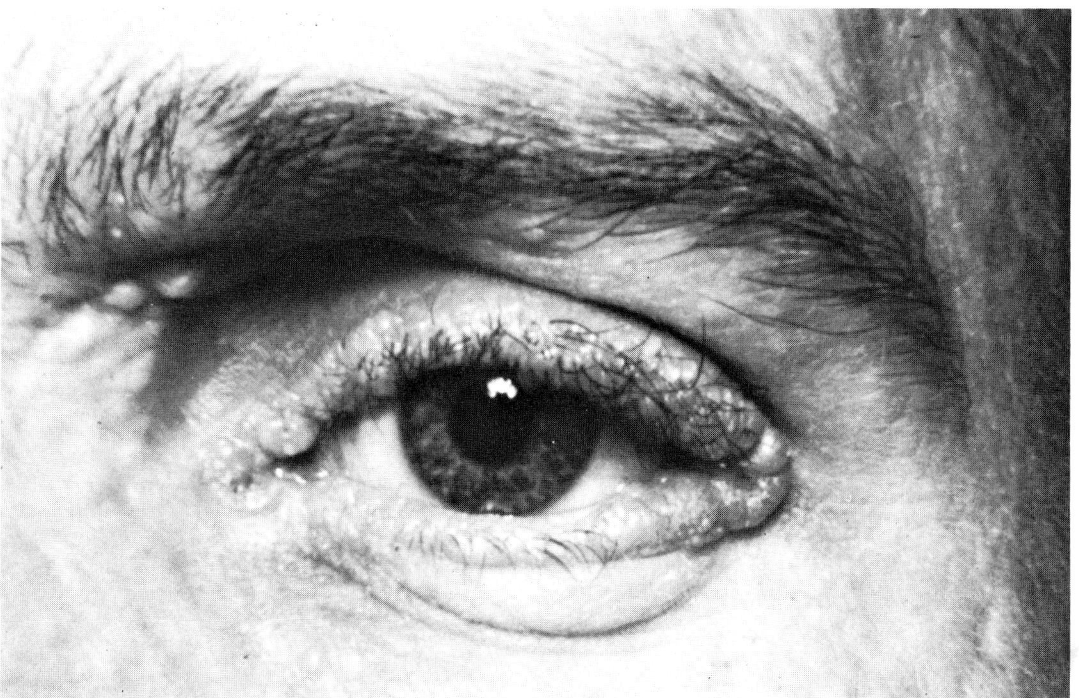

Figure 4–11. Lipoid proteinosis. Characteristic nodules on lid margins. (Courtesy of Dr. Richard Caplan.)

mouth, thereby producing a condition simulating syphilis. The tongue may be firm and woody and difficult to extrude, a condition which mimics amyloidosis. Plaques and nodules can also be found on gums, soft palate, uvula, frenulum, and floor of the mouth.

Hoarseness secondary to vocal cord involvement is a clinical feature in virtually every case, and if not present, the diagnosis of lipoid proteinosis is in doubt (Fig. 4–12).[75]

Respiratory obstruction resulting from severe laryngeal involvement and dysphagia caused by pharyngeal infiltration can complicate this disorder. Deposition of the glycoprotein in the rectal and genital mucosae has also been reported. Many individuals with this disease have aplasia or hypoplasia of the lateral upper incisors.

The abnormal glycoprotein can also be found in other organs.[76] Within the brain the glycoprotein becomes calcified and produces bilateral opacifications, which can be seen lateral to and just above the dorsum sellae on radiographic examination. The calcification occurs around the capillaries in the hippocampal gyri of the temporal lobes.[77] In a few patients, these findings were coincident with epilepsy. Involvement of the oral mucosa can occlude Stensen's duct and produce parotid gland enlargement. The abnormal glycoprotein has also been found in the esophagus, stomach, trachea, vagina, testes, eye, pancreas, bladder, kidney, lymph nodes, and striated muscle. Chromosomal analyses have been normal in the few cases that have been studied.[76]

Many patients are first diagnosed after they have reached adulthood, but the disease is probably present from birth. Although the data are not complete, it appears that the prognosis of this disorder is good and that the individual's longevity is normal.

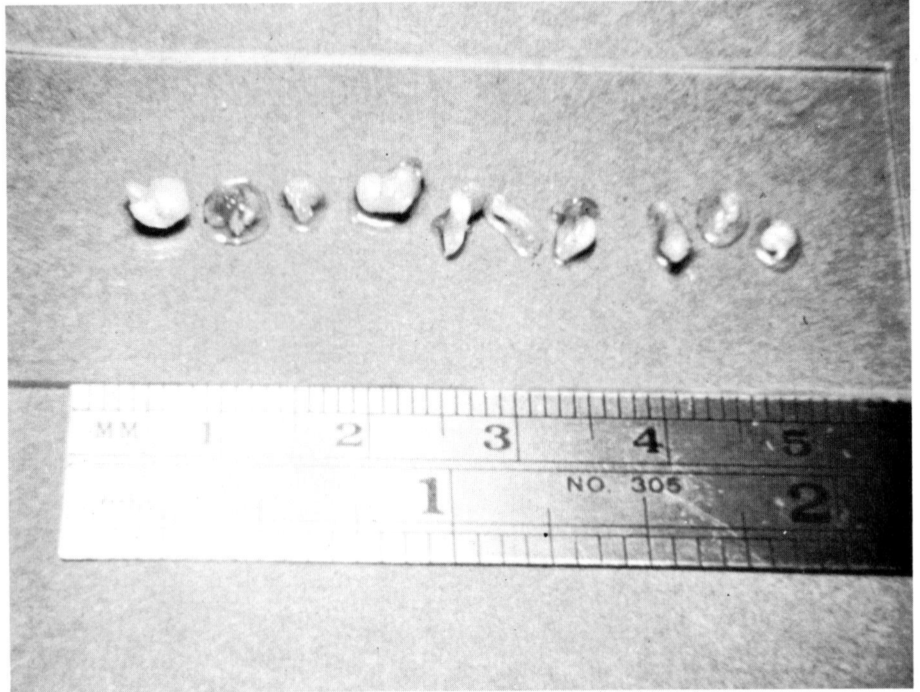

Figure 4–12. Lipoid proteinosis. Nodules removed from vocal cords. (Courtesy of Dr. Richard Caplan.)

During the individual's early childhood the evolution of the cutaneous lesions is different from that of adulthood. Small vesicles producing ulcers and varioliform scars on the face, neck, hands, and feet are the rule. Hemorrhagic bullae can also spontaneously develop. This scarring persists into adult life. Although photosensitivity is not thought to be a feature of lipoid proteinosis, the bullae, with resultant varioliform scars, do appear predominantly in light-exposed areas.[78]

In some instances, two photosensitivity disorders, hydroa vacciniforme and erythropoietic protoporphyria, have been confused with lipoid proteinosis because perivascular hyaline material resembling that found in lipoid proteinosis can also be found in these photosensitivity diseases.[79]

REFERENCES

1. Lichtenstein, L.: Histiocytosis X: integration of eosinophilic granuloma of bone, "Letterer-Siwe Disease" and "Schüller-Christian Disease" as related manifestations of a single nosologic entity. Arch. Pathol., *56*:84, 1953.
2. Bluefarb, S. M.: The systemic reticuloendothelial granulomas. *In* Bluefarb, S. M. (ed.): Cutaneous Manifestations of the Reticuloendothelial Granulomas. Charles C Thomas, Springfield, Ill., 1960, p. 115.
3. Lever, W. F.: Histopathology of the Skin. 5th edition. J. B. Lippincott, Philadelphia, 1975, pp. 371–376.
4. Batson, R., Shapiro, L., Christie, A., and Riley, H. D., Jr.: Acute non-lipid disseminated reticuloendotheliosis. Am. J. Dis. Child., *90*:323, 1955.
5. Avery, M. E., McAfee, J. G., and Guild, H. G.: The course and prognosis of reticuloendotheliosis (eosinophilic granuloma, Schüller-Christian disease, and Letterer-Siwe disease). Am. J. Med., *22*:636, 1957.
6. Lane, C. W., and Smith, M. G.: Cutaneous manifestations of chronic idiopathic lipoidosis (Hand-Schüller-Christian disease). Arch. Dermatol. Syph., *39*:617, 1939.
7. Braunstein, G. D., and Kohler, P. O.: Endocrine manifestations of histiocytosis. Am. J. Pediatr. Hematol./Oncol., *3*:67, 1981.
8. Braunstein, G. D., and Kohler, P. O.: Pituitary function in Hand-Schüller-Christian disease. Evidence for deficient growth-hormone release in patients with short stature. N. Engl. J. Med., *286*:1225, 1972.
9. Lieberman, P. H., Jones, C. R., Dargeon, H.

W. K., and Begg, C. F.: A reappraisal of eosinophilic granuloma of bone, Hand-Schüller-Christian syndrome and Letterer-Siwe syndrome. Medicine, *48*:375, 1969.

10. Mancer, J. F. K.: Histiocytosis X: Pathology. *In* Godden, J. O. (ed.): Cancer in Childhood. Plenum Press, New York, 1973, p. 113.
11. Meyer, E.: Hand-Schüller-Christian disease or eosinophilic xanthomatous granuloma. Am. J. Med., *15*:130, 1953.
12. Avioli, L. V., Lasersohn, J. T., and Lopresti, J. M.: Histiocytosis X (Schüller-Christian disease): a clinico-pathological survey, review of ten patients and the results of prednisone therapy. Medicine, *42*:119, 1963.
13. Braunstein, G. D., Raiti, S., Hansen, J. W., and Kohler, P. O.: Response of growth-retarded patients with Hand-Schüller-Christian disease to growth hormone therapy. N. Engl. J. Med., *292*:332, 1975.
14. Sonley, M. J., and Ghavimi, F.: Histiocytosis X: Management. *In* Godden, J. O. (ed.): Cancer in Childhood. Plenum Press, New York, 1973, p. 128.
15. Vogel, J. M., and Vogel, P.: Idiopathic histiocytosis: a discussion of eosinophilic granuloma, the Hand-Schüller-Christian syndrome, and the Letterer-Siwe syndrome. Semin. Hematol., *9*:349, 1972.
16. Basset, F., and Turiaf, J.: Identification par la microscopie electronique de particules de nature probablement virale dans les lesions granulomateuses d'une histiocytose X pulmonaire. C. R. Acad. Sci. (Paris), *261*:3701, 1965.
17. Nezelof, C., Basset, F., and Rousseau, M. F.: Histiocytosis X. Histogenetic arguments for a Langerhans cell origin. Biomedicine, *18*:365, 1973.
18. Wolff, K.: The Langerhans cell. Curr. Probl. Dermatol., *4*:79, 1972.
19. Yassin, T. M. A., and Toner, P. G.: Langerhans cells in the human oesophagus. J. Anat., *122*:435, 1976.
20. Hashimoto, K., and Tarnowski, W. M.: Some new aspects of the Langerhans cell. Arch. Dermatol., *97*:450, 1968.
21. Basset, F., Soler, P., Wyllie, L., Mazin, F., and Turiaf, J.: Langerhans' cells and lung interstitium. Ann. N.Y. Acad. Sci., *278*:599, 1976.
22. Feuerman, E. J., and Sandbank, M.: Histiocytosis X with skin lesions as the sole clinical expression. Acta Dermatovenereol., *56*:269, 1976.
23. Altman, J., and Winkelmann, R. K.: Xanthoma disseminatum. Arch. Dermatol., *86*:582, 1962.
24. Thannhauser, S. J.: Lipidoses. Diseases of the Intracellular Lipid Metabolism. 3rd ed., Grune & Stratton, New York, 1958, p. 370.
25. Cited by Altman, J., and Winkelmann, R. K.: Xanthoma disseminatum (reference 23). Arch. Dermatol., *86*:582, 1962.
26. Griffith, J. P. C.: Xanthoma tuberosum with early jaundice and diabetes insipidus. Arch. Pediatr., *39*:297, 1922.
27. Weidman, F. D., and Freeman, W.: Xanthoma tuberosum: two necropsies disclosing lesions of the central nervous system and other tissues. Arch. Dermatol. Syph., *9*:149, 1924.
28. Weidman, F. D., and Stokes, J., Jr.: Extensive xanthoma tuberosum in childhood due to infectious cirrhosis of the liver. Development of xanthomatous changes in laparotomy and other scars. Am. J. Dis. Child., *53*:1230, 1937.
29. Stickler, G. B., and Pinkel, D.: Reticuloendotheliosis complicated by xanthomatous biliary cirrhosis. Report of a case. Gastroenterology, *36*:702, 1959.
30. Altman, J., and Winkelmann, R. K.: Xanthomatous cutaneous lesions of histiocytosis X. Arch. Dermatol., *87*:164, 1963.
31. Thannhauser, S. J., *op. cit.*, p. 392, (case XLII).
32. Fleischmajer, R., and Hyman, A. B.: Juvenile giant cell granuloma (nevoxanthoendothelioma). *In* Fleischmajer, R.: The Dyslipidoses. Charles C Thomas, Springfield, Ill., 1960, p. 329.
33. Gartmann, H., and Tritsch, H.: Klein-und Grossknotiges Naevoxanthoendotheliom. Bericht ¨uber 13 Beobachtungen. Arch. Klin. Exp. Dermatol., *215*:409, 1963.
34. Sanders, T. S.: Intraocular juvenile xanthogranuloma (nevoxanthoendothelioma): survey of 20 cases. Am. J. Ophthalmol., *53*:455, 1962.
35. Cogan, D. G., Kuwabara, T., and Parke, D.: Epibulbar nevoxanthoendothelioma. Arch. Ophthalmol., *59*:717, 1958.
36. Hadden, O. B.: Bilateral juvenile xanthogranuloma of the iris. Br. J. Ophthalmol., *59*:699, 1975.
37. Helwig, E. B.: Juvenile xanthogranuloma. Proceedings of the 9th meeting of the Pacific Dermatologic Society, 1957, p. 25.
38. Lottsfeldt, F. I., and Good, R. A.: Juvenile xanthogranuloma with pulmonary lesions. Pediatrics, *33*:233, 1964.
39. Webster, S. B., Reister, S. C., and Harman, L. E.: Juvenile xanthogranuloma with extracutaneous lesions. Arch. Dermatol., *93*:71, 1966.
40. Newell, G. B., Stone, O. J., and Mullins, J. F.: Juvenile xanthogranuloma and neurofibromatosis. Arch. Dermatol., *107*:262, 1973.
41. Rodriguez, J., and Ackerman, A. B.: Xanthogranuloma in adults. Arch. Dermatol., *112*:43, 1976.
42. Davies, M. E., and Marks, R.: Multiple xanthogranulomata in an adult. Br. J. Dermatol., *97*(Suppl. 15):70, 1977.
43. Ref. Nos. 8 & 9 cited in Rodriguez, J., and Ackerman, A. B.: Xanthogranuloma in adults. Arch. Dermatol., *112*:43, 1976.
44. Orkin, M., Goltz, R. W., Good, R. A., Michael, A., and Fisher, I.: A study of multicentric reticulohistiocytosis. Arch. Dermatol., *89*:640, 1964.
45. Barrow, M. V., and Holubar, K.: Multicentric reticulohistiocytosis. A review of 33 patients. Medicine, *48*:287, 1969.
46. Gold, R. H., Meltzer, A. L., Mirra, J. M.,

Weinberger, H. J., and Killebrew, K.: Multicentric reticulohistiocytosis (lipoid dermatoarthritis). An erosive polyarthritis with distinctive clinical roentgenographic and pathologic features. Am. J. Roentgenol., *124*:610, 1975.
47. Krey, P. R., Comerford, F. R., and Cohen, A. S.: Multicentric reticulohistiocytosis. Fine structural anslysis of the synovia and synovial fluid cells. Arthritis Rheum., *17*:615, 1974.
48. Barrow, M. V.: The nails in multicentric reticulohistiocytosis. Arch. Dermatol., *95*:200, 1967.
49. Barrow, M. V., Sunderman, F. W., Jr., Hackett, R. L., and Colvin, W. S.: Identification of tissue lipids in lipoid dermatoarthritis (multicentric reticulohistiocytosis). Am. J. Clin. Pathol., *47*:312, 1967.
50. Purvis, W. E., III, and Helwig, E. B.: Reticulohistiocytic granuloma ("reticulohistiocytoma") of the skin. Am. J. Clin. Pathol., *24*:1005, 1954.
51. Montgomery, H.: Benign and malignant dermal neoplasms. J.A.M.A., *150*:1182, 1952.
52. Urbach, F., Koblenzer, C. C., and Ramasoota, T.: Multicentric reticulohistiocytosis. Arch. Dermatol., *95*:232, 1967.
53. Farber, S., Cohen, J., and Uzmann, L. L.: Lipogranulomatosis — a new lipoglycoprotein storage disease. J. Mount Sinai Hosp. NY, *24*:816, 1957.
54. Zellerstrom, R.: Disseminated lipogranulomatosis (Farber's disease). Acta Paediatr., *47*:501, 1958.
55. Abul-Haj, S. K., Martz, D. G., Douglas, W. F., and Geppert, L. J.: Farber's disease. J. Pediatr., *61*:221, 1962.
56. Dulaney, J. T., Milunsky, A., Sidbury, J. B., Hobolth, N., and Moser, H. W.: Diagnosis of lipogranulomatosis (Farber disease) by use of cultured fibroblasts. J. Pediatr., *89*:59, 1976.
57. Amirhakimi, G. H., Haghighi, P., Ghalambor, M. A., and Honari, S.: Familial lipogranulomatosis (Farber's disease). Clin. Genet., *9*:625, 1976.
58. Iwamori, M., and Moser, H. W.: Above-normal urinary excretion of urinary ceramides in Farber's disease, and the characterization of their components by high-performance liquid chromatography. Clin. Chem., *21*:725, 1975.
59. Rutsaert, J., Tondeur, M., Vamos-Hurwitz, E., and Dustin, P.: The cellular lesions of Farber's disease and their experimental reproduction in tissue culture. Lab. Invest., *36*:474, 1977.
60. Moser, H. W., Prensky, A. L., Wolfe, H. J., and Rosman, N. P.: Farber's lipogranulomatosis: report of a case and demonstration of an excess of free ceramide and ganglioside. Am. J. Med., *47*:869, 1969.
61. Sugita, M., Dullaney, J. T., and Moser, H. W.: Ceramidase deficiency in Farber's disease (lipogranulomatosis). Science, *178*:1100, 1972.
62. Harlan, W. R., Jr., and Still, W. J. S.: Hereditary tendinous and tuberous xanthomatosis without hyperlipidemia. N. Engl. J. Med., *278*:416, 1968.
63. Schimschock, J. R., Alvord, E. C., Jr., and Swanson, P. D.: Cerebrotendinous xanthomatosis. Clinical and pathologic studies. Arch. Neurol., *18*:688, 1968.
64. Truswell, A. S., and Pfister, P. J. V. S.: Cerebrotendinous xanthomatosis. Br. Med., J., *1*:353, 1972.
65. Pastershank, S. P., Yip, S., and Sodhi, H. S.: Cerebrotendinous xanthomatosis. J. Can. Assoc. Radiol., *25*:282, 1974.
66. Kearns, W. P., and Wood, W. S.: Cerebrotendinous xanthomatosis. Arch. Ophthalmol., *94*:148, 1976.
67. Salen, G.: Cholestanol deposition in cerebrotendinous xanthomatosis. A possible mechanism. Ann. Intern. Med., *75*:843, 1971.
68. Setoguchi, T., Salen, G., Tint, G. S., and Mosbach, E. H.: A biochemical abnormality in cerebrotendinous xanthomatosis. J. Clin. Invest., *53*:1393, 1974.
69. Tint, G. S., and Salen, G.: Evidence for the early reduction of the 24, 25, double bond in the conversion of lanosterol to cholesterol in cerebrotendinous xanthomatosis. Metabolism, *26*:721, 1977.
70. Laymon, C. W., and Hill, E. M.: Hyalinosis cutis et mucosae. Arch. Dermatol., *75*:55, 1957.
71. Burnett, J. W., and Marcy, S. M.: Lipoid proteinosis. Am. J. Dis. Child., *105*:81, 1963.
72. Hofer, P.-A., Ek, B., Goller, H., Laurell, H., and Lorentzon, R.: A clinical and histopathological study of twenty-seven cases of Urbach-Wiethe disease. Acta Pathol. Microbiol. Scand., Section A., Suppl. 245:1974.
73. McCusker, J., and Caplan, R.: Lipoid proteinosis (lipoglycoproteinosis). A histochemical study of two cases. Am. J. Pathol., *40*:599, 1962.
74. Heyl, T., and de Kock, D.: A chromatographic study of skin lipids in lipoid proteinosis. J. Invest. Dermatol., *42*:333, 1964.
75. Grosfeld, J. C. M., Spaas, J., Van de Staak, W. J. B. M., and Stadhouders, A. M.: Hyalinosis cutis et mucosae (lipoid proteinosis, Urbach-Wiethe). Dermatologica, *130*:239, 1965.
76. Caplan, R. M.: Visceral involvement in lipoid proteinosis. Arch. Dermatol., *95*:149, 1967.
77. Holtz, K.: Uber Gehirn-und Augenveranderungen bei Hyalinosis Cutis et Mucosae (Lipoidproteinose) mit Autofsiebefund. Arch. Klin. Exp. Dermatol., *214*:289, 1962.
78. Heyl, T.: Lipoid proteinosis I. The clinical picture Br. J. Dermatol., *75*:465, 1963.
79. Peterka, E., Fusaro, R., and Goltz, R.: Erythropoietic protoporphyria II. Histological and histochemical studies of cutaneous lesions. Arch. Dermatol., *92*:357, 1965.

5

Multiple Myeloma and the Other Dysproteinemias

The dysproteinemias are characterized by abnormalities — involving either overproduction or underproduction — in the synthesis of gamma globulin. The protein abnormalities in these disorders are described in terms of immunoglobulin classes: IgG, IgA or IgM.[1,2] Each of the three main immunoglobulin classes is composed of heterogeneous, but closely related, gamma globulins which migrate together on electrophoresis.

The basic molecular structure of the immunoglobulins has been determined and the various immunoglobulins and their component parts are now being used as a basis for classification of the dysproteinemic states. Two additional classes are recognized: IgD, which appears to act along with IgM as the primary receptor for antigen on B-lymphocytes, and IgE, the reaginic antibody of atopy.

The molecular structures of the various immunoglobulins are similar: each molecule is made up of heavy (H) and light (L) polypeptide chains, which are synthesized separately and then assembled. IgG, the molecule most studied, and IgA both have two H and two L chains. IgG and IgA have molecular weights of 160,000 and 170,000, respectively, and sedimentation constants of 7S. IgM, a more complex molecule, has a molecular weight of 900,000 and a sedimentation constant of 19S. In addition, this molecule is made up of five subunits, each of which contains two H and two L chains. All of the immunoglobulins contain a carbohydrate prosthetic group. The carbohydrate content ranges from 3 per cent in IgG to 7 per cent of IgA, 11 per cent in IgE, 12 per cent in IgM, and 13 per cent in IgD. IgG contains the least with 3 per cent. IgG crosses the placental barrier readily, while IgM and IgA show insignificant passage.

Figure 5–1 is a diagram of the organization of the basic monomeric unit of all immunoglobulins and their subunits. One L chain and one H chain are held together by a disulfide bond, and two such units are joined via the H chains by two pairs of disulfide bonds. The overall structure is Y-shaped. All L chains in the carboxyl terminal half have identical amino acid sequences which are referred to as the constant portion, C_L. All N-terminal halves of L chains have different amino acid sequences from one another, and are called the variable portion, V_L. The H chain has one variable (V_H) and three homologous constant regions (C_H1, C_H2, and C_H3). Each of the variable and constant regions contains a 55 to 60 amino acid sequence pulled into a loop by a disulfide bond (Fig. 5–2). Enzymatic digestion of an immunoglobulin molecule occurs in the hinge peptide

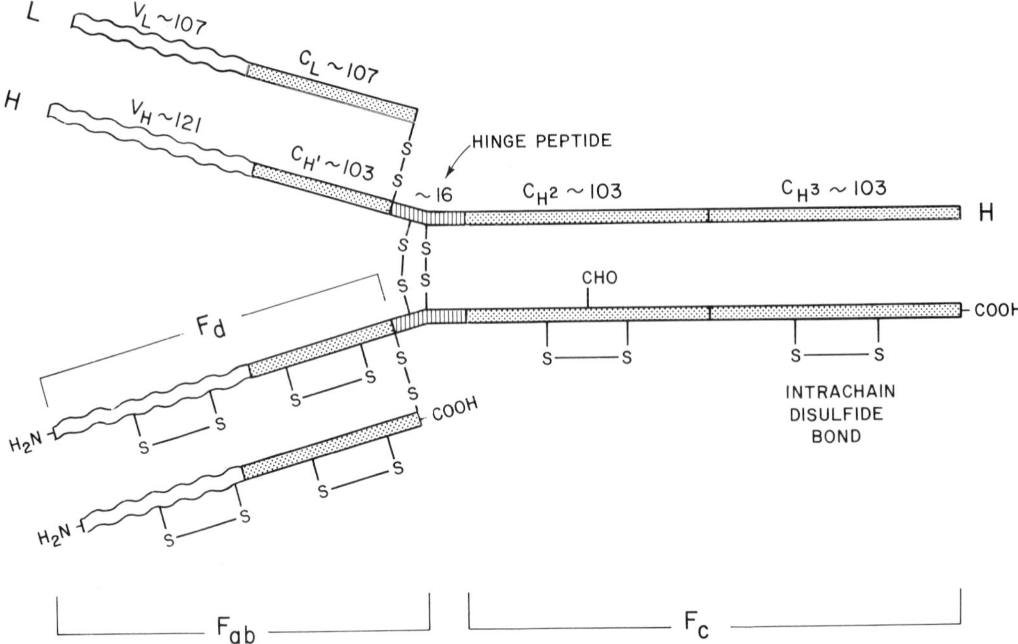

Figure 5–1. Diagram of the organization of the basic monomeric unit of all immunoglobulins and their subunits.

region, which is a 9 to 16 amino acid sequence in the zone of the two disulfide bonds joining the H chains. Enzymatic digestion with papain produces three pieces. Two are identical and contain the antibody-combining site. This fragment is called Fab and is made up of an L chain and half of the H chain joined together by a disulfide bond. The variable regions in both chains are responsible for the activity of the antibody-combining site. The third piece is called the Fc fragment (crystallizable) and represents a dimer of the carboxyl terminal half of the H chain. The Fc portion lacks a combining site, but has the functional properties of complement fixation, and placental transport. The H chain portion of the Fab fragment is called Fd.

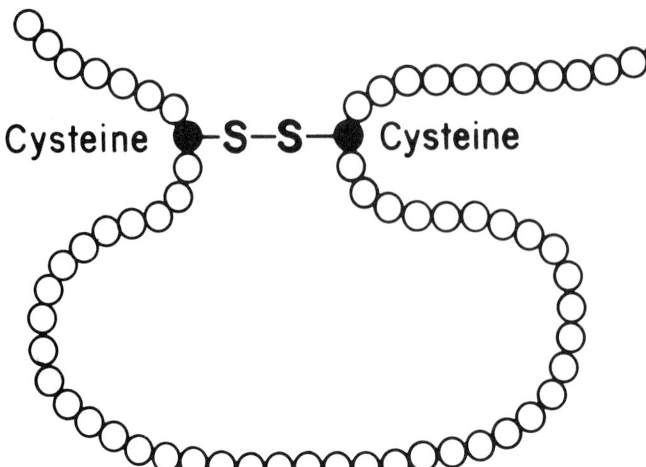

Figure 5–2. Diagram of variable and constant regions of immunoglobulin molecule. Each circle represents an amino acid in the polypeptide chain.

All immunoglobulins contain L chains of two antigenic types: kappa or lambda. The three classes of immunoglobulins are distinguished on the basis of the antigenic differences of their H chains. The H chains of IgG (called γ) have four antigenic subtypes (IgG1, IgG2, IgG3, and IgG4); IgA (α), two subtypes (IgA1 and IgA2); and IgM (μ), two subtypes (IgM1 and IgM2). IgD and IgE have configurations similar to those of the other immunoglobulins but appear to have only one subclass of H chain, δ and ϵ.

An individual immunoglobulin molecule has either kappa or lambda chains. The immunoglobulins of healthy individuals show the following distribution: 60 per cent kappa, 30 per cent lambda, and 10 per cent of unknown antigenic type.

The dysproteinemias to be considered in this chapter show (1) an increased synthesis of all immunoglobulin classes; (2) an increased production of a single molecular immunoglobulin species (paraprotein), often with a marked diminution of the other immunoglobulins; or (3) a selective increase or decrease of one or more classes.

The first variety, represented by hypergammaglobulinemia, shows a broad gamma globulin band on electrophoresis. This finding is nonspecific and occurs in many diverse situations, including hyperglobulinemic purpura of Waldenström.

The second type includes the *M component diseases*. A single prominent *narrow* band appears anywhere from the very slow gamma globulin region to the faster alpha-1 zone on the electrophoretic pattern. Often the paraprotein may also be found in the urine.

In individual cases, the M component represents a single homogeneous immunoglobulin species belonging to either IgG, IgA, IgM, or rarely, IgD, and having only kappa or lambda chains. Four instances of an IgE M component have been reported.[3] In rare instances two M components can be present in the same patient. The important M component diseases are multiple myeloma, macroglobulinemia of Waldenström, heavy chain diseases, light chain disease, amyloidosis, and papular mucinosis (lichen myxedematosus, scleromyxedema). The term *plasma cell dyscrasias* was coined by Osserman to encompass these pathologic conditions that seem to represent an unbalanced proliferation of the cells that normally synthesize immunoglobulins.

The third category includes the antibody deficiency syndromes.

DIFFUSE HYPERGAMMAGLOBULINEMIA

The disorders most commonly responsible for an overall increase in serum gamma globulins include lupus erythematosus, rheumatoid arthritis, Sjögren's syndrome, polyarteritis nodosa and related angiitides, sarcoidosis, chronic liver disease, ulcerative colitis, regional ileitis, Hashimoto's thyroiditis, and chronic infections caused by bacteria, viruses, fungi, and protozoa. Although all of the immunoglobulins are usually elevated in these chronic diseases, IgG accounts for most of the rise.

In 1943, Waldenström described three cases of purpura in association with hyperglobulinemia, and since then many cases have been reported in the literature.[4] The clinical appearance and course of hyperglobulinemic

PLATE 14

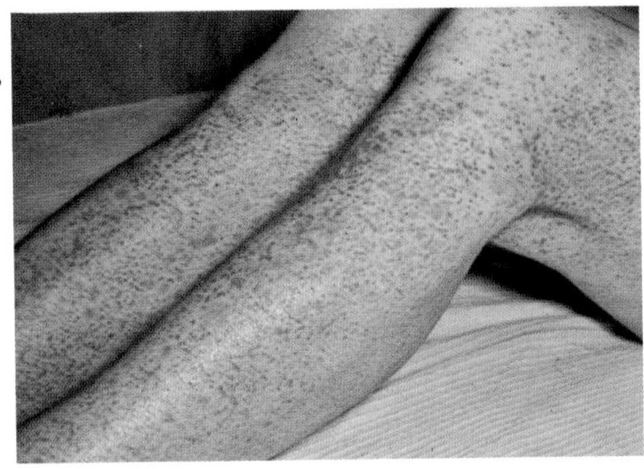

A, Waldenström's hyperglobulinemic purpura.

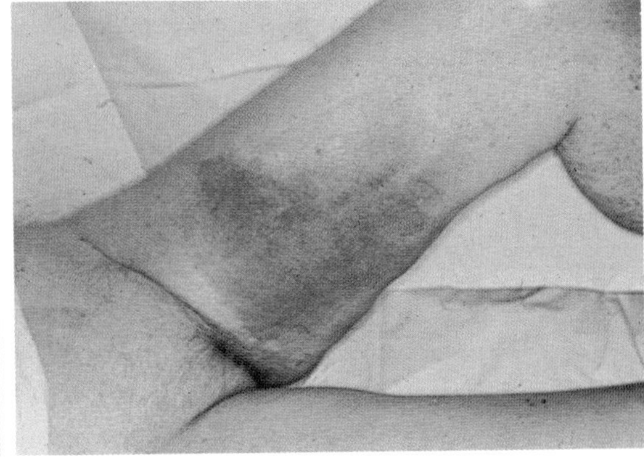

B, Multiple myeloma. Cellulitis on thigh produced by *Cryptococcus neoformans*.

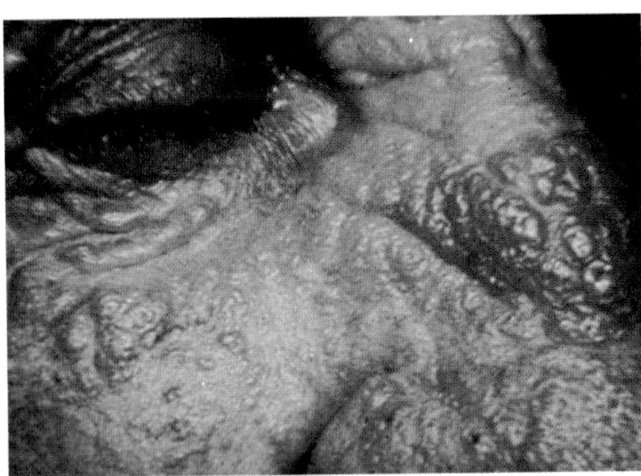

C, Primary amyloidosis. Cutaneous lesions. (Courtesy of Dr. Thomas Kugelman.)

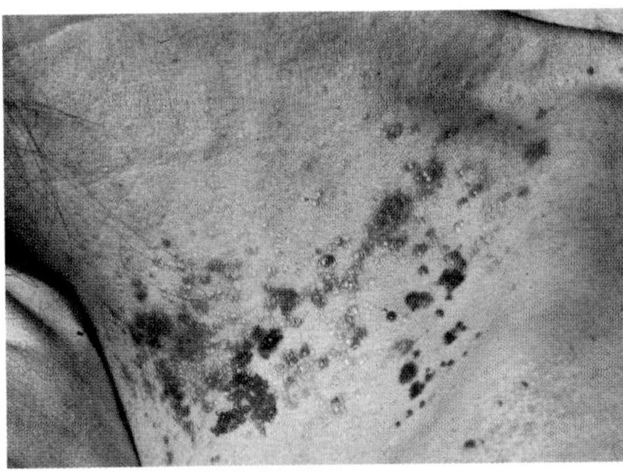

D, Primary amyloidosis. Skin of neck showing numerous translucent waxy papules, some of which have become hemorrhagic. (From Medicine [Balt.], *31*:381, 1952. Courtesy of Dr. Robert Goltz.)

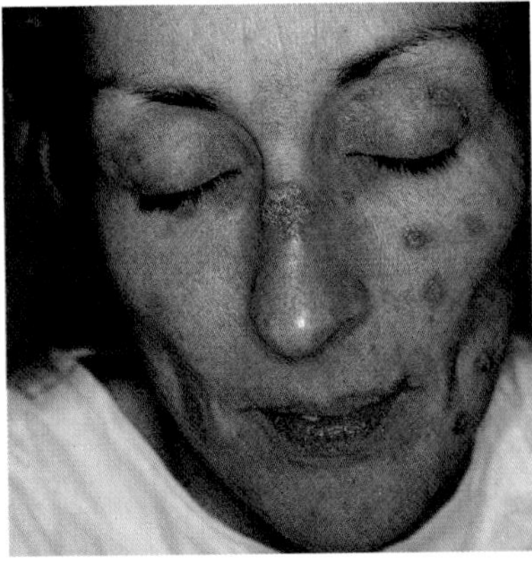

E, Lupus erythematosus (LE). Discoid lesions on nose and cheeks.

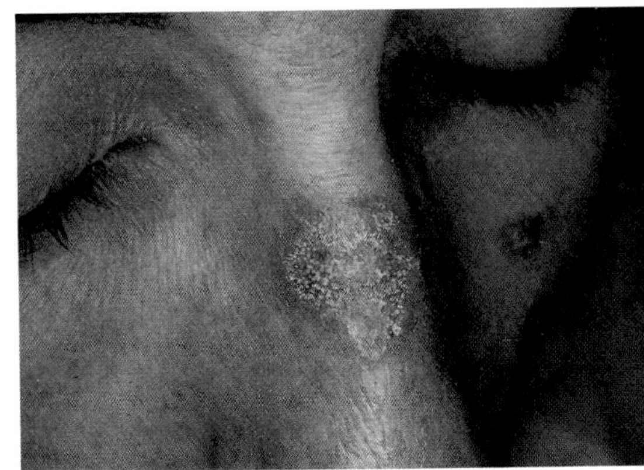

F, LE. Close-up of discoid lesions on nose of patients shown in *E*. Fine scale with follicular plugging.

purpura is relatively clear-cut. It can be seen in association with Sjögren's syndrome, sarcoidosis, neoplasia, and lupus erythematosus; however, in different series no underlying disease was found in 10 to 50 per cent of the cases.[5-7]

This syndrome develops in adults of all ages but occurs in females more frequently than in males. The purpura develops primarily on the legs as nonelevated petechiae that range in size from 1 to 4 mm (Plate 14*A*). Often they arise in crops. Ecchymoses do not occur, but the petechiae can become confluent. Regression of the petechiae may be complete, or hemosiderin deposits may remain. Arthralgias may accompany the petechial eruption. It is characteristic for the hemorrhagic rash to be brought on by prolonged standing, walking, or wearing of tight undergarments (Fig. 5–3). Paresthesias may precede the appearance of the eruption, but in general the rash is asymptomatic. Scarring is not produced as the lesions resolve. Although purpura occurs primarily on the lower extremities, minor trauma can produce petechiae on the arms, and in rare cases the trunk and the soles of the feet can be affected. The petechial eruption is probably correlated with the increased capillary fragility detected in most cases. The disorder can be chronic with fresh efflorescences occurring for a period of several years at intervals that range from a day to a month. In one of our cases, this syndrome preceded the appearance of systemic lupus erythematosus by 14 years.

Most of the hypergammaglobulinemia results from circulating intermediate-sized complexes with sedimentation coefficients ranging between 7S and 19S.[8] These large complexes are composed of IgG–anti-

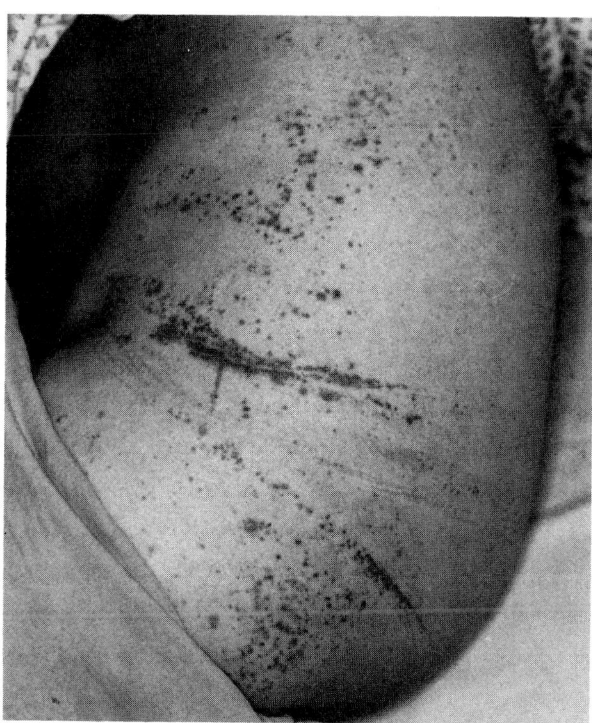

Figure 5–3. Hyperglobulinemic purpura. Tight underclothing produced the purpuric eruption on the waist and upper thigh in this patient.

IgG molecules, which in sufficient quantities can produce increase in serum viscosity. A hyperviscosity syndrome can develop in such situations.[9] The discovery that the anti-IgG globulins are of the IgG class also explains why patients with this syndrome have an IgG rheumatoid factor rather than the IgM type found in rheumatoid arthritis.

Biopsies of the purpuric lesions have shown either a necrotizing angiitis or a nonspecific mild chronic inflammatory reaction about the vessels. The pathogenesis of the purpura could be related to vascular damage from sludging secondary to hyperviscosity or to the deposition of complexes within vascular walls producing an Arthus or serum sickness–like reaction. However, immunofluorescence studies have usually not shown immunoglobulins and complement in and around the vascular walls. In addition, it is currently believed that complexes larger than 19S are required to produce necrotizing vasculitis (see Chap. 8). Additional studies are required to resolve these points.

Capra et al. demonstrated that the anti-IgG globulin in two-thirds of their 16 sera was monoclonal.[8] This is a potentially important observation, because the development of a polyclonal anti-IgG globulin might suggest an underlying connective tissue disease, while a monoclonal moiety might point to the eventual development of a myeloproliferative disorder. One of our patients had hyperglobulinemic purpura for 12 years prior to the development of an IgA myeloma (see p. 229). Two similar case reports are found in the literature.[8]

I would favor the restriction of the term *purpura hyperglobulinemia* to those cases in which the petechiae are *flat*, occur after exertion or standing, appear in crops, and resolve without scarring even though hemosiderin may be left behind.

The progressive pigmentary dermatoses (purpura simplex, Schamberg's disease, Majocchi's disease) might be confused with purpura hyperglobulinemia, but serum protein abnormalities are not present, and the clinical picture of fine red-brown puncta within circumscribed brownish areas is not usually seen in purpura hyperglobulinemia. The lesions of Schamberg's disease occur as discrete patches, even when the disorder is generalized, in contrast to purpura hyperglobulinemia, in which the petechiae are always diffuse (see p. 431).

DISEASES WITH M COMPONENT

When large series of patients with M components are studied, several associated disorders are customarily found.[10-12] Multiple myeloma accounts for 30 to 50 per cent of the cases; Waldenström's macroglobulinemia, 15 per cent; primary amyloidosis, 2.5 to 5 per cent; lymphomas, leukemia, and cancer, 5 to 10 per cent; assorted benign conditions, 25 to 30 per cent; and some normal individuals who never develop a detectable associated illness, 0.1 to 0.8 per cent. The cancers most frequently found are those of the breast, colon, lung, stomach, and prostate. Benign conditions constitute a significant proportion of the associated illnesses, but the pathogenetic relationship to the M component, if any, is not clear. The commonest disorders include arteriosclerotic heart disease, diabetes mellitus, duodenal ulcer, chronic infections, especially of the urinary tract, chronic hepatic and biliary tract diseases, and advanced age.

Myeloma

Multiple myeloma is a neoplasm of plasma cells and is characterized by discrete osteolytic lesions associated with pain and pathologic fractures, plasma cell infiltration of bone marrow, anemia, hepatosplenomegaly, and lymphadenopathy. Intensive study of the Bence Jones urinary protein and of the "myeloma" spikes produced by the plasma cells on electrophoresis has been responsible for the current breakthrough in knowledge of the structure and function of the immunoglobulins: the M component in approximately 70 per cent of patients with myeloma is IgG; in 28 per cent, IgA; and in two per cent, IgD.[10, 13-15] IgE has been detected in four cases.[3] Kappa chains are found in two-thirds of the IgA and IgG paraproteins. Almost all of the IgD M components are lambda in type. Bence Jones proteins are pure L chains and are excreted in the urine as disulfide bonded dimers (Fig. 5–4). They have the same antigenic group (kappa or lambda) present in the serum M component and can be detected in about 50 per cent of cases. In some myelomas, the only detectable monoclonal immunoglobulins may be kappa or lambda L chains as in the series of Stone and Frenkel.[16] Twenty per cent of their 35 patients had associated amyloidosis — twice the prevalence usually found in myeloma. The courses of these seven patients were dominated by the clinical features of primary systemic amyloidosis rather than by the typical findings of myeloma.

The high concentration of paraproteins is associated with a marked decrease in the other immunoglobulins. An increased susceptibility of the host to bacterial infections, especially pneumococcal pneumonia, results from the decreased levels of normal immunoglobulins.

The cutaneous manifestations of myeloma are related to the following conditions: (1) specific plasma cell infiltrates in the skin and adjacent tissues; (2) amyloidosis, found in 10 per cent of the cases; (3) cryoglobulinemia, found in 5 per cent of the cases; and (4) nonspecific reaction patterns.

Specific Infiltrations. Plasmacytomas, or collections of malignant plasma cells, usually develop initially within the bone marrow and then erode into the skin to produce tender bluish subcutaneous masses. Cutaneous nodules of plasma cells, unrelated to bony lesions, have been reported but are very uncommon, and they display no morphologic features that would suggest the correct diagnosis.[17]

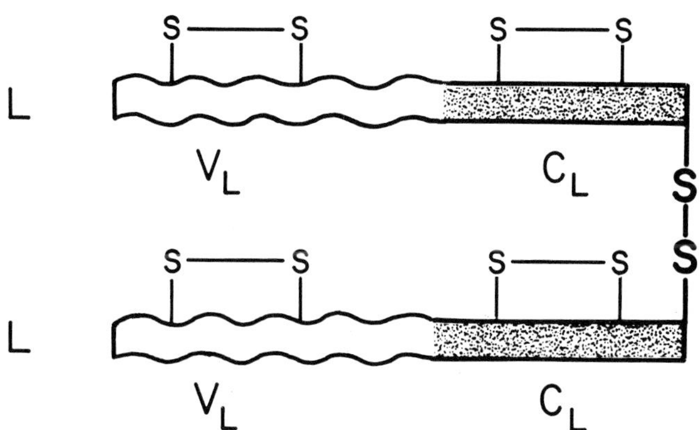

Figure 5–4. Diagram of organization of light chains. V_L and C_L are variable and constant regions, respectively.

Solitary plasmacytomas can exist for many years before they disseminate and before the typical course of myeloma begins. Extramedullary plasmacytomas develop most commonly in the upper respiratory passages, but they can also arise in the gastrointestinal tract and in the thyroid.

Amyloidosis. Amyloidosis associated with myeloma and primary amyloidosis have an identical distribution: the skin, tongue, blood vessels, gastrointestinal tract, and heart. The cutaneous features of amyloidosis in myeloma and in other diseases are considered in Chapter 6.

Cryoglobulinemia. Cryoglobulinemia occurs most commonly in myeloma (in about 5 per cent of the cases) and less frequently in Waldenström's macroglobulinemia. Cryoglobulins may also be found with carcinomas of the breast and colon; with leukemias and lymphomas; and in diseases associated with diffuse hyperglobulinemia, such as bronchiectasis, rheumatic fever, kala-azar, polyarteritis nodosa, lupus erythematosus, rheumatoid arthritis, and subacute bacterial endocarditis.[18]

The presence of cryoglobulin can be detected easily by separating the serum or plasma from a blood sample at 37°C and allowing it to cool overnight in a tube at 4°C. The cryoprotein will form a globule at the bottom of the tube and will dissolve when rewarmed.

By studying purified cryoglobulins with immunoelectrophoretic techniques, Brouet et al. have classified cryoglobulins into three groups.[19] Type I cryoglobulins are composed of monoclonal immunoglobulins — IgM and IgG and rarely IgA. This was the type first recognized in clinical medicine by Lerner and Watson.[20] Type II cryoglobulins are mixed cryoglobulins with a monoclonal component, usually IgM, which possesses antibody activity against polyclonal IgG. IgG-IgG and IgA-IgG cryoglobulins are uncommon. Type III cryoglobulins are mixed polyclonal immunoglobulins combined with non-immunoglobulin molecules such as lipoprotein or the C1q component of complement. Types II and III cryoglobulins also behave as immunoglobulin–anti-immunoglobulin immune complexes. In their study of 86 patients, Brouet et al. found that 25 per cent of the cryoglobulins were Type I, 25 per cent Type II, and 50 per cent Type III.

Type I occurred chiefly in myeloma and Waldenström's macroglobulinemia. Type II cryoglobulins were uncommon in myeloma, but were present in 50 per cent of patients with macroglobulinemia. Type III did not occur in the immunoproliferative diseases.

Cold sensitivity is often associated with Type I cryoglobulins. Mottling of skin, blotchy cyanosis on exposure to cold, and Raynaud's phenomenon with or without gangrene are common. Urticaria which becomes hemorrhagic, especially upon rewarming, is a characteristic feature. Thromboses of the retinal veins and gelation of endolymph, which produces deafness, have also been described. Epistaxis, stomatitis, pharyngitis, bleeding gums, and retinal bleeding have also been ascribed to the presence of cryoglobulins.[21] However, in those instances in which myeloma was the underlying disease, it is possible that bleeding could have been related to undetected amyloidosis or a hyperviscosity syndrome.

The most common finding in patients with cryoglobulinemia is

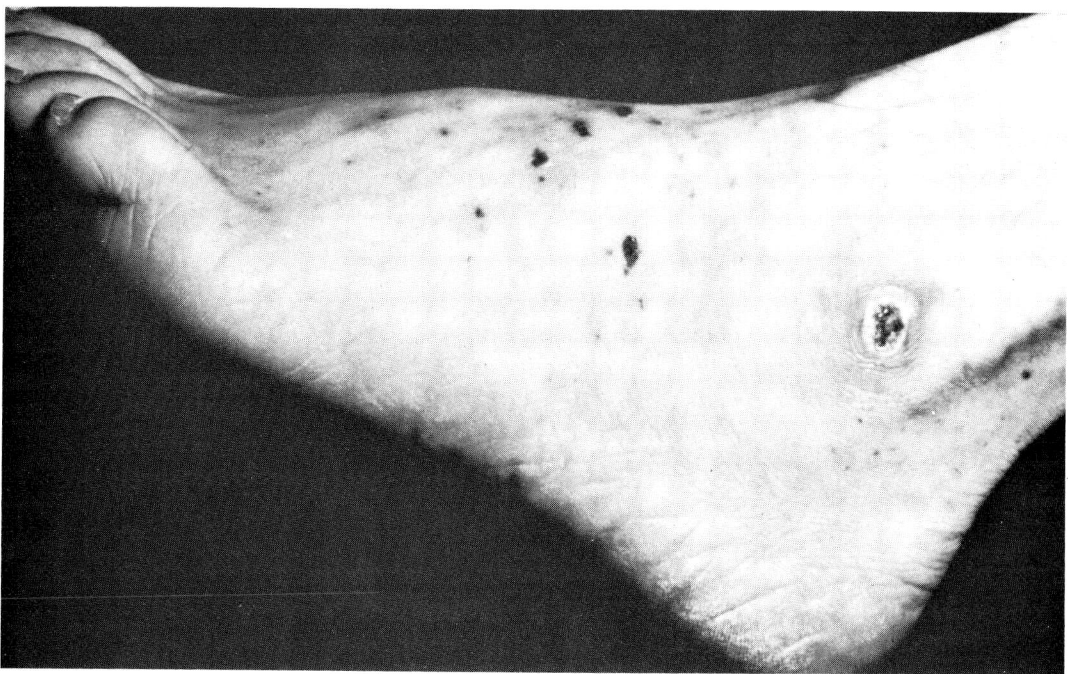

Figure 5–5. Cryoglobulinemia. Ulcerations and purpura around the ankles are characteristic of this entity.

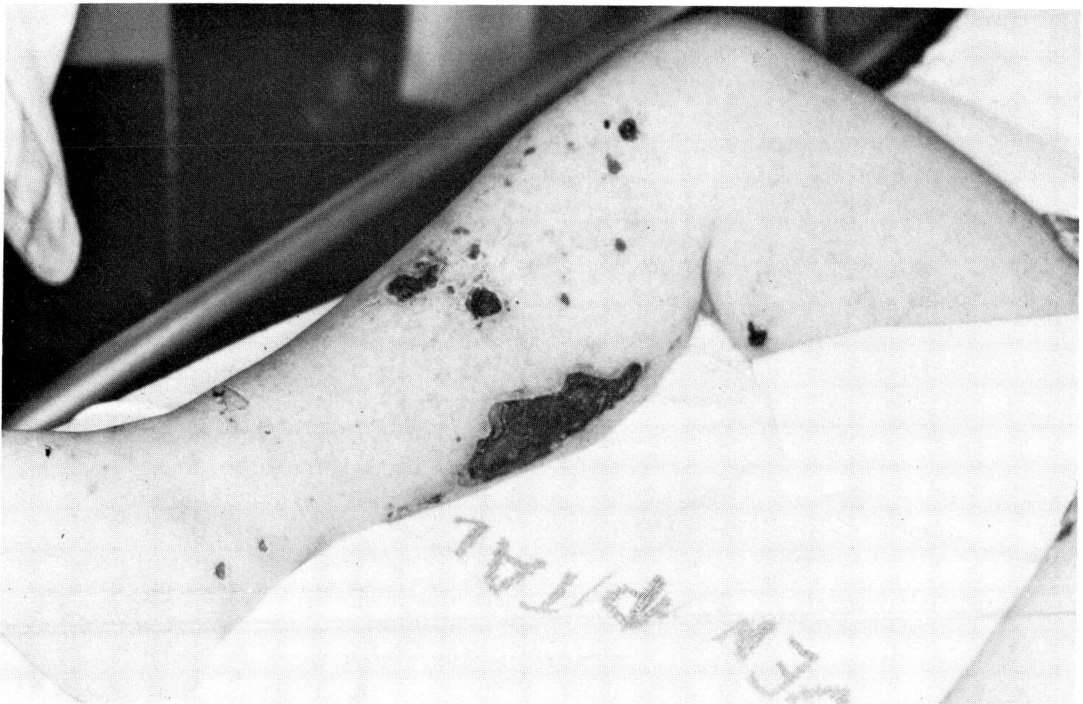

Figure 5–6. Cryoglobulinemia. The eruption began as large hemorrhagic bullae that broke within 24 hours to produce these ulcerations. This patient had multiple myeloma.

ulceration that occurs about the ankles, hands, and occasionally the ears, upon prolonged exposure to cold (Fig. 5–5). The lesions can begin as hemorrhagic bullae which quickly break and leave large denuded areas as illustrated in Figure 5–6. In this instance the patient had myeloma with cryoglobulinemia. The hemorrhagic bullae and ulcerations were the presenting signs of her disease. The ulcers healed completely after several weeks. Cryoglobulinemia can be diagnosed via a biopsy of the edge of an ulcer. Eosinophilic material, presumed to be cryoprotein, can be found within small vessels.[22] Vascular obstruction by cryoprotein is believed to produce the cutaneous hemorrhagic blisters and ulcers.

Although the clinical signs and symptoms attributed to cryoglobulinemia were described before the phenomenon of mixed cryoglobulinemia was recognized, it is likely that they do correlate with Type I cryoglobulins rather than with Types II and III, as judged by the preliminary clinical observations detailed by Brouet et al. Prospective studies in this regard need to be performed.

Types II and III cryoglobulins can behave as immune complexes and produce small vessel vasculitis in the skin as well as immune complex nephritis. Types II and III cryoglobulins are found in leukemias, lymphomas, systemic lupus erythematosus, autoimmune hemolytic anemia, Sjögren's syndrome, periarteritis nodosa, rheumatoid arthritis, many systemic infections, and essential cryoglobulinemia. Type I cryoglobulins occurred only infrequently in the autoimmune diseases.[19] However, monoclonal cryoglobulins sometimes behave as immune complexes to produce glomerulonephritis and nephrotic syndrome.[23]

Cold urticaria by itself is an uncommon feature of cryoglobulinemia; of the 431 cases of cryoglobulinemia collected in the literature, only 15 exhibited cold urticaria.[24] An unusual situation was described by Volpé et al. The patient experienced cold urticaria associated with chills and fever for 25 years. Subsequently, purpura appeared in the hives. The protocol did not state whether there was a family history of this type of urticaria, which is usually familial. This patient also exhibited melena, hemoptysis, and deafness, which were attributed to cryoglobulinemia. Laboratory studies showed that his blood sludged and that the red blood cells aggregated after exposure to cold.[25] These clinical phenomena have to be restudied and correlated with the recent advances in our understanding about the nature of cryoglobulins.

Nonspecific Reaction Patterns. Nonspecific pallor secondary to anemia is common in the late stages of myeloma. Because of a decrease in effective immunoglobulins, bacterial infections, including cutaneous ones, are common. An unusual case, though, is shown in Plate 14*B*. This patient with myeloma was thought to have a bacterial cellulitis on her thigh. However, a skin biopsy revealed a cryptococcal infection. At autopsy, cryptococcal meningitis was found.

Purpura develops secondary to thrombocytopenia or amyloidosis of cutaneous vessels in otherwise normal-appearing skin. Purpura hyperglobulinemia preceding the diagnosis of myeloma by 10 to 14 years has been described in two cases.[26, 27] Ulcerations about the ankle arise not only secondary to cryoglobulinemia but can also be a result of unsuspected amyloidosis of vessels or peripheral nerves. Pemphigoid has been described in association with multiple myeloma by Kingery and Montes.[28]

Acquired ichthyosis, usually associated with lymphoma, has also been reported. One of our patients developed generalized dryness of the skin six months before myeloma was diagnosed. The unique features of his eruption are shown in Figure 5–7. He developed horny follicular spicules on his nose and cheeks. The spicules often surrounded a fine hair and could be extracted easily. Histologic examination revealed normal sebaceous glands and an absence of inflammation in the dermis. Hyperkeratosis was found within the follicle itself and probably was related to the xerotic skin. We have not found a previous description of a similar eruption coincident with myeloma.

Myeloma has been reported with hypercholesterolemia in the absence of xanthomas; cases of myeloma and xanthomas without hyperlipemia or hypercholesterolemia have also been described.[13, 29] Savin reported the fourth instance of myeloma associated with hyperlipemia and xanthomas in a patient from the Yale-New Haven Medical Center.[26]

The patient was a 68-year-old white woman who had hyperglobulinemic purpura for 14 years (Plate 14*A*). Her petechiae appeared in crops, were flat, and were associated with arthralgias. The purpura was aggravated by prolonged exercise and standing. Four years before she died, tuberous xanthomata appeared over both heels, and the bouts of purpura diminished in severity and frequency. She never developed an arcus or xanthelasma. Symptoms of angina pectoris developed one year later. She was found to have extremely high serum levels of cholesterol, fatty acids, and triglycerides, but there were no findings consistent with the common lipidoses. The family history was negative for heart disease, diabetes mellitus, xanthomatosis, and purpura. Lipid studies of two sisters, a son, and a daughter were normal. These abnormal lipid findings suggested the possibility of myeloma to her physicians. A bone marrow examination showed 50 to 60 per cent atypical plasma cells characteristic of the disease. The patient died of a myocardial infarction, and the diagnosis of myeloma was confirmed at autopsy. The myeloma was of the IgA type. The degree of atherosclerotic change

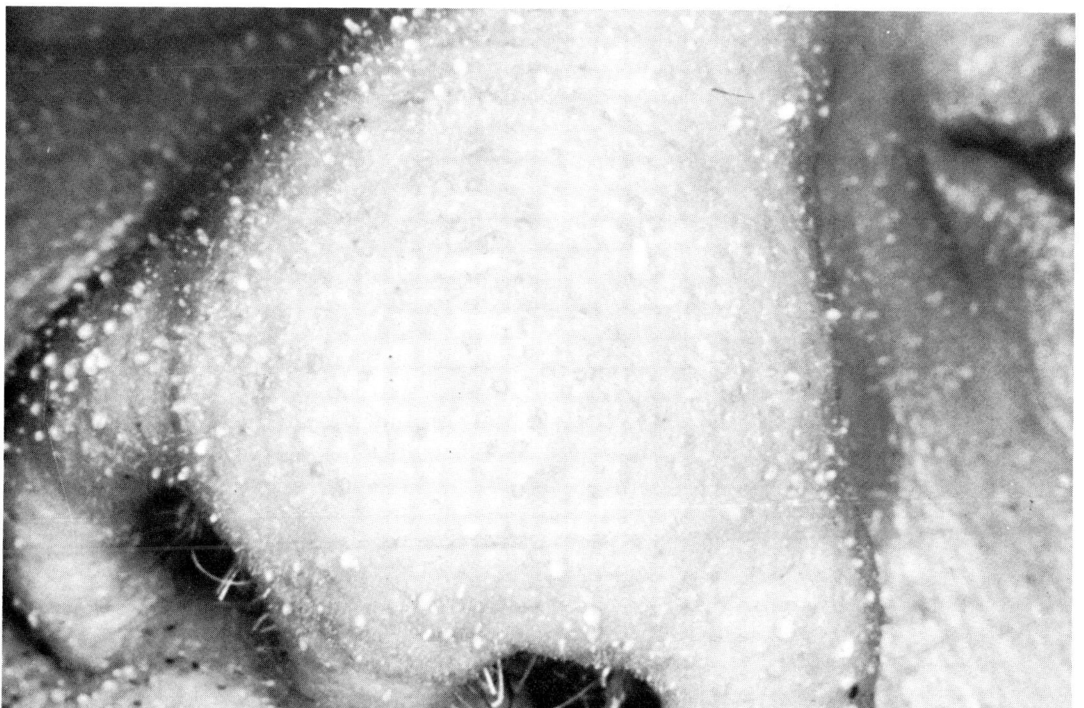

Figure 5–7. Multiple myeloma. Hyperkeratotic spicules in hair follicles.

within the great vessels was considered normal for a person of this age, an unexpected finding in view of the high serum lipid levels. Electrophoretic analysis revealed an elevated beta-2-globulin, and ultracentrifugation analysis revealed markedly elevated beta lipoprotein and decreased alpha lipoprotein. It was postulated that the hyperplastic plasma cells were producing a lipogenic protein which caused the elevated serum lipids and which was secondarily responsible for the xanthomas.

In the three similar patients — one man and two women, 59 to 68 years old — the course of the myeloma was long; there were elevated levels of beta lipoprotein; Bence Jones proteinuria was absent; and there was a normal degree of atherosclerosis in spite of hyperlipidemia.[26]

Lynch and Winkelmann reviewed the problems of generalized normolipemic flat xanthomas in relation to systemic disease.[30] Although any area of skin can be involved, the sides of the neck, the upper trunk, and scars are the sites of predilection (Figs. 5–8 and 5–9; Plate 12*C*). Two of their patients developed leukemia, but 8 of 16 adult patients terminated in myeloma.

An unusual syndrome has been reported from Japan in persons who have myeloma manifested by a *localized osteosclerotic* bone lesion. The clinical features include diffuse hyperpigmentation, anasarca or pitting edema of the legs, hypertrichosis of the anterior thighs and knees, and a sensorimotor polyneuropathy.[31] Men have gynecomastia and are impotent, and women are amenorrheic. In some patients the skin of the chest feels thickened because of edema. Diabetes mellitus and/or primary hypothyroidism are often present. Successful therapy of the bony myeloma lesion has been associated with marked improvement in the signs and

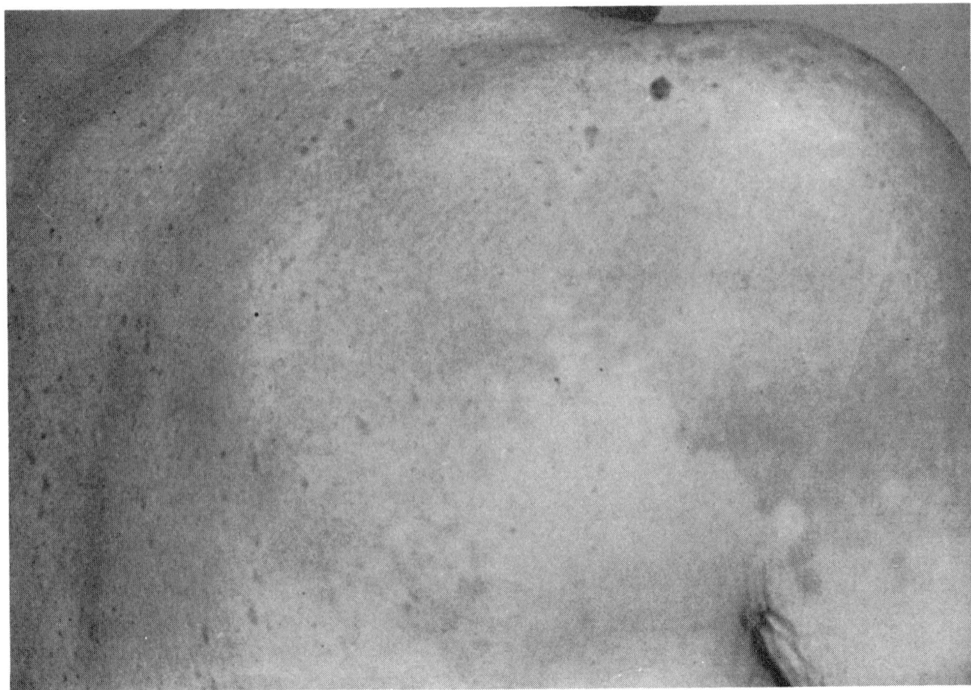

Figure 5–8. Normolipemic flat xanthomas. Same patient as in Plate 12*C*.

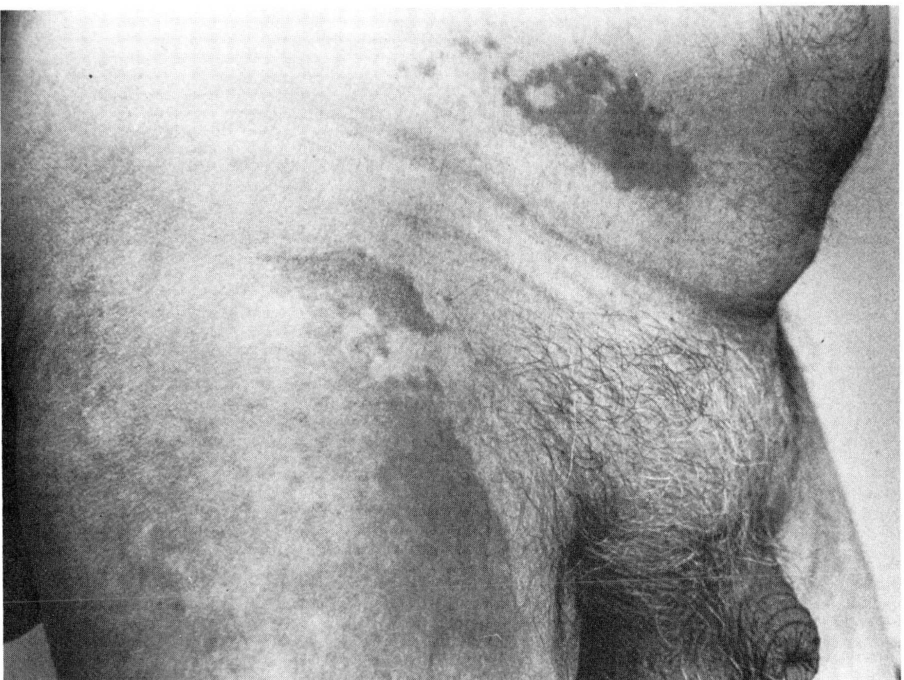

Figure 5–9. Normolipemic flat xanthomas. Same patient as in Plate 12*C*.

symptoms of this syndrome. This entity has recently been reported in the United States. The identical syndrome has also been described in persons without myeloma.[32] The pathogenesis of this disorder is unknown.

Other M Component Diseases

M components can be found in elderly patients without any sign or subsequent development of myeloma. Such cases have been classified as benign monoclonal gammopathies. M components can be detected in 3 per cent of the individuals over 70 years old.[33]

Heavy chain disease (HCD) was described by Franklin et al. and by Osserman and Takatsuki in five patients having the clinical features of hepatosplenomegaly, lymphadenopathy, fever, and elevated serum uric acid.[34, 35] The patients exhibited no evidence of bone involvement, and the M component was shown to be the Fc heavy chain fragment of IgG. Since then, at least 30 patients have been recognized, but not all have been studied in detail.[36] Heavy chain diseases involving IgA and IgM have also been recognized, and the three heavy chain diseases have been designated as γHCD, αHCD, and μHCD.

In γHCD, most patients are elderly and only four of the 30 have been under 40 years of age. Two patients had soft tissue tumors of the face. A biopsy of one tumor showed noncaseating epithelioid cell granulomas surrounded by lymphocytes and plasma cells. Eight of 20 patients developed unusual erythema and edema of the palate and uvula, which often gave rise to respiratory difficulties (Fig. 5–10). The edema and swelling of the mucosa lasted for only a few days and subsided spontaneously. This has been attributed to the characteristic waxing and waning of

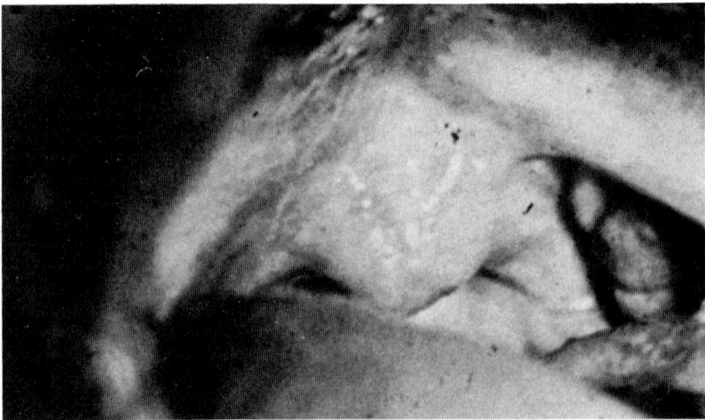

Figure 5–10. Heavy chain disease. Swollen uvula. (From Zawadzki, Z.: Rheumatoid arthritis terminating in heavy-chain disease. Ann. Intern. Med., *70*:335, 1969.)

lymphadenopathy in this disease. The predominant clinical features in all cases have resembled malignant lymphoma without skeletal involvement: a proliferation of the plasma cell and "reticulum" cell series, a clinical pattern of malignant lymphoma, and an abnormal production of heavy chain fragments of IgG with a decreased synthesis of normal immunoglobulins.

Structural studies have shown that the γHCD proteins consist of at least four types. Type 1 shows partial deletion of the Fd fragment with an intact hinge peptide region and Fc portion. Type II consists of a γ chain without the hinge region. Type III is a γ chain with a partial deletion of the Fd region and complete deletion of the hinge zone. Type IV represents fragments that could have resulted from proteolysis at the hinge region or position 100 from the N-terminal end of the γ chain — areas that are known to be very labile to a number of different enzymes.

Three patients had benign courses, two developed plasma cell leukemia terminally, and the rest had histologic changes that were considered to be a neoplasm of plasma cells, "reticulum cells," and lymphocytes. Survival from the time of onset of symptoms ranged from four months to over five years. Bacterial pneumonia and sepsis were the cause of death in all cases.

Alpha-HCD is an analogous disorder that had originally been called "Mediterranean-type abdominal lymphoma" but has been reported from other parts of the world as well. The predominant features are a diffuse lymphoma-like proliferation of abnormal appearing plasma cells, lymphocytes, and "reticulum" cells in the lamina propria of the small intestine, mesentery, and abdominal lymph nodes. The bone marrow shows a moderate increase in plasma cells, and the bones show moderate diffuse osteoporosis without destructive lesions.[36] Clinically, the patients have chronic diarrhea and malabsorption unresponsive to gluten deprivation. Villous atrophy of the mucosa is present. The disease generally pursues a progressive and fatal course, although remissions have occurred. The disease is present in the younger age group, in contrast to γHCD, and spares the liver, spleen, and other lymphoid organs. In two children, the disease involved the respiratory tract instead of the small intestine.[36, 37] Clubbing is a frequent finding in αHCD. Retardation of growth and expression of secondary sex characteristics are also common.[38]

The αHCD proteins contain at least the entire Fc fragment and hinge region. It has not yet been possible to determine whether or not a portion of the Fd fragment is present.

Mu-HCD is rare. Only three individuals with this disorder have been reported and all had longstanding chronic lymphatic leukemia. The spleen, liver, and abdominal nodes were primarily involved, and peripheral lymphadenopathy was insignificant. The μHCD proteins have not been as well characterized as the others, but they appear to be almost complete μ chains except for deletion of a portion of the Fd region.[36]

Macroglobulinemia of Waldenström is characterized by malignant proliferation of lymphocytoid cells with IgM as the M component.[39-41] The disease is seen most frequently in men past the age of 50. Lymphadenopathy, splenomegaly, and hepatomegaly develop in 20 to 40 per cent of patients, producing a clinical pattern resembling a malignant lymphoma or lymphatic leukemia. In 10 to 15 per cent of the patients, Bence Jones proteinuria is also present. Examination of the bone marrow reveals cells with features of plasma cells and lymphocytes, but osteolytic lesions are rare. In a few cases osteolytic lesions were present, and the bone marrow showed malignant plasma-like cells; however, the M component was IgM, thereby indicating a close relationship to myeloma.[42]

The patient with macroglobulinemia typically complains of weakness, fatigue, and anorexia, and often develops epistaxes, retinal hemorrhages, oral and gastrointestinal bleeding, and leg ulcers. Neurological signs and symptoms are also common and include headache, dizziness, true vertigo, nystagmus, somnolence, coma, seizures, and deafness caused by thromboses of veins in the inner ear. All of these signs and symptoms are believed to be related to high blood viscosity produced by the increased levels of IgM. Hyperviscosity has also been associated with aggregated IgG in classic myeloma.[43, 44] Features similar to macroglobulinemia — mucosal hemorrhage, retinal vein engorgement, and bleeding — were observed in these cases. The mechanism by which hyperviscosity promotes bleeding is not understood, but alterations in platelet function are believed to be contributory factors.[44]

Cryoglobulinemia is also a feature of this disease and is associated with Raynaud's phenomenon, cold urticaria, and vascular occlusion producing gangrene after exposure to cold. The carpal tunnel syndrome may develop as in myeloma, but the etiology has not been established, although amyloid deposition is suspected.

The most recent addition to M component disease is papular mucinosis (lichen myxedematosus, scleromyxedema), a curious and rare dermatosis produced by the deposition of mucin in the skin.[45] Although not fatal, the disease can be disfiguring and severely disabling. The deposits of mucin occur in two major morphologic forms. In the first, one sees discrete erythematous or yellowish papules, sometimes lichenoid, sometimes conical, present in a disseminated symmetrical fashion on the face, neck, and upper arms (Figs. 5–11 and 5–12). The scalp, chest, and back are less frequently involved. The papules may be arranged in linear or in confluent patches (Fig. 5–13). In less severely involved individuals, the eruption may be confined to a small area in the form of papules, urticarial plaques, or small nodules.[46, 47] The skin does not feel indurated. I would favor calling this expression of the disease papular mucinosis or lichen myxedematosus.

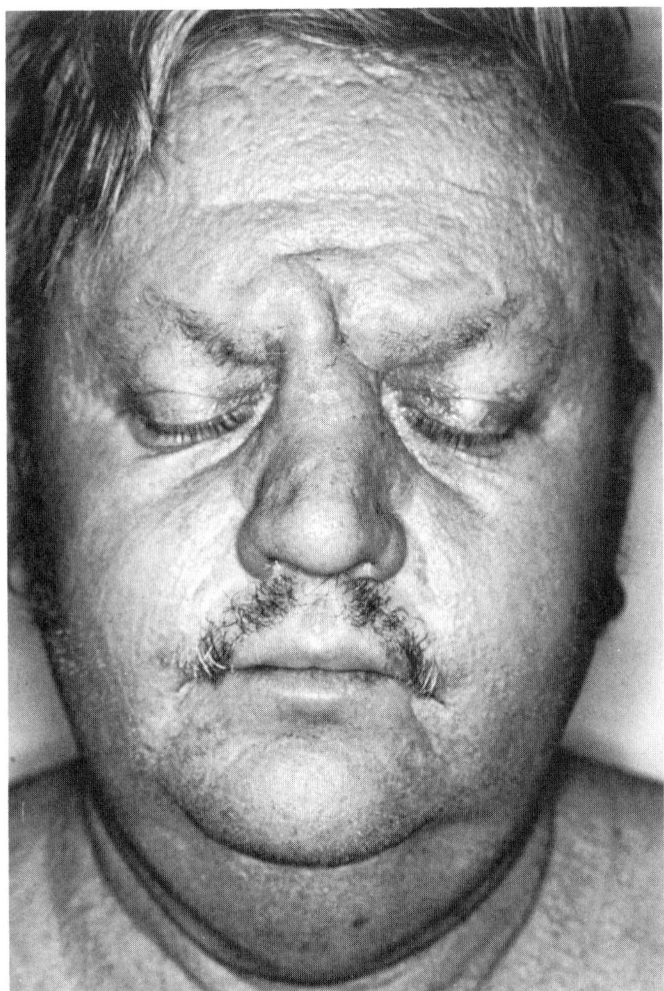

Figure 5–11. Lichen myxedematosus. Same patient as in Figures 5–12 and 5–13. The facial skin was not indurated.

As a second manifestation of this disorder, the papules may coalesce into plaques, especially on the face, where they produce a leonine facies or exaggerated furrows that simulate acromegaly or myxedema (Figs. 5–14 to 5–18). The skin over large areas of the body becomes brawny and indurated, with a resultant loss of mobility of the arms, legs, and hands. Individuals may have difficulties opening their mouths or changing their facial expression. This form of the disease ought to be called scleromyxedema.

Histological examination of the skin reveals a dermal deposition of mucin, chiefly hyaluronic acid, indistinguishable from that seen in hypothyroidism and pretibial myxedema in conjunction with a proliferation of stellate and fusiform fibroblasts in numbers larger than are usually seen in those two conditions. The deposits of mucin and proliferation of fibroblasts are limited to the upper dermis in some cases but are distributed throughout the dermis and subcutaneous fat in others.

The M component in papular mucinosis is a markedly basic globulin

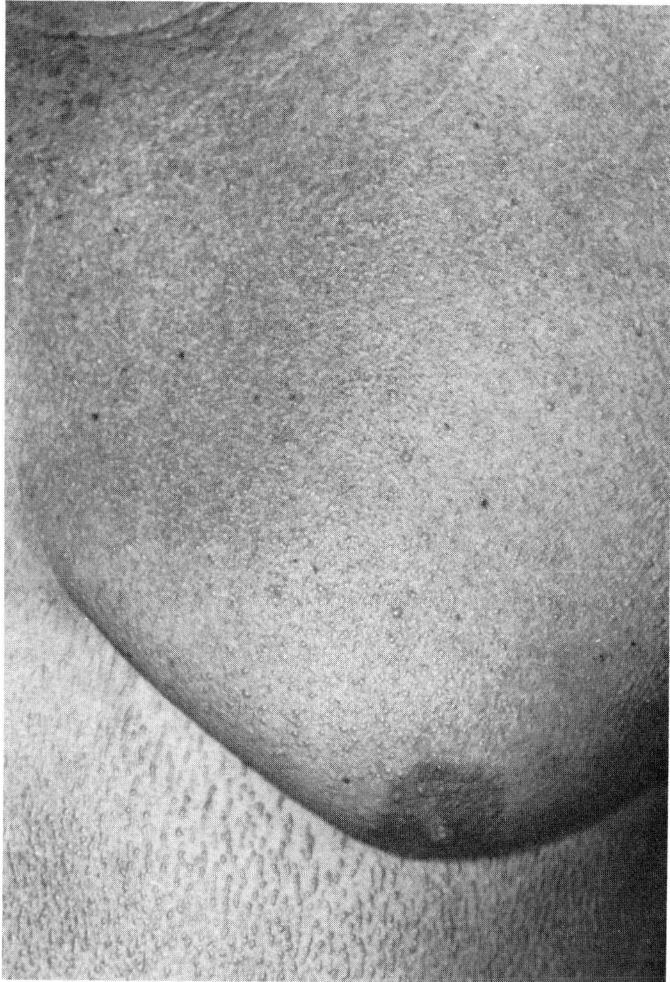

Figure 5–12. Lichen myxedematosus.

which migrates very slowly at the very end of the gamma globulin peak, a behavior similar to that of euglobulin.

This paraprotein has been found in most but not all cases of scleromyxedema.[48] (Localized forms of papular mucinosis do not seem to be accompanied by a paraprotein.[47]) These patients have not developed myeloma. All of the M proteins described have been IgG with lambda chains — in contrast to myeloma — except for four cases in which the IgG had kappa chains.[49] In the case report by Kitamura et al. the M component was an IgG, lambda class, with a molecular weight of 110,000 (normal 160,000) because a significant portion of the Fd fragment had been deleted from the molecule.[50]

IgG can be demonstrated in involved dermis by direct immunofluorescence in most cases, but the relationship between this deposition and the increase in acid mucopolysaccharides is unclear. IgG may be present in the dermis in the absence of detectable M component in the serum.[48] James et al. proposed that the M component might be an antibody directed against mucin.[51] Harper and Rispler recently demonstrated increased DNA synthesis and cell proliferation of normal human fibroblasts in cultures incubated with serum from affected individuals. This

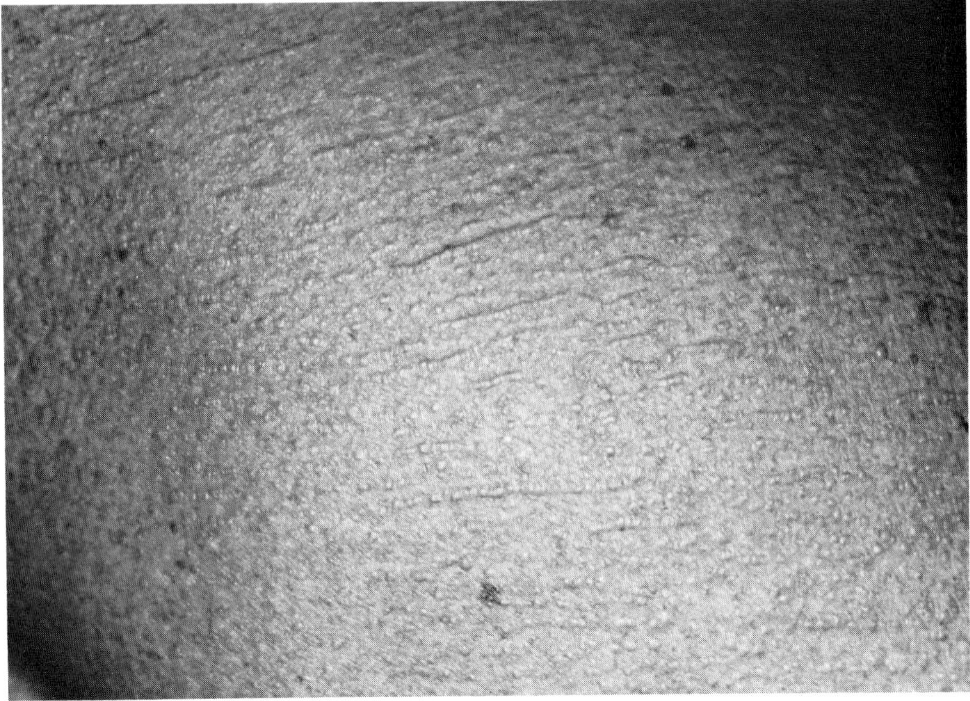

Figure 5–13. Lichen myxedematosus. Papules are arranged in linear or confluent patches.

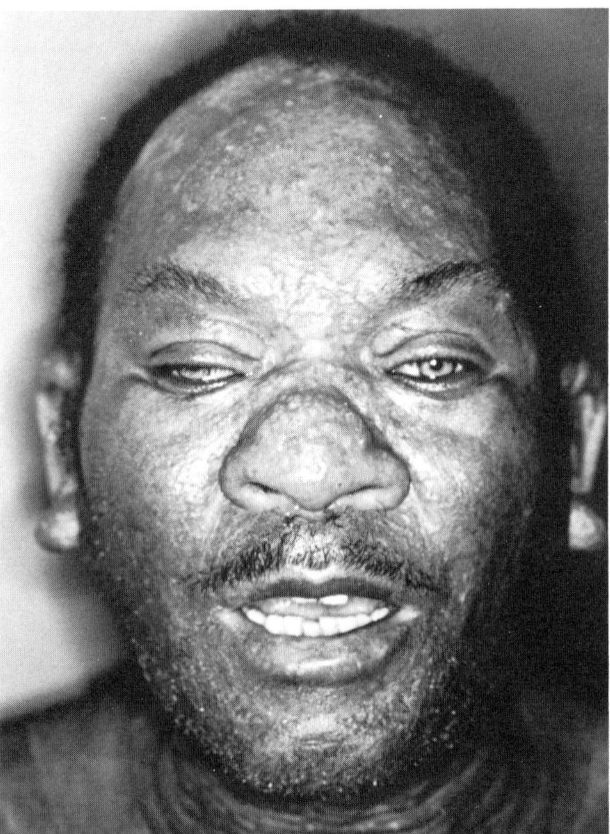

Figure 5–14. Scleromyxedema. Papules coalesce in plaques producing leonine facies or exaggerated furrows simulating acromegaly or myxedema.

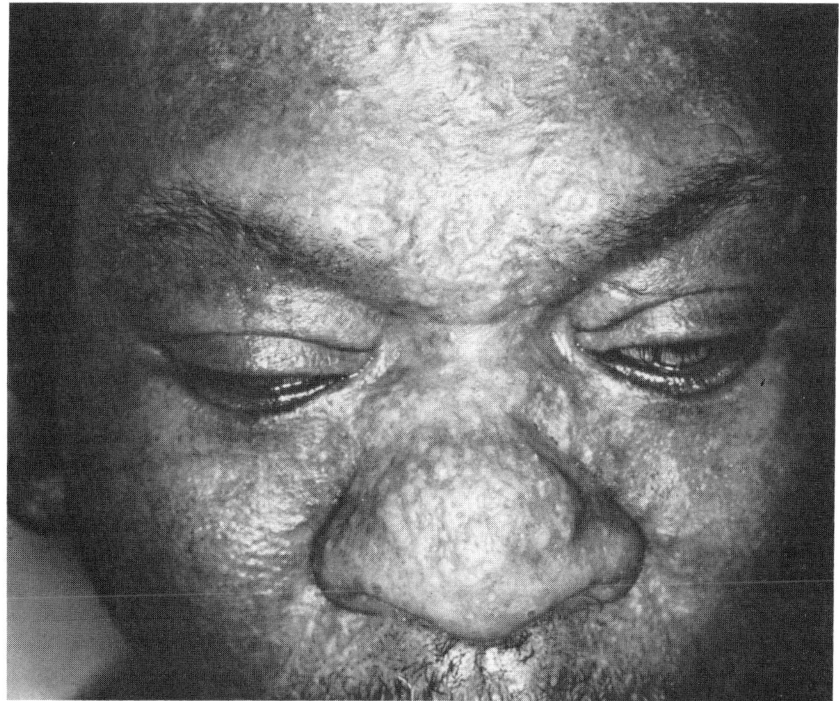

Figure 5–15. Scleromyxedema. Close-up of papules in Figure 5–14.

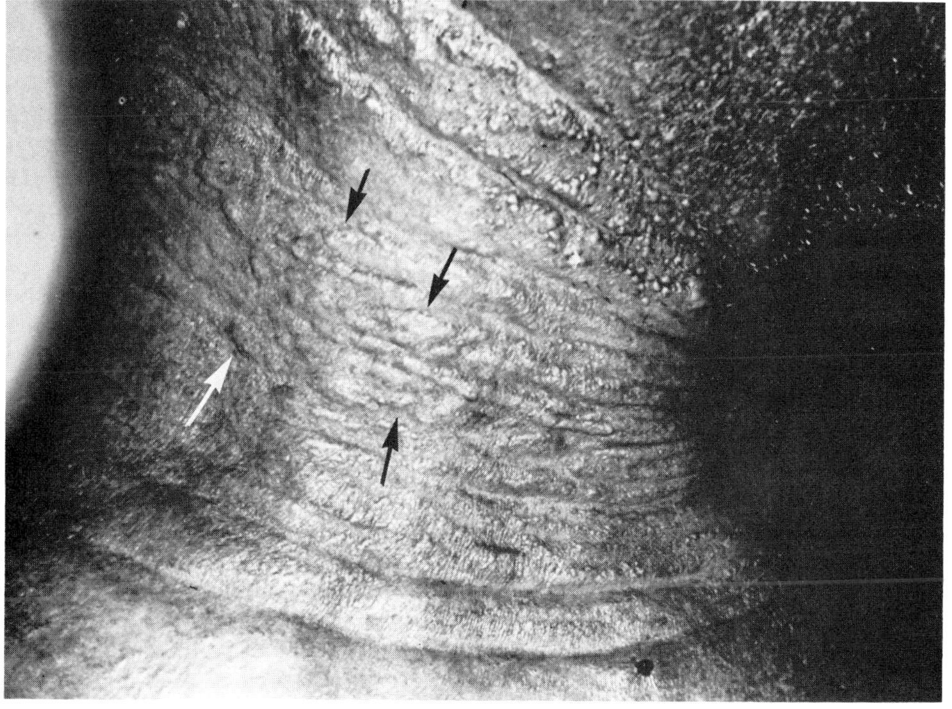

Figure 5–16. Scleromyxedema. Close-up of papules on neck (arrows). Same patient as in Figure 5–14.

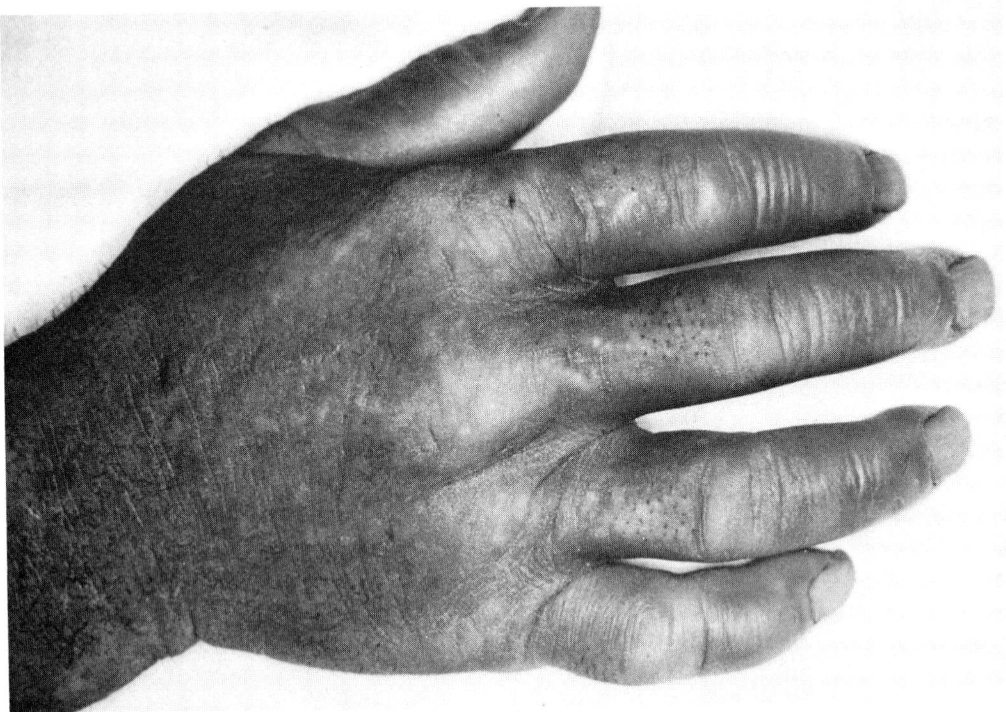

Figure 5–17. Scleromyxedema. Swollen brawny indurated hands of patient in Figure 5–14.

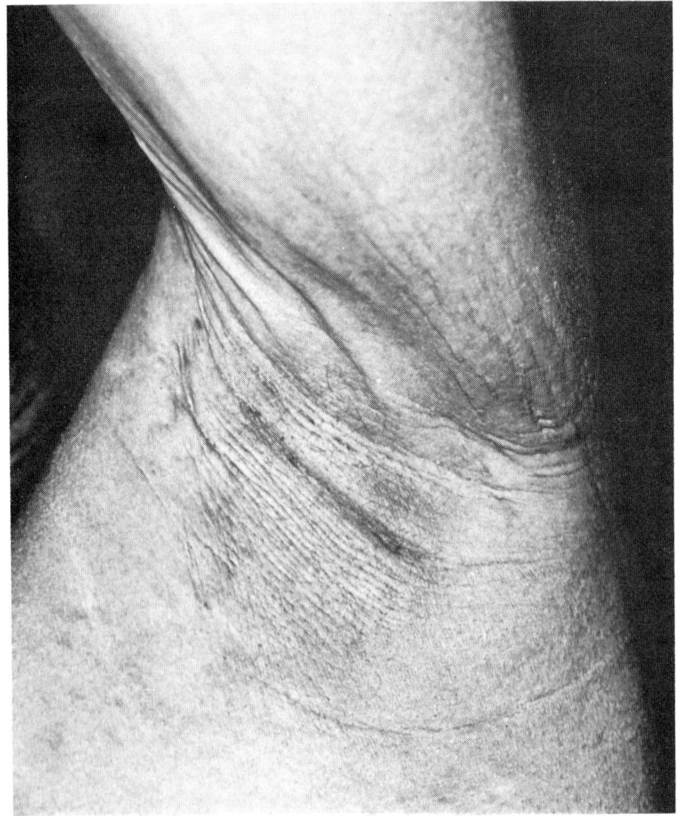

Figure 5–18. Scleromyxedema. Furrowed, slightly pendulous skin of upper arm and axilla in patient shown in Figure 5–14.

stimulatory activity was not associated with the IgG paraprotein, suggesting that additional systemic factors may be important in the pathogenesis of lichen myxedematosus–scleromyxedema.[52] An analogous serum factor appears to be important in the pathogenesis of pretibial myxedema (see p. 632).

Two case reports with autopsy studies have been cited as providing support for the systemic and occasionally fatal nature of this disease, because mucin accompanied by fibroblastic proliferation was found in the perivascular spaces and connective tissues of many organs.[53, 54] However, a review of the clinical course and skin lesions in these two cases suggests to me that Degos' disease is a better diagnosis than lichen myxedematosus. The natural history of papular mucinosis–lichen myxedematosus–scleromyxedema has not been fully delineated. The three terms have been used interchangeably in the literature, so it is unclear whether there is a correlation between the extent of mucin deposition, clinical appearance of the eruption, and the presence of the paraprotein. Although it is generally assumed that the three terms correspond to variants of the same disorder, it is important to determine whether this assumption is correct. By categorizing the syndromes into three varieties — localized papular mucinosis, papular mucinosis (lichen myxedematosus), and scleromyxedema — it should be possible to answer the questions about course, extent of mucin deposition, prognosis, association with paraprotein, and response to therapy.

The following three patients illustrate the spectrum of papular mucinosis and some of the problems involved in establishing an exact diagnosis. Figures 5–14 to 5–18 show one of our patients who had polymyositis in addition to scleromyxedema. He was barely able to open his mouth because of the cutaneous infiltration. In addition, he had severe hoarseness and dysphagia, unrelated to his myositis. Direct laryngoscopy and esophagoscopy revealed an infiltrated appearance of the mucosa and submucosa of the vocal cords and esophagus. This was presumed to be caused by deposition of mucin, which had previously been demonstrated in biopsies of muscle and rectal mucosa. There was complete lack of peristalsis in the esophagus as demonstrated by ciné x-ray studies. Polymyositis-dermatomyositis and scleromyxedema have been reported together twice before.[55] Our patient is an example of scleromyxedema with systemic deposition of mucin.

Figures 5–12 and 5–13 show a 50-year-old man with a papular eruption involving the entire skin except for the tibial surfaces. The skin was not indurated. Histologic examination revealed mucin confined to the papillary dermis. Immunoglobulins were not demonstrated in the dermis by direct immunofluorescence, nor did he have an M component. He fits into the category of papular mucinosis (lichen myxedematosus), rather than scleromyxedema.

Figures 5–19 and 5–20 illustrate the case of a 50-year-old woman with a four-month history of intermittent pain in the left knee, leg, and ankle. Swelling and discomfort of both feet from heels to toes occurred at the same time. The size of the feet had increased considerably so that she could no longer wear her shoes. Two years earlier, she was diagnosed as having Lyme arthritis because she had developed erythema chronicum migrans.

On physical examination, there was an indurated swelling of both

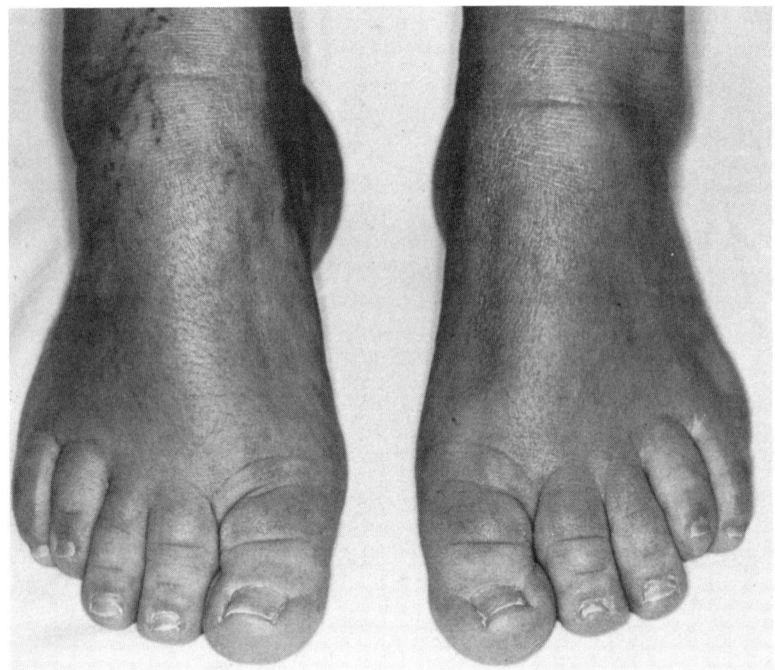

Figure 5–19. Papular mucinosis. Indurated swelling from heels to tip of toes, producing increase in size of feet.

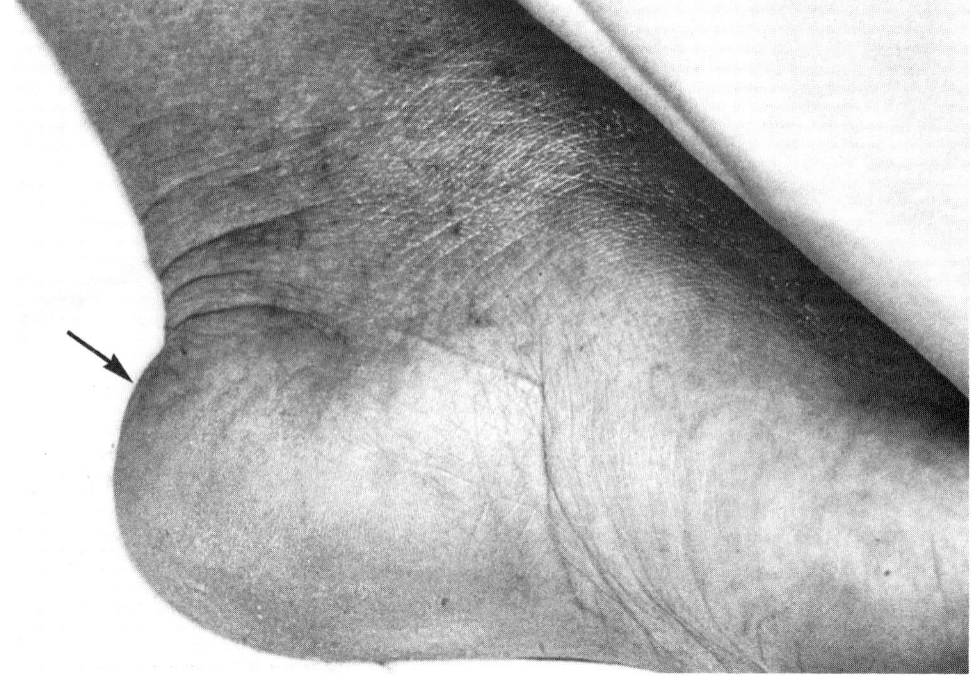

Figure 5–20. Papular mucinosis. Same patient as in Figure 5–19. Indurated nodular swelling of heels (arrow).

feet from the heels to the tips of the toes. Beneath both breasts were reddish-brown petechiae and small purpuric spots measuring 1 to 3 mm. Except for the feet, the skin felt normal. There were no lichenoid papules or other lesions elsewhere on the skin. Biopsies taken from the purpuric area, heel, and side of the foot all showed the deposition of mucin throughout the dermis and fat accompanied by a marked proliferation of dermal fibroblasts. Additional studies failed to demonstrate an M component, immunoglobulins in the dermis by direct immunofluorescence, long acting thyroid stimulator (LATS) in the serum, or evidence of thyroid disease. Cutaneous amyloidosis was excluded by appropriate histochemical stains.

This patient displays an unusual morphologic expression of cutaneous mucinosis. The mucin deposition was as deep as in our patient with scleromyxedema, but the serologic marker and dermal immunoglobulin deposition were absent. Clinically, the mucinosis appeared to be limited to the feet and could have been categorized as the localized form of papular mucinosis, but skin biopsies showed that the deposition of mucin was generalized as well as deep. The localized form of papular mucinosis can evolve into the generalized lichenoid form as described by Montgomery and Underwood.[56] Long-term observations may clarify the current clinical picture in our patient. These three patients illustrate the spectrum of papular mucinosis and some of the problems involved in nosology.

ANTIBODY DEFICIENCY SYNDROMES

Patients with congenital and acquired agammaglobulinemia and hypogammaglobulinemia show increased susceptibility to bacterial infections such as pyoderma, recurrent sinusitis, and pneumonia leading to progressive bronchiectasis. Plate 12*D* illustrates one of the several recurrent episodes of erysipelas in a woman who developed agammaglobulinemia of unknown etiology when she was 55 years old. Increased susceptibility to viral infections does not occur. In children below the age of 15 years who have a primary immunodeficiency disease, there is an increased prevalence of lymphoreticular malignancy. The risk of death from these neoplasms is about 100 times normal.[58]

An unusual syndrome of adult-acquired hypogammaglobulinemia with noncaseating epithelioid granulomas in the skin, lung, and liver has been reported. Primary agammaglobulinemia can evolve into malignant lymphoma, and acquired agammaglobulinemia and hypogammaglobulinemia are commonly associated with lymphomatous disease.[59, 60]

The Louis-Bar syndrome (ataxia-telangiectasia) is inherited as an autosomal recessive trait. Neurologic and immunologic abnormalities coupled with striking telangiectasia on the face, ears, and bulbar conjunctivae are the main features of this disorder (see p. 538). The immunologic deficits include a decreased capacity to manifest cellular immunity and abnormal levels of serum immunoglobulins. In 70 per cent of patients with ataxia-telangiectasia, serum IgA is diminished or undetectable; in 30 per cent, serum IgG is low. Although various combinations of immunoglobulin abnormalities have been observed, the isolated deficiency of IgA is the most common.[61]

Chronic and recurrent sinopulmonary infections are frequently, but not invariably, found in this syndrome. Children with this complication usually develop a progressive bronchiectasis and eventually die of respiratory insufficiency and pneumonia. The sinopulmonary infections can be correlated in part with the low levels or absence of IgA in the respiratory tract secretions.[62] The level of IgA in the bronchial secretions parallels that found in the blood. Lymphomas often develop in children who survive into their late teens and early twenties.

Solitaire reviewed the neuropathologic literature of ataxia-telangiectasia and reported autopsy findings in two of his own patients. On the basis of these data, he concluded that the neurologic disease in the Louis-Bar syndrome represents a spinocerebellar atrophy of unknown pathogenesis. The vascular and immunologic disturbances in this illness appear to be unrelated to the neurologic abnormalities.

Solitaire also observed bizarre nuclear changes in the cells of the anterior pituitary. Similar observations have been made by others. These cytologic findings may be related to the gonadal dysgenesis which is being recognized as another feature of ataxia-telangiectasia. Follicular agenesis in the ovary has been discovered in some patients, and secondary sex characteristics have failed to develop in others.[63]

The Wiskott-Aldrich syndrome is a recessively inherited sex-linked disorder which is characterized by the following: a generalized eczematous eruption that mimics atopic dermatitis; thrombocytopenia, which is responsible for petechiae, ecchymoses, and gastrointestinal bleeding; and recurrent major infections such as pneumonia, otitis media, and meningitis. Isohemagglutinins are absent and the serum level of IgM is low. The cause of the eczema is unknown, but the thrombocytopenia appears to be produced by increased destruction of abnormal platelets.[64] The infectious agents have included viruses, bacteria, fungi, and *Pneumocystis carinii*. Most of the affected children have died within the first few years of life because of infection or hemorrhage. Many of those who have survived into later childhood have developed lymphoreticular malignancy.[65]

Cooper et al. have shown that children with the Wiskott-Aldrich syndrome are unable to produce antibodies against pneumococcal polysaccharide and Witebsky substances A and B. Their sera also lack naturally occurring Forssman antibodies, which are directed against another polysaccharide antigen. Yet these children are able to generate antibodies against bacterial, viral, and simple protein antigens.[63] Thus it appears that the primary immunologic deficiency in these patients resides in their inability to respond to polysaccharide antigens.

Cooper and associates also demonstrated that early in this disease, the thymus and the accumulations of thymus-dependent lymphocytes in peripheral lymphoid tissues are normal. With time, however, a depletion of lymphocytes in the circulation, lymph nodes, and spleen occurs. This depletion of the thymus-dependent lymphocytes is accompanied by the development of a deficiency in cell-mediated immunologic functions.

REFERENCES

1. Putnam, F. W.: Immunoglobulin structure: variability and homology. Science, *163*:633, 1969.
2. Solomon, A., and McLaughlin, C. L.: Immunoglobulin structure determined from products of plasma cell neoplasms. Semin. Hematol., *10*:3, 1973.
3. Weiner, E. D., Camelli, R., Showel, J., Osmand, A. P., Sasseti, R. J., and Gewurz, H.: IgE myeloma presenting with classic myeloma features. J. Allergy Clin. Immunol., *58*:373, 1976.
4. Waldenström, J.: Clinical methods for determination of hyperproteinemia and their practical value for diagnosis. Nord. Med., *20*:2288, 1943.
5. Strauss, W. G.: Purpura hyperglobulinemia of Waldenström. Report of a case and review of the literature. N. Engl. J. Med., *260*:857, 1959.
6. Hambrick, G. W., Jr.: Dysproteinemic purpura of the hypergammaglobulinemic type. Arch. Dermatol. *77*:23, 1958.
7. Kyle, R. A., Gleich, G. J., Bayrd, E. D., and Vaughn, J. H.: Benign hypergammaglobulinemic purpura of Waldenström. Medicine, *50*:113, 1971.
8. Capra, J. D., Winchester, R. J., and Kunkel, H. G.: Hypergammaglobulinemic purpura. Studies on the unusual anti-γ-globulins characteristic of the sera of these patients. Medicine, *50*:125, 1971.
9. Blaylock, W. M., Waller, M., and Normansell, D. E.: Sjögren's syndrome: hyperviscosity and intermediate complexes. Ann. Intern. Med., *80*:27, 1974.
10. Waldenström, J.: Studies on "abnormal" serum globulins (M components) in myeloma, macroglobulinemia and related diseases: clinical diagnosis and biochemical findings in material of 296 sera with M-type narrow γ globulins. Acta Med. Scand. *170* (Suppl. 367):110, 1961.
11. Ameis, A., Ko, H. S., and Pruzanski, W.: M components — a review of 1242 cases. Can. Med. Assoc. J., *114*:889, 1976.
12. Pick, A. I., Schoenfeld, Y., Skvaril, F., Schreibman, S., Frohlichman, R., Weiss, H., and Pinkhas, J.: Symptomatic (benign) monoclonal gammopathy — a study of 100 patients. Ann. Clin. Lab. Sci., *7*:335, 1977.
13. Osserman, E. F., and Takatsuki, K.: Plasma cell myeloma: gamma globulin synthesis and structure. Review of biochemical and clinical data with description of newly-recognized and related syndrome. Medicine (Balt.), *42*:357, 1963.
14. Kyle, R. A.: Multiple myeloma. Review of 869 cases. Mayo Clin. Proc., *50*:29, 1975.
15. Jancelewicz, Z., Takatsuki, K., Sugai, S., and Pruzanski, W.: IgD multiple myeloma, review of 133 cases. Arch. Intern. Med., *135*:87, 1975.
16. Stone, M. J., and Frenkel, E. P.: The clinical spectrum of light chain myeloma. A study of 35 patients with special reference to the occurrence of amyloidosis. Am. J. Med., *58*:601, 1975.
17. Levin, H. A., Freeman, R. G., Smith, F. E., and Lane, M.: Multiple extramedullary plasmacytomas. Arch. Dermatol. *96*:456, 1967.
18. Lerner, A. B., Barnum, C. P., and Watson, C. J.: Studies on cryoglobulins II. Spontaneous precipitation of protein from serum at 5° C in various disease states. Am. J. Med. Sci., *214*:416, 1947.
19. Brouet, J.-C., Clauvel, J.-P., Danon, F., Klein, M., and Seligmann, M.: Biologic and clinical significance of cryoglobulins. Am. J. Med., *57*:775, 1974.
20. Lerner, A. B., and Watson, C. J.: Studies of cryoglobulins. I. Unusual purpura associated with presence of a high concentration of cryoglobulins. Am. J. Med. Sci., *214*:410, 1947.
21. Bluefarb, S. M.: Cutaneous manifestations of multiple myeloma. Arch. Dermatol. Syph., *72*:506, 1955.
22. Ellis, F. A.: The cutaneous manifestations of cryoglobulinemia. Arch. Dermatol. *89*:690, 1964.
23. Bengtsson, U., Larsson, O., Lindstedt, G., and Svalander, C.: Monoclonal IgG cryoglobulinemia with secondary development of glomerulonephritis and nephrotic syndrome. Q. J. Med., *44*:491, 1975.
24. Costanzi, J. J., and Coltman, C. A., Jr.: Kappa chain cold precipitable immunoglobulin G (IgG) associated with cold urticaria I. Clinical observations. Clin. Exp. Immunol., *2*:167, 1967.
25. Volpé, R., Bruce-Robertson, A., Fletcher, A. A., and Charles, W. B.: Essential cryoglobulinemia. Am. J. Med., *20*:533, 1956.
26. Savin, R. C.: Hyperglobulinemic purpura terminating in myeloma, hyperlipemia and xanthomatosis. Arch. Dermatol., *92*:679, 1965.
27. Rogers, W. R., and Welch, J. D.: Purpura hyperglobulinemia terminating in multiple myeloma. Arch. Intern. Med., *100*:478, 1957.
28. Kingery, F. A. J., and Montes, L. F.: A non-acantholytic bullous dermatosis associated with multiple myeloma. Arch. Dermatol., *78*:293, 1958.
29. Short, M. H.: Multiple myeloma with xanthoma formation. Arch. Pathol., *77*:400, 1964.
30. Lynch, P. J., and Winkelmann, R. K.: Generalized plane xanthoma and systemic disease. Arch. Dermatol., *93*:639, 1966.
31. Iwashita, H., Ohnishi, A., Asada, M., Kanazawa, Y., and Kuroiwa, Y.: Polyneuropathy, skin hyperpigmentation, edema, and hypertrichosis in localized osteosclerotic myeloma. Neurology, *27*:675, 1977.
32. Trentham, D. E., Masi, A. T., and Marker, H. W.: Polyneuropathy and anasarca: evidence for a new connective tissue syn-

drome and vasculopathic contribution. Ann. Intern. Med., *84*:271, 1976.

33. Hällén, J.: Discrete gamma globulin (M-) components in serum. Clinical study of 150 subjects without myelomatosis. Acta. Med. Scand., *180*(Suppl. 462): 1966.
34. Franklin, E. C., Lowenstein, J., Bigelow, B., and Meltzer, M.: Heavy chain disease: a new disorder of serum gamma globulins. Report of the first case. Am. J. Med., *37*:332, 1964.
35. Osserman, E. F., and Takatsuki, K.: Clinical and immunochemical studies of four cases of heavy (Hγ^2) chain disease. Am. J. Med., *37*:351, 1964.
36. Frangione, B., and Franklin, E. C.: Heavy chain disease: clinical features and molecular significance of the disordered immunoglobulin structure. Sem. Hematol., *10*:53, 1973.
37. Stoop, J. W., Ballieux, R. E., Hijmans, W., and Zegers, B. J. M.: Alpha chain disease with involvement of the respiratory tract in a Dutch child. Clin. Exp. Immunol., *9*:625, 1971.
38. Talbane, S., Talbane, F., and Cammon, M.: Mediterranean lymphoma with alpha heavy chain monoclonal gammopathy. Cancer, *38*:1989, 1976.
39. Dutcher, T. F., and Fahey, J. L.: The histopathology of the macroglobulinemia of Waldenström. J. Nat. Cancer Inst., *22*:887, 1959.
40. Rosen, F.: The macroglobulins. N. Engl. J. Med., *267*:491, 1962.
41. Krajny, M., and Pruzanski, W.: Waldenström's macroglobulinemia: review of 45 cases. Can. Med. Assoc. J., *114*:899, 1976.
42. Osserman, E. F.: Plasma cell myeloma. II. Clinical aspects. N. Engl. J. Med., *261*:952, 1006, 1959.
43. Smith, E., Kochwa, S., and Wasserman, C. R.: Aggregation of IgG globulin *in vivo* I. The hyperviscosity syndrome in multiple myeloma. Am. J. Med., *39*:35, 1965.
44. Bloch, K. J., and Maki, D. G.: Hyperviscosity syndromes associated with immunoglobulin abnormalities. Sem. Hematol., *10*:113, 1973.
45. de Graciansky, P., Boulle, S., Boulle, M., and Gutkow, M.: Lichen myxoedemateux. Sem. Hop. Paris, *33*:254, 1957.
46. Perry, H. O., Kierland, R. R., and Montgomery, H.: Plaque-like form of cutaneous mucinosis. Arch. Dermatol., *82*:980, 1960.
47. Coskey, R. J., and Mehregan, A.: Papular mucinosis. Int. J. Dermatol., *16*:741, 1977.
48. Howsden, S. M., Herndon, J. H., Jr., and Freeman, R. G.: Lichen myxedematosus. A dermal infiltrative disorder responsive to cyclophosphamide therapy. Arch. Dermatol., *111*:1325, 1975.
49. Danby, F. W., Danby, C. W. E., and Pruzanski, W.: Papular mucinosis with IgG (k) M component. Can. Med. Assoc. J., *114*:920, 1976.
50. Kitamura, W., Matsuoka, Y., Miyagawa, S., and Sakamoto, K.: Immunochemical analysis of the monoclonal paraprotein in scleromyxedema. J. Invest. Dermatol., *70*:305, 1978.
51. James, K., Fudenberg, H., Epstein, W. L., and Shuster, J.: Studies on a unique diagnostic serum globulin in papular mucinosis (lichen myxedematosus). Clin. Exp. Immunol., *2*:153, 1967.
52. Harper, R. A., and Rispler, J.: Lichen myxedematosus serum stimulates human skin fibroblast proliferation. Science, *199*:545, 1978.
53. McCuistion, C. H., and Schoch, E. P., Jr.: Autopsy findings in lichen myxedematosus. Arch. Dermatol., *74*:259, 1956.
54. Perry, H. O., Montgomery, H., and Stickney, J. M.: Further observation on lichen myxedematosus. Ann. Intern. Med., *53*:955, 1960.
55. Johnson, B. L., Horowitz, I. R., Charles, C. R., and Cooper, D. L.: Dermatomyositis and lichen myxedematosus. A clinical histopathological and electron microscopic study. Dermatologica, *147*:109, 1973.
56. Montgomery, H., and Underwood, L. J.: Lichen myxedematosus (differentiation from cutaneous myxedema or mucoid states). J. Invest. Dermatol., *20*:213, 1953.
57. Rosen, F.: The primary immunodeficiencies: dermatologic manifestations. J. Invest. Dermatol., *67*:402, 1976.
58. Kersey, J. H., Spector, B. D., and Good, R. A.: Cancer in children with primary immunodeficiency diseases. J. Pediatr., *84*:263, 1974.
59. Zinneman, H. H., Hall, W. H., and Heller, B. I.: Acquired agammaglobulinemia. Report of 3 cases. J.A.M.A., *156*:1390, 1954.
60. Pearce, K. M., and Perinpanayagam, M. S.: Congenital idiopathic hypogammaglobulinemia. Arch. Dis. Child., *32*:422, 1957.
61. Peterson, R. D. A., and Good, R. A.: Ataxia-telangiectasia. *In* Immunologic Deficiency Diseases in Man. Birth defects original article series. The National Foundation. New York, *4*:370, 1967.
62. South, M. A., Cooper, M. D., Wollheim, F. A., and Good, R. A.: The IgA system. II. The clinical significance of IgA deficiency: studies in patients with agammaglobulinemia and ataxia-telangiectasia. Am. J. Med., *44*:168, 1968.
63. Solitaire, G. B.: Louis-Bar's syndrome (ataxia-telangiectasia). Anatomic considerations with emphasis on neuropathologic observations. Neurology, *18*:1180, 1968.
64. Cooper, M. D.: Functional deficiency of a B-cell subline; prime immunologic abnormality in the Wiskott-Aldrich syndrome ? J. Invest. Dermatol., *67*:431, 1976.
65. Cooper, M. D., Chase, H. P., Lowman, J. T., Krivit, W., and Good, R. A.: Immunologic defects in patients with Wiskott-Aldrich syndrome. *In* Immunologic Deficiency Diseases in Man. *op. cit.*, p. 378.

6

Amyloidosis

A major breakthrough in our understanding of amyloidosis has occurred within the past 15 years.[1,2] Earlier, amyloid was considered an ill-defined mixture of different proteinaceous substances that appeared as a homogeneous, extracellular, eosinophilic material in histological sections. These deposits replaced the tissue within an organ and compromised or destroyed its function. Amyloid was identified in tissues by its ability to be stained with Congo red and to exhibit green birefringence with this dye when viewed through polarizing lenses. In addition, amyloid stained metachromatically with crystal violet. In 1959, electron microscopic studies revealed that amyloid was fibrillar and within three to five years, the amyloid fibrils were isolated in relatively pure form from tissues for examination by electron microscopy, x-ray diffraction, and infrared spectroscopy. However, the fibrils were insoluble and relatively resistant to proteolytic digestion, thereby thwarting attempts at chemical analysis. In the late 1960's there was general agreement that amyloid was a protein unrelated to the immunoglobulins.[1]

Traditionally, amyloidosis has been divided into primary and secondary types. In the primary type, when there is no underlying disease, amyloid is found in the gastrointestinal tract, heart, tongue, skin, muscle, and blood vessels. Amyloidosis associated with myeloma has an identical distribution. Secondary amyloidosis is associated with chronic infectious, inflammatory, and neoplastic diseases, such as tuberculosis, leprosy, ileitis, osteomyelitis, bronchiectasis, rheumatoid arthritis, renal cell cancer, Hodgkin's disease, and dermatomyositis, and involves the kidney, liver, and spleen. It became evident in the early 1960's that this classification was no longer warranted. The differences in the staining reaction of amyloid in primary and secondary amyloidosis were not distinct. When studied by electron microscopy, the amyloid was fibrillar and identical in both, and there was an overlap in the pattern of organ involvement by amyloid in the two types. A simplified and more pragmatic classification of amyloidosis was proposed by Cohen.[3]:

1. Generalized amyloidosis associated with a recognized predisposing disease.
2. Generalized amyloidosis in the absence of a recognized predisposing disease.
3. Generalized amyloidosis on a familial basis.
4. Localized amyloidosis.

Beginning in 1969, reports of successful attempts to solubilize the amyloid fibril in order to extract the major protein fraction for chemical

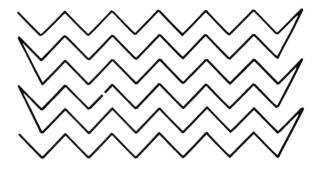

Figure 6–1. Diagram of "cross-β" pleated sheet conformation. Each line represents a polypeptide chain that is folded at its ends in an antiparallel fashion.

identification began to appear.[2] At the same time, x-ray diffraction and infrared spectroscopic studies clearly demonstrated that all amyloid fibrils studied, whether primary or secondary in type, were made up of polypeptide chains that had a cross β-pleated sheet conformation and were folded in an antiparallel fashion (Fig. 6–1). The diagnostic staining properties of amyloid resided not in its chemical composition but rather in its physical conformation. Any polypeptide that forms cross β-pleated sheets will appear as "amyloid" when viewed by electron and light microscopy and develop birefringence after staining with Congo red. At least three major groups of polypeptides have been found to be capable of forming amyloid, and they form the basis for some of the amyloidosis syndromes. A classification of amyloidosis based upon chemical composition, cellular origin, and mechanism of deposition of the fibrillar protein will eventually be possible, as proposed by Glenner and Page.[2] The following working classification attempts to combine the above principles with current information about the chemical composition of the various amyloids.

1. Primary amyloidosis associated with myeloma, monoclonal gammopathy, macroglobulinemia, heavy chain diseases, and other neoplasms of the lymphoid system.
2. Secondary amyloidosis associated with chronic suppurative, granulomatous, and inflammatory diseases.
3. Hereditofamilial forms of amyloidosis.
4. Amyloidosis localized to organs without any systemic involvement.
5. Amyloidosis of endocrine organs.
6. Amyloidosis associated with aging.
7. Amyloidosis localized to the skin.

In primary amyloidosis associated with myeloma and the other plasma cell dyscrasias, the amyloid fibril has as its major protein component either an intact L chain, the N-terminal fragment of the L chain (the variable region V_L), or both (see Fig. 5–4). The amino acid sequences of these amyloids are identical to the Bence-Jones proteins found in the urine or serum of the same patient. Lambda L chains are found more frequently than kappa L chains as the major protein component of amyloid. Only certain L chains appear to be amyloidogenic. Although the molecular basis for this transformation is not understood, it is not thought to be directly related to the amino acid sequences in the V_L.[2]

In secondary amyloidosis and in the amyloidosis of familial Mediterranean fever, the only hereditofamilial syndrome studied to date, the major component is a unique protein called AA (amyloid A), which is unrelated to the immunoglobulins.[2] It is believed to be a fragment of a larger serum protein called SAA (serum amyloid A). By analogy, the protein component in primary amyloidosis is now referred to as AL (amyloid L chain). Currently hypotheses propose that both the AL and AA proteins arise by lysosomal enzymatic degradation of the parent molecules within macrophages in the setting of immunologic stimulation. The reader is referred to the papers of Cohen et al.,[1,4] Glenner and Page,[2] and Franklin and Zucker-Franklin[5] for a more thorough discussion of proposed mechanisms.

Plaques and tumors of amyloid can develop in certain organs without there being systemic involvement. The respiratory tract (larynx, trachea, bronchi, and lungs), bladder, and eye are the most common sites. In all of these areas, one finds masses of amyloid in association with plasma cells, histiocytes, and lymphocytes. It has been suggested that local monoclonal plasma cells are producing the immunoglobulin component of amyloid. In support of this proposal, amyloid from a case of nodular amyloidosis of the lung was shown to be composed primarily of the N-terminal fragment of a monoclonal lambda L chain.[2] The amyloid casts in myeloma kidneys appear to be produced through the degradation of myeloma proteins by lysosomal enzymes in renal tubules.[6]

The third major class of amyloid protein is found in certain hormone-secreting tumors. Insulin-producing islet cell tumors of the pancreas are associated with amyloid deposits in the islets of Langerhans, and amyloid is found within the stroma of medullary carcinomas of the thyroid, a distinctive tumor found in both MEN type 2 and MEN type 3 (see p. 22). Both insulin and glucagon can develop cross β-pleated sheet configurations *in vitro*, and in so doing, they exhibit the staining characteristics of amyloid with Congo red. Insulin has been demonstrated by immunofluorescence to be present in the amyloid deposits found in the pancreatic islets. Similarly, calcitonin, the hormone secreted by medullary carcinoma of the thyroid, can be demonstrated by immunofluorescence within the amyloid of that tumor. However, chemical proof is not yet available. Therefore, polypeptide endocrine hormones possessing the capacity to form cross β-pleated sheets are potentially amyloidogenic.

Amyloid deposits develop in the brain, pancreas, heart, and aorta with age. The deposition is believed to be a manifestation of aging. However, nothing is yet known about the chemical nature of this variety of amyloid.

Amyloid limited to the skin is also considered to be a distinct entity. In lichen and macular amyloidosis, the amyloid is present as small deposits in the dermal papillae. There is no involvement of blood vessels as in the other categories of amyloidosis listed above, and tumor formation does not occur. The nature of this amyloid has not yet been elucidated.

A tumefactive form of cutaneous amyloidosis is recognized and is a rare form of amyloidosis.[7] Most of the cases have not been associated with systemic involvement, and in those that have, no details have been given other than that "follow-up information disclosed evidence of systematic amyloidosis."[7] In the tumefactive lesions the dermis and subcutaneous tissues are infiltrated with amyloid. The large blood vessels may also be severely affected, and there may be an infiltrate of plasma cells and giant cells as well as foci of calcification. I believe this entity belongs under category four of the classification.

Amyloid can be divided into two basic types, AL and AA proteins (exclusive of the type found in endocrine tumors). All AA proteins are accompanied by small amounts of immunoglobulin L chain–related proteins. Amyloid may also contain small amounts of complement derivatives, fibrinogen, lipoprotein, and polysaccharides. Amyloid also contains a minor constituent, the P component, a donut-shaped structure that is identical to a 9.5S glycoprotein found in human serum. This molecule can aggregate into rods, but it is not part of the amyloid fibril, does not stain with Congo red, and its function in amyloid is as yet unknown.

The classification proposed above takes into account the various syndromes and the nature of amyloid as we currently understand them. Although exceptions can be cited, I believe that this classification is a useful one for an overview of amyloid. The distinction between AL and AA proteins is not absolute. Two patients with amyloidosis secondary to inflammatory diseases have been found to have AL protein, and two patients with amyloidosis apparently unrelated to any inflammatory disease have had AA protein.[2] However, if further studies continue to indicate that the AL and AA proteins correlate reasonably well with the two basic types of amyloidosis syndromes, then the value of such a classification increases.

CLINICAL MANIFESTATIONS

Primary systemic amyloidosis and myeloma-associated amyloidosis have identical clinical patterns both in their cutaneous manifestations and in their organ distribution. Both entities have M components, and often Bence-Jones proteins can be demonstrated in the serum and urine. In myeloma clinically significant amyloidosis has developed in 4 to 20 per cent of the patients,[8, 9] with the greater percentage occurring in those whose M component consisted of L chains.[10] Primary systemic amyloidosis with M component ought to be considered identical to benign monoclonal gammopathy with amyloidosis, because the immunoglobulin and plasma cell abnormalities are comparable.[1, 11] In the series of 236 cases of amyloidosis reported by Kyle and Bayrd, 56 per cent were primary, 26 per cent were related to myeloma, 9 per cent were localized, 8 per cent were secondary, and 1 per cent was familial. Thus, over 80 per cent of the patients had a plasma cell dyscrasia.[12]

Cutaneous amyloidosis, other than lichen amyloidosis, is a sign of myeloma-associated amyloidosis or primary systemic amyloidosis, and almost never a manifestation of secondary amyloidosis or the heredi-tofamilial type.[13, 14] The rare tumefactive form probably represents localized disease.[7] Although chronic suppurative and infectious diseases most commonly are associated with the development of secondary amyloidosis producing hepatomegaly and renal disease, occasionally a dermatosis may be the underlying cause. In 5 of 100 patients with secondary amyloidosis, the associated disorders included hidradenitis suppurativa, stasis ulcers, psoriatic arthritis, dystrophic epidermolysis bullosa, and an extensive basal cell carcinoma that had eroded into the skull and meninges.[15]

In amyloidosis associated with myeloma or benign monoclonal gammopathy, the mucocutaneous surfaces are involved in approximately 30 to 40 per cent of the cases.[14-16] The gingivae appear thickened, nodular, and spongy but actually are friable and bleed easily after minor trauma. Diffuse deposition of amyloid in the tongue produces a smooth, pale, and atrophic macroglossia, and spotty involvement results in erythematous nodules and papules. Induration, with symmetrical enlargement of the tongue, is most frequently observed, and the tongue may protrude (Fig. 6–2). The enlargement can be sudden or gradual and is usually painless. Along the edges of such enlarged tongues, there may be scalloped indentations produced by the teeth (Fig. 6–3). Pale red or yellow papules and plaques can arise on the buccal, conjunctival, nasal, vaginal, and anal mucosae. The lips may be swollen, with areas of nodularity. Purpura develops in all of these sites after minor trauma. It is uncommon for the larynx and trachea to be involved, but when they are, obstruction can result.

Cutaneous amyloidosis usually presents as 1-mm to 2-cm, superficial translucent waxy yellow and pink elevated lesions. Sites of predilection are the eyelids, nasolabial folds, perioral and periumbilical areas, sides of the neck, upper chest, axillae, and other intertriginous areas, including the perineum (Plate 14*C*). Less often, amyloid deposition can produce deep subcutaneous nodules, pedunculated tumors simulating condyloma-

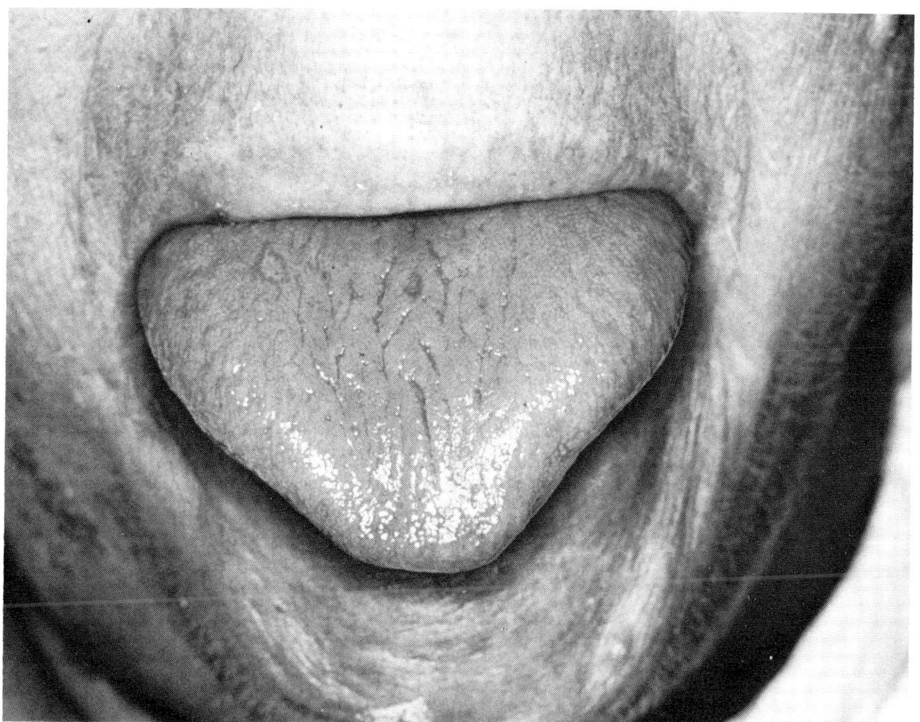

Figure 6–2. Generalized amyloidosis. Enlarged tongue in patient with multiple myeloma.

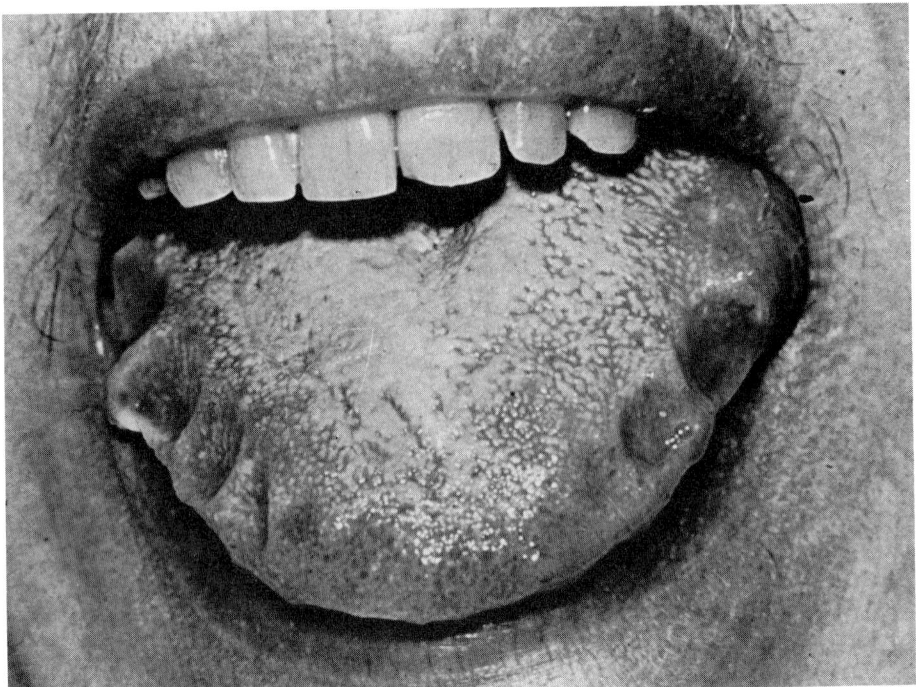

Figure 6–3. Generalized amyloidosis. Enlarged tongue with scalloped indentations produced by teeth in patient with myeloma. (Courtesy of Dr. Zbigniew Zawadzki).

ta, and papules arising over the extensor surfaces of the fingers. The cutaneous lesions are often mistaken for vesicles because of their shiny and translucent quality, but close inspection reveals their solid nature. Rubbing and pinching produce bleeding, which converts the yellow and the pink of the nodules into purple, reddish-brown, and dark amber colors (Plate 14*D*). Bleeding occurs readily because amyloid is deposited in the vessel walls as well as focally within the dermis. "Pinch purpura" is the term applied to this technique of detecting amyloid in the skin. Purpura may appear in the absence of clinically obvious skin lesions, but a biopsy will reveal amyloidosis of the vessel walls.

Although cutaneous amyloidosis tends to be papular and nodular, large indurated yellow and pink plaques can develop on the chest, abdomen, hands, and perineal area, thereby simulating the appearance of scleroderma. Pruritus is unusual in cutaneous amyloidosis. Diffuse amyloid infiltration of the hands and feet can produce nonpitting edema. Diffuse facial involvement simulates myxedema: coarse features, lack of wrinkling, and rigid facial expression. The pinnae may be swollen, and alopecia can develop from cutaneous infiltration in the scalp, eyebrows, axillary region, and pubic area. A deep erythema may accompany the facial infiltration.

Figures 6–4 and 6–5 and Plate 12*E* and *F* show myeloma-associated amyloidosis of the hand simulating sclerodactyly. The plaque on the thumb and a papule on the palm have become purpuric because of rubbing.

In three patients the extensive deposition of amyloid in the dermis was accompanied by trauma-induced blistering, sometimes with hemor-

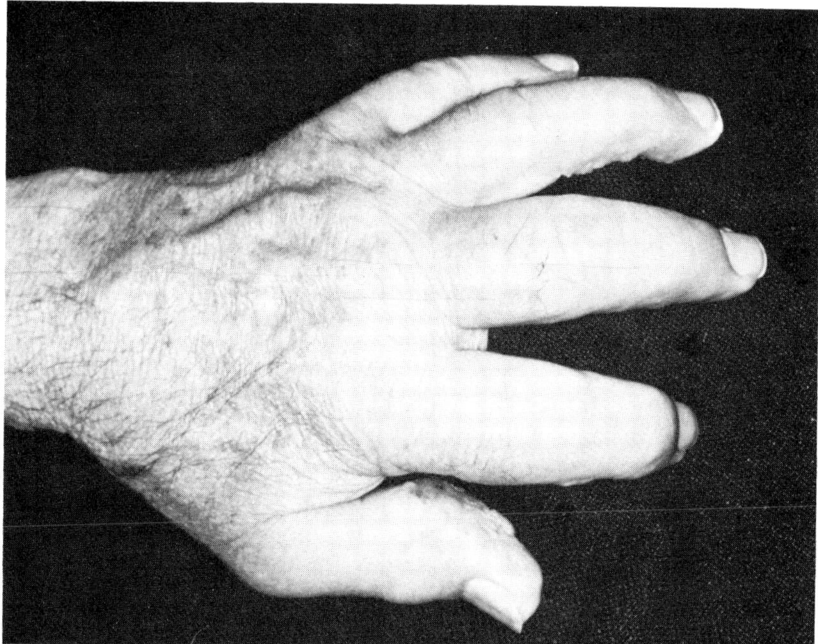

Figure 6–4. Generalized amyloidosis with swelling of hand simulating sclerodactyly. Same patient as in Figure 6–5 and Plate 12*E,F*.

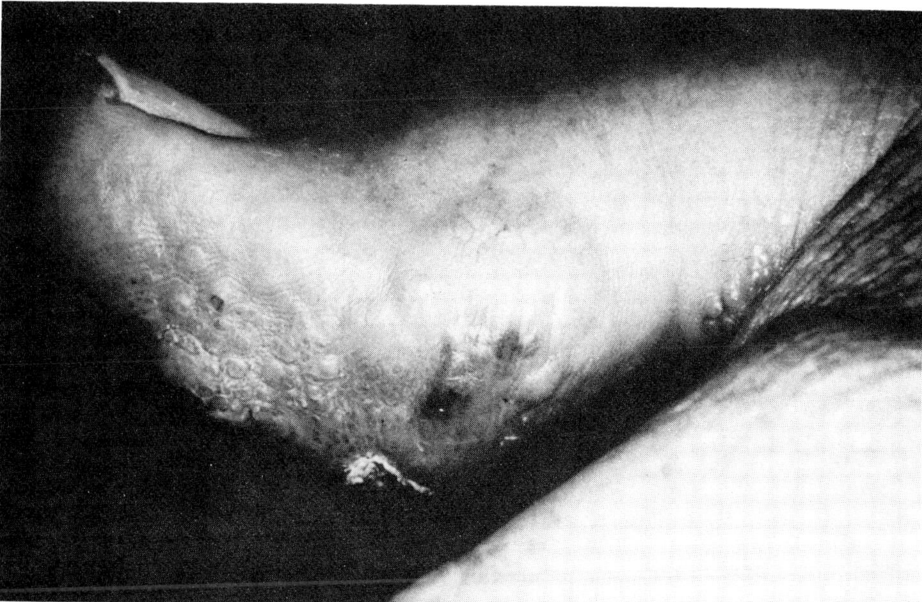

Figure 6–5. Generalized amyloidosis. Papules and plaques of amyloid that have developed spots of purpura secondary to trauma.

rhage. The split occurred through the amyloid deposits in the upper dermis. The skin appeared clinically *normal* and healed with formation of milia. These patients had been diagnosed as having epidermolysis bullosa acquisita before the true nature of the disease was discovered.[17]

Rubinow and Cohen[14] have recently confirmed and reemphasized an observation made by Brownstein and Helwig,[13] namely that a punch biopsy of clinically normal skin will be diagnostic in 50 per cent of patients with primary systemic amyloidosis. Rubinow and Cohen also studied 12 patients with secondary amyloidosis related to chronic inflammatory and infectious diseases. Two of the individuals had skin involvement clinically: one had focal petechiae and purpura on the chest and extremities and the other displayed easy bruisability over the limbs. Biopsies of involved and normal skin in the first patient and of normal skin in the second individual showed amyloid deposits in cutaneous blood vessels. Biopsies of normal skin in three of the remaining 10 patients without clinically involved skin showed amyloid deposits in the dermis and fat and around sweat glands but *not* in blood vessels. The diagnostic specificity of amyloid deposition in only extravascular sites was not established because there were no controls in this study. Nevertheless, punch biopsies should be carried out on the normal skin of patients suspected of having primary systemic amyloidosis because a yield of 50 per cent may obviate the need for a biopsy of less accessible tissues such as the liver, kidney, tongue, gingiva, and buccal and rectal mucosae.

Several syndromes of hereditofamilial amyloidosis are recognized. The constellation of peripheral neuropathy with painless ulcers and the eventual loss of fingers and toes, carpal tunnel syndrome, malabsorption, vitreous opacities, and cardiac involvement is found among certain Portuguese and other ethnic groups. In 21 Swedish patients with this type of familial amyloidosis, Lither noted that almost all of them had skin changes indistinguishable from those found in diabetes mellitus: hyperpigmented atrophic scars (diabetic dermopathy) and spontaneous blisters (bullosis diabeticorum).[20] Amyloid was present in the walls of the cutaneous blood vessels of these patients.

Sephardic Jews afflicted with familial Mediterranean fever (periodic disease) have an unusually high incidence of amyloid nephropathy (see p. 577). Severe amyloid heart disease is the salient feature in another group of families.[21] The syndrome of recurrent urticaria ushered in with fever and chills in adolescence and followed by progressive deafness and amyloid nephropathy in adulthood has been described in several English families.[22]

The hereditofamilial disorders differ from the more common generalized amyloidosis by the absence of macroglossia and palpable peripheral nerves. Vitreous opacities produced by amyloid deposition are frequent in hereditofamilial types and rare in generalized amyloidosis; conversely, cutaneous involvement is uncommon in the hereditary varieties. Other abnormalities of the pupil and iris have been noted in patients with familial amyloidosis: segmental paralysis of the irides and scalloped pupillary margins.[23]

Lichen amyloidosus is a chronic, intensely pruritic dermatosis that develops primarily on the lower extremities but which can occur on the arms and back. It is *not* associated with systemic amyloidosis. The eruption is composed of discrete hemispherical papules that often appear

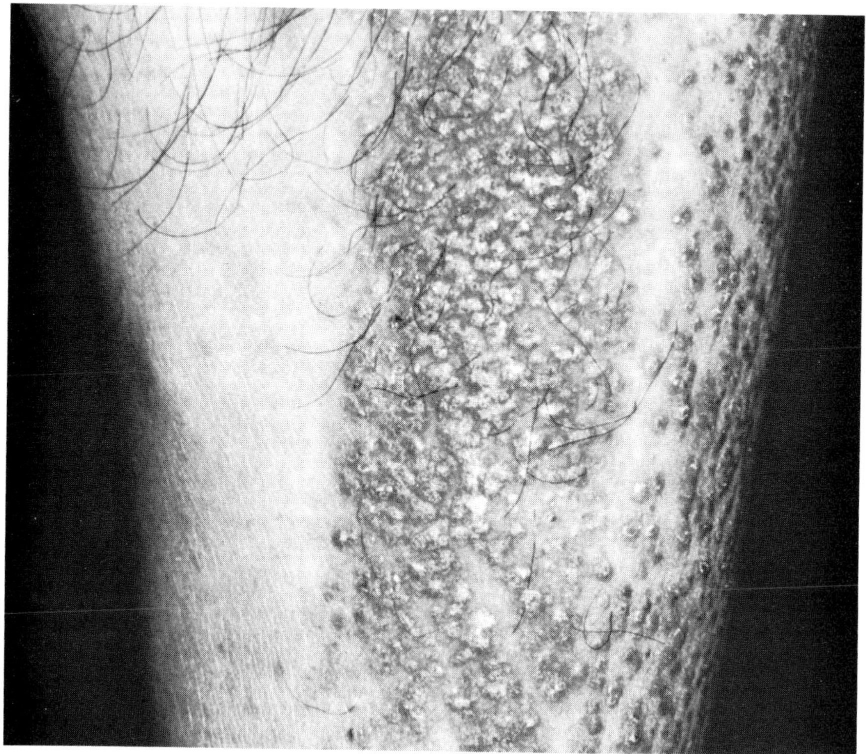

Figure 6–6. Lichen amyloidosus on shin. Characteristic gray verrucose papules.

translucent and vary from flesh tones to pink and brown. The papules can remain discrete or coalesce into plaques having slightly irregular or highly verrucose surfaces (Fig. 6–6). Masses of amyloid are deposited only within the dermal papillae and not in vascular walls or below the level of the papillary dermis, as in generalized amyloidosis.[24, 25]

Macular amyloidosis is a variant of the lichenoid form and has the same histologic findings. It is not unusual for a patient to have both forms of the disease, and occasionally the macular variety becomes papular and assumes the characteristic appearance of lichenoid amyloidosis.[26, 27] The macular variety is also pruritic and has the same cutaneous distribution as the lichenoid form. It is composed of oval, often poorly delineated, brown to grayish-brown patches made up of closely aggregated macules or minute papules. Sometimes these small macules produce whorled patterns of hyperpigmentation. Macular amyloidosis may be confused clinically with ichthyosis, stasis dermatitis, or pigmented purpuric eruptions of the lower extremities, depending upon the extent and distribution of involvement. Although almost all instances of lichenoid and macular amyloidosis are sporadic, there have been seven reports of a familial variety of the disease that is identical to the sporadic form.[27]

The chemical nature of the amyloid and the reasons for its accumulation in this disorder are not known. It is likely that the pruritus is the initial manifestation of amyloid deposition and that, in time, the accumulation becomes clinically apparent. On the other hand, the possibility that amyloid may be produced and deposited as a result of persistent rubbing and scratching of either normal skin or an antecedent pruritic dermatitis has not been excluded.

REFERENCES

1. Cohen, A. S., and Cathcart, E. S.: Amyloidosis and immunoglobulins. Adv. Intern. Med., *19*:41, 1974.
2. Glenner, G. C., and Page, D. L.: Amyloid, amyloidosis, and amyloidogenesis. Int. Rev. Exp. Pathol., *15*:1, 1976.
3. Cohen, A. S.: Amyloidosis. N. Engl. J. Med., *277*:522, 574, 628, 1967.
4. Cohen, H. J., Lessin, L. S., Hallal, J., and Burkholder, P.: Resolution of primary amyloidosis during chemotherapy. Studies in a patient with nephrotic syndrome. Ann. Intern. Med., *82*:466, 1975.
5. Franklin, E. C., and Zucker-Franklin, D.: Current concepts of amyloid. Adv. Immunol., *15*:249, 1972.
6. Tan, M., and Epstein, W.: Polymer formation during the degradation of human light chain and Bence-Jones proteins by an extract of the lysosomal fraction of normal human kidney. Immunochemistry, *9*:9, 1972.
7. Brownstein, M. H., and Helwig, E. B.: The cutaneous amyloidoses. I. Localized forms. Arch. Dermatol., *102*:8, 1970.
8. Kyle, R. A.: Multiple myeloma. Review of 869 cases. Mayo Clin. Proc., *50*:29, 1975.
9. Jancelewicz, Z., Takatsuki, K., Sugai, S., and Pruzanski, W.: IgD multiple myeloma. Review of 133 cases. Arch. Intern. Med., *135*:87, 1975.
10. Stone, M. J., and Frenkel, E. P.: The clinical spectrum of light chain myeloma. A study of 35 patients with special reference to the occurrence of amyloidosis. Am. J. Med., *58*:601, 1975.
11. Pruzanski, W., and Katz, A.: Clinical and laboratory findings in primary generalized and multiple-myeloma-related amyloidosis. Can. Med. Assoc. J., *114*:906, 1976.
12. Kyle, R. A., and Bayrd, E. D.: Amyloidosis: review of 236 cases. Medicine, *54*:271, 1975.
13. Brownstein, M. H., and Helwig, E. B.: The cutaneous amyloidoses. II. Systemic forms. Arch. Dermatol., *102*:20, 1970.
14. Rubinow, A., and Cohen, A. S.: Skin involvement in generalized amyloidosis. A study of clinically involved and uninvolved skin in 50 patients with primary and secondary amyloidosis. Ann. Intern. Med., *88*:781, 1978.
15. Brownstein, M. H., and Helwig, E. B.: Systemic amyloidosis complicating dermatoses. Arch. Dermatol., *102*:1, 1970.
15a. Goltz, R. W.: Systematized amyloidosis. A review of the skin and mucous membrane lesions and a report of 2 cases. Medicine (Balt.), *31*:381, 1952.
16. Rukavina, J. G., Block, W. D., Jackson, C. E., Falls, H. F., Carey, J. H., and Curtis, A. C.: Primary systemic amyloidosis. Review and experimental, genetic and clinical study of 29 cases with particular emphasis on the familial form. Medicine (Balt.), *35*:239, 1956.
17. Muller, S. A., Sams, W. M., Jr., and Dobson, R. L.: Amyloidosis masquerading as epidermolysis bullosa acquisita. Arch. Dermatol., *99*:739, 1969.
18. Andrade, C.: Peculiar form of peripheral neuropathy: familiar atypical generalized amyloidosis with special involvement of peripheral nerves. Brain, *75*:408, 1952.
19. Horta, J. da S., Filipe, I., and Durante, S.: Portuguese polyneuritic familial type of amyloidosis. Pathol. Microbiol., *27*:809, 1964.
20. Lither, F.: Skin lesions of the legs and feet and skeletal lesions of the feet in familial amyloidosis with polyneuropathy. Acta Med. Scand., *199*:197, 1976.
21. Fredericksen. T., Gotzsche, H., Harboe, N., Kiaer, W., and Mellemgaard, K.: Familial primary amyloidosis with severe amyloid heart disease. Am. J. Med., *33*:328, 1962.
22. Muckle, T. J., and Wells, M.: Urticaria, deafness and amyloidosis: new hereditofamilial syndrome. Q. J. Med., *31*:235, 1962.
23. Lessell, S., Wolf, P. A., Benson, M. D., and Cohen, A. S.: Scalloped pupils in familial amyloidosis. N. Engl. J. Med., *293*:914, 1975.
24. Anekoji, K., and Irisawa, K.: Five cases of lichen amyloidosis. Arch. Dermatol., *84*:759, 1961.
25. Hashimoto, K., Gross, B. G., and Lever, W. F.: Lichen amyloidosis: histochemical and electron microscopic studies. J. Invest. Dermatol., *45*:204, 1965.
26. Brownstein, M. H., Hashimoto, K., and Greenwald, G.: Biphasic amyloidosis: link between macular and lichenoid forms. Br. J. Dermatol., *88*:25, 1973.
27. Vasily, D. B., Bhatia, S. G., and Uhlin, S. R.: Familial primary cutaneous amyloidosis. Arch. Dermatol., *114*:1173, 1978.

7

Connective Tissue (Rheumatic) Diseases

The connective tissue diseases — lupus erythematosus (LE), dermatomyositis, and scleroderma — exhibit a wide variety of skin markings. Probably more cutaneous signs exist in this group of disorders than in any other. Some markings are specific for one of these clinical entities, whereas other markings merely indicate the presence of a connective tissue disease.

Only recently has it been appreciated that this group of disorders can occur in mixed and undifferentiated forms. A patient may have combinations of typical LE and scleroderma, dermatomyositis and scleroderma, or myositis and LE. In an individual case there may be enough evidence of cutaneous and multisystem involvement to indicate the presence of a connective tissue disorder, but insufficient findings to label a specific disease.

Reactivity of the vascular system, ranging from telangiectasia through vivid violaceous coloring and vasospastic phenomena to necrotizing arteritis, is the outstanding feature of these diseases and acts as a common link in three seemingly disparate disorders.

The degree of cutaneous involvement in LE, dermatomyositis, and scleroderma is not necessarily proportional to the extent of visceral involvement. Severe disease may be accompanied by skin lesions that are either subtle or florid, and sometimes there may be no skin lesions at all. On the other hand, a similar spectrum of lesions may occur in the absence of any systemic involvement.

LUPUS ERYTHEMATOSUS

Lupus erythematosus occurs almost four times as often in women as in men. Black women develop LE three times more frequently than white women, and during the childbearing years, 15 to 49, their mortality rate is three times greater. Although black men develop LE 1.5 times more often than white men, the data are inconclusive as to whether they also incur a higher mortality rate.[1] In early adulthood, the prevalence of, and mortality from, SLE are also higher in Puerto Rican women than in white women.[2] The peak incidence in children occurs between 11 and 13 years of age, and the disease is rare before the age of 3 years. Most adults are affected before the age of 40, but the onset has been seen as late as 70 years. Fibrinoid degeneration of connective tissue with variable degrees of inflammation is the characteristic histologic finding in LE. Nearly

Table 7–1. Signs, Symptoms, and Laboratory Findings in LE[3–8, 16]

Weight loss	70%	Renal involvement	50-70%
Fever	86-100%	Psychoses	10-30%
Skin lesions	50-90%	Seizures	7-30%
Arthralgias	70-90%	Photosensitivity	11-50%
Arthritis	12-30%	Raynaud's phenomenon	10-30%
Lymphadenopathy	30-70%	Chronic urticaria	7%
Splenomegaly	8-40%	False positive serology	20-30%
Hepatomegaly	30-40%	LE cell phenomenon	70-90%
Cytoid bodies (fundus oculi)	24%	Antinuclear antibodies	90%
Pleurisy	50-60%	Leukopenia (WBC <4500)	70%
Pleural effusion	16-60%	Thrombocytopenia	10-30%
Lupus pneumonitis	20%	Hemolytic anemia	2-10%
Cardiac involvement	50-70%	Normocytic normochromic anemia	60%
Gastrointestinal involvement	10-50%		

every organ in the body runs the risk of involvement, resulting in the impressive array of signs and symptoms listed in Table 7–1.[3-8, 16]

The spectrum of LE varies from an acute fulminant disease of a few months' duration to a chronic smoldering process lasting more than 30 years. A single organ or system may be involved for many years before others are similarly affected, thereby revealing the true nature of the disorder. Thus epilepsy, arthritis, idiopathic thrombocytopenic purpura, or chronic glomerulonephritis may be the sole manifestation of LE before the disease is diagnosed.

The skin may be the sole organ of involvement in a patient's lifetime, or it may precede the involvement of other systems by any period up to 30 years.[9] The term *discoid LE* has been applied to cases in which there is only cutaneous involvement. The classic discoid lesion is a scaly erythematous atrophic plaque. The debate about whether discoid LE and systemic LE are different entities is no longer a major issue, and most investigators agree that discoid LE and systemic LE are manifestations of the same disorder.[10, 11] At one pole are individuals with disease confined to the skin (discoid LE) and at the other are patients with severe systemic disease that is often fatal because of progressive nephritis. Between these extremes one observes patients with graded degrees of systemic involvement in whom discoid skin lesions are frequently present. Some of the evidence indicating that discoid LE and systemic LE are part of a spectrum includes the following: antinuclear antibodies and biologic false positive reactions are found in both varieties[10-12]; patients with systemic LE may have classic discoid lesions, clinically and histologically; 30 to 50 per cent of discoid LE patients intermittently exhibit abnormal laboratory findings such as leukopenia, elevated sedimentation rate, and mild anemia[9, 11, 13]; the conversion rate from discoid LE to systemic LE varies from 2 to 10 per cent in various series (average 4.2 per cent)[9, 13-18]; fatigue and weakness, as encountered in systemic LE, may be the only indication of systemic involvement in a case of discoid LE; and, finally, some patients with systemic LE develop discoid lesions when they enter remission.

A better terminology would be cutaneous LE and systemic LE. One cannot determine from the clinical or histologic examination of a discoid-appearing lesion whether or not there is systemic involvement. Only a complete history and physical examination, as well as appropriate laboratory testing, will help settle this point. If all these data are normal, the patient can be considered to have cutaneous LE, which is usually a benign disease with a good prognosis and a normal lifespan.

The skin is involved at some time during the course of the disease in almost all patients. In most cases the cutaneous lesions are either specific for LE clinically and histologically, or they at least indicate a connective tissue disorder. Markings may be transient or persistent. They will indicate the true disorder underlying seemingly classic cases of idiopathic thrombocytopenic purpura, epilepsy, rheumatoid arthritis, migratory polyarthritis, hemolytic anemia, psychoses, and chronic renal disease.

There are two commonly held misconceptions about the cutaneous signs of LE: first, it is thought that the most common lesion is an erythematous (*butterfly* or *batwing*) flush over the malar and nasal areas; and second, telangiectasia alone is believed to be characteristic of the disease in this butterfly distribution. The malar or butterfly flush is neither specific for LE nor its most frequent sign. Moreover, the presence of telangiectasia without the accompanying features of scaling, atrophy, or erythema is never a marker of LE.

One of the basic cutaneous lesions of LE is the discoid type: a well-demarcated elevated firm red-purple plaque which shows scaling, atrophy, and fine telangiectasia (Plates 14*E*, *F*, and 15*A*). At times the openings of the hair follicles are dilated and plugged with scales. All of these characteristic features may not be present in every lesion, but the distinctive scaling, violaceous color, and atrophy always occur together.

Usually the scale is thin and fine, but sometimes it can be heavy and lamellar and resemble the scaling of ichthyosis and psoriasis. If the scale is thick enough, it can be lifted in one piece (Figs. 7–1 and 7–2). The undersurface has follicular projections that resemble carpet tacks. This is a characteristic sign of LE. Occasionally, however, this phenomenon can be observed with scales in seborrheic dermatitis and pemphigus foliaceus.

Atrophy in a plaque is indicated by a smooth surface devoid of the normal skin lines or by a surface characterized by delicate wrinkling (Plate 15*B*, *C*). This latter sign can be brought out by gently pinching the lesion. As the plaque evolves, this epidermal atrophy is often followed by a loss of dermal tissue. Sharply punched out atrophic lesions are the final result (Fig. 7–3). Partial or complete loss of pigmentation or hyperpigmentation, or both, frequently accompany the development of atrophy (Plate 15*D*).

Occasionally the discoid plaques may resemble the lesions of psoriasis (Plate 15*E*, *F*). However, this latter diagnosis can be easily excluded by looking for epidermal atrophy in the lesions, a finding that is never present in the eruptions of psoriasis. Rarely the discoid lesion may be markedly elevated and have a verrucose surface. These plateau-like lesions have been called LE hypertrophicus (Plate 16*A*) (see p. 292 for further discussion.)

Discoid plaques may be single or multiple. The malar regions are usually involved, but they need not be. The lesions can be asymmetrical. Cutaneous surfaces — especially the legs, arms, hands, fingers, chest, and abdomen — may be extensively affected (Fig. 7–4). Diagnostic lesions of atrophy, scaling, and dyspigmentation are frequently found on the scalp and in the ears (Fig. 7–5). These areas should be inspected

Text continued on page 262

PLATE 15

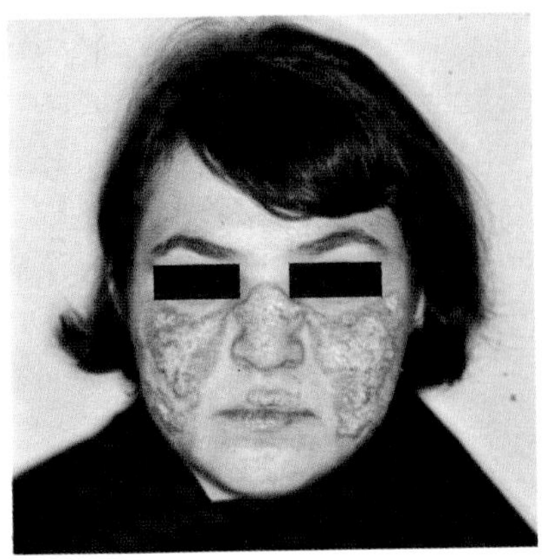

A, LE. Discoid lesions in butterfly distribution.

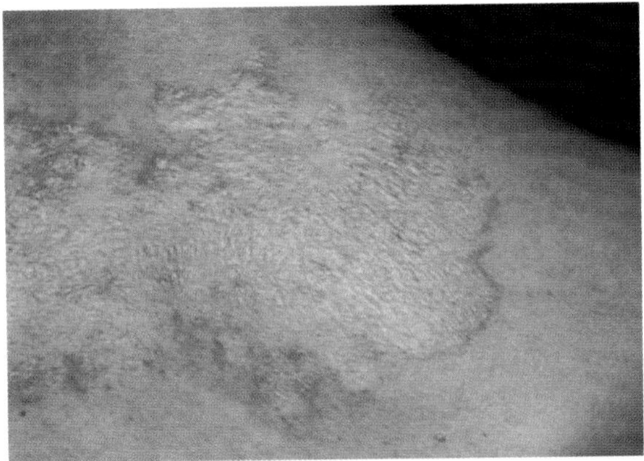

B, LE. Close view of discoid lesion to demonstrate atrophy: delicate wrinkling and hypopigmentation of skin.

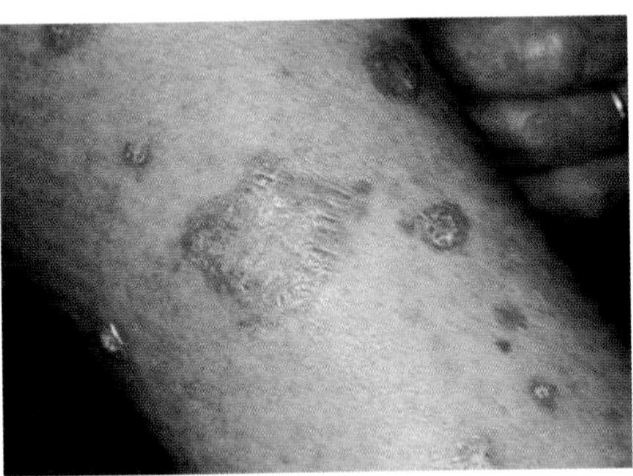

C, LE. Close view of discoid lesions.

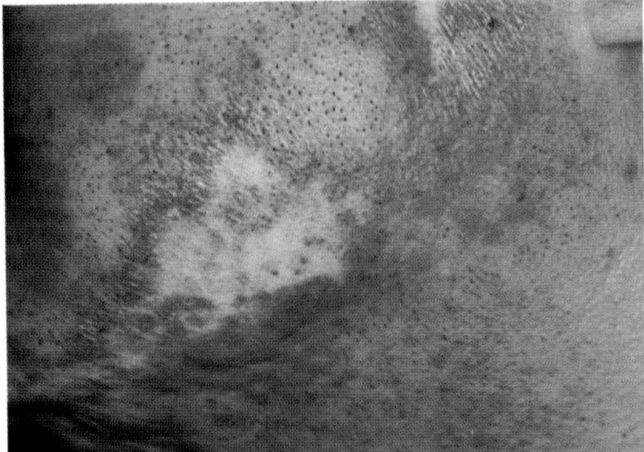

D, LE. Discoid lesion with hypopigmented atrophic inactive center and active erythematous border.

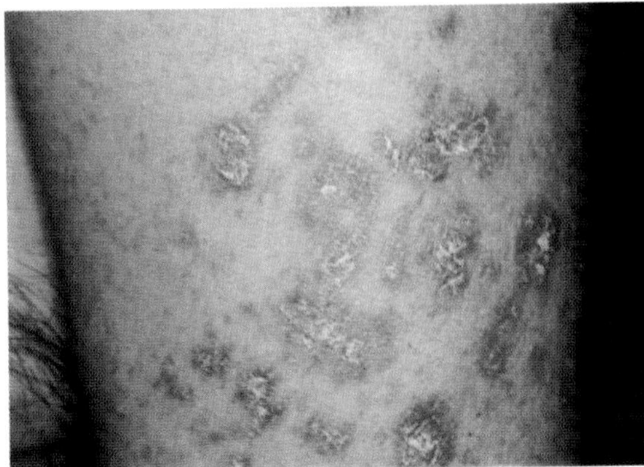

E, LE. Psoriasiform lesions. Atrophy is present in some areas.

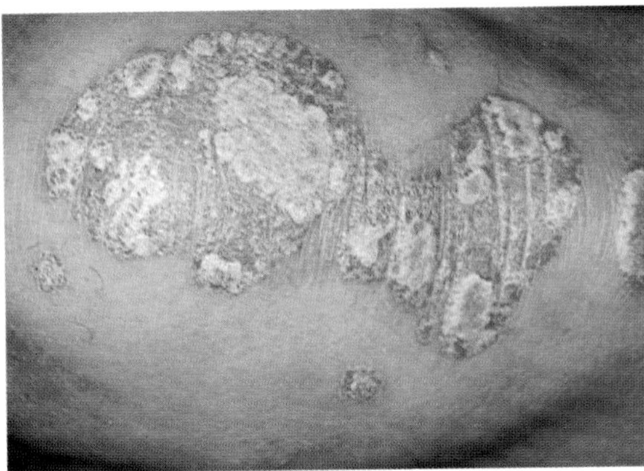

F, Psoriasis. Compare with *E*. Atrophy never occurs in a plaque of psoriasis.

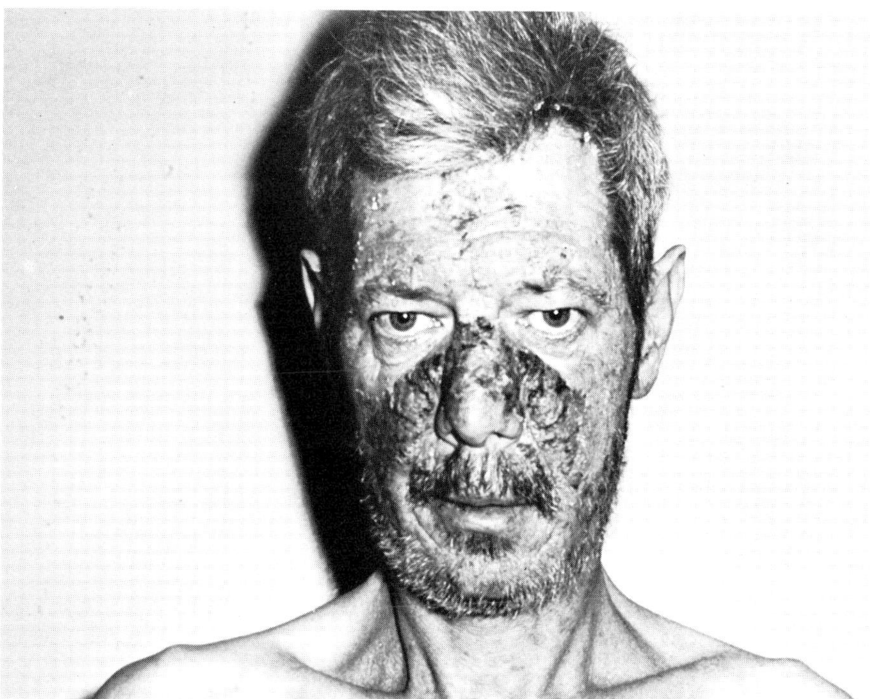

Figure 7–1. Lupus erythematosus (LE). Unusually heavy scale in butterfly distribution.

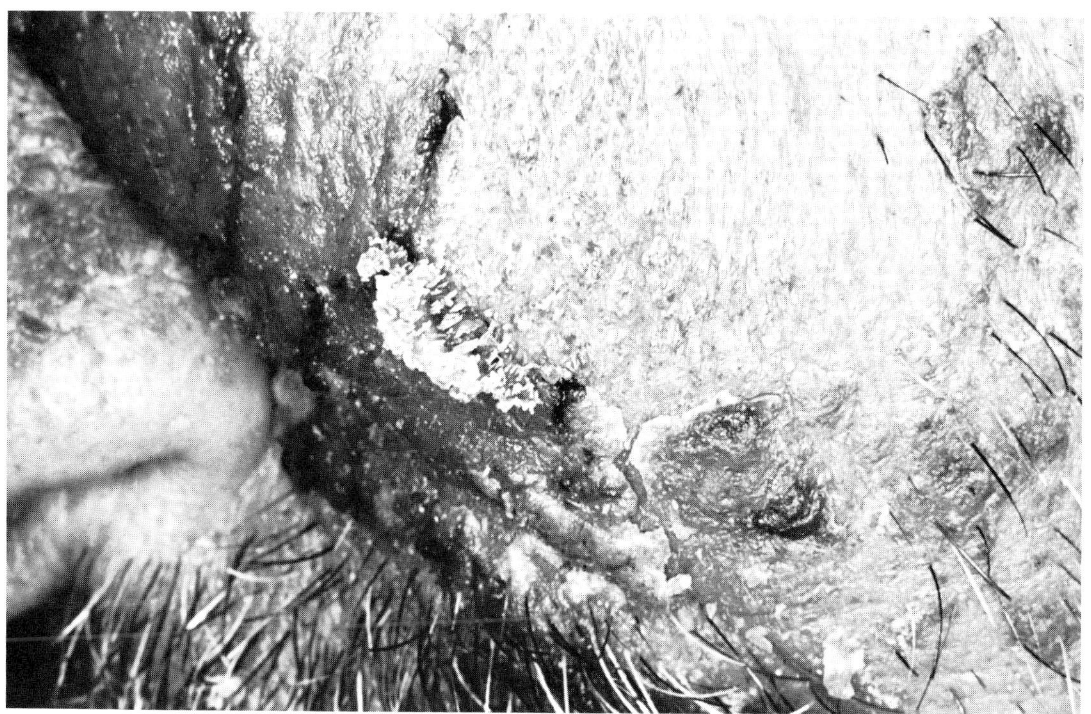

Figure 7–2. LE. Carpet tack sign demonstrated. The scale shown in Figure 7–1 has been carefully pulled off in order to exhibit its undersurface.

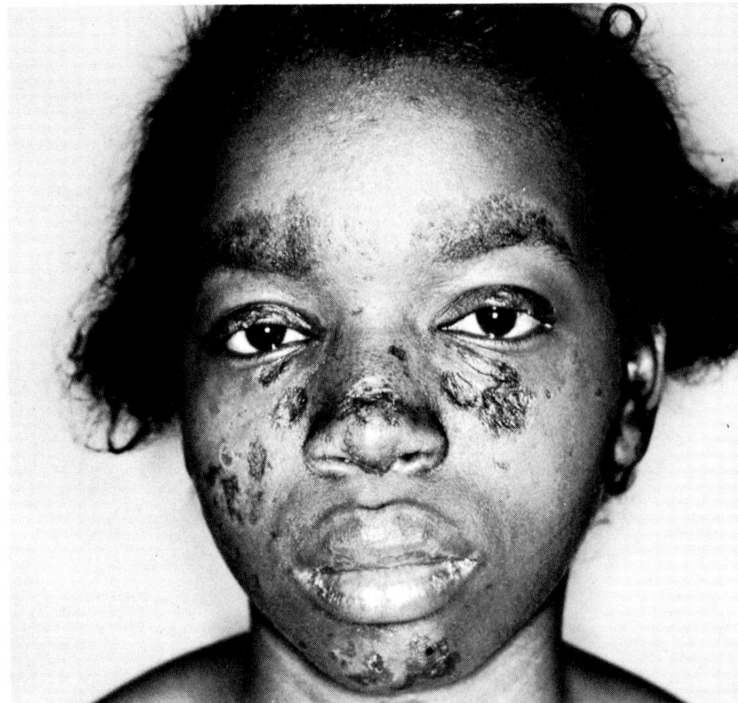

Figure 7–3. LE. Discoid lesions. Sharply punched out areas of atrophy.

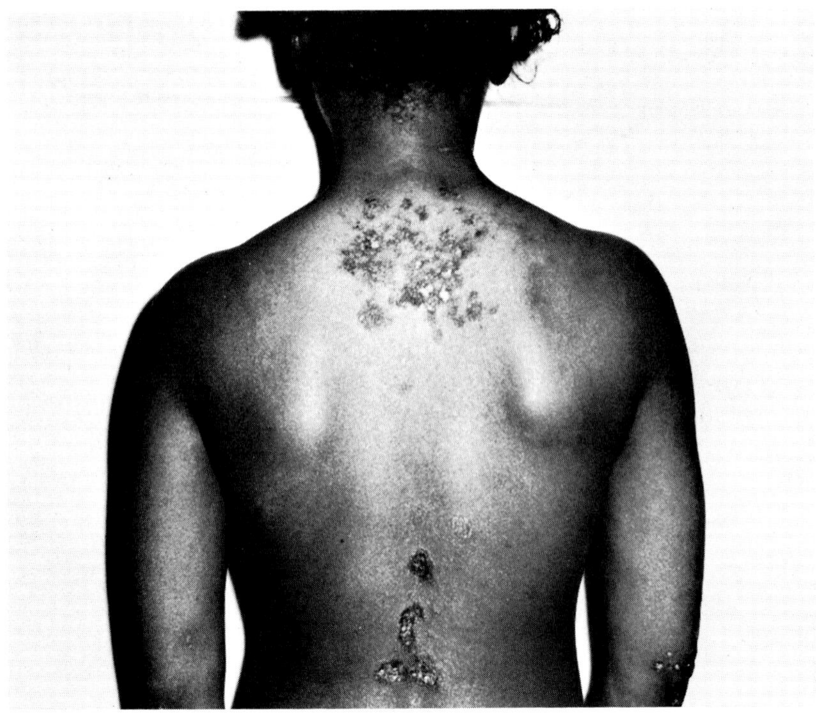

Figure 7–4. LE. Discoid lesions on trunk.

PLATE 16

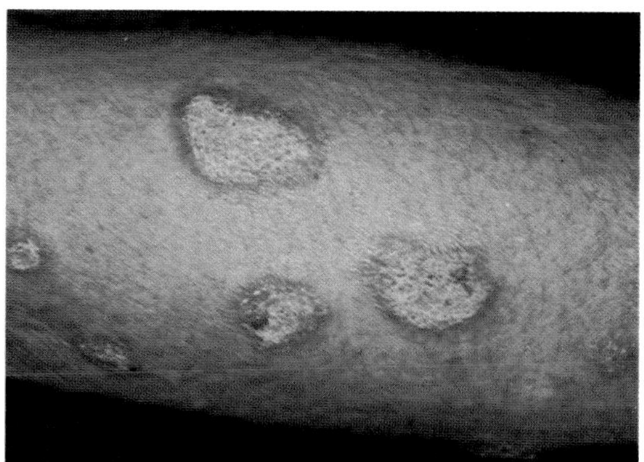

A, Verrucose lesion of LE called *lupus hypertrophicus*.

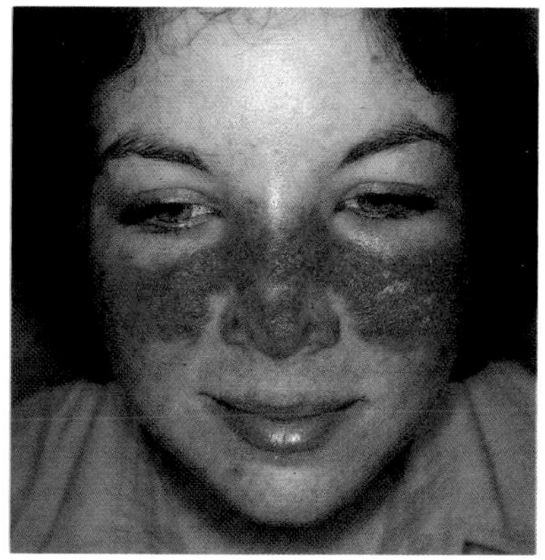

B, LE. Discoid lesions in a woman with systemic LE.

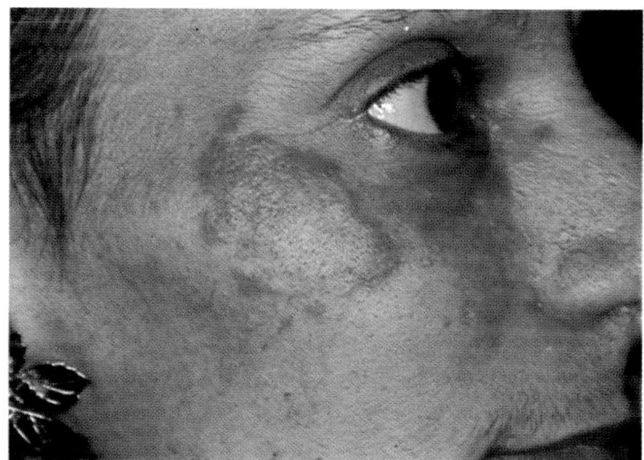

C, LE. Urticarial plaque which can persist for months.

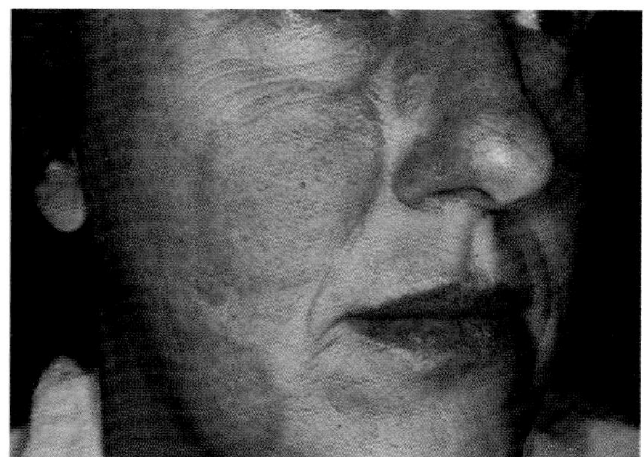

D, LE. Urticarial plaque.

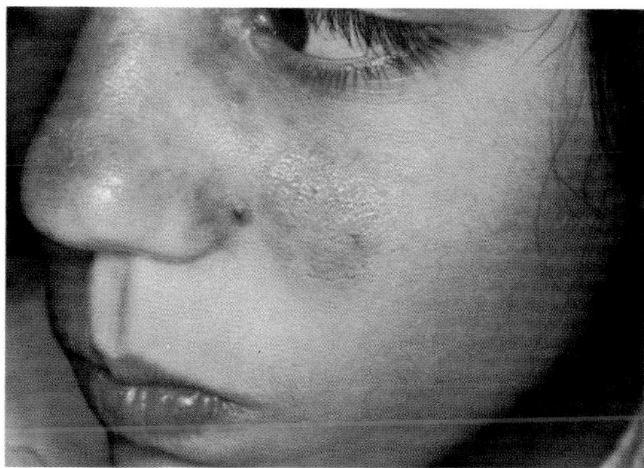

E, LE. Type of urticarial plaque frequently seen in acute systemic LE.

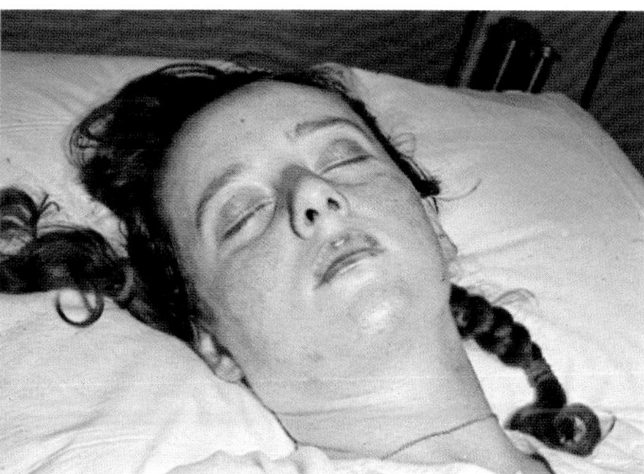

F, Systemic LE. Transient violaceous urticarial lesions over right mandible. They were present only during acute attack. Note patches of erythema on lips and malar areas.

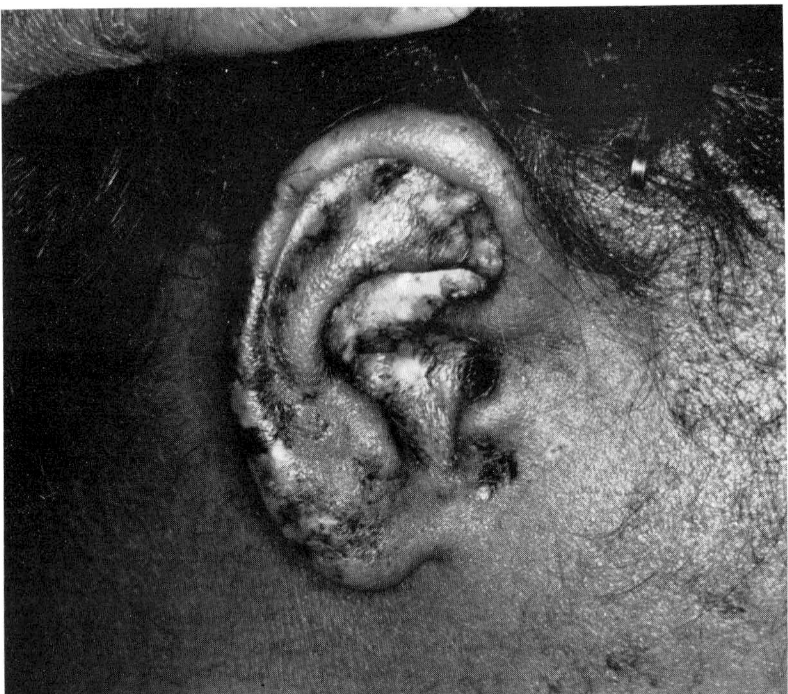

Figure 7–5. LE. Typical lesions on ear showing atrophy, dyspigmentation, and telangiectasia.

carefully; they may be the only sites of involvement. The sides of the neck and other exposed parts of the skin should also be searched for hypopigmented atrophic flat spots that have resulted from spontaneously resolving lesions. The eyelid margins may also be involved, and there may be an associated conjunctivitis if the inflammatory reaction is severe. Longstanding lesions of the lids produce epilation. A silvering or whitening of the vermilion border of the lips is a pathognomonic sign of LE; it is often misdiagnosed and treated as leukoplakia, but the hyperkeratotic features characteristic of this premalignant lesion are not present. Discoid lesions may also affect the lips (Figs. 7–6 to 7–8).

The buccal and nasal mucosae often disclose a silvery-white scarring which may ulcerate (Figs. 7–9, 7–10 and 7–13). One can also see punched-out erosions in the absence of scar formation. Nasal septal perforation is an uncommon complication of LE. However, mucosal lesions are not necessarily a sign of systemic involvement or severe illness, because they are often found in patients with cutaneous LE. The gingivae may appear red, edematous, friable, and eroded, or they may exhibit silvery-white changes similar to those on the buccal mucosa. The tongue may be similarly affected. These whitish cicatrizing plaques must be distinguished from the oral lesions of lichen planus, which have a reticulated pattern in their fully developed form (Fig. 7–12). The earliest lesions of oral lichen planus are usually simple rings with short radiating spines that produce a lacy pattern on confluence (Fig. 7–11). The palate and tongue may be diffusely involved by lichen planus (Fig. 7–14). Lichen planus may also cause ulceration, but the presence of the typical violaceous flat-topped polygonal papules of lichen planus elsewhere on the body indicates the correct diagnosis. Leukoplakia of the mouth shows hyperkeratosis. Bite marks from the impingement of the molars on the

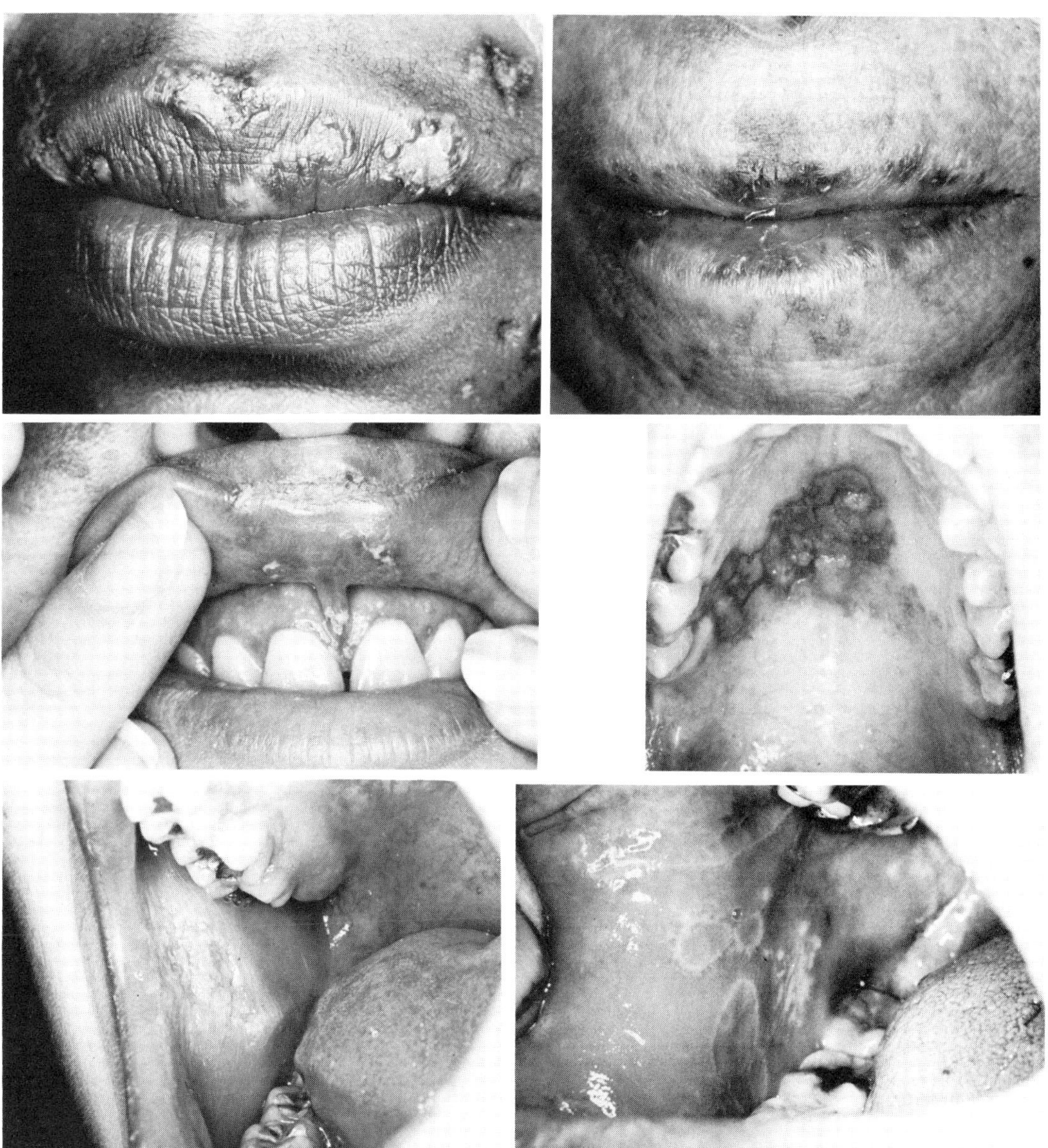

Figure 7–6. Top left. LE. Discoid lesions on lips.

Figure 7–7. Top right. LE. Discoid lesions on lips.

Figure 7–8. Center left. LE. Discoid lesions on lips.

Figure 7–9. Center right. LE. Palatal ulcerations.

Figure 7–10. Botton left. LE. Silvery white scarring with ulceration.

Figure 7–11. Bottom right. Lichen planus. Buccal lesions consist of coalescing rings, each of which has short radiating spines. The rings produce a reticulated pattern in their fully developed form (Fig. 7–12).

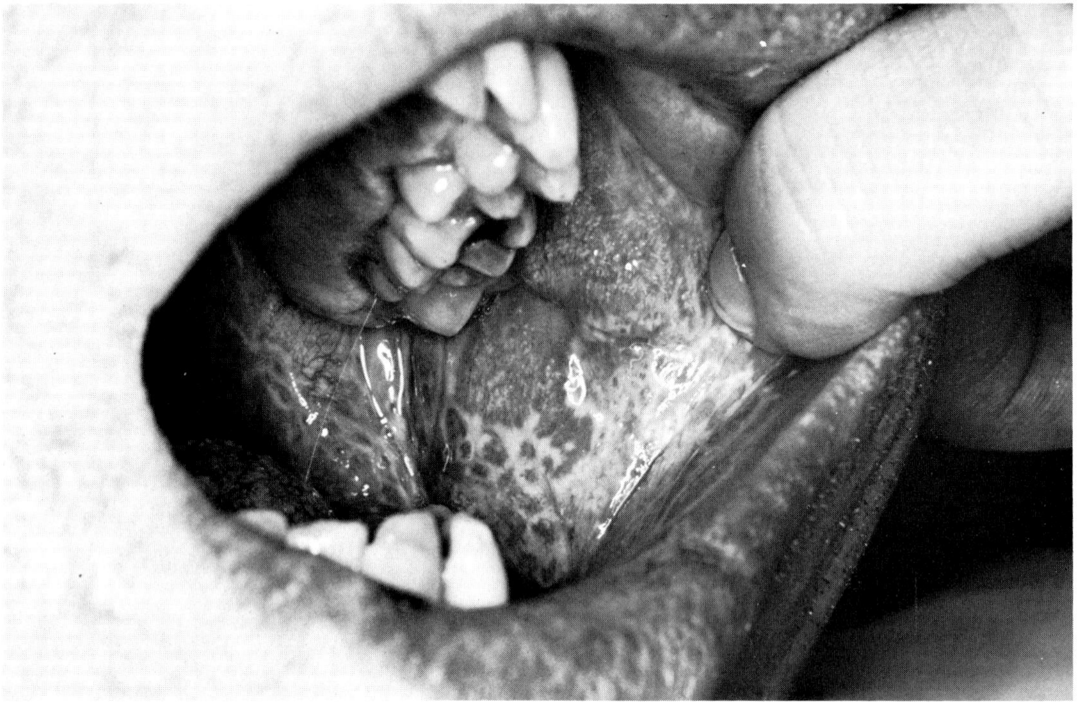

Figure 7–12. Lichen planus. The oral lesions of lichen planus have a reticular (lacy) pattern.

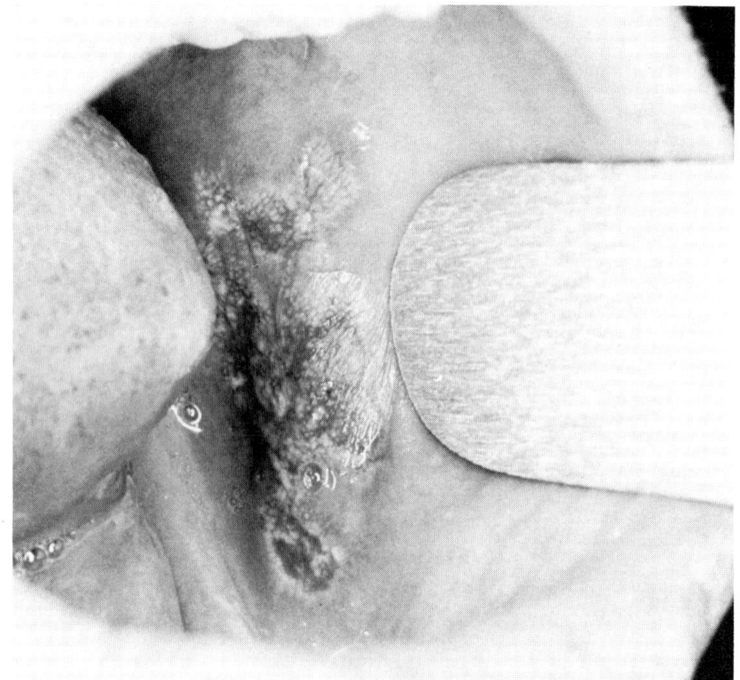

Figure 7–13. LE. Silvery white scarring plaque with ulceration.

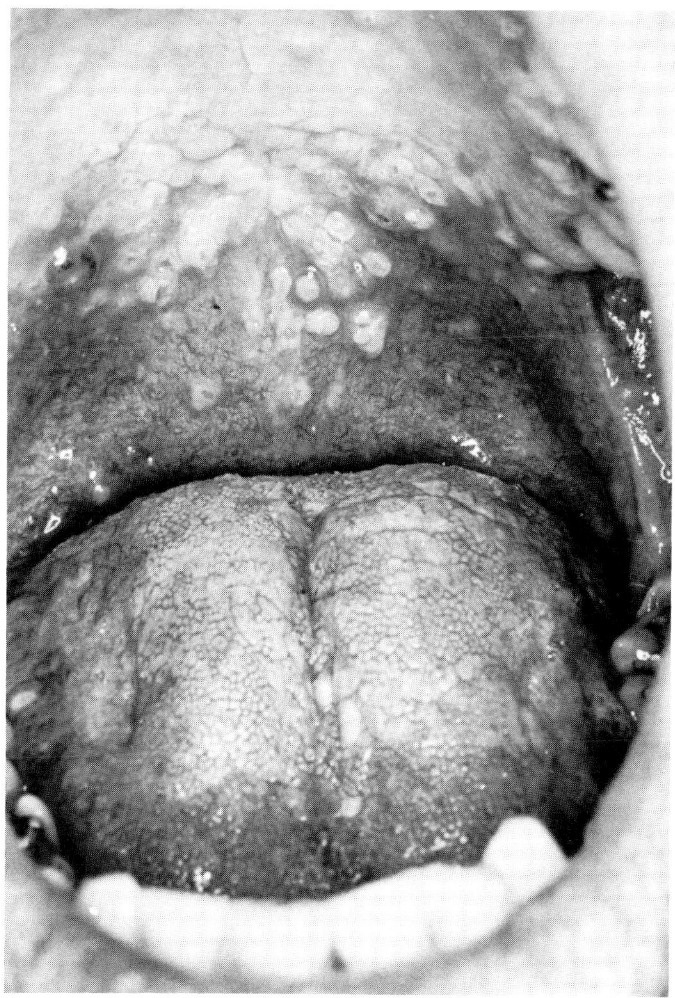

Figure 7–14. Lichen planus. Diffuse involvement of tongue and palate.

buccal mucosa must also be considered in the differential diagnosis. The histopathology of the oral lesions of LE is essentially identical to that found in the cutaneous discoid lesions.[18]

Follicular plugging is seen primarily on the face and scalp where the pilosebaceous units are most numerous and most highly developed (Fig. 7–15). Plugging is also produced by the focal accumulation of scale in pits and depressions in the skin that are unrelated to hair follicles. The fingers and palms are the sites most commonly involved by this process. LE lesions are almost always asymptomatic.

Lupus profundus is a name that has been applied to a form of panniculitis which occurs in approximately 2 per cent of patients with cutaneous or systemic LE.[19] The subcutaneous lesions develop as well-defined firm nodules and plaques measuring up to several centimeters (Figs. 7–16 to 7–18). They are generally asymptomatic and only rarely tender. They may develop beneath typical lupus lesions, but usually the overlying skin is clinically normal or simply erythematous (Plate 17*A*). The lesions of lupus profundus may persist for years. Areas of predilection are the forehead, cheeks, upper arms, and buttocks. In two patients with longstanding cutaneous LE, lupus profundus presented as discrete breast nodules that simulated breast carcinoma on a mammogram.[20] When the panniculitis resolves, it leaves behind depressed areas similar to those observed in Weber-Christian panniculitis and in exceptional instances, depressions resembling lipoatrophy (Fig. 7–19). Nonspecific trauma has appeared to induce lesions in some patients. Ulceration may develop spontaneously in the nodules, but more frequently it follows a biopsy procedure or intralesional injection of corticosteroids. However, the lesions and ulcerations usually respond favorably to antimalarial therapy.[19, 20] Histologically lupus profundus is characterized by a perivascular lymphocytic infiltration about dermal and subcutaneous vessels without accompanying fat necrosis. The infiltrate may extend into the fat lobules, and the septa of the fat may show hyalinization with foci of calcification.[21]

Severe scarring can produce horrible disfigurement in patients with LE. In a few cases, skin cancers have arisen in the scars, as they more commonly do in the cicatrices of burns and the lupus vulgaris form of cutaneous tuberculosis (Fig. 7–20). With progressive atrophy, hyperpigmentation with or without hypopigmentation develops and is very striking in dark-skinned individuals (Fig. 7–21). Pigmentary changes sometimes may be reversed with therapy. It is important to treat individuals with cutaneous LE in order to prevent disfigurement and the rare sequelae of skin cancers arising in the scars.

The lesions of LE can mimic those of cutaneous tuberculosis (lupus vulgaris) if they form plaques with elevated erythematous borders and severe central scarring as shown in Plate 17*B*. This patient had several such lesions in addition to marked involvement of the palms and vulva (Figs. 7–22 and 7–23).

In summary, the discoid plaque is pathognomonic of LE. It occurs in both cutaneous and systemic LE, and only a careful history, a physical examination, and appropriate laboratory tests will distinguish the two states (Plate 16*B*).

The next most common type of lesion is the reddish-purple urticarial plaque which is relatively fixed in shape and time and does not undergo

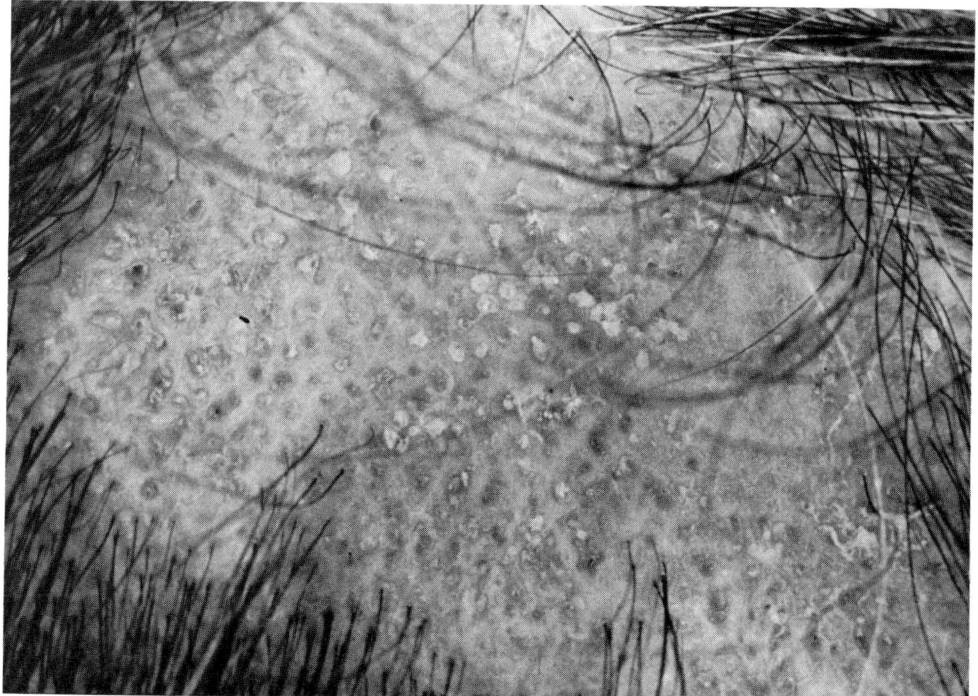

Figure 7–15. LE. Alopecia with follicular plugging. Follicular openings are dilated and filled with scale.

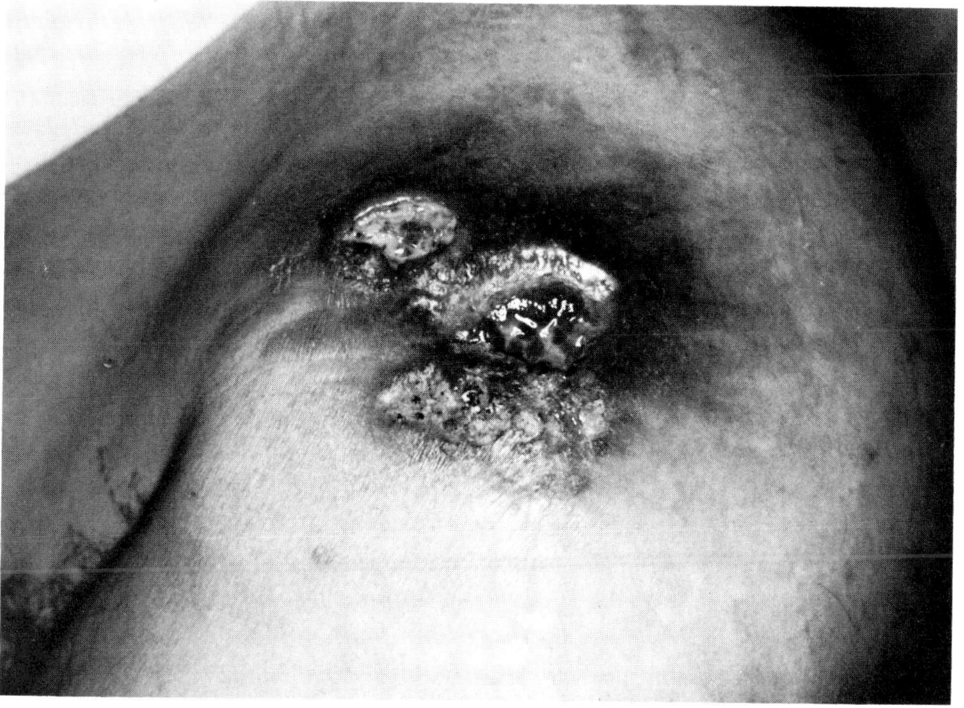

Figure 7–16. Lupus profundus with ulceration.

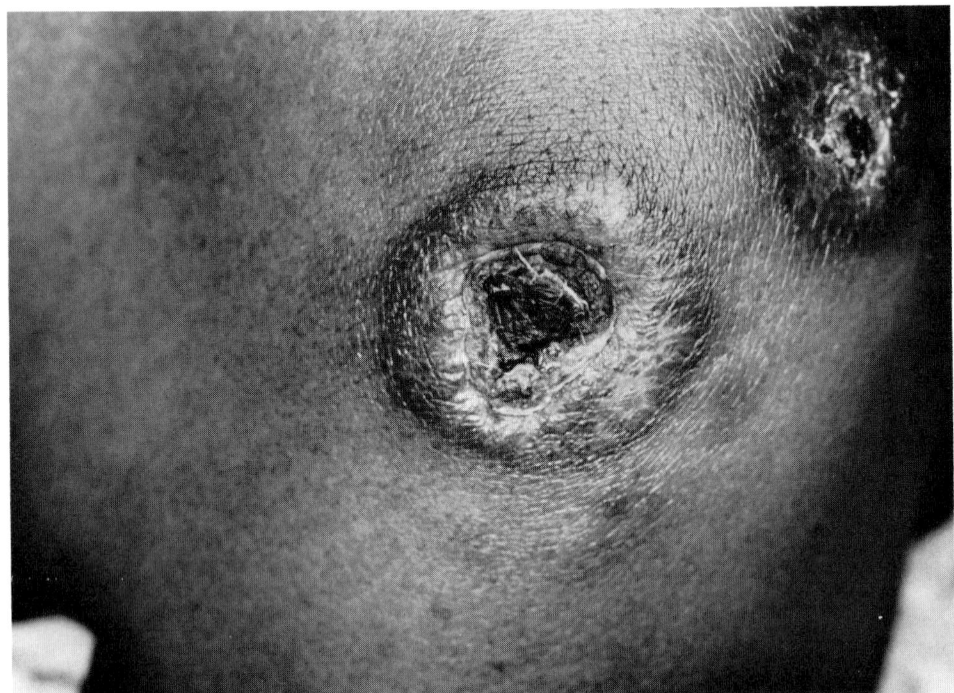

Figure 7–17. Lupus profundus with ulceration.

atrophy or scaling (Plate 16*C*, *D*, *E*). It looks like a fixed hive and is usually on the face. It may be asymmetrical or occur in a butterfly distribution. The urticarial plaque occurs in both cutaneous and systemic LE. It should be distinguished from polymorphous light eruption and from Jessner's benign lymphocytic infiltration of the skin. Small solitary lesions can be confused with sarcoidosis, lymphoma, or insect bites. A biopsy may be necessary to determine the correct diagnosis. Examination of such a skin lesion by direct immunofluorescence for the presence of immunoglobulins and complement at the dermal-epidermal junction (lupus band test) is useful in a diagnostically difficult case that could represent a light eruption or Jessner's disease. Immunoreactants are not found at the dermal-epidermal junction in polymorphous light eruption and Jessner's disease.[22] In addition, increased amounts of acid mucopolysaccharides are deposited in the dermis of LE lesions but not in those of light eruptions.[23]

In the systemic form of the disease, a more acute reaction is seen in the skin: violaceous urticarial papular lesions that last only a few days and are probably related to the activity of the disease (Plate 16*F*). They look like hives except for their violaceous color, and they disappear without scarring. These lesions most likely represent a more acute stage of the urticarial plaque just described.

Lesions often described and illustrated in textbooks are the malar flush with edema, erythema, and prominent telangiectasia. Vesiculation, superficial ulceration, and crusting develop if the edema is severe (Plate 18*A*).

Periorbital edema with a violaceous hue and telangiectasia may be present, and the neck and V area of the chest may also be purple-red. Although these changes are seen in systemic LE, they are observed more

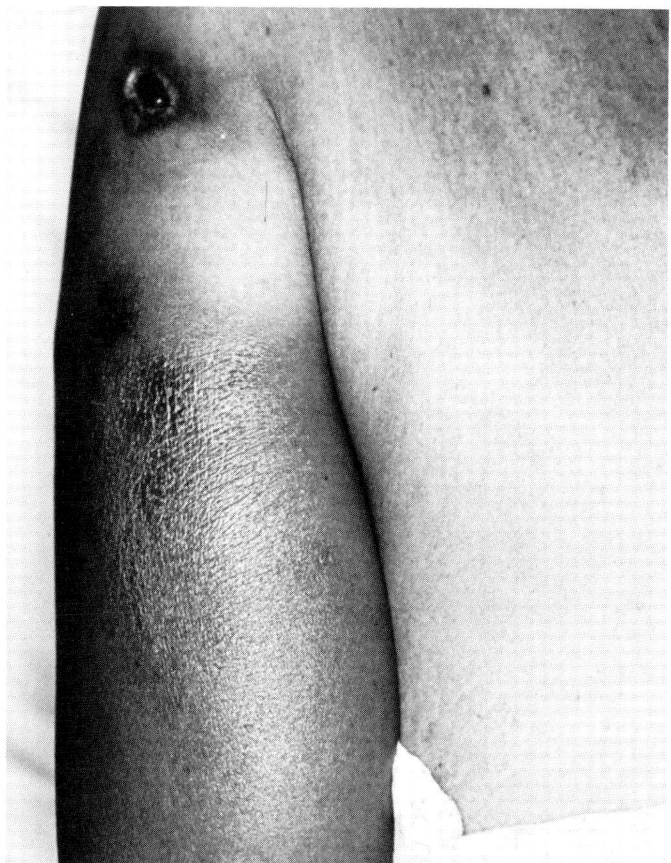

Figure 7–18. Lupus profundus. Large plaque involving mid-upper arm.

frequently in dermatomyositis. It is sometimes difficult to distinguish between LE and the early stage of dermatomyositis when striking cutaneous changes are present and when myositis is minimal. Examination of the skin by direct immunofluorescence may be helpful here also. Immunoreactants are not found at the dermal-epidermal junction in dermatomyositis.[22]

Three unusual types of lesions have been observed in eight of our patients. Three people developed plaques with an edematous elevated border; the remainder of the plaque was either hyperpigmented or normal in color (Plate 19*A*). Atrophy and scaling were absent except in one small area, but telangiectasia was present. Two other patients had an eruption mimicking the iris lesions of erythema multiforme; however, atrophy and fine scaling were present. Three patients had arciform lesions (Fig. 7–24; Plate 18*F*). The classic histologic changes of LE were found in the biopsy specimens from these seven patients.

Sontheimer et al. have grouped these arciform lesions and the psoriasiform plaques described earlier under the rubric of subacute cutaneous LE.[24] Twenty-seven patients out of a total of 299 had such eruptions. The annular lesions may remain individual or may coalesce to form polycyclic gyrate patterns. The eruption of subacute cutaneous LE tends to occur on the face, neck, upper part of the back and chest, shoulders, and extensor surfaces of the arms and hands. The inner

Text continued on page 277

PLATE 17

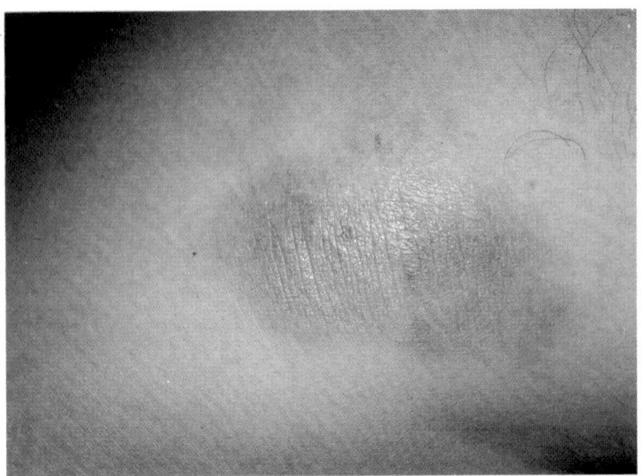

A, Lupus profundus. Induration extending to subcutis with overlying induration.

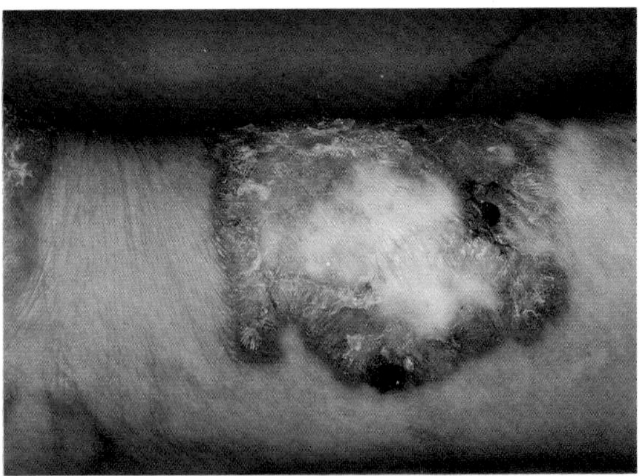

B, Discoid LE lesion resembling lupus vulgaris.

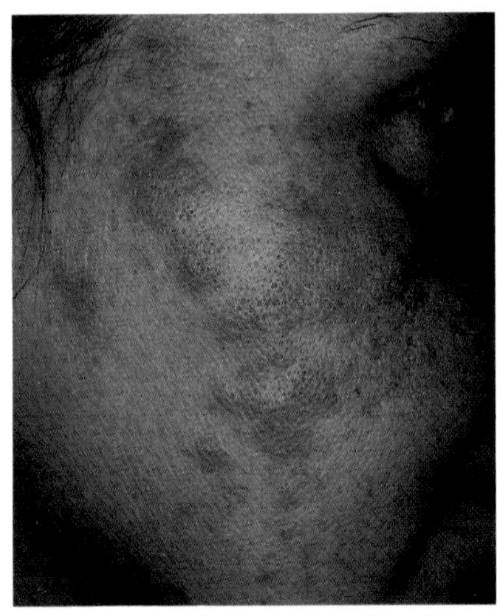

C, Jessner's disease. Benign lymphocytic infiltration of skin. Firm pink to red plaques.

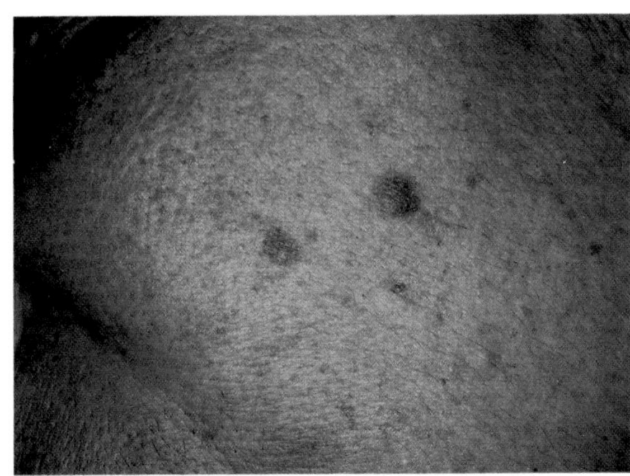

D, Granuloma faciale. Red-brown papules and nodules which lack scale and atrophy.

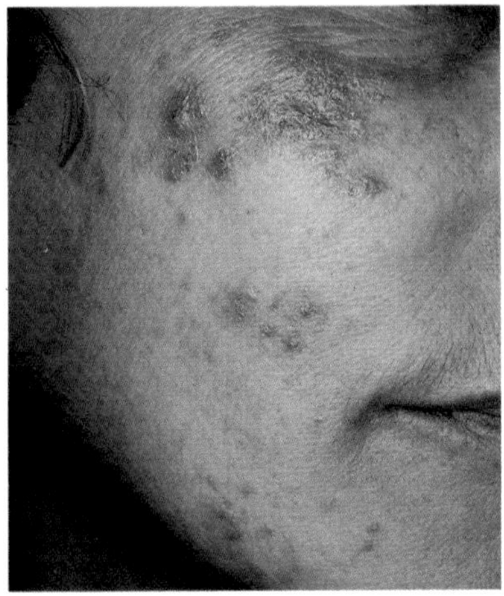

E, Acne rosacea. Erythematous papules and pustules.

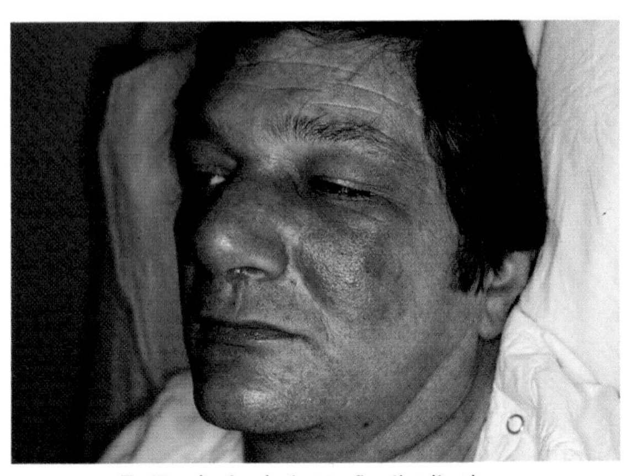

F, Erysipelas in butterfly distribution.

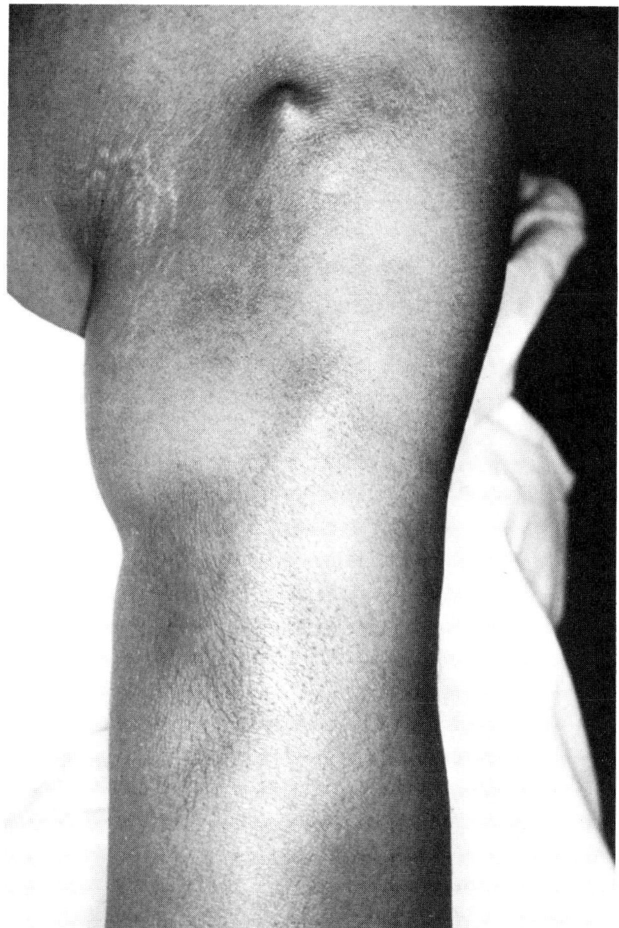

Figure 7–19. Lupus profundus. Resolution of lesions may be followed by lipoatrophy.

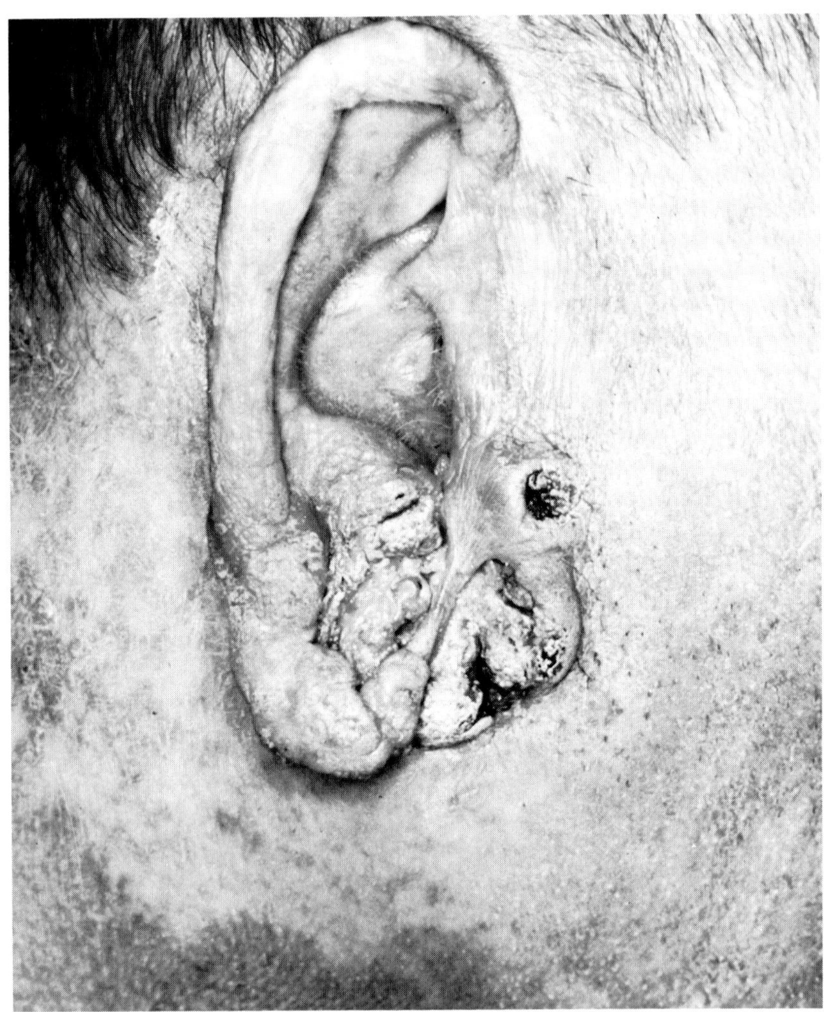

Figure 7–20. LE. This patient with LE developed a squamous cell carcinoma arising in a discoid lesion that involved his ear lobe.

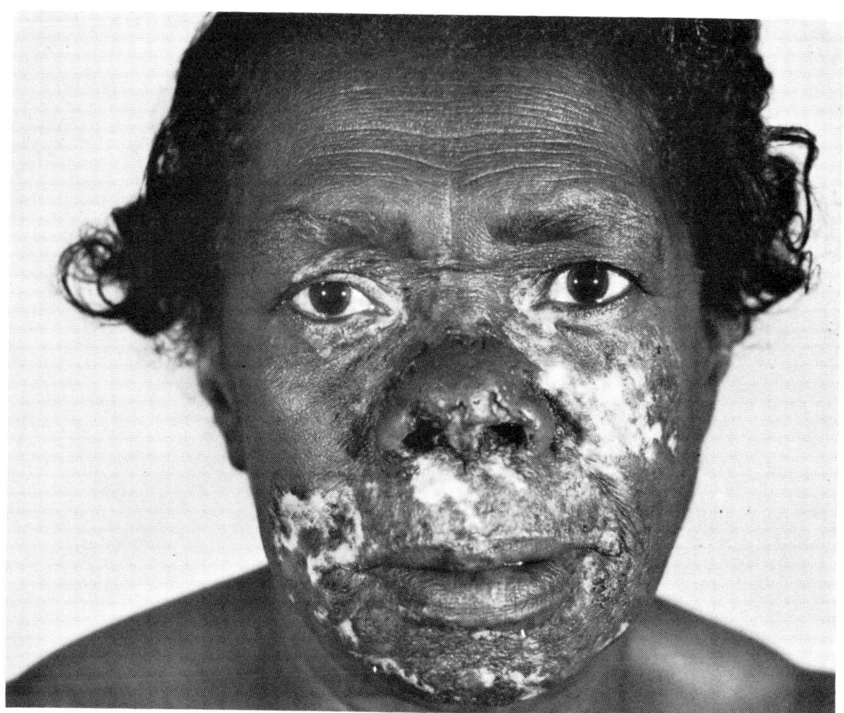

Figure 7–21. LE. Severe destructive scarring and pigment loss.

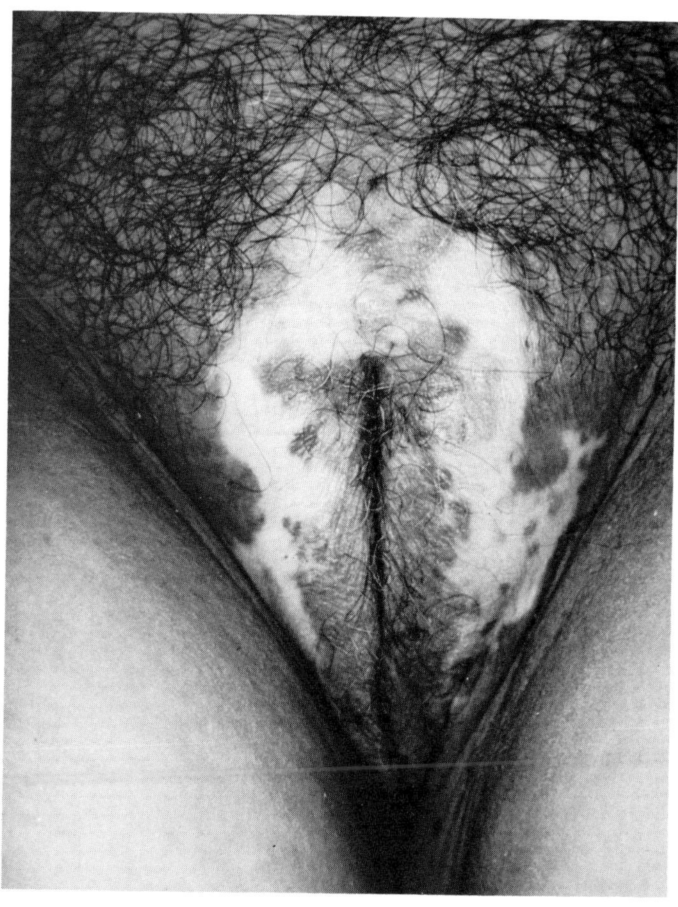

Figure 7–22. LE. Discoid lesions involving vulva.

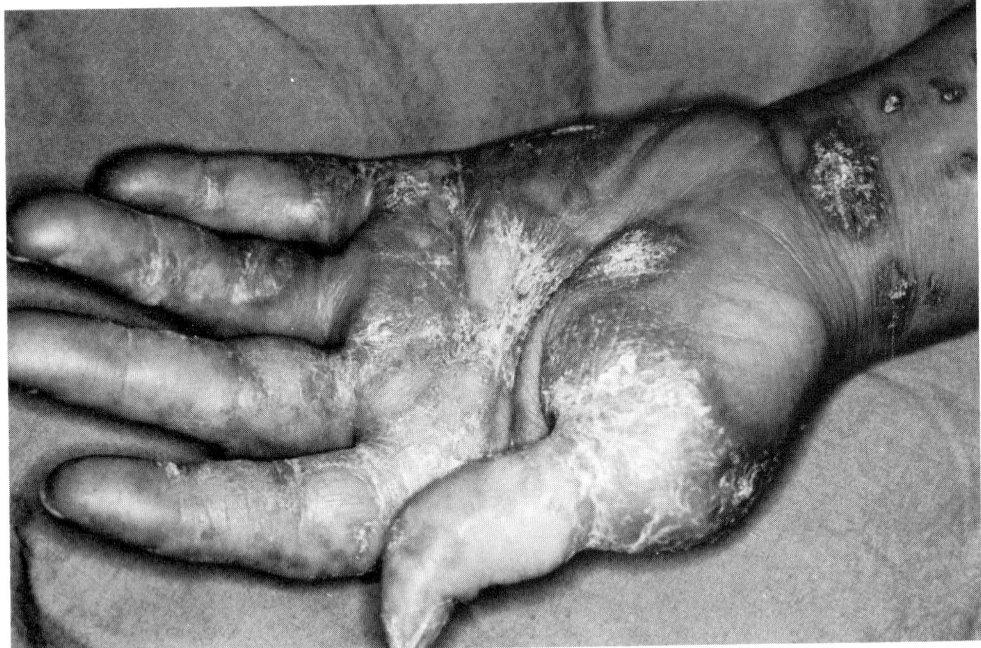

Figure 7–23. LE. Discoid lesions on palms.

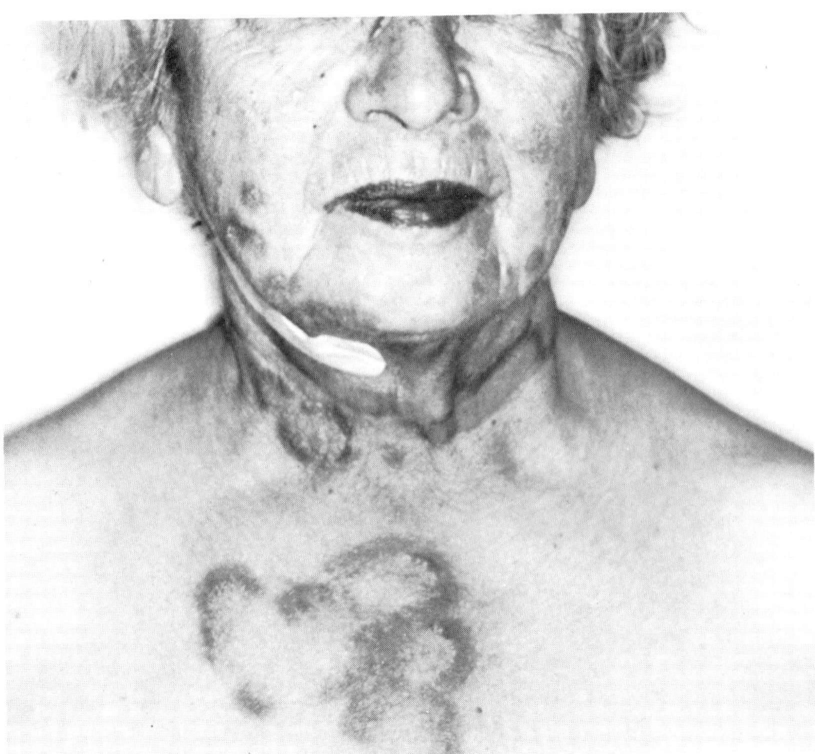

Figure 7–24. LE. Unusual polycyclic lesions which showed the typical histopathology of LE.

PLATE 18

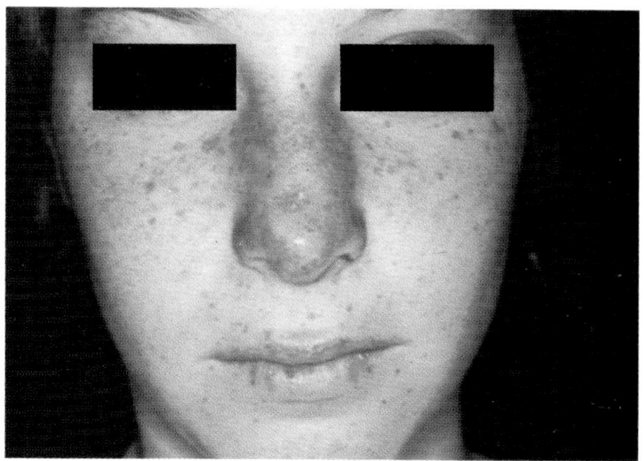

A, Acute systemic LE. Eruption over the nose is erythematous and edematous. Superficial ulceration with crust formation may occur in such acute lesions.

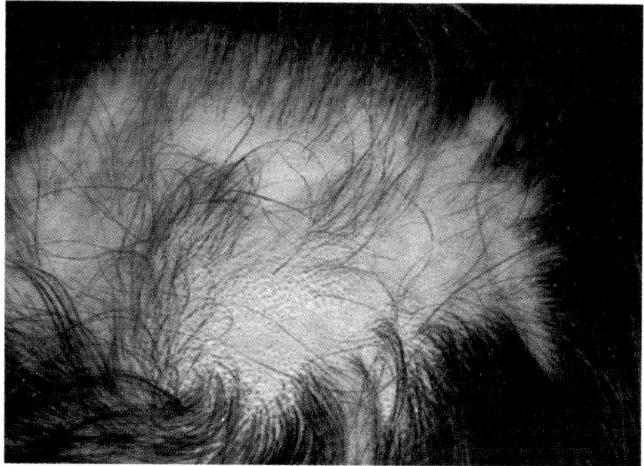

B, LE. Area of alopecia shows atrophy, dyspigmentation, and erythema identical to discoid lesions elsewhere.

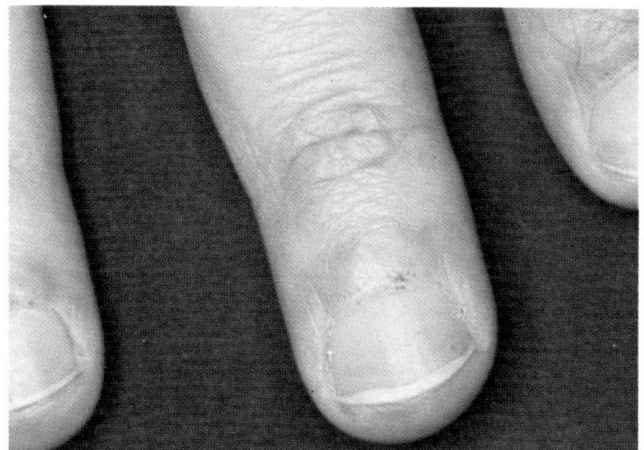

C, Cuticular telangiectasia with periungual erythema. Characteristic of the connective tissue disorders.

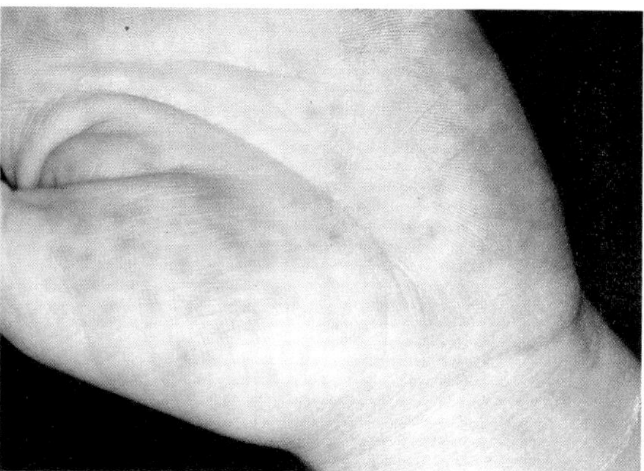

D, Papular telangiectasis on palms characteristic of LE.

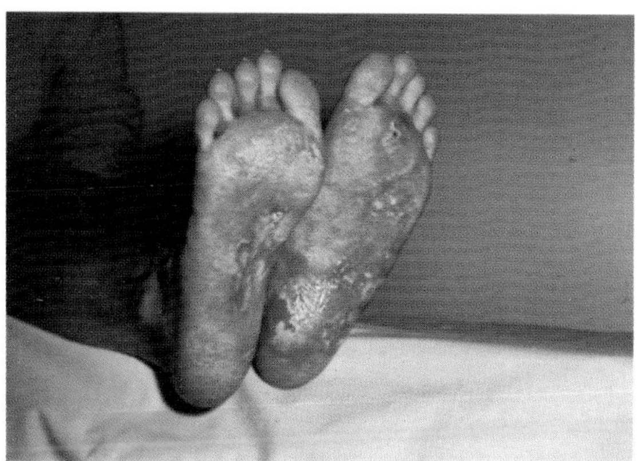

E, LE, Plantar ulcerations — unusual manifestation. LE/LP overlap syndrome.

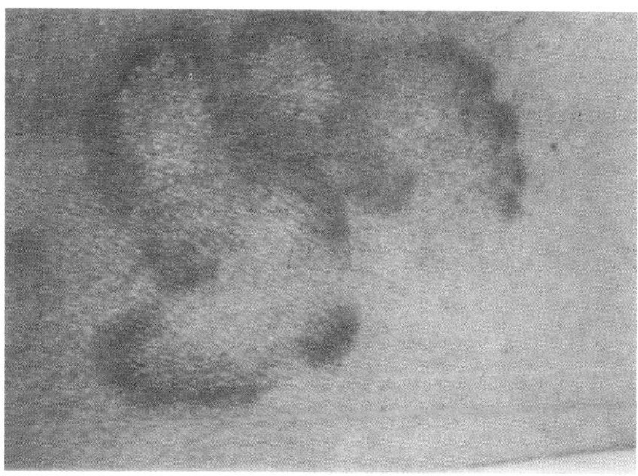

F, LE. Arciform lesions.

PLATE 19

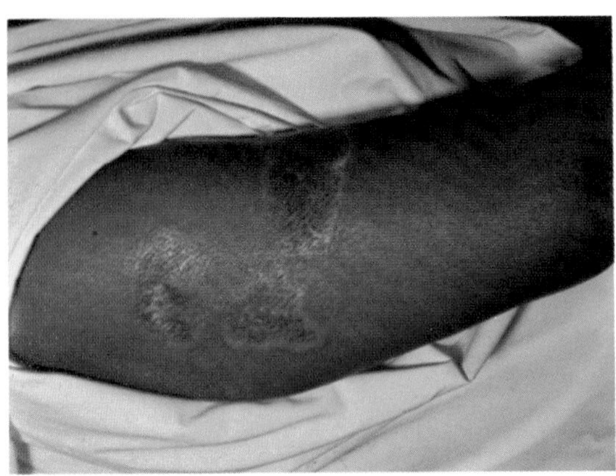

A, LE, Oval lesions with relatively clear centers and elevated borders. One lesion shows a small area of atrophy and scaling in the center.

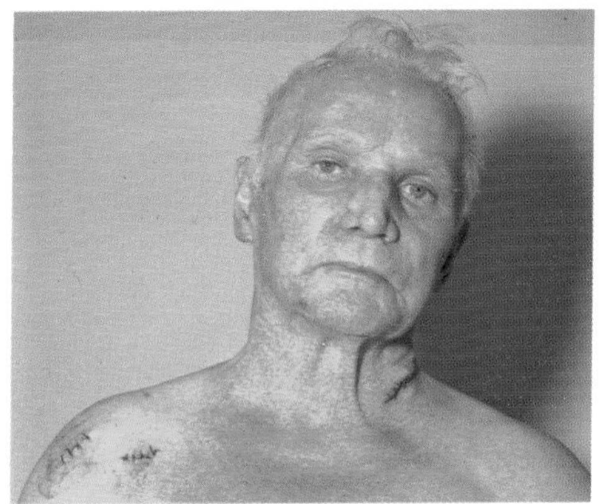

B, Dermatomyositis. Characteristic violaceous color on face and V of neck.

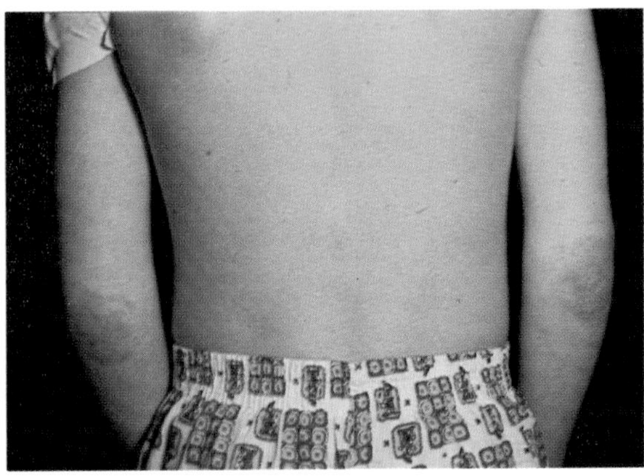

C, Dermatomyositis. Characteristic erythema and scaling over the elbows.

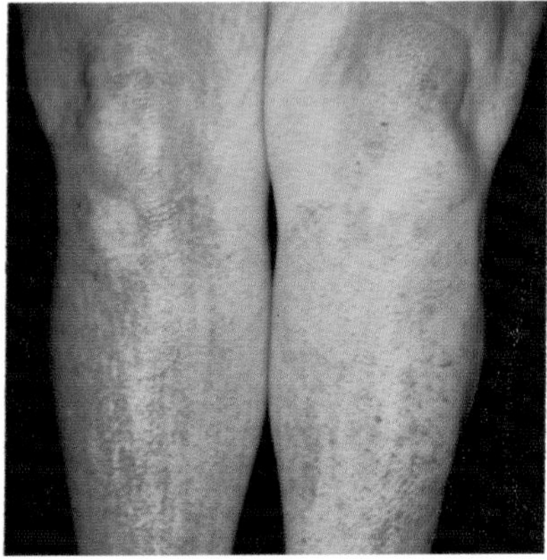

D, Dermatomyositis. Marked edema in addition to erythema and scaling over the knees. Linear lesions were produced by scratching because of associated marked pruritus.

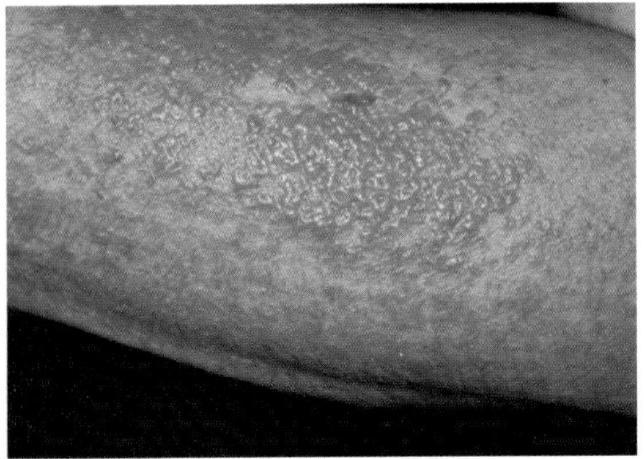

E, Dermatomyositis. Same patient as in *D*. Vesiculation produced by marked edema in skin lesions simulated an acute contact dermatitis.

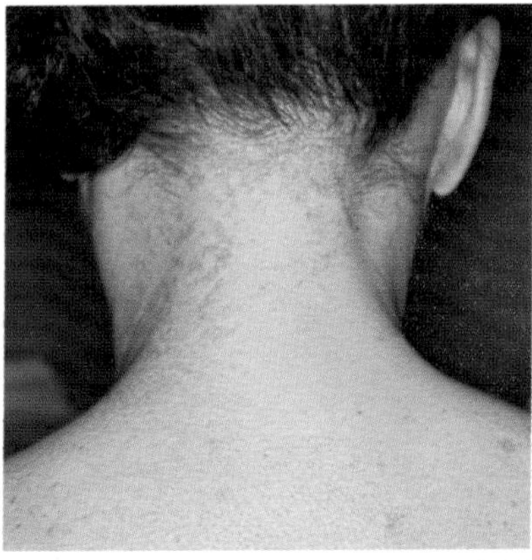

F, Dermatomyositis. Erythema along the hairline.

aspects of the arms, axillae, lateral surfaces of the trunk, and the areas below the waist are generally spared. The centers of the annular lesions are often telangiectatic and hypopigmented with a grayish color. The borders are red, have a superficial scale, and in my experience are slightly elevated. Although these lesions may be present for many years, they do not lead to significant dermal atrophy after resolution. However, the hypopigmentation and telangiectasia persist for prolonged periods, although repigmentation tends to occur eventually. Almost half of their 27 patients had clinical and serological evidence of mild systemic involvement — arthralgias, fever, malaise. Central nervous system involvement occurred in 19 per cent but was not severe. Renal disease was present in 11 per cent and was mild. Sontheimer et al. propose that patients with subacute cutaneous LE are a subset who generally have an illness intermediate in severity between discoid LE and severe systemic LE.

Alopecia is an extremely important marker (Fig. 7–25; Plate 18*B*). Hair may be lost in single or multiple patches that are well-demarcated and exhibit the classic changes of LE: atrophy, erythema, scaling, telangiectasia, and plugging. These lesions are often discovered by the hairdresser or barber. Scarring alopecia is so characteristic of LE that such lesions must be considered those of LE until proved otherwise.

In the differential diagnosis, a previous bacterial infection of the scalp must be ruled out. Infection by the fungus *Trichophyton tonsurans* may closely mimic the alopecia of LE. Alopecia areata is distinguished by the absence of erythema, atrophy, and scaling in a well-circumscribed area of hair loss. Pseudopelade, a rare noninflammatory alopecia with atrophy, could be confused with an inactive atrophic LE lesion. Infrequently, sarcoidosis and metastatic carcinoma produce scarring alopecia. A biopsy would determine the correct diagnosis in these situations.

Diffuse thinning of the scalp hair can be seen in LE. If the patient becomes very ill, a generalized shedding of scalp hair may ensue about three months later, because the stress of acute illness has caused the germinative cells in many of the hair bulbs to pass prematurely from the anagen (growing) phase into the telogen (resting) phase. When the anagen phase resumes three months later, the new growing hairs expel the old resting hairs that have been retained in the follicles, producing a temporary alopecia (telogen effluvium). The same mechanism is responsible for the transient alopecia following pregnancy and any severe febrile illness, drug reaction, or emotional stress.

However, diffuse thinning of the hair sometimes occurs in the normal-appearing scalp of a patient with LE who is not severely ill. In two of our patients, a biopsy of the scalp revealed microscopic lesions of LE. On the other hand, the entire scalp in LE may show redness, scaling, and scattered areas of atrophy. The presence of atrophy rules out a severe seborrheic dermatitis of the scalp, which may also be associated with thinning hair..

A receding frontal hairline with broken hairs has been dubbed "lupus hair" (Fig. 7–26). Increased fragility of the hair from unknown causes produces this disheveled appearance.

Although telangiectasia is a very important feature of LE lesions, it is significant in its own right. Three types of vascular changes are reliable signs of connective tissue disease: linear telangiectasia at the base of the

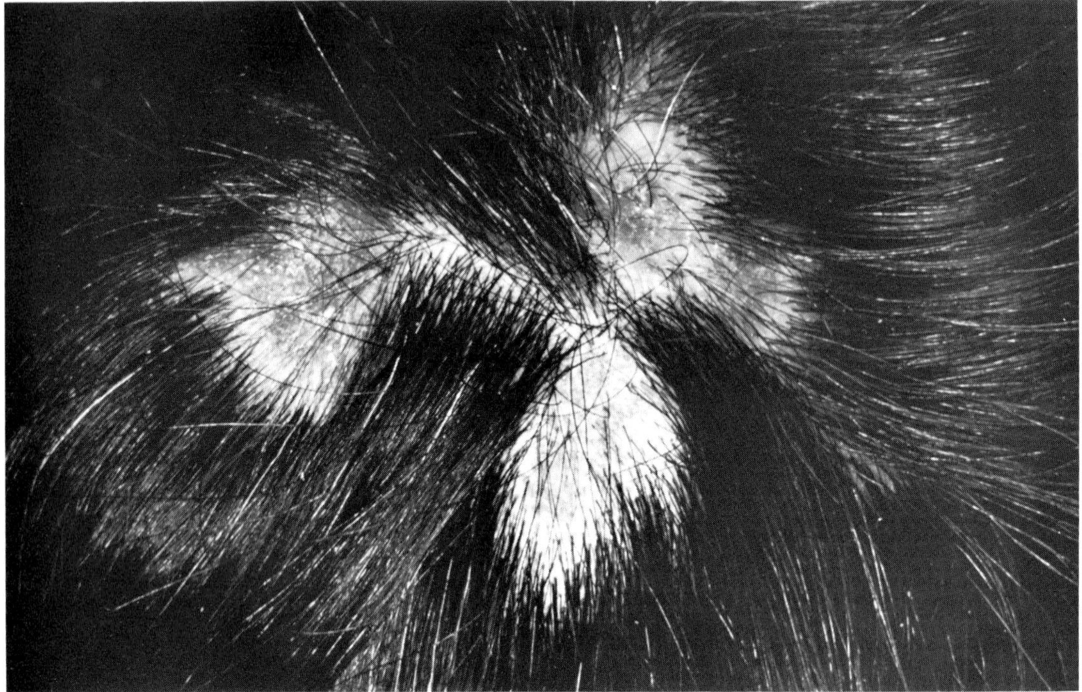

Figure 7–25. LE. Scarring alopecia showing the characteristic erythema, atrophy, scaling, and telangiectasia.

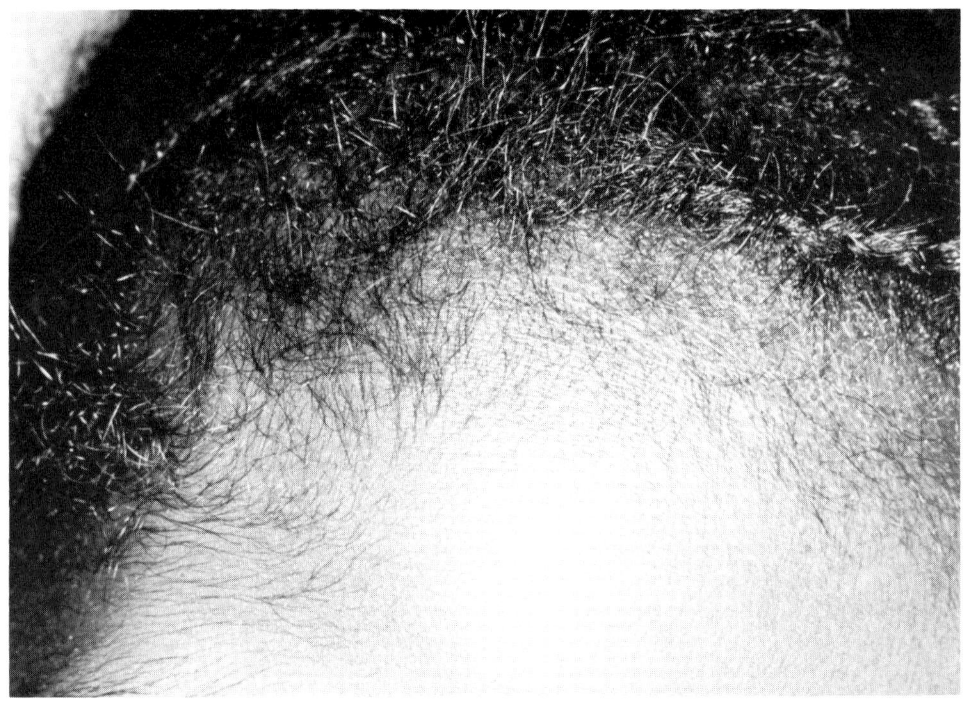

Figure 7–26. Lupus hair. Receding frontal hairline with broken hairs.

nail, erythematous polyangular macules, and palmar-digital papular telangiectasia.

In most cases of systemic LE, scleroderma, and dermatomyositis, short linear telangiectases are visible in the posterior nail fold and contiguous cuticle (Plate 18*C*). The telangiectases are sometimes seen only in the cuticles. These dilated vessels represent the capillary loops of the dermal papillae, which are oriented parallel to the skin surface in these sites and are abnormally enlarged so that they can be seen without the aid of a capillary microscope. Within the cuticle, the telangiectatic vessels often become thrombosed, producing black rather than red lines. In LE and dermatomyositis, the periungual skin at the base of the nail is usually diffusely red as well. Linear telangiectasia on the posterior nail fold and cuticle is seen in only four diseases: LE, dermatomyositis, scleroderma, and rheumatoid arthritis. It probably does not occur in more than 5 per cent of cases of rheumatoid arthritis. Trauma rarely produces such changes. Only one hand or only one or two fingers may be affected. A hand lens may be needed to see linear telangiectasia in its earliest stage.

In blond, fair-skinned individuals, the capillaries normally present on the posterior nailfold can sometimes be seen, but they are easily distinguished from those observed in the connective tissue disorders because they are thinner, less red, and not thrombosed.

Telangiectasia may assume the form of flat, red, irregular, and polyangular lesions which are found primarily on the face and hands. Such lesions are called telangiectatic mats and are seen almost exclusively in scleroderma (Plates 20*F* and 21). However, I have seen them develop in a patient with sclerodermatomyositis after the myositis underwent remission and the sclerodermatous features of Raynaud's phenomenon and sclerodactyly developed. I have also seen several such lesions on the fingertips of two patients with systemic LE (Fig. 7–27). Many such lesions in an individual should alert the physician to the possibility of an underlying connective tissue disorder.

Discrete papular telangiectasia on the palms and fingers is a characteristic sign of systemic LE (Plate 18*D*; Fig. 7–28). Palmar erythema of liver disease and pregnancy is not papular and does not extend onto the fingers as it does in LE. We have biopsied the palmar lesions in four patients with systemic LE. In two, a necrotizing (leukocytoclastic) angiitis was found. IgG and C3 were found in the vascular walls by direct immunofluorescence. In the other two, only dilated telangiectatic vessels without inflammatory cells or other histologic abnormalities were present. All four patients had clinically identical-appearing lesions which had been present for one to three weeks.

In the absence of scaling, induration, and epidermal atrophy, ordinary telangiectasia consisting of discrete dilated vessels on the cheeks, nose, or elsewhere on the body should not be used as an indicator of connective tissue disease.

Diffuse erythema, with or without scaling, is sometimes observed over the interphalangeal and large joints and the periorbital tissues. However, these changes are much more commonly associated with dermatomyositis than with LE.

Necrotizing vasculitis involving the dermal vessels is common in systemic LE and may be accompanied by cryoglobulins of the mixed

PLATE 20

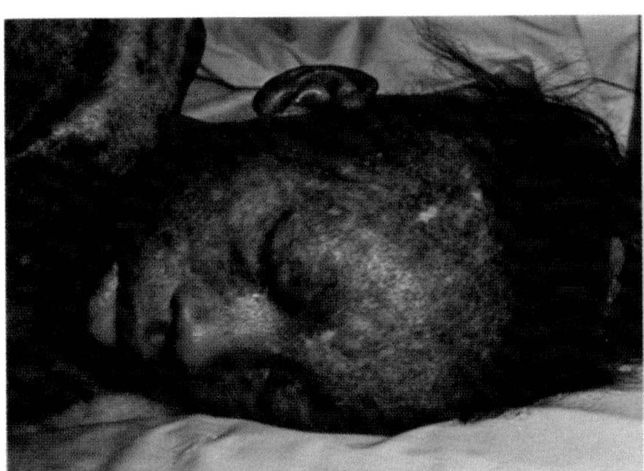

A, Dermatomyositis. Poikilodermatous phase of skin lesion.

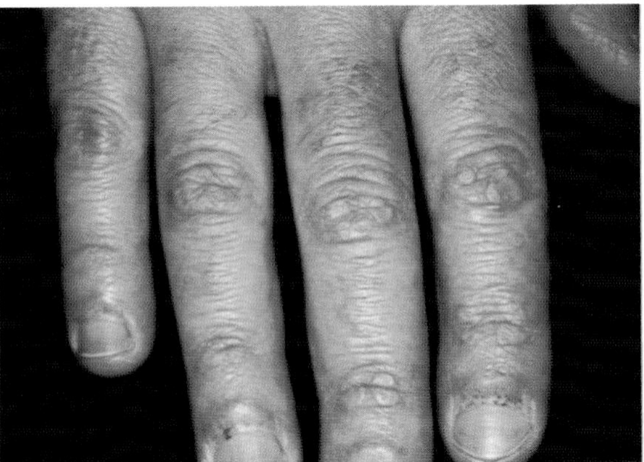

B, Dermatomyositis. Gottron's sign. Flat-topped violaceous papules over knuckles are a pathognomonic sign of dermatomyositis. Cuticular telangiectasia is also present in this patient.

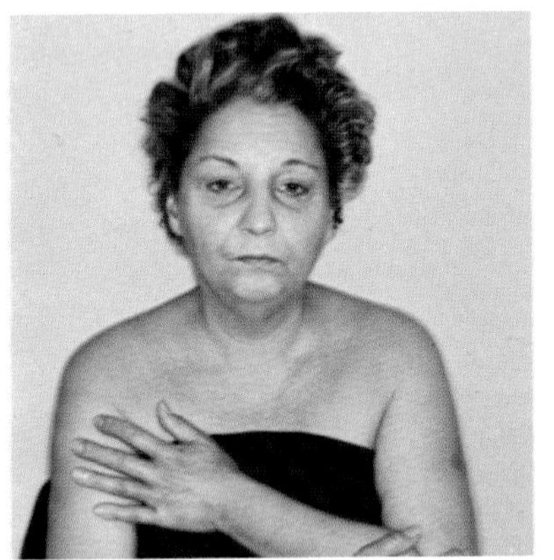

C, Scleroderma. Addisonian hyperpigmentation. Skin has not yet become sclerotic.

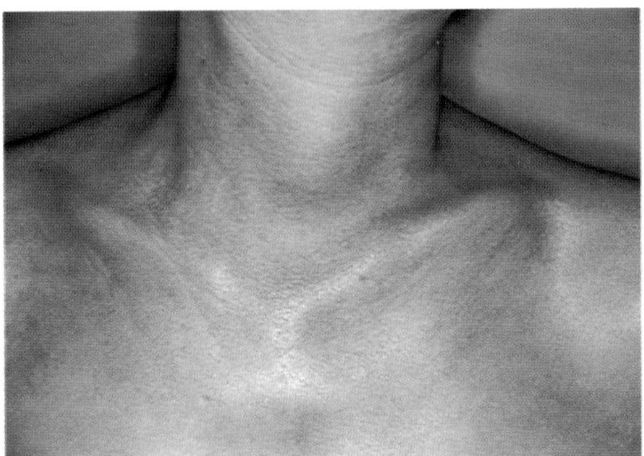

D, Scleroderma. Diffuse variety of scleroderma which begins centrally on chest.

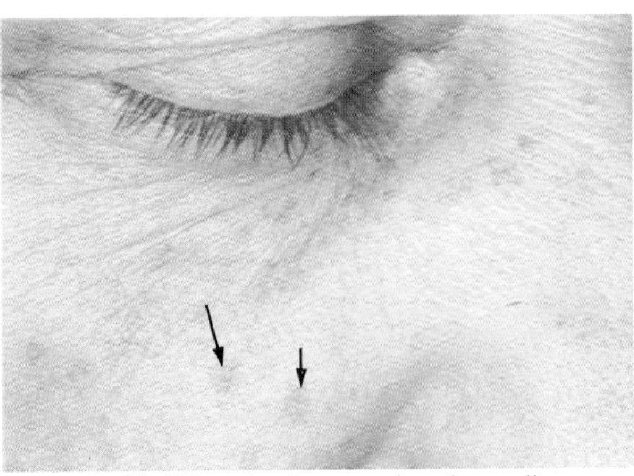

E, Undifferentiated connective tissue disease. Two faint red polyangular mats are present above the nasolabial fold (arrows).

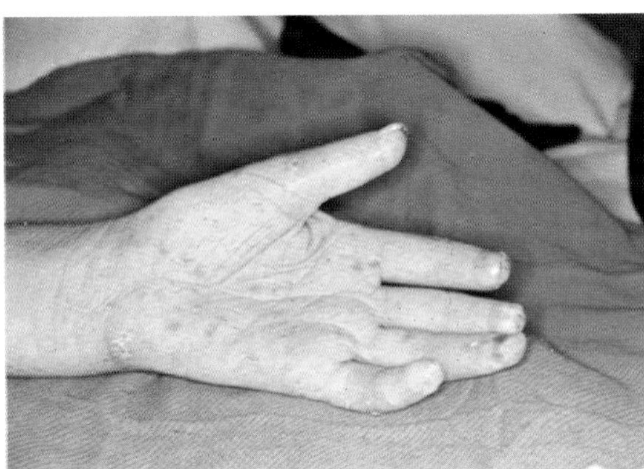

F, Scleroderma. Polyangular telangiectatic mats characteristic of scleroderma. Sclerodactyly also present.

PLATE 21

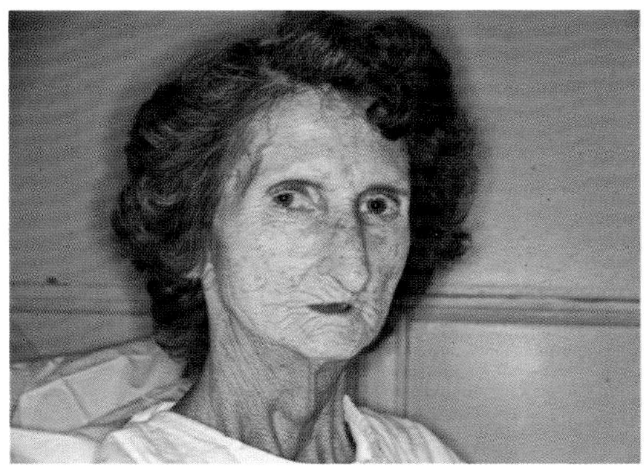

A, Scleroderma. Pinched facies caused by shrinkage of tissues, not cutaneous sclerosis. Telangiectatic mats on face.

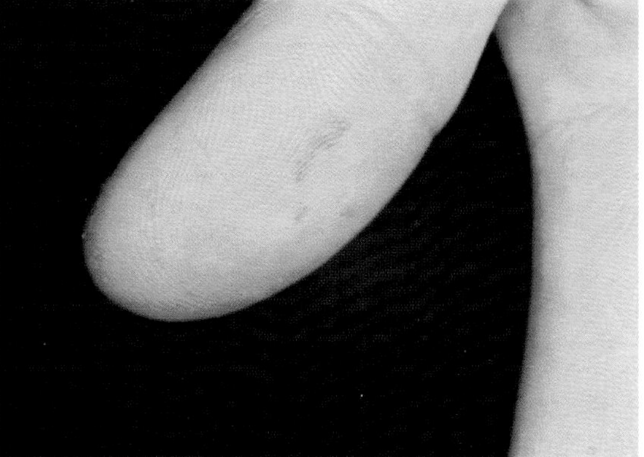

B, Scleroderma. Telangiectatic mats.

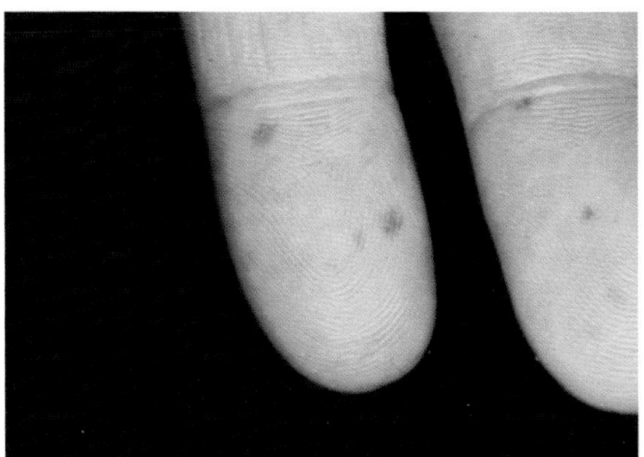

C, Scleroderma. Telangiectatic mats.

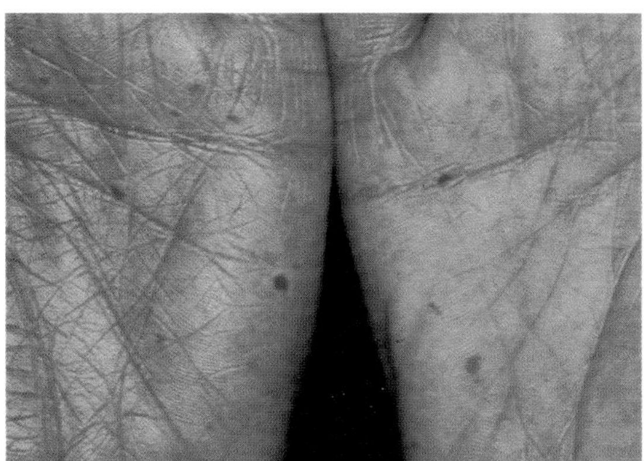

D, Scleroderma. Telangiectatic mats.

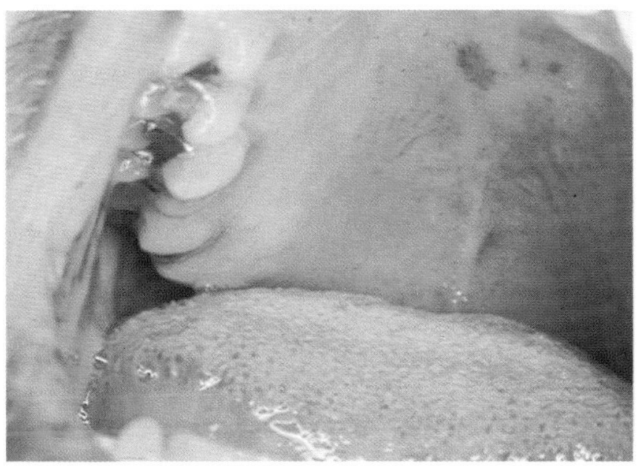

E, Scleroderma. Telangiectatic mats on palate.

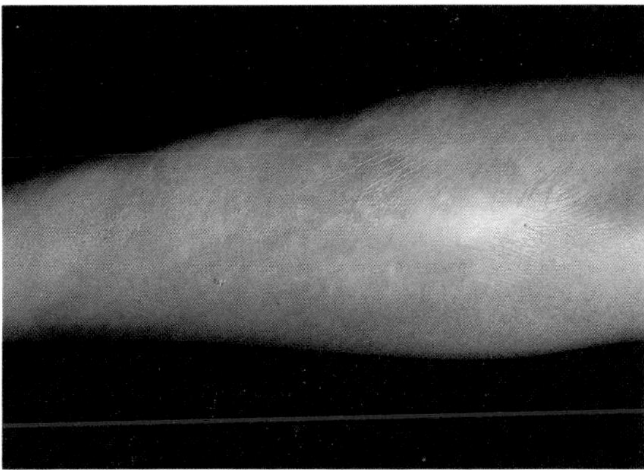

F, Morphea. Indurated plaque with typical yellow-ivory color on arm.

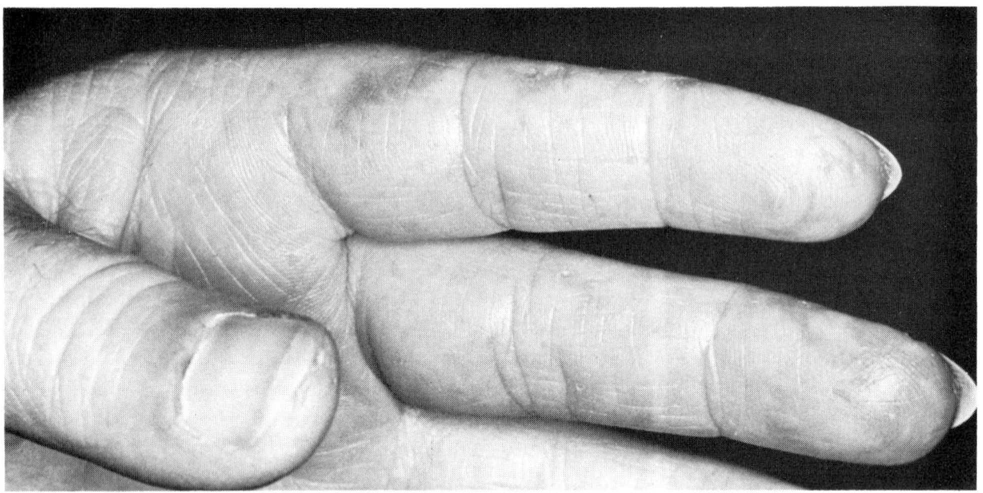

Figure 7–27. LE. Telangiectatic mats. Rare manifestation of LE.

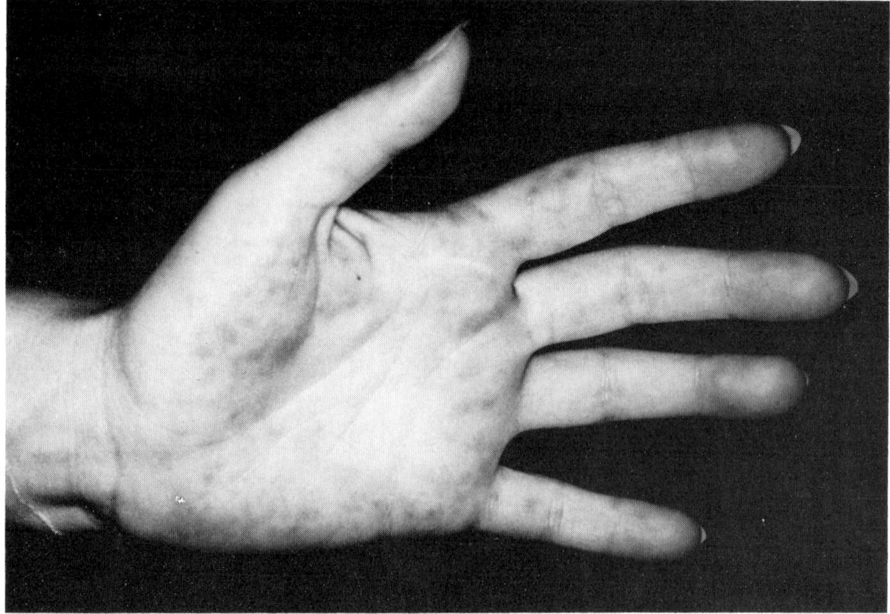

Figure 7–28. LE. Discrete papular telangiectasia on palms and fingers is characteristic sign of SLE.

type. The cutaneous lesions are identical to those found in leukocytoclastic angiitis and include palpable purpura, hemorrhagic bullae, and ulcerations (see Chapter 8). A special presentation of vasculitis in LE is livedo reticularis with ulceration. Livedo reticularis is a persistent reddish-blue to cyanotic-appearing reticulated vascular pattern that may be present on the trunk and extremities (see p. 437). Although it may occur in young children and adults without obvious cause (cutis marmorata), its association with ulcerations of the leg is often a sign of an underlying small or large vessel vasculitis. The vasculitic changes are found only in the ulcers. The reticulation is produced by slowing of the blood flow in the superficial capillaries secondary to vasospasm of the underlying arterioles.[25] These two vasculitic presentations may precede the appearance of serologic and other diagnostic evidence of LE by several years.

Figure 7–29 illustrates erythematous and purulent nodules on the buttocks which were initially misdiagnosed as a staphylococcal pyoderma but were subsequently shown to be a small vessel (leukocytoclastic) angiitis. The patient also had erythematous papules on the fingers (Fig. 7–30). These lesions were the presenting feature of systemic LE in this patient. Fever, polyarthritis of the hands and knees, a normochromic normocytic anemia, and positive antinuclear antibody completed the clinical picture.

Raynaud's phenomenon occurs in 30 per cent of cases of LE and may precede the onset of the disease by months or years, as it does in scleroderma. Raynaud's phenonemon is also a feature of dermatomyositis. Digital gangrene and ulceration may be produced by severe Raynaud's phenomenon in any of the three connective tissue disorders, although this complication is most frequently found in scleroderma. Focal digital gangrene (Fig. 7–31) can also be produced by necrotizing angiitis. Figures 7–32 and 7–33 show digital gangrene in a 15-year-old girl with

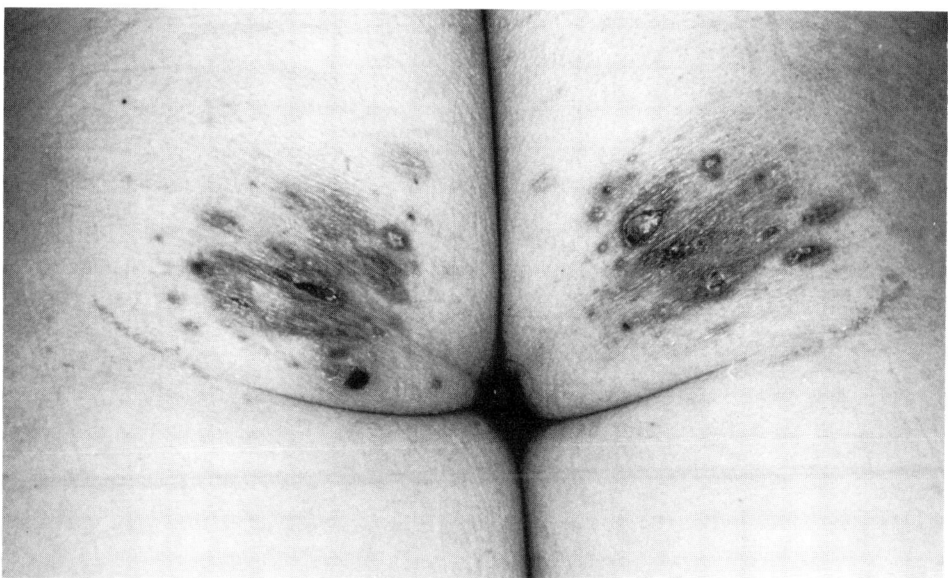

Figure 7–29. LE. Leukocytoclastic vasculitis on buttocks produced erythematous and purulent nodules simulating staphylococcal pyoderma

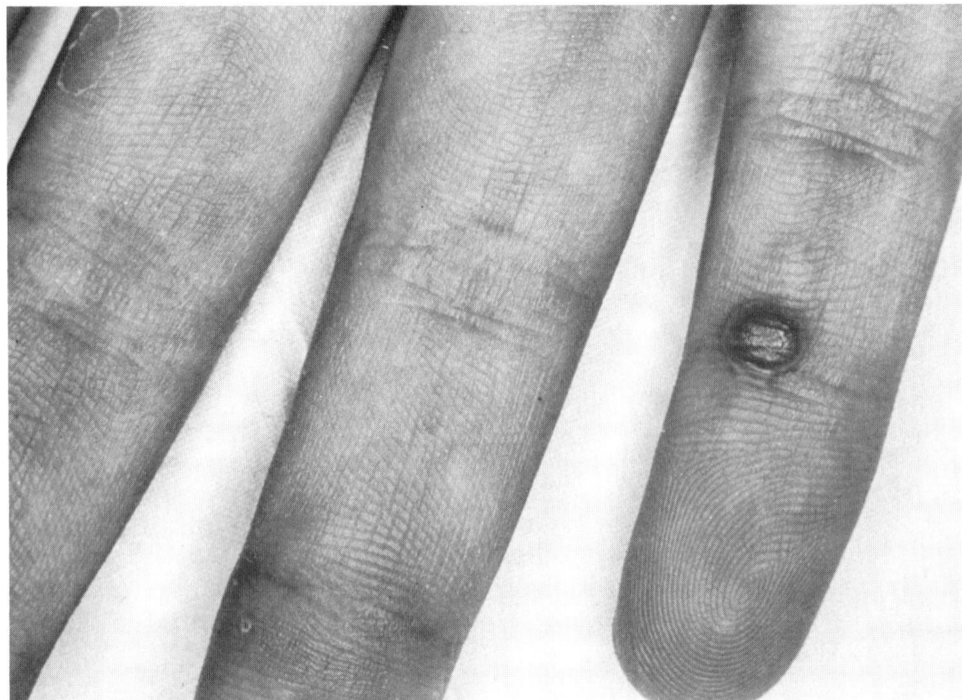

Figure 7–30. LE. Erythematous papules on fingers produced by leukocytoclastic vasculitis in patient shown in Figure 7–29.

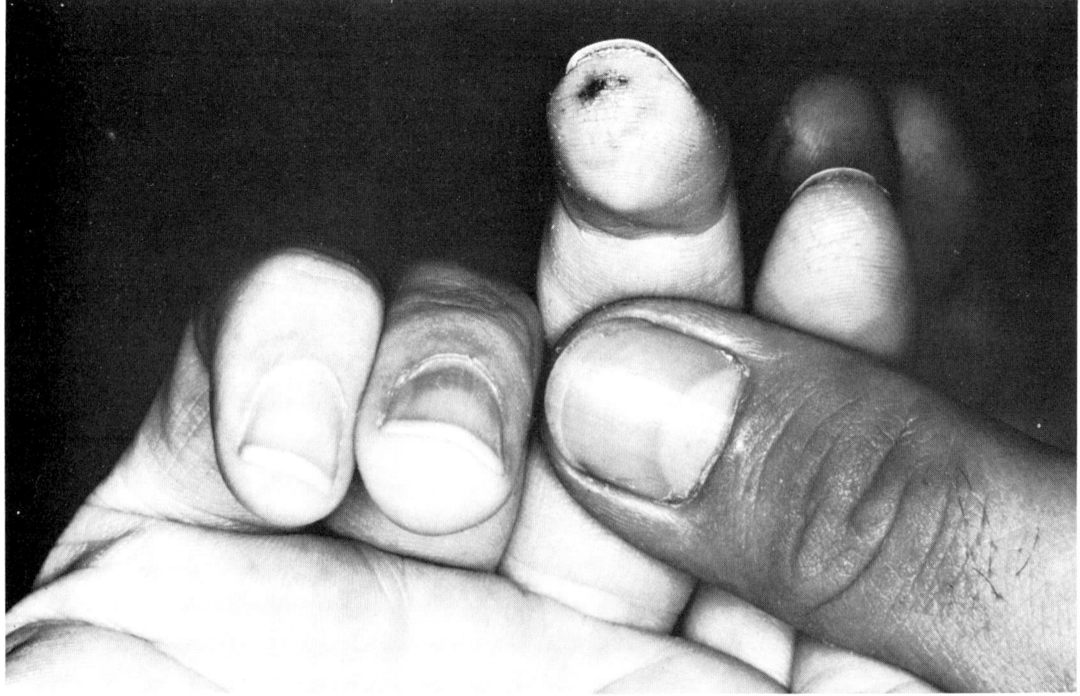

Figure 7–31. LE. Focal digital gangrene produced by an arteritis occurring during the course of LE.

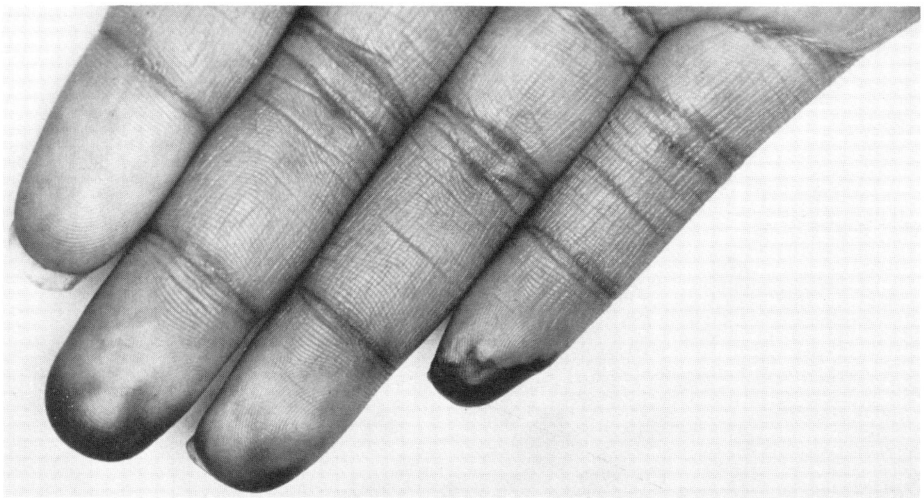

Figure 7–32. LE. Digital gangrene produced by chronic vasospasm of brachial arteries.

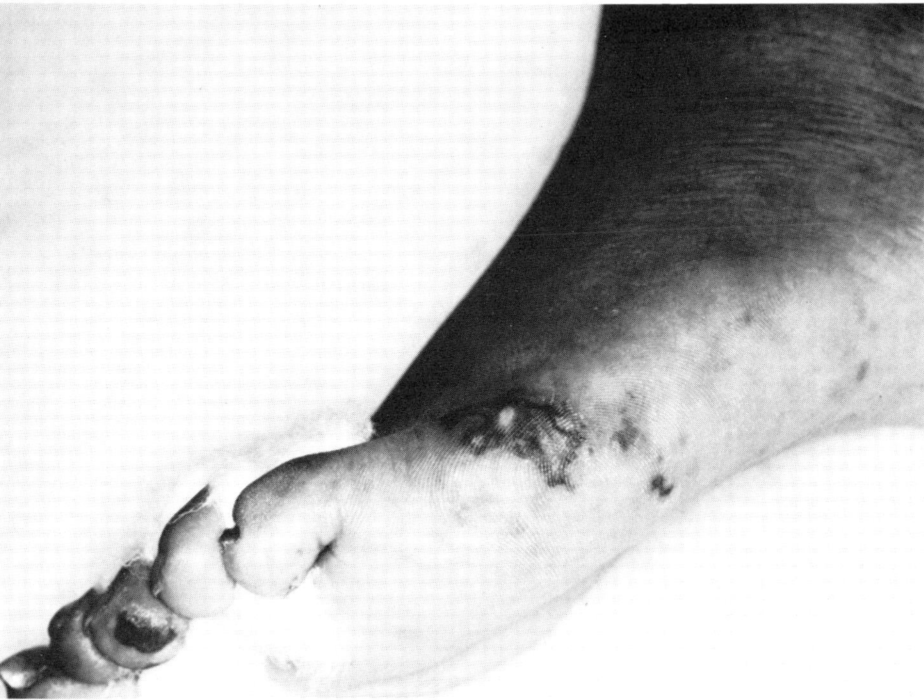

Figure 7–33. LE. Gangrene of feet and toes secondary to chronic vasospasm of femoral arteries in patient shown in Figure 7–32.

systemic LE; the gangrene was produced by chronic vasospasm of the brachial arteries as demonstrated by an arteriogram. Gangrene of the toes developed secondary to vasospasm of the femoral arteries. These complications developed while she was in the hospital and asymptomatic from her Raynaud's phenomenon. Chronic vasospasm of arteries in the extremities should be considered in the differential diagnosis of conditions producing digital gangrene.

Chilblain, or pernio, has also been responsible for producing slightly tender, cyanotic to reddish-blue nodules on the toes of three of our patients with systemic LE. The lesions developed during the winter and disappeared in the summer, only to recur in the following winters. Chilblain represents cold-induced, chronic vasospasm of digital vessels akin to Raynaud's phenomenon and should not be confused with necrotizing vasculitis (see Chapter 8). Millard and Rowell observed that chilblain was present in 17 of their 150 patients. The fingers, toes, heels, and calves were affected.[26] Although 3 of the 17 patients developed systemic involvement 5, 8, and 18 years after the onset of cutaneous LE, there were no data to suggest that the appearance of chilblain could be used as a prognostic indicator in this disorder.

Urticaria has been found in 7 to 22 per cent of the cases of LE in four large series[3, 27-29] and is often related to increased activity of the disease. Angioneurotic edema of the face and limbs can also occur. Chronic urticaria may be the presenting manifestation of LE but is uncommon. Erythema multiforme may also be an expression of increased disease activity in LE. Although erythema nodosum has been reported,[30] it is not clear whether it was a manifestation of LE or a coincidental association. In our experience erythema nodosum has not been associated with LE.

O'Loughlin et al. have recently re-examined the phenomenon of urticarial lesions in systemic LE.[28] They found that in 11 of 12 cases in which the urticarial lesions were biopsied, 9 disclosed a necrotizing vasculitis. In addition, immunoglobulins and complement were present at the dermal-epidermal junction in all, and in the dermal blood vessels in 50 per cent of the biopsy specimens. They also found immunoreactants in the dermal blood vessels in 50 per cent of biopsies from uninvolved skin. This is not surprising, because Braverman and Yen demonstrated that in patients with necrotizing angiitis, circulating immune complexes can be found in normal-appearing skin by direct immunofluorescence and electron microscopy.[31] Although palpable purpura is the most common manifestation of necrotizing vasculitis, in a small percentage of individuals nonpurpuric urticarial lesions are observed.[32] Thus, it appears that urticaria in systemic LE is usually the cutaneous expression of the underlying circulating immune complexes and not simply a manifestation of the ordinary variety of chronic urticaria, which is characterized by a banal, sparse, perivascular lymphocytic infiltrate.

Both clear and hemorrhagic blisters arising from urticarial bases may appear during the active phase of systemic LE. In one case, the hemorrhagic blisters were found to contain LE cells,[33] and in another case, hematoxylin bodies.[34] Although about 30 cases of bullous LE to date have been reported in the literature,[34] only a few presented data adequate to determine the nature of these bullous dermatoses. It is clear that in some cases, the hydropic degeneration of the basal cell layer plus the upper dermal edema was severe enough to produce a subepidermal blister with elevation of the epidermis.[35] This would be a true instance of bullous LE. We have seen such examples in three patients who had urticarial lesions surmounted by small bullae that could be confused with erythema multiforme or bullous pemphigoid.

However, six cases of bullous LE described in the literature have been reported as showing either intraepidermal blisters without acantholysis[27, 33, 34] or subepidermal blister formation.[36-38] In the latter category, the histology was said to be compatible with either erythema multiforme or bullous pemphigoid. Circulating antibodies to the basement membrane zone of the epidermis were present in one case,[36] absent in a second,[37] and not evaluated in a third (case 3[38]). Immunoreactants were present at the dermal-epidermal junction in the first two cases, but were not studied in the third case. The first case satisfies the diagnostic criteria for bullous pemphigoid.[36] The second case,[37] although labeled bullous LE, provided no histologic evidence for that diagnosis. The immunofluorescent findings in the second case could just as easily support a diagnosis of erythema multiforme arising in the otherwise normal skin of a patient with systemic LE where a postive band test is frequently found.[22] A diagnosis in the third case cannot be made because of insufficient data. The pathogenesis and significance of the intraepidermal blisters in three cases are unknown. More information is needed to understand the lesions of bullous LE.

An unusual bullous eruption was seen in one of our patients with systemic LE.

In 1963, an 18-year-old white woman was diagnosed as having cutaneous LE on her face. No systemic disease was detected and the eruption spontaneously disappeared after a time. In 1969, immediately postpartum, she developed acute pericarditis with effusion and lupus nephritis confirmed by renal biopsy. She was treated with prednisone and azathioprine. In 1972, she began to develop recurrent episodes of bullae which arose from urticarial plaques. Biopsies showed the histological changes of erythema multiforme. Initially the eruption was controlled by prednisone and she enjoyed remissions from her blistering disease for a few weeks at a time. With each new episode, the eruption became more extensive and severe. In January, 1973, the eruption developed a new quality. Minor trauma induced blisters that broke easily and spread to produce larger denuded areas of skin. She was referred to the Yale-New Haven Medical Center in May, 1973, at which time 40 per cent of her skin surface was denuded because of the traumatically induced bullae. Biopsies again showed the histology of erythema multiforme. There was no evidence of necrotizing vasculitis or lupus erythematosus. Immunofluorescent studies were not performed. Porphyria cutanea tarda was excluded by normal urinary porphyrin studies. She was treated as a burn patient because of the extensive denudation (Fig. 7–34), but new bullae continued to erupt. Two weeks after admission she developed gram-negative sepsis and a shock lung. She died of cardiac arrest.

The bullous eruption in this patient seemed to be erythema multiforme at the onset but later assumed features of epidermolysis bullosa and toxic epidermal necrolysis. Drugs did not seem to be implicated in the etiology of this eruption. This case report is included because of the unusual course and behavior of the bullous eruption.

Purpura and petechiae occur and may be related to thrombocytopenia, to vasculitis, or, in treated cases, to prolonged steroid therapy. Petechiae may appear on the hard palate in patients with thrombocytopenia.

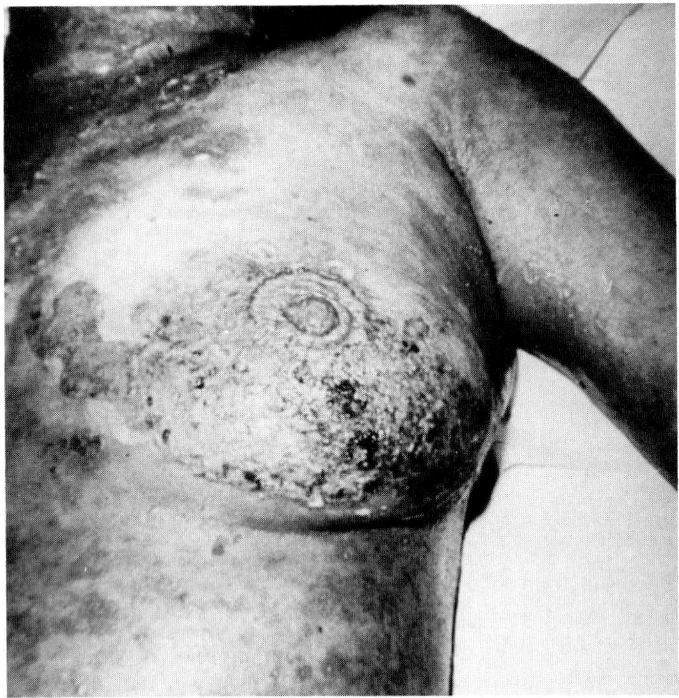

Figure 7–34. Unusual blistering disease with features of toxic epidermal necrolysis and epidermolysis bullosa in a patient with SLE.

Calcinosis cutis, which had not been thought to occur in LE, has been reported at least 11 times since 1961. Soft tissue calcification developed in subcutaneous tissue, muscle, and periarticular structures in patients with longstanding disease (average duration 9.8 years).[39]

Although the arthritis of LE is usually nondeforming, in some instances it resembles rheumatoid arthritis and may be associated with transient subcutaneous nodules about the proximal interphalangeal joints, elbows, dorsa of the wrists, extensor surfaces of the extremities, and occiput. The nodules, which are usually nontender and cartilaginous in consistency, have the histologic features of a rheumatoid nodule. These nodules have also been observed on the palm and fingers.[40]

Figures 7–35 and 7–36 show subcutaneous nodules in a patient with systemic LE and arthritis. The nodules were present on the face, hands, and flexor and extensor surfaces of the forearms. They disappeared following therapy with antimalarial drugs.

Sjögren's syndrome has been associated with LE as well as with scleroderma and dermatomyositis. Thrombophlebitis also has been considered an associated feature of LE. A few patients have exhibited generalized hyperpigmentation. LE lesions can arise in areas of trauma (Koebner phenomenon). Curiously, though, this phenomenon happens only in sun-exposed areas of the skin.[41]

In summary, most of the skin markings of LE are either specific for this disease or for a connective tissue disorder. Only a minority of patients with LE have nonspecific features such as leg ulcers, purpura, and thrombophlebitis.[27]

Although an abnormal immune mechanism is thought to play a

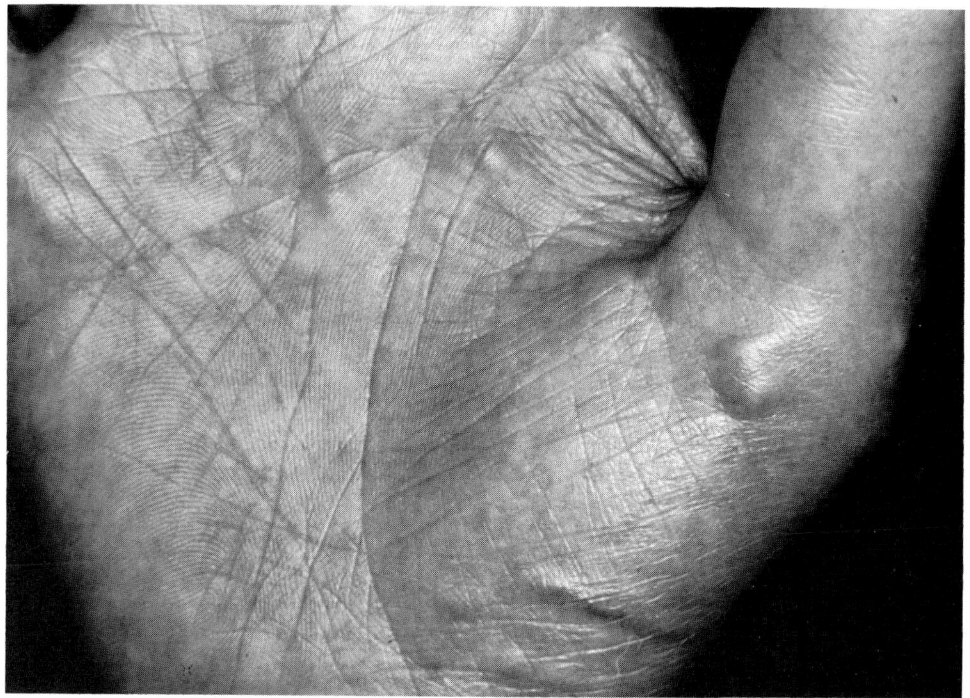

Figure 7–35. LE. Subcutaneous rheumatoid nodules on palm.

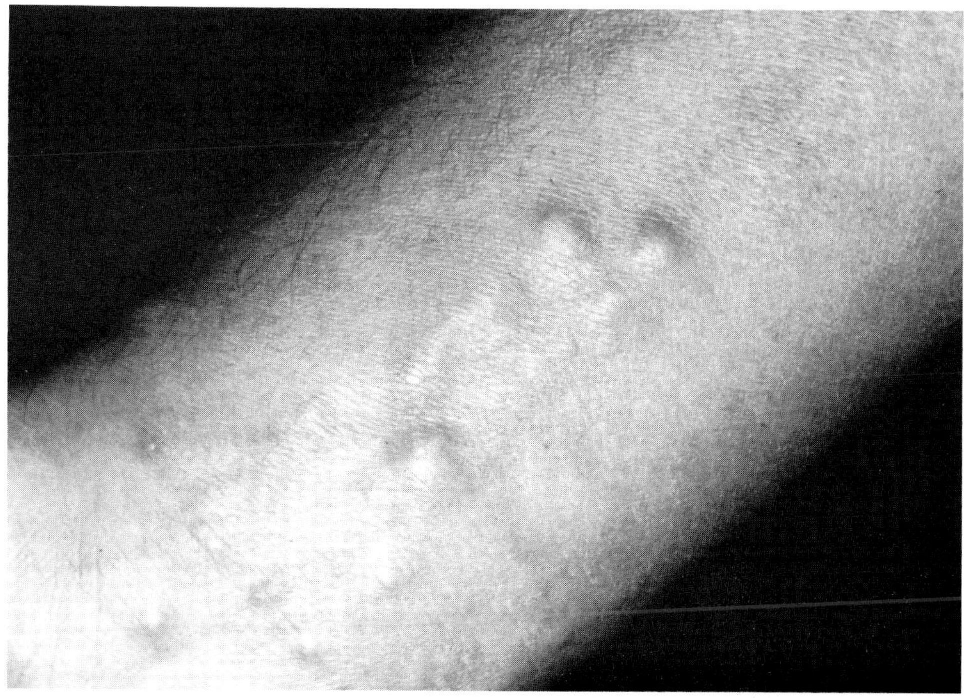

Figure 7–36. LE. Subcutaneous rheumatoid nodules on flexor forearm.

decisive role in the pathogenesis of LE, several factors may exacerbate the disease. Recognition and control of these factors will prove helpful in the management and therapy of LE. Drug reactions may initiate or exacerbate the disease. The onset may be associated with pregnancy, usually either in the first trimester or post partum. Major surgical procedures also can exacerbate the disease process.

Photosensitivity reactions are common and important (Fig. 7–37). Many patients with LE exhibit photosensitivity at some time during the course of illness. The fact that sun sensitivity is not a presenting feature or an early sign in the disease does not mean that it will never be a problem. Photosensitivity reactions include the production of specific atrophic scaling plaques, fixed urticarial plaques, transient urticarial papules, and a persistent violaceous flush over the face and V of the neck. Any exposed area of skin may be affected. The lesions may persist for hours, days, or weeks.

The cutaneous lesions are not a serious problem in themselves. However, photosensitivity reactions may cause a fatal exacerbation of the disease. All patients with LE must protect themselves against sunlight whether or not they have a history of photosensitivity. If possible, potentially photosensitizing drugs, such as phenothiazines and chlorothiazides, should not be used.

Although most photosensitive patients react to the sunburn (UV-B) portion of the ultraviolet spectrum, some are sensitive to the blue-green radiation emitted by fluorescent lamps.[42] Photosensitivity reactions tend to crop up in summer and early fall rather than in the spring; reactions occurring in the spring are characteristic of the polymorphous light

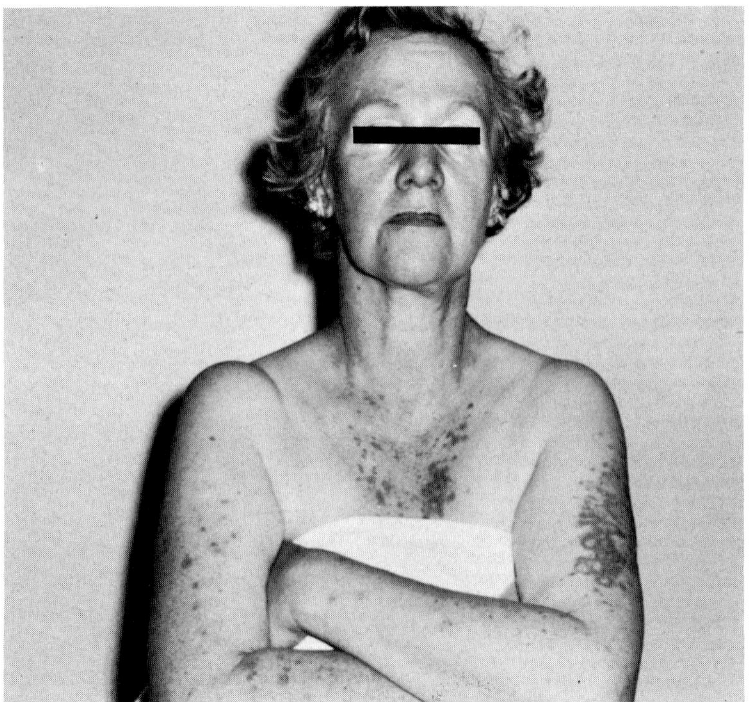

Figure 7–37. LE. Patient with photosensitivity. Discoid lesions developed in sun-exposed areas after each episode of photosensitivity.

reactor. The importance of photosensitivity reactions in a patient may often be judged by determining the extent of lesions on the sun-exposed, versus the covered, parts of the body.

In the differential diagnosis of the urticarial plaque of LE, two disorders must be considered: polymorphous light eruption and benign lymphocytic infiltration of skin (Jessner's syndrome). Polymorphous light eruption is a true physical allergy. Susceptible individuals react to the first strong rays of sunlight each year, usually in March or April. As spring and summer progress and as a tan is acquired, these individuals usually become less reactive to the sun. The urticarial plaque form of this disorder is clinically indistinguishable from that of LE. Polymorphous light reactors can also develop eczematous lesions. However, this pattern is not seen in LE and does not enter into the differential diagnosis. Biopsy of the urticarial plaque is not always helpful in distinguishing between LE and polymorphous light eruptions because of the very similar, and at times identical, histologic features.

The histopathologic features of the skin lesions in LE are hyperkeratosis, epidermal atrophy, hydropic degeneration of the basal cell layer, and a lymphocytic infiltrate in the dermis around the blood vessels and appendages. The histologic changes of light eruptions are usually characterized by perivascular lymphocytic infiltration and parakeratosis *and a normal-appearing epidermis.* In some instances, however, LE may show parakeratosis, and light eruptions may show epidermal atrophy and hydropic degeneration of the basal cell layer. It is sometimes necessary to observe a patient for several seasons before it is possible to decide whether the person has LE or a polymorphous light eruption. Nail fold or mat telangiectasia or mucous membrane lesions would be helpful signs if they were present. The finding of immunoreactants at the dermal-epidermal junction and the deposition of increased amounts of acid mucopolysaccharides in the dermis would establish the diagnosis of LE over a light eruption.[22, 23]

Benign lymphocytic infiltration of skin (Jessner) poses other problems. This is a relatively new clinical entity, and it is a syndrome rather than a specific disease. The typical marking is an asymptomatic discrete *pink* to *reddish-brown* papule or plaque which tends to extend peripherally, leaving a clear center (Plate 17*C*). Single or multiple lesions of firm consistency may be present. Their surface is smooth, and their disappearance is not associated with scarring. They are usually located on the face, but they may be found elsewhere, lasting from a few weeks to many years and resolving spontaneously. The *nonviolaceous* color, the lack of atrophy and scaling, and the configuration distinguish these lesions from those of LE. A dense perivascular lymphocytic infiltrate in the dermis and a normal-appearing epidermis (changes closely resembling polymorphous light eruption) are the histopathologic features of this disorder. The annular lesions produced by Jessner's syndrome are mimicked only rarely by LE. In a recent study from the Mayo Clinic, 9 of 23 patients with this syndrome believed that their lesions were related to sun exposure.[43] Two of the nine had LE, and this eruption of Jessner's disease appeared during the course of LE. The other 7 were thought to have a light sensitivity. The remaining 14 patients had lesions that lasted from 2 weeks to 30 years and were unrelated to sun exposure. We have also seen a patient with typical lesions of Jessner's syndrome (confirmed by biopsy) on the elbows and typical lesions of LE located elsewhere. It is clear that Jessner's syndrome may be evoked by sunlight, may occur during the course of LE, and may also act as a disorder *sui generis*.

In the differential diagnosis of facial erythematous plaques and papules with and without atrophy, three other conditions in addition to LE, light eruptions, and Jessner's syndrome have to be considered: lupus vulgaris, granuloma faciale, and sarcoidosis.

Lupus vulgaris produces much more scarring and atrophy than does LE. It usually begins as a solitary papule or nodule that slowly extends peripherally leaving a scarring atrophic center resembling radiodermatitis. At the periphery of the lesion, one can see smooth yellow-brown nodules by means of diascopy. In this procedure a glass slide is pressed on the granulomatous nodules; this obliterates their superficial vascular supply and demonstrates their characteristic apple-jelly color. Fortunately this disease is now rare in the United States (see Chapter 18).

Granuloma façiale is characterized by smooth nonatrophic *reddish-brown* papules and nodules that are found almost exclusively on the face (Plate 17*D*). The basic abnormality is a vasculitis with eosinophils and mononuclear cells surrounding the vessels. The etiology of granuloma faciale is unknown. It behaves as a benign disease.[44]

Sarcoidosis may show purplish plaques and papules without scale or atrophy. These three disorders can be easily differentiated by histologic examination.

Seborrheic dermatitis should not be confused with LE. Yellow greasy scales with variable erythema are seen in the nasolabial folds, about the eyes, ears, hairline, eyebrows, and lid margins. Atrophy is never present.

Acne rosacea is sometimes mistaken for LE (Plate 17*E*). Although there is telangiectasia over the malar area and nose, it is coarse and not of as fine a quality as that found in LE. The erythematous papular lesions of rosacea tend to be concentrated in the central part of the face. The skin is very oily. There are often pustules — a finding never seen in LE — and a rhinophyma may be present. In early cases of rosacea, the differential diagnosis may be difficult.

Erysipelas may involve the face in a butterfly distribution (Plate 17*F*). Differentiation from LE is easily made by the clinical and laboratory findings of a bacterial infection. The lesion of erysipelas is warm and never shows atrophy, scaling, or telangiectasia.

At least 16 patients have now been described in whom the clinical, histopathologic, and immunofluorescent features of the cutaneous lesions show overlapping features of LE and lichen planus (LP).[45-47] The term LE/LP overlap has been applied to this syndrome because it has not been possible to make an unequivocal diagnosis of either disorder in these patients. An analysis of this syndrome is presented to help clarify the problem.

The cutaneous lesions have been described as *atrophic* patches and plaques which are livid red to violaceous. In at least half of the reported cases, a uniform depigmentation or hypopigmentation also is present in these same areas. The patches and plaques have arisen chiefly on the backs of the hands and feet, including the nailfolds, and on the palms and soles. Much less frequently, they have been present on the trunk, face, and scalp. In a few patients, the plaques have ulcerated or developed transient bullae. The description of the plaques has included terms such as *atrophic, verrucoid,* and *scaling,* which means that the plaques must have had a smooth or irregular surface with varying amounts of scale. Pruritus has not been a feature of the lesions, but pain and tenderness have been present in many. The cutaneous lesions have persisted for as long as 20 years in some individuals, and have generally been refractory to treatment. Two individuals had whitish to red reticulated patches on the oral mucosa. In almost half the patients, the nailplates have been permanently lost.

The striking histologic feature has been a dense bandlike (lichenoid) infiltrate composed of lymphocytes and histiocytes that is closely applied to the dermal-epidermal junction and is associated with changes in the basal cells that have been described as varying from liquefaction degeneration to lysis and dissolution.[45] Immunofluorescent studies have demonstrated ovoid bodies staining for immunoglobulins and complement at the dermal-epidermal junction.

Although it appears to be difficult to make an unequivocal diagnosis of either LE or LP in these patients because the histologic findings strongly suggest LP and the immunofluorescent pattern is consistent with either disease, the overall evidence clearly favors cutaneous LE: none of the affected individuals has had typical lesions of LP elsewhere, but two have had discoid LE lesions of the scalp[45]; histologically, the characteristic "saw tooth" pattern of the epidermis in LP has not been described or illustrated in any report; an increased granular cell layer has been inconstantly present in individual lesions; and the bandlike infiltrate, which has been described as both cell-rich and cell-poor (the former typical of LP and the latter characteristic of LE), varies in its composition within individual lesions and among different lesions from the same patient[45]; although considerable emphasis has been placed on the immunofluorescent pattern involving ovoid bodies, this is a nonspecific finding, since it has also been seen in some cases of dermatomyositis, mycosis fungoides, and fixed drug eruption[48]; in four patients, immunofluorescent studies demonstrated a faint linear band of immunoglobulins and complement characteristic of LE, in addition to ovoid bodies, at the dermal-epidermal junction[45]; one reported case of this overlap syndrome eventually developed systemic LE[46]; and in another patient, the presence of type II cryoglobulins was correlated with activity of the skin lesions.[47] This individual also had a deficiency of C4 for unexplained reasons.

Too much emphasis has been placed on the presence of the bandlike infiltrate and too little on the *absence* of the other histologic features of LP in these cutaneous lesions. In addition, in most cases, the clinical appearance of the cutaneous lesions, either by description or illustration, has been characteristic of LE; only in a minority would there be clinical confusion between hypertrophic LP and LE.

The clinical and histological features of the lesions in the LP/LE syndrome are virtually identical to those of lupus hypertrophicus (Plate 16A). Uitto et al. recently described an additional seven patients with cutaneous LE who had classic discoid lesions on the scalp and face and hypertrophic nodules and plaques on the extremities.[49] They emphasized that the verrucous hyperkeratotic lesions could be nodular or plaque-like with keratinous plugs in the centers, thereby simulating keratoacanthomas or hypertrophic lichen planus. The histopathology and immunofluorescent findings in their patients were identical to those described in the LE/LP syndrome. None of the seven patients had oral or nail involvement or the *atrophic* skin lesions. However, it should be reemphasized that only about half the reported patients have had nail involvement and fewer have had oral lesions. The term *atrophic,* used to describe the cutaneous lesions in the overlap syndrome, is misleading because it was used to describe the surface of plaques and not the presence of macular or flat lesions. Loss of nail plates and nailbed atrophy should not be considered an unacceptable feature of cutaneous LE, since we readily accept the presence of depressed scars in discoid lesions and permanent alopecia in scalp lesions resulting from scarring following lymphocytic infiltration in these sites. Why should the cells of the nail matrix be exempt from permanent damage when the overlying posterior nailfold and contiguous dermis are so floridly involved?

The bandlike infiltrate that mimics one of the histologic features of lichen planus in both lupus hypertrophicus and in the LE/LP overlap may simply be a reflection of the chronicity of the lymphocytic infiltration. The following case report supports this hypothesis.

A 44-year-old white man had been suffering from recurrent episodes of polyarthralgias and polyarthritis associated with crops of painful red plaques and nodules on the hands, feet, fingers, and toes for four years (Figs. 7–38 and 7–39). The central portions of some lesions were hyperkeratotic. Both the joint disease and skin lesions would remit for weeks to months following short courses of oral steroids. Biopsies of three plaques that had been present for six to eight weeks following one of these attacks showed changes compatible with hypertrophic lichen planus. There was no serologic or other cutaneous evidence of LE. Following a remission of nine months produced by oral steroids, he once again developed polyarthritis, including an effusion in the left knee, and cutaneous nodules and plaques. Biopsies from two nodules only five and ten days old revealed the classic

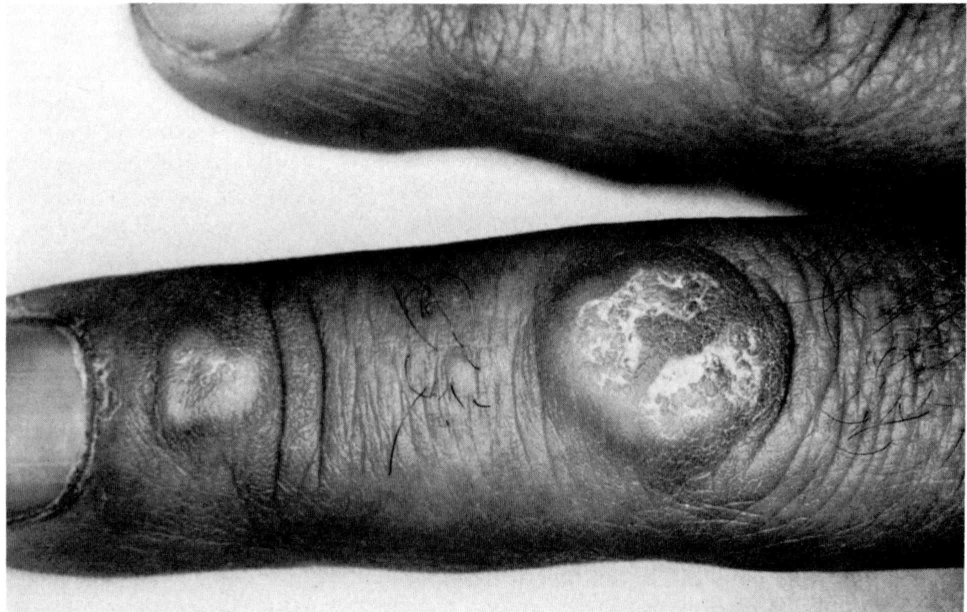

Figure 7–38. LE/LP overlap syndrome. Red plaques and nodules with atrophic scaly surface.

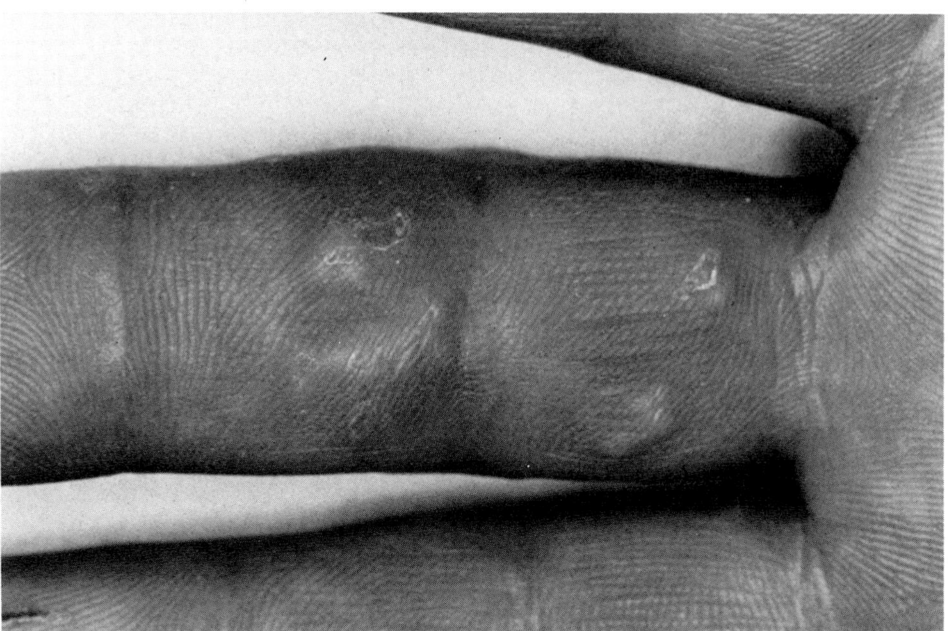

Figure 7–39. LE/LP overlap syndrome.

changes of LE, but not of hypertrophic LP as had been found in the chronic lesions. This case is believed to represent mild systemic LE with joint involvement and the cutaneous lesions of lupus hypertrophicus.

It is highly unlikely that patients with the LE/LP overlap have two diseases, as suggested by Romero et al.[45] However, such a coincidence will be found occasionally, and this may have been the case in Thormann's patient who had unequivocal evidence of LP clinically and histologically, in association with a biological false positive serology, a positive test for rheumatoid factor, and a low titer of antinuclear antibody.[50]

Another example of the confusion between LE and LP is illustrated by the patient shown in Plate 18*E*. This 41-year-old woman had a 20-year history of recurring ulcerations of both soles that developed following a generalized erythroderma occurring after sun exposure. Biopsies of the ulcerations were interpreted as representing LP on one occasion and LE on another. She also had whitish patches on the buccal mucosa which had histologic features suggestive of LP. However, on two separate occasions during her course she developed an erythematous papular eruption on her extremities which showed the histological features of LE. Immunofluorescent studies of the plantar ulceration and the eruption on the extremities revealed neither a fluorescent linear band nor ovoid bodies. Our patient has never exhibited any of the serological abnormalities of LE, but her sister has systemic LE.

Current Concepts

Our understanding of the nature of LE has expanded tremendously during the past decade because of information derived from study of the New Zealand mouse models (NZB, NZB/NZW hybrids) which mimic the human disease in almost every respect. The search for analogous findings in man has resulted in the following current hypotheses for the human disease: viral infections are a possible etiologic factor[51-55] that, in genetically predisposed individuals[56-62] with an altered cellular immunity (reduction in functional activity of suppressor T cells),[63] results in the development of circulating immune complexes of the DNA–anti-DNA type, which produce tissue inflammation and injury.[64, 65] In addition, immunological reactivity is significantly influenced by sex hormones.[66]

A few of the observations and experiments underlying these hypotheses are as follows. In mice, the gene(s) determining complement protein synthesis and resistance to viral infections are closely linked to both the histocompatibility and immune response genes. The major histocompatibility locus (HLA) on chromosome 6 in man is currently thought to be similar to the H-2 region of the mouse.[67-70] A number of genetically determined complement deficiency syndromes have been described, among which C2 deficiency is the most common.[60] Cutaneous LE and mild systemic LE-like syndromes (fever, arthralgias, low incidence and low titers of anti-DNA antibodies, infrequent positive lupus band tests, and rare instances of renal disease) are commonly associated with these complement deficiency syndromes, especially the C2 variety. It is currently proposed that a deficiency of the early components of complement or a deficiency of the postulated closely linked immune response gene(s) or others determining viral resistance may be responsible for the predisposition to the lupus-like syndromes through increased susceptibility to viral infections.[60, 71]

The New Zealand mouse model represents a disorder in which a genetically predisposed host is infected with a type C RNA virus. The virus and its corresponding antibody contribute to the immune deposits in the nephritic kidneys of NZB and NZB/NZW hybrid mice.[72] DNA–anti-DNA antibody complexes also are major contributors to the immune deposits in the nephritic kidneys of these mice.[55] Genetic factors appear to play a significant role in human LE based upon studies involving families and twins.[59] Similarly, environmental factors appear to be acting in concert with genetic predisposition in human LE. Close consanguineous household contacts of patients with LE have a much higher incidence of anti-RNA antibodies than nonconsanguineous household contacts or consanguineous relatives with infrequent patient contact.[51] The presence of these antibodies to double-stranded RNA strengthens the hypothesis that an environmental agent, probably a virus, is important in the pathogenesis of LE.

The clinical observations that women in the childbearing age have a higher prevalence of LE than men have long suggested that sex hormones may play an important role in the development of autoimmunity. Male NZB/NZW hybrids have a significantly longer survival than females, and castration of the male significantly accelerates mortality to the rate found in females.[73] Castration of males in other hybrid mouse strains predisposes to the development of naturally occurring autoantibodies to thymocytes.[58] These murine studies imply that male sex hormones suppress the development of autoimmunity and that castration removes this effect.

A detailed review of the experiments and observations underlying the current concepts of LE is provided in references 51, 55–67, 71, and 73 for the interested reader.

There is consensus that circulating immune complexes of the DNA–anti-DNA antibody type are responsible for producing the major manifestations of lupus: nephritis, cerebritis, cutaneous vasculitis, serositis, and polyarthritis. Generally, but not invariably, elevated levels of anti-DNA antibodies, as measured by radioimmunoassay techniques, correlate well with disease activity. Hypocomplementemia, measured either as total hemolytic complement (CH_{50}) or as C3 or C4, in association with elevated levels of anti-DNA antibodies, usually indicates active renal disease. However, this combination may be found with an extensive lupus rash, vasculitis, or central nervous system involvement in the absence of active renal disease.[74] Elevated levels of anti-DNA antibody may on occasion be found in the absence of clinically active disease.[64]

A variety of antinuclear antibodies are found in patients with systemic LE: antibodies against nucleoprotein, histone, single- and double-stranded DNA, nuclear RNA protein, nucleolar RNA, and single- and double-stranded RNA. A presumed non-nucleic acid nuclear antigen called Sm and the two cytoplasmic antigens La and Ro, all named after the patients in whom they were first identified, have also been detected in patients with systemic LE. Ro has been studied more extensively than La. In a survey of 5000 sera by Maddison et al., anti-Ro antibodies were found in 72 patients.[75-77] Diagnoses of systemic LE were made in 58 (81 per cent), Sjögren's syndrome in four (16 per cent), and rheumatoid arthritis in two, scleroderma in one, cutaneous vasculitis in one, and nonrheumatic diseases in six. Two of the four patients with Sjögren's syndrome also had polymyositis and another one had rheumatoid arthritis. Thus, the presence of anti-Ro antibodies has a high predictive value for systemic LE and may also be a marker for Sjögren's syndrome. These investigators also found that 37 of 140 patients with LE and 10 of 25 individuals with Sjögren's syndrome had anti-Ro antibodies. These 37 patients with LE differed from the typical individual with systemic LE only by exhibiting a much higher prevalence of a photosensitive malar eruption, Sjögren's syndrome, and rheumatoid factor.

Among the 140 patients were 16 individuals who had a striking photosensitive malar eruption that clinically and histologically was diagnostic of LE. However, repeated tests for antinuclear antibody were consistently negative. Rheumatoid factor was present in all, and polyarthritis eventually developed in 50 per cent. One of these individuals eventually developed antinuclear antibody four years after the onset of LE. Seven of the 16 patients have died and in six, the cause of death was directly related to rapidly progressive lupus nephritis. Significant quantities of anti-Ro antibodies were detected in the glomerular eluates at autopsy in two patients, thus supporting a pathogenetic role for Ro–anti-Ro immune complexes in the nephritis.

The Ro antigen appears to identify a subset of LE patients who seem to have only marked photosensitivity as a manifestation of their disease. Clinical and laboratory evidence of systemic involvement is lacking.[76] However, after varying periods of time, measured in years, a significant number have developed polyarthritis and irreversible renal failure. Ro-positive individuals need to be carefully followed.

The lupus rash in cutaneous and systemic LE, however, is not a manifestation of cutaneous vasculitis. Although the pathogenesis has not been established, it is likely that cell-mediated immunity is operative because of the marked lymphocytic perivascular and periappendageal infiltrates in the dermis. Examination of cutaneous lupus lesions by immunofluorescent methods to detect immunoglobulins and complement has proved to be a useful diagnostic and prognostic procedure. More than 90 per cent of the rashes in cutaneous and systemic LE have immunoglobulins and complement deposited linearly in a granular or solid band at the dermal-epidermal junction (lupus band test).[22, 78] The band test is negative in the normal-appearing skin in cutaneous LE. In systemic LE, the band test will be positive 50 per cent of the time in normal-appearing, light-protected skin, and 50 to 95 per cent positive in normal-appearing but light-exposed skin. The band test can be helpful in detecting systemic involvement in patients with primarily cutaneous lesions, or in supporting a diagnosis of LE in patients with extracutaneous disease suspected of being LE. The band test performed on normal skin has also been proffered as a likely indicator of renal disease. Although this application is still controversial, the bulk of evidence indicates that a positive band test is found more frequently in association with renal disease, especially the more severe forms, than in the absence of renal disease. In addition, other studies have suggested that band tests showing deposits of IgA in nonlesional skin are usually associated with disease activity,[79] and that deposits of IgG alone or in combination with any other immunoglobulin are linked with greater disease activity, more severe renal disease, or greater mortality than if only IgM is present.[22, 80] The components of the alternative complement pathway (properdin and factor B) have been found almost as frequently as the components of the classic pathway (Clq and C4) at the dermal-epidermal junction of lesional and nonlesional skin.[79]

Deposition of immune reactants at the dermal-epidermal junction does not play a role in the pathogenesis of the lupus lesion. In well-controlled studies, the immunoglobulins and complement did not appear for seven weeks to six months after the clinical lesions developed.[81] In the New Zealand mouse model a positive band test develops about two months after circulating antinuclear antibodies and glomerular immune deposits can be detected.[82] The experimental evidence strongly suggests that the deposition of immunoreactants results from circulating antinuclear antibodies that combine with DNA released from epidermis damaged by ultraviolet irradiation,[83] rather than from circulating antigen-antibody complexes that lodge there because of increased vascular permeability in the upper dermis.

Neonatal LE has been reported in approximately 15 patients thus far.[84, 85] The neonates have developed erythematous macular lesions, sometimes scaly, primarily on the face and scalp, and less frequently on the trunk and extremities. The periorbital areas are especially affected. The lesions have the histologic features of lupus erythematosus and in one of two patients studied, the lupus band test was positive.[85] In virtually all the children the cutaneous lesions have spontaneously disappeared by one to two years of age and only rarely has it been necessary to treat them for the skin lesions. Systemic features of LE were present in three children who developed anemia, thrombocytopenia, and hepatosplenomegaly, which either disappeared spontaneously after several months or responded to treatment with corticosteroids. One infant died of systemic LE at four years. One child whose disease spontaneously remitted at age five months developed mild systemic LE with membranous glomerulonephritis at age 19 years.[86] However, the maternal influences must be very important, because in 10 instances the mothers have had either LE, rheumatoid arthritis, or an undifferentiated connective tissue disease before, during, or after the pregnancy. Does the stress of birth induce LE in a genetically predisposed neonate? The mere passage of the LE cell factor into the infant via the cord blood does not produce LE in children, nor does the LE cell factor adversely affect cells in tissue culture.[85]

Drugs may also induce an LE-like syndrome characterized by fever, malaise, arthralgias, arthritis, pleuritis, and pericarditis. Renal disease is almost never a feature of this syndrome and rashes are rare. The drugs implicated in this event include hydralazine, procainamide, isoniazid, anticonvulsants, chlorpromazine, and penicillamine.[87, 88] The antinuclear antibodies that develop in drug-induced LE, except for the syndrome produced by hydralazine, are directed against nucleoprotein, denatured DNA, or single-stranded DNA, but not native DNA as in typical LE.[89] Hydralazine-induced lupus, however, is associated with antibodies both to the drug and to native DNA.[90] Some individuals carry an autosomal recessive gene that affects the specific enzyme activity of an N-acetyl transferase in the liver responsible for metabolism of hydralazine, isoniazid, procainamide, and other drugs. Those who are slow acetylators are at higher risk than fast acetylators in developing drug-induced lupus.

LE is also associated with the porphyria syndromes, but the reasons are not known. At least 24 such patients have been reported.[91] In 18 patients, porphyria cutanea tarda was associated with cutaneous or systemic LE; in four individuals acute intermittent porphyria was associated with systemic LE; in one individual acute intermittent porphyria was associated with cutaneous LE; and in one patient variegate porphyria accompanied cutaneous LE. They may occur together or follow one another by intervals as long as eight years. No set pattern or order has been noted. The therapeutic use of antimalarials and estrogens, including the contraceptive pill, may precipitate an attack of porphyria cutanea tarda in either its latent or active phase.

DERMATOMYOSITIS

Polymyositis is a necrotizing inflammatory disease of unknown etiology involving striated muscle. When skin manifestations accompany the disorder, it is called dermatomyositis. In series describing polymyositis-dermatomyositis, approximately 60 per cent of cases have skin markings.[92, 93] Muscle weakness is the dominant symptom, and in its absence, with rare exceptions, the diagnosis should not be made.

Histologic examination of affected striated muscles in polymyositis reveals striking pathologic findings: mononuclear cell infiltrates, widespread necrosis, regeneration and phagocytosis of single muscle fibers, and proliferation of sarcolemmal nuclei. Calcification and fibrosis of muscle may develop as a result of these destructive changes. A less severe form of muscular inflammation producing myalgias is common in LE, scleroderma, rheumatoid arthritis, and rheumatic fever. Any set of muscles, with or without weakness, may be affected and the histological findings are similar to, but much less severe than, those seen in polymyositis.[94, 95] However, myositis in the form of polymyositis or dermatomyositis may accompany scleroderma, LE, and rheumatoid arthritis to produce mixed connective tissue (overlap) syndromes. Although a biopsy of muscle may show pathologic features of an inflammatory myopathy in an individual case, this finding alone should not be used to change the diagnosis of an otherwise typical case of LE or scleroderma to dermatomyositis. Walton and Adams' 1958 classification of myositis[94] need only be modified slightly to include all the clinical syndromes currently recognized. Although childhood dermatomyositis has been included as a separate entity in a recent classification,[93] the basis for its inclusion is controversial at present.

Group 1 — Polymyositis.

Group 2 — Polymyositis with variable degrees of skin involvement (dermatomyositis). Other features of connective tissue disease may be present, but they play a minor role in the individual case.

Group 3 — Polymyositis and dermatomyositis in association with an underlying neoplasm. This group is indistinguishable from group 2.

Group 4a — Myositis as a minor feature of LE, scleroderma, rheumatoid arthritis, and rheumatic fever. In these diseases there may be muscle pain and tenderness with or without weakness. The histologic features of myositis may be found in clinically normal muscle.

Group 4b — Polymyositis or dermatomyositis as a major feature of another connective tissue disease (overlap syndrome).

Group 5 — Childhood dermatomyositis associated with vasculopathy.

There is no correlation between the extent of skin markings and the degree of muscle involvement in dermatomyositis. Some patients with dermatomyositis have severe cutaneous involvement and minimal (but definite) muscle disease, or vice versa. We have seen a 13-year-old white girl with the classic cutaneous changes of dermatomyositis present for 10 years in the absence of clinical or enzymatic evidence of muscle disease. In another patient, a 16-year-old girl with the characteristic eruption of dermatomyositis without evidence of myositis, oral and topical corticosteroid therapy had no effect on the rash, which spontaneously disappeared after two years.

The natural history of polymyositis and dermatomyositis is variable: the course may be acute and fulminant, with death occurring in less than a year; it may be recurrent with long remissions; it may require constant corticosteroid therapy for control with relapse occurring whenever medication is discontinued; it may pursue a slowly progressive course lasting 10 or more years; or in a few cases it may remit spontaneously and permanently.

Dermatomyositis may begin as early as one year of age or as late as 70 years. At least 15 per cent of cases are seen in children less than 15 years old. It is more common in females. Although the proximal muscles of the extremities and girdle muscles are primarily affected, the distal musculature is not exempt. Muscle disease usually begins insidiously with swelling, tenderness, and pain. These findings are not always present, but muscle weakness is a constant feature. Striated muscles of the pharynx, esophagus, thoracic wall, diaphragm, and myocardium are involved in decreasing order of frequency. Ocular muscles are not commonly affected. Muscular fasciculations, an extremely rare finding, were observed in one of our patients. A myasthenia gravis–like syndrome has been noted in a few cases.

The patient may experience difficulty in walking up or down stairs, getting up from a chair, or lifting his head from a pillow. Dysphagia resulting from involvement of pharyngeal and upper esophageal muscles and dysphonia related to abnormalities of the palatal muscles are common. When the disease is severe, food is regurgitated through the nose. In some patients muscle involvement is quite minimal and the disease runs a relatively benign course without development of cutaneous calcification or contractures.

If muscle destruction has been severe, extensive calcification of muscle and skin develops two to three years after the onset of the disease. Calcification develops more commonly in children than in adults. It is more widespread and plaque-like than in scleroderma, in which calcification is focal, limited to the skin, and appears much later in the course of the disease.[96] Cutaneous calcification in LE is uncommon.[39]

The extent of muscle atrophy and contractures observed in dermatomyositis depends not only upon the inflammation and necrosis of muscles but also upon therapy. Contractures are seen almost exclusively in patients who have not had the benefit of physical therapy, a modality that is most important in treating dermatomyositis (Fig. 7–40).

Although skin markings usually precede muscle involvement by a variable period of time, they may develop after the onset of polymyositis. When skin markings precede myositis, the interval is generally three to six months, but it may be as long as four years. In its early stages, dermatomyositis can be confused with LE because of cutaneous and extracutaneous features common to both. In its late stages, it may be difficult to distinguish from scleroderma. Nevertheless it is usually possible to separate LE, dermatomyositis, and scleroderma. This is important because of differences in therapy and prognosis. Overlapping signs and symptoms of these three diseases are discussed more fully later.

There are fewer clinically distinctive skin markings in dermatomyositis than in LE. However, the characteristic distribution and mode of

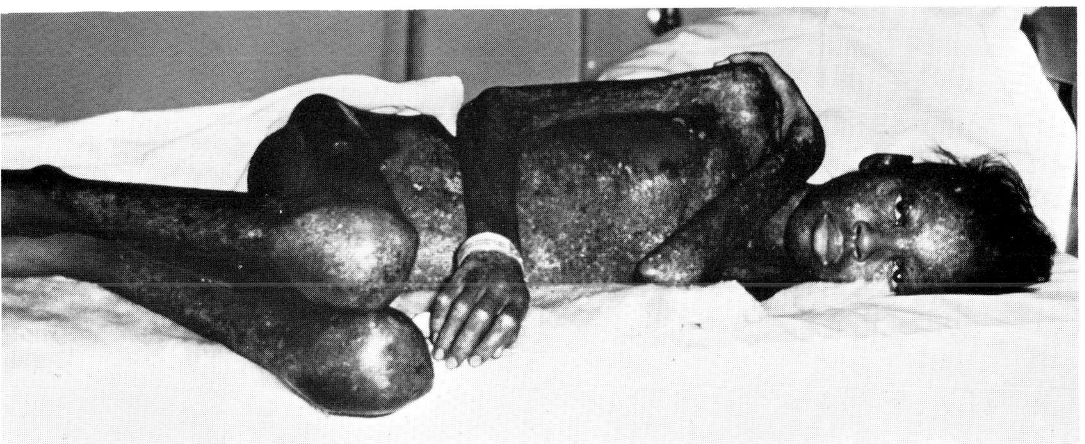

Figure 7–40. Dermatomyositis. Severe muscle atrophy and contractures.

spread in dermatomyositis compensate for the lack of specific lesions. Histologic examination of cutaneous lesions in dermatomyositis usually discloses a nonspecific inflammatory reaction in the dermis. In a few instances, changes similar to those seen in acute LE have been observed.

The development of skin lesions in dermatomyositis falls into two patterns, although overlapping occurs (Plate 19*B–F*). Most of the lesions are flat, violaceous, scaling, and nonatrophic. Pruritus is a frequent complaint.

In the first pattern of development, the patient notes *transient* blotchy violaceous macules over the trunk, the extremities, and on the face, especially over the malar regions. Scaling, if present, is of fine quality. The lesions may be urticarial. Diagnoses of seborrheic dermatitis, contact dermatitis, or "allergy" are usually made. Arthralgia, polyarthritis, and edema and stiffness of the hands are common signs and symptoms during this period. Later the cutaneous changes become more extensive; persistent facial edema develops, often in a butterfly pattern. The swelling is usually red or purplish-red. The periorbital tissues or only the lid margins may become edematous and violaceous ("heliotrope"). (Plate 22*A*, Fig. 7–41) Telangiectasia punctuates many of the lesions. Atrophy is never present initially.

Characteristically, a fine scaly erythema appears over the extensor surfaces of both the large and the interphalangeal joints. The hands may show a blotchy violaceous color with or without fine scaling on the dorsal and palmar surfaces (Figs. 7–42 to 7–45). These cutaneous features, usually transient at the onset, become fixed as the disease progresses;

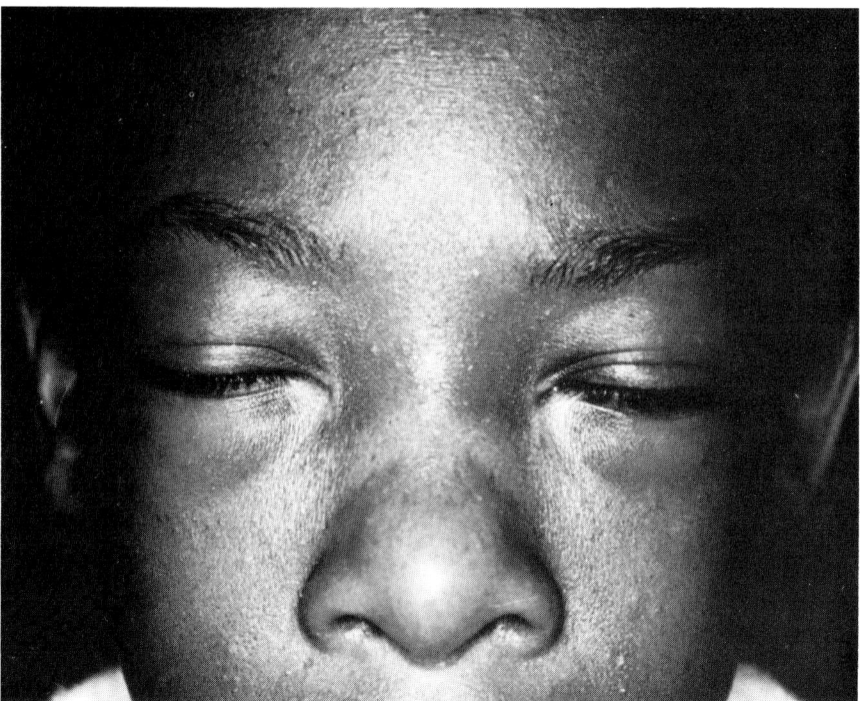

Figure 7–41. Dermatomyositis. Periorbital edema.

PLATE 22

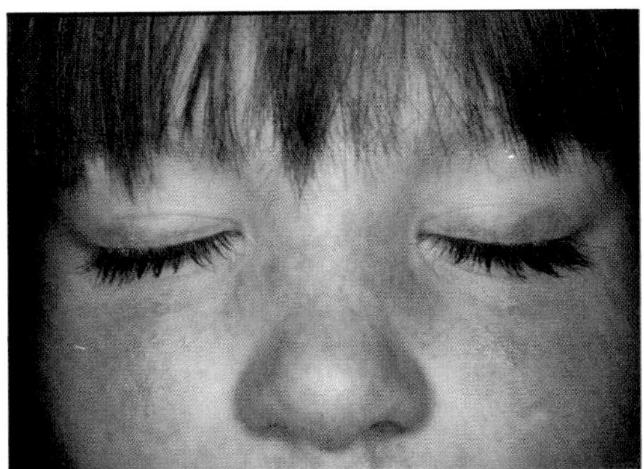

A, Dermatomyositis. Heliotrope color of lid margins.

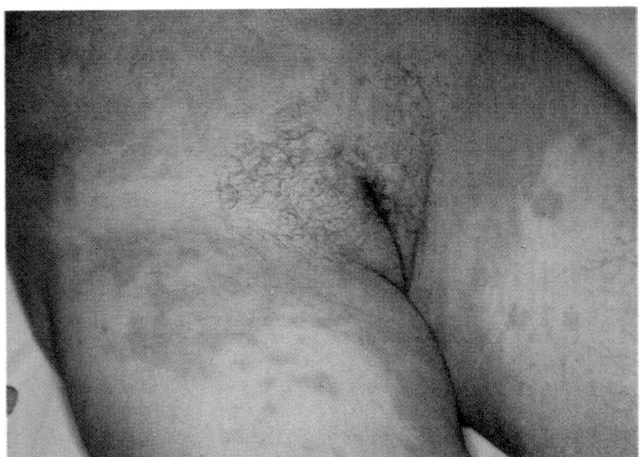

B, Morphea. Generalized, discrete violaceous patches without edema or induration.

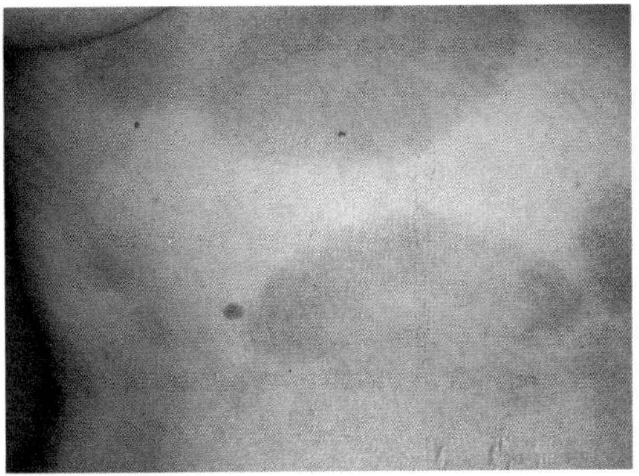

C, Morphea. Discrete erythematous patches without edema or induration. A violaceous inflammatory border is present.

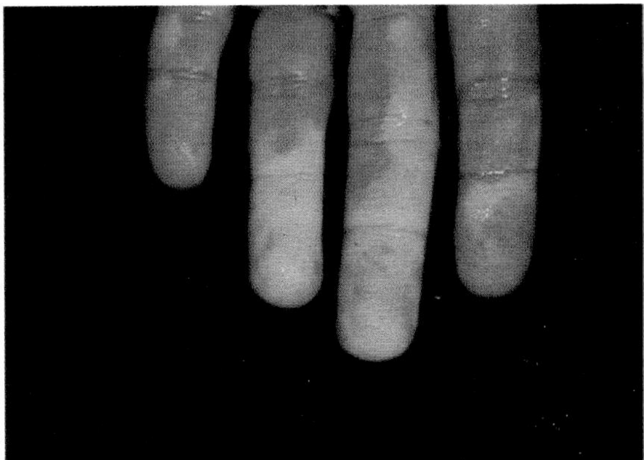

D, Raynaud's phenomenon showing phase of blanching. Note irregular areas of involvement.

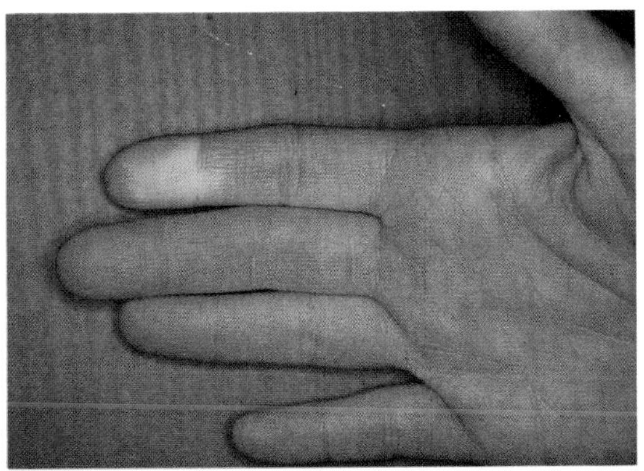

E, Raynaud's phenomenon. Blanching confined to distal phalanx of index finger.

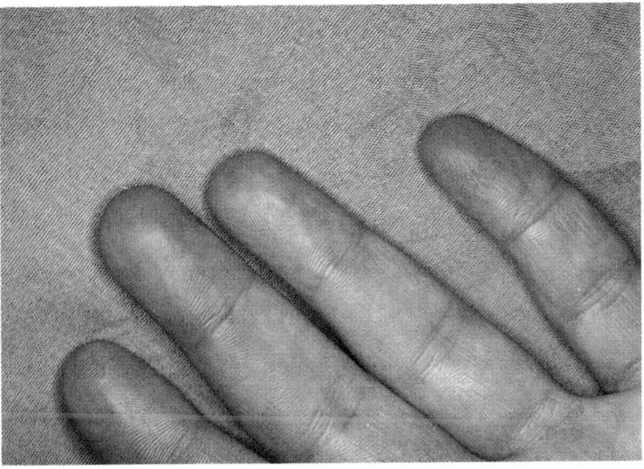

F, Raynaud's phenomenon. Cyanosis of finger tips.

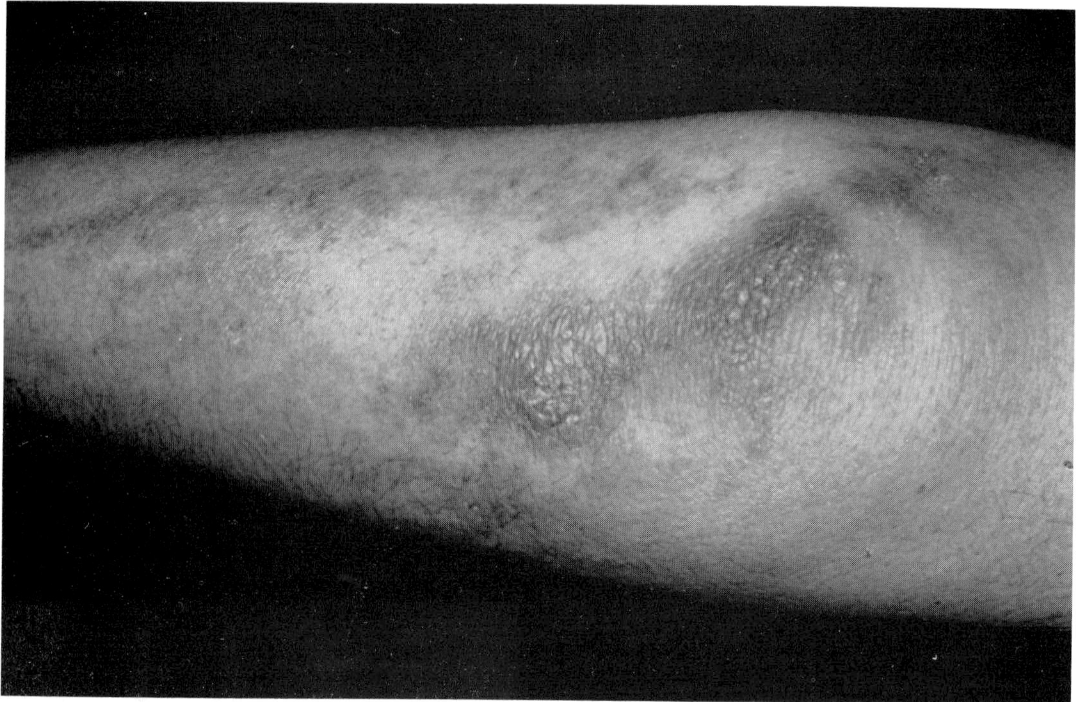

Figure 7–42. Dermatomyositis. Characteristic erythema and scaling over extensor surfaces of the elbow.

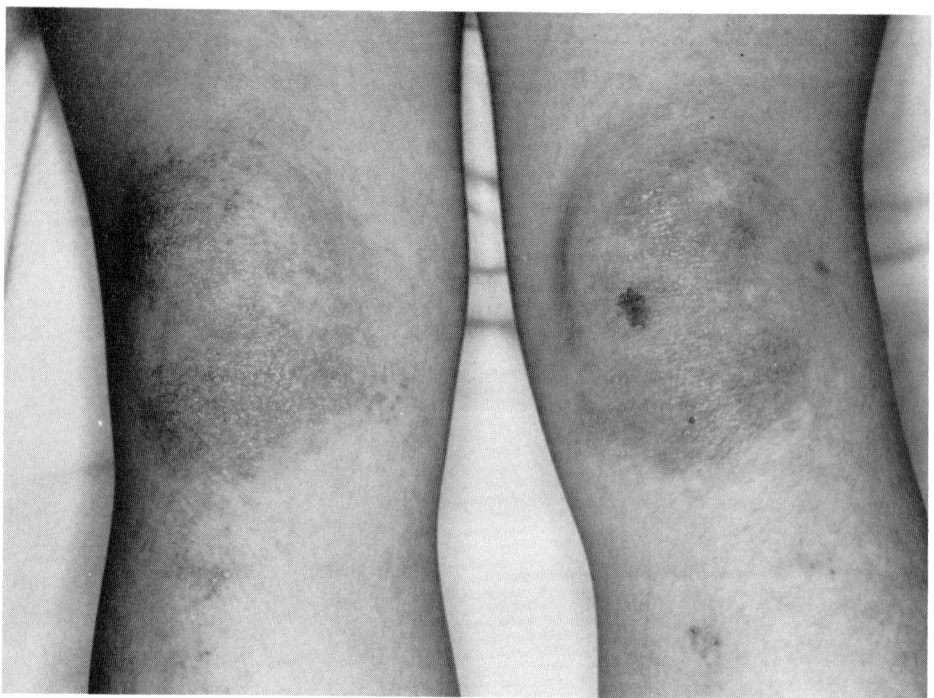

Figure 7–43. Dermatomyositis. Violaceous scaly patches on knees.

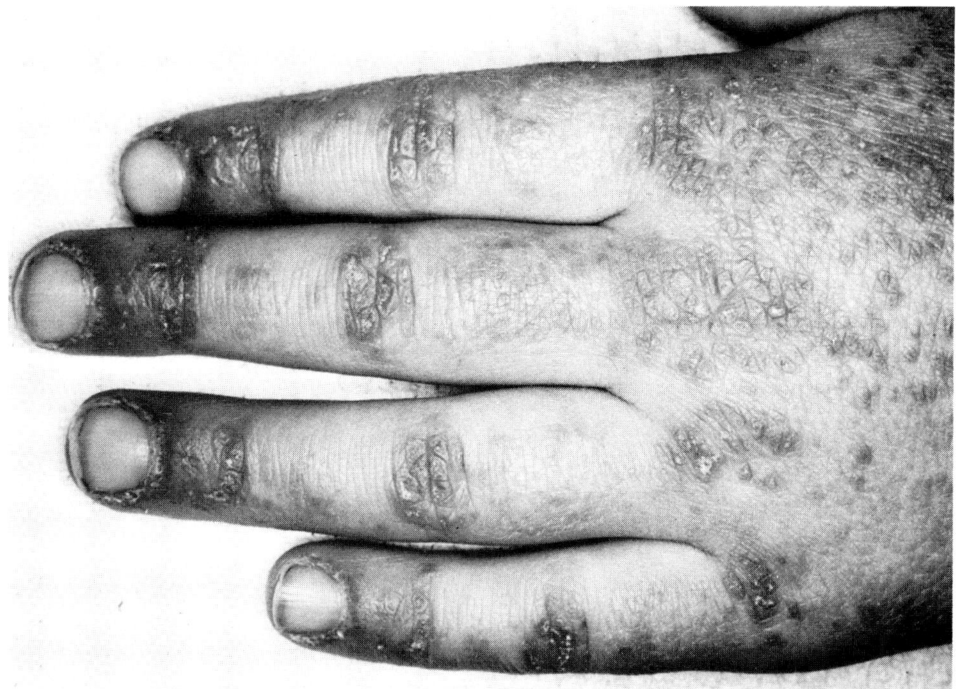

Figure 7–44. Dermatomyositis. Violaceous scaly patches on knuckles. Gottron's sign.

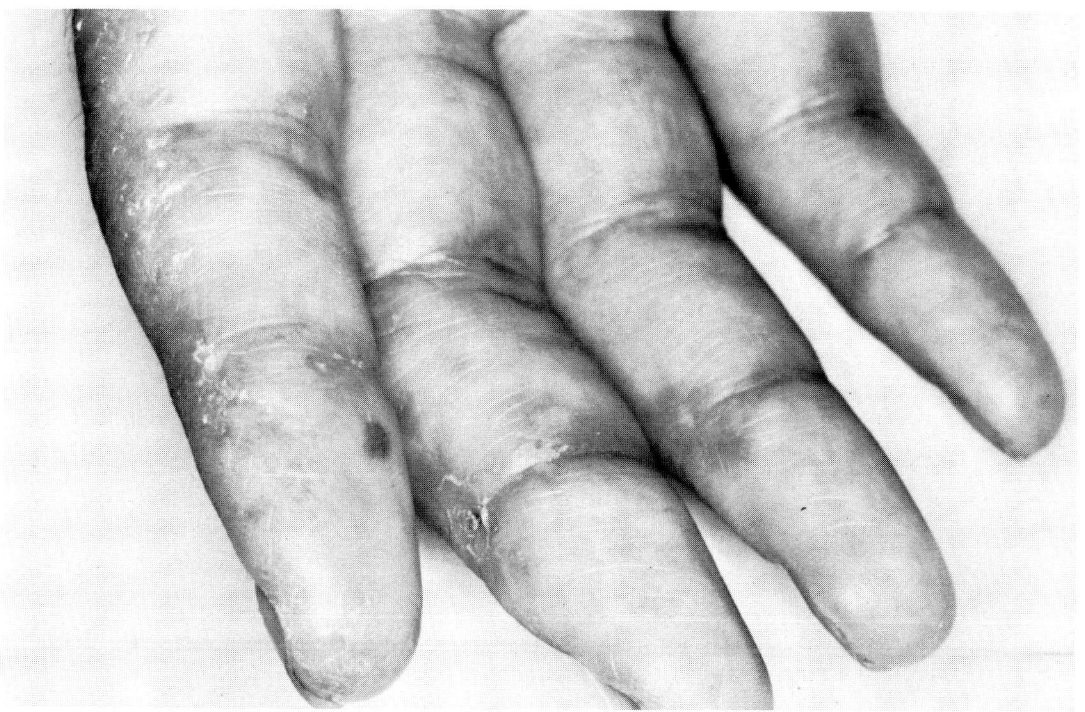

Figure 7–45. Dermatomyositis. Erythema and scaling on hand.

they may evolve over a three- to six-month or even a four-year period before muscle weakness becomes evident.

All the skin markings described above are also seen in LE. However, they appear as presenting signs in dermatomyositis much more frequently than in LE. Cutaneous involvement tends to be more extensive in dermatomyositis. Scaly erythema over the major joints and the dorsal interphalangeal joints is seen much more often in dermatomyositis than in LE. When the dorsum of the hands is involved in LE, the skin over the dorsal interphalangeal joints is usually spared. The scaly atrophic plaque (discoid lesion), diagnostic of LE, is never seen in dermatomyositis.

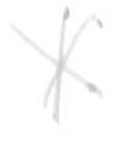

In the second pattern of development, widespread persistent involvement of the skin occurs within a few weeks. The face, V of the neck, and other sun-exposed areas are characteristically affected with a confluent, sometimes scaly, violaceous, and telangiectatic efflorescence. Edema may be a prominent feature of the lesions and may, because of epidermal-dermal separation, give rise to vesicles and bullae (Plate 19*D*, *E*). A contact dermatitis may be simulated. The scalp may be erythematous and scaly, and the hairline and nape of the neck are often involved (Plate 19*F*). Although seborrheic dermatitis is usually diagnosed, the striking purple color and the distribution of lesions in light-exposed areas are never seen in seborrheic dermatitis. Violaceous periorbital edema of varying severity is almost always present. Ulceration in the folds of the upper lids may accompany the swelling. As these vasodilatory changes become fixed, a new picture develops; namely, poikiloderma vasculare atrophicans: a finely speckled pattern of hyperpigmented and hypopigmented macules, one to two millimeters in size and interspersed with fine telangiectasia and cutaneous atrophy (Plate 20*A*). Poikiloderma, which represents a late state, is seen almost exclusively in dermatomyositis, never in scleroderma, and only rarely in LE. Poikilodermatomyositis is a term sometimes used to describe this stage of the disease. Even though the term *poikiloderma vasculare atrophicans* is also used to describe the skin manifestations of pre–mycosis fungoides, dermatomyositis and mycosis fungoides would never be confused because of their other distinguishing features.

With the onset of myositis, edema localized to the skin and the subcutaneous tissue over the affected muscles may occur. Although the edema may be massive enough to produce vesicles and bullae, usually the skin merely exhibits brawny thickening. Hypertrichosis may develop in areas of previous cutaneous involvement.

Periungual erythema and linear telangiectasia on the posterior nailfold and on the cuticle, with or without thromboses, are seen in almost all cases. In six patients, Samitz noted that in addition to nailfold erythema and telangiectasia, the cuticle may be thickened, hyperkeratotic, and irregular, as one might see following picking or overzealous manicuring.[98] The cuticular changes were observed in the absence of erythema and clinically detectable telangiectasia, and resolved and reappeared in parallel with disease activity in some of these patients. We have seen identical cuticular changes in scleroderma.

A pathognomonic sign in dermatomyositis is the Gottron papule: a violaceous flat-topped lesion over the dorsal interphalangeal joints which usually occurs late in the disease in about one third of the patients.[99] Cutaneous atrophy, telangiectasia, and hypopigmentation develop in the site when the papule resolves; the scaly erythema over the major joints is

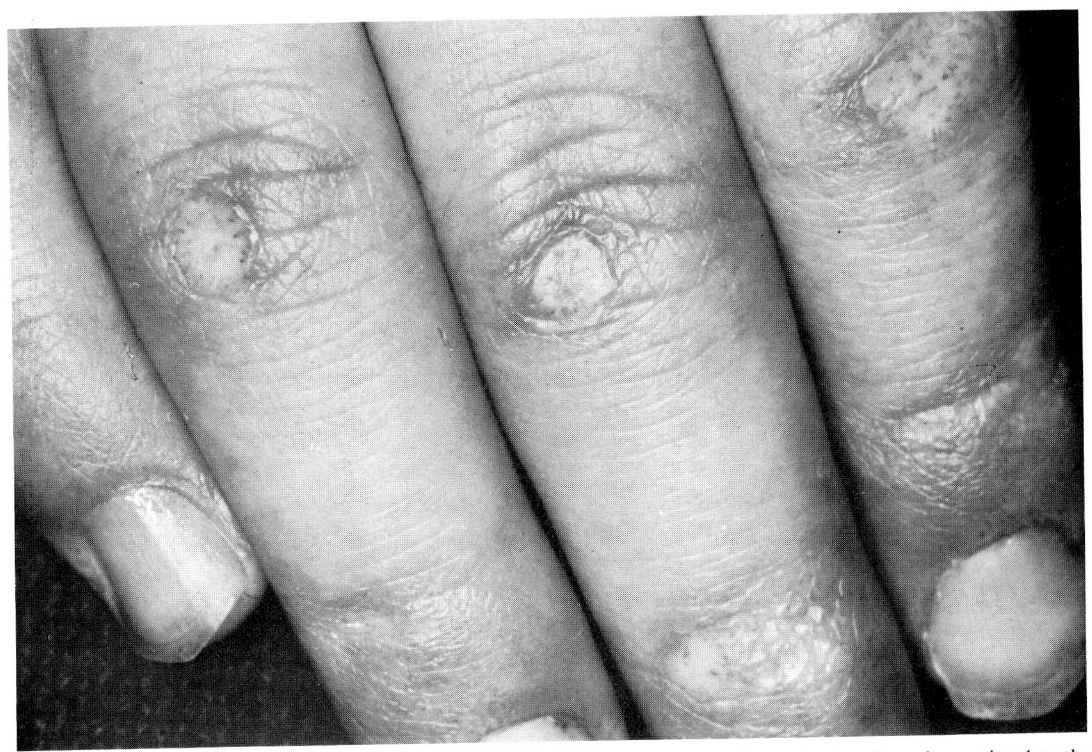

Figure 7–46. Dermatomyositis. Gottron's sign. Hypopigmentation, atrophy, and telangiectasia restricted to the knuckles.

replaced by similar changes (Fig. 7–46; Plate 20*B*). When the Gottron papule is present early in the course of the disease, it serves as a diagnostic marker for dermatomyositis. Its specificity for dermatomyositis and polymyositis is supported by its absence in uncomplicated cases of systemic LE and scleroderma and by the following case report of one of our patients.

A 21-year-old woman developed polymyositis affecting the muscles of the shoulder and hip girdles six months after the onset of scleroderma. The myositis responded promptly to prednisone therapy and after three years of low dose maintenance therapy, the prednisone was discontinued without recurrence of the polymyositis. Sometime between 6 and 12 months after discontinuation of steroid therapy, she developed Gottron's papules (Fig. 7–47). For three years, as of 1978, she has continued in remission without therapy. The Gottron papules have resolved, leaving atrophic patches behind on the knuckles.

Occasionally a diffuse lichenoid eruption occurs that may be mistaken for a lichen planus–like drug reaction or for lichen planus itself. However, this eruption is seen on both the extensor and flexor surfaces of the extremities and does not have the typical Wickham's striae of lichen planus.

Photosensitivity is also a feature of dermatomyositis and may be partly responsible for the lesions on the face, V of the neck, and other exposed areas. Erythema of the palate and the buccal mucosa, with and without ulceration, and whitish patches on the buccal mucosa and tongue, similar to those seen in LE, have been observed.[100] Varying degrees of alopecia are also found in dermatomyositis.

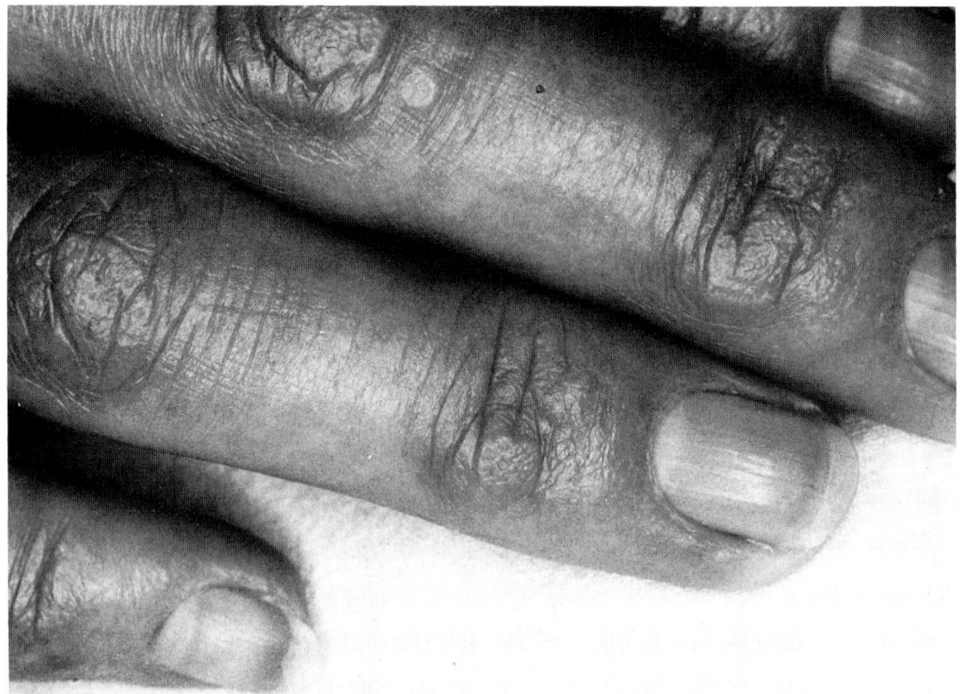

Figure 7–47. Gottron's papules in patient with scleroderma and polymyositis.

Raynaud's phenomenon occurs in 10 to 20 per cent of individuals with dermatomyositis. Some patients will develop sclerodactyly, cutaneous sclerosis, hyperpigmentation and depigmentation characteristic of scleroderma six months to three years after the onset of dermatomyositis. This variety of the disease has been called sclerodermatomyositis.[101] The myositis may be mild or inactive when this stage of the illness becomes prominent. Although this may simply be an example of an overlap syndrome, the improvement or the inactivity of the myositis, which is frequently present when the sclerodermatous features develop, makes this a discrete clinical entity. One can distinguish these cases by looking for the Gottron papules or their atrophic residua over the dorsal interphalangeal joints (Fig. 7–48). The patient shown in this figure had developed dermatomyositis six months before the sclerodermatous features developed. The myositis remitted spontaneously at the end of six months and was soon forgotten by successive house officers who listed her as a patient with scleroderma for the next eight years in the hospital's medical records.

The differential cutaneous and laboratory features of LE, dermatomyositis, and scleroderma are summarized in Table 7–2.

The course of dermatomyositis in children is different from that in adults.[96, 102] Children rarely have Raynaud's phenomenon, but they tend to have more inflammation and necrosis of muscle with consequently more calcification. A respiratory illness often precedes the onset of dermatomyositis in children, but this sequence is not common in adults. In our series, dermatomyositis seemed to develop after a reaction to penicillin that was prescribed for two adults with upper respiratory

Table 7–2. DIFFERENTIAL CUTANEOUS AND LABORATORY FEATURES OF THE COLLAGEN DISORDERS

	LE	Dermatomyositis	Scleroderma
Periungual erythema	+++	+++	0
Cuticular telangiectasia	+++	+++	+++
Gottron's papules on knuckles	0	+	0
Raynaud's phenomenon	++	++	+++
Sclerodactyly with hyper-pigmentation	+	++	+++
Poikiloderma	rare	+++	0
Calcinosis cutis	rare	+++	++
Erythema on extensor surfaces	+	+++	0
Violaceous color in exposed areas	++	+++	0
Myositis	+	+++	+
Pruritus	0	++	+
Leukopenia	+++	+	0
Increased erythrocyte sedimentation rate	+++	++	+
LE cell phenomenon	+++	rare	rare
Antinuclear factor	+++	++	++

Note: +, ++, and +++ indicate the relative frequencies of the listed features among the disorders; +++ indicates the highest frequency, and 0 indicates the absence of that feature.

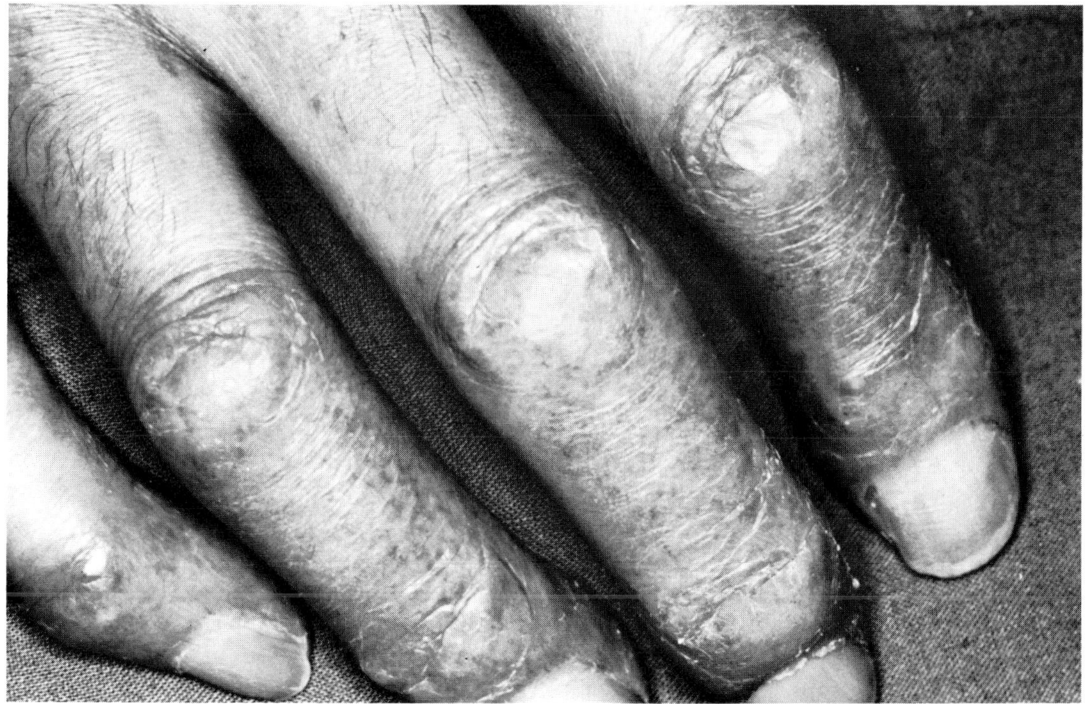

Figure 7–48. Sclerodermatomyositis. Skin over knuckles is atrophic and wrinkled, not tight and hidebound as in scleroderma.

infections. In adults the disease usually begins in a healthy-appearing individual without any obvious antecedent illness.

The incidence of mortality in childhood and adult dermatomyositis has ranged from 25 to 60 per cent in the literature.[96, 103, 104] However, in the past decade the aggressive use of corticosteroids has markedly reduced mortality and morbidity and increased functional recovery, even though the total duration of the disease may not have been shortened.[105-107] The cause of death in dermatomyositis is directly related to the consequences of muscle weakness or sepsis in those patients without cancer, and usually to the metastatic effects of the malignancies in those so affected. Dysphagia with regurgitation results in aspiration pneumonitis. Weakness of the diaphragm and thoracic muscles results in respiratory insufficiency and inevitable pneumonitis. Myocarditis with congestive heart failure is a rare cause of death. In one of our cases extensive amyloidosis of the liver, spleen, and kidney was found at autopsy. A similar case is cited in the literature.[108]

Ulceration of the gastrointestinal tract with perforation unrelated to oral steroid therapy was the cause of death in the majority of children in Cook's series.[102] Although this feature has been found only rarely in other series,[105, 107] it served as the impetus for studies implicating a vasculopathy as the underlying pathogenetic mechanism in the childhood form of the disease[109, 110] and for considering it a special entity in the most recently proposed classification of dermatomyositis.[93] However, the cutaneous eruption and clinical features of the myositis in children are indistinguishable from those in adults, including the cases in Cook's and Banker's series.[102, 109, 110]

The differential diagnosis of dermatomyositis includes LE, trichinosis, scleroderma, rheumatoid arthritis, and muscular dystrophy. With the exception of LE, the other disorders are readily discernible on the basis of history, physical examination, and laboratory findings.

Dermatomyositis is associated with neoplasms in adults. Malignancy has been reported three times in childhood dermatomyositis: a 5½-year-old boy developed dermatomyositis three months after the onset of acute leukemia[102]; an 11-year-old girl was found to have a chromophobe adenoma of the pituitary two years after the onset, but six months after complete remission of dermatomyositis[108]; and a 17-year-old male developed the disease in association with a widespread malignancy involving liver, spleen, and mediastinum. The neoplasm could be categorized no better than "reticuloendotheliosis."[111]

The prevalence of neoplasia in adults with dermatomyositis varies from 6 to 50 per cent and is more common in dermatomyositis than pure polymyositis. In one series the incidence was 50 per cent when only patients over the age of 40 years were considered.[112] In our group of 63 patients, 15 of 40 adults (37.5 per cent) over the age of 37 had an associated malignancy. All types of neoplasms, including lymphomas, sarcomas, and melanomas, have been noted. Carcinomas of the breast and lung are the most common. In our cases, carcinomas of the prostate, bladder, anorectal junction, breast, lung, and cecum and a carcinoid of the pylorus were found.

One of our patients developed *only the cutaneous eruption* of dermatomyositis as a manifestation of an underlying lung cancer. Some patients with an associated neoplasm have a fiery red suffusion superimposed on the more chronic erythematous lesions of dermatomyositis. This suffusion, called *malignant erythema*, may be obliterated by diascopy, thus revealing the more chronic skin lesions of dermatomyositis.[101] In a few patients, successful treatment of the underlying neoplasm has led to complete remission of the dermatomyositis. The exact incidence of such improvement is not known, but many clinicians have seen one or two such cases.

It is imperative that all adults with dermatomyositis be investigated for an underlying malignancy. Usually the neoplasm and dermatomyositis appear together. However, dermatomyositis has been reported as long as three to eight years before, and five years after, the detection of a malignancy.[113] In those cases in which dermatomyositis has improved following treatment of the malignancy, a relapse may herald recurrence of the tumor or metastatic spread.

Bohan and colleagues published two comprehensive papers dealing with dermatomyositis and polymyositis.[93, 114] The first was a critical review of the literature, which led them to categorize our current knowledge about three disorders into *fact, fancy,* and *fiction.*[114] Their main criticism dealt with poor documentation of the natural history of the disease, and the lack of generally accepted diagnostic criteria and suitable classifications which resulted in studies inadequate to properly evaluate laboratory tests, prognostic factors, and therapy. The purported association between malignancy and dermatomyositis also came under attack because of the lack of rigorous statistical evaluation. Their second paper, published two years later, was a computer-assisted analysis of all these factors in their 153 patients.[93] The results of their second study reaffirmed most of the previous conventional wisdom, including therapeutic modalities, which had been compiled and accepted by experienced clinicians. Many items listed as *fancy* in the first paper were elevated to *fact* in the second. One important item of *fiction* became *fancy*: namely that adults with dermatomyositis-polymyositis should be evaluated for occult malignancy.

Bohan et al. stressed that the most useful criteria for diagnosis were proximal muscle weakness, elevated serum enzymes, electromyographic and muscle biopsy abnormalities and the classic skin rash of dermatomyositis. However, if other diagnostic criteria were met, the diagnosis of dermatomyositis and polymyositis could still be made in the presence of normal serum enzymes, normal electromyography, normal muscle biopsy, and even normal muscle strength. I concur with these conclusions.

Four instances of endocrine disease following dermatomyositis by 6 to 8 years have been described. Cushing's syndrome developed in three patients.[115, 116] One had extensive calcinosis that resolved when the Cushing's syndrome became active. Pochi presented an interesting case before the New England Dermatological Society in 1966. A 16-year-old white girl developed dermatomyositis at age 5. At age 13, acanthosis nigricans appeared, followed by generalized hirsutism and amenorrhea. A bilateral ovarian wedge resection for polycystic ovaries was performed at age 16. The significance of the association between dermatomyositis and endocrine disease is unknown.

Pathogenesis

Cell-mediated hypersensitivity appears to play a major role in the pathogenesis of dermatomyositis and polymyositis. Currie et al. demonstrated that homogenates of whole skeletal muscle, but not of liver or kidney, stimulated these patients' lymphocytes to undergo blast transformation; that their peripheral blood lymphocytes were cytotoxic to cultures of human fetal skeletal muscle; and that serum from these patients and lymphocytes from individuals with other muscle wasting diseases did not react in these ways.[117, 118] Johnson et al. showed that minced autologous muscle induced peripheral blood lymphocytes of these patients to produce lymphotoxin that was cytotoxic to human fetal skeletal muscle monolayers; in two individuals, whose muscle specimens were rich in mononuclear cell infiltrates, lymphotoxin was produced by the incubation *in vitro* of the muscle tissue itself; the lymphotoxin had the same chromatographic properties as purified lymphotoxin; methyl prednisolone inhibited the action of lymphotoxin on monolayers of fetal muscle; and in one patient with dermatomyositis and carcinoma of the breast, neither the breast tissue nor tumor stimulated peripheral lymphocytes to produce lymphotoxin, while homogenate of muscle did.[119] Dawkins and Mastiglia confirmed these various studies with quantitative techniques and found that lymphocytes from patients with active myositis induced damage within 18 hours in monolayers of chick-embryo muscle, but not in chick-embryo fibroblast cultures. They also showed that lymphocytes from individuals on high doses of prednisone or azathioprine showed low levels of cytotoxicity, while those on low dose prednisone exhibited high levels of cytotoxicity, strongly suggesting that adequate treatment of polymyositis requires the suppression of lymphocyte-induced myotoxicity.[120]

Thus, lymphocyte- and lymphokine-mediated tissue injury could account for the pathologic features in adult dermatomyositis and polymyositis: widespread degeneration of single muscle fibers, phagocytosis of disintegrating fibers, and varying degrees of intramuscular infiltration with mononuclear inflammatory cells. Regenerative activity, indicated by basophilia of the hyaline content of the muscle fiber and proliferation of sarcolemmal nuclei, accompanies these inflammatory destructive changes. (It needs to be emphasized that significant vascular changes and abnormalities that might be caused by vascular disease are conspicuously lacking in the histopathologic picture.[95]) It appears likely that lymphocyte-mediated tissue damage is a primary rather than a secondary event in polymyositis-dermatomyositis because this mechanism has not been found in other muscle diseases such as muscular dystrophy, trauma, and polyneuropathies.[121, 122]

Questions that need to be answered in regard to cell-mediated hypersensitivity in this disorder are (1) does muscle contain a specific autoantigen and (2) is there an immunogenic infectious agent, or an antigen that cross-reacts with an infectious agent, to which the polymyositis patient is sensitized? In one case of dermatomyositis with breast carcinoma, there was no cross-reaction between muscle and tumor tissue when measured by lymphocyte stimulation tests.[119] All of the experiments dealing with cell-mediated hypersensitivity have been performed in adult patients, so that their applicability to cases of childhood dermatomyositis, while highly likely, has not been established.

The pathogenesis of childhood dermatomyositis is in need of considerable study and may include more than one mechanism. Banker and Victor originally proposed that a vasculopathy was responsible for the tissue damage in childhood dermatomyositis. Their cases were clinically indistinguishable from those of adult dermatomyositis, except for the presence of ulcerative lesions of the gastrointestinal tract that resulted in hemorrhage and perforation leading to death.[109] They described infarction of skeletal muscle caused by arteries and veins exhibiting intimal proliferation, fibrin thrombi, fibrinoid necrosis of vascular walls, and intramural and perivascular accumulation of neutrophils and mononuclear cells. The histological features of single muscle necrosis and regenerative activity found in adult cases were not observed. Identical vascular changes were found in the skin, gastrointestinal tract, fat, and small nerves. Thus, the vasculopathy closely resembled an immune complex disorder such as periarteritis nodosa. In a later paper, Banker restudied the problem with the aid of electron microscopy in another group of children.[110] Her conclusions were that the primary event was endothelial cell degeneration and regeneration followed by platelet and fibrin thrombus formation leading to infarction of muscle in the absence of perivascular inflammatory cells. These later findings were not confirmed by Ludatscher et al.[123]

There is no doubt that a vasculitis plays a major role in a minority of children with dermatomyositis. However, the majority have clinical features and muscle biopsy abnormalities indistinguishable from those in adults. None of the 11 children in Bohan's series had histological evidence of vasculitis on muscle biopsy but four adults did.[93] Gastrointestinal bleeding occurred in one of 34 children in Sullivan's series[105] and in one of 23 in Miller's,[124] but the pathologic basis for the bleeding was not determined. In two other series totalling 41 children, gastrointestinal bleeding and perforation did not occur.[106, 107] Whitaker and Engel found deposition of immunoglobulins and complement in the vessels of skeletal muscle more frequently in children than in adults with dermatomyositis.[125] However, the presence of immunoreactants was not associated with fibrin thrombi, perivascular and intramural inflammatory cells, or muscle necrosis. Circulating immune complexes can lodge in vascular walls without producing clinical lesions.[31] It is not unusual for more than one immunological mechanism to be active in an individual. Studies of tuberculin-type skin tests have shown that cell-mediated hypersensitivity can be preceded by an Arthus reaction. The conflicting clinical observations about childhood dermatomyositis can be reconciled by recognizing that in some patients the immune complex mechanism producing vasculitis is more important than the cell-mediated mechanism. Gastrointestinal bleeding and perforation would dominate the clinical picture, and infarction of skeletal muscle would obscure any evidence of cell-mediated tissue damage.

A febrile illness sometimes precedes the onset of childhood dermatomyositis, suggesting a possible viral etiology. In support of this observation, viral particles characteristic of a picornavirus such as Coxsackie have been found by electron microscopy in skeletal muscles of adults with dermatomyositis.[126, 127] Travers et al. reported rising titers of neutralization antibodies to a specific serotype of Coxsackie B virus in four adults with polymyositis and dermatomyositis.[128] The interval between the onset of symptoms and the highest titer ranged from two to seven months. Antibodies to viruses and other infectious agents were sought but not found: adenovirus, cytomegalic virus, herpes simplex, influenza A and B, measles, mumps, parainfluenza 1 and 3, psittacosis, respiratory syncytial virus, varicella-zoster, *Coxiella burnetti*, type 2, and mycoplasma. Preliminary reports of increased frequency of HLA-B8 in children and adults and HLA-B14 in adults with dermatomyositis suggest that there may be a predisposition to this disease.[129-131] One possibility includes increased susceptibility to an infectious agent or an altered immune response to such an agent.

The mechanism underlying the relationship between dermatomyositis and cancer is unknown. Individuals with dermatomyositis and cancer are able to produce antibodies to their tumors, but there is no evidence that they are causally related to the myopathy. In two patients with dermatomyositis and cancer who were tested by the Prausnitz-Küstner technique, wheal and flare reactions were transferred to normal individuals given serum and tumor extracts from the patients.[132, 133] In another patient, there was no cross-reactivity between muscle and breast carcinoma when evaluated by lymphocyte stimulation tests.[119]

At least three patients have developed dermatomyositis after having been apparently cured of their cancer. te Lintum and Goedbloed described a 67-year-old woman whose disease began seven months after successful therapy for breast cancer.[134] One of our patients, a 55-year-old woman, developed dermatomyositis six months after a uterine cancer was successfully treated, and in another, a 60-year-old woman, the disease appeared three years after curative resection of a breast carcinoma. The induction of cell-mediated hypersensitivity during cancer growth with subsequent clinical expression is a likely explanation for this phenomenon, considering the complex interactions of suppressor and helper T cell subpopulations. Weston and Thorne observed a profound T lymphopenia in one patient with dermatomyositis and cancer, whereas in two control patients with dermatomyositis in the absence of cancer the level of circulating T lymphocytes was normal.[135] This observation merits further study, since it may prove useful in detecting the presence of an underlying malignancy.

SCLERODERMA

Of the three connective tissue diseases, scleroderma is the easiest to diagnose. Cutaneous involvement is only one facet of this disorder. *Progressive systemic sclerosis* and *viscerocutaneous collagenosis* have been proposed as more accurate terms to describe the fibrosis, or increased deposition of collagen, in the heart, lung, gastrointestinal tract, kidney, joints, and skin. Although the term *scleroderma* was coined in 1847 by Gintrac, it has received world-wide acceptance only since 1865.[136] It is unlikely that this term will be supplanted by more accurate terminology, since it concisely and simply denotes a well-known clinical and pathologic entity.

As our understanding of scleroderma developed, it became apparent that the disease could appear in one of two forms; *acrosclerosis* or *diffuse scleroderma*.[137] Acrosclerosis, accounting for 85 to 95 per cent of all cases of scleroderma, was characterized by cutaneous sclerosis of the digits (sclerodactyly) and Raynaud's phenomenon. Diffuse scleroderma exhibited rapid progression, affecting the trunk and extremities within weeks to months, frequently in the absence of vasospastic phenomena.[137-140] The two types of scleroderma were thought to be different because acrosclerosis seemed to have a relatively long and benign course, whereas diffuse scleroderma was rapidly fatal. This concept is not entirely correct. Acrosclerosis may run a course identical in both duration and severity to that of diffuse scleroderma. Visceral involvement is the same in both. The only value of this classification, which is still in use, is that it describes the mode of onset and the distribution of lesions in a particular case; it also connotes the extremely poor prognosis associated with *diffuse scleroderma*. In a series from the Mayo Clinic, 74 per cent of the patients with acrosclerosis survived for five years, whereas only 17 per cent of the patients with diffuse scleroderma were alive after this interval.[137] In acrosclerosis, the ratio of women to men is approximately three to one, but in diffuse scleroderma it is more nearly equal.[138, 140]

Medsger et al., in their series of 309 patients, classified the extent of cutaneous sclerosis into *restricted* (sclerodactyly or acrosclerosis limited to hands or feet, with or without facial involvement) and *nonrestricted* involvement (acrosclerosis plus involvement of arms, legs, or trunk). The *nonrestricted* category was defined only by extent of cutaneous involvement. Rapidity of cutaneous spread was not used as a differential point as in the *diffuse scleroderma* of Tuffanelli and Winkelmann[138] and Barnett and Coventry.[140] Nonrestricted sclerodermatous skin change was also associated with a poorer prognosis, not *per se*, but because of its more frequent linkage with internal organ involvement.[141] Rapidity of cutaneous spread by itself, however, might be an indicator of poor prognosis, but this factor was not evaluated in this series.[141] Although scleroderma is uncommon in children, its natural history is identical to that in adults.[142]

Three additional large series comprising 734 cases and employing life table methodology have provided us with useful data concerning prognosis and survival.[141, 143, 144] This information, which is listed in Table 7–3, emphasizes the following points. The presence of renal, cardiac, and pulmonary involvement at the time of initial diagnosis is associated with greatly reduced survivorship. (Renal involvement was defined as rapidly progressive renal failure, or proteinuria greater than 3.5 grams per day, or persistent cellular casts. Cardiac involvement was characterized by any one of the following: congestive heart failure, pericarditis, or EKG abnormalities, and pulmonary disease by active pleuritis, pulmonary hypertension, abnormal diffusion capacity, or radiographic evidence of fibrosis.) The following features of the disease were not associated with reduced survivorship: involvement of esophagus, small and large bowel, joints, or muscles; Raynaud's phenomenon, hypertension, telangiectases, elevated erythrocyte sedimentation rate, hyperglobulinemia, antinuclear antibody, and rheumatoid factor. However, in men over age 50, an elevated sedimentation rate was associated with reduced survival. When renal disease developed, it was either present at the time of initial diagnosis or appeared within the first year in 50 per cent of those affected. In Bennett's series, 73 per cent of patients over 40 years of age died within the first six years. In the series of Medsger and Masi, the greatest

Table 7–3. SURVIVAL STATISTICS FOR SCLERODERMA

	Number of Patients	**Per Cent Surviving After Initial Diagnosis at Years of Follow-up** *1*	*2*	*3*	*5*	*7*	*10*
Winkelmann[137] (not life table analysis)	605	–	–	–	70	–	59
Sackner[139]	65	70	–	–	34	27	–
Bennett[143]	67	–	–	–	73	–	50
diagnosis made before age 40		–	–	–	95	–	70
diagnosis made after age 40		–	–	–	50	–	30
Medsger	309	–	–	–	48	35	–
diagnosis made before age 45		85	75	70	60	55	–
diagnosis made after age 45		73	65	55	40	20	–
survival in absence of 3 prognostic factors (lung, cardiac, renal) at time of diagnosis		87	81	75	65	56	–
presence of lung involvement alone		81	72	56	40	27	–
presence of cardiac involvement alone*		58	50	35	25	5	–
presence of renal disease alone†		0	0	0	0	0	–
female under 45 years		97	–	90	86	80	–
male under 45 years		89	–	76	67	67	–
female over 45 years		88	–	77	66	47	–
male over 45 years		73	-	54	43	34	–
White females without 3 factors, under 45		–	–	–	–	80	–
White males without 3 factors, under 45		–	–	–	–	67	–
White females without 3 factors, over 45		–	–	–	–	47	–
White males without 3 factors, over 45		–	–	–	–	34	–
Medsger[144]	358						
male VA pts. overall – under 50 yr.‡		82	75	64	55	46	–
male VA pts. overall – over age 50 yr.‡		56	45	36	29	22	–
male VA pts. in absence of 3 prognostic factors under 50		95	91	78	68	53	–
male VA pts, in absence of 3 prognostic factors under 50		67	58	52	46	26	–
male VA pts. overall – absence of 3 prognostic factors at time of diagnosis		87	80	73	62	46	–
overall – presence of lung involvement only		67	58	47	35	35	–
overall – presence of cardiac involvement only		44	35	32	23	15	–
overall – presence of renal involvement only§		0	0	0	0	0	–

– Data not available.

*Association with lung involvement did not make statistics worse.

†All 16 patients died within several months of diagnosis.

‡Greatest decrease in survival occurred in first two years, then slope was equal in two groups.

§All patients with renal involvement at entry died within 10 months. Patients who developed renal decrease later in course were eliminated from further analysis.

decrease in survivorship occurred in the first two years, and women had a slightly better survivorship than men, even though the disease develops three times more often in women than in men.

However, the long-term course in an individual case of scleroderma cannot be predicted, making the evaluation of therapy difficult.

Some observers, including myself, believe that the spectrum of scleroderma can be extended further.[143, 145, 146] Raynaud's disease in the majority of cases probably represents the mildest form of scleroderma and imperceptibly merges with the stage of sclerodactyly and the more severe forms of scleroderma.

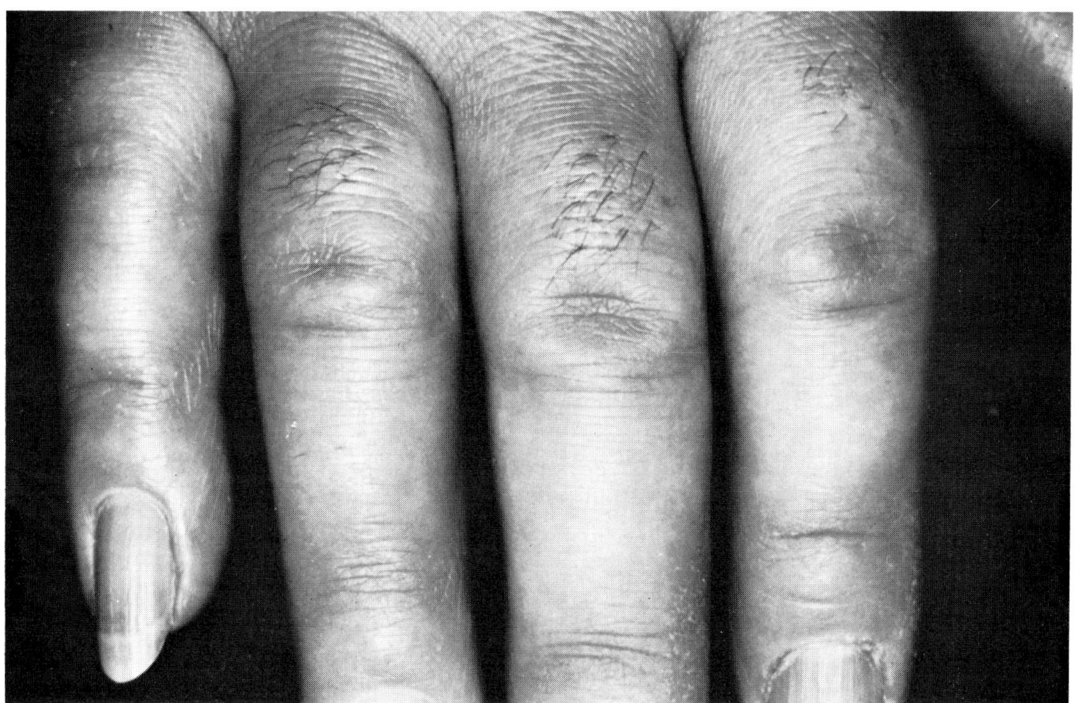

Figure 7–49. Scleroderma. Edematous phase of sclerodactyly.

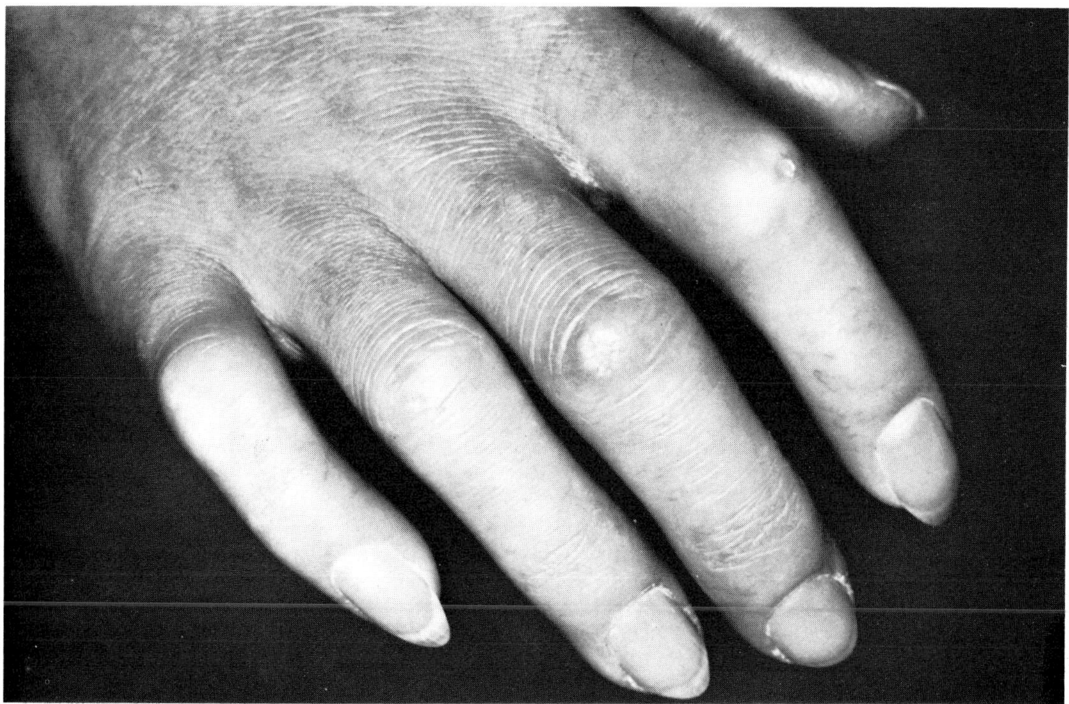

Figure 7–50. Scleroderma. More advanced stage of sclerodactyly. Skin over knuckle of index finger is ulcerated.

Scleroderma (acrosclerosis) is often ushered in by arthralgia or arthritis, which may mimic rheumatoid arthritis. The skin may not harden for weeks or months following these early signs and symptoms. Transient and recurrent edema of the extremities, especially of the hands, often precedes the sclerodermatous changes. Sclerosis can also begin insidiously without obvious swelling. Typical sclerodactyly is the usual outcome: tapered fingers with shiny hidebound skin (Figs. 7–49 to 7–52). Such changes may develop within a few months or more slowly over a period of many years. The sclerosis often spreads to the proximal portions of the extremities and to the chest, face, and scalp. Edema may also precede the sclerosis in these areas. In the patient shown in Figure 7–53, facial edema has persisted for three years without the development of sclerosis, even though the hands and forearms have become sclerodermatous. As the skin becomes taut, contractures of the large and small joints may develop. In the hand, a claw deformity is typically produced. Several factors enter into the formation of contractures: skin tightness, muscular atrophy caused by disuse, muscular fibrosis, and sclerosis of the synovia itself.[147, 148]

The striking pigmentary disturbances of scleroderma appear in three patterns: generalized hyperpigmentation or a darkening of exposed regions and the mucous membranes, which simulates adrenal insufficiency (Fig. 7–54; Plate 20*C*); focal hyperpigmentation and hypopigmentation in areas of sclerosis (Fig. 7–55); and patches of perifollicular pigmentation appearing on a background of complete pigment loss, which mimics a patch of repigmenting vitiligo. The vitiligo-like changes are most commonly found on the upper chest and back, but they may be seen on the

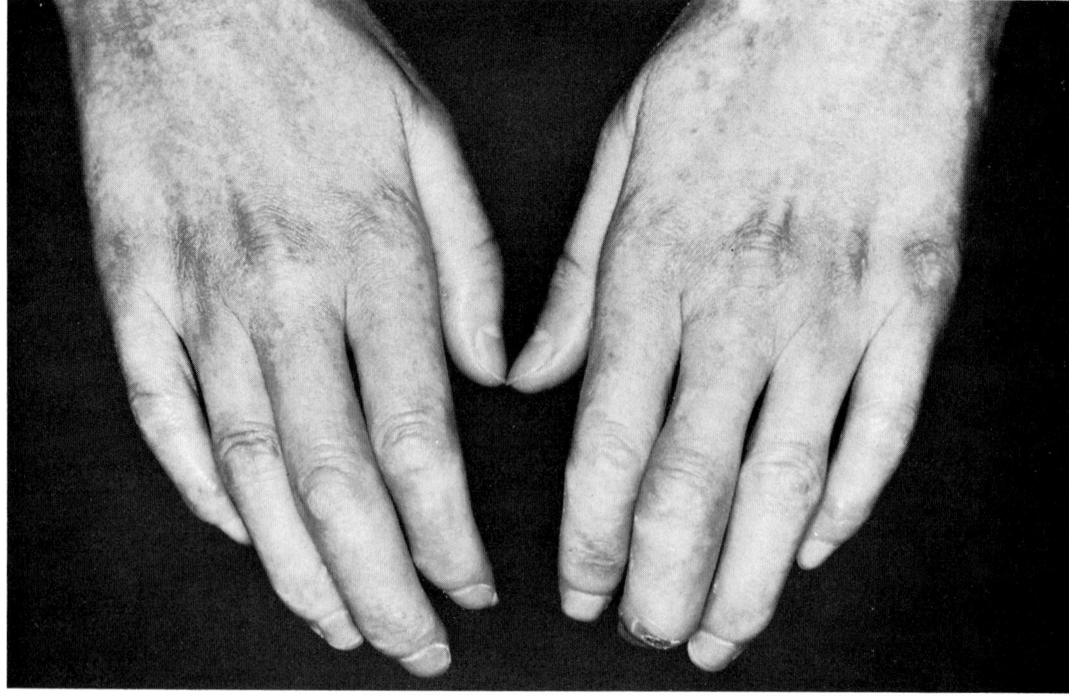

Figure 7–51. Scleroderma. Advanced sclerodactyly. Focal areas of hyper- and hypopigmentation in areas of cutaneous sclerosis.

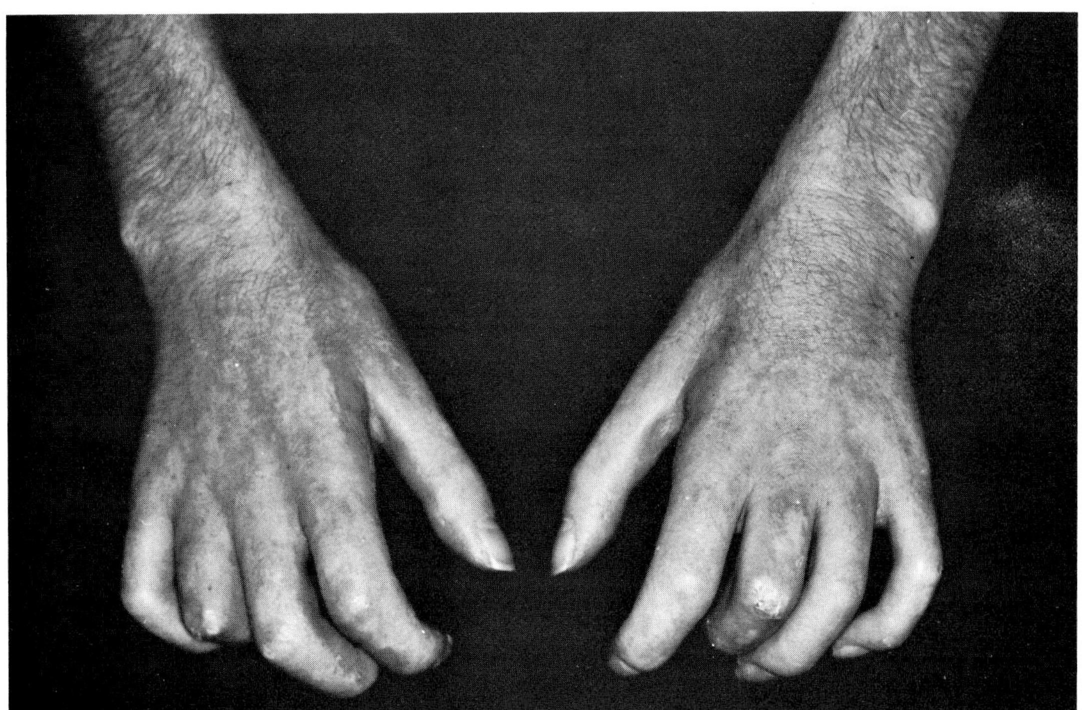

Figure 7–52. Scleroderma. Severe sclerodactyly with flexion contractures. Focal areas of hypo- and hyperpigmentation in areas of sclerosis.

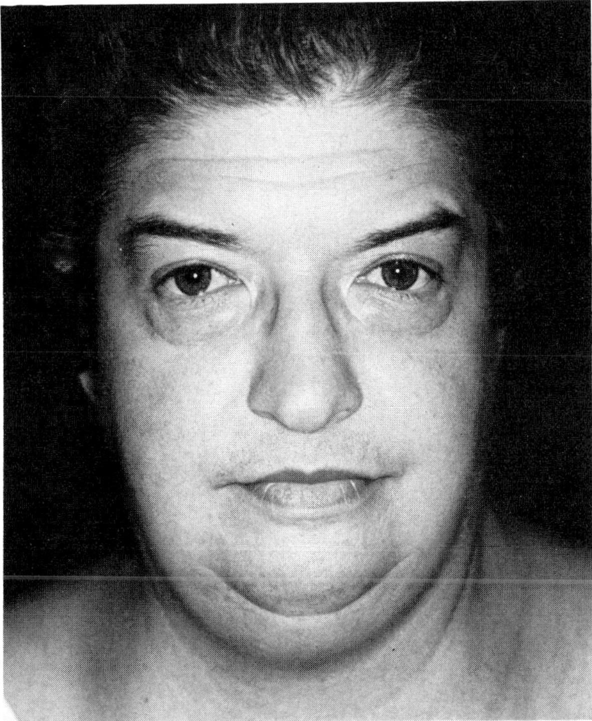

Figure 7–53. Scleroderma. Persistent facial swelling.

scalp, hairline, dorsa of the hands and forearms, and on the pinnae (Figs. 7–56 to 7–58).

The Addisonian type of pigmentation is not restricted to regions of sclerosis and develops in the presence of normal adrenal cortical function. Immunoreactive beta-MSH activity has been excluded as the cause of Addisonian hyperpigmentation in scleroderma.[149] In one of our patients it preceded the other signs of scleroderma by six months. Pruritus is often associated with this type of hyperpigmentation in scleroderma. The focal hyperpigmentation and hypopigmentation that develop in areas of sclerosis are probably postinflammatory changes. The vitiligo-like pigmentation probably is a variant of ordinary vitiligo. The pigment disturbance occurs in areas of normal skin, and in one of our patients there was complete repigmentation following treatment with psoralens and sunlight, which is prescribed for ordinary vitiligo. Dr. Sidney Klaus in our department has shown that the histological features of these lesions are indistinguishable from those of ordinary vitiligo when they are examined in epidermal sheets treated with DOPA.[149a]

Raynaud's phenomenon, present in almost every case of acrosclerosis, varies from mild vasospasm without permanent changes in the skin to severe episodic vascular insufficiency producing ulceration or gangrene of the fingertips (Fig. 7–59; Plate 23*B*). Small pitted scars on the fingertips, representing the mildest changes produced by Raynaud's phenomenon, are diagnostic of the vasospastic disorder (Fig. 7–60). During the course of acrosclerosis, there may be a gradual resorption of bone in the terminal phalanges, resulting in short blunt fingers. Nail growth is usually not affected, although sometimes the nails may curve downward and grow

Text continued on page 325

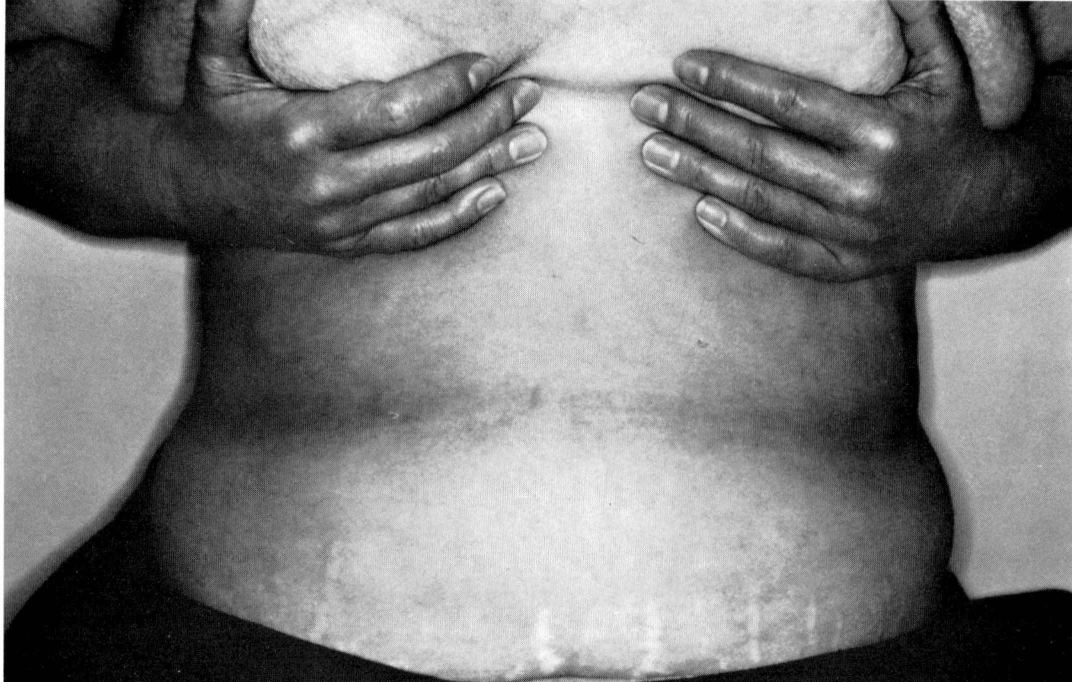

Figure 7–54. Scleroderma. Hyperpigmentation mimicking adrenal insufficiency. Cutaneous sclerosis has not yet developed in this patient. Generalized pruritus was present, and adrenal cortical function was normal.

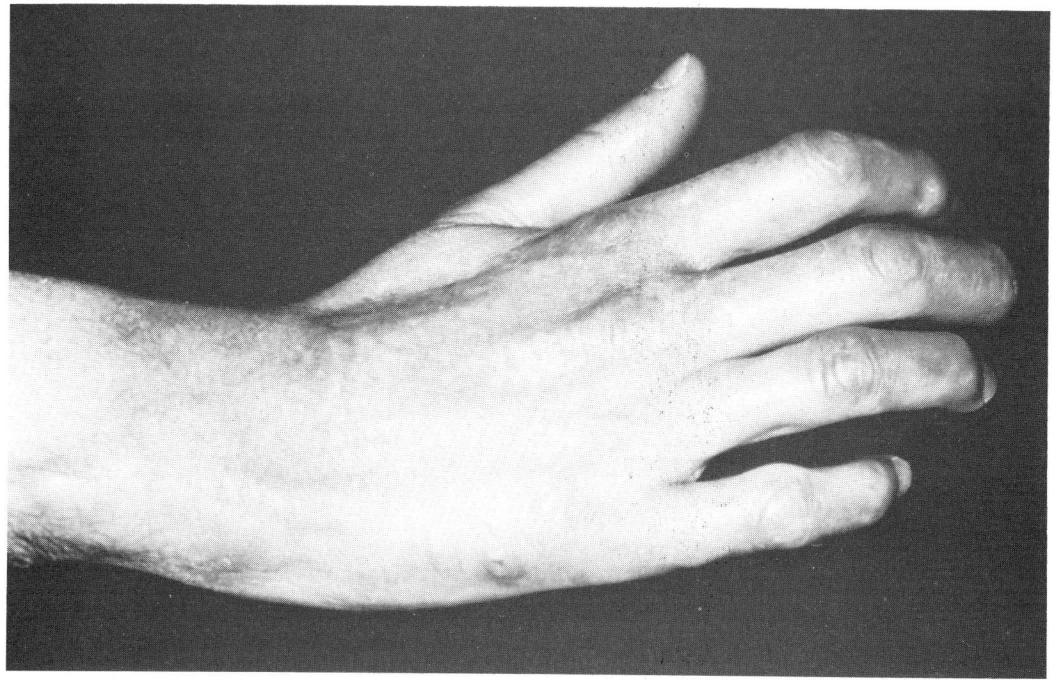

Figure 7–55. Scleroderma. Focal areas of hyper- and hypopigmentation in areas of cutaneous sclerosis.

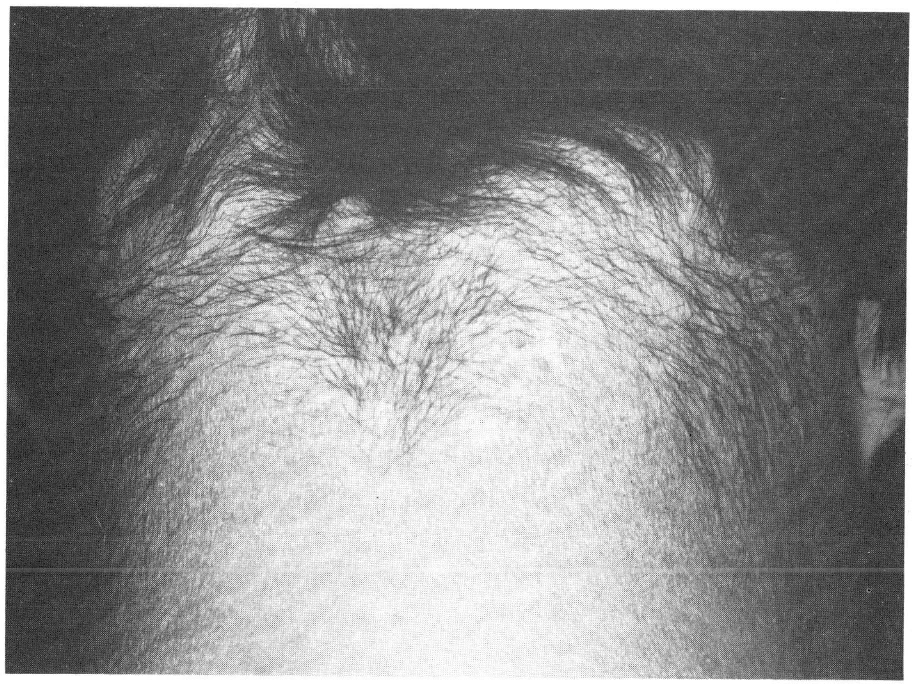

Figure 7–56. Scleroderma. Vitiligo-like depigmentation along hair line.

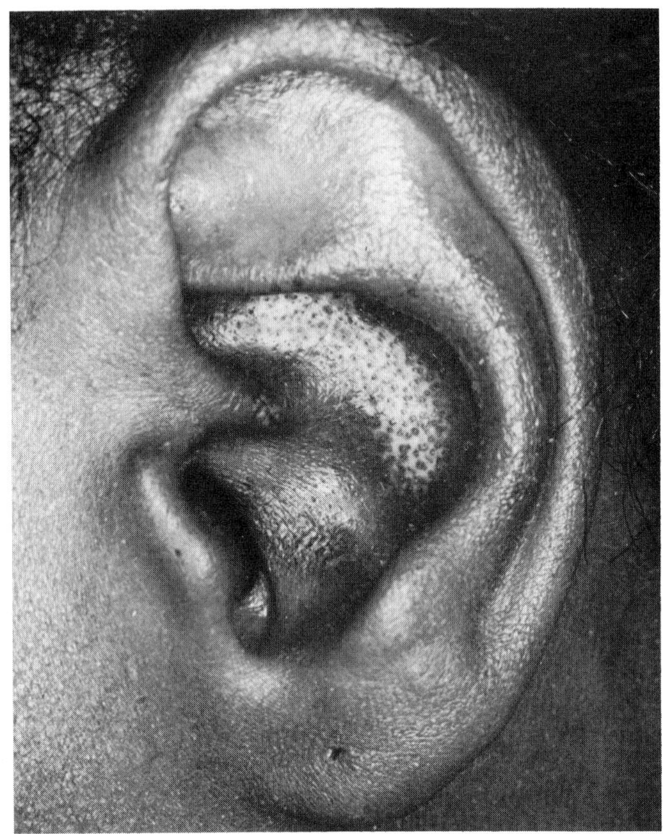

Figure 7–57. Scleroderma. Vitiligo-like depigmentation in pinna.

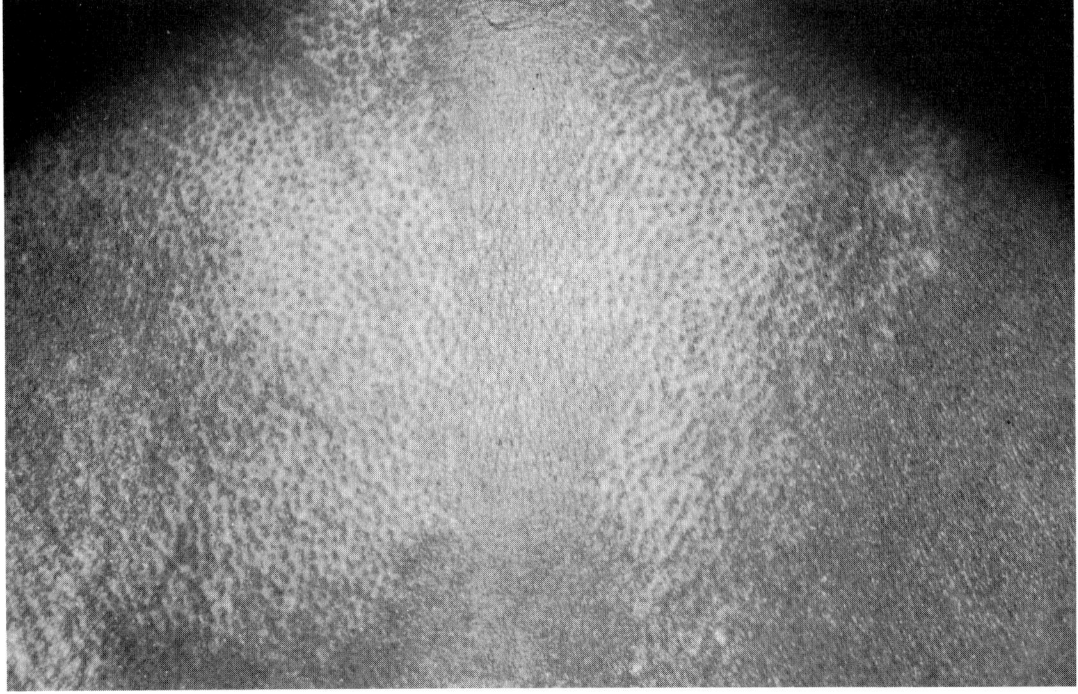

Figure 7–58. Scleroderma. Areas of pigment loss with only perifollicular pigment remaining. This lesion resembles repigmenting vitiligo.

PLATE 23

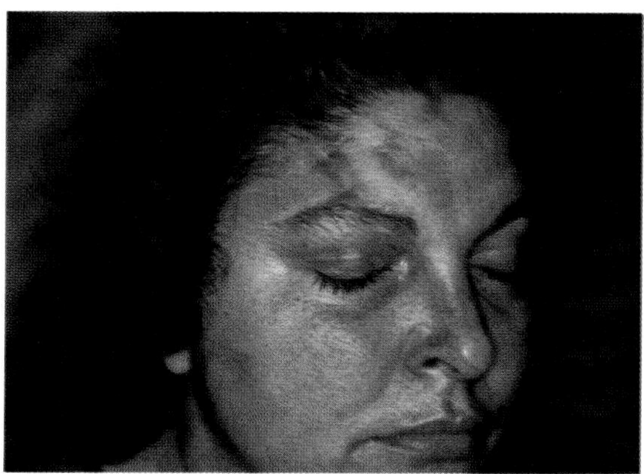

A, Morphea. Coup de sabre variety beginning over right eye and skipping to the right ala nasi. Mucosal involvement of upper lip is shown in Figure 7–82.

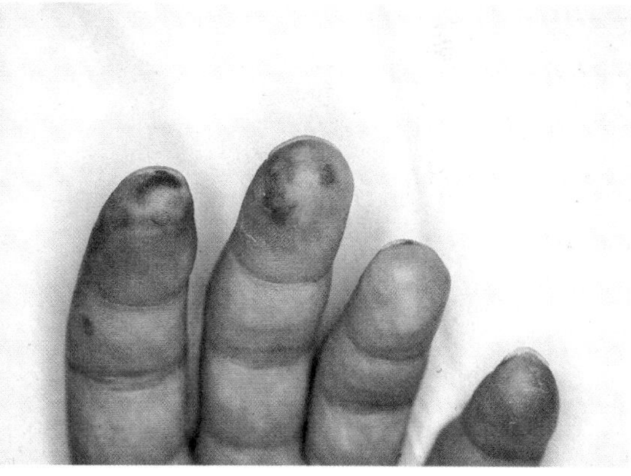

B, Raynaud's phenomenon. Focal gangrene developing in cyanotic finger tips of patient shown in Plate 22*F*.

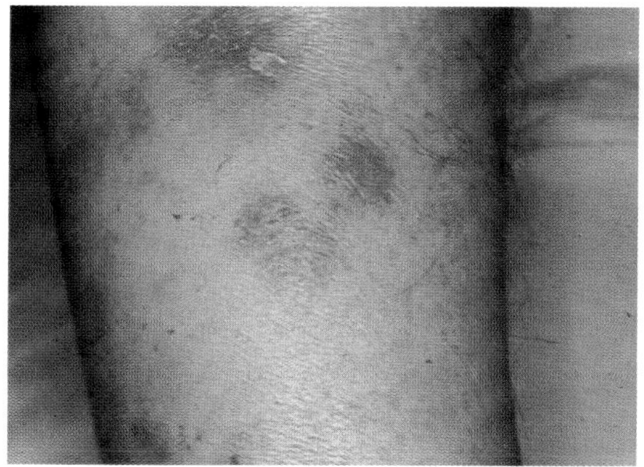

C, Wegener's granulomatosis with involvement of the subcutaneous fat, resulting in a nodular panniculitis.

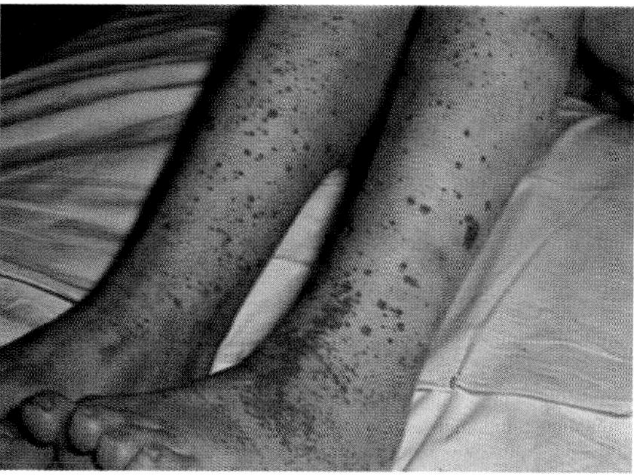

D, Leukocytoclastic angiitis. Erythematous macules and urticarial lesions becoming purpuric.

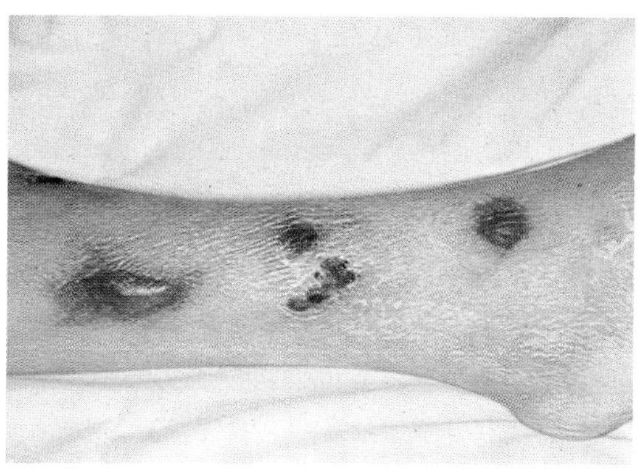

E, Leukocytoclastic angiitis. Hemorrhagic bullae appeared each time the patient ingested aspirin.

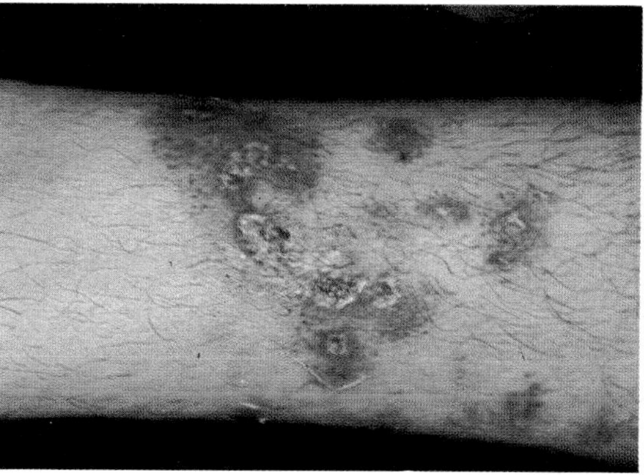

F, Leukocytoclastic angiitis. Purpura and ulceration.

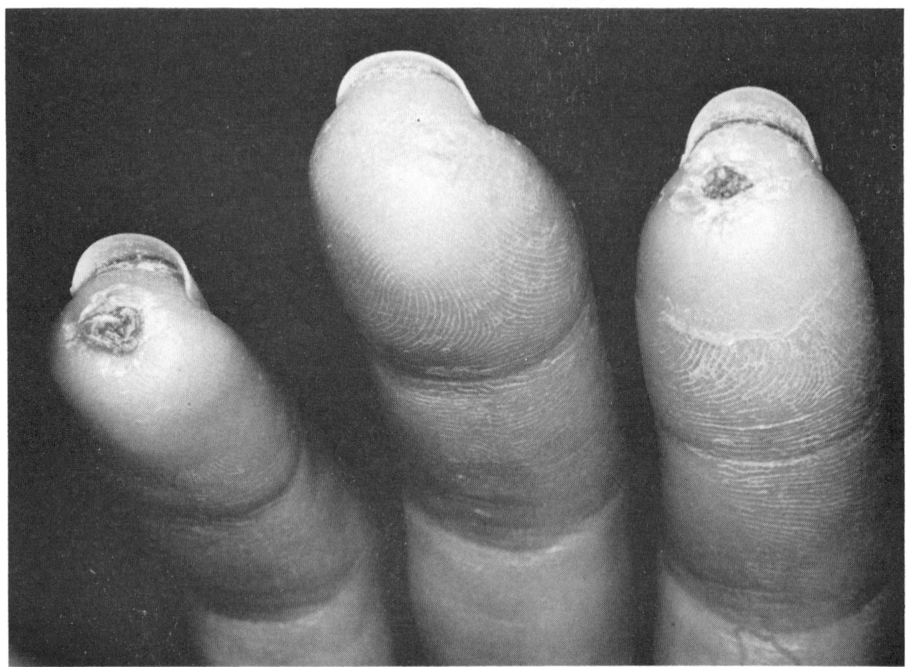

Figure 7–59. Scleroderma. Raynaud's phenomenon producing ulceration of fingertips.

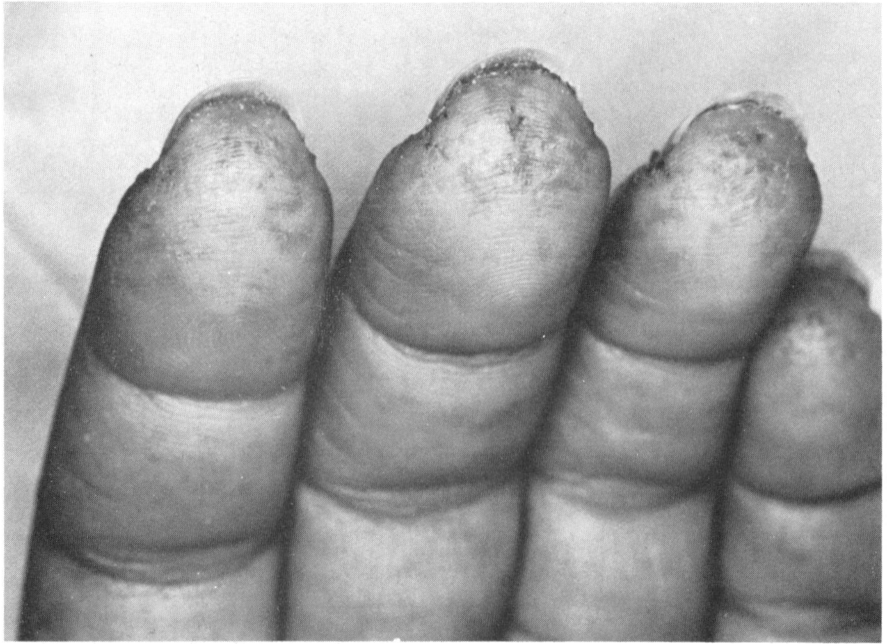

Figure 7–60. Scleroderma. Raynaud's phenomenon producing pitted scars on fingertips.

over the fingers. Ulcerations of the fingertips, toes, knuckles, and ankles, especially the malleoli, are common. Chronic vascular insufficiency and trauma contribute to tissue destruction. Radiographic examination sometimes discloses small areas of calcification at the base and borders of the ulcer. It is not clear whether the calcification is a cause or a result of the ulceration.

Calcinosis cutis is usually seen late in the course of scleroderma; this is in contrast to its early appearance in dermatomyositis. Calcium is deposited in small foci primarily about the major joints and on the fingers; it is not disabling, as in dermatomyositis, but it is often painful (Figs. 7–61 and 7–62). This complication of scleroderma has been called the Thibierge-Weisenbach syndrome. The yellow-to-white firm nodules of calcium eventually erode through the surface of the skin and discharge their contents. Patients often pluck the calcium to obtain relief from the painful inflammation associated with its deposition. Erysipelas and cellulitis frequently arise at these open areas of calcinosis.

There are two characteristic facies in scleroderma. Only one is related to cutaneous sclerosis. In its extreme form, the sclerodermatous process produces a facial pattern consisting of a fixed stare, a permanent grimace, and a wrinkle-free brow (Fig. 7–63). The mouth cannot be opened widely and the forehead cannot be wrinkled. In the other facies, unrelated to cutaneous sclerosis, the patient has a pinched nose, small mouth with thin lips, and sunken cheeks (Plate 21*A*). The lower half of the face seems small. Sclerosis has never taken place; the skin feels normal, and it is likely that the changes are caused by shrinkage of the tissues.

In diffuse scleroderma, the uncommon variety, cutaneous sclerosis begins over the chest and spreads centrifugally to the head and extremi-

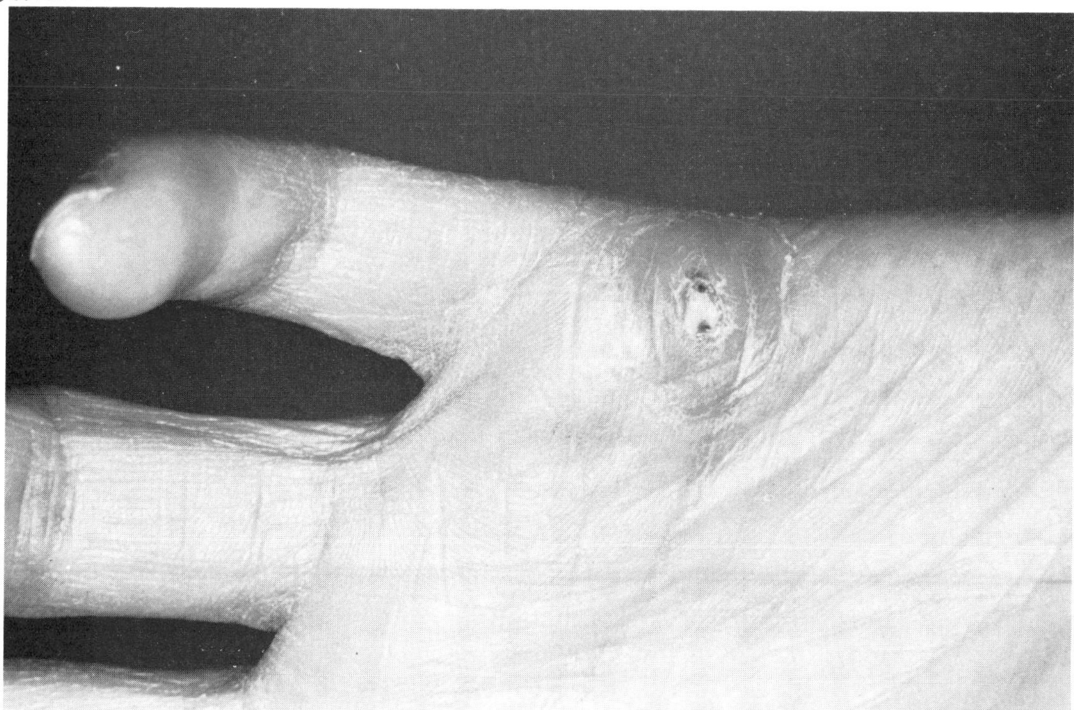

Figure 7–61. Scleroderma. Calcinosis cutis on palm and finger tip.

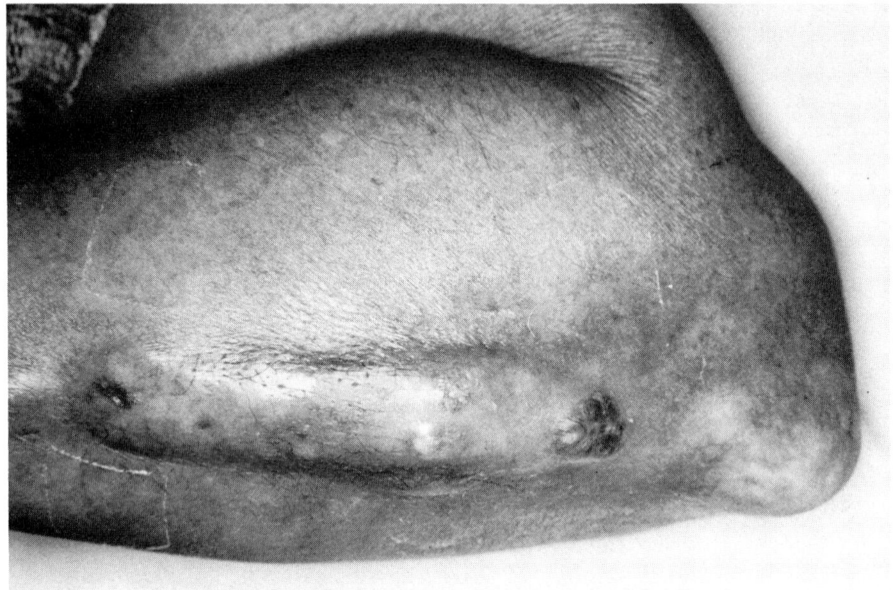

Figure 7–62. Scleroderma. Calcinosis cutis on elbow.

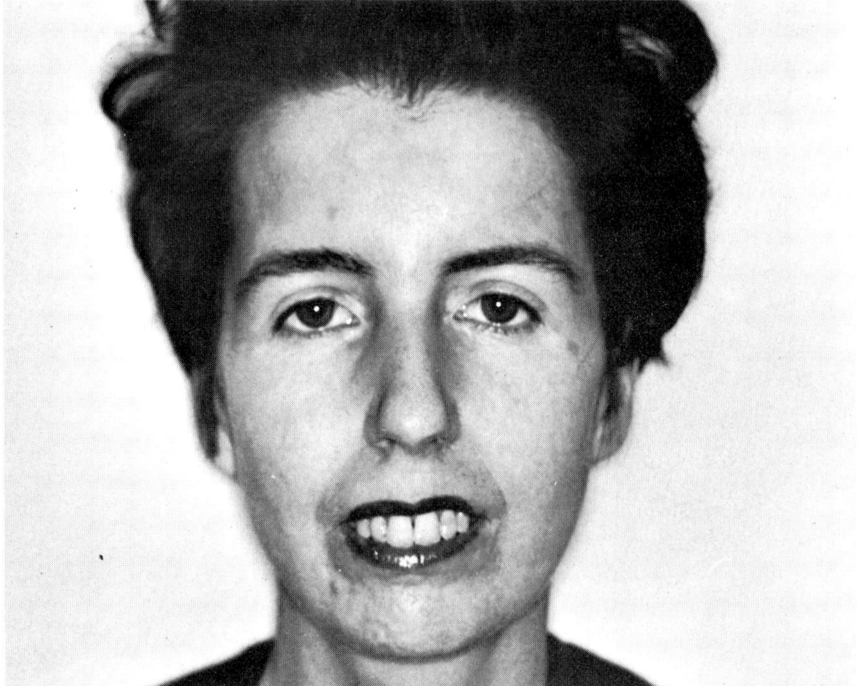

Figure 7–63. Scleroderma. Typical facies produced by hardening of the skin.

ties (Plate 20*D*). Edema may precede the development of sclerosis. The areas of sclerosis are characteristically yellowish-brown and waxy. The course of the disease is usually so rapid that there is not enough time for sclerodactyly to develop. Raynaud's phenomenon is uncommon in diffuse scleroderma; otherwise, this form of the disease is identical to acrosclerosis both in visceral involvement and in cause of death.

Photosensitivity does not occur in scleroderma, nor is there violaceous coloring in any of the cutaneous lesions. In most cases of scleroderma, linear telangiectasia, identical to that found in LE and dermatomyositis, is present on the nailfolds (Fig. 7–64). Ulceration and superficial infection of the cuticle also occur, but periungual erythema is rare.

Sharply defined telangiectatic macules of linear, oval, square, and multiangular configurations are commonly found on the face, hands, lips, and buccal mucosa (Plates 20*F* and 21*A–E*; Figs. 7–65 and 7–66). They usually vary from pink to bright red and range in size from 1 to 5 mm, but in exceptional patients they may be as large as 1 to 2 cm. Close inspection reveals delicate telangiectatic vessels in some; in others only a homogeneous erythema can be seen. The edges of these flat lesions may be sharp or slightly fuzzy. The diagnostic feature of this type of telangiectasia resides in its shape and not in the character of its vessels. *Telangiectatic mats* would be an appropriate name for these lesions. Although telangiectasia is a feature of all three connective tissue diseases, telangiectatic mats are seen almost exclusively in scleroderma. I have also observed them in cases of sclerodermatomyositis. In two patients with systemic LE, irregularly shaped telangiectatic macules were present on the fingers (Fig. 7–27).

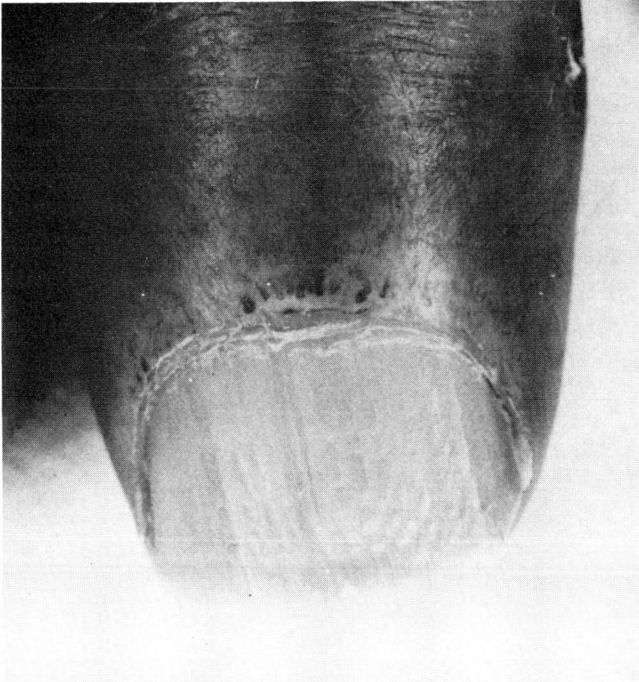

Figure 7–64. Scleroderma. Linear telangiectasia is present on the posterior nailfold and extends onto the cuticle. Periungual erythema is absent.

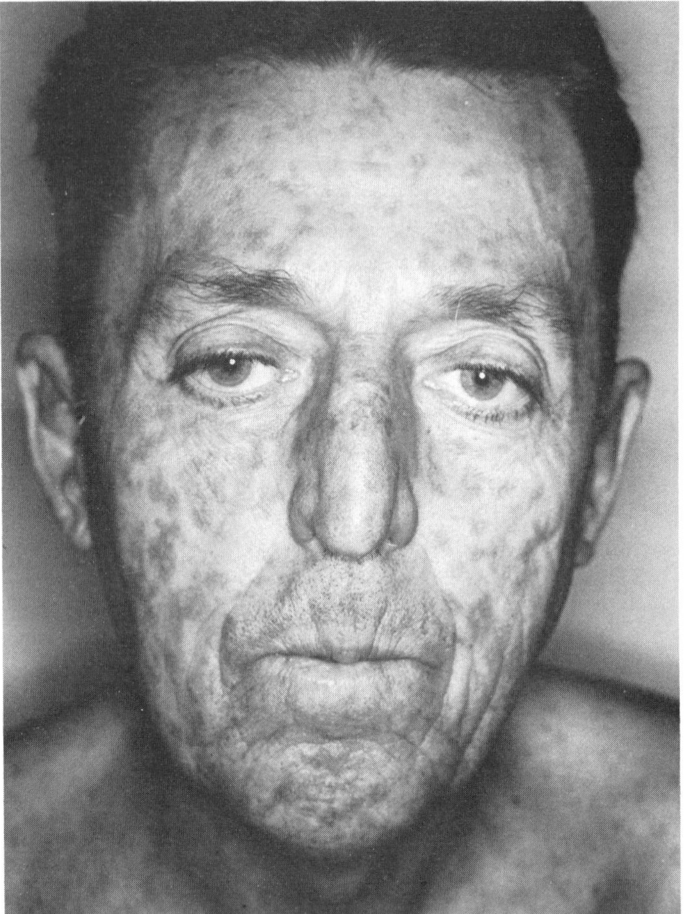

Figure 7–65. Scleroderma. Giant telangiectatic mats occurring on nonsclerotic skin of face.

Telangiectasia of the nail fold and telangiectatic macules seem to be specific for the connective tissue disease. In some patients they are the only cutaneous expression of these disorders. Angiomas indistinguishable from those found in Rendu-Osler-Weber disease may also be seen in scleroderma (see CRST syndrome, p. 335).

The gastrointestinal tract and the lungs are the two organ systems most frequently affected by sclerosis. Dysphagia develops in most cases and eventually leads to emaciation, weight loss, and aspiration pneumonitis. In scleroderma, dysphagia occurs because of abnormal functioning of the neural-smooth muscle system; this dysfunction is present only in the distal two thirds of the esophagus. In dermatomyositis, dysphagia is caused by disease of the striated muscle in the pharynx and proximal one third of the esophagus. On x-ray examination, the esophagus is atonic and dilated. Sclerosis of the submucosa and the atrophy of smooth muscle in the muscularis layer with subsequent replacement by fibrous tissue take place in the esophagus and elsewhere in the gastrointestinal tract. Recent studies, however, clearly indicate that these histopathologic findings are not primarily responsible for the abnormalities of esophageal function: diminution in amplitude of peristaltic waves with their eventual disap-

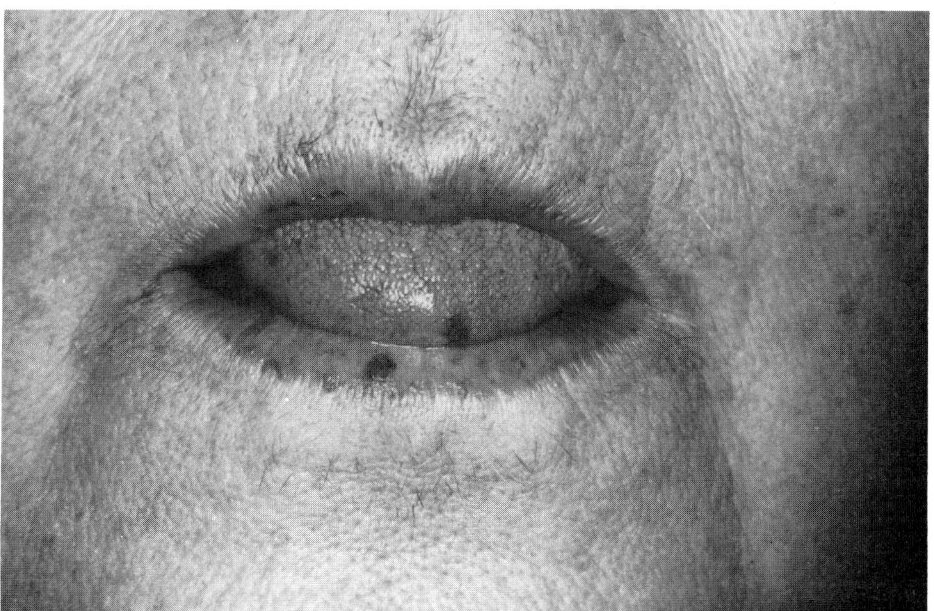

Figure 7–66. Scleroderma. Telangiectatic mats on tongue and lips.

pearance in the distal one half to two thirds of the esophagus and the development of an incompetent lower esophageal sphincter (LES). The physiological disturbance of hypomotility precedes any observable changes in the smooth muscle or collagen of the submucosa.[150]

Cohen et al. reinvestigated this problem with pharmacological and hormonal agents having known mechanisms of action to determine whether differences in response existed between those agents that act directly upon smooth muscle and those that work indirectly through the neuromuscular junction.[151] Four groups of patients were studied: (1) persons with Raynaud's phenomenon in the absence of a connective tissue disorder; (2) scleroderma patients with normal and abnormal peristalsis in the distal esophagus; (3) nonsclerodermatous patients with isolated LES incompetence; and (4) normal individuals as controls. Each person served as his own control by having the physiologic LES pressure measured manometrically before and after testing with each of the following agents: gastrin I, which acts through the neural release of acetylcholine; edrophonium, a cholinesterase inhibitor that enhances the effect of released acetylcholine; and methacholine, which acts directly on the muscle through cholinergic receptors.

These investigators found that there was an abnormality of response to compounds that acted indirectly through cholinergic nerves at a time when the response to direct muscle stimulation by a cholinergic compound was preserved. The results of these studies defined three groups of individuals. Group I consisted of 15 persons with Raynaud's disease or scleroderma who had normal esophageal peristalsis. They reacted normally to methacholine, which stimulates smooth muscle directly, and to the anticholinesterase, edrophonium, but displayed a moderately reduced response to gastrin I, which stimulates the nerve to release acetylcholine. This finding suggests that patients with Raynaud's phenomenon, either as an idiopathic condition or in association with scleroderma, have a latent abnormality in esophageal function based on cholinergic nerve dysfunction. Group II consisted of 15 patients with scleroderma and abnormal peristalsis who responded normally to methacholine but poorly to edrophonium and gastrin I, indicating that while the smooth muscle could be stimulated normally and directly, the neural component of acetylcholine release was abnormal. Group III was composed of two individuals with scleroderma and abnormal peristalsis who responded neither to direct muscle stimulation with methacholine nor to indirect stimulation with edrophonium and gastrin I. It is likely that muscle atrophy was present in these two patients, because a third individual with scleroderma, not part of this study, who also failed to respond to all three agents had marked atrophy of esophageal smooth muscle on examination at autopsy. The individuals with incompetent LES reacted like the normal controls to the three agents. These experiments strongly suggest that "autonomic dysfunction" is responsible for the hypomotility and that defective neural smooth muscle innervation is responsible for the subsequent smooth muscle atrophy that is followed by fibrous tissue replacement. However, histologic studies of the neural elements in the esophagus have not revealed any abnormalities.[152]

Aperistalsis of the esophagus has been correlated with the presence of Raynaud's phenomenon both in healthy individuals and in those with other collagen disorders, including systemic LE.[152] Although one customarily employs the esophageal motility test as a diagnostic test for scleroderma, a detected abnormality in function actually represents an association with Raynaud's phenomenon and not scleroderma. However, since most instances of Raynaud's phenomenon are found in scleroderma, the abnormal motility test proves to be a highly probable but not strictly pathognomonic sign of the disease.

Functional and histological abnormalities of the small intestine and colon are identical to, but much less frequent than, those in the esophagus. When the small bowel is involved, the patient often complains of cramps, diarrhea, and vague abdominal distress, and he may develop malabsorption. When the large colon is involved, the loss of peristalsis can lead to obstruction with perforation. A characteristic radiographic finding by barium enema is broad-mouthed diverticula.

In the past, pulmonary insufficiency was attributed to restricted movement of the chest wall by the hidebound skin over the thorax, but this explanation is incorrect.[146] Approximately 95 per cent of patients with scleroderma have abnormal pulmonary function tests: reduced vital capacity, impaired gaseous diffusion, low lung compliance suggesting stiffening of the alveoli, and pulmonary hypertension. Objective studies show that the skin of the chest wall does not mechanically restrict respiratory movements.

Although impaired CO diffusion capacity is used as the earliest and most sensitive indicator of pulmonary involvement in scleroderma, recent studies by Guttadauria et al. suggest that small airway disease as detected by elevated residual volumes may be an earlier abnormality.[153] They have proposed that the diffusion abnormality, which is believed to be caused by a ventilation-perfusion mismatching, is actually related in part to small airway disease. They pointed out that in scleroderma, there is smooth muscle atrophy and loss of elastic tissue in the bronchiolar wall. The resulting bronchiolectasia produces intermittent expiratory obstruction to air flow and widespread formation of small cysts in the pulmonary parenchyma. Interstitial fibrosis causes additional anatomic narrowing of the small airways. Mononuclear cell infiltrates and peribronchiolar edema of undetermined etiology precede the bronchiolar wall abnormalities.

The triad of pulmonary hypertension, Raynaud's phenomenon, and telangiectasia without obvious cutaneous signs of scleroderma has been reported many times.[154] This combination undoubtedly represents the CRST variant of scleroderma.[155] It seems likely that the pulmonary hypertension in scleroderma and its variant, CRST, is related to vasomotor overactivity of the pulmonary vasculature because of its frequent occurrence in the absence of pulmonary fibrosis. The arterial intimal proliferation in the pulmonary arteries in scleroderma and the CRST syndrome is identical to that found in the digital arteries of patients with Raynaud's phenomenon, whether on an idiopathic basis or in association with scleroderma, and to that found in the interlobular arteries of scleroderma kidney whether or not hypertension is present. These same pathological changes of arterial intimal proliferation with or without myxoid changes have also been found in sclerodermatous lung in the absence of clinically apparent pulmonary hypertension or pulmonary fibrosis.[156] It appears that the obliterative arterial small vessel disease is one of the pathogenetic factors in scleroderma and that it may very well be produced by a chronically and/or intermittently increased vasoconstrictor tone acting upon these vessels.[146]

Twenty-five to 50 per cent of patients with scleroderma in different series have had clinical pulmonary impairment.[137, 141] X-rays of the chest indicate fibrosis with and without cyst formation and linear streaks at the bases of the lungs. Eight instances of alveolar cell carcinoma have been reported in sclerodermatous lungs.[157] Although this neoplasm is not specific for scleroderma and can appear with pulmonary fibrosis from any cause, the possible development of alveolar cell carcinoma in any patient with severe sclerodermatous pulmonary disease should be kept in mind.

Myocardial fibrosis is frequently found at autopsy and is likely responsible for secondary degeneration of the A-V bundle, resulting in bundle branch block and other arrhythmias.[156] Occasionally, EKG changes characteristic of myocardial infarction may be found, even though the patient has had no signs or symptoms of such an event (Fig. 7–67).[158] The distinctive obliterative vascular changes have also been found in the small coronary arteries and arterioles and are likely responsible for the asymptomatic infarction pattern.

About 20 per cent of patients with scleroderma die from renal failure. If one applies the criteria of proteinuria, hypertension, and azotemia, then 45 per cent of individuals with scleroderma have been shown to exhibit some evidence of renal involvement.[159] In a series of 210 patients from Columbia-Presbyterian Medical Center, the mortality rate over 20 years for individuals without any of these clinical signs was only 10 per cent compared to 63 per cent for those with signs of renal involvement.[159] In this series, proteinuria alone occurred in 45 per cent of patients, and in another 45 per cent, there were varying combinations of hypertension, proteinuria, and azotemia *without* hypertension. In those with proteinuria alone, the mortality rate over 20 years was 47 per cent, compared with 76

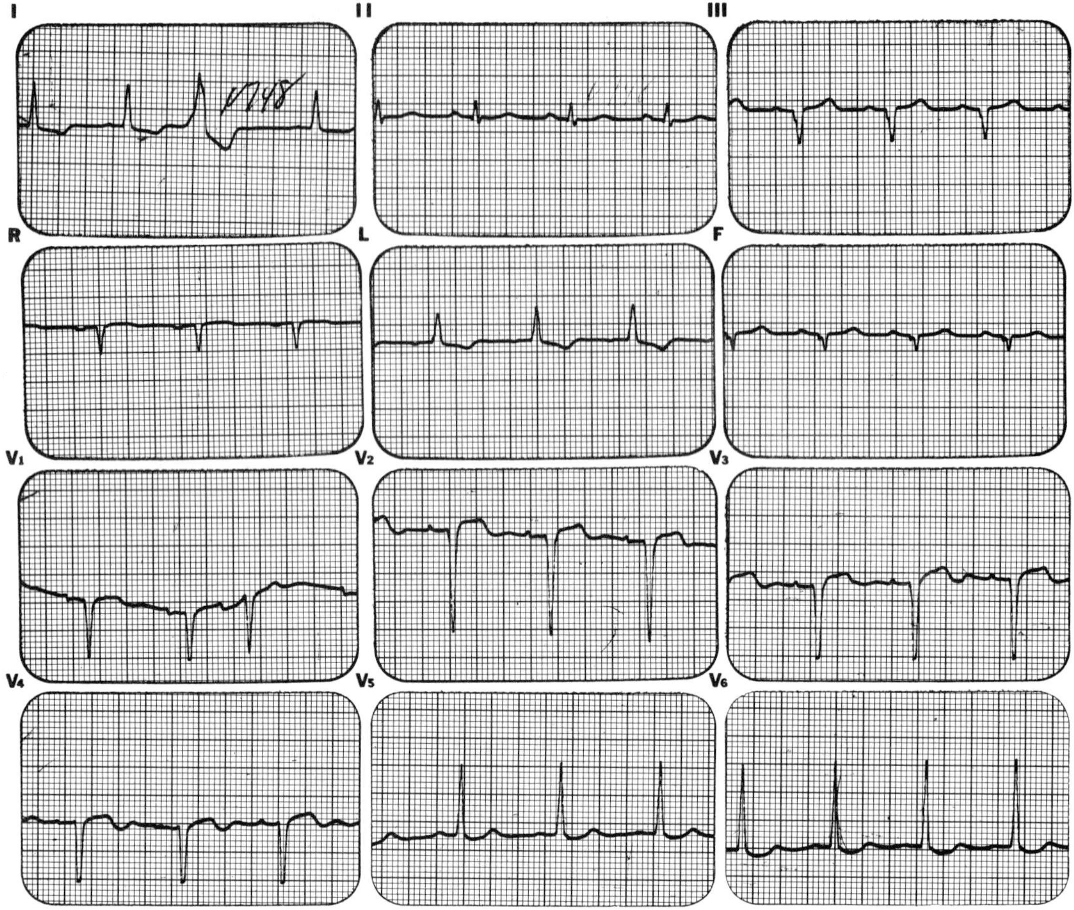

Figure 7–67. Scleroderma. EKG showing changes of old inferior and anteroseptal myocardial infarction in 23-year-old woman who had no previous or current signs or symptoms of cardiac disease.

per cent in whom the proteinuria was associated with hypertension or azotemia or both. The causes of death in those with proteinuria alone was not cited. In this series, the mean time for renal involvement as defined above was 2.3 years after onset of the illness.

Two clinical patterns of oliguric renal failure occur in scleroderma. In one, renal insufficiency is associated with the sudden development of malignant hypertension leading to death within a few weeks to months and occurs in 2.5 to 7 per cent of patients.[137, 159] In the other pattern, renal insufficiency is often precipitated by an episode of heart failure, pericardial effusion, abdominal surgery, dehydration, or intercurrent infection in an individual who has had mild chronic hypertension or has been normotensive for many years with signs of renal involvement. The acute insult produces decreased renal arterial perfusion, which irreversibly compromises an already depressed renal function. Left-sided cardiac failure may occur in association with these two syndromes of renal failure.

Raynaud's phenomenon involving the renal arteries is believed to be the major pathogenetic mechanism in the renal disease. The evidence may be summarized as follows: 76 per cent of all deaths from renal failure occurred in fall and winter; decreased renal cortical blood flow was found in the presence of vasospasm of larger renal vessels; renal cortical blood could be increased significantly by instillation of the potent vasodilator aminophylline into the renal artery; and induced cutaneous Raynaud's phenomenon was associated with a significant reduction in renal cortical blood flow in patients with scleroderma but not in normal individuals.[159] The interlobular arteries of the kidney show intimal proliferation with deposition of mucopolysaccharides producing luminal narrowing, identical to the vascular changes found in the lung, digital vessels, and heart. These vascular changes were present in both hypertensive and normotensive individuals and are not the changes of malignant hypertension. The arterioles distal to the interlobular arteries and the glomeruli showed ischemic necrosis and fibrin deposits that are indistinguishable from those seen in malignant hypertension.

The obliterative intimal vascular lesions are not related to hypertension but appear to be intrinsic to the disease process. Increased levels of plasma renin activity have usually but not invariably been associated with hypertension in scleroderma. In one study, the sudden appearance of increased renin activity was often but not always associated with rapid renal deterioration.[160] It is believed that vasoconstriction of the renal vessels plus luminal narrowing from intimal proliferation of interlobular arteries leads to release of renin and generation of angiotensin II, which produces hypertension and probably additional vasoconstriction. Thus, sudden exacerbations of Raynaud's phenomenon, episodes of hypotension, or congestive heart failure may produce total occlusion of interlobular arteries by additional vasoconstriction on an already narrowed lumen. The cellular anoxia distal to this blockade may prevent the vessels from reopening after restoration of normal perfusion pressure or termination of the initiating vasospasm. The failure of cortical small arteries to reopen after periods of occlusion may explain the proteinuria, azotemia, and rapidly progressive renal failure in some patients with sclerodermal renal disease.

Rapidly progressive renal failure may not be totally irreversible, as indicated by four recent case reports.[161, 162] Prolonged and intensive medical antihypertensive therapy has produced reversal of renal failure and the return of blood pressure to normal levels. In one patient, Raynaud's phenomenon disappeared, again suggesting that renal vasospasm is an important factor in the pathogenesis of the renal disease.[162]

A prospective study employing renal biopsies in nine *normotensive* patients without evidence of renal disease showed the presence of definite early intimal proliferation in four individuals and milder changes in two others.[163] Plasma renin activity was elevated in three of the four individuals with prominent vascular lesions, in one of two with the mild vascular lesions, and in none of two with normal renal biopsies. Cold pressor tests in the four patients with prominent vascular lesions caused an abnormally increased elevation of plasma renin activity, supporting the hypothesis that a decrease in the renal cortical blood flow results in release of renin.[159] In this particular study, renin elevation was not associated with rapid deterioration of renal function during the 10 to 18 months of observation. Complement without immunoglobulins or inflammatory cells was found in the renal vessels by immunofluorescence. This important study also strengthens the hypothesis that obliterative arterial disease is an important pathogenetic mechanism in scleroderma. Sokoloff had suggested in 1952 that Raynaud's phenomenon occurred in the kidney in scleroderma and might be responsible for the renal lesions.[164]

Polymyositis producing progressive clinical weakness of proximal muscles and accompanied by elevated serum levels of muscle enzymes is an accompanying feature of a minority of patients with scleroderma. These patients require and usually respond to oral corticosteroid therapy. However, there exists a larger group of patients with mild nonprogressive proximal muscle weakness who have normal or slightly elevated serum levels of muscle enzymes and require no therapy. Their electromyographic examinations show polyphasic motor unit potentials of normal amplitude and duration, and their muscle biopsies show interstitial fibrosis and variation in muscle fiber diameter without active inflammation. It is important to distinguish between this "simple myopathy" of scleroderma and the complication of true polymyositis.[165] This myopathy would be part of the spectrum of myositis seen in group 4a patients in the classification of dermatomyositis (p. 300).

X-ray examination of the teeth discloses a widening of the periodontal space in 30 per cent of patients with scleroderma. Laboratory tests are not as helpful in scleroderma as they are in LE and dermatomyositis. Clinical and laboratory data from four large series of cases of scleroderma are summarized in Table 7–4.[137, 140, 141, 166]

The natural history of scleroderma is unpredictable. Of 209 living patients surveyed by the Mayo Clinic, 59 had improved, 90 were unchanged, and 54 had become worse; in 6 patients, the disease process had disappeared completely.[137] The evaluation of therapy in scleroderma must take these statistics into consideration.

Currently, physiotherapy and general supportive care are the best

Table 7–4. Clinical and Laboratory Data from Four Large Series of Cases of Scleroderma[137, 140, 141, 166]

Presenting Symptoms	Per Cent
Raynaud's phenomenon	47
Cutaneous sclerosis	30
Articular disability	12
Visceral Manifestations	
Raynaud's phenomenon	90
Esophageal involvement	64–74
Pulmonary involvement	25–50
Cardiac involvement	7–55
Renal involvement	7–20
Articular disability	27–56
Myositis	17–32
Laboratory Studies	
Increased ESR	43–72
False positive serology	1.4
Rheumatoid factor	16–40
Hypergammaglobulinemia	27–50
Serum antinuclear factor	36–70
LE cell phenomenon	5

forms of therapy for scleroderma, since there are no agents that have been shown to consistently influence the course of the cutaneous sclerosis or visceral involvement. Only recently has there been an encouraging therapeutic advance in sclerodermal renal disease in which intensive antihypertensive therapy seems to have reversed and improved the disease process in four patients.[161, 162]

CRST Syndrome

The tetrad of calcinosis cutis, Raynaud's phenomenon, sclerodactyly, and telangiectasia resembling that of Rendu-Osler-Weber disease was designated *CRST syndrome* by Winterbauer in 1964.[167] The vascular lesions, obvious on the face, lips, tongue, oral and nasal mucosae, and hands, have also been observed in the stomach, colon, and bladder. Although bleeding from the oral cavity did not develop in any of Winterbauer's patients, two individuals had melena and hematuria. Abnormal esophageal motility patterns similar to those seen in scleroderma were recorded in most of his patients, and some had cutaneous sclerosis as well. Rodnan has suggested renaming this syndrome CREST, in order to emphasize the esophageal dysfunction.[168]

The predominance of the disorder in women, the lack of genetic transmission, and the absence of bleeding are evidence against this syndrome's being a hybrid between Rendu-Osler-Weber disease and scleroderma. The CRST syndrome represents a relatively benign form of scleroderma that tends to remain stable or pursue a very slow progressive course in most individuals. Uncommonly, disease activity may quicken, leading to severe disability or death. In Rodnan's series of 90 patients, 79 per cent were alive 20 or more years after the onset of the illness.[168]

There is a good reason to continue using the term CRST syndrome instead of scleroderma, because it emphasizes the diagnostic telangiectatic mat. The original report of CRST syndrome described the telangiectases as being identical to those seen in hereditary hemorrhagic telangiectasia. However, inspection of the published photographs and examination of my own cases show that most patients with the CRST syndrome display the sharply defined, broad telangiectatic mats characteristic of scleroderma.

It is of more than academic importance to distinguish between these telangiectatic mats and the vascular lesions of hereditary hemorrhagic telangiectasia. The broad angiomatous macule is virtually pathognomonic of scleroderma and is not a diagnostic feature of Rendu-Osler-Weber disease. Patients with scleroderma may have telangiectases indistinguishable from those in Rendu-Osler-Weber disease, but they are in the minority. Less than 10 per cent of our patients with the CRST syndrome have had such telangiectatic lesions (Figs. 7–68 and 7–69). The morphologic features of these two types of telangiectasia are described in more detail on pages 536 and 537 and in Plates 21 and 29.

Visceral scleroderma without cutaneous involvement is a well-accepted entity.[169, 170] In the past, the absence of cutaneous sclerosis was the criterion for making this diagnosis. However, on the basis of our current studies it is possible that in some cases Raynaud's phenomenon with telangiectasia may have been present without the significance of the vascular lesions being appreciated. I have observed patients with proven

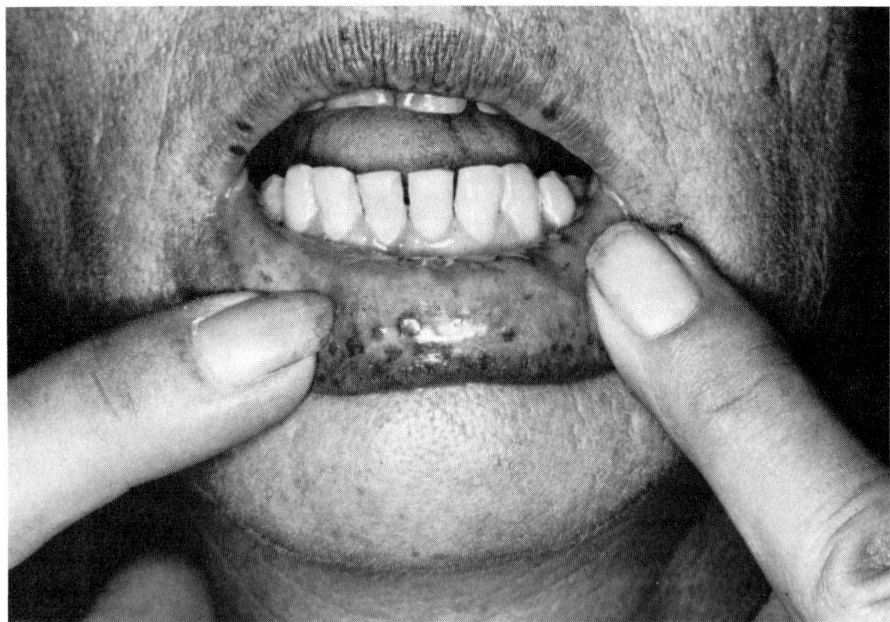

Figure 7–68. Scleroderma. Telangiectases characteristic of hereditary hemorrhagic telangiectasia in patient with CRST syndrome.

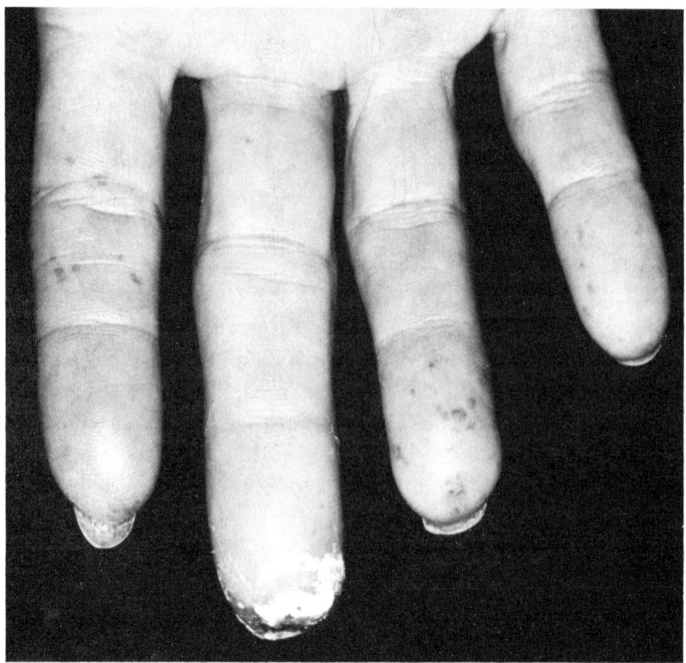

Figure 7–69. Scleroderma. Telangiectases characteristic of hereditary hemorrhagic telangiectasia on fingers of patient shown in Figure 7–68. Fingertip ulceration secondary to Raynaud's phenomenon covered by zinc oxide.

visceral scleroderma whose only cutaneous findings were Raynaud's phenomenon and one or more of the following: sclerodactyly, telangiectasia, and calcinosis. Different combinations of these findings can be summarized in the alphabetical shorthand of the CRST syndrome as RS, RT, RST, and CRT. Telangiectasia is as significant as cutaneous sclerosis in the clinical diagnosis of scleroderma.

The CRST syndrome may be found in association with primary biliary cirrhosis, although the relationship between them is not known.[168, 171] Because hyperpigmentation and pruritus, which are two of the hallmarks of primary biliary cirrhosis, can also be seen in scleroderma, it seemed possible that such patients might have latent primary biliary cirrhosis, since no other reason has yet been found to explain these findings.[151] Testing for antimitochondrial antibodies, which are characteristic of primary biliary cirrhosis, is one approach to this problem. Thus far we have been able to study only one such patient with hyperpigmentation and pruritus. Antimitochondrial antibodies were not found and liver function tests were normal.

Visceral scleroderma sine scleroderma is illustrated by one of our patients.

The patient is a 38-year-old woman who had mild Raynaud's phenomenon for many years. At age 30, she developed swelling of her fingers in the early morning which disappeared by the end of the day. Over the course of the next two years, these episodes became less severe. At age 32, cutaneous edema of the shoulders, arms and face suddenly appeared. The edema of the shoulders and extremities subsided after two weeks but the facial edema persisted, being worse in the morning and lessening by evening. Mild erythema accompanied the facial edema, suggesting diagnoses of LE and dermatomyositis, but no specific diagnoses could be made.

On examination at the Yale-New Haven Medical Center, three months later, she was noted to have marked swelling of the face. She had no cutaneous edema elsewhere. Her skin felt normal and there were no telangiectases. The history of Raynaud's phenomenon, swelling of the fingers, and facial edema suggested the diagnosis of scleroderma. Positive laboratory findings included an abnormal esophageal motility study (loss of peristalsis in mid-and lower esophagus and abnormally low LES pressure), and biopsy evidence of scleroderma in skin from forearm, deltoid, and submandibular areas (homogenization of collagen in lower dermis and replacement of subcutis by collagen). Over the next six years, the facial edema slowly subsided so that by age 38 her facial appearance had returned almost to normal. The Raynaud's phenomenon had responded to treatment with Dibenzyline and had not been a significant problem since age 36.

At age 38, approximately one month before being reevaluated at Yale, she once again developed facial edema but on this occasion it was accompanied by sacral and pedal edema and a weight gain of 26 pounds. She was found to have a pleural and pericardial effusion but was not thought to be in congestive heart failure. EKG showed abnormally low voltage and nonspecific T wave abnormalities. Her fluid retention was corrected by diuretics alone. Further evaluation revealed that esophageal motility was still abnormal, but the LES pressure was now in the low normal range. Biopsies of skin adjacent to the areas biopsied six years earlier showed histological evidence of scleroderma. Her skin felt normal, however, and no telangiectases were present. Serologic tests including those for antinuclear antibody and extractable nuclear antigen (ENA) were normal. Pulmonary function tests, including evaluation of diffusion capacity, have been normal during her course.

This patient is reported here because of her unusual presentation and course. Her scleroderma has manifested itself by facial and peripheral edema, Raynaud's phenomenon, abnormal esophageal motility, pleural and pericardial effusions, EKG abnormalities and histological but not clinical evidence of scleroderma.

Differential Diagnosis

Seven other disorders with varying degrees of cutaneous induration must be differentiated from scleroderma: scleredema adultorum, scleromyxedema, porphyria cutanea tarda, lichen sclerosus et atrophicus, acroosteolysis, eosinophilic fasciitis, and morphea. The histopathologic, clinical, and historical aspects of these seven diseases allow easy differentiation from one another and from scleroderma.

The striking feature of scleredema adultorum is firm nonpitting edema of the face, neck, and trunk; the hands and feet are spared. This edema often follows an infection and may persist for a few months or for years. The edema, which is caused by increased amounts of acid mucopolysaccharide, may impart a peau d'orange appearance, a marking never seen in scleroderma. Scleredema is frequently associated with diabetes mellitus.

Scleromyxedema is a rare disease that closely resembles scleredema. However, the excessive deposition of acid mucopolysaccharides in the dermis, which is responsible for the induration, produces a papular and nodular appearance of the involved skin (see p. 233).

In porphyria cutanea tarda, cutaneous induration and pigmentary changes clinically and histologically indistinguishable from morphea may develop over sun-exposed parts of the body. However, other characteristic features such as blistering, skin fragility, scarring, milia, liver disease, and abnormal urinary uroporphyrin excretion are also usually present and facilitate the correct diagnosis (see p. 687).

Lichen sclerosus et atrophicus is strictly a cutaneous disease. When present on the trunk and extremities, it is confused most often with morphea (Figs. 7–70 to 7–72); when the vulva is involved, the disorder is sometimes erroneously called kraurosis vulvae (Fig. 7–73). Involvement of the perineum (vulva and perianal area) produces the pattern of a white figure eight. *Balanitis xerotica obliterans* is the term used for involvement of the glans penis and urethral mucosa in men (Fig. 7–74). Lichen sclerosus et atrophicus sometimes coexists with morphea. The lesions consist of white to yellowish macules and firm papules that may coalesce into large indurated plaques. They are not premalignant. As the lesions evolve, induration gives way to atrophy and wrinkling. The formation of central depressions, called delling, may be found in the papules and scattered throughout the plaques. Sometimes it is possible to see hyperkeratotic plugs and scaling in the follicular openings of the lesions. Bullae may develop spontaneously or following minor trauma in areas of lichen sclerosus et atrophicus. Figures 7–70 to 7–72 and 7–75 show one of our patients with extensive bullous lichen sclerosus et atrophicus. The histopathology of the various types of lesions in this patient was identical and showed the characteristic subepidermal edematous zone in conjunction with homogenization of the collagen in the dermis and fat indistinguish-

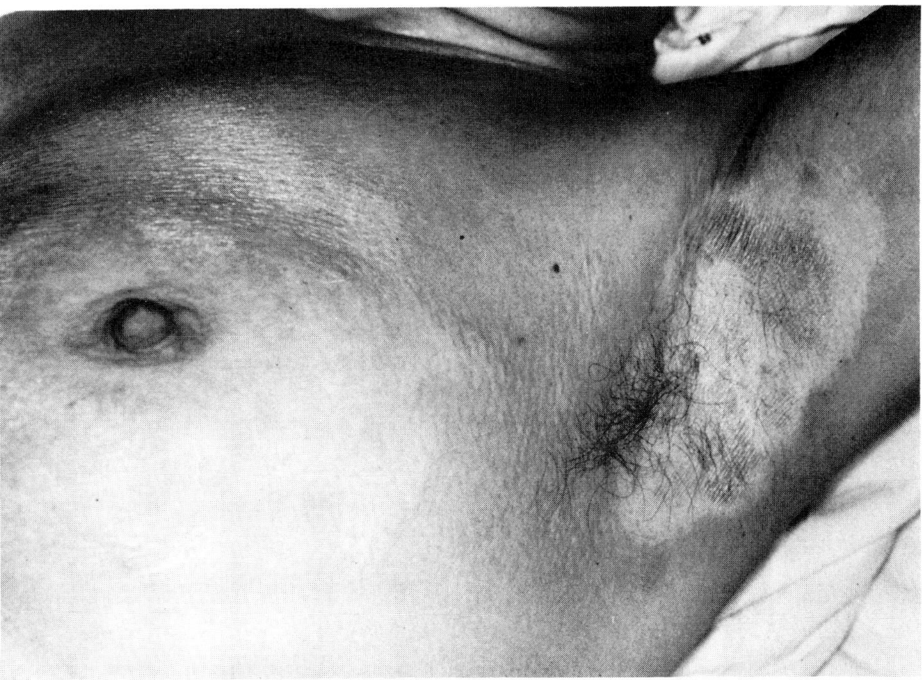

Figure 7–70. Lichen sclerosus et atrophicus involving axillae and breasts.

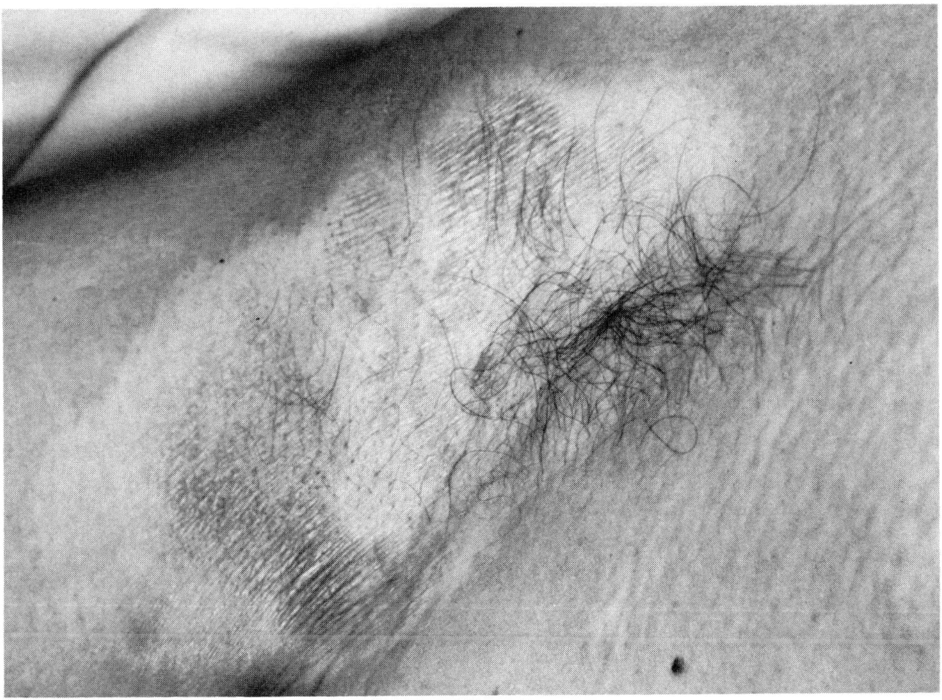

Figure 7–71. Lichen sclerosus et atrophicus. Close-up of axillary lesion shown in Figure 7–70. Skin is depigmented and shows parchment-like wrinkling.

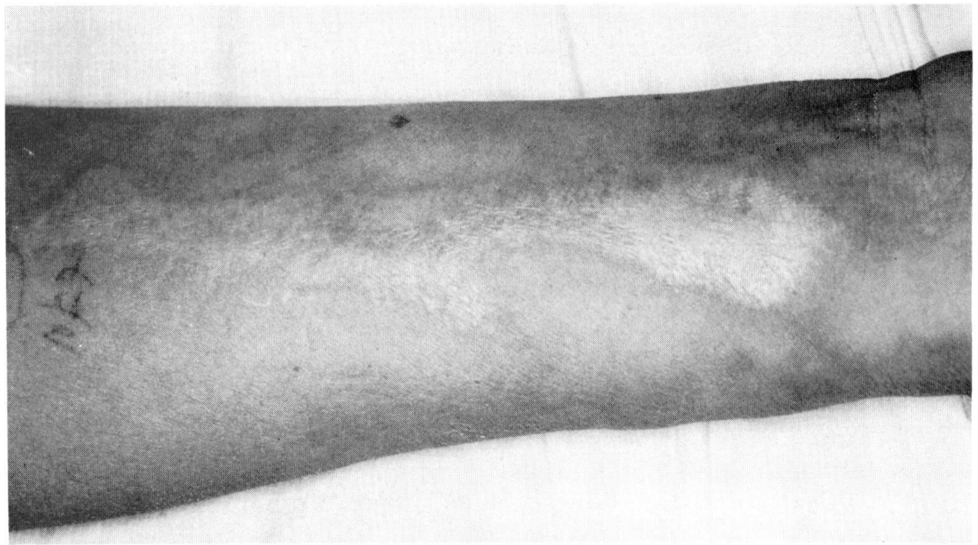

Figure 7–72. Lichen sclerosus et atrophicus on forearm of patient shown in Figure 7–70 simulating morphea.

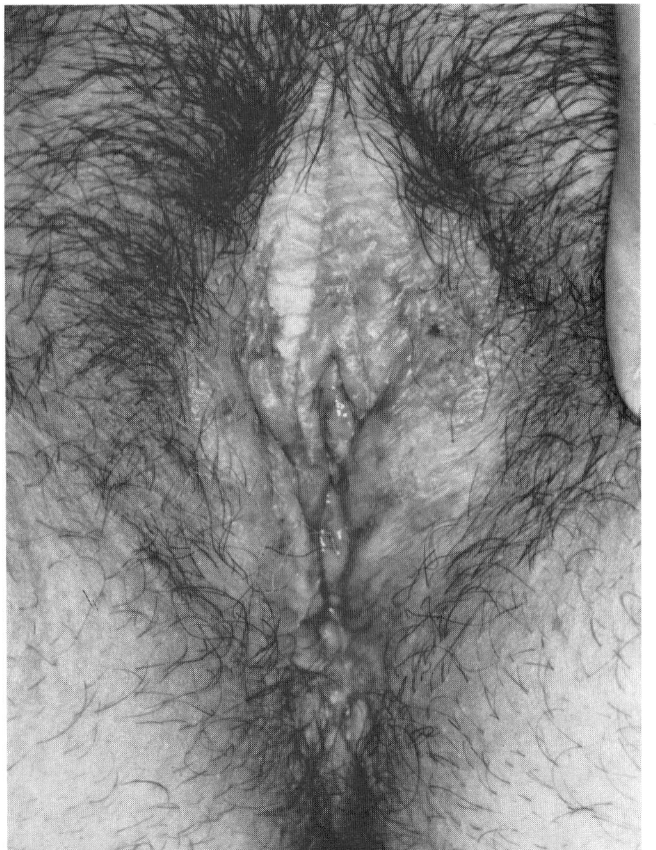

Figure 7–73. Lichen sclerosus et atrophicus involving vulva.

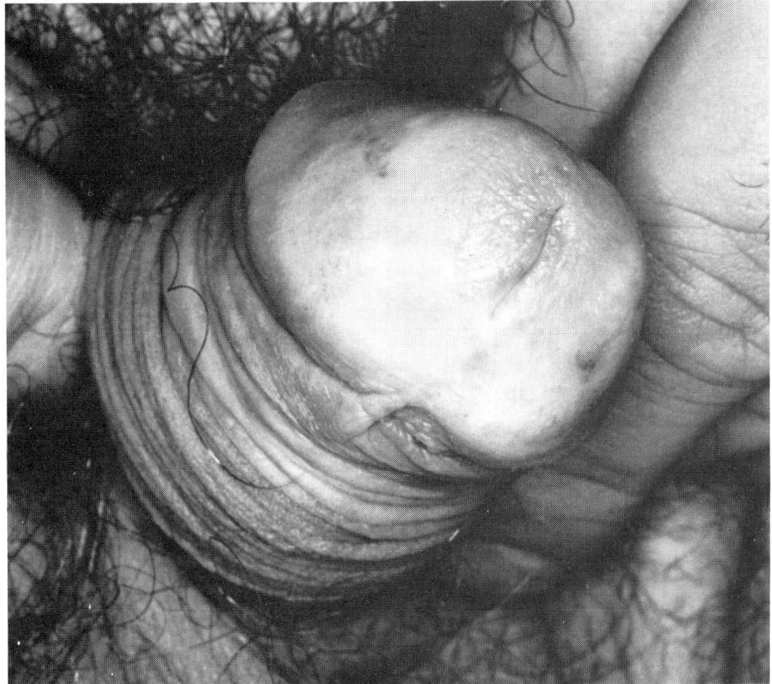

Figure 7–74. Lichen sclerosus et atrophicus on glans penis (balanitis xerotica obliterans).

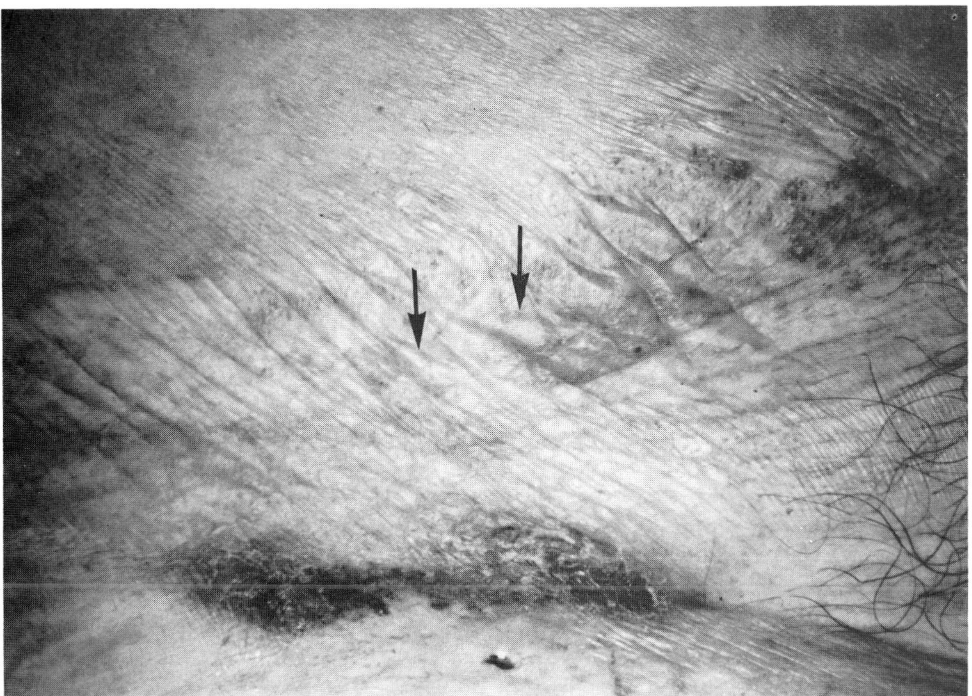

Figure 7–75. Lichen sclerosus et atrophicus in the inguinal and suprapubic areas. Bullous form. Arrows indicate two of several bullae present.

able from that seen in scleroderma or morphea. Patients reported in the past to have bullous morphea probably had lichen sclerosus et atrophicus.

Occupational acroosteolysis is an uncommon disorder developing in individuals working in the manufacture of polyvinyl chloride.[172] Almost all the cases have occurred in workers who clean the autoclaves or reactors in which polyvinyl alcohol and vinyl chloride have been mixed with a number of other chemicals and heated in the absence of oxygen to produce polyvinyl chloride. About 3 per cent of reactor cleaners have developed this disorder, which is presumed to be caused by exposure to one of the incompletely polymerized compounds.

The disorder has appeared one month to three years after exposure. The symptoms include Raynaud's phenomenon and swelling of the hands followed by thickening of the skin over the hands and wrists, especially over the flexor and extensor tendons. In extensive cases, the forearm skin up to the elbows has been involved. The feet may be affected. The thickened skin has a finely papular, nodular, or lobular (ropelike) quality and is fixed to the underlying subcutaneous tissue. There may be some limitation of motion in the fingers because of these cutaneous changes. Telangiectases are not present, and esophageal and pulmonary function is normal. In spite of the cutaneous induration, hair is present. Raynaud's phenomenon has developed in most of the affected individuals. The skin may remain pale or blue and be painful even when not exposed to cold.

X-rays show lytic lesions in the center of the distal phalanges of the hands, leaving the tuft and base intact. The ulna, radius, and sacroiliac joints may also be involved. In scleroderma one sees destruction of the distal phalangeal tuft. In spite of the extensive destruction of bone, the individuals have no symptoms referable to the musculoskeletal system. The bones eventually heal with digital shortening after exposure is discontinued. As far as it is known, the skin lesions have persisted. Histologically, there is disruption and fragmentation of collagen and elastic fibers with new collagen formation in the dermis. However there is no homogenization of collagen or other features resembling scleroderma. This disorder has also been reported in a woman without any occupational exposure. Her hands and the alveolar process of the jaw were affected.[173]

Eosinophilic fasciitis (diffuse fasciitis with eosinophilia, Shulman syndrome) is a newly described entity characterized by pain and swelling of extremities followed by cutaneous induration.[174, 175] The hands, fingers, face, trunk, and, in two cases, single extremities have been affected.[176] The indurated skin has a puckered, dimpled, or cobblestone appearance (Fig. 7–76) and may have a yellowish or erythematous hue. Approximately 30 cases have now been reported (many in abstracts), and men have accounted for almost three quarters of the cases. In many patients, the syndrome has developed following an episode of strenuous exercise. Eosinophilia and hypergammaglobulinemia have been present in almost every case and may spontaneously disappear.[177] Antinuclear antibody and rheumatoid factor have been present in only three patients,[178] and Raynaud's phenomenon in one.[179]

The major pathologic finding is thickening and inflammation of the fascial layer between the subcutaneous fat and muscle, but there is also widening and inflammation of the septa in the subcutaneous fat.[180] Acid mucopolysaccharide, probably as hyaluronic acid, is also found in the tissues.[180] Lymphocytes and plasma cells are the predominant inflammatory cells in both areas, and in a few cases eosinophils have been present as well.[175] Deposition of IgG and complement have been found in the fascial lesion in a minority of cases.[174, 175]

As the disease progresses, the skin becomes tightly bound down, producing limitation of motion in contiguous joints such as the wrists, elbows, and shoulders. However, synovial inflammation is also a feature of this syndrome and may partly account for the flexion contractures of large joints, as well as those of the small joints of the hands and fingers when the latter are not affected by cutaneous swelling and induration.[178, 179] Oral steroid therapy has usually produced a prompt resolution of the skin lesions and restoration of joint mobility to normal, but in a few cases, the hide-bound skin has persisted in spite of joint improvement.[177, 180]

It is not clear whether diffuse fasciitis is a variant of scleroderma, and only longer follow-up observations will be able to resolve this problem. The features suggesting that it is a unique syndrome are the male predominance, low incidence of serologic abnormalities, the distinctive fascial lesion, and prompt response of cutaneous edema to oral steroid therapy. Features favoring a relationship to scleroderma include histologic findings of scleroderma in late cutaneous lesions,[177, 178] eosinophilia in blood and skin lesions in 18 to 20 per cent of patients with scleroderma and morphea,[181] and widening and inflammation in subcutaneous fat septa similar to those seen in scleroderma.[180] In addition, Caperton et al. reported in two abstracts that morphea and diffuse fasciitis coexisted in their patients; relapses occurred several months after discontinuing steroids; and diffuse fasciitis appeared in one patient with scleroderma involving lungs and esophagus.[177, 178] Biopsies of the deep fascia need to be performed in scleroderma and morphea to determine whether diffuse fasciitis with eosinophilia is a unique disease or a variant of scleroderma.

Figure 7–76 illustrates a patient seen at the Yale-New Haven Medical Center whose diffuse fasciitis was associated with a small cell lymphoproliferative disorder exhibiting plasmacytic differentiation and producing an antibody-mediated aplastic anemia.[182] Excessive exercise consisting of house painting and rowing exercises antedated the development of the diffuse fasciitis. The cutaneous induration and limitation of joint movement responded dramatically to steroid therapy.

Morphea usually arises as flesh-colored or erythematous edematous plaques that evolve into waxy and shining lesions that range in color from ivory to yellow-white and feel firm or indurated (Plate 21*F*; Fig. 7–77). A violaceous or lilac-tinged inflammatory border may be present around such indurated lesions and is frequently associated with peripheral enlargement of the plaques. Hyperpigmentation may develop in lesions of long duration (Fig. 7–78). In some cases, morphea may arise as single or multiple flat purplish-red patches without edema or induration and may remain in this state for several months to several years before spontaneously resolving (Plate 22*B*, *C*). The violaceous inflammatory border is not seen in scleroderma.

The lesions of morphea vary from a few millimeters in the *guttate* variety to several centimeters in the more usual *plaque* variety. Solitary or multiple plaques may be present. A fusion of many lesions results in

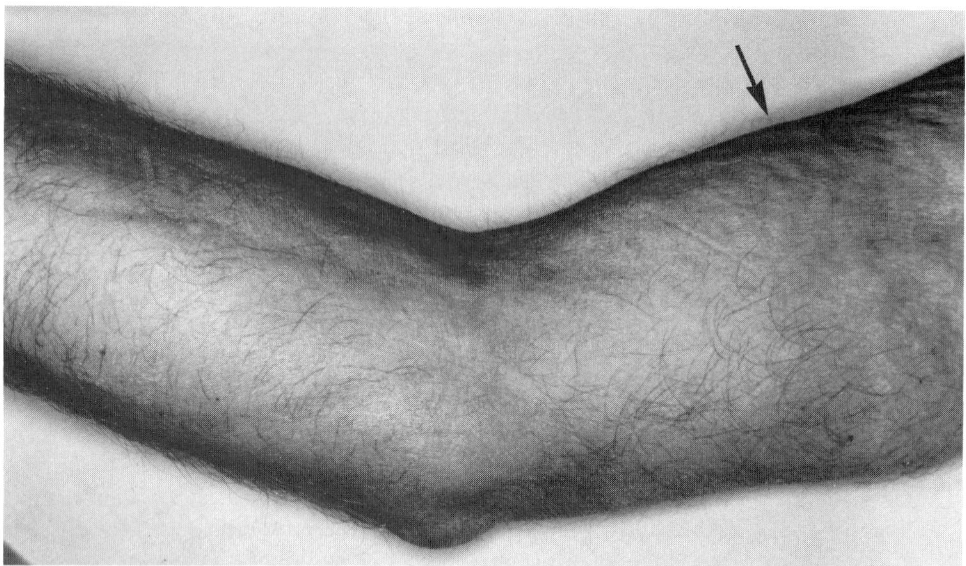

Figure 7–76. Eosinophilic fasciitis. Indurated skin has a puckered, dimpled, or cobblestone appearance (arrow).

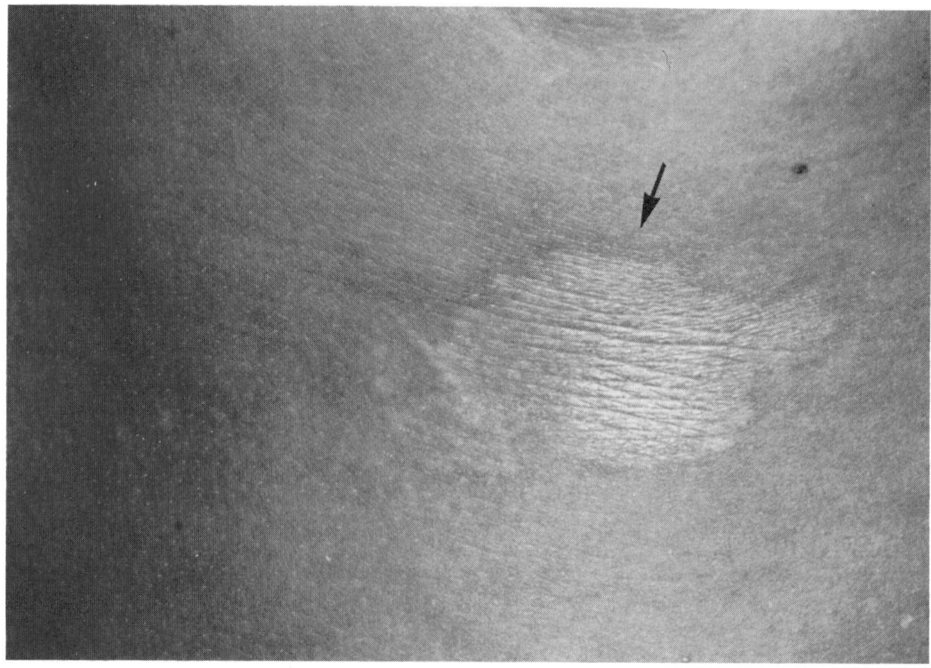

Figure 7–77. Morphea with violaceous border (arrow).

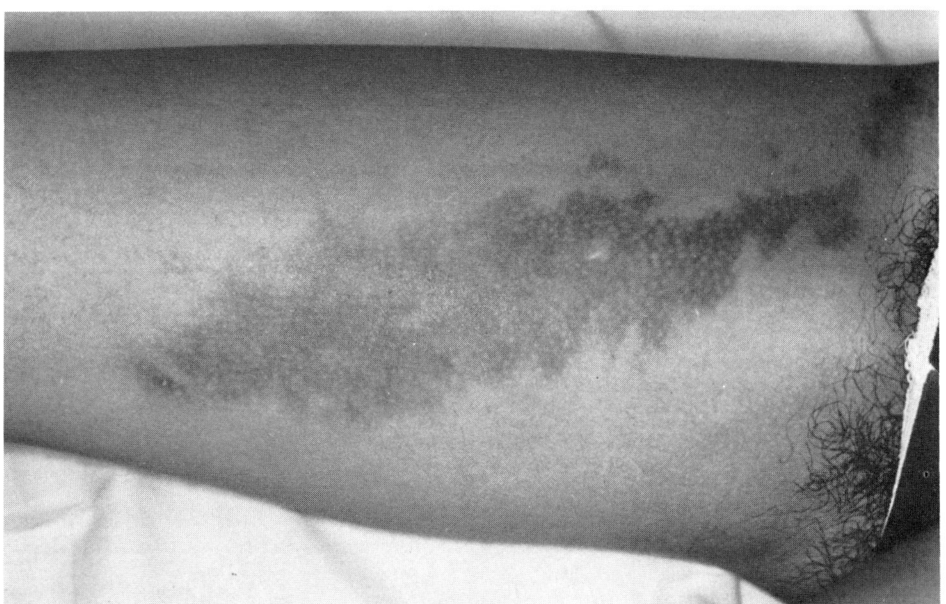

Figure 7–78. Morphea with hyperpigmentation.

generalized morphea in which the entire face or trunk may be affected. Linear morphea occurs primarily in children. An entire limb may show a narrow or broad band of morphea (Figs. 7–79 and 7–80). Edema of the lower extremity may precede the onset of a unilateral lesion. Linear morphea may affect subcutaneous fat, muscle, and fascia (pansclerosis) and may cause contracture of the limb. Examination of the muscle discloses histologic evidence of myositis that is indistinguishable from that seen in scleroderma. Atrophy of the subcutaneous tissues, including the bone, often develops and results in shortening of the limb. In some cases atrophy of one entire side of the body occurs. Surgery and physiotherapy are often necessary to correct existing contractures. Calcinosis cutis is associated with linear morphea.

Figure 7–81 illustrates linear morphea forming an almost complete circumferential band around the lower third of the breast of a 16-year-old girl. The lesion spontaneously resolved without leaving any deformity 12 months later.

The pansclerosis found in some cases of linear scleroderma may occur in a generalized fashion as guttate, plaque, or linear lesions on the trunk, extremities, face, and scalp. This syndrome has been named *disabling pansclerotic morphea of children* by Diaz-Perez et al.[182a] In several children the syndrome began as linear scleroderma before becoming generalized. The age of onset has ranged from 1 to 14 years, and most of the affected children have been girls. The musculoskeletal involvement produces marked disability in the form of flexion contractures of the hands, feet, elbows, and knees; tiptoe gait because the frequently involved Achilles tendon becomes shorter; and musculoskeletal atrophy of extremities. The pansclerosis of the skin and soft tissues is sometimes progressive. Two children have died after four and nine years of progres-

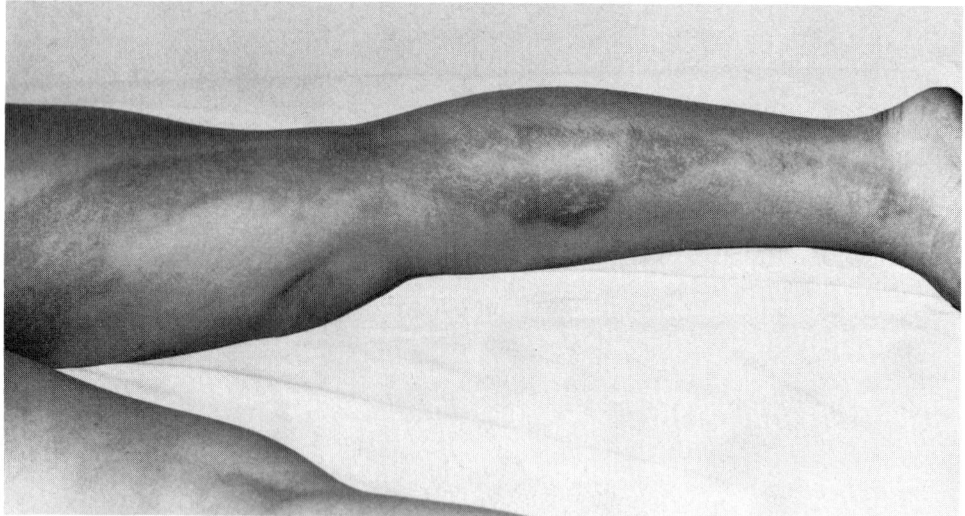

Figure 7–79. Linear morphea involving leg.

sive disease. One child was found dead in bed from unknown causes, and the other died of bronchopneumonia. However, the natural history of this syndrome remains to be defined.

En coup de sabre is a spectacular variation of linear morphea which appears specifically on the face (Fig. 7–82; Plate 23*A*). It originates in the frontoparietal region of the scalp on one side of the midline and is often associated with alopecia. The lesion extends vertically onto the face, does not follow any dermatome, and may leave areas of normal skin in its linear path. In patients with extensive involvement, the oral mucous membrane may be affected. The skin may be depressed, appear ivory to yellowish-white, and feel either indurated or normal. Not only is there

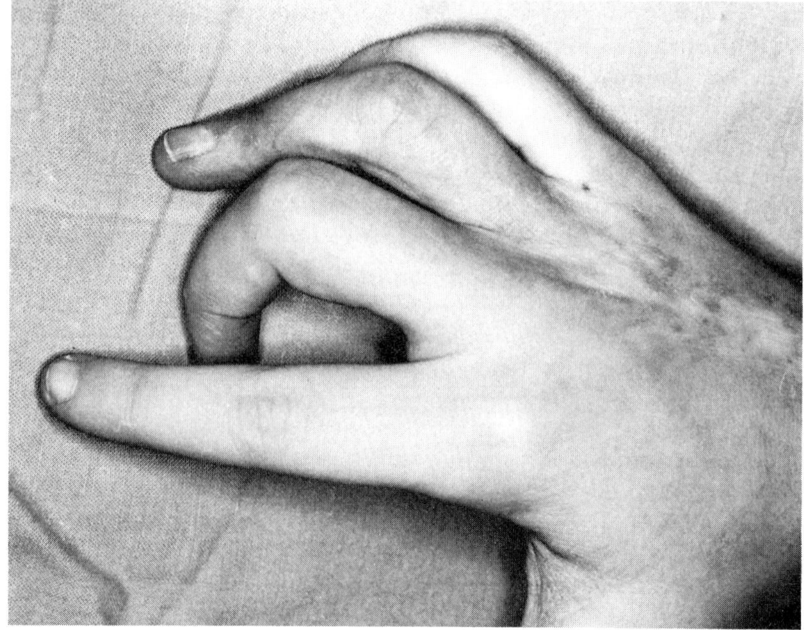

Figure 7–80. Linear morphea involving hand to produce flexion contracture of finger.

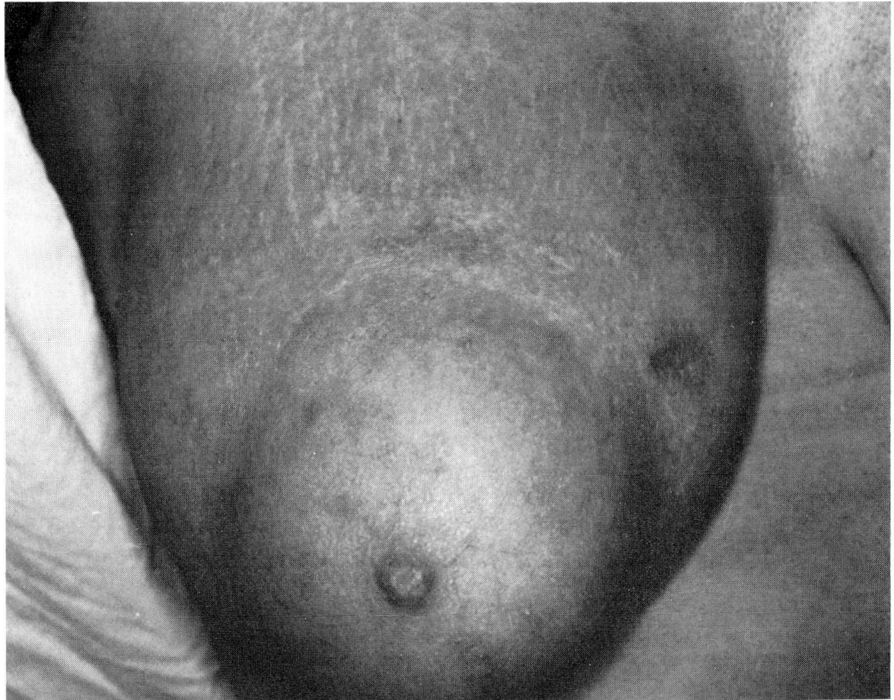

Figure 7–81. Linear morphea producing a circumferential band around the lower third of the beast.

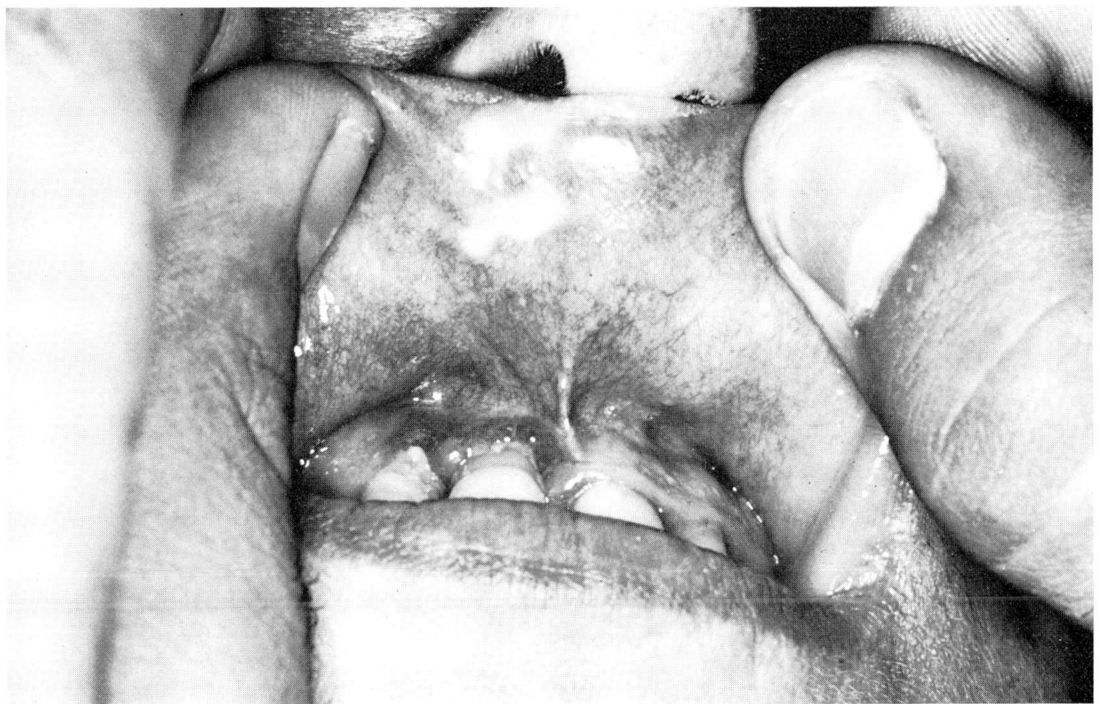

Figure 7–82. Morphea (coup de sabre). The mucosa of the upper lip is affected. See Plate 23*A* for the other components of this lesion in this patient. Gingiva overlying right incisor is atrophic.

atrophy of the subcutaneous fat, but there may also be similar involvement of the facial muscles and bones. The mechanism by which these tissues are involved is not known. *En coup de sabre* may represent an abortive form of progressive facial hemiatrophy (Parry-Romberg syndrome). Figures 7–83 to 7–88 show sequential changes in a youngster with the Parry-Romberg syndrome. He also had multiple lesions of morphea on the trunk, neck, and scalp. Focal atrophy of the gingiva exposed the base of a tooth. There was no evidence of bony or muscular atrophy in this youngster. The clinical picture was produced solely by atrophy of the subcutaneous fat.

The linear and guttate or linear and plaque varieties of morphea may appear together in the same individual. The histopathology of morphea is identical to that seen in scleroderma except that the dermal perivascular infiltrate is more prominent in the early lesions of morphea, perhaps accounting for the inflammatory lilac border.

The relationship between morphea and scleroderma is neither completely understood nor agreed upon. All clinicians seem to believe that morphea is essentially a benign disease that resolves spontaneously in a few months to a few years. Some investigators feel that morphea is a limited form of scleroderma. However, morphea does not bear the same relation to scleroderma that cutaneous LE bears to systemic LE. Many cases of systemic LE begin with discoid lesions, but it is extremely rare for scleroderma to develop with the lesions of morphea.

A few cases have been observed in which morphea coexisted with acrosclerosis, intestinal scleroderma, and sclerodermatous involvement of the heart, lung, and esophagus.[183, 184] In one series, scleroderma developed in 2 out of 44 cases of generalized morphea.[185] and in another series, scleroderma developed in 6 out of 111 cases of various forms of morphea, including the linear variety.[186] Most patients with morphea are not reported in the literature, so the incidence of such transformation is undoubtedly very low.

Plate 22*B* illustrates one of our patients who had morphea and visceral scleroderma. This 63-year-old woman had Raynaud's phenomenon, telangiectatic mats on her fingers, lips, and face, pericardial effusion, and positive tests for antinuclear antibody and rheumatoid factor. She had extensive purplish-red patches without edema or induration over her thighs and lower trunk. In the center of one such area on her right flank there was an indurated yellowish plaque. Histological examination of the purplish red patches and the yellowish plaque revealed the typical changes of scleroderma. She did not have any other cutaneous evidence of scleroderma: sclerodactyly, cutaneous sclerosis, or puffy fingers.

In 235 cases of morphea from the Mayo Clinic, data were presented which suggested that morphea might be a systemic disorder.[185] Arthralgia occurred in 45 per cent of the patients, migraine in 15 per cent (the incidence in population being 1 to 5 per cent), abdominal pain of unknown etiology in 12 per cent, and Raynaud's phenomenon in 4 per cent. In two families, siblings had scleroderma. Abdominal pain, migraine, and linear scleroderma developed simultaneously at puberty in six patients. Abnormal electroencephalograms have been detected in 60 per cent of the patients with morphea and in 39 per cent of those with scleroderma.[187] Jablonska et al. described abnormal sensory chronaxy values in morphea and scleroderma.[188] Ansell described nine children, some with

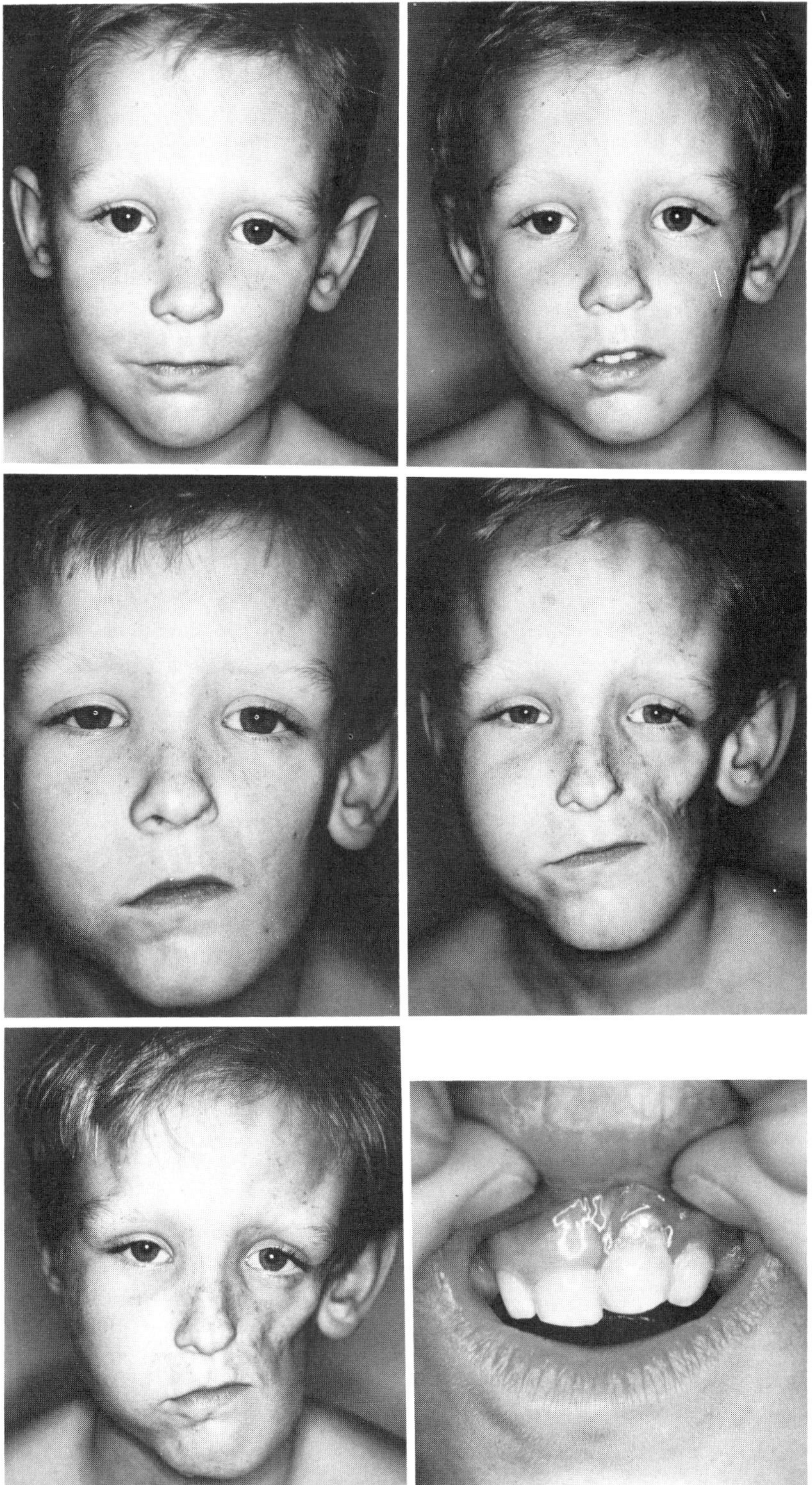

Figure 7–83. Top left. Parry-Romberg syndrome. Figures 7–83 to 7–88 show sequential changes in a youngster with this variant of morphea. May, 1974.

Figure 7–84. Top right. Parry-Romberg syndrome. Oct., 1974.

Figure 7–85. Center left. Parry-Romberg syndrome. Feb., 1976.

Figure 7–86. Center right. Parry-Romberg syndrome. Nov., 1978.

Figure 7–87. Bottom left. Parry-Romberg syndrome, Nov., 1979.

Figure 7–88. Bottom right. Parry-Romberg syndrome. Focal atrophy of gingiva exposed base of a tooth.

morphea and some with linear scleroderma, who had chronic polyarthritis manifested by joint stiffness and occasionally soft tissue swelling around the joints. The sedimentation rate was normal in eight of the nine; rheumatoid factor, negative in all; and antinuclear antibody positive in four, in the absence of elevated anti-DNA antibodies or abnormalities in serum complement levels.[189] Evidence of systemic involvement was present in several of the 14 children with *disabling pansclerotic morphea* reported from the Mayo Clinic.[182a] The following abnormalities were found: polyclonal hypergammaglobulinemia in 10 of 11 children; peripheral eosinophilia in 9 of 10; elevated erythrocyte sedimentation rate in 8 of 13; positive antinuclear antibody tests in 2 of 11; and false positive serologic tests for syphilis in 2 of 9. In addition, the CO diffusion capacity was decreased in 5 of 7; chest x-ray showed basilar fibrosis in 2 of 14; periodontal membrane thickening was present in one; and decreased motility of the lower two-thirds of the esophagus was detected in another. The preceding data suggest that morphea is more than a cutaneous disorder and bears more than a casual relationship to scleroderma.

However, as already stated, the transformation of morphea to scleroderma is exceedingly rare. It has been argued that in such instances scleroderma with morphea-like lesions had been present from the beginning of the disease. Regardless of the interpretations, a rare case will convert to scleroderma.

For many years it was postulated that morphea occurring on the back and legs was associated with spina bifida occulta and a neurotropic mechanism was suggested for the genesis of the morphea. It is now agreed that spina bifida occulta is a common radiographic finding and that its association with morphea is coincidental. However, a rarer bone disorder, melorheostosis, has been described in morphea as well as in vascular anomalies of the skin and in neurofibromatosis.[190] The radiographic appearance shows roughening of one surface of the long bones of the limbs, a picture like that of wax flowing down the side of a candle.

Raynaud's Phenomenon

Because of its significant relationship to underlying disease, Raynaud's phenomenon merits as thorough an investigation, in any patient, as does erythema multiforme, erythema nodosum, or acanthosis nigricans. Paroxysmal vasospasm of the digits is called *Raynaud's phenomenon* when an associated disorder exists and *Raynaud's disease* when idiopathic. Recent evidence, however, suggests that *Raynaud's disease* may represent a mild form of scleroderma (see later).

Raynaud's phenomenon is an episodic vascular insufficiency of the digital arteries which is often precipitated by an abrupt exposure to a cooler temperature and by emotional stress. Rarely, no precipitating factor can be detected. A characteristic, triphasic reaction of pallor, cyanosis, and hyperemia develops symmetrically. Initially the fingers and toes become white as arterial vasoconstriction produces blanching with pain, numbness, and sometimes increased sweating. As vasoconstriction lessens, blood trickles into a vascular bed in which the venous outflow is partially obstructed because of vasospasm.[191] The resulting stagnant blood flow causes cyanosis. Complete vasodilatation of the arteries and venules and the probable opening of arteriovenous shunts result in a striking reactive hyperemia with sensation of tingling, burning, and at times mild swelling of the hands (Plate 22*D*, *E*, *F*).

The triphasic reaction occurs in only two thirds of the patients. In some individuals, the blanching or cyanotic phases are so brief that cyanosis and rubor or pallor and rubor constitute the clinical expressions of Raynaud's phenomenon. In a few patients, only pallor or only cyanosis develops. When recovery from the abnormal vascular response is slow, pallor, cyanosis, and hyperemia may develop in adjacent areas of skin. An attack may be stopped when the patient immerses his hands in warm water or when he enters a very warm room.

Raynaud's phenomenon occurs predominantly in females and is usually bilateral, although in a few cases it has been unilateral for two to five years before becoming bilateral. The distal phalanges are more frequently and severely involved than the middle and proximal segments. A single digit or only portions of digits may be affected. The nose, lips, tongue, cheeks, ears, and chest are uncommon sites of disease.[192] Episodes of Raynaud's phenomenon take place from a few times a day to several times a year. As the vasospastic process becomes more severe, attacks may occur during the summer on a cool evening as well as in the winter. Raynaud's phenomenon may remain mild and stable or pursue a rapidly progressive course. Moderate to severe Raynaud's phenomenon is frequently associated with intimal proliferation of the digital arteries that reduces the caliber of the lumen.[193, 194] The compromised lumina are further reduced in size by increased vasoconstrictor tone and often by superimposed thromboses that develop in such damaged digital arteries. These factors in varying combinations are responsible for the focal areas of digital scarring and gangrene (Plate 23*B;* Figs. 7–59 and 7–60). However, massive gangrene is not a feature of Raynaud's phenomenon per se; it usually is a manifestation of acute thromboses or embolization.

Raynaud's phenomenon occurs in several settings. It is present in almost every case of scleroderma (acrosclerosis), in 10 to 30 per cent of patients with systemic LE and dermatomyositis, and in a minority of individuals as an idiopathic disorder of variable severity.

Raynaud's phenomenon is associated with the cervical rib and scalenus anticus syndromes, thromboangiitis obliterans, arteriosclerosis obliterans, atherosclerosis of the aortic arch, atrial myxoma with peripheral embolization, cold injury, and accidental or surgical trauma to the vessels of an extremity. The normal vasoconstrictive tone further reduces the blood flow in these occlusive vascular disorders to precipitate the triphasic color reaction. The development of Raynaud's phenomenon in a male, in individuals over 50 years of age, or in an atypical fashion is strongly suggestive of such an underlying disease.

Pneumatic hammer disease, now rare in the United States but still common in the mining industries of Canada and northern Europe, is another cause of Raynaud's phenomenon. Pneumatic hammers, operating with low frequency–high amplitude vibrations, sensitize the digital vessels of susceptible persons to cold. Reasons for susceptibility are unknown. Any form of activity, including chronic squeezing or pounding with the palm of one's hand, that causes repeated trauma to the palmar arches or digital arteries may produce significant vasospasm and eventually, occlusive arterial disease.[195, 196] Individuals prone to suffer from this type of vascular injury include stone cutters, chain saw users, riveters, pianists, typists, hand ball enthusiasts, and even obstetricians who rely excessively on outlet forceps and bowlers who use ill-fitting balls.[197] In one study, narrowing and occlusion of the digital arteries were found in all 14 pedestal grinders studied by arteriography.[196]

Sclerodactyly and severe trophic skin changes are rare sequelae of vibration-induced injury, but nerve damage producing sensory loss and weakness of hand muscles is common.[198] In its early stages, vibration-induced Raynaud's phenomenon may be reversible in approximately 25 per cent of individuals if they change jobs.[199] In one worker who did develop digital gangrene, the digital arteries showed extensive intimal proliferation with luminal narrowing and fibrin and platelet thrombi in some areas.[195] Nerem calculated that shear stress to the walls of digital arteries could rise to abnormally high levels from the vibratory frequencies usually produced by a jackhammer.[200] Fry demonstrated that shear stress of such magnitude can produce endothelial cell damage that increases with duration of the stress: endothelial cell swelling, necrosis, and eventual disintegration, leaving the basement membrane and underlying structures exposed to the circulation.[201]

Clumping or sludging of red blood cells in response to cold has been held responsible for Raynaud's phenomenon in cryoglobulinemia, polycythemia vera, and in disorders with high titers of circulating cold agglutinins.[202] The loss of blood fluidity in response to the cold produces a true mechanical block. Ergotism also has been associated with Raynaud's phenomenon. However, intoxication with arsenic and lead has not been shown unequivocally to produce this disorder.

Maurice Raynaud was not the first to describe the intermittent color changes in the skin in response to cold and emotional stress or the development of digital gangrene in the absence of *demonstrable* occlusive arterial disease. Eponymic honor was bestowed, however, because he reemphasized these occurrences and was the first to point out that repeated severe vasospastic attacks could lead to scarring and gangrene of the fingertips. Raynaud was unaware that occlusive arterial diseases (thromboangiitis obliterans and arteriosclerosis obliterans) and scleroderma could be associated with vasospastic phenomena in their early stages. Unknowingly, he included such cases in his series. Thirty-nine years later, in 1901, Jonathan Hutchinson recognized that several diseases were associated with vasospastic phenomena. He proposed that *Raynaud's phenomenon* be substituted for *Raynaud's disease* and be qualified by terms denoting its cause. Unfortunately, Raynaud's disease continued to be applied willy-nilly to all cases with color changes and gangrene without any attention to the possible presence of an underlying disorder. It was not until 1932 that the clinical chaos surrounding the vasospastic disorder finally ended. In that year, Allen and Brown reemphasized the distinction between Raynaud's disease and Raynaud's phenomenon, They required the following five criteria for the diagnosis of *Raynaud's disease*: the vasospastic phenomenon must (1) be precipitated by cold or emotional stress, (2) occur bilaterally, (3) be accompanied by minimal or no gangrene, (4) take place in the absence of any predisposing or underlying disorders, and (5) be present for at least two years.[203]

Although these five principles were extremely useful, recent studies into connective tissue disease and the vasospastic phenomenon necessitate their revision. The presence of Raynaud's phenomenon for two years with no detectable underlying disorder does not unequivocally differentiate it from Raynaud's disease.

Gifford and co-workers applied these five criteria to 756 case records of Raynaud's phenomenon seen at the Mayo Clinic and found that 377 cases conformed to the diagnosis of Raynaud's disease.[204] Mailed questionnaires were used to follow up 280 cases. A connective tissue disorder developed in 5 per cent of the patients 4 to 15 years after the Raynaud's phenomenon had begun. Farmer et al. studied 71 individuals with Raynaud's phenomenon and sclerodactyly from this same series[205] and found that three patients developed scleroderma 5 to 15 years later. Gifford noted that 30 per cent of patients with Raynaud's disease eventually developed sclerodactyly.[206] Farmer observed that digital scarring and ulcerations developed in half of his patients with Raynaud's phenomenon and sclerodactyly. In Gifford's series, the Raynaud's phenomenon spontaneously improved or completely disappeared in 40 per cent and 10 per cent of the cases, respectively. Gifford and Farmer interpreted their data to indicate that the five principles could be applied with great accuracy to distinguish Raynaud's disease from Raynaud's phenomenon and that Raynaud's disease with sclerodactyly should not be included in the spectrum of scleroderma.

Contrary data have been obtained by Jablonska,[207] Stava,[145] and de Takats,[202] who observed over 160 patients with Raynaud's phenomenon for more than 10 years. Jablonska and Stava followed 130 patients with Raynaud's phenomenon and scleroderma; de Takats followed 66 cases of Raynaud's phenomenon associated with various disorders. Scleroderma developed in more than 50 per cent of their patients 2 to 34 years after the vasospastic phenomenon began. De Takats was able to pinpoint an underlying disorder in each of the 66 patients in his series: collagen disease in 38 (scleroderma in 34, LE in 3, and dermatomyositis in one); peripheral vascular disease in 20; sludged blood syndrome in 4; and central vasomotor nervous discharge in 4.

This last group of 4 patients, in which Raynaud's phenomenon was attributed to central vasomotor overactivity, lends some support to Raynaud's original theory that central autonomic overactivity is responsible for the vasospastic phenomenon. These four patients suffered from hyperhidrosis, tachycardia, anxiety, and crying spells. All four had electroencephalographic abnormalities characterized by 6 and 14 per second high voltage positive spike activity bilaterally over the parietal and occipital lobes.

De Takats believes that sympathectomy is successful only in patients with peripheral vascular disease and central vasomotor discharge. Patients with scleroderma may derive temporary benefit from sympathectomy, but invariably, Raynaud's phenomenon recurs. Although digital ulcerations may heal, the cutaneous sclerosis progresses unabatedly without even temporary improvement.

The personal observations and more sophisticated studies of Jablonska, Stava, and de Takats probably account for the differences between their data and those of Gifford and Farmer. The data of the latter team may be interpreted differently. Raynaud's disease may develop into clinically obvious scleroderma in only 5 per cent of the cases; this is analogous to the conversion rate of cutaneous LE to systemic LE. A restudy of these patients by more modern techniques might reveal a much higher conversion rate. The more recent studies by Jablonska et al. indicate that the course of scleroderma is usually more benign as the interval lengthens between the onset of Raynaud's phenomenon and cutaneous sclerosis. But some patients with slowly progressive scleroderma suddenly deteriorate rapidly and die. The percentage of spontaneous improvement in Raynaud's disease demonstrated in the studies made by Gifford and Farmer is similar to that in scleroderma itself.

It seems most likely that the spectrum of scleroderma extends from Raynaud's disease without sclerodactyly through the RS, RT, RST, and CRST syndromes to classic scleroderma with diffuse cutaneous involvement. In all of these stages, visceral involvement may be minimal, or severe. There may be involvement of the internal organs in the absence of skin changes or in the presence of only cuticular telangiectasia. In some individuals, pulmonary hypertension associated with Raynaud's phenomenon is a manifestation of scleroderma.[154]

Raynaud's phenomenon is certainly the harbinger of connective tissue disease as well as an accompaniment of peripheral vascular disorders, a reflection of central nervous system abnormalities, and a manifestation of sludged blood syndromes. Is there such an entity as Raynaud's disease, and if so, how frequently does it occur? The studies of Gifford and Farmer have been interpreted as showing that Raynaud's disease is more common than Raynaud's phenomenon. However, the studies of Jablonska, Stava, and de Takats have indicated that Raynaud's phenomenon secondary to an underlying disease is more common, and in de Takat's series a related cause was found in all 66 patients. A more recent retrospective study of 137 individuals by Velayos et al. indicated that about 80 per cent of persons with Raynaud's phenomenon had an associated disease and in 20 per cent no etiology was discovered.[208] Approximately 42 per cent of individuals had a connective tissue disease and 38 per cent had associated peripheral vascular disease, cold injury, or trauma. To obtain a more accurate assessment of the prevalence of primary Raynaud's disease, one needs to carry out a prospective study with appropriate methods of initial investigation and a careful follow-up based on personally conducted interviews and examinations. The evaluation should include inspection of the skin and mucous membranes for the three types of telangiectases described previously, esophageal motility and pulmonary function tests, cardiovascular and musculoskeletal examinations, and serological and immunological tests appropriate for connective tissue disorders. The first step in this direction has been taken by Porter et al., who evaluated 100 consecutive patients with Raynaud's phenomenon. This group was felt to be a representative sample of the population from which they were drawn.[209] Eighty-one had a definite or strongly suspected connective tissue disease, with scleroderma, CRST, or the sclerodermatous component of an overlap syndrome accounting for 41 per cent of the cases and LE, 16 per cent. No disease was found in 19 patients, but 14 of the 19 had single serologic abnormalities. Porter et al. did not find any associated peripheral vascular diseases in their patients. They proposed replacing the terms *Raynaud's disease* and *phenomenon* with *Raynaud's syndrome* because they regard any patient with this vasospastic disorder as being at high risk for an associated autoimmune disease. My own personal experience supports this view.

Raynaud's phenomenon is not responsible for cutaneous sclerosis or sclerodactyly. These may occur independently of each other, or Raynaud's phenomenon may antedate or appear after sclerosis has begun. Coffman has shown that although there is decreased capillary blood flow in the fingers of patients with scleroderma and Raynaud's phenomenon, the capillary blood flow is normal in the sclerodermatous involved skin of the forearms.[210]

The differential diagnosis of Raynaud's phenomenon includes acrocyanosis, which is characterized by coolness and persistent cyanosis of the hands and feet, unrelieved by increasing the environmental temperature. It occurs primarily in women but is not associated with sclerodactyly, dystrophic cutaneous changes, or any known illness. Landis and Lewis have shown that arteriolar spasm in the affected areas, and not spasm of the digital arteries as in Raynaud's phenomenon, is responsible for acrocyanosis.[211]

The mechanism underlying Raynaud's phenomenon is still unresolved. Although Raynaud originally stressed that systemic vasomotor overactivity was the principal cause, Lewis has shown by a series of simple but elegant clinical experiments that a local "fault" in the digital arteries is responsible for the cold-induced vasospasm.[191] Although systemic vasoconstriction adds to the locally generated vasmotor tone, Lewis did not believe that the systemic tone was excessive in these patients. He showed that the digital arteries themselves were sensitive to cold and remained so after sympathectomy, as well as after local anesthesia of the ulnar nerve. Physiological abnormalities involving serotonin and catecholamines have been proposed but not proven as the basis for Raynaud's phenomenon.[212, 213]

Some individuals complain of cold and numbness in their hands without color changes in the winter season. Hunt has called this *hereditary cold fingers*. Allen, Barker, and Hines believe that such cases may represent the mildest form of Raynaud's phenomenon.[214] In their experience, a few of the affected individuals developed typical Raynaud's phenomenon later in life. In certain families, there are some members with vasospastic phenomena and others with a tendency to cold hands and feet. Lewis has also recorded case histories of patients who have developed Raynaud's phenomenon following a history of cold fingers, or cold fingers followed by chilblain, or after chilblain alone.[191] A spectrum of cold sensitivity exists, but whether this represents quantitative progression or qualitative change remains to be determined.

It is clear that in digital Raynaud's phenomenon, locally generated vasospastic stimuli are paramount, with systemic vasoconstrictor tone playing a minor role.[191] However, in some patients the body must be chilled in order to produce the phenomenon because immersion of the hands in ice water alone is unsuccessful. A systemic vasoconstrictor tone is needed to bring about additional luminal reduction to produce the clinical phenomenon — a practical point to remember when one attempts to verify a history of Raynaud's phenomenon. However, locally generated stimuli from exposure to cold do not seem to be applicable to cases in which the tongue is affected along with the hands[192] or in the pulmonary and renal circulations in which vasospasm has been shown to occur.

Systemic vasoconstrictor tone must be important in these situations, and the digital arteries may represent an exception, where local influences predominate.

Pathogenetic Mechanisms

In the past decade, a considerable amount of information has been generated in regard to scleroderma. The disease may be viewed from three points: collagen synthesis, immunologic abnormalities, and generalized vascular disease.

It is now clear that the hidebound and firm consistency of sclerodermatous skin is produced by newly synthesized collagen that replaces most or all of the subcutaneous fat, thereby tethering the skin to the underlying tissues.[215] Skin fibroblasts from patients with scleroderma synthesize more collagen in culture than normal fibroblasts and this difference can be propagated in culture for as many as 15 generations.[216, 217] Fibroblasts from the lower dermis and subcutis are more active than those from the upper dermis.[217, 218] In normal skin, there is no functional difference between upper and lower dermal fibroblasts.[217]

Krieg et al. reported that the procollagen peptides, the aminoterminal extension peptides from procollagen, are capable of regulating normal fibroblastic synthesis of collagen through feedback inhibition. They also claimed that the addition of procollagen peptides to the culture medium of scleroderma fibroblasts restored excessive collagen synthesis almost to normal without affecting the formation of other proteins. This work, if confirmed by others, would suggest that the mechanism for the regulation of collagen synthesis by feedback inhibition remains intact in scleroderma fibroblasts.[219] In some patients, the sclerodermatous skin softens and returns to normal, suggesting that there may be reestablishment of normal feedback inhibition following activation of skin fibroblasts. The stimulus for increased production of collagen by dermal and subcutaneous fibroblasts is unknown, but recent observations suggest that sensitized lymphocytes may play a role.

A marked lymphocytic infiltrate is present in the subcutis and lower dermis of early sclerodermatous lesions,[220] and most of the lymphocytes have been shown to be T cells.[221] Johnson and Ziff have shown that phytohemagglutinin-stimulated normal lymphocytes produce a soluble factor that stimulates embryonic lung fibroblasts in culture to produce collagen.[222] Kondo et al. demonstrated that circulating lymphocytes from some patients with scleroderma react to extracts of both normal and sclerodermatous skin with formation of migration inhibitory factor (MIF).[221] Stuart et al. showed that such lymphocytes produce a chemotactic factor for monocytes when they are cultured in the presence of purified normal human skin collagen, skin collagen from lathyritic chicks, and the alpha-polypeptide chains of collagen. Blast transformation also occurred in some of these experiments.[223] The possibility of cell-mediated hypersensitivity in scleroderma is further strengthened by reports of individuals with chronic graft-versus-host reactions following bone marrow transplants who have developed cutaneous changes histologically and clinically indistinguishable from scleroderma and morphea.[224-226]

The role of cell-mediated hypersensitivity in the pathogenesis of scleroderma is far from established, but it is a promising avenue for further research. Some questions to be answered are (1) is it a primary or secondary event? (2) is it the sole explanation for cutaneous and pulmonary sclerosis? (3) is the cell-mediated mechanism specific for scleroderma? The studies summarized above showed that the lymphocytes in only 10 of 16 patients with scleroderma and in only one of 10 with CRST syndrome reacted to extracts of normal and sclerodermatous skin with MIF formation.[221] In the study by Stuart et al., lymphocytes in 11 of 12 patients with scleroderma reacted to collagen stimulation with formation of chemotactic factor for monocytes, but only three showed blast transformation.[223] This reactivity may not be limited to scleroderma, because nine of 16 patients with systemic LE showed blast transformation to collagen and two of four patients with rheumatoid arthritis produced monocyte chemotactic factor in response to stimulation by collagen.[223] The serological abnormalities of rheumatoid factor, antinuclear antibody, hyperglobulinemia, and antinucleolar and anti–smooth muscle antibodies do not appear to participate directly in the pathogenesis of the disease. They may simply reflect an abnormal immune system in which cell-mediated hypersensitivity can develop.

The generalized vascular disease of scleroderma is characterized by intimal proliferation with narrowing of the lumen. It is frequently present and primarily affects the pulmonary, coronary, digital, and renal interlobular arteries. These vascular changes are indistinguishable from those seen in idiopathic Raynaud's disease. The intimal proliferation in the digital arteries and the subsequent development of superimposed thromboses correlate fairly well with the severity of the Raynaud's phenomenon and probably with the total duration of the process.[194] The intimal proliferation could be the end result of the reparative processes following repeated and prolonged endothelial cell damage secondary to Raynaud-induced tissue ischemia or other noxious factors.

In support of such an hypothesis, one can cite the experiments of Willms-Kretschmer and Majno, who showed that transient ischemia for as long as six hours can be produced in rat and rabbit skin without any subsequent or significant dermal necrosis.[227] However, profound endothelial cell injury develops in the microcirculatory vessels within the ischemic area. The endothelial cells swell and form blebs that narrow and occlude the lumen. Fry had shown that the vibrational energy from jackhammers produced severe endothelial cell damage.[201] Gertz et al. induced basilar and coronary artery vasospasm in the cat by various methods: mechanical stroking, electrical stimulation, introduction of autologous blood into adjacent tissue spaces, or partial ligation with sutures.[228] They demonstrated marked endothelial cell damage by scanning electron microscopy within 15 minutes of initiation of the stimulus. Thromboses subsequently developed at points of maximum constriction. The mechanism of endothelial cell damage was attributed to an increase in the mechanical shear forces of the blood that develop at acutely narrowed arterial segments. Most recently, Kahaleh and LeRoy found a factor in the sera of 11 of 21 patients with scleroderma that can be cytotoxic and inhibitory to the growth of endothelial cells in culture.[229] In one patient, this factor disappeared with improvement in the disease. The thromboses in the digital arteries may be secondary to such endothelial cell damage or to a hypercoagulable state that appears to exist in some patients.[230, 231]

Similarly, the telangiectases in scleroderma could represent vascular proliferation in the capillary portion of the microcirculation in response to repeated endothelial cell damage and subsequent repair following tissue ischemia. Fleischmajer et al. have shown by electron microscopy that endothelial cell injury with luminal obstruction can be seen in many of the upper dermal capillaries in the early cutaneous lesions of scleroderma.[232] By autoradiography, they demonstrated increased mitotic activity of endothelial cells and pericytes in these same vessels. It is probably not a coincidence that the mat and nailfold telangiectases appear only in areas where Raynaud's phenomenon has been described — face, tongue, lips, hands, and upper chest. These telangiectases are often present in nonsclerotic skin, as demonstrated in the CRST syndrome, indicating that they are not related to the development of cutaneous sclerosis. The dilated and giant capillary loops detected by capillary microscopy on the fingers and dorsa of the hands in patients with scleroderma, dermatomyositis, and Raynaud's syndrome[233] could be explained in the same way.

Although arterial vasospasm in scleroderma is usually considered to be limited to the digital arteries and to be synonymous with Raynaud's phenomenon, it also occurs in larger vessels much more frequently than we have appreciated. Figures 7–32 and 7–33 illustrate a patient with systemic LE who had persistent brachial and femoral artery vasospasm that produced digital gangrene of the hands and feet without symptoms of Raynaud's phenomenon. Pulmonary and renal artery vasospasm producing pulmonary hypertension and renal disease, respectively, are analogous processes. Porter et al. demonstrated by arteriography that resting vasospasm, in addition to organic blocks, is present in the digital arteries of scleroderma patients with Raynaud's phenomenon.[209]

The following unitary hypothesis is proposed for the pathogenesis of scleroderma. A systemic vasoconstrictor tone is responsible for the vasospasm producing pulmonary hypertension, renal and cardiac disease, and, coupled with local influences, it is responsible for Raynaud's phenomenon. Repeated and prolonged vasospastic episodes result in both tissue ischemia and endothelial cell damage, with subsequent repair leading to intimal proliferation. The tissue ischemia and necrosis in the presence of an abnormal immune system facilitates the development of cell-mediated hypersensitivity so that sensitized lymphocytes become capable of stimulating fibroblasts to produce cutaneous and pulmonary fibrosis. The basis for the vasoconstrictor tone is unknown, but it could represent an abnormality of neural smooth muscle innervation which produces both vascular vasospasm and gastrointestinal peristaltic dysfunction. In the gastrointestinal tract, the abnormality in innervation leads to atrophy and disappearance of smooth muscle. Although the plasma levels of serotonin and catecholamines have been shown to be normal in scleroderma, the basic defect might be an abnormality of their receptors on the smooth muscle in vessels and gastrointestinal tract.

Vasospasm is a feature common to the three connective tissue diseases and takes the form of Raynaud's phenomenon, livedo reticularis, and chilblain-like lesions. Livedo reticularis is a vasospastic disorder of arterioles that histologically shows endarteritis. Although it is most commonly found in systemic LE, it can also be seen in scleroderma. Chilblain-like lesions affecting the toes and sides of the feet are also a manifestation of systemic LE.

MIXED AND UNDIFFERENTIATED CONNECTIVE TISSUE DISORDERS

Not every instance of a connective tissue disease can be diagnosed as LE, dermatomyositis, or scleroderma; overlap, transitional, and incomplete or undifferentiated cases also occur. The major clinical manifestations of two or three connective tissue disorders may coexist actively in the same patient to produce a *mixed* or *overlap* syndrome. The connective tissue disease may seemingly be transformed into another to produce a *transitional* case. Some illnesses do not differentiate sufficiently as they evolve and allow only the diagnosis of *undifferentiated* or *incomplete* connective tissue disease. One will observe patients who develop individual connective tissue diseases sequentially over the course of several years. For example, one of our patients, a 50-year-old man with dermatomyositis, developed scleroderma four years after his dermatomyositis entered remission. Another man, 55 years old, had cutaneous LE limited to the vermilion border of the lower lip and adjacent skin for 10 years. Coincident with a spontaneous remission of these lesions, he developed polymyositis involving the shoulder and hip girdles. After three years of therapy with prednisone and methotrexate, the polymyositis entered remission. However, coincident with this event he developed a diffuse patchy nonscarring alopecia, puffy hands, and mild Raynaud's phenomenon (Figs. 7–89 and 7–90). A biopsy of the scalp showed the histological features of LE. There was no serological evidence of systemic LE.

The most common mixed connective tissue disease joins the major features of dermatomyositis and scleroderma. Combinations of LE and

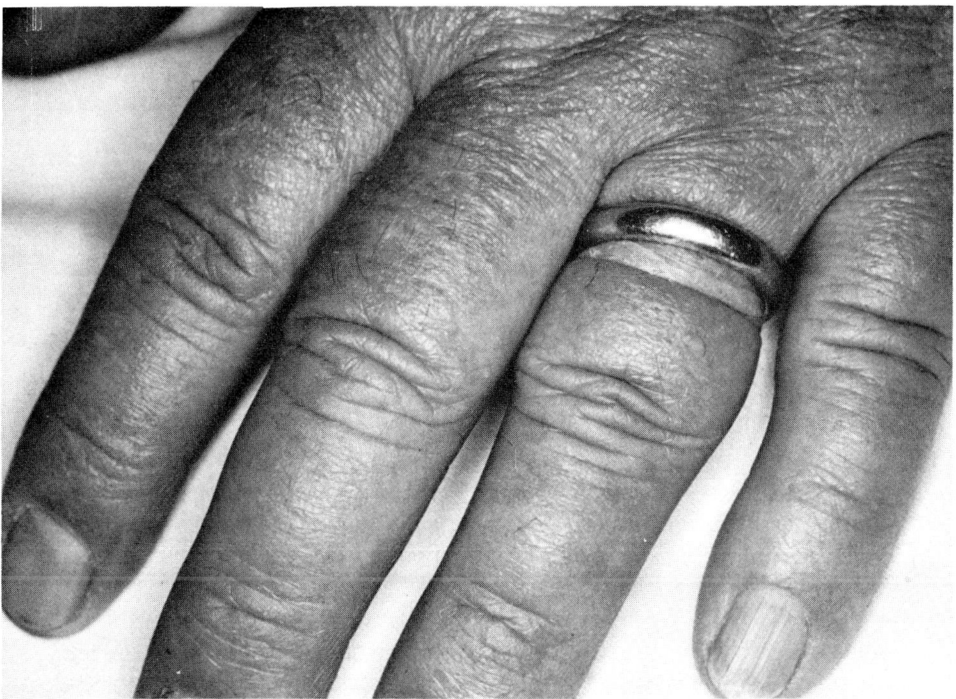

Figure 7–89. Puffy hands in patient with overlap syndrome of LE and polymyositis.

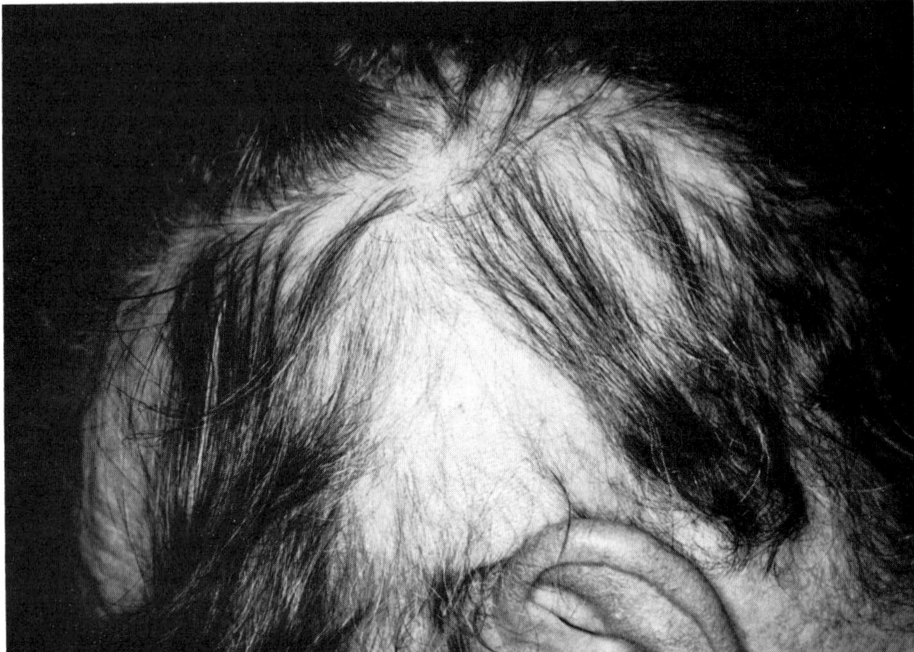

Figure 7–90. Alopecia in patient shown in Figure 7–89.

scleroderma and LE and dermatomyositis appear much less frequently. Linear morphea with LE, as well as discoid LE and scleroderma, has also been described. Of 727 patients with scleroderma studied at the Mayo Clinic, 36 had features of dermatomyositis, 5 of 96 patients tested had positive LE cell tests, 7 had Sjögren's syndrome, 31 had rheumatoid arthritis, and 10 had false positive serologic reactions for syphilis.[137]

In 1972, Sharp et al. defined a new rheumatic syndrome that they called Mixed Connective Tissue Disease (MCTD).[234] The initial report described 25 patients whose major clinical features included arthralgias and mostly nondeforming arthritis, puffy hands producing sausage-shaped or sclerodactyly-like fingers (Fig. 7–91), Raynaud's phenomenon, abnormal esophageal motility function, and polymyositis. More than two thirds of the patients had signs and symptoms combining the features of scleroderma and dermatomyositis. The remainder of the group had additional features compatible with LE: fever, serositis, hepatosplenomegaly, anemia, leukopenia, hypergammaglobulinemia, and positive LE cell tests. Anti-DNA antibodies were present only in a minority. After more patients were reported, it was realized that Sjögren's syndrome, pulmonary fibrosis, and abnormal pulmonary function tests showing restrictive lung disease and decreased diffusion capacity were also part of the syndrome.[235] Many patients developed deforming arthritis mimicking rheumatoid arthritis.[236] All of the individuals had antinuclear antibody in their sera, which showed a speckled nuclear immunofluorescent pattern. The antinuclear antibody, however, was not directed against DNA or nucleoprotein as usually seen in LE, but was reactive against a soluble extractable nuclear antigen (ENA) which eventually was shown to be composed of at least two antigens — RNP, a ribonucleoprotein and Sm, another soluble nuclear macromolecule. Both appeared to exist *in vivo* as a molecular complex.[237] RNP was found in all cases of MCTD, and Sm

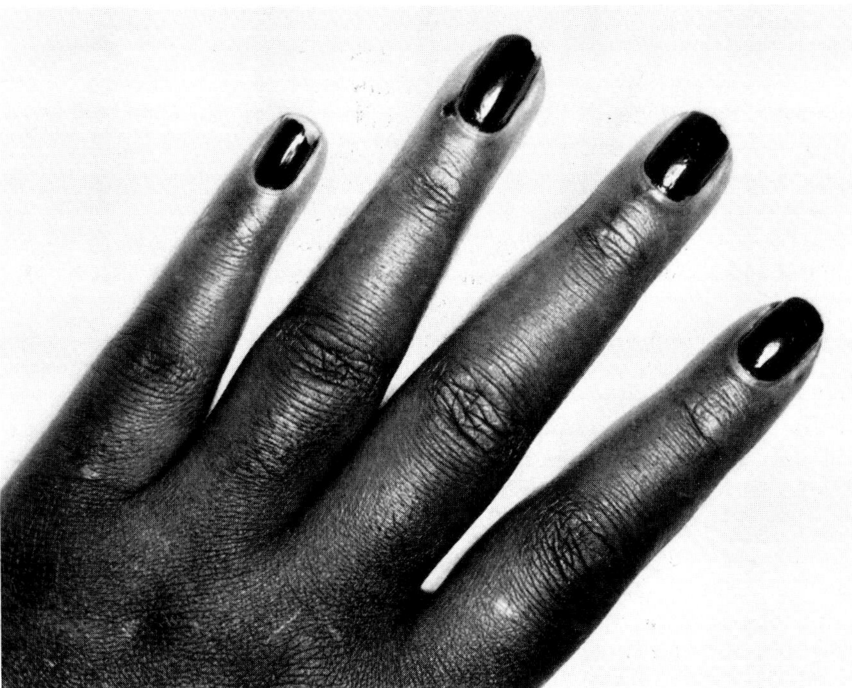

Figure 7–91. Puffy hands producing the appearance of sclerodactyly in patient with MCTD defined by high titer of anti-RNP antibody.

was detected chiefly in systemic LE, although occasionally both were present in some patients. By definition, MCTD could be diagnosed only by finding anti-RNP antibody in a patient's serum, in a titer greater than 1:1000 and usually ranging from 1:40,000 to greater than 1:1,000,000.

MCTD seemed to have a more benign course than other connective tissue diseases; to be more responsive to steroid therapy in all its aspects, including the swelling and thickening of the digital skin; and to be associated with a much lower prevalence of renal disease and central nervous system involvement than lupus erythematosus. Renal disease developed in about 10 per cent of patients with MCTD.

Over 200 cases with anti-RNP antibody have been reported, and all varieties of connective tissue syndromes and diseases have been found to be associated with this antibody: overlap syndromes of scleroderma and polymyositis, scleroderma and LE, and scleroderma, LE, and dermatomyositis. In addition, patients with classic cases of systemic LE, cutaneous LE, scleroderma, dermatomyositis, and rheumatoid arthritis have also had anti-RNP antibody.[238, 239] The varieties of syndromes also included patients with overlap features of two or three diseases at the onset as well as individuals with a single disorder who developed one or more additional connective tissue diseases over the course of several years.

With experience, it has become evident that the syndrome does not necessarily have a benign course, nor is it always very responsive to steroid therapy. The sclerodermatous features do not always disappear with steroid treatment, and more advanced disease may respond poorly to treatment. Autopsy studies in children and adults have shown that the vascular changes characteristic of scleroderma — arterial intimal proliferation — are present in many organs.[240] The syndrome may have a poorer prognosis in children than in adults.[241] The anti-RNP antibody is clearly a marker for a syndrome that exhibits an increased frequency of Raynaud's phenomenon, puffy hands, and myositis, while Sm is usually associated with the clinical features of systemic LE. Anti-RNP antibody plays no role in the pathogenesis of the disorder, because it remains in unvarying high titer during disease activity and remission.[235, 238] Although MCID is considered to be a distinct entity because of the presence of RNP, the clinical syndrome also exists in the absence of the antibody,[238, 242] and is otherwise indistinguishable from many of the overlap syndromes one normally encounters.

MCTD is considered to be important because of the low prevalence (10 per cent) of associated renal disease compared to the high frequency (over 50 per cent) in systemic LE. It has been proposed that the presence of anti-RNP antibody may be protective against the development of renal disease. However, it does not exert protection, if anti-DNA antibodies are also present in the serum.[243] The methods of data collection need to be modified in order to be certain that the development of renal disease is low in MCTD. Only MCTD patients with a systemic LE component should be compared with patients with classic systemic LE, because the majority of MCTD patients have scleroderma-dermatomyositis features in which clinical renal disease is not common. The means of diagnosing renal disease need to be uniform, since the frequency will be greater in studies utilizing renal biopsies than in those employing only urinalyses and renal function tests. Two recent reports have indicated prevalence rates for renal disease of 20 and 40 per cent in MCTD.[241, 244] None of the large studies to date has provided information about the clinical features of MCTD in individual patients so that one is unable to discern whether there is a pattern that distinguishes those who develop renal disease from those who do not.

The clinical characteristics of MCTD have been defined by retrospective studies. Given a group of patients with the clinical features of MCTD, one does not yet know what percentage will have anti-RNP antibody. Features that should make one particularly suspicious of MCTD are Raynaud's phenomenon in association with puffy hands and arthralgias; Raynaud's phenomenon arising in the course of systemic LE; patchy nonscarring alopecia, swollen fingers, and Raynaud's phenomenon[239]; and speckled epidermal nuclear fluorescence for IgG in direct immunofluorescent studies of clinically normal skin. In a series of 20 patients with such immunofluorescent findings, 15 had anti-RNP antibody. Eight patients had cutaneous lesions of LE. Sclerodermatous features of Raynaud's phenomenon, pigmentary disturbances as illustrated in Figure 7–58, and swollen hands occurred in 13, 10, and 7 of the patients, respectively. Nonscarring, diffuse spotty alopecia was present in 10 individuals and myositis occurred in three.[239]

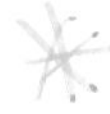

In our own small series, a total of 60 blood samples from suspected cases of MCTD have been submitted by physicians from the Yale-New Haven Medical Center over the past two years. Eleven cases were found to have anti-RNP antibody by hemagglutination and immunodiffusion methods performed in the immunology reference laboratory at Scripps Clinic.

The 11 cases are briefly summarized:

Case 1. B.G. 26-year-old black female. RNP titer 1:82,000, Sm 1:2580, Discoid LE lesions, face and chest; puffy fingers and hands, simulating sclerodactyly; proximal myositis; *absent* Raynaud's phenomenon; membranous glomerulonephritis diagnosed by renal biopsy; anti-DNA antibodies, 61 per cent binding (normal less than 20 per cent); and pulmonary diffusion capacity abnormally depressed.

Case 2. M.H. 30-year-old white female. RNP titer 1:80,860, Sm, negative. Fever and deforming polyarthritis diagnosed as rheumatoid arthritis. Developed polymyositis one year later, requiring prednisone and methotrexate for control. Raynaud's phenomenon present. Renal disease absent.

Case 3. Y.K. 16-year-old black female. RNP titer 1:1,000,000, Sm, 1:1280. Systemic LE with pleural and pericardial effusion, polyserositis, Raynaud's phenomenon, and vasospasm of brachial and femoral arteries producing digital gangrene (Figs. 7–32 and 7–33). No evidence of renal disease. DNA-binding, 7 to 19 per cent, in multiple tests.

Case 4. A.M. 22-year-old white female. RNP titer greater than 1:1,000,000, Sm, 1:1,000,000. Systemic LE with pleuropericarditis, polyarthralgias, and mild proliferative glomerulonephritis. DNA binding 42 to 72 per cent in multiple tests. Raynaud's phenomenon present.

Case 5. R.S. 34-year-old white female. RNP titer 1:40, Sm negative. Systemic LE with discoid lesions and Raynaud's phenomenon. Pulmonary hypertension secondary to pulmonary artery vasospasm. Lung biopsy showed absence of fibrosis and presence of arterial intimal proliferation. Arthralgias, myalgias, and thrombocytopenic purpura. Renal disease present as membranous glomerulonephritis. DNA-binding 14 to 20 per cent in multiple tests.

Case 6. L.B. 34-year-old black female. RNP titer greater than 1:5120, Sm negative. Polymyositis, pulmonary fibrosis, and fatigue. Absence of Raynaud's phenomenon and renal disease. DNA-binding 2 per cent.

Case 7. P. W. 32-year-old white female. RNP titer, greater than 1:640, Sm, negative. Systemic LE with seizures, arthritis, discoid lesions, and scarring alopecia. Polymyositis and Raynaud's phenomenon present. Diffuse proliferative glomerulonephritis. DNA-binding 38 per cent.

Case 8. L.D. 54-year-old male. RNP titer, 1:40,960; Sm negative. Swollen hands, Raynaud's phenomenon, and myositis. Absence of renal disease. DNA binding 0 per cent.

Case 9. J.L. 24-year-old white male. RNP titer. 1:8, Sm 1:16. Systemic LE with widespread discoid lesions on face, arms, and trunk in light-exposed areas. Absence of Raynaud's phenomenon. Diffuse proliferative glomerulonephritis. DNA-binding 55 to 70 per cent, in multiple tests.

Case 10. R.N. 28-year-old white male. Proteinuria secondary to membranous glomerulonephritis developed at age 20. Postive antinuclear antibody found at age 22. Vasospasm of branchial arteries producing loss of radial pulses and cold hands led to finding of RNP titer 1/320. Sm negative at age 28. DNA binding 2 to 15 per cent, in multiple tests. Working diagnosis, lupus nephritis.

Case 11. I.B. 64-year-old white female. Onset at age 55 of acrosclerosis, Raynaud's phenomenon, and polymyositis. Spontaneous improvement in polymyositis over next two years, while scleroderma progressed to produce pulmonary fibrosis, esophageal dysfunction with dysphagia and stricture formation, malabsorption secondary to small bowel involvement, and development of sacculations in the colon. She had persistent leukopenia of 3000 to 4000 during nine-year course. During last year of illness, polymyositis became worse. Studies at this time revealed antinuclear antibody titer 1:512 (homogeneous pattern), rheumatoid factor 1:2560, DNA binding capacity 83 per cent, RNP titer greater than 1:1,000,000, Sm, 1:647,680. Renal disease absent. Patient died suddenly from bilateral pulmonary hemorrhage of unknown etiology. Autopsy revealed pulmonary fibrosis with arterial intimal proliferation. Kidneys showed arteriolar nephrosclerosis without any evidence of lupus or sclerodermal renal disease. There was no evidence of vasculitis and the muscles showed a chronic active myositis. The smooth muscle in the gastrointestinal tract was atrophic and replaced by fibrous tissue.

These brief case reports highlight two aspects of MCTD that have not been emphasized before. Four of the 11 patients had significant antibody titers to both RNP and Sm. Case reports in the literature have, with rare exceptions, described patients with RNP antibodies only. In the series of Farber and Bole, four of 44 patients had both antibodies, 13 had anti-RNP only, and 27 anti-Sm only.[238] Of the four patients with both, three had systemic LE and one had polymyositis. In the cooperative group study reported by Sharp et al., 100 patients had only anti-RNP, and 27 anti-Sm antibodies.[245] However, there were seven patients cited under *Methods* who had significant titers of both, but they were excluded from the clinical analysis reported in the paper. In the series of Prystowsky and Tuffanelli, seven of 30 patients with RNP antibody also had significant titers of anti-SM, as judged by the fact that they were still greater than 1:200 after treatment with ribonuclease.[246] The clinical features of all these patients were grouped by percentage so that one does not know the natural history and clinical characteristics of any of the patients exhibiting both antibodies. Our data suggest that any amount of anti-Sm antibody may negate the putative protective effect of anti-RNP antibody against the development of renal disease. Singsen et al. pointed out that in their series of 10 children with MCTD, only two children had both anti-Sm and anti-RNP antibodies.[241] These two children, who also did not have anti-DNA antibodies, had the most marked renal involvement. Their clinical features were those of scleroderma-polymyositis. In none of the studies dealing with a correlation between renal disease and MCTD has there been any attempt to determine whether anti-Sm antibody plays a role in the prevalence of renal disease. The impression has been promulgated that when anti-Sm and anti-RNP antibodies occur together, the anti-RNP is "usually present in lesser amounts."[235]

Our cases emphasize a second point: four cases had low titers of anti-RNP (Cases 5, 7, 9, and 10). Tan and Rodnan found that in 12 of 56 patients with scleroderma, RNP was present in a titer of less than 1:1000.[247] The significance of these low titers is not clear, since the typical MCTD patient has titers greater than 1:1000.

The patients in our series had tests for ENA performed because they had features suggesting either mixed or undifferentiated connective tissue syndromes. Only one patient was found with anti-Sm (titer greater than 1,000,000) in the absence of anti-RNP antibody. She is a 30-year-old white female with systemic LE, discoid lesions, photosensitivity, nephritis, polymyositis, and schizophrenia. Raynaud's phenomenon is absent.

Our other 48 cases with negative anti-RNP and anti-Sm antibodies had connective tissue syndromes clinically indistinguishable from the positive cases summarized above. In this small prospective study, approximately 18 per cent of patients suspected of having MCTD were found to have anti-RNP antibody as the major serologic abnormality.

The patient shown in Figures 7–89 and 7–90 developed spotty, clinically nonscarring alopecia, swollen hands, and mild Raynaud's phenomenon after a long history of cutaneous LE, followed by polymyositis. RNP and Sm antigens were not present. This patient had the cutaneous features of MCTD emphasized by Gilliam and Prystowsky but without the serologic markers.[239] Biopsy of an area of alopecia disclosed lymphocytic infiltration around vessels and hair follicles typical of LE. The epidermis was normal.

The question has been raised whether MCTD is a distinct entity or a variant of LE.[248, 249] The latter has been suggested because Sm antigen is found chiefly in patients with LE; Sm and RNP exist as a molecular complex in calf thymus extract[237]; anti-Sm and anti-RNP antibodies occasionally coexist in patients' sera; and anti-RNP antibody alone may be found in 12 to 25 per cent of LE sera.[245, 249, 250] On the other hand, anti-RNP and anti-Sm antibodies alone or together have been reported often enough in patients with scleroderma, polymyositis, juvenile rheumatoid arthritis, Sjögren's syndrome, sclerodermatomyositis as well as in cutaneous and systemic LE, and MCTD,[238, 239, 243, 245, 251] that it is equally likely for them to be nonspecific markers of connective tissue disease, similar to the false positive serologic reaction to syphilis. The titers of anti-RNP and anti-Sm antibodies with rare exceptions do not change in relation to disease activity.[238, 251] In the cooperative multicenter study involving 100 patients with positive RNP tests, 74 had MCTD, but 12 had systemic LE; eight, scleroderma; and six, less well-defined connective tissue disease. Of 27 with positive tests for Sm, 23 had systemic LE; two, MCTD; one, scleroderma; and one, dermatomyositis.[245]

Overlap syndromes without anti-RNP antibody are more common than those with such antibody. Conclusive evidence has yet to be presented that MCTD has a different prognosis or significance from similar overlap syndrome without anti-RNP antibody. Careful long-term observations, precise measurements of serological abnormalities including anti-RNP and anti-Sm antibodies, uniform methods for detecting renal disease, and publication of detailed findings in prototypical patients are necessary to determine these points conclusively. The natural history and the full spectrum of MCTD and its status as an independent entity or as a variant of LE remain to be established. However, the major contribution of MCTD has been to draw the clinician's attention to the frequent occurrence of overlap and undifferentiated connective tissue syndromes, in much the same way that the CRST syndrome has alerted physicians to the frequency and diagnostic value of telangiectases in scleroderma.

A goal of those interested in the rheumatic diseases is to be able to correlate patterns of autoantibodies with specific disorders and syndromes. Precise molecular identification of the antigens involved is necessary. A major breakthrough and advance toward this goal have been accomplished by Michael Lerner, an MD/PhD candidate at Yale, and Professor Joan Steitz and their colleagues. They have demonstrated that anti-Sm serum selectively precipitates six small nuclear RNA molecules and that anti-RNP serum selectively precipitates two of these six.[252] The small RNA molecules range in size from 95 to 196 nucleotides. Antigenicity of these RNA molecules depends upon their being complexed with specific proteins. Each of the RNA protein complexes has a molecular weight of 175,000 and exists as an independent entity. The sites of the antigenic determinants for Sm and RNP on these RNA protein complexes are not known. The two small RNA molecules in the RNP antigen are closely related and differ by only a few nucleotides in the middle of the molecules. The Ro antigen has been identified as a group of cytoplasmic RNA protein complexes, and La as a group of nuclear RNA protein complexes.[253] The analytic techniques employed in these experiments should be capable of precisely identifying all the macromolecules against which patients with connective tissue diseases produce antibodies.

The following case reports are those of patients seen *before* the era of MCTD. They are included to stress the variability of overlap, transitional, and undifferentiated connective tissue syndromes.

The following brief case history is an example of a mixed connective tissue disorder in which the two components were equally active:

A 47-year-old white woman had had LE since the age of 27. Pericarditis with effusion and arthritis of the wrists, fingers, and knees were the initial manifestations. A false positive serology was discovered during one or her pregnancies. Recurrent abdominal pain simulating acute surgical emergencies occurred during her pregnancies. On one occasion an exploratory laparotomy for suspected acute cholecystitis was performed, but no abnormalities were found. LE cell tests were positive at age 37. When she was 46, the patient noted the onset of Raynaud's phenomenon and increased pigmentation of the face, upper chest, forearms, and hands in association with a thickening of the skin in these areas (Fig. 7–92). A

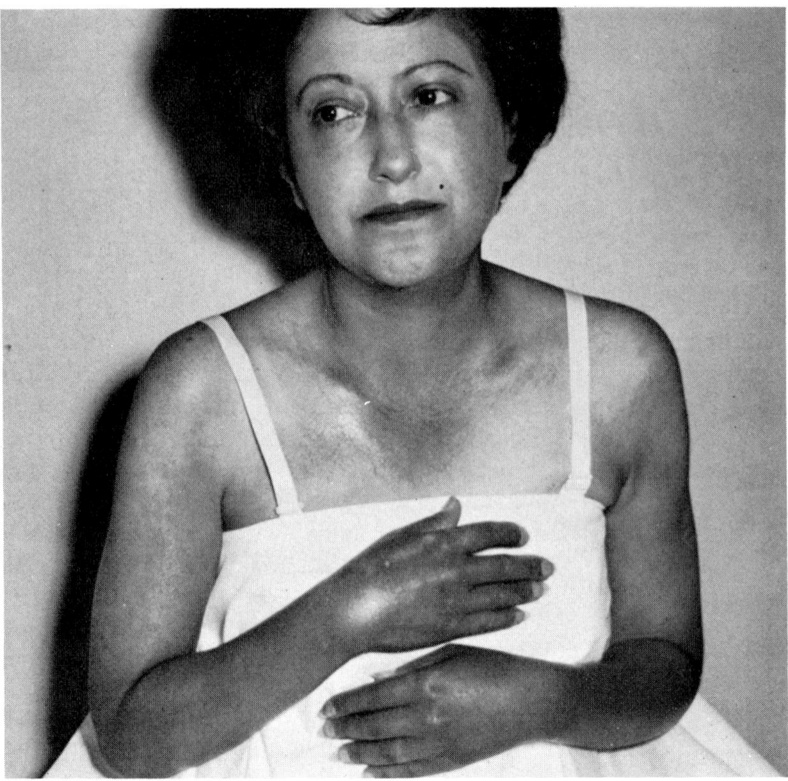

Figure 7–92. This patient has both LE and scleroderma. Note the Addisonian pigmentation. Adrenal cortical function was normal in this woman.

recent scar also became darker. The hard palate, buccal mucosa, and lips showed hyperpigmentation, although these findings had been first noted seven years previously. Adrenal cortical function studies ruled out Addison's disease. The patient also had Coombs'-positive hemolytic anemia. Prednisone therapy was necessary to keep her illness under control.

This patient illustrates a mixed syndrome of LE and scleroderma and an associated spectacular hyperpigmentation similar to Addison's disease.

The following case report illustrates the transitional type of connective tissue disorder:

A 69-year-old white woman had suffered from fatigue, extreme muscle weakness, and edema of the hands, feet, and periorbital tissues since the age of 62. Arthralgias, a dusky color of the hands, Gottron's papules, and cuticular telangiectasia were also present. The illness lasted about nine months, at which time the patient's muscular strength returned. With the improvement in her general state she noted the onset of Raynaud's phenomenon and increased pigmentation with sclerodermatous changes of the face, forearms, and hands. Calcinosis of the fingers developed, along with contractures of the hands and elbows, for the next six and one half years. During this time sclerodermatous features predominated, and signs and symptoms of dermatomyositis were relatively inactive. The only stigmata of dermatomyositis were the atropic and telangiectatic patches over the knuckles (Fig. 7–48) and a patch of poikiloderma on the midback.

In this instance, acute dermatomyositis lasting for only nine months was the presenting feature of illness. The sclerodermatous phase ensued and became the striking clinical feature of the malady. The woman's appearance was so striking that she was considered to have scleroderma. The initial features of her illness had been forgotten. Some people call this variety of disease sclerodermatomyositis.

Another transitional case is summarized in the following history:

A 6-year-old black boy had an onset of fever, edema of the hands and feet, erythema, and scaling of the face and extensor surfaces of the major joints two weeks after an upper respiratory infection that had been treated with penicillin. He also complained of pain in the leg muscles and large joints. The rash on his face was erythematous, scaling, and atrophic. Biopsy results were characteristic of LE. Laboratory findings included hypergammaglobulinemia, leukopenia, and an elevated sedimentation rate; but the LE cell preparation was negative. Cuticular telangiectasia was noted. Oral prednisone therapy resulted in prompt subsidence of his signs and symptoms. Nine months later his condition flared; he had profound weakness of the neck and abdominal muscles, atrophic hypopigmented areas over the elbows and ankles, Gottron's papules on the knuckles, and heliotrope-colored eyelids. Muscle biopsy, SGOT, and LDH enzyme levels all confirmed dermatomyositis. An increase in prednisone therapy resulted in marked improvement. Over the following two years, extensive calcification developed in his paraspinous, gluteal, and subscapular muscles.

The initial features of this illness resembled LE very closely. The later signs and symptoms were unequivocally those of dermatomyositis. Kierland has described the reverse situation in a 10-year-old girl who initially developed acute dermatomyositis confirmed by muscle biopsy, electromyograms, and SGOT enzyme levels. She also had leukopenia, increased sedimentation rate, hypergammaglobulinemia, and negative LE cell test. Within a year, the LE cell test became positive. Pericarditis and pleuritis ensued. She died of cardiac failure two years after the onset of her illness.[254]

There are patients who exhibit some of the signs and symptoms characteristic of connective tissue disease but in whom it is not possible to assign a specific diagnosis. Raynaud's phenomenon, livedo reticularis, violaceous edema of the hands and feet, erythema and scaling over the extensor surfaces of the major joints, cuticular telangiectasia, telangiectatic macules, psychiatric symptoms, and arthralgia are the most common features in the undifferentiated type of connective tissue disease. The following case report is illustrative of this entity:

A 45-year-old white woman had suffered from stiffness and arthralgias of her fingers, knees, wrists, and shoulders since the age of 42. She also complained of Raynaud's phenomenon, recurrent headaches, lightheadedness, and fear of leaving her house and being in crowds. She sought the aid of many physicians, all of whom thought she had a psychiatric disorder. She was first seen at the Yale-New Haven Hospital when she was 45, at which time she exhibited erythema and scaling over the knees, elbows, and periorbital tissues. Her hands were slightly puffy and violaceous. The only abnormal laboratory finding was an elevated sedimentation rate. LE cell tests were negative, and a muscle biopsy did not show evidence of myositis. During the next four years, oral prednisone therapy in the range of 10 to 15 milligrams per day controlled all the signs and symptoms except for the Raynaud's phenomenon and psychiatric complaints. Whenever oral steroids were discontinued, skin rash, headache, and arthralgia promptly returned. Myositis or evidence of other organic involvement never developed. She did show telangiectatic macules on her face and cuticular telangiectasia one year before she died (Plate 20*E*). Six months before death, malignant hypertension and uremia developed. Autopsy examination revealed lupus nephritis.

This patient had the signs and symptoms of connective tissue disease which, at the onset of her illness, most closely resembled the cutaneous features of dermatomyositis. Subsequently, the telangiectasia characteristic of a connective tissue disorder developed. Autopsy revealed lupus nephritis with hematoxylin bodies. No other organs were involved.

THE THYMUS AND CONNECTIVE TISSUE DISORDERS

The thymus gland plays a significant role in the development of immunologic competence in guinea pigs, mice, and rabbits.[255] A genetic disorder identical to LE occurs in NZB mice (see p. 296). A number of thymic abnormalities are associated with autoimmune diseases, agammaglobulinemia, and lymphoreticular malignancy in man.

Approximately one third of the individuals with congenital and acquired agammaglobulinemia develop an illness indistinguishable from rheumatoid arthritis one to eight years after the onset of this immunologic deficiency.[256] Four other patients have been described as having a dermatomyositis-like syndrome in which the striking feature was marked induration of tissues with contractures, not muscular weakness.[102] In a case reported by Page et al. a youngster died of a malignant lymphoma two and a half years after the onset of the dermatomyositis-like illness. In retrospect, these cases actually may have represented eosinophilic fasciitis occurring on a background of malignancy, as in the case from Yale reported by Hoffman et al.[182] Diffuse necrotizing arteritis was present in another case of agammaglobulinemia. A 15-month-old boy with this immunologic aberration was reported to have suddenly developed scleroderma, which then resolved over the succeeding 18 months. However, his history and course were more consistent with scleredema than scleroderma.[258]

Thymoma and thymic hyperplasia with formation of germinal centers have been detected in biopsy specimens from patients with myasthenia gravis and LE. Antinuclear factors and antimuscle antibodies are found in the sera of many patients with myasthenia gravis. Both illnesses have been coincident in nine patients. In a few instances LE has appeared after thymectomy for myasthenia gravis.[259] Ulcerative colitis, which may also be a disorder of autoimmunity, has been associated with LE[260] and scleroderma.[261]

The frequency of leukemia and lymphoma is increased in patients with congenital and acquired agammaglobulinemia. LE with malignant lymphoma has been seen in four instances[267] and the combination of Sjögren's syndrome and lymphoma has been observed in seven.[263]

The increased risk of lymphoma in Sjögren's disease appears to be associated with parotid swelling, splenomegaly, and lymphadenopathy — all indicators of extensive lymphoproliferation. Such patients ought to be followed closely for the development of lymphoma.

REFERENCES

1. Kaslow, R. A., and Masi, A. T.: Age, sex, and race effects on mortality from systemic lupus erythematosus in the United States. Arthritis Rheum., *21*:473, 1978.
2. Siegel, M., and Lee, S. L.: The epidemiology of systemic lupus erythematosus. Sem. Arthritis Rheum., *3*:1, 1973.
3. O'Loughlin, S., Schroeter, A. L., and Jordon, R. E.: A study of lupus erythematosus with particular reference to generalized discoid lupus. Br. J. Dermatol., *99*:1, 1978.
4. Shearn, M. A., and Pirofsky, B.: Disseminated lupus erythematosus. Arch. Intern. Med., *90*:790, 1952.
5. Jessar, R. A., Lamont-Havers, W., and Ragan, C.: Natural history of lupus erythematosus disseminatus. Ann. Intern. Med., *38*:717, 1953.
6. DuBois, E. L.: The effect of L. E. cell test on the clinical picture of systemic lupus erythematosus. Ann. Intern. Med., *38*:1265, 1953.
7. Feinglass, E. J., Arnett, F. C., Dorsch, C. A., Zizic, T. M., and Stevens, M. B.: Neuropsychiatric manifestations of systemic lupus erythematosus: diagnosis, clinical spectrum, and relationship of other features of the disease. Medicine, *55*:323, 1976.
8. Walravens, P. A., and Chase, H. P.: The prognosis of childhood systemic lupus erythematosus. Am. J. Dis. Child., *130*:929, 1976.
9. Rothfield, N., March, C. H., Miescher, P., and McEwen, C.: Chronic discoid lupus erythematosus: a study of 65 patients and 65 controls. N. Engl. J. Med., *269*:1155, 1963.
10. Tuffanelli, D. L.: Lupus erythematosus. Arch. Dermatol., *106*:553, 1972.
11. Prystowsky, S. D., Herndon, J. H., Jr., and Gilliam, J. N.: Chronic cutaneous lupus erythematosus (DLE) — A clinical and laboratory investigation of 80 patients. Medicine, *55*:183, 1975.
12. Peterson, W. C., Jr., and Gokcen, M.: Antinuclear factors in chronic discoid lupus erythematosus. Arch. Dermatol., *86*:783, 1962.
13. DuBois, E. L., and Martel, S.: Discoid lupus erythematosus: an analysis of its systemic manifestations. Ann. Intern. Med., *44*:482, 1956.
14. Haserick, J. R.: Modern concepts of systemic lupus erythematosus: a review of 126 cases. J. Chron. Dis., *1*:317, 1955.
15. Storck, H. Von, and Berzups, S.: Über Lupus erythematodes unter besonderer Berucksichtigung des Uberganges von lokalisierten in generalisierte Formen. Dermatologica, *124*:142, 1962.
16. Harvey, A. M., Shulman, L. E., Tumulty, P. A., Conley, C. L., and Schoenrich, E. H.: Systemic lupus erythematosus: review of the literature and clinical analysis of 138 cases. Medicine, *33*:291, 1954.
17. Scott, A., and Rees, E. G.: The relationship

of systemic lupus erythematosus and discoid lupus erythematosus: a clinical and hematological study. Arch. Dermatol., *79*:422, 1959.
18. Shklar, G., and McCarthy, P. L.: Histopathology of oral lesions of discoid lupus erythematosus. Arch. Dermatol., *114*: 1031, 1978.
19. Tuffanelli, D. L.: Lupus erythematosus panniculitis (profundus). Clinical and immunologic studies. Arch. Dermatol., *103*:231, 1971.
20. Harris, R. B., and Winkelmann, R. K.: Lupus mastitis. Arch. Dermatol., *114*:410, 1978.
21. Winkelmann, R. K.: Panniculitis and systemic lupus erythematosus. J.A.M.A., *211*:472, 1970.
22. Monroe, E. W.: Lupus band test. Arch. Dermatol., *113*:830, 1977.
23. Panet-Raymond, G., and Johnson, W. C.: Lupus erythematosus and polymorphous light eruption. Arch. Dermatol., *108*:785, 1973.
24. Sontheimer, R. D., Thomas, J. R., and Gilliam, J. N.: Subacute cutaneous lupus erythematosus. Arch. Dermatol., *115*: 1409, 1979.
25. Barker, N. W., Hines, E. A., Jr., and Craig, W. McK.: Livedo reticularis: A peripheral arteriolar disease. Am. Heart J., *21*:592, 1941.
26. Millard, L. G., and Rowell, N. R.: Chilblain lupus erythematosus (Hutchinson). A clinical and laboratory study of 17 patients. Br. J. Dermatol., *98*:497, 1978.
27. Tuffanelli, D. L., and DuBois, E. L.: Cutaneous manifestations of systemic lupus erythematosus. Arch. Dermatol., *90*:377, 1964.
28. O'Loughlin, S., Schroeter, A. L., and Jordon, R. E.: Chronic urticaria-like lesions in systemic lupus erythematosus. Arch. Dermatol., *114*:879, 1978.
29. Estes, D., and Christian, C. L.: The natural history of systemic lupus erythematosus by prospective analysis. Medicine, *50*:85, 1971.
30. Tumulty, P. A.: Clinical course of systemic lupus erythematosus. J.A.M.A., *156*:947, 1954.
31. Braverman, I. M., and Yen, A.: Demonstration of immune complexes in spontaneous and histamine-induced lesions and in normal skin of patients with leukocytoclastic angiitis. J. Invest. Dermatol., *64*:105, 1975.
32. Soter, N. A., Austen, K. F., and Gigli, I: Urticaria and arthralgias as manifestations of necrotizing angiitis (vasculitis). J. Invest. Dermatol., *63*:485, 1974.
33. Tromovitch, T. A., and Hyman, A. B.: Systemic lupus erythematosus with hemorrhagic bullae. Arch. Dermatol., *83*:910, 1961.
34. Stone, J. A., and Leavell, U. W., Jr.: Unusual cells in lupus erythematosus bullae. Arch. Dermatol., *112*:1753, 1976.
35. Lever, W. F.: Histopathology of the Skin. 4th ed. J. B. Lippincott, Philadelphia, 1967, p. 455.
36. Kumar, V., Binder, W. L., Schotland, E., Beutner, E. H., and Chorzelski, T. P.: Coexistence of bullous pemphigoid and systemic lupus erythematosus. Arch. Dermatol., *114*:1187, 1978.
37. Pedro, S. D., and Dahl, M. V.: Direct immunofluorescence of bullous systemic lupus erythematosus. Arch. Dermatol., *107*:118, 1973.
38. Jordon, R. E., Muller, S. A., Hale, W. L., and Beutner, E. H.: Bullous pemphigoid associated with systemic lupus erythematosus. Arch. Dermatol., *99*:17, 1969.
39. Quismorio, F. P., Dubois, E. L., and Chandor, S. B.: Soft-tissue calcification in systemic lupus erythematosus. Arch. Dermatol., *111*:352, 1975.
40. Bywaters, E. G. L.: A variant of rheumatoid arthritis characterized by recurrent digital pad nodules and palmar fasciitis closely resembling palindromic rheumatism. Ann. Rheum. Dis., *8*:1, 1949.
41. Lodin, A.: Discoid lupus erythematosus and trauma. Acta Dermatovenereol., *43*:142, 1963.
42. Lamb, J. H., Jones, P. E., Rebell, G., and Alston, H. D.: Sensitivity to fluorescent (blue-green) light. Arch. Dermatol., *77*:519, 1958.
43. Gottlieb, B., and Winkelmann, R. K.: Lymphocytic infiltration of skin. Arch. Dermatol., *86*:626, 1962.
44. Johnson, W. C., Higdon, R. S., and Helwig, E. B.: Granuloma faciale. Arch. Dermatol., *79*:42, 1959.
45. Romero, R. W., Nesbitt, L. T., Jr., and Reed, R. J.: Unusual variant of lupus erythematosus or lichen planus. Arch. Dermatol., *113*:741, 1977.
46. Copeman, P. W. M., Schroeter, A. L., and Kierland, R. R.: An unusual variant of lupus erythematosus or lichen planus. Br. J. Dermatol., *83*:269, 1970.
47. Januson, T. H., Cooper, N. M., and Epstein, W. V.: Lichen planus and discoid lupus erythematosus. Overlap syndrome associated with cryoglobulinemia and hypocomplementemia. Arch. Dermatol., *114*:1039, 1978.
48. Ueki, H.: Hyaline bodies in subepidermal papillae. Immunohistochemical studies in several dermatoses. Arch. Dermatol., *100*:610, 1969.
49. Uitto, J., Santa-Cruz, D. J., Eisen, A. Z., and Leone, P.: Verrucous lesions in patients with discoid lupus erythematosus. Br. J. Dermatol., *98*:507, 1978.
50. Thormann, J.: Ulcerative lichen planus of the feet. A case in which the serological findings suggested systemic lupus erythematosus. Arch. Dermatol., *110*:753, 1974.
51. DeHoratius, R. J., Pillarisetty, R., Messner, R. P., and Talal, N.: Antinucleic acid antibodies in systemic lupus erythematosus patients and their families. J. Clin. Invest., *56*:1149, 1975.

52. Block, S. R., and Christian, C. L.: The pathogenesis of systemic lupus erythematosus. Am. J. Med., *59*:453, 1975.
53. Phillips, P. E.: The virus hypothesis in systemic lupus erythematosus. Ann. Intern. Med., *83*:709, 1975.
54. Markenson, J. A., and Phillips, P. E.: Type C viruses and systemic lupus erythematosus. Arthritis Rheum., *21*:266, 1978.
55. Talal, N.: Autoimmunity and lymphoid malignancy in New Zealand mice. *In* Progress in Clinical Immunology, edited by R. S. Schwartz. Grune and Stratton, New York *2*:101, 1974.
56. Braverman, I. M.: Study of autoimmune disease in New Zealand mice. I. Genetic features and natural history of NZB, NZY, and NZW strains and NZB/NZW hybrids. J. Invest. Dermatol., *50*:483, 1968.
57. Datta, S. K., and Schwartz, R. S.: Genetics of expression of xenotropic virus and autoimmunity in NZB mice. Nature, *263*:412, 1976.
58. Raveché, E. S., Steinberg, A. D., Klassen, L. W., and Tjio, J. H.: Genetic studies in NZB mice. J. Exp. Med., *147*:1487, 1978.
59. Arnett, F. C., and Shulman, L. E.: Studies in familial systemic lupus erythematosus. Medicine, *55*:313, 1976.
60. Agnello, V.: Complement deficiency states. Medicine, *57*:1, 1978.
61. Schur, P. H.: Pathophysiology of rheumatic diseases. Arthritis Rheum., *21*:500, 1978.
62. Reinertson, J. L., Klippel, J. H., Johnson, A. H., Steinberg, A. D., Decker, J. L., and Mann, D. L.: B-lymphocyte alloantigens associated with systemic lupus erythematosus. N. Engl. J. Med., *299*: 515, 1978.
63. Waldmann, T. A., Blaese, R. M., Broder, S., and Krakauer, R. S.: Disorders of suppressor immunoregulatory cells in the pathogenesis of immunodeficiency and autoimmunity. Ann. Intern. Med., *88*:226, 1978.
64. Bardana, E. J., Harbeck, R. J., Hoffman, A. A., Pirofsky, B., and Carr, R. I.: The prognostic and therapeutic implications of DNA:anti-DNA immune complexes in systemic lupus erythematosus (SLE). Am. J. Med., *59*:515, 1975.
65. Davis, J. S., Godfrey, S. M., and Winfield, J. B.: Direct evidence for circulating DNA/anti-DNA complexes in systemic lupus erythematosus. Arthritis Rheum., *21*:17, 1978.
66. Masi, A. T., and Kaslow, R. A.: Sex effects in systemic lupus erythematosus. Arthritis Rheum., *21*:480, 1978.
67. Ochs, H. D., Rosenfeld, S. I., Thomas, E. D., Giblett, E. R., Alper, C. A., Dupont, B., Schaller, J. G., Gilliland, B. C., Hansen, J. A., and Wedgwood, R. J.: Linkage between the gene (or genes) controlling synthesis of the fourth component of complement and the major histocompatibility complex. N. Engl. J. Med., *296*:470, 1977.
68. Caldwell, J. L.: Genetic regulation of immune responses. *In* Basic and Clinical Immunology. 2nd ed., edited by H. H. Fundberg, D. P. Stites, J. L. Caldwell, and J. V. Wells. Lange Medical Publications, Los Altos, Calif., 1978, p. 155.
69. Perkins, H. A.: The human major histocompatibility complex (MHC). *In* Basic and Clinical Immunology, *op. cit.*, p. 165.
70. Klein, J.: Genetic control of virus susceptibility. *In* Biology of the Mouse Histocompatibility-2 Complex. Springer-Verlag, New York, 1975, p. 389.
71. Daniels, C. A., Borsos, T., Rapp, H. J., Synderman, R., and Notkins, A. L.: Neutralization of sensitized virus by purified components of complement. Proc. Nat. Acad. Sci., *65*:528, 1970.
72. Yoshiki, T., Mellors, R. C., Strand, M., and August, J. T.: The viral envelope glycoprotein of murine leukemic virus and the pathogenesis of immune complex glomerulonephritis of New Zealand mice. J. Exp. Med., *140*:1011, 1974.
73. Roubinian, J. R., Papoian, R., and Talal, N.: Androgenic hormones modulate autoantibody responses and improve survival in murine lupus. J. Clin. Invest., *59*:1066, 1977.
74. Singsen, B. H., Bernstein, B. H., King, K. K., and Hanson, V.: Systemic lupus erythematosus in childhood: correlations between changes in disease activity and serum complement levels. J. Pediatr., *89*:358, 1976.
75. Maddison, P., Mogavero, H., Provost, T. T., and Reichlin, M.: The clinical significance of autoantibodies to a soluble cytoplasmic antigen in systemic lupus erythematosus and other connective tissue diseases. J. Rheumatol., *6*:189, 1979.
76. Provost, T. T.: Subsets in systemic lupus erythematosus. J. Invest Dermatol., *72*:110, 1979.
77. Provost, T. T., Ahmed., A. R., Maddison, P. J., and Reichlin, M.: Antibodies to cytoplasmic antigens in lupus erythematosus. Serologic marker for systemic disease. Arthritis Rheum., *20*:1457, 1977.
78. Schrager, M. A., and Rothfield, N. F.: The lupus band test. Clinics Rheum. Dis., *1*:597, 1975.
79. Schrager, M. A., and Rothfield, N. F.: Clinical significance of serum properidin levels and properidin deposition in the dermal-epidermal junction in systemic lupus erythematosus. J. Clin. Invest., *57*:212, 1976.
80. Sontheimer, R. D., and Gilliam, J. N.: A reappraisal of the relationship between subepidermal immunoglobulin deposits and DNA antibodies in systemic lupus erythematosus: a study using the crithidia luciliae immunofluorescence anti-DNA assay. J. Invest. Dermatol., *72*:29, 1979.
81. Cripps, D. J., and Rankin, J.: Action spectra of lupus erythematosus and experi-

mental immunofluorescence. Arch. Dermatol., *107*:653, 1973.

82. Gilliam, J. N., Hurd, E. R., and Ziff, M.: Subepidermal deposition of immunoglobulin in NZB/NZW F_1 hybrid mice. J. Immunol., *114*:133, 1975.
83. Natali, P. G., and Tan, E. M.: Experimental skin lesions in mice resembling lupus erythematosus. Arthritis Rheum., *16*: 579, 1973.
84. Soltani, K., Pacernick, L. J., and Lorincz, A. L.: Lupus erythematosus-like lesions in newborn infants. Arch. Dermatol., *110*:435, 1974.
85. Vonderheid, E. C., Koblenzer, P. J., Ming, P. M. L., and Burgoon, C. F., Jr.: Neonatal lupus erythematosus. Arch. Dermatol., *112*:698, 1976.
86. Fox, J. R., Jr., McGuiston, H., and Schoch, E. P., Jr.: Systemic lupus erythematosus. Association with previous neonatal lupus erythematosus. Arch. Dermatol., *115*:340, 1979.
87. Blomgren, S. E.: Drug-induced lupus erythematosus. Sem. Hematol., *10*:345, 1973.
88. Omenn, G. S.: Drug-induced lupus-like syndromes: a pharmacogenetic relationship. Arthritis Rheum., *21*:322, 1978.
89. Alarcón-Segovia, D.: Drug-induced systemic lupus erythematosus and related syndromes. Clinics Rheum. Dis., *1*:573, 1975.
90. Hahn, B. H., Sharp, G. C., Irvin, W. S., Kantor, O. S., Gardner, C. A., Bagby, M. K., Perry, H. M., Jr., and Osterland, C. K.: Immune responses to hydralazine and nuclear antigens in hydralazine-induced lupus erythematosus. Ann. Intern. Med., *76*:365, 1972.
91. Cram, D. L., and Tuffanelli, D. L.: Lupus erythematosus and porphyria. Arch. Dermatol., *108*:779, 1973.
92. Pearson, C. M.: Patterns of polymyositis and their response to treatment. Ann. Intern. Med., *59*:827, 1963.
93. Bohan, A., Peter, J. B., Bowman, R. L., and Pearson, C. M.: A computer-assisted analysis of 153 patients with polymyositis and dermatomyositis. Medicine, *56*:255, 1977.
94. Walton, J. N., and Adams, R. D.: Polymyositis. E. and S. Livingstone, Ltd., Edinburgh, 1958.
95. Adams, R. D., Denny-Brown, D., and Pearson, C. M.: Diseases of Muscle. A Study in Pathology. 2nd ed. Hoeber, New York, 1962.
96. Muller, S. A., Winkelmann, R. K., and Brunsting, L. A.: Calcinosis in dermatomyositis. Arch. Dermatol., *79*:669, 1959.
97. Krain, L. S.: Dermatomyositis in six patients without initial muscle involvement. Arch. Dermatol., *111*:241, 1975.
98. Samitz, M. H.: Cuticular changes in dermatomyositis. Arch. Dermatol., *110*:866, 1974.
99. Gottron, H.: Hautveränderungen bei Dermatomyositis. Comptes-rendu du Huitième Congrès International de Dermatologie et de Syphilologie, Copenhagen, 1930, p. 826. Cited by Keil, H.: Dermatomyositis and systemic lupus erythematosus. Arch. Intern. Med., *66*:109, 1940.
100. Keil, H.: The manifestations in the skin and mucous membranes in dermatomyositis with special reference to the differential diagnosis from systemic lupus erythematosus. Ann. Intern. Med., *16*:828, 1942.
101. Winkelmann, R. K.: The cutaneous diagnosis of dermatomyositis, lupus erythematosus, and scleroderma. N. Y. J. Med., *63*:3080, 1963.
102. Cook, C. D., Rosen, F. S., and Banker, B. Q.: Dermatomyositis and focal scleroderma. Pediatr. Clin. North Am., *10*:979, 1963.
103. Sheard, C., Jr., and Knoepfler, P. T.: Dermatomyositis and the incidence of associated malignancy. Arch. Dermatol., *75*:224, 1957.
104. Bitnum, S., Daeschner, C. W., Jr., Travis, L. B., Dodge, W. F., and Hoops, H. C.: Dermatomyositis. J. Pediatr., *64*:101, 1964.
105. Sullivan, D. B., Cassidy, J. T., and Petty, R. E.: Dermatomyositis in the pediatric patient. Arthritis Rheum., *21*:327, 1978.
106. Rose, A. L.: Childhood polymyositis. A follow-up study with special reference to treatment with corticosteroids. Am. J. Dis. Child., *127*:518, 1974.
107. Kornreich, H., Koster, K., and Hanson, V.: The rheumatic diseases in adolescence. Pediatr. Clin. North Am., *20*:911, 1973.
108. Sunde, H.: Dermatomyositis in children. Acta Paediatr., *37*:287, 1949.
109. Banker, B. Q., and Victor, M.: Dermatomyositis (systemic angiopathy) of childhood. Medicine, *45*:261, 1966.
110. Banker, B. Q.: Dematomyositis of childhood, ultrastructural alterations of muscle and intramuscular blood vessels. J. Neuropathol. Exp. Neurol., *34*:46, 1975.
111. Sheldon, J. H., Young, F., and Dyke, S. C.: Acute dermatomyositis associated with reticuloendotheliosis. Lancet, *1*:82, 1939.
112. Arundell, F. D., Wilkinson, R. D., and Haserick, J. R.: Dermatomyositis and malignant neoplasms in adults: survey of twenty years' experience. Arch. Dermatol., *82*:772, 1960.
113. Barnes, B. E.: Dermatomyositis and malignancy. A review of the literature. Ann. Intern. Med., *84*:68, 1976.
114. Bohan, A., and Peter, J. B.: Polymyositis and dermatomyositis. N. Engl. J. Med., *292*:344, 403, 1975.
115. Christianson, H. B., Brunsting, L. A., and Perry, H. O.: Dermatomyositis. Arch. Dermatol., *74*:581, 1956.
116. Curtis, A. C.: Discussion of case presentation at Chicago Dermatological Society. Arch. Dermatol., *71*:416, 1955.
117. Currie, S., Saunders, M., Knowles, M., and Brown, A. E.: Immunological aspects of polymyositis. The in vitro activity of lym-

phocytes on incubation with muscle antigen and with muscle cultures. Q. J. Med., New Series, *40*:63, 1971.

118. Mastaglia, F. L., and Currie, S.: Immunological and ultrastructural observations on the role of lymphoid cells in the pathogenesis of polymyositis. Arch. Neuropathol., *18*:1, 1971.
119. Johnson, R. L., Fink, C. W., and Ziff, M.: Lymphotoxin formation by lymphocytes and muscle in polymyositis. J. Clin. Invest., *51*:2435, 1972.
120. Dawkins, R. L., and Mastaglia, F. L.: Cell-mediated cytotoxicity to muscle in polymyositis. Effect of immunosuppression. N. Engl. J. Med., *288*:434, 1973.
121. Whitaker, J. N., and Engel, W. K.: Mechanisms of muscle injury in idiopathic inflammatory myopathy. N. Engl. J. Med., *289*:107, 1973.
122. Dawkins, R. L., and Mastaglia, F. L.: Reply to reference 121. N. Engl. J. Med., *289*:108, 1973.
123. Ludatscher, R., Gellei, B., Guershoni, G., and Benderley, A.: Small blood vessel involvement in childhood dermatomyositis. Isr. J. Med Sci., *13*:20, 1977.
124. Miller, J. J., III: Late progression in dermatomyositis in childhood. J. Pediatr., *83*:543, 1973.
125. Whitaker, J. N., and Engel, W. K.: Vascular deposits of immunoglobulin and complement in idiopathic inflammatory myopathy. N. Engl. J. Med., *286*:333, 1972.
126. Chou, S. M., and Gutmann, L.: Picornavirus-like crystals in subacute polymyositis. Neurology, *20*:205, 1970.
127. Mastaglia, F. L., and Walton, J. N.: Coxsackie virus–like particles in skeletal muscle from a case of polymyositis. J. Neurol. Sci., *11*:593, 1970.
128. Travers, R. L., Hughes, G. R. V., Cambridge, G., and Sewell, J. R.: Coxsackie B neutralization titers in polymyositis/dermatomyositis. Lancet, *1*:1268, 1977.
129. Pachman, L. M., Jonasson, L. M., O'Cannon, R. A., and Freedman, J. M.: Increased frequency of HLA-B8 in juvenile dermatomyositis. Lancet, *2*:1238, 1977.
130. Behan, W. M. H., Behan, P. O., and Dick, H. A.: HLA-B8 in polymyositis. N. Engl. J. Med., *298*:1260, 1978.
131. Cumming, W. J. K., Hudgson, P., Lattimer, D., Sussman, M., and Wilcox, C. B.: HLA and serum complement in polymyositis. Lancet, *2*:978, 1977.
132. Grace, J. T., Jr., and Dao, T. L.: Dermatomyositis in cancer: a possible etiological mechanism. Cancer, *12*:648, 1959.
133. Curtis, A. C., Heckaman, J. H., and Wheeler, A. H.: Study of the autoimmune reaction in dermatomyositis. J.A.M.A., *178*:571, 1961.
134. te Lintum, J. C. A., and Goedbloed, R.: Poikilodermatomyositis. Dermatologica, *148*:52, 1974.
135. Weston, W. L., and Thorne, E. G.: Profound T lymphopenia in dermatomyositis with cancer. N. Engl. J. Med., *291*:208, 1974.
136. Guntrac, E.: Note sur la sclérodermie. Rev. Med. Chir. (Paris), *2*:263, 1847. Quoted by Rodnan, G. P., and Bendek, T. F.: An historical account of the study of progressive systemic sclerosis (diffuse scleroderma). Ann. Intern. Med., *57*:305, 1962.
137. Tuffanelli, D. L., and Winkelmann, R. K.: Systemic scleroderma. Arch. Dermatol., *84*:359, 1961.
138. Tuffanelli, D. L., and Winkelmann, R. K.: Diffuse systemic scleroderma; a comparison with acrosclerosis. Ann. Intern. Med., *57*:198, 1962.
139. Sackner, M. A.: Scleroderma. Grune and Stratton, Inc., New York, 1966, pp. 147–149.
140. Barnett, A. J., and Coventry, D. A.: Scleroderma. 1. Clinical features, course of illness and response to treatment in 61 cases. Med. J. Aust., *1*:992, 1969.
141. Medsger, T. A., Jr., Masi, A. T., Rodnan, G. P., Benedek, T. G., and Robinson, H.: Survival with systemic sclerosis (scleroderma). A life-table analysis of clinical and demographic factors in 309 patients. Ann. Intern. Med., *75*:369, 1971.
142. Cassidy, J. T., Sullivan, D. B., Dabich, L., and Petty, R. E.: Scleroderma in children. Arthritis Rheum., *21*:351, 1978.
143. Bennett, R., Bluestone, R., Holt, P. J. L., and Bywaters, E. G. L.: Survival in scleroderma. Ann. Rheum. Dis., *30*:581, 1971.
144. Medsger, T. A., Jr., and Masi, A. T.: Survival with scleroderma — II: a life table analysis of clinical and demographic factors in 358 male U.S. veteran patients. J. Chron. Dis., *26*:647, 1973.
145. Stava, Z.: The problem of interrelation between diffuse generalized scleroderma, acrosclerosis, Raynaud's phenomenon and Raynaud's disease. Dermatologica, *118*:1, 1959.
146. Sackner, M. A., Akgun, N., Kimbel, P., and Lewis, D. H.: The pathphysiology of scleroderma involving the heart and respiratory system. Ann. Intern. Med., *60*:611, 1964.
147. Rodnan, G. P.: The nature of joint involvement in progressive systemic sclerosis (diffuse scleroderma). Ann. Intern. Med., *56*:422, 1962.
148. Schumacher, H. R., Jr.: Joint involvement in progressive systemic sclerosis (scleroderma): a light and electron microscopic study of synovial membrane and fluid. Am. J. Clin. Pathol., *60*:593, 1973.
149. Smith, A. G., Holti, G., and Shuster, S.: Immunoreactive beta-melanocyte-stimulating hormone and melanin pigmentation in systemic sclerosis. Br. Med. J., *2*:733, 1976.

149a. Klaus, Sidney. Personal communication.

150. Treacy, W. L., Baggenstoss, A. H., Slocumb, C. H., and Code, C. F.: Scleroderma of the esopaghus. Ann. Intern. Med., *59*:351, 1963.

151. Cohen, S., Fisher, R., Lipshutz, W., Turner, R., Myers, A., and Schumacher, R.: The pathogenesis of esophageal dysfunction in scleroderma and Raynaud's disease. J. Clin. Invest., *51*:2663, 1972.

152. Stevens, M. B., Hookman, P., Siegel, C. I., Esterly, J. R., Shulman, L. E., and Hendrix, T. R.: Aperistalsis of the eosphagus in patients with connective tissue disorders and Raynaud's phenomenon. N. Engl. J. Med., *270*:1218, 1964.

153. Guttadauria, M., Ellman, H., Emmanuel, G., Kaplan, D., and Diamond, H.: Pulmonary function in scleroderma. Arthritis Rheum., *20*:1071, 1977.

154. Celoria, G. C., Friedell, G. H., and Sommers, S. C.: Raynaud's disease and primary pulmonary hypertension. Circulation, *22*:1055, 1960.

155. Salerni, R., Rodnan, G. P., Leon, D. F., and Shaver, J. A.: Pulmonary hypertension in the CREST syndrome variant of progressive systemic sclerosis (scleroderma). Ann. Intern. Med., *86*:394, 1977.

156. D'Angelo, W. A., Fries, J. F., Masi, A. T., and Shulman, L. E.: Pathologic observations in systemic sclerosis (scleroderma). A study of fifty-eight autopsy cases and fifty-eight matched controls. Am. J. Med., *46*:428, 1969.

157. Montgomery, R. D., Stirling, G. A., and Hamer, N. A. J.: Bronchiolar carcinoma in progressive systemic sclerosis. Lancet, *1*:586, 1964.

158. Piper, W. N., and Helwig, E. G.: Progressive systemic sclerosis: visceral manifestations in generalized scleroderma. Arch. Dermatol., *72*:535, 1955.

159. Cannon, P. J., Hassar, M., Case, D. B., Casarella, W. J., Sommers, S. C., and LeRoy, E. C.: The relationship of hypertension and renal failure in scleroderma (progressive systemic sclerosis) to structural and functional abnormalities of the renal cortical circulation. Medicine, *53*:1, 1974.

160. Gavras, H., Gavras, I., Cannon, P. J., Brunner, H. R., and Laragh, J. H.: Is elevated plasma renin activity of prognostic importance in progressive systemic sclerosis? Arch. Intern. Med., *137*:1554, 1977.

161. Mittick, P. D., and Feig, P. U.: Control of hypertension and reversal of renal failure in scleroderma. N. Engl. J. Med., *299*:871, 1978.

162. Wasner, C., Cooke, C. R., and Freis, J. F.: Successful medical treatment of scleroderma renal crisis. N. Engl. J. Med., *299*:873, 1978.

163. Kovalchik, M. T., Guggenheim, S. J., Silverman, M. H., Robertson, J. S., and Steigerwald, J. C.: The kidney in progressive systemic sclerosis. A prospective study. Ann. Intern. Med., *89*:881, 1978.

164. Sokoloff, L.: Some aspects of the pathology of collagen diseases. Bull. N.Y. Acad. Med., *32*:760, 1952.

165. Clements, P. J., Furst, D. E., Campion, D. S., Bohan, A., Harris, R., Levy, J., and Paulus, H. E.: Muscle disease in progressive systemic sclerosis. Arthritis Rheum., *21*:62, 1978.

166. Rodnan, G. P.: A review of recent observations and current theories on the etiology and pathogenesis of progressive systemic sclerosis (diffuse scleroderma). J. Chron. Dis., *16*:929, 1963.

167. Winterbauer, R. H.: Multiple telangiectasia, Raynaud's phenomenon, sclerodactyly and subcutaneous calcinosis. A syndrome mimicking hereditary hemorrhagic telangiectasia. Bull. Hopkins Hosp., *114*:361, 1964.

168. Rodnan, G. P., Medsger, T. A., Jr., and Buckingham, R. B.: Progressive systemic sclerosis —CREST syndrome: Observations on natural history and late complications in 90 patients. Arthritis Rheum., *18*:423, 1975.

169. Crown, S.: Visceral scleroderma without skin involvement. Br. Med. J., *2*:1541, 1961.

170. Rodnan, G. P., and Fennell, R. H., Jr.: Progressive systemic sclerosis *sine* scleroderma. J.A.M.A., *180*:665, 1962.

171. Reynolds, T. B., Denison, E. K., Frankl, H. D., Lieberman, F. L., and Peters, R. L.: Primary biliary cirrhosis with scleroderma, Raynaud's phenomenon and telangiectasia. Am. J. Med., *50*:302, 1971.

172. Markowitz, S. S., McDonald, C. J., Fethiere, W., and Kerzner, M. S.: Occupational acroosteolysis. Arch. Dermatol., *106*:219, 1972.

173. Meyerson, L. B., and Meier, G. C.: Cutaneous lesions in acroosteolysis. Arch. Dermatol., *106*:224, 1972.

174. Shulman, L. E.: Diffuse fasciitis with eosinophilia: a new syndrome? Trans. Assoc. Am. Phys., *88*:70, 1975.

175. Rodnan, G. P., DiBartolomeo, A., Medsger, T. A., and Barnes, E. L.: Eosinophilic fasciitis —report of six cases of a newly recognized scleroderma-like syndrome. Arthritis Rheum., *18*:422, 1975.

176. Lupton, G. P., and Goette, D. K.: Localized eosinophilic fasciitis. Arch. Dermatol., *115*:85, 1979.

177. Caperton, E. M., Hathaway, D. E., and Dehner, L. P.: Morphea, fasciitis and scleroderma with eosinophilia: a broad spectrum of disease. Arthritis Rheum., *19*:792, 1976.

178. Caperton, E. M., and Hathaway, D. E.: Scleroderma with eosinophilia and hypergammaglobulinemia. The Shulman syndrome. Arthritis Rheum., *18*:391, 1975.

179. Bennett, R. M., Herron, A., and Keough, L.: Eosinophilic fasciitis. Ann. Rheum. Dis., *36*:354, 1977.

180. Shewmake, S. W., Lopez, A., and McGlamory, J. C.: The Shulman syndrome. Arch. Dermatol., *114*:556, 1978.

181. Fleischmajer, R., Jacotot, A. B., Shore, S., and Binnick, S. A.: Scleroderma, eosinophilia, and diffuse fasciitis. Arch. Dermatol., *114*:1320, 1978.

182. Hoffman, R., Dainiak, N., Sibrack, L., Pober, J. S., and Waldron, J. A., Jr.: Antibody-mediated aplastic anemia and diffuse fasciitis. N. Engl. J. Med., *300*:718, 1979.
182a. Diaz-Perez, J. L., Connolly, S. M., and Winkelmann, R. K.: Disabling pansclerotic morphea of children. Arch. Dermatol., *116*:169, 1980.
183. Jablonska, S., Bubnow, B., and Szczepanski, A.: Morphea: is it a separate entity or a variety of scleroderma? Dermatologica, *125*:140, 1962.
184. Leinwand, I., Duryee, A. W., and Richter, M. N.: Scleroderma. Ann. Intern. Med., *41*:1003, 1954.
185. Christianson, H. B., Dorsey, C. S., O'Leary, P. A., and Kierland, R. R.: Localized scleroderma. Arch. Dermatol., *74*:629, 1956.
186. Curtis, A. C., and Jansen, T. G.: The prognosis of localized scleroderma. Arch. Dermatol., *78*:749, 1958.
187. Stava, Z., and Stein, J.: Electroencephalography in scleroderma. Dermatologica, *123*:375, 1961.
188. Jablonska, S., Bubnow, B., and Lukasiak, B.: Auswertung von Chronaxiemessungen bei Sklerodermie. Dermatol. Wochenschr., *136*:821, 1957.
189. Ansell, B. M.: Scleroderma. Arthritis Rheum., *21*:363, 1978.
190. Morris, J. M., Samelson, R. L., and Cooley, C. L.: Melorheostosis. J. Bone Joint Surg. [Amer.] *45A*:1191, 1963.
191. Lewis, T.: Experiments relating to the peripheral mechanism involved in spasmodic arrest of the circulation in the fingers, a variety of Raynaud's disease. Heart, *15*:7, 1929.
192. Giunta, J. L.: Raynaud disease with oral manifestations. Arch. Dermatol., *111*:78, 1975.
193. Lewis, T.: The pathological changes in the arteries supplying fingers in warm-handed people and in cases of so-called Raynaud's disease. Clin. Sci., *3*:287, 1938.
194. Lewis, T., and Landis, E. M.: Further observations upon a variety of Raynaud's disease; with specific reference to arteriolar defects and to scleroderma. Clin. Sci., *3*:329, 1938.
195. Walton, K. W.: The pathology of Raynaud's phenomenon of occupational origin. *In* The Vibration Syndrome, edited by W. Taylor. Academic Press, London, 1974, p. 109.
196. James, P. B., and Galloway, R. W.: Brachial arteriography in vibration induced white finger. *In* Taylor, W., *op. cit.*, p. 195.
197. Schatz, I. J.: Vibration-induced white finger. Lancet, *1*:151, 1976.
198. Taylor, W.: The vibration syndrome: introduction. *In* Taylor, W., *op. cit.*, p. 1.
199. Stewart, A. M., and Goda, D. F.: Vibration syndrome. Br. J. Indust. Med., *27*:19, 1970.
200. Nerem, R. M.: Vibration-induced arterial shear stress. The relationship to Raynaud's phenomenon of occupational origin. Arch. Environ. Health, *26*:105, 1973.
201. Fry, D. L.: Acute vascular endothelial changes associated with increased blood velocity gradients. Circ. Res., *22*:165, 1968.
202. De Takats, G., and Fowler, E. F.: Raynaud's phenomenon. J.A.M.A., *179*:1, 1962.
203. Allen, E. V., and Brown, G. E.: Raynaud's disease: a critical review of minimal requisites for diagnosis. Am. J. Med. Sci., *183*:187, 1932.
204. Gifford, R. W., Jr., and Hines, E. A., Jr.: Raynaud's disease among women and girls. Circulation, *16*:1012, 1957.
205. Farmer, R. G., Gifford, R. W., Jr., and Hines, E. A., Jr.: Raynaud's disease with sclerodactylia. Circulation, *23*:13, 1961.
206. Gifford, R. W., Jr.: Arteriospastic disorders of extremities. Circulation, *27*:970, 1963.
207. Jablonska, S., Bubnow, B., and Szczepanski, A.: Diffuse scleroderma and Raynaud's disease. Br. J. Dermatol., *74*:174, 1962.
208. Velayos, E. E., Robinson, H., Porciuncula, F. U., and Masi, A. T.: Clinical correlation analysis of 137 patients with Raynaud's phenomenon. Am. J. Med. Sci., *262*:341, 1971.
209. Porter, J. M., Bardana, E. J., Jr., Baur, G. M., Wesche, D. H., Andrasch, R. H., and Rosch, J.: The clinical significance of Raynaud's syndrome. Surgery, *80*:756, 1976.
210. Coffman, J. D.: Skin blood flow in scleroderma. J. Lab. Clin. Med., *76*:480, 1970.
211. Lewis, T., and Landis, E. M.: Observations upon the vascular mechanism in acrocyanoses. Clin. Sci., *3*:229, 1938.
212. Kontos, H. A., and Wasserman, A. J.: Effect of reserpine in Raynaud's phenomenon. Circulation, *39*:25, 1969.
213. Sapira, J. D., Rodnan, G. P., Scheib, E. T., Klaniecki, T. S., and Rizk, M.: Studies of endogenous catecholamines in patients with Raynaud's phenomenon secondary to progressive systemic sclerosis. Am. J. Med., *52*:330, 1972.
214. Allen, E. V., Barker, N. W., and Hines, E. A.: Peripheral Vascular Disease. W. B. Saunders Company, Philadelphia, 1946, p. 198.
215. Fleischmajer, R.: The pathophysiology of scleroderma. Int. J. Dermatol., *16*:310, 1977.
216. LeRoy, E. C.: Increased collagen synthesis by scleroderma skin fibroblasts in vitro. A possible defect in the regulation or activation of the scleroderma fibroblast. J. Clin. Invest., *54*:880, 1974.
217. Buckingham, R. B., Prince, R. K., Rodnan, G. P., and Taylor, F.: Increased collagen accumulation in dermal fibroblast cultures from patients with progressive systemic sclerosis (scleroderma). J. Lab. Clin. Med., *92*:5, 1978.

218. Perlish, J. S., Bashey, R. L., Stephens, R. E., and Fleischmajer, R.: Connective tissue synthesis by cultured scleroderma fibroblasts. Arthritis Rheum., *19*:891, 1976.
219. Krieg, T., Hörlein, D., Wiestner, M., and Müller, P. K.: Amino terminal extension peptides from type I procollagen normalize excessive collagen synthesis of scleroderma fibroblasts. Arch. Dermatol. Res., *263*:171, 1978.
220. Fleischmajer, R., Perlish, J. S., and Reeves, J. R. T.: Cellular infiltrates in scleroderma skin. Arthritis Rheum., *20*:995, 1977.
221. Kondo, H., Rabin, B. S., and Rodnan, G. P.: Cutaneous antigen-stimulating lymphokine production by lymphocytes of patients with progressive systemic sclerosis. J. Clin. Invest., *58*:1388, 1976.
222. Johnson, R. L., and Ziff, M.: Lymphokine stimulation of collagen accumulation. J. Clin. Invest., *58*:240, 1976.
223. Stuart, J. M., Postlethwaite, A. E., and Kang, A. H.: Evidence for cell-mediated immunity to collagen in progressive systemic sclerosis. J. Lab. Clin. Med., *88*:601, 1976.
224. Lawley, T. J., Peck, G. L., Moutsopoulos, H. M., Gratwohl, A. A., and Deisseroth, A. B.: Scleroderma. Sjögren-like syndrome, and chronic graft-versus-host disease. Ann. Intern. Med., *87*:707, 1977.
225. VanVloten, W. A., Scheffer, E., and Dooren, L. J.: Localized scleroderma-like lesions after bone marrow transplantation in man. A chronic graft-versus-host reaction. Br. J. Dermatol., *96*:337, 1977.
226. Furst, D., Clements, P., Graze, P., Gale, R., and Roberts, N.: A syndrome resembling progressive systemic sclerosis (PSS) following bone marrow transplantation — a model for PSS? Arthritis Rheum., *21*:557, 1978.
227. Willms-Kretschmer, K., and Majno, G.: Ischemia of the skin. Electron microscopic study of vascular injury. Am. J. Pathol., *54*:327, 1969.
228. Gertz, S. D., Gotsman, M. S., Merin, G., Blaumanis, O. R., Pasternak, R. C., and Nelson, E.: Endothelial cell damage and thromboses following partial coronary arterial constriction: relevance to the pathogenesis of myocardial infarction. Isr. J. Med. Sci., *14*:384, 1978.
229. Kahaleh, M. B., and LeRoy, E. C.: Specific endothelial cell injury produced by scleroderma serum in vitro. Arthritis Rheum., *21*:567, 1978.
230. Gratwick, G. M., Kelin, R., Sergent, J. S., and Christian, C. L.: Fibrinogen turnover in progressive systemic sclerosis. Arthritis Rheum., *21*:343, 1978.
231. Silverman, M., Kovalchik, M. T., and Steigerwald, J. C.: Coagulation abnormalities and possible relationship to renal disease in progressive systemic sclerosis. Arthritis Rheum., *21*:592, 1978.
232. Fleischmajer, R., Perlish, J. S., Shaw, K. V., and Pirozzi, D. J.: Skin capillary changes in early systemic scleroderma. Arch. Deramtol., *112*:1553, 1976.
233. Maricq, H. R., Spencer-Green, G., and LeRoy, E. C.: Skin capillary abnormalities as indicators of organ involvement in scleroderma (systemic sclerosis) Raynaud's syndrome and dermatomyositis. Am. J. Med., *61*:862, 1976.
234. Sharp, G. C., Irvin, W. S., Tan, E. M., Gould, R. G., and Holman, H. R.: Mixed connective tissue disease — an apparently distinct rheumatic disease syndrome associated with a specific antibody to an extractable nuclear antigen (ENA). Am. J. Med., *52*:148, 1972.
235. Sharp, G. C.: Mixed connective tissue disease — overlap syndromes. Clinics Rheum. Dis., *1*:561, 1975.
236. Halla, J. T., and Hardin, J. G.: Clinical features of the arthritis of mixed connective tissue disease. Arthritis Rheum., *21*:497, 1978.
237. Mattioli, M., and Reichlin, M.: Physical association of two nuclear antigens and mutual occurrence of their antibodies: the relationship of the Sm and RNA protein (Mo) systems in SLE sera. J. Immunol., *110*:1318, 1973.
238. Farber, S. J., and Bole, G. C.: Antibodies to components of extractable nuclear antigen. Arch. Intern. Med., *136*:425, 1976.
239. Gilliam, J. N., and Prystowsky, S. D.: Mixed connective tissue disease syndrome. Cutaneous manifestations of patients with epidermal nuclear staining and high titer serum antibody to ribonuclease-sensitive extractable nuclear antigen. Arch. Dermatol., *113*:583, 1977.
240. Singsen, B. H., Landing, B., Wolfe, J. F., Bernstein, B., Oxenhandler, R. W., Sharp, G. C., and Hanson, V.: Histologic evaluation of mixed connective tissue disease in children and adults. Arthritis Rheum., *21*:593, 1978.
241. Singsen, B. H., Kornreich, H. K., Koster-King, K., Brink, S. J., Bernstein, B. H., Hanson, V., and Tan, E. M.: Mixed connective tissue disease in children. Arthritis Rheum., *21*:355, 1978.
242. Sharp, G. C.: Mixed connective tissue disease. Bull. Rheum. Dis., *25*:828, 1975.
243. Parker, M. D.: Ribonucleoprotein antibodies: frequency and clinical significance in systemic lupus erythematosus, scleroderma, and mixed connective tissue disease. J. Lab. Clin. Med., *82*:769, 1973.
244. Bennett, R. M., and Spargo, B. H.: Immune complex nephropathy in mixed connective tissue disease. Am. J. Med., *63*:534, 1977.
245. Sharp, G. C., Irvin, W. S., May, C. M., Holman, H. R., McDuffie, F. C., Hess, E. V., and Schmid, F. R.: Antibodies to ribonucleoprotein and Sm antigens in rheumatic diseases. N. Engl. J. Med., *295*:1149, 1976.
246. Prystowsky, S. D., and Tuffanelli, D. L.: Speckled (particulate) epidermal nuclear IgG deposition in normal skin: correlation

of clinical features and laboratory findings in 46 patients with a subset of connective tissue disease characterized by antibody to extractable nuclear antigen (ENA). Arch. Dermatol., *114*:705, 1978.

247. Tan, E. M., and Rodnan, G. P.: Profile of antinuclear antibodies in progressive systemic sclerosis (PSS). Arthritis Rheum., *18*:430, 1975.
248. Reichlin, M.: Problems in differentiating SLE and mixed connective-tissue disease. N. Engl. J. Med., *295*:1194, 1976.
249. Reichlin, M., and Mattioli, M.: Correlation of a precipitin reaction to an RNA protein antigen and a low prevalence of nephritis in patients with systemic lupus erythematosus. N. Engl. J. Med., *286*:908, 1972.
250. Mattioli, M., and Reichlin, M.: Characterization of a soluble nuclear ribonucleoprotein antigen reactive with SLE sera. J. Immunol., *107*:1281, 1971.
251. Hamburger, M., and Hodes, S.: The clinical significance of anti-Sm and anti-RNP antibodies. Arthritis Rheum., *18*:384, 1975.
252. Lerner, M. R., and Steitz, J. A.: Antibodies to small nuclear RNA's complexed with proteins are produced by patients with systemic lupus erythematosus. Proc. Nat. Acad. Sci., *76*:5495, 1979.
253. Lerner, M. R., Boyle, J. A., Mount, S. M., Weliky, J. L., Wolin, S. A., Hardin, J. A., and Steitz, J. A.: Personal communication.
254. Kierland, R. R.: The collagenoses: transitional forms of lupus erythematosus, dermatomyositis and scleroderma. Mayo Clin. Proc., *39*:53, 1964.
255. Good, R. A., Peterson, R. D. A., and Gabrielson, A. E.: The thymus and central lymphoid tissue in immunobiology. Bull. Rheum. Dis., *15*:351, 1964.
256. Gitlin, D., Rosen, F. S., and Janeway, C. A.: Undue susceptibility to infection. Pediatr. Clin. North Am., *9*:405, 1962.
257. Page, A. R., Hansen, A. E., and Good, R. A.: Occurrence of leukemia and lymphoma in patients with agammaglobulinemia. Blood, *21*:197, 1963.
258. Van Gelder, D. W.: Clinical significance of alterations in gamma globulin levels. Southern Med. J., *50*:43, 1957.
259. Alarcón-Segovia, D., Galbraith, R. F., Maldonado, J. E., and Howard, F. M., Jr.: Systemic lupus erythematosus following thymectomy for myasthenia gravis. Lancet, *2*:662, 1963.
260. Alarcón-Segovia, D., Herskovic, T., Dearing, W. H., Bartholomew, L. G., Cain, J. C., and Shorter, R. G.: Lupus erythematosus cell phenomenon in patients with chronic ulcerative colitis. Gut, *6*:39, 1965.
261. De Luca, V. A., Jr., Spiro, H. M., and Thayer, W. R.: Ulcerative colitis and scleroderma. Gastroenterology, *49*:433, 1965.
262. Nilsen, L. B., Missal, M. E., and Condemi, J. J.: Appearance of Hodgkin's disease in a patient with systemic lupus erythematosus. Cancer, *20*:1930, 1967.
263. Kassan, S. S., Thomas, T. L., Moutsopoulos, H. M., Hoover, R., Kimberly, R. P., Budman, D. R., Costa, J., Decker, J. L., and Chused, T. M.: Increased risk of lymphoma in sicca syndrome. Ann. Intern. Med., *89*:888, 1978.

8

The Angiitides

The clinician applies the terms *angiitis* and *vasculitis* to syndromes produced by necrotizing inflammation that involves blood vessels without specifying the type of vessel. It would be more precise to use the terms *arteritis* and *venulitis* for involvement of arterial and venular vessels, respectively. The size of the vessel, its anatomic site, and the severity of the inflammatory and necrotic response determine the clinical signs and symptoms. The almost infinite combinations of size, site, and severity have resulted in many syndromes and many classifications. There are multiple etiologies for this group of disorders, and currently it is believed that deposition of circulating immune complexes in vascular walls is the major pathogenetic mechanism in most cases.

The histopathologic criteria for the diagnosis of angiitis or vasculitis, as defined by light microscopy, include the following: necrosis of vascular walls and surrounding perivascular tissue, usually accompanied by material having the staining qualities of fibrinoid; presence of a marked cellular infiltrate, in the vascular wall and perivascular zone, composed predominantly of neutrophils, but also containing lymphocytes, eosinophils, and other mononuclear cells; and the finding of fine basophilic droplets, termed *nuclear dust*, within the necrotic areas of the vessel wall and surrounding tissues. The nuclear dust is produced by distintegration of neutrophilic nuclei (leukocytoclasis). It is not essential to demonstrate extravasated erythrocytes in histologic sections in order to make the diagnosis of necrotizing vasculitis. Erythrocytes may be difficult to find in tissue specimens conventionally sectioned in a vertical plane, when they are present in small numbers.

The size of the vessels involved in these syndromes ranges from arteries having calibers the size of hepatic and coronary vessels to venules, arterioles, and capillaries. The inflammatory process of the vascular wall is accompanied by a proliferation and swelling of endothelial cells, which result in the reduction of the lumen and, sometimes, in thrombosis.

In some of the disorders to be discussed, the necrosis may be accompanied by the formation of granulation tissue, granulomas, or giant cells. Fibrosis and luminal obstruction can be the end result of these pathologic processes in the vascular walls.

The terms angiitis and vasculitis are properly applied only to necrotizing inflammation and should not be used to describe the perivascular lymphocytic accumulations that frequently occur with many cutaneous drug reactions and with other dermatoses such as pityriasis rosea, eczematous dermatitis, photodermatitis, and lupus erythematosus. In these disorders, the vessel walls remain intact and there is no necrosis. There may be endothelial swelling and a marked perivascular cuffing by lymphocytes, but neutrophils, nuclear dust, and fibrinoid material are absent. Also, *angiitis* includes neither endarteritis and endophlebitis, which are characterized by endothelial swelling and intimal thickening as seen in diabetes mellitus and scleroderma, nor secondary necrotizing vasculitis, which results from malignant hypertension or from infection or infarction in the immediate area of blood vessels.

Historical analysis is of immense help in trying to understand the complexities of the angiitides. Zeek has been instrumental in clarifying much of the confusion surrounding the necrotizing vasculitides; her lucid expositions should be read by everyone interested in this problem.[1-3]

Periarteritis nodosa was described by Kussmaul and Maier in 1866. The disorder that they reported was a necrotizing arteritis of muscular arteries whose caliber was that of the coronary and hepatic vessels. Both necrotizing and healing lesions were present in the affected arteries. About 70 cases were reported between 1866 and the early 1920's. In the succeeding 15 years an additional 400 cases were recorded; however, many did not conform to the original description by Kussmaul and Maier. Apparently the diagnosis of periarteritis nodosa was also being applied to necrotizing inflammation involving arterioles, venules, and capillaries.[1] The signs and symptoms of this small vessel arteritis (microscopic periarteritis nodosa) were extremely variable, and the relationship of the published cases to one another was further obscured because either the cutaneous or the systemic manifestations were emphasized, depending upon whether the dermatologist or the internist reported the case.

At least nine different names have been assigned to the entity of small vessel angiitis. Zeek called this disorder hypersensitivity angiitis because seven of her ten patients became sick and died following a reaction to oral sulfonamides administered for an infectious illness.[2] Experimental work in the 1930's and 1940's supported Zeek's choice of terms because animals sensitized to bacterial antigens and foreign proteins, including horse serum, developed a necrotizing arteritis of small blood vessels rather than of the large muscular arteries. The small vessel arteritis in experimental serum sickness and the Arthus reaction is produced by the deposition of antigen-antibody complexes in the vascular walls.

There is now considerable evidence to support such an underlying mechanism in small vessel vasculitis, especially in serum sickness, some drug reactions, systemic LE, rheumatoid arthritis, and many chronic bacterial and viral infections. However, in many cases no underlying hypersensitivity disorder can be identified, and in only a minority of cases can an etiology be determined. It seems, therefore, preferable to refer to small vessel angiitis by its histopathologic descriptive term — leukocytoclastic angiitis — rather than by an etiologic or pathogenetic term, such as hypersensitivity angiitis, until we know more about the causes and mechanisms of this entity.

While Zeek was clarifying the problem of classic periarteritis nodosa versus *microscopic* periarteritis nodosa, two other syndromes of necrotizing vasculitis were being defined: allergic granulomatosis of Churg and Strauss, and Wegener's granulomatosis.

The most useful classification of necrotizing angiitis and the one that best correlates the clinical and pathologic features is still Zeek's original grouping, which is reproduced here with only minor modifications.[3] Zeek divided the necrotizing vasculitides into six types, five of which have significant cutaneous manifestations and are discussed in this chapter. The sixth type, rheumatic arteritis, is primarily a histopathologic entity that is discovered at autopsy in the lungs and hearts of patients who have died of fulminant rheumatic fever. The five types of necrotizing arteritis are:

1. periarteritis nodosa
2. allergic granulomatosis
3. Wegener's granulomatosis
4. leukocytoclastic angiitis (hypersensitivity angiitis)
5. giant cell arteritis

This classification, which is based upon the *type* and *size* of the involved vessel and the *histologic pattern* of the accompanying inflammation, encompasses most of the patients with vasculitic syndromes. However, exceptional cases will be found, especially individuals who have evidence of both large and small vessel involvement (categories 1 and 4).[4, 5] Such exceptions do not invalidate the classification. Although clinical and experimental evidence indicates that immune complex deposition can produce small and large vessel vasculitis, we still do not understand the nature of the physical and chemical properties of complexes that determine sites of localization.

PERIARTERITIS NODOSA

In 1866, Kussmaul and Maier reported the prototype case, which involved a young man who had fever, pallor, weakness, muscle pain, abdominal colic, paresthesias, tachycardia, hematuria, and albuminuria and who died within a few months.[6]

Muscular arteries the size of the hepatic and coronary vessels are primarily affected in this disease, but occasionally the small muscular arteries in the subcutaneous tissue are involved as well. The necrotizing process usually begins in a sector of the vessel wall and frequently extends to involve the entire circumference. However, occurrences of the inflammation and necrosis are spotty and affect only small segments of the arteries. The sites of predilection are the branching points of the arteries. Veins are involved only when adjacent arteries are severely affected. Arterioles are involved very rarely.

All the elements of the vascular wall — intima, media, and adventitia — are eventually involved in the necrotizing inflammation, which is composed of neutrophils, eosinophils, and lymphocytes. Thrombosis is an eventual accompaniment to the severe mural inflammation. The acute inflammatory reaction is followed by the generation of granulation tissue and, eventually, by fibrosis. In periarteritis nodosa, both acute and healing vascular lesions are found in biopsy and autopsy material. This finding is essential to the diagnosis.

The severe destruction of the vessel wall leads to aneurysmal dilatation that can be seen macroscopically at autopsy as nodules at the bifurcation points of affected vessels or by angiography of visceral organs that are not readily amenable to biopsy during life. The use of angiography to demonstrate aneurysms in patients with systemic vasculitis is becoming an important diagnostic procedure. The aneurysms can also be detected as subcutaneous nodules during a physical examination of the skin. If the aneurysms are not filled with thrombi, the swellings may pulsate. Nodules may be present in large numbers, and they follow the course of the artery. These nodes are responsible in part for the name of the disease, which actually should be called "panarteritis" because all three layers of the arterial wall are affected. "Panarteritis" is preferable to "polyarteritis" as the correct term for this disorder because the latter means "involvement of many vessels" without conveying any sense of the nature of the vascular pathology. However, "periarteritis" has been used for such a long time that it is unlikely that it will be replaced by a more accurate term.

Because the mural involvement is spotty, a random biopsy of deep vessels may miss the diagnostic histopathology. Even when a characteristic cutaneous lesion is sampled, the tissue specimen may have to be sectioned serially in order to find acute and healing lesions. In necrotizing vasculitis affecting venules and capillaries (leukocytoclastic angiitis), only acute necrotic lesions without evidence of healing or thrombosis are found.

In periarteritis nodosa, the arteries tend to be affected at their branching points, near their mesenteric attachments to the bowel, and in the hila of viscera. The tissues most frequently involved are the myocardium, mesenteric vessels, kidneys, muscles, and the vasa vasorum of peripheral nerves. The pulmonary arteries are spared, but the bronchial arteries can be affected.

The arterial involvement in periarteritis nodosa produces, by means of ischemia, the following signs and symptoms of this illness: glomerulosclerosis, rather than necrotizing glomerulitis, as the cause of renal failure; hypertension; myocardial infarction; muscle pain; intestinal infarction with bleeding and pain; and peripheral neuropathy. Arthralgias and rheumatoid-like arthritis are characteristic features of the disease. Involvement of the central nervous system can produce organic brain syndrome, confusion, and delirium, but it is a minor feature of the illness. The lungs are spared in the classic form of the disease. Periarteritis develops in both adults and children and runs an identical course in both age groups.[7, 8]

In many articles and books, asthma and other pulmonary abnormalities accompanied by eosinophilia are cited as features of periarteritis nodosa. However, such cases represent instances of leukocytoclastic angiitis (*microscopic* periarteritis nodosa), allergic granulomatosis, or Wegener's granulomatosis. For instance, Rose and Spencer reviewed over 100 cases of periarteritis nodosa and were able to divide them into two groups: those with pulmonary disease and those without pulmonary disease.[9] Many of the case histories of patients with lung involvement were typical of allergic granulomatosis and Wegener's granulomatosis, although they were not then recognized as such by the authors.

Rose and Spencer[9] and Knowles et al.[2] pointed out that at least 85 per cent of individuals with periarteritis nodosa do not survive for more than 6 to 12 months, although exceptional patients have survived for 8 to 11 years, and some individuals have entered a spontaneous remission after 3 months to 7 years. More recently, Sack et al. reviewed the clinical courses of 40 patients with periarteritis nodosa.[10] Of those who succumbed to the disease, 78 per cent did so in the first three months after diagnosis. However, the five-year survival was 57 per cent. Frohnert and Sheps had reported 48 per cent five-year survivals in 1967.[11] This improvement in survival is most likely related to the more vigorous steroid therapy employed in the past two decades. Sack et al. noted in their series that peripheral neuropathy, muscle involvement, and older age at onset of disease were bad prognostic signs. However, myocardial disease, central nervous system involvement, and hypertension were not invariably bad signs. Australia antigen (hepatitis B viral antigen) was found in only 6 per cent of their patients, although it has been reported to be as high as 37 to 55 per cent in other series.[12, 13] They also found that renal arteriograms for detection of small renal artery aneurysms and biopsies of muscle or testis, whether or not there was clinical involvement in those sites, were useful diagnostic procedures.

In Rose and Spencer's series, renal failure was responsible for deaths in 65 per cent of the patients, myocardial infarction in 15 per cent, and gastrointestinal tract or nervous system involvement in the remaining patients. Hypertension develops during renal insufficiency, but it does not seem to be the cause of the arteritis in the renal vessels. The causes of death were the same in the series of Sack et al.[10]

Cutaneous manifestations are said to occur in 20 to 25 per cent of patients with periarteritis.[14, 15] All types of lesions — ranging from purpura, bullae, and livedo reticularis to ulcerated nodules, urticaria, and maculopapular eruptions — have been described, but many of these reports were actually cases of leukocytoclastic angiitis that were mistakenly diagnosed as periarteritis nodosa.

The only valid cutaneous signs of periarteritis nodosa seem to be the following: subcutaneous nodules that are no larger than 5 to 10 mm and that follow the course of the arteries, ulceration resulting from infarction, peripheral gangrene of fingers and toes, and ecchymoses resulting from the rupture of aneurysms and weakened walls of necrotic arteries. Tender red subcutaneous nodules in a linear distribution were present on the soles, calves, or tibial surfaces in one series of children with periarteritis.[7] Although livedo reticularis can be a major manifestation of periarteritis nodosa,[7, 16] most reports of this eruption in association with alleged cases of periarteritis have actually been examples of leukocytoclastic angiitis, as can be verified by examining the photomicrographs or written descriptions of the histopathology.[17-21]

Classic periarteritis involving only the skin is a rare occurrence. In the past, periarteritis nodosa was considered to be a single disease of unknown etiology. It has become evident that there are several etiologies for this disorder and it would be more appropriate to speak of the "syndrome of periarteritis nodosa secondary to a specific etiology," where that is known. Periarteritis nodosa can be associated with chronic hepatitis B antigenemia,[12, 13] abuse of the drug methamphetamine,[22] and rheumatoid arthritis.[23] It has developed as a late sequela of mixed cryoglobulinemia,[24] and following beta-streptococcal infections.[8] The pathogenesis of this syndrome involves the deposition of immune complexes within the vessel wall and will be discussed in relation to the other angiitides later in this chapter.

In the past decade, vasculitic syndromes have been described in which the pathologic findings resemble those of periarteritis but lack some important features. In one type, the histologic changes are those of an *acute* necrotizing inflammation, often with thrombosis, of muscular arteries similar in size to those affected in periarteritis. However, healing or scarring lesions are not present in the vessels. Some authors have considered these histologic findings to be part of the spectrum of periarteritis because of the size and type of involved vessel; others have felt that the pathologic picture represents a histologic point on a continuous spectrum, and that the classification of the vasculitides may be too inflexible to apply to all clinical situations. In support of this latter viewpoint, one can cite the pathologic findings in patients with chronic hepatitis B antigenemia whose vasculitic syndromes are clinically similar but whose vascular lesions range histologically from classic periarteritis through *acute* necrotizing inflammation in muscular arteries to leukocytoclastic angiitis involving dermal venules.[25] These *acute* lesions have been found in vasculitic syndromes following beta-streptococcal infections in both children and adults.[26, 27] Sergent and Christian reported seven cases following serous otitis media by two weeks to ten months.[28]

Diaz-Perez and Winkelmann found these *acute* necrotizing lesions in 31 children and adults.[27] The arteritis was confined to the subcutis and adjacent dermis and was interpreted as being diagnostic of periarteritis nodosa. Diaz-Perez and Winkelmann designated this syndrome, which appears to have a benign but relapsing course, as the cutaneous form of periarteritis nodosa. The cutaneous lesions consisted of patches of livedo reticularis and erythematous nodules, which were most commonly found on the lower extremities but also involved other areas such as the head, neck, buttocks, and scapulae. In almost all of their patients, subcutaneous red tender nodules, 0.5 to 2 cm in size, appeared first and became dusky as they healed. Nodules tended to be grouped and appear in crops and only rarely followed the course of arteries. Pain was the most characteristic symptom. Livedo reticularis developed around the nodules later, producing a characteristic picture of patchy livedo reticularis with nodule formation. The patches of livedo were likened to the "star-bursts" of exploding sky rockets. With subsequent exacerbations of the disease, new nodules would develop in the areas of livedo.

Ulcerations were common. They tended to have irregular borders and were surrounded by a halo of livedo reticularis. They did not arise from the nodules, but from areas of skin that had previously developed hemorrhage and necrosis as a consequence of ischemia produced by the underlying vasculitis.

None of these patients had evidence of systemic involvement with periarteritis, but they did have prolonged, relapsing courses that could be controlled and put into remission for varying periods of time with moderate doses of oral corticosteroids. Exacerbations were accompanied by arthralgias and myalgias in many patients and by fever in a few. In some patients arthralgias were associated with periarticular erythema and edema, but joint involvement was never demonstrated. The involved extremities became painful during these flares.

In three patients, pharyngitis or an upper respiratory infection preceded the initial episode and the subsequent flares. The disease was controlled by sulfonamides and by penicillin in four patients, again suggesting that bacterial infections, probably beta-streptococcal, are important initiating factors in some cases of periarteritis. Tests for rheumatoid factor, antinuclear antibody, cryoglobulins, VDRL, and serum complement levels were normal in these individuals. None of the five patients tested had evidence of hepatitis B antigenemia.

This distinctive syndrome of cutaneous periarteritis nodosa has also been observed in association with regional enteritis. Nine persons have been reported with this combination.[28a–28c] In some the activities of the bowel disorder and the vasculitis paralleled each other, while in others they did not.

Figure 8–1 demonstrates the patchy livedo in a 16-year-old girl with this syndrome. Her disease was kept under control with 5 mg of prednisone per day for two years. Following discontinuation of the prednisone, she has continued to remain in complete remission for the past two years.

It is important to emphasize that the livedo reticularis in this syndrome appears after the nodules have developed and evolved and is present only in the areas where the nodules are. The common variety of livedo reticularis has a more extensive distribution and precedes nodule or ulcer formation when it is associated with leukocytoclastic angiitis, systemic LE, and classic periarteritis nodosa (see p. 437).

The identical arteritic lesion can also be found in Cogan's syndrome, which is characterized by the combination of a nonsyphilitic interstitial keratitis with bilateral hearing loss and vertigo.[29] Approximately 72 per cent of the patients have had one or more of the following: gastrointestinal bleeding, generalized lymphadenopathy, hypertension, myositis, arthralgias, arthritis, splenomegaly, and eosinophilia. In 10 per cent, acute fulminant aortic insufficiency has developed. Of 53 patients with this

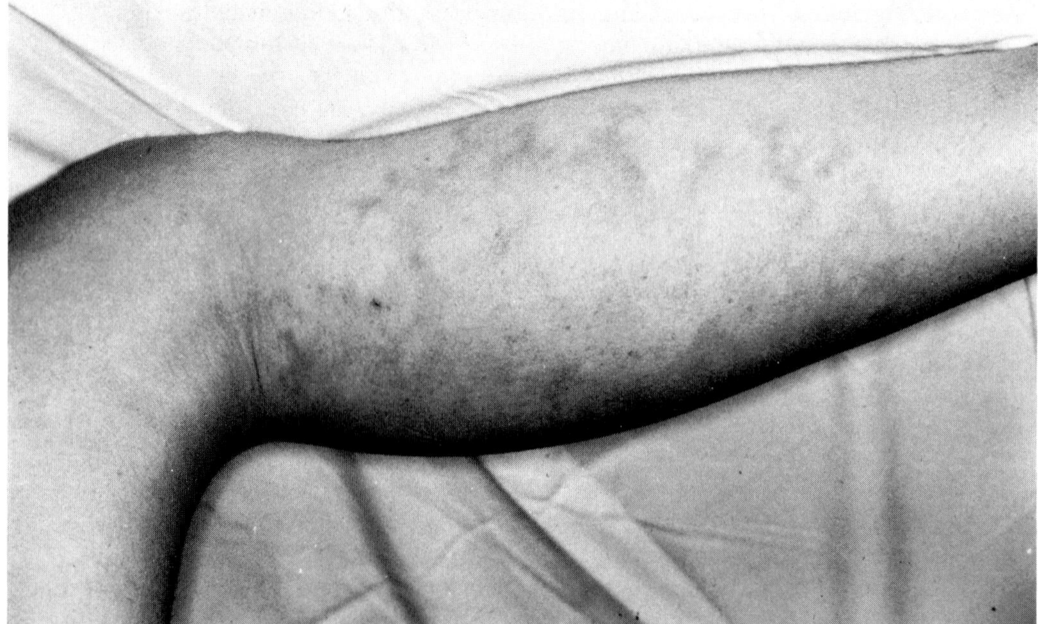

Figure 8–1. Cutaneous periarteritis nodosa of calf. Patchy livedo reticularis (star-burst pattern) on posterior and lateral leg.

syndrome, 18 have had biopsies of various tissues. Ten of the 18 have had necrotizing vasculitis that was diagnosed as classic periarteritis nodosa, small vessel vasculitis (leukocytoclastic), or an *acute* necrotizing arteritis as described above. Cogan's syndrome may be part of a more generalized disease in which the heart and blood vessels are primarily involved.

Mucocutaneous lymph node syndrome (Kawasaki's disease) is an acute febrile illness characterized by distinctive oral and cutaneous lesions and cervical lymphadenopathy that develops primarily in children under two years of age (see p. 865). Approximately 1 to 2 per cent of children have died suddenly in the third or fourth week of the illness from myocardial arrhythmias or infarction produced by an arteritis of the coronary arteries. Other major arteries — bronchial, brachial, iliac, splenic, pancreatic, hepatic, mesenteric, and paratracheal — have shown identical changes. It is now agreed that Kawasaki's disease is identical to *infantile* periarteritis nodosa. The pathology in the blood vessels closely resembles that of *classic* periarteritis nodosa, but there are some differences: the pathologic process appears to begin in the vasa vasorum and involve the major vessels secondarily; fibrinoid deposition is not found in the major vessels, perhaps for that reason; and the vessels affected are usually extraparenchymal.[30-32]

Until more is known about the etiologies of the vasculitic syndromes, my own bias is to group disorders by pathologic findings held in common and size of affected vessel. Presumably there are some common pathogenetic factors underlying the above syndromes that are responsible for initiating necrotizing inflammation in muscular arteries.

ALLERGIC GRANULOMATOSIS

Allergic granulomatosis, sometimes called allergic angiitis and granulomatosis, was described by Churg and Strauss in 1951.[33] Their report was based on 13 patients, most of whom were studied at necropsy. Since then, several patients have been diagnosed ante mortem.[34-36]

This illness resembles periarteritis nodosa in that identical-sized muscular arteries are affected; also, similar organs are involved: heart, spleen, kidney, gut, pancreas, gallbladder, and liver. But here the similarity ends.

Pulmonary involvement in the form of asthma is the striking initial manifestation of allergic granulomatosis. The asthmatic phase is accompanied by hypereosinophilia and fever and can persist for a few months to 10 years before diffuse angiitis with multiple organ involvement develops. Characteristically the asthma spontaneously remits or abates before the angiitic phase. Three years was the average duration of the asthmatic phase in Churg and Strauss' cases.

The histopathology is different from that of periarteritis nodosa. When healing occurs in allergic granulomatosis, granulomas develop in the vessel wall and extravascularly. The lesions are characterized by large numbers of eosinophils, giant cells, and plasma cells. The muscular vessels in the fat and at the junction between the dermis and the subcutis are affected. Occasionally the arterioles in the dermis may be similarly affected; consequently, in some patients a skin biopsy can establish the diagnosis.

In the majority of the cases reported by Churg and Strauss, the vessels in the skin and the subcutaneous fat were involved. The cutaneous lesions consisted of deep nodules, purpura, and erythematous "macular and papular eruptions." Pustules were also reported.

In the arteritic phase, arthralgias, peripheral neuropathy, convulsions, coma, and pericarditis with effusion occurred. Almost every affected patient has had abdominal pain, bloody diarrhea, hypertension, and mild hematuria and albuminuria. The most frequent cause of death was congestive heart failure secondary to myocardial damage from the arteritis. In the series of Churg and Strauss, the duration of the arteritic phase ranged from 3 to 60 months; the average was 20 months. Oral corticosteroids, with or without azathioprine, have produced remissions in several cases.[34-36]

Although the etiology of allergic granulomatosis is not known and its nosologic niche is not agreed upon, for the present it deserves to be classified as a separate entity among the angiitides.

WEGENER'S GRANULOMATOSIS

In 1936 and 1939, on the basis of three cases Wegener delineated the syndrome that bears his name. In 1954 Godman and Churg reviewed the problem and added seven cases of their own.[37] Their criteria for the anatomic diagnosis of this illness are currently used.

Wegener's granulomatosis is accompanied by fever, malaise, and weight loss. It is characterized by the triad of necrotizing granulomas in the upper and lower respiratory tract; necrotizing angiitis that affects medium-sized arteries and veins, arterioles, venules, and probably capillaries in the lungs and other organs; and focal necrotizing glomerulitis that sometimes develops into a granulomatous glomerulonephritis. Renal failure is the most frequent cause of death in this illness. Arthralgias with morning stiffness is a complaint of some patients. The histopathologic features of the angiitis resemble both classic periarteritis nodosa with acute and healed lesions and leukocytoclastic angiitis.

The granulomas develop independently of the angiitis and are composed of a necrotic center surrounded by granulation tissue infiltrated with plasma cells, lymphocytes, and giant cells. Neutrophils and histiocytes are present in small numbers. Eosinophils and epithelioid cells are almost never present, a feature that distinguishes these granulomas from those found in allergic granulomatosis. An infectious etiology for this syndrome has not been demonstrated.

The granulomas arise primarily within the respiratory tract, but they may be found occasionally in other viscera such as the spleen, liver, lymph nodes, kidney, prostate, and epididymis. The granulomas frequently develop in the nose, thereby causing obstruction, and within the sinuses in association with purulent sinusitis. Involvement of the trachea, bronchi, and larynx, including the vocal cords, is not unusual; frequently the granulomas produce enormous ulcerated mucosal lesions at these sites. When the pulmonary parenchyma is involved, the granulomas grossly may simulate primary and metastatic lung cancer, pale infarcts, and abscesses. The granulomas may have diameters as large as 6 or 7 cm. These respiratory lesions often produce symptoms of cough, dyspnea, and chest pain, thus bringing the patient to the attention of a physician. However, sometimes the pulmonary involvement is asymptomatic and discovered only on a screening chest film.

Mucocutaneous involvement is a prominent feature of Wegener's granulomatosis and occurs in at least half of the patients.[38] The nasal granulomas may appear as crusting, bleeding, nonhealing sores at the nostrils or on the septum (Fig. 8–2). One of our patients developed a flesh-colored nodule at the nostril whenever the disease became active (Fig. 8–3). The nodule never ulcerated and always disappeared without leaving a scar when the disease remitted after appropriate therapy. Granulomas can arise in the middle ear and produce purulent drainage in the ear canal. Other types of mucosal involvement that have been reported include extensive gingivitis with necrosis of the alveolar ridge (Fig. 8–4), palatal ulcers with perforation, and ulceration of the tongue.

Skin lesions occur in 30 to 50 per cent of cases.[38-40] They are often present initially or develop early in the course of the disease, whose general activity they may parallel. Two basic types of lesions are found: (1) Petechiae, purpura, or ecchymoses, sometimes in association with ulcerations or blisters. Although they are present chiefly on the legs, they may also be found on the trunk, face, and upper limbs. Histologic examination shows necrotizing vasculitis affecting the medium-sized vessels in the dermis and fat. (2) Papules and nodules, 1 to 5 cm in diameter, may appear on the extremities, elbows, forearms, trunk, neck, and upper chest. They may be tender. Histologically, one usually finds a granulomatous vasculitis involving the dermis and subcutaneous fat. Fauci et al. described one patient with necrotizing papules on the finger

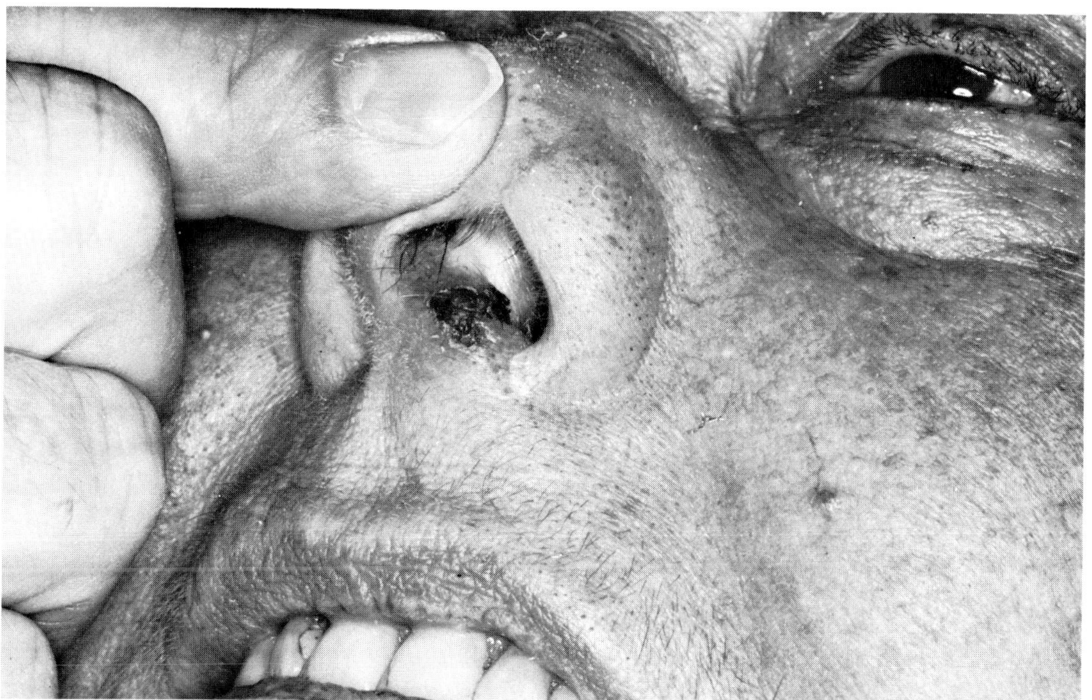

Figure 8–2. Wegener's granulomatosis. Characteristic septal ulceration.

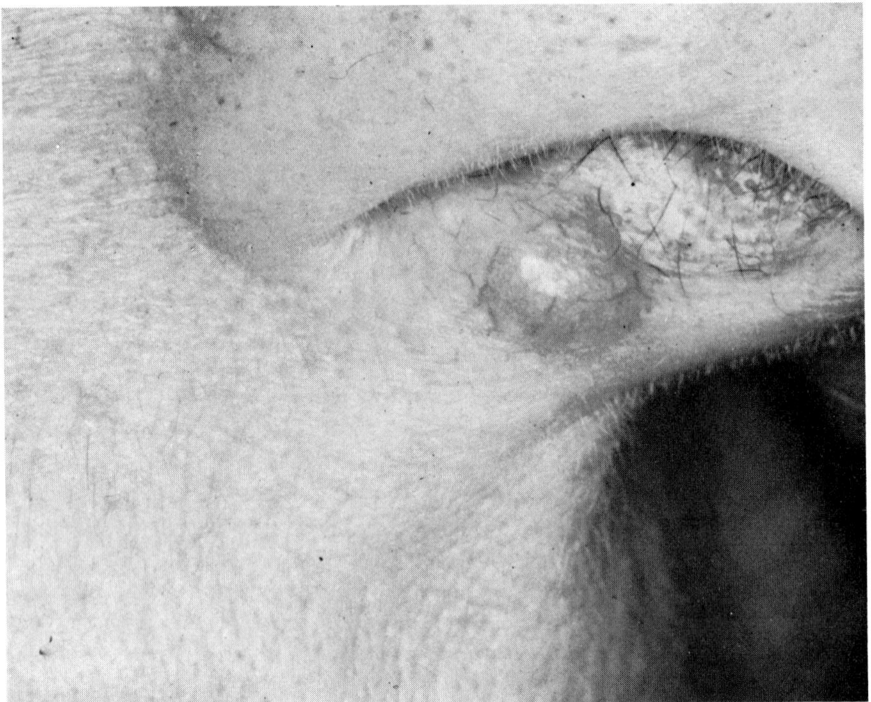

Figure 8–3. Wegener's granulomatosis. With almost every exacerbation of the disease, this patient developed a nodule at the nostril. The lesion did not ulcerate and always disappeared when the illness was brought under control by corticosteroids or ACTH.

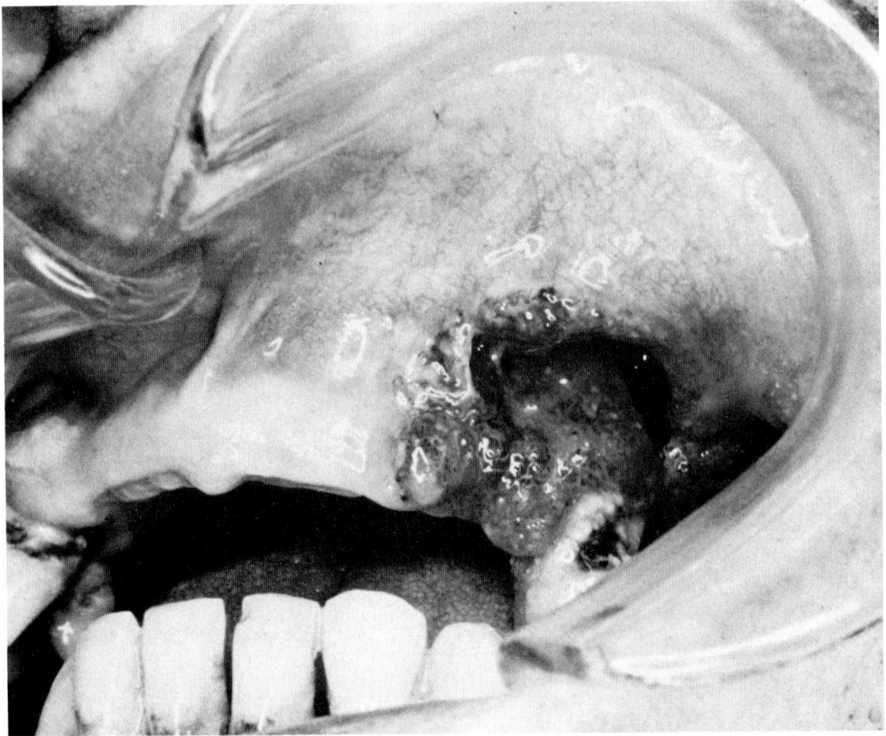

Figure 8–4. Wegener's granulomatosis involving the alveolar ridge. (Courtesy of Dr. Hubert Merchant.)

tips and another with subcutaneous nodules in whom biopsies showed granulomas without obvious vasculitis.[39] Kraus reported similar findings in a patient who developed papulopustules and necrotic papules over the fingers and elbows and in a scar from a previous muscle biopsy.[41] Ulcerations secondary to vasculitis may develop in the absence of purpura or nodules. Livedo reticularis or cutaneous nodules following the course of blood vessels have not been reported in association with Wegener's syndrome.

The eyes are affected in 40 to 50 per cent of individuals with Wegener's disease: conjunctivitis, episcleritis, corneoscleral ulceration, uveitis, retinal artery thrombosis, proptosis, and pseudotumor of the orbit. These abnormalities result from focal vasculitis involving the anterior ciliary and retinal vessels and those in the ocular muscles; from granuloma formation in the cornea and ciliary bodies; and from inflammatory changes spreading from granulomatous inflammation occurring within the contiguous paranasal sinuses.[42]

Over 200 cases of Wegener's granulomatosis have been recorded in the literature.[39] Men are affected almost 1.5 times as often as women. Although most cases appear in the fourth and fifth decades, the disease has been diagnosed in a 3-month-old infant and in a 75-year-old man. The illness is invariably fatal, if untreated, and 80 per cent of patients have survived for only 5 to 12 months. Only 10 per cent have lived for longer than two years.[39] However, in many cases, long-term remissions and even cures have been achieved following treatment with cyclophosphamide.[39, 43]

Carrington and Liebow collected and studied 16 cases of Wegener's granulomatosis in which the pathology was confined primarily to the lungs.[44] Extrapulmonary lesions did occur in seven of these patients, but significant renal disease was present in none. Five of eight patients were still alive after two years, and (at the time of the report) three patients were still living after four to fifteen months. Six had died of pulmonary involvement or complications of therapy with corticosteroids, and two had died of causes unrelated to Wegener's syndrome. The histologic features in these 16 cases were identical to those found in the complete syndrome. Limited forms of the disease do occur, and these appear to have a better prognosis than the classic disorder.

One of the women included in Carrington and Liebow's series (Case 3) first came under our care in 1962.

The illness began at the age of 55 with the development of tender red nodules on the legs in association with fever and malaise (Plate 23*C*). One year later she sought medical attention at the Yale-New Haven Dermatology Clinic. A clinical diagnosis of panniculitis of the Weber-Christian type was made, and a biopsy seemed to confirm this impression. A routine chest film revealed a coin lesion that was believed to be a lung cancer. An exploratory thoracotomy revealed multiple nodules of Wegener's granulomatosis; and a review of the skin biopsy discovered a necrotizing arteritis in the fat, which was the underlying cause of the panniculitis. The patient's main problem then became one of recurrent deep ulcers over the ankles; these ulcers were always preceded by tenderness and the livid color of ischemia (Fig. 8–5). ACTH, corticosteroids, and methotrexate have been used successfully at different times for treatment of her disease. Renal involvement never developed. In 1969, she began treatment with weekly doses of 50 mg methotrexate given I.M. and promptly entered a remission. Over the next four

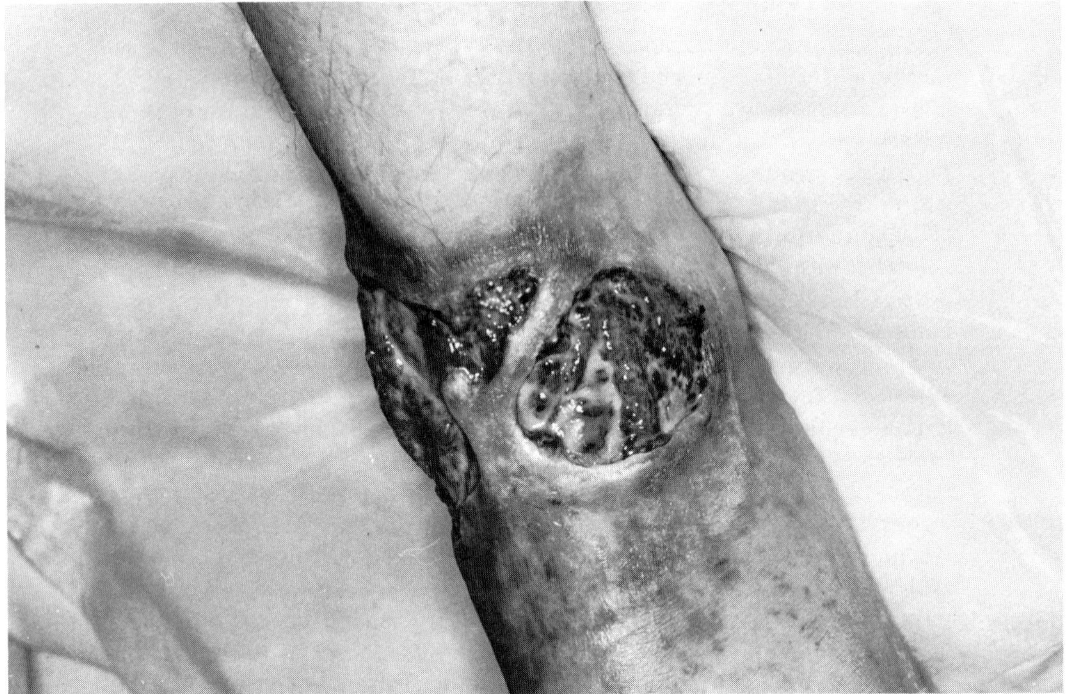

Figure 8–5. Wegener's granulomatosis. Angiitis in this illness produced the extensive ulceration about the ankle.

years, her disease remained suppressed by weekly oral doses (15 to 25 mg). Methotrexate was discontinued in 1973 because of the development of cirrhosis believed to be caused by the antimetabolite. Her disease flared, and the methotrexate was cautiously reinstituted after a course of oral cyclophosphamide had proved ineffective. Her disease responded again to methotrexate and she remained in remission from 1974 to 1975. She died in September, 1975, from cryptococcal meningitis. At autopsy the only evidence of active disease was the presence of granulomatous vasculitis in a few small cutaneous nodules.

Wegener's granulomatosis seems to be sufficiently distinct from periarteritis nodosa and allergic granulomatosis to be classified as a separate entity among the angiitides. However, there are three case reports of patients who appear to have had an illness combining the features of Wegener's granulomatosis and allergic granulomatosis.

Lethal midline granuloma is a clinical term to describe those entities that can produce progressive destructive ulcerations of the central part of the face. The initial lesions arise in the nose, sinuses, palate, or pharynx. There is general agreement that epithelial tumors, conventional malignant lymphomas, and syphilis can produce this noma-like destruction. However, three disorders are more commonly found. The first is polymorphic reticulosis or midline malignant reticulosis, a malignant lymphoma displaying a pleomorphic and polymorphous histologic pattern.[45] Malignant-appearing "reticulum" cells and lymphocytes are enmeshed in an intense mixed infiltrate of normal inflammatory cells that sometimes can obscure the tumor cells. For this reason multiple and repeated biopsies are often required to establish the correct pathologic diagnoses. The second entity, idiopathic midline granuloma, is characterized histologically by a non-neoplastic granulomatous tissue reaction without evidence of arteritis.[38, 46] Both disorders respond to local x-ray therapy but not to chemotherapy.[47] In view of the difficulties encountered at times in finding tumor cells in midline malignant reticulosis, because of the accompanying normal inflammation and tissue necrosis, it is possible that idiopathic midline granuloma is actually identical to midline malignant reticulosis. The third entity is Wegener's granulomatosis. A major controversy exists as to whether localized Wegener's disease is a rare cause[39, 48] or a usual cause[49-51] of lethal midline granuloma. The choice of treatment becomes critical because Wegener's granulomatosis responds to chemotherapy, while midline malignant reticulosis and idiopathic midline granuloma respond only to local x-irradiation.[47, 48]

In 1972, Liebow, Carrington, and Friedman described a new entity, lymphomatoid granulomatosis, which bore a striking resemblance to Wegener's granulomatosis.[49] The disease was twice as frequent in men as in women. The average age of onset was 30 to 60 years, but it ranged from eight and one-half years to the seventies. Although the lungs were primarily involved in this entity, the skin, kidney, liver, and nervous system, both central and peripheral, were often affected as well. The lymph nodes, spleen, and bone marrow were usually spared. Patients frequently consulted their physicians because of varying combinations of fever, cough, and dyspnea. Chest x-rays rev aled nodular lesions peripherally in both lower lung fields. The nodules tended to be more numerous, smaller, and less well defined than those seen in Wegener's disease. The nodules also tended to wax and wane. Small pleural effusions and cavitation were common. Histologically, one saw massive proliferation of lymphoreticular cells — some plasmacytoid and many exhibiting marked atypia — within and surrounding blood vessel walls. Within the lung parenchyma, this massive proliferation was associated with necrosis. The angiitis and granulomatous inflammation seen in Wegener's disease were reproduced in lymphomatoid granulomatosis, but the normal inflammatory cells were replaced by malignant-appearing cells of the lymphoreticular system. Ultrastructural studies have shown that the abnormal cells do not resemble those of mycosis fungoides, histiocytic lymphoma, histiocytosis X, or leukemic reticuloendotheliosis, thereby further strengthening this disorder as a distinct clinicopathologic entity.[52]

Although lymphomatoid granulomatosis was not considered to be a frank malignant lymphoma, the prognosis was poor: 40 per cent had died one year later and 65 per cent four years later. In 13 per cent of patients, the disease did progress to involve the lymph nodes and other reticuloendothelial tissues and behaved as a lymphoma. However, most patients died from pulmonary hemorrhage secondary to cavitation or from other consequences of lung and central nervous system involvement. The histologic changes found in the lung also occurred in the skin and other affected organs.

The skin was involved in 45 per cent of patients and was often the first sign of the disease. The cutaneous lesions took the form of erythematous macules, papules, plaques, or nodules that sometimes ulcerated. In one of our patients, a 26-year-old white woman, the lesions were 5- to 8-mm red papules that arose suddenly, developed central necrosis, and disappeared, leaving behind a scar with fine wrinkling over the course of approximately two weeks (Figs. 8–6 to 8–9).

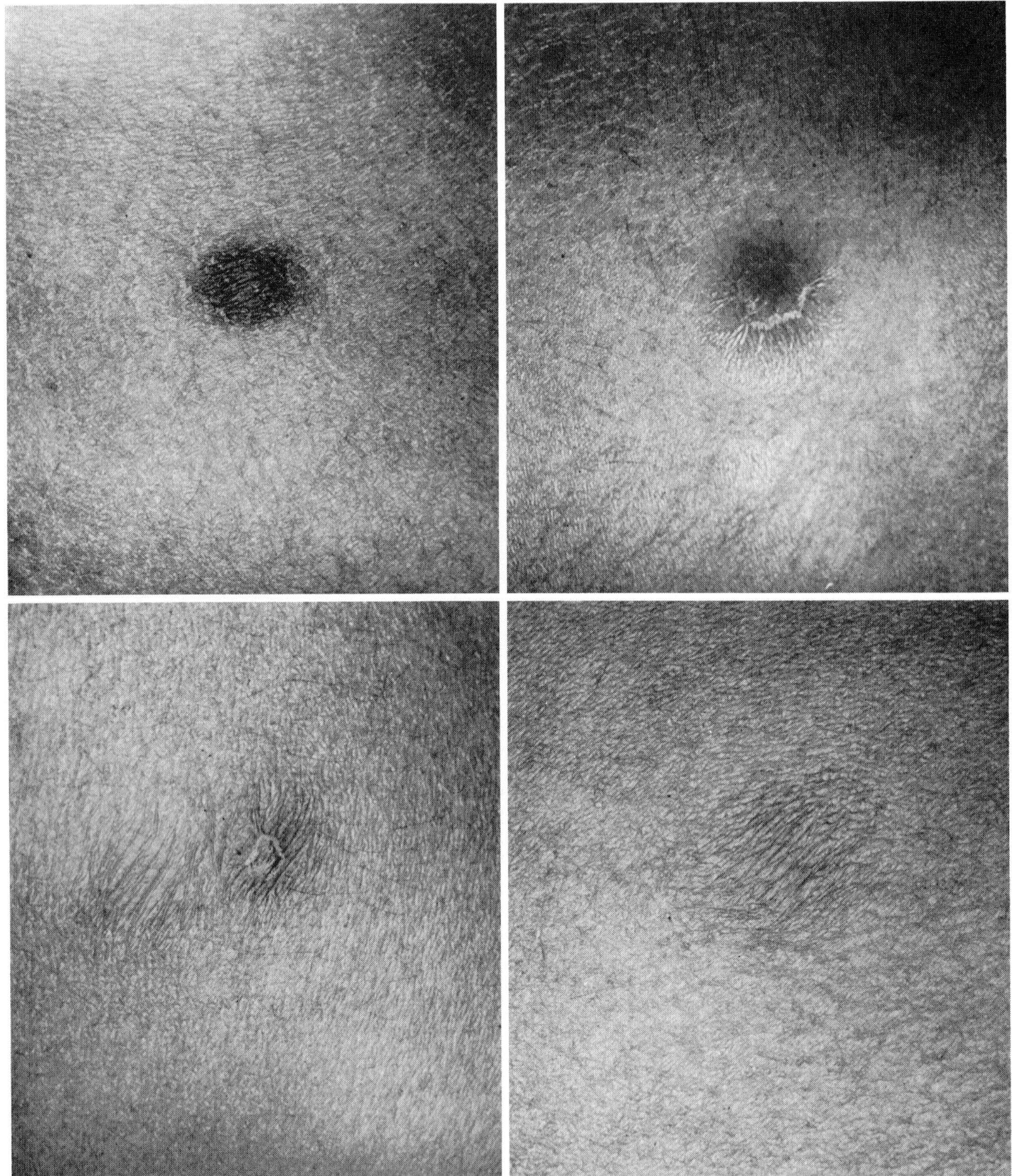

Figure 8–6. Top left. Lymphomatoid granulomatosis. Figs. 8–6 to 8–9 show the evolution of the erythematous papules in this patient. Initial papule.

Figure 8–7. Top right. Papule undergoing necrosis.

Figure 8–8. Bottom left. Necrotic papule healing.

Figure 8–9. Bottom right. Residual scar is characterized by fine wrinkling.

Other features of the disease include arthralgias, peripheral neuritis, ataxia, diplopia, and cranial nerve palsies. Nodules develop in the kidney but glomerulitis does not. In one patient, fever, diplopia, and ataxia were present for six months before the characteristic pulmonary nodules appeared.[53]

It is important to recognize this entity because in its advanced phase it is not responsive to chemotherapy, as Wegener's disease is.

Israel et al. defined another group of patients who showed some histologic features of both Wegener's granulomatosis and lymphomatoid granulomatosis.[50] The disease was limited to the lungs except for one patient who had cutaneous nodules. The lung lesions showed nodular collections of *mature* lymphocytes and plasma cells. Angiitis and necrosis were less pronounced than in Wegener's disease. He designated this entity "benign lymphocytic angiitis and granulomatosis." The disorder may transform after long intervals into lymphomatoid granulomatosis. In the early phase it is responsive to chemotherapy; in the transformed phase, it is not.

LEUKOCYTOCLASTIC ANGIITIS

The most frequently encountered variety of necrotizing vasculitis is leukocytoclastic angiitis (Figs. 8–10 and 8–11). Venules and postcapillary venules in the skin and internal organs are affected by an acute necrotizing inflammatory process that differs in the several following ways from those which occur in periarteritis nodosa: all the vascular lesions are of the same age, and there is no healing phase; vessels within organs, rather than those at the hilum of a viscus, are affected; exudative and hemorrhagic, rather than ischemic, phenomena are responsible for the clinical signs and symptoms; and small, rather than large, vessels are involved. The clinical syndromes associated with periarteritis nodosa, Wegener's granulomatosis, allergic granulomatosis, and temporal arteritis are much more uniform and display a much narrower spectrum of manifestations than do the syndromes associated with leukocytoclastic angiitis.

The multitude of syndromes and names that have been applied to this small vessel disease has certainly not been helpful to a further understanding of its etiology and pathogenesis. The description and reporting of small vessel angiitis have been made primarily by dermatologists, internists, and pathologists. The dermatologists have viewed these cases from the standpoint of the skin manifestations and have described the various syndromes under the following names: arteriolitis allergica (Ruiter), dermatitis nodularis necrotica (Werther), nodular dermal allergid (Gougerot and Duperrat), and the mono-penta-symptom complexes (Gougerot). All of these entities have the same histopathology and cutaneous manifestations.

On the other hand, the internist and pathologist have looked at the problem of small vessel angiitis through its systemic manifestations and the findings at necropsy. In many instances the skin lesions have probably been overlooked; and when they have been observed and described, their significance has not been fully appreciated. The internists and pathologists have described leukocytoclastic angiitis under the following names: allergic angiitis, systemic allergic vasculitis (McCombs),

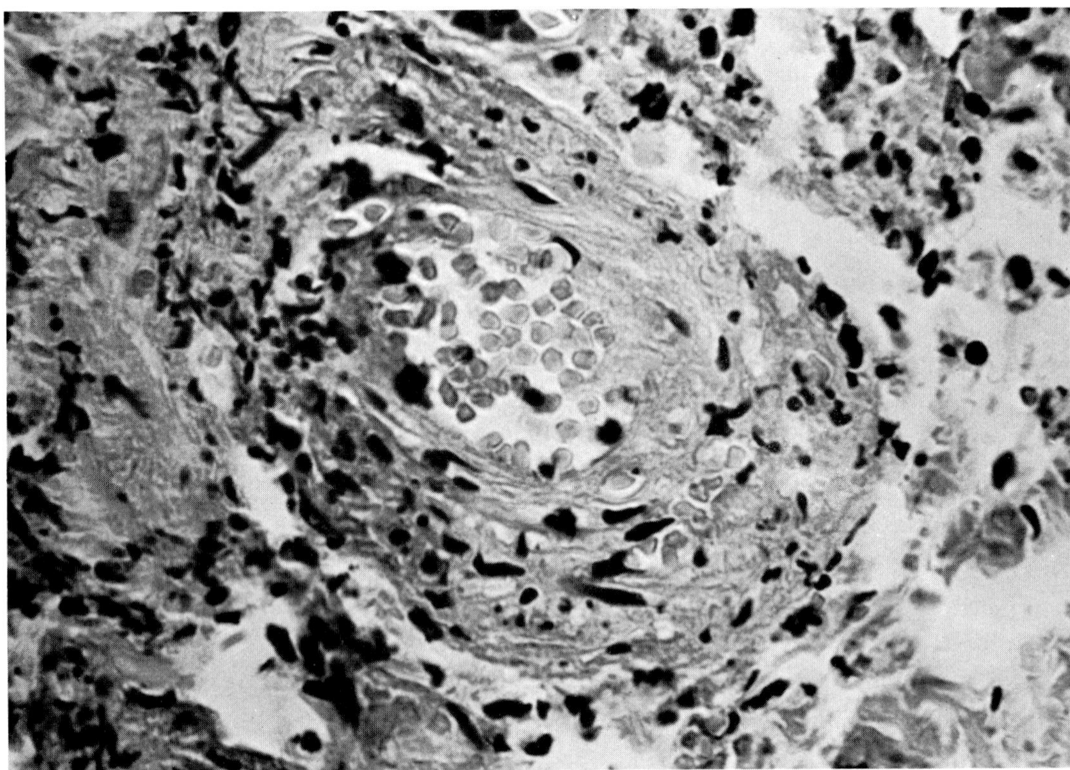

Figure 8–10. Leukocytoclastic angiitis. Fibrinoid necrosis of vascular wall and perivascular tissue. Polymorphonuclear leukocytes comprise most of the cells within the vessel wall and surrounding area. Disintegrating nuclei of the leukocytes produce nuclear dust. Note lack of thrombi. Hematoxylin and eosin. × 400.

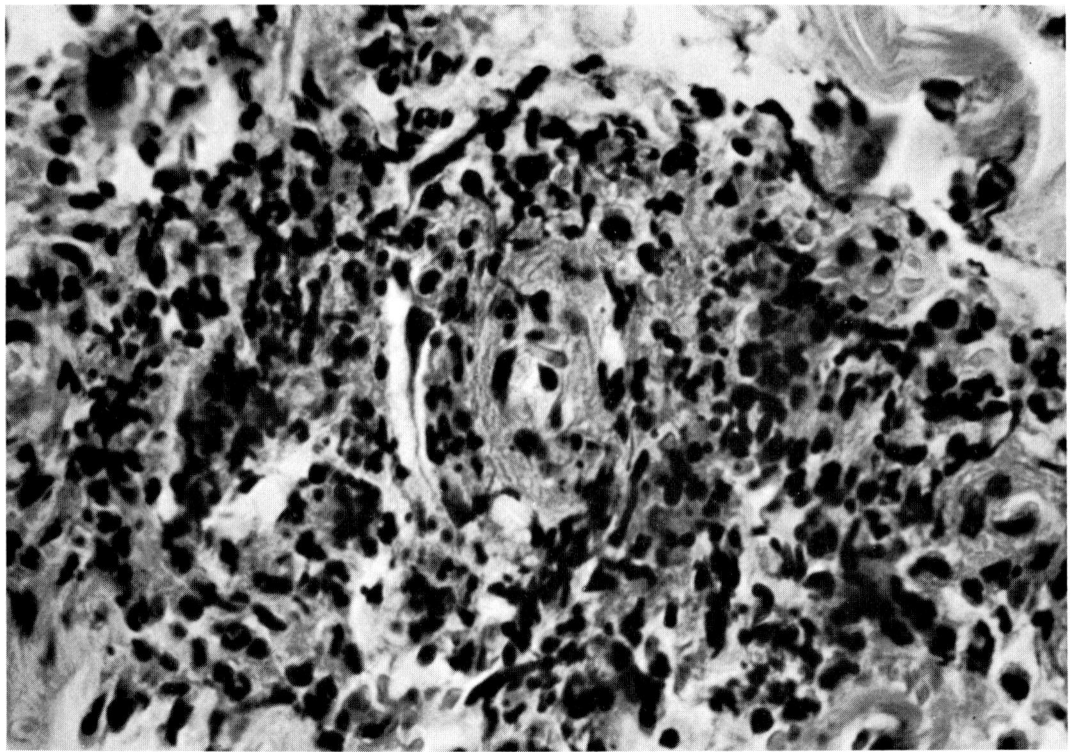

Figure 8–11. Leukocytoclastic angiitis. Histopathology. Hematoxylin and eosin. × 400.

hypersensitivity angiitis (Zeek), anaphylactoid purpura (Schönlein-Henoch purpura), and microscopic periarteritis nodosa. The cutaneous lesions and the histopathology in these systemic disorders are identical to those in the previously enumerated dermatologic disorders.

Leukocytoclastic angiitis produces two major syndromes: Schönlein-Henoch disease, occurring primarily in children and young adults; and cutaneous-systemic angiitis. The cutaneous manifestations of both entities relate to the distribution of the affected vessels. In most cases the postcapillary venules and venules of the upper dermis are involved, and the blood vessels in the mid-dermis, lower dermis, and fat are not affected. However, in a minority of cases of cutaneous-systemic angiitis, similar-sized vessels in the mid-dermis, at the dermal-subcutaneous junction, and within the fat are affected by the same necrotizing process.

Cutaneous Manifestations

The development and appearance of cutaneous lesions in leukocytoclastic angiitis depend upon several factors. Exudation and hemorrhage into the skin are the prominent clinical features. Purpura is almost always present in the cutaneous lesions and is usually accompanied by evidence of increased vascular permeability. Therefore purpura, when present, is almost always *palpable*. Petechiae and purpura associated with thrombocytopenia are *flat*. This is an important differential point. *Flat* purpura is an extremely uncommon manifestation of vasculitis.

The postcapillary venule — the segment of the microcirculation that immediately follows the capillary bed — is the primary site of involvement in leukocytoclastic angiitis. This segment lies in a horizontal plexus in the upper dermis just below the epidermal layer. The blood that diffuses out from these inflamed vessels produces *oval* or *circular* purpuric spots that usually coalesce into larger oval, circular, or polycyclic patches. By contrast, in periarteritis nodosa, necrotizing inflammation with thrombosis affects large arterial vessels in the deep dermis and fat. The combination of inflammation and thromboses with deeply situated vessels produces a hemorrhagic infarction in the overlying dermis, which appears clinically as *irregularly* outlined, indurated, or edematous patches of purpura.

The exudative and inflammatory components in leukocytoclastic angiitis account for the evolution of the cutaneous lesions. Within a few hours of their development, erythematous macules become edematous and assume an urticarial appearance. Shortly thereafter they become grossly purpuric (Figs. 8–12 and 8–13; Plate 23*D*). Only rarely do the erythematous macules and urticarial papules disappear without ever becoming purpuric. In a few patients, these urticarial lesions have persisted for 24 to 72 hours before disappearing and have been diagnosed as chronic urticaria (Fig. 8–14).[54] Sometimes, instead of becoming uniformly purpuric, the red macule or papule develops a spot of purpura in its center and a ring of stippled petechiae on its periphery (Fig. 8–15).

If the inflammatory component is very severe, an inordinate amount of edema forms in the upper dermis and causes the epidermis to rise and form a hemorrhagic blister (Fig. 8–16; Plate 23*E*). The blisters may break and leave denuded areas. Thrombosis may develop because of the

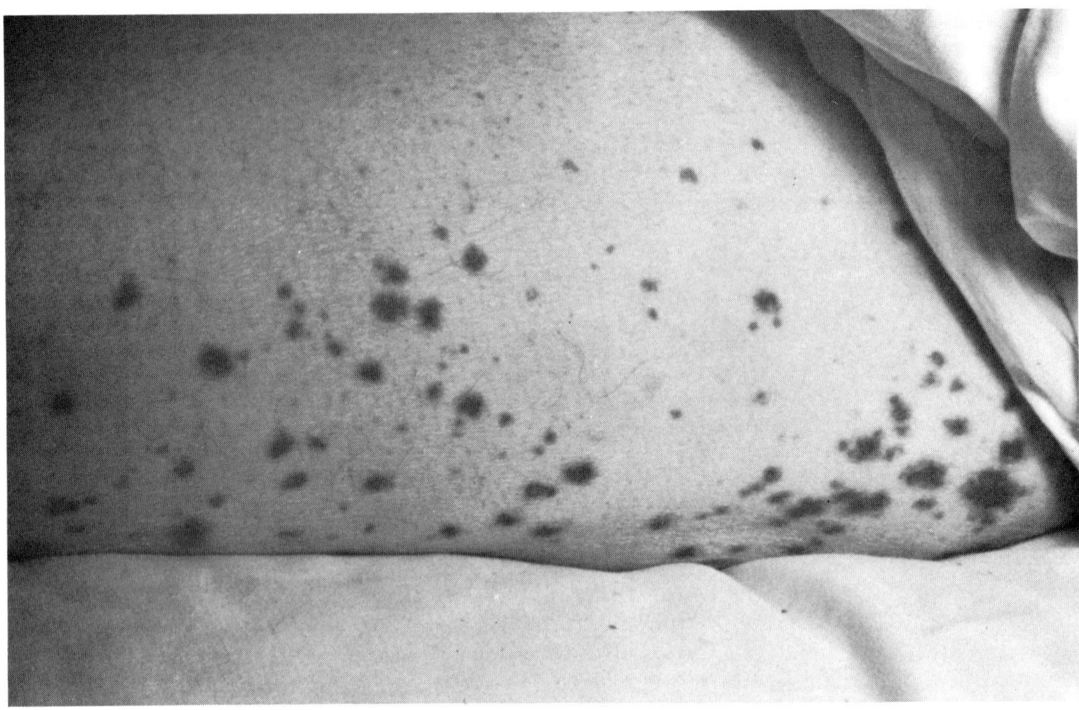

Figure 8–12. Leukocytoclastic angiitis. Macules have become urticarial and hemorrhagic.

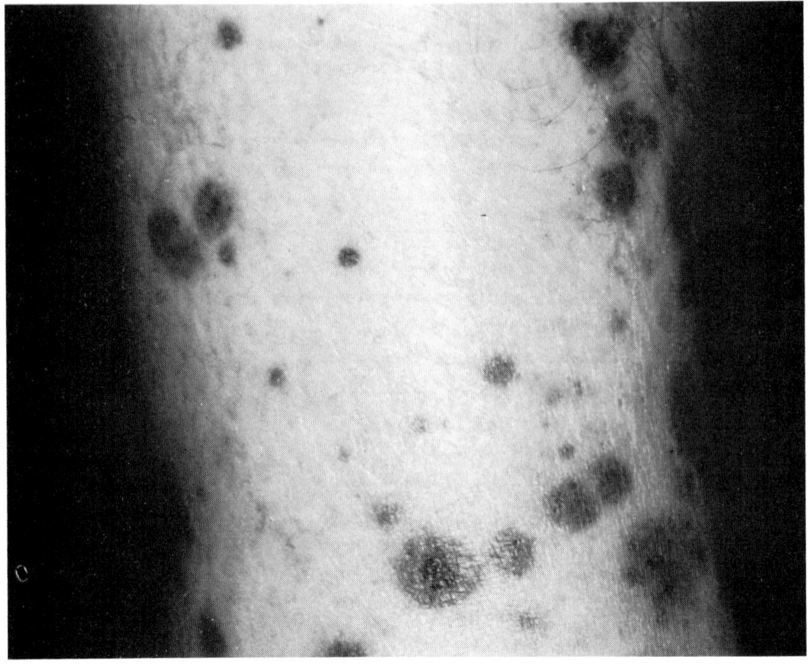

Figure 8–13. Leukocytoclastic angiitis. Purpuric edematous lesions.

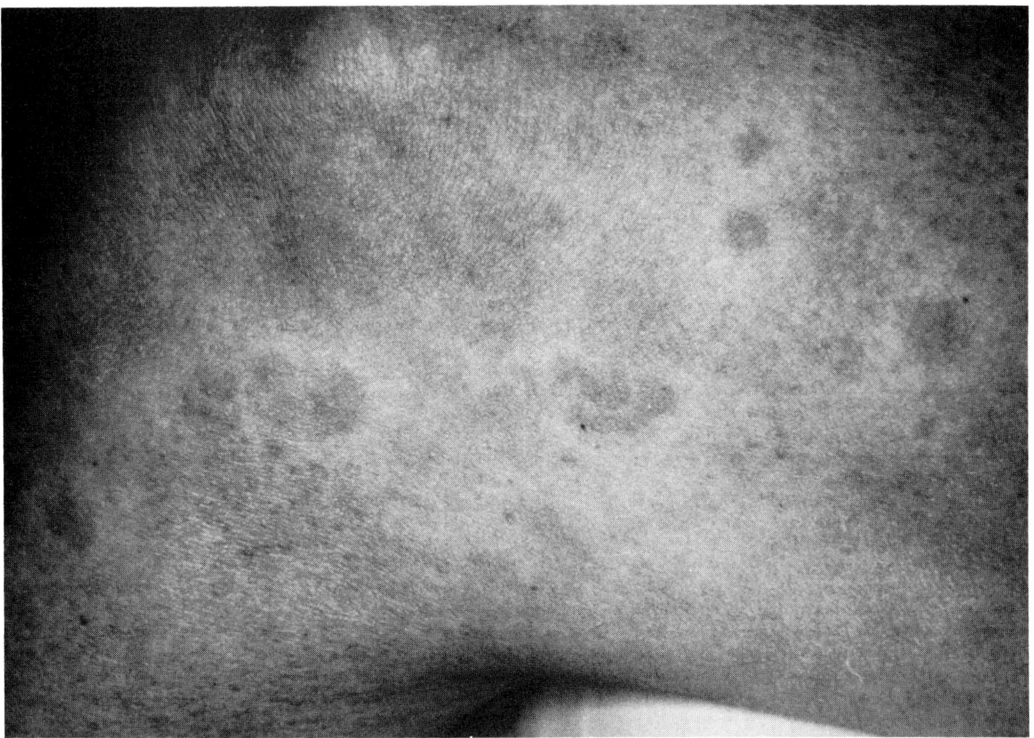

Figure 8–14. Urticarial vasculitis. Clinically the lesions are morphologically indistinguishable from ordinary urticaria, but histologically they show the features of leukocytoclastic vasculitis.

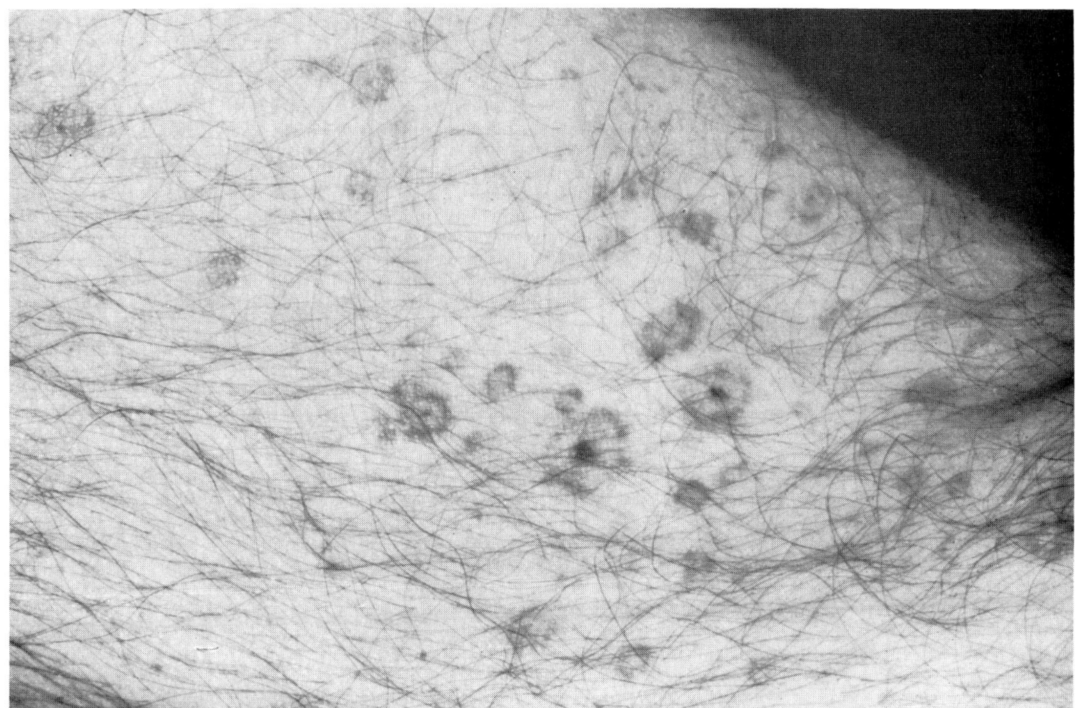

Figure 8–15. Leukocytoclastic angiitis. The lesions in this patient were made up of rings formed by petechiae around a hemorrhagic center.

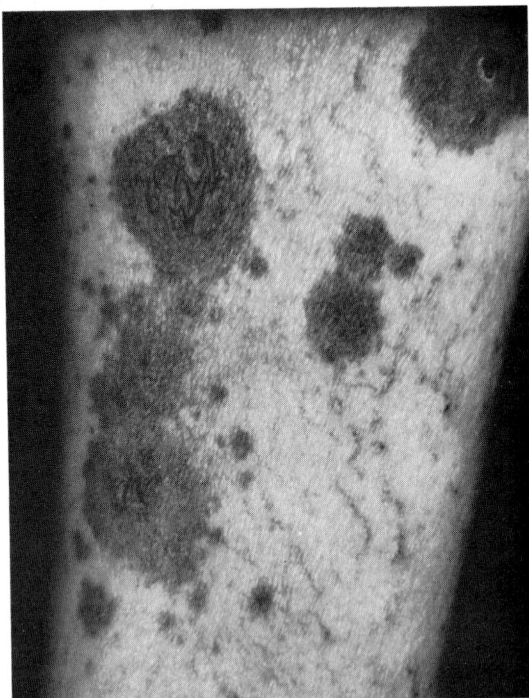

Figure 8–16. Leukocytoclastic angiitis. Hemorrhagic partially collapsed bullae.

marked inflammation in the vascular wall, but this is an unusual event. Rather, one often sees endothelial cell swelling that drastically narrows the lumen. Ulceration developing on a purpuric or erythematous base is the consequence of such luminal narrowing, and scarring is usually the sequel (Figs. 8–17 to 8–19; Plate 23*F*). In exceptional cases, the numbers of neutrophils migrating through the vascular walls into the perivascular tissues may be so enormous that they produce macroscopic pustules simulating abscesses or folliculitis (Figs. 7–29 and 8–20). Leukocytoclastic angiitis may also manifest itself as dusky red papules that persist for one to three weeks before resolving (Fig. 7–30).

Figures 8–21 to 8–26 illustrate a spectrum of lesions affecting areas uncommonly involved by leukocytoclastic vasculitis.

Although the small vessels in the deep dermis are affected less often, involvement of these vessels does occur and can produce a red nonpurpuric intradermal nodule that may be tender but rarely ulcerates. Though not produced by a vasculitis, livedo reticularis is an important sign of an underlying leukocytoclastic angiitis. Livedo reticularis may be associated with red tender intradermal nodules up to 1 or 2 cm in size, and this combination represents a unique sign of leukocytoclastic angiitis.[18-21] The significance of livedo reticularis will be discussed in more detail later.

All of the lesions described above, except for livedo reticularis, characteristically arise in crops, persist for one to four weeks, and usually subside spontaneously, either with or without scarring, depending upon the severity of the necrotizing process. All of the lesions, including livedo reticularis, appear initially on the lower legs and ankles and tend to remain localized. Edema of the legs and ankles is frequently present as well. During the course of the disease, the various eruptions may also

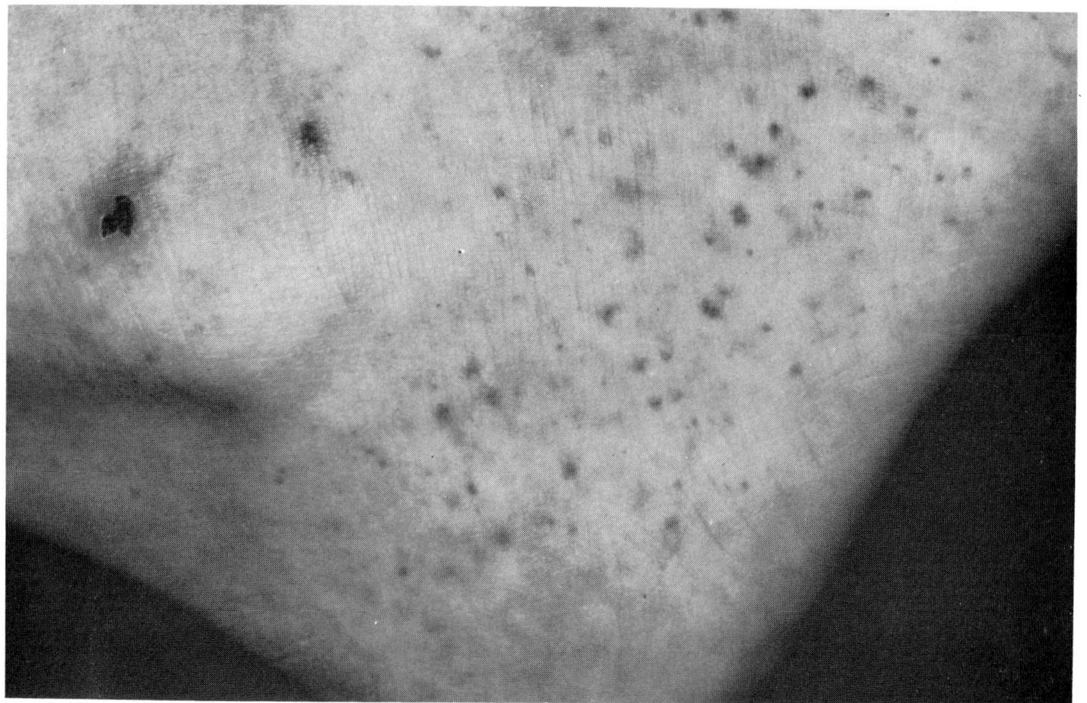

Figure 8–17. Leukocytoclastic angiitis. Purpura and ulceration.

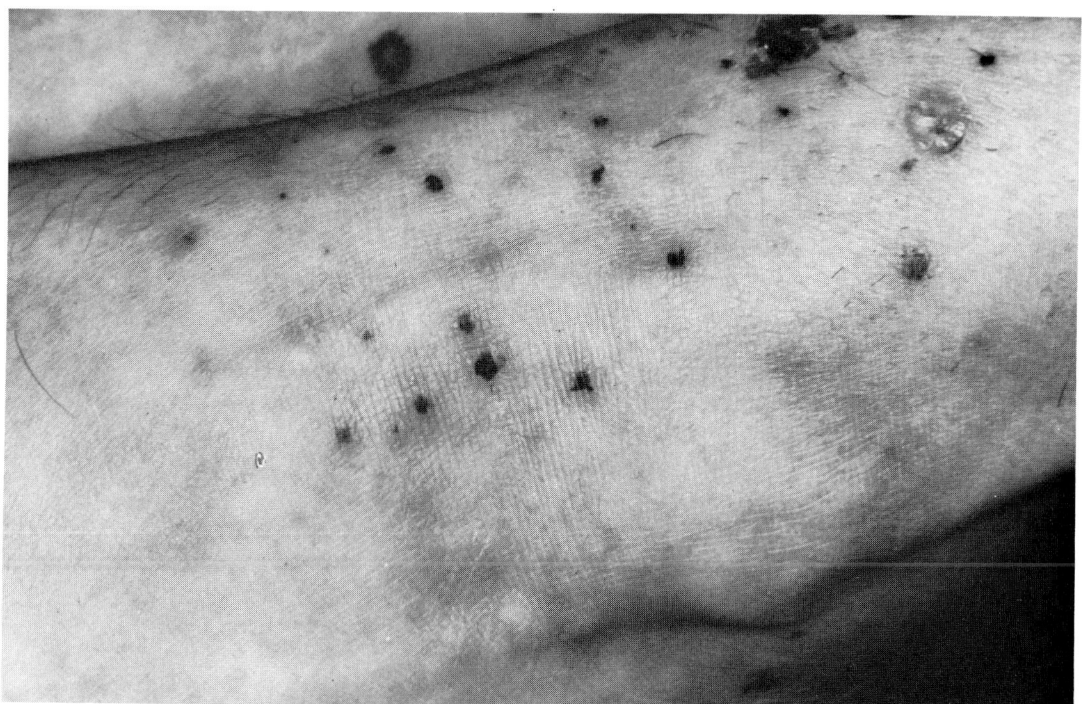

Figure 8–18. Leukocytoclastic angiitis. Purpura and ulceration.

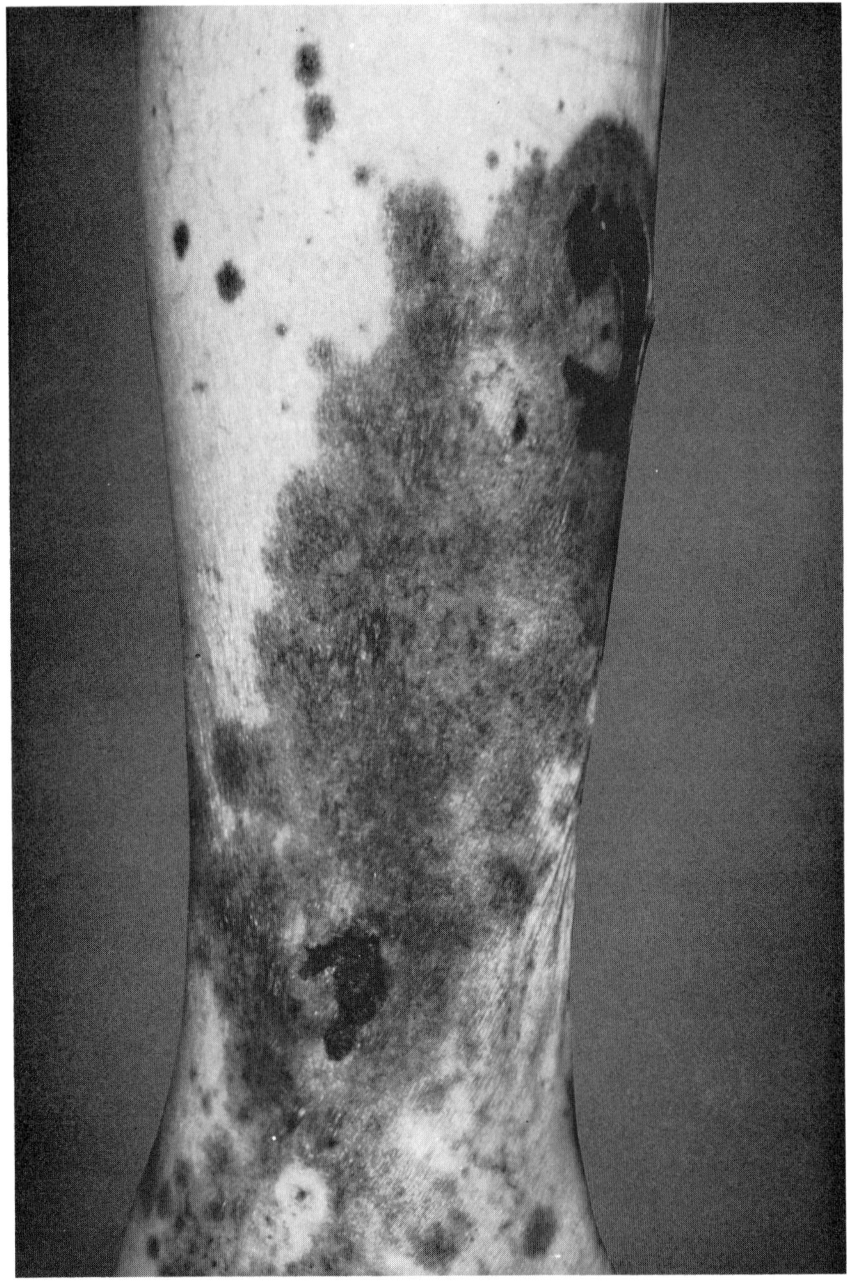

Figure 8–19. Leukocytoclastic angiitis. Purpura and ulceration. Note that the smallest areas of purpura are oval and as they coalesce they produce larger areas of purpura with polycystic borders.

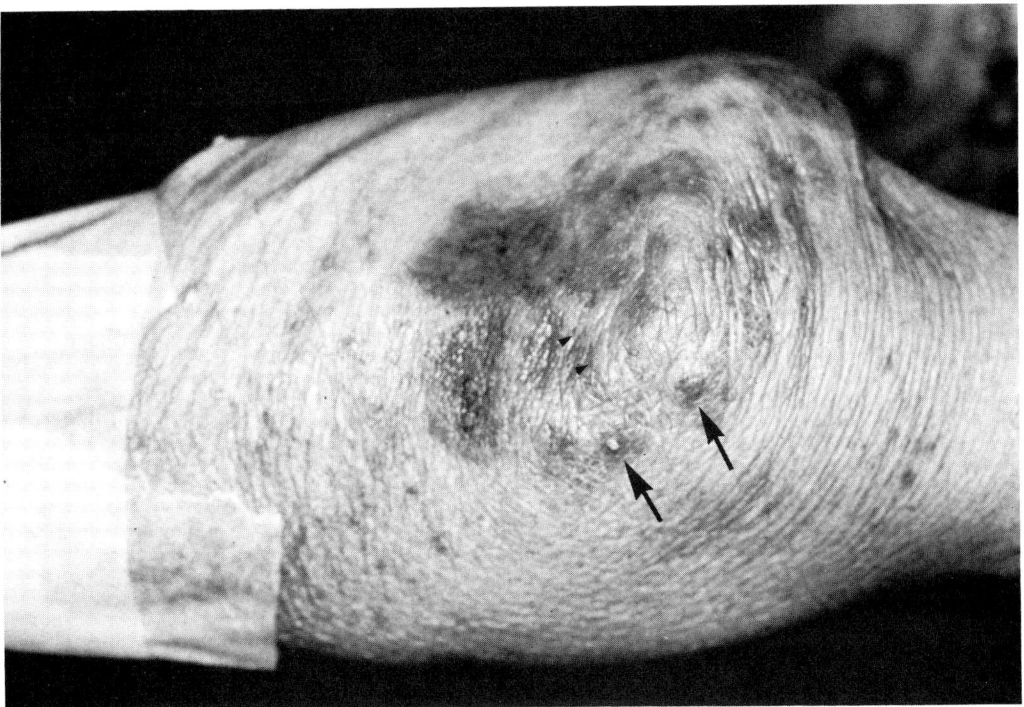

Figure 8–20. Leukocytoclastic vasculitis. Massive migration of neutrophils can produce pustular lesions as illustrated over this patient's elbow (arrows).

appear on the arms, hands, trunk, face, ears, and even in the mouth. However, this spreading is only a minor facet of leukocytoclastic angiitis; its presence does not detract from the significance of the striking localization of lesions on the lower extremities.

Erythema elevatum diutinum (EED) is a rare entity that has been considered merely a dermatologic curiosity. However, a more careful evaluation indicates that this disorder is a chronic indolent manifestation of leukocytoclastic angiitis.[4, 55-57] EED is characterized by erythematous papules, nodules, or plaques that appear chiefly over the extensor surfaces of the knees, elbows, and small joints of the hands (Figs. 8–27 to 8–29). The buttocks, lower legs, and pinnae of the ears are involved less frequently. The lesions sometimes have a purplish, brown, or yellowish hue and may be painful when they first erupt. Vesicles, bullae, and ulcerations may develop in the center of the lesions. The natural history of an individual spot is unpredictable: it may persist indefinitely, disappear completely, or appear and disappear chronically in the same site. Individual lesions may coalesce to form irregular, arcuate, or gyrate patterns.[57] Following resolution they often leave hypo- or hyperpigmented atrophic spots. The differential diagnosis of the lesions in EED includes granuloma annulare, recurrent febrile neutrophilic dermatosis (Sweet), xanthoma, and multicentric reticulohistiocytosis. However, EED can be easily distinguished from them on the basis of the histologic findings.

Occasionally one sees individuals with the classic palpable purpura of leukocytoclastic angiitis developing at sites characteristic of EED.

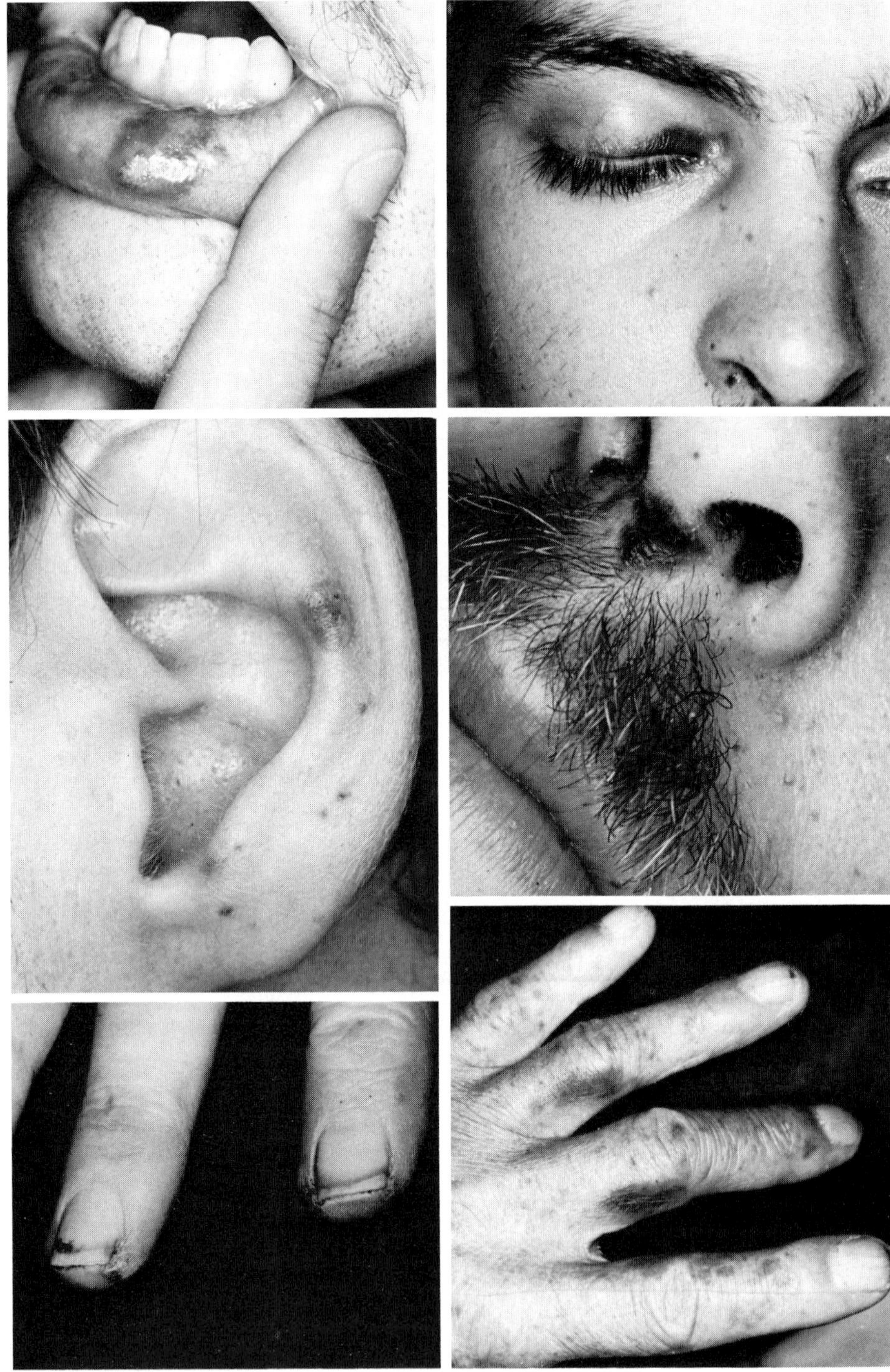

Figure 8–21. Top left. Leukocytoclastic vasculitis affecting lip.

Figure 8–22. Top right. Leukocytoclastic vasculitis of eyelid.

Figure 8–23. Center left. Leukocytoclastic vasculitis affecting pinna.

Figure 8–24. Center right. Leukocytoclastic vasculitis involving nostril.

Figure 8–25. Bottom left. Leukocytoclastic vasculitis of finger tips.

Figure 8–26. Bottom right. Leukocytoclastic vasculitis affecting fingers.

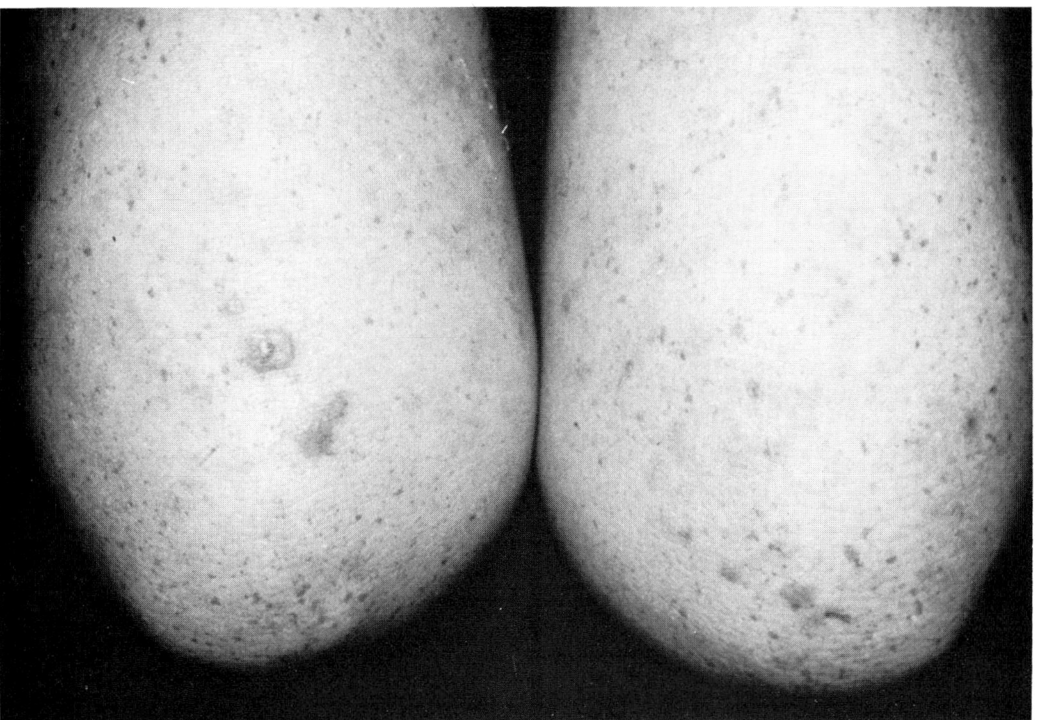

Figure 8–27. Erythema elevatum diutinum. Reddish brown papules on elbow.

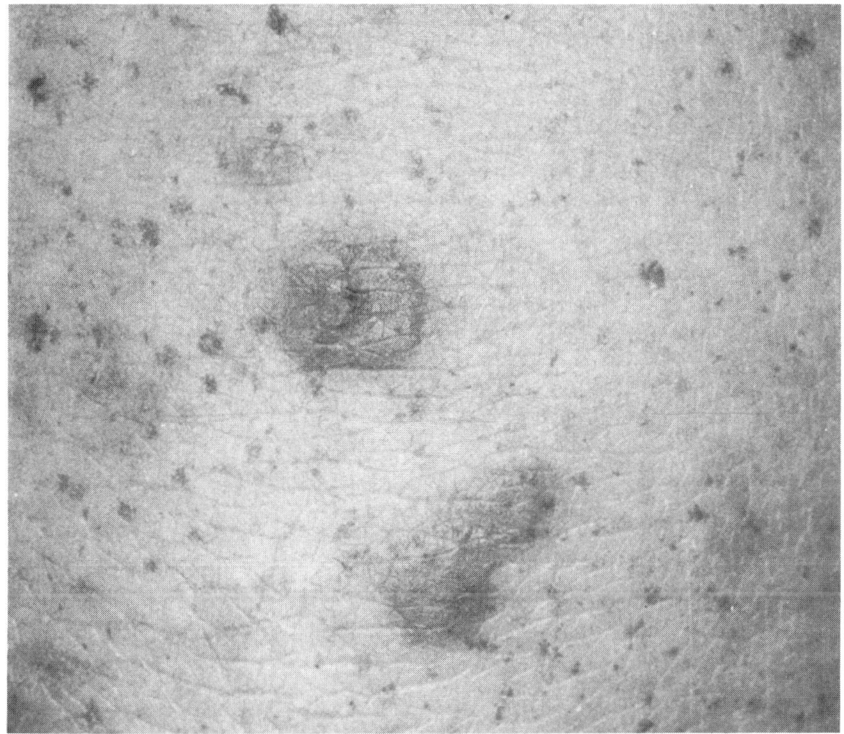

Figure 8–28. Erythema elevatum diutinum. Close-up of EED lesions in Figure 8–27.

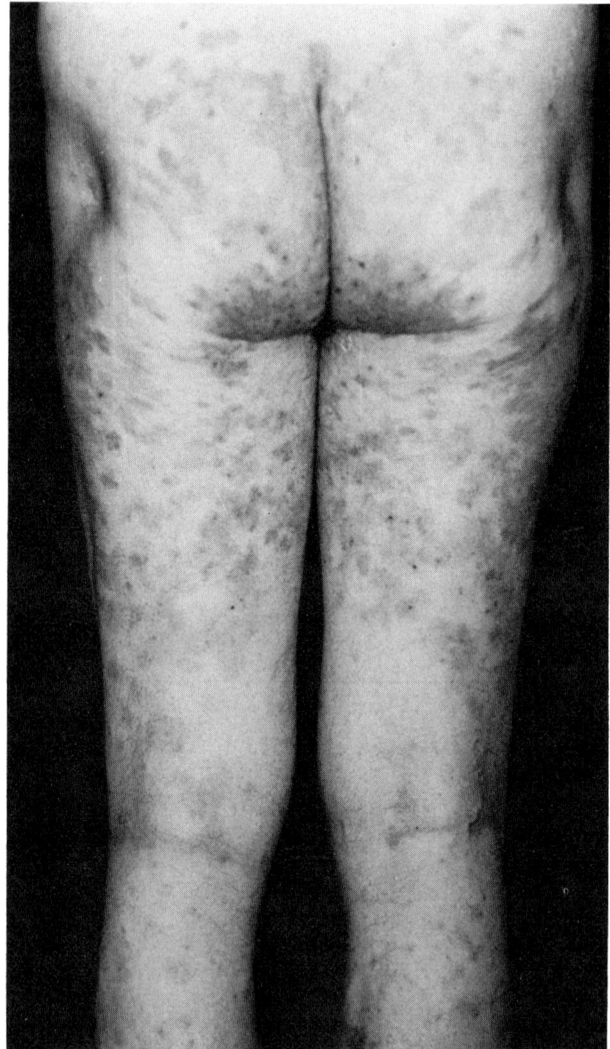

Figure 8–29. Erythema elevatum diutinum. Papules and plaques involving buttocks and posterior thighs.

(Figs. 8–30 and 8–31). In Schönlein-Henoch purpura, the vasculitic lesions commonly develop on the buttocks and extensor surfaces of the limbs as in EED. Winkelmann and Ditto described a patient (Case 11) with the typical lesions of EED who also developed urticarial papules and vesicles of acute leukocytoclastic angiitis.[4]

The acute lesion of EED exhibits the typical changes of leukocytoclastic angiitis. In its chronic phase, a hyaline PAS-positive mantle and an organized histiocytic infiltrate develop perivascularly, but nuclear dust is still present. In the late stage, extensive dermal fibrosis is present. Lipids, primarily as cholesterol esters, may be deposited both intracellularly and extracellularly in the chronic lesions of EED — the true identity of the dermatosis known as extracellular cholesterosis.

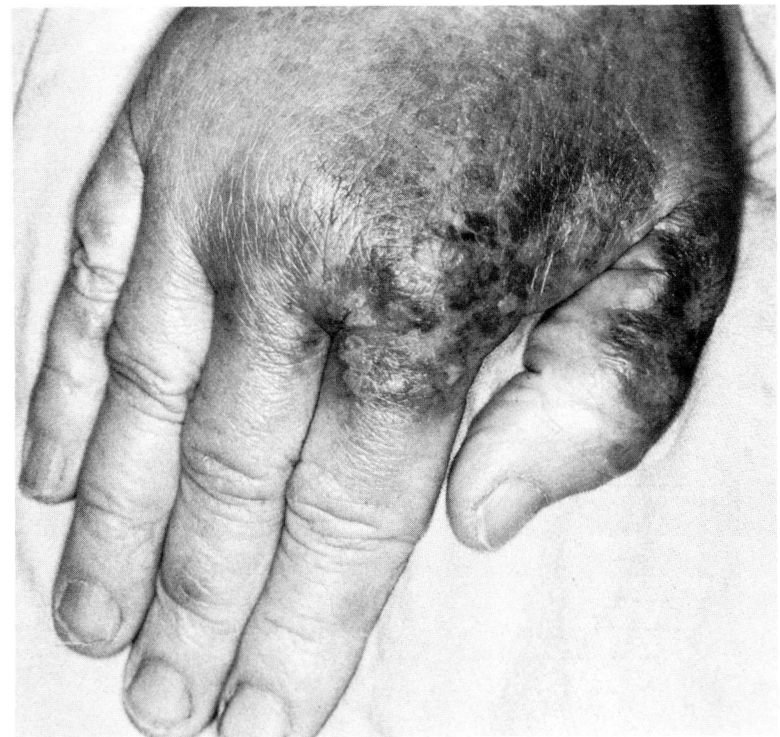

Figure 8–30. Leukocytoclastic vasculitis developing at sites characteristic of EED.

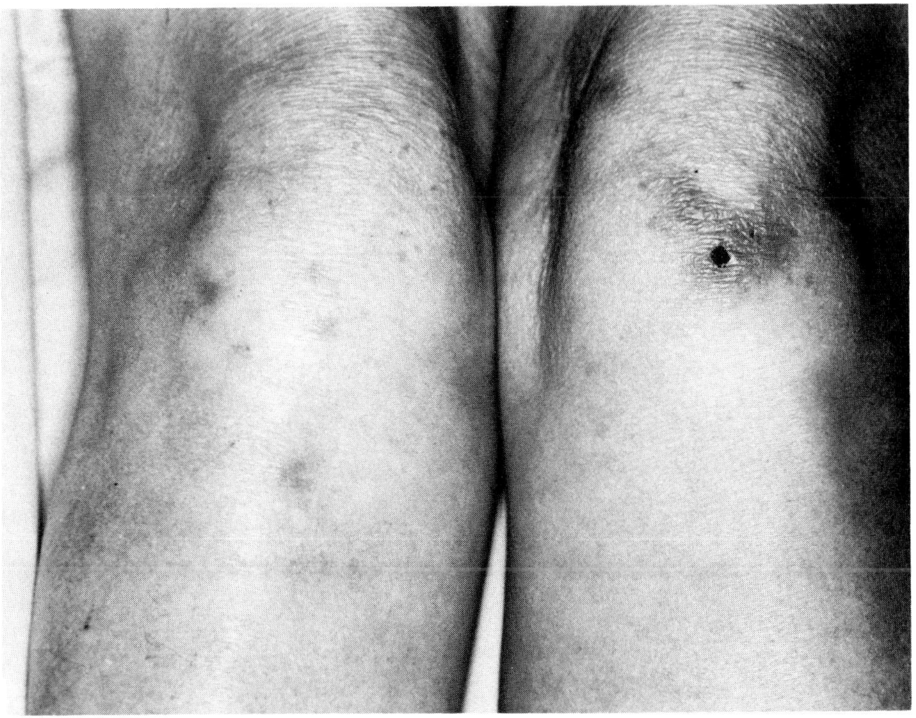

Figure 8–31. Leukocytoclastic vasculitis arising at sites characteristic of EED.

Clinical Manifestations

Schönlein-Henoch Purpura. The Schönlein-Henoch syndrome occurs primarily in children and young adults and more often in boys than in girls.[58-60] Synonyms for this illness are anaphylactoid purpura, allergic purpura, and hemorrhagic capillary toxicosis. The histopathology is a leukocytoclastic angiitis involving the blood vessels in the dermal papillae and upper dermis. Deeper vascular involvement in the dermis of fat does not occur. The disease has a peak incidence during March, April, and May. An upper respiratory infection often precedes its onset by one to three weeks.

Headache, anorexia, and fever frequently usher in the illness. These symptoms are followed by pain in the abdomen and joints, purpuric eruptions, and evidence of renal involvement. Abdominal colic with purpura (Henoch's purpura) may occur in the absence of joint pain with purpura (Schönlein's purpura), although they are both present in the complete syndrome. Cutaneous hemorrhage can also develop without joint or gastrointestinal involvement and can be the sole manifestation of any attack. Usually the disease is limited to a single episode that lasts from 4 to 6 weeks, but in 40 per cent of the cases, recurrences ensue within a few weeks of the initial attack. The total duration of the illness can be from several months to two years.

The skin lesions usually begin as red macules that become urticarial and then purpuric within a day, although some lesions may not become hemorrhagic but may simply resolve after the urticarial phase. When the inflammation and exudation are severe, hemorrhagic vesicles, bullae, and ulcers develop. The sites of predilection are the extensor surfaces of the limbs, the buttocks, back, and, on occasion, the face. The oral mucosa can also be affected. The purpura may be limited to the skin over painful joints. Bleeding occurs in the presence of a normal number of platelets.

Children less than three years old initially tend to develop edema of the scalp, hands, feet, and periorbital tissues. The edema arises in the absence of renal or cardiac disease and probably reflects an increased capillary permeability resulting from the underlying vasculitis. In Allen's series, this type of edema did not occur in children over eight years old.[60] Older children have more gastrointestinal and renal involvement than the younger ones. In Allen's series of 131 patients, renal disease occurred in 25 per cent of children under two years of age, but in 50 per cent of children over two years of age; and gastrointestinal bleeding and pain were present in 25 per cent of children under two years of age, but in 75 per cent of children over two years of age. The abdominal pain is usually a colic; it may be localized anywhere in the abdomen; and it is commonly associated with vomiting and melena. Bleeding occurs in the submucosa and subserosa of the gut, but intussusception is uncommon. The focal mucosal ulceration and hemorrhage produced by the vasculitis is responsible for the bleeding and pain. Epistaxis and gingival, subarachnoid, pulmonary, and cerebral bleeding are rare manifestations of anaphylactoid purpura.[61]

Single or multiple joints can be affected, and often the pain flits from one articulation to another. The knees and ankles are most frequently affected. Articular swelling, tenderness, and effusions are uncommon. Synovial hemorrhage is the cause of the joint pain.[62] Articular symptoms persist for a few days and are frequently recurrent.

Renal involvement is the most serious complication of this disease. Microscopic hematuria occurs during the acute phase of the illness in 20 to 70 per cent of the children.[63] Proteinuria without hematuria does not occur. Death from renal failure is uncommon, but mild renal impairment, such as hematuria, proteinuria, decreased concentrating ability, and diminished creatinine clearance, was detected for at least four to six years in 16 to 28 per cent of children initially affected by nephritis.[60, 61] It is not known how many patients develop chronic renal insufficiency after an episode of Schönlein-Henoch purpura, but it is believed to be less than 10 per cent.[61, 63]

Schönlein-Henoch disease frequently follows a respiratory infection whose etiologic agents have not been identified. Gairdner isolated beta-streptococci in more than 50 per cent of his patients and showed that subsequent streptococcal infections could provoke a relapse.[58] Allen also believed that a preceding beta-streptococcal infection was a predisposing factor in 30 per cent of his patients, but conclusive proof was not established.[60] Other studies have failed to demonstrate a definite correlation between beta-streptococcal infections and Schönlein-Henoch disease.[64, 65] Although streptococcus-induced disease may not account for the majority of cases, it is a significant factor in individual cases, just as it appears to be in some cases of periarteritis nodosa, leukocytoclastic angiitis, and EED. Viral infections are thought to be the important etiologic events, although none has been specifically identified. Food allergy, including food and drug additives, are documented but rare causes of anaphylactoid purpura. The food additives have included benzoates and the azo dyes tartrazine, Sunset Yellow, and New Coccine. Aspirin has been demonstrated to be a cause in a few patients.[59]

Cutaneous-Systemic Angiitis. I have chosen the term *cutaneous-systemic angiitis*, rather than any of the nine previously enumerated synonyms, to describe the second of the two major syndromes found in patients with small vessel vasculitis that affects the skin and internal organs. This term emphasizes the clinical features of this syndrome without implying either etiology or pathogenesis. The eruptions associated with cutaneous-systemic angiitis have been described earlier in this chapter and are illustrated in Figures 8–12 to 8–31 and in Plates 23*D, E, F* and 24*A, B*.

Small vessel vasculitis is a syndrome. It occurs both as an idiopathic disorder and as a manifestation of an underlying illness such as a connective tissue disease, a malignancy, or a drug reaction. When associated with a specific disease, the symptoms of the vasculitis are frequently masked or overshadowed by the associated disorder. The description that follows relates primarily to the idiopathic disorder, and it is presented in some detail because this aspect of vasculitis is generally not extensively discussed in articles reviewing this subject.

The clinical manifestations of this syndrome form a spectrum. At one pole are patients with primarily cutaneous involvement, and at the other pole are individuals with visceral involvement and minimal or absent angiitis in the skin. Persons with significant involvement of both skin and internal organs complete the spectrum. Both sexes are affected equally. Although the disease begins most often in individuals between 30 and 60 years old, it is not unusual for it to appear in children, young adults, and those over 60.

PLATE 24

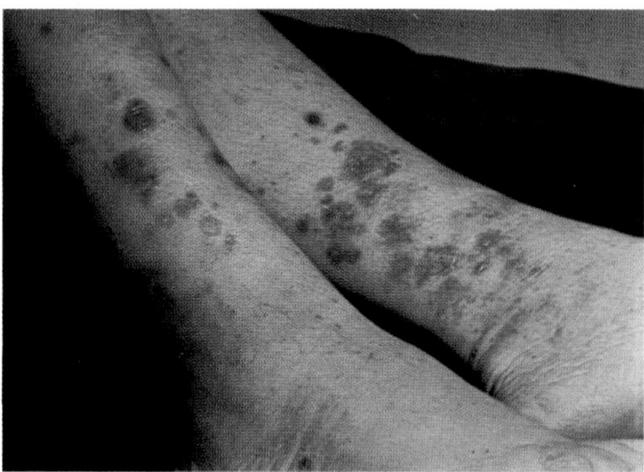

A, Leukocytoclastic angiitis. Hemorrhagic blisters. Hyperpigmented scars indicate previous crops of similar lesions.

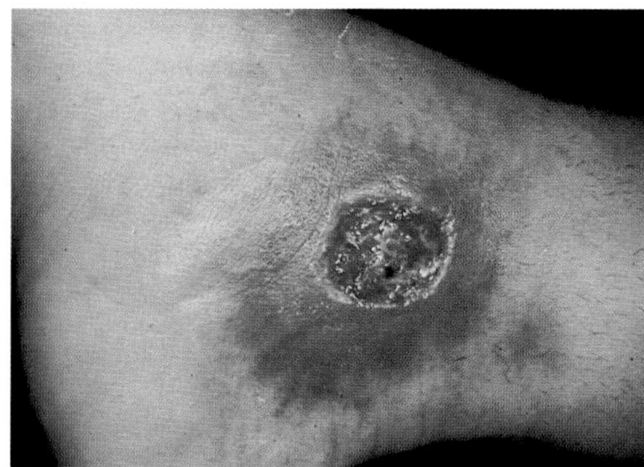

B, Leukocytoclastic angiitis producing ulceration.

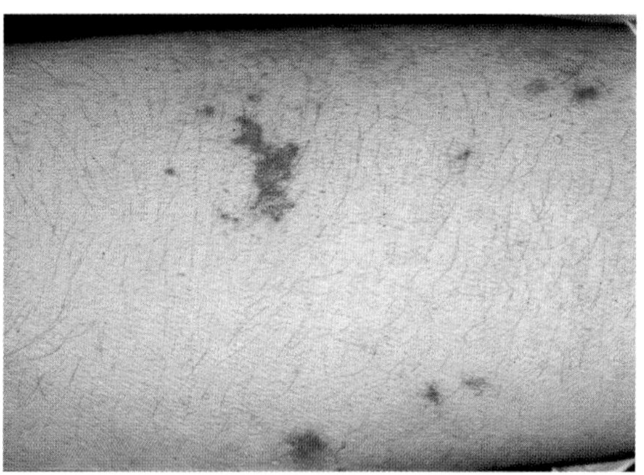

C, Meningococcemia. Characteristic purpuric lesions are gun-metal gray, indurated, and have irregular margins.

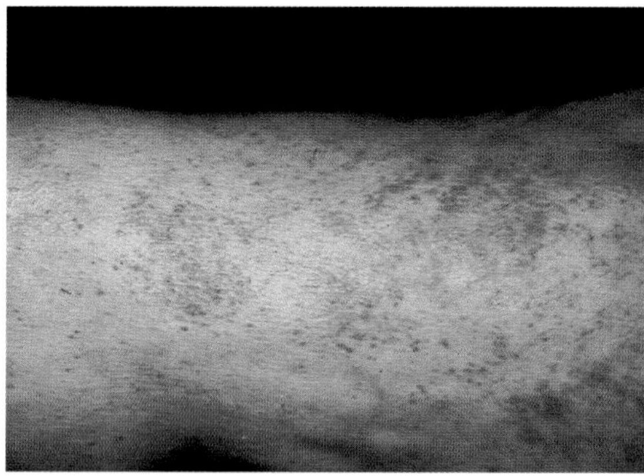

D, Schamberg's disease. Fine red petechiae on a background of brown hemosiderin.

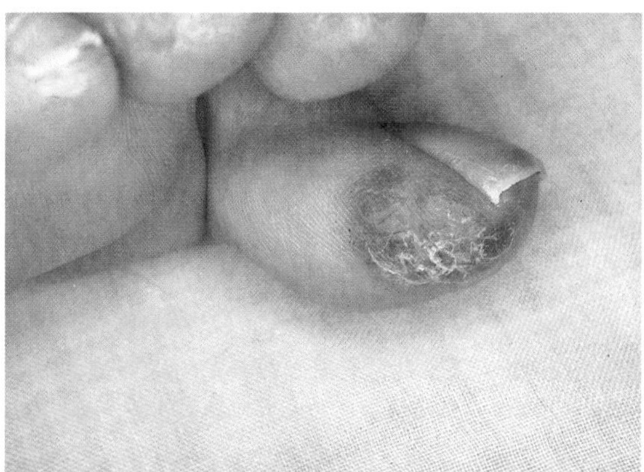

E, Chilblains. Purplish tender nodules in pulp of toe.

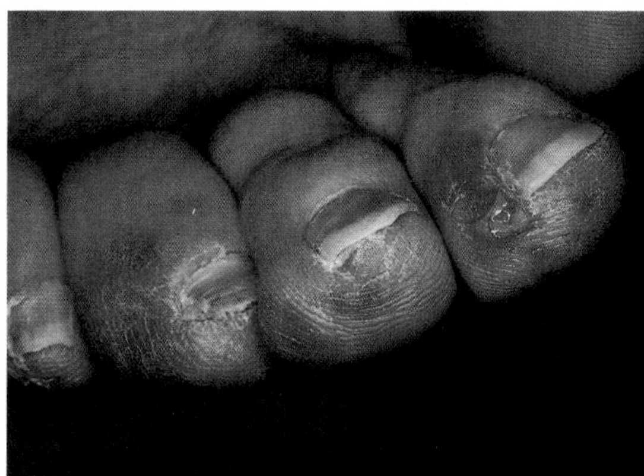

F, Chilblains. Purplish tender nodules in pulps of toes.

Winkelmann and Ditto reported the clinical and pathologic findings in 36 individuals with leukocytoclastic angiitis.[4] Cutaneous involvement was the sole manifestation of the disease in five cases. In twelve of the patients, visceral angiitis preceded cutaneous angiitis by four days to two years, the average being six months. In nine patients, the skin and viscera were affected simultaneously, and in ten patients, skin involvement preceded visceral involvement — by as long as four years in one patient; the intervals for the other nine patients were not stated.

Systemic involvement takes many forms. The arthritis and arthralgia that often accompany an acute attack can persist between episodes. In this respect the arthropathy resembles that of the connective tissue diseases and differs from that of Schönlein-Henoch purpura. Myalgia with stiffness and weakness is a common complaint. Renal involvement occurs frequently. The course and ultimate fate of patients with mild proteinuria and microscopic hematuria in the presence of normal renal function have not been determined, but observations thus far indicate that these renal abnormalities can persist for months or years without progressive renal failure; patients who do succumb usually die from chronic, rather than acute, renal insufficiency. The nephrotic syndrome is a rare manifestation of renal involvement. Histologic examination of the kidneys by percutaneous biposy or autopsy reveals focal necrotizing glomerulitis or diffuse glomerulonephritis. Peripheral neuropathy, rather than central nervous system involvement, is another manifestation of this syndrome. However, the central nervous system can be affected and patients may have headaches, delirium, mental confusion, diplopia, and even brain stem symptoms. When angiitis involves the lungs, the patient may cough, be short of breath, or cough up blood. Asymptomatic pulmonary infiltrates, which are detected by routine chest films, also occur. Vasculitis in the gastrointestinal tract can produce abdominal pain, diarrhea, melena, and hematemesis. Congestive heart failure, arrhythmias, and pericarditis can develop from myocardial angiitis. Table 8–1 summarizes the frequency of systemic involvement in six important series.[2, 4, 66-69]

The acute episodes of vasculitis are invariably ushered in by fever, malaise, joint pains, and myalgia. These signs and symptoms may be

Table 8–1. MANIFESTATIONS OF LEUKOCYTOCLASTIC ANGIITIS

Series	Knowles and Zeek⁺	O'Duffy et al.⁺	Winkelmann and Ditto*	McCombs*†	Wilkinson*	Ramsay and Fry*§
Number of patients	10	11	36	72	23	21
Organ involvement (in per cent)						
Lungs	40	55	20	30	Δ	–
Gastrointestinal tract	40	55	15	10	22	–
Nervous system	50	64	20	25	–	–
Skin	40	45	100	50	100	–
Joints	20	45	50	50	Δ	–
Kidneys	100	100	60	30	38	33
Heart	10	64	–	–	–	–

⁺Autopsy study.
*Studied during life.
†Seventeen of 72 patients had periarteritis nodosa. Organ involvement in two varieties of angiitis not separated in paper.
ΔOrgans affected but frequency not stated.
§Only renal involvement cited.

either mild or severe. The eruption appears on the legs in crops, persists from one to four weeks, often heals with scarring, and recurs at intervals of days or months. Edema of the legs and ankles may accompany the cutaneous lesions; it is partly responsible for the frequent misdiagnosis of thrombophlebitis in these patients. The illness can continue in this fashion for weeks, months, or years. Gougerot reported a case of a patient in whom the disease had been chronically present for 30 years.[70]

Visceral involvement may already exist at the onset of the disease, or it may arise at any time during its course. Even with a moderate degree of systemic disease, the affected person usually does not look chronically ill.

The longest observation period of a significant number of patients with marked cutaneous involvement is only 11 years, and in the majority of patients, this period is probably considerably less. Exact statistics were not published in the two most important papers dealing with this topic.[4, 66] Based upon the brief case histories published in these articles, it is clear that patients with only cutaneous involvement at the onset may develop a progressive fatal disease. The disorder is unpredictable, partly because the natural history has yet to be completely chronicled.

Patients whose disease runs a fulminant course that leads to renal insufficiency make up the other end of the spectrum of cutaneous-systemic angiitis. Cutaneous lesions of angiitis have occurred in about 40 per cent of such patients, but the eruptions have not been emphasized in case reports, nor has their significance been realized during life.[2, 4, 67] Some clinicians still make a diagnosis of *hypersensitivity angiitis of Zeek* in such patients, because they assume it to be a distinct type of necrotizing vasculitis. Unfortunately, the severity of the systemic involvement has overshadowed the cutaneous eruption, which is the morphologic and histologic link between the primarily cutaneous and the purely systemic varieties of this disorder.

Zeek coined the term *hypersensitivity angiitis* on the basis of the clinical course and autopsy findings in 10 patients.[2] All of them had died of uremia within one month after the onset of their illness. Seven of the 10 individuals had been treated with sulfonamides for different types of infections, but in the remaining three patients, the precipitating cause was not found. The small vessels of the lungs, gut, nervous system, kidneys, and myocardium showed necrotizing angiitis that Zeek recognized as distinct from the changes of periarteritis nodosa. Four of the 10 patients had purpura, bullae, or a generalized maculopapular eruption. Arthralgias occurred in some patients. One of Zeek's patients may have had SLE that was triggered by the administration of sulfonamides, since a butterfly erythema of the face was present in addition to the purpura on the extremities.

Since the publication of Zeek's observations, the term *hypersensitivity angiitis* has been applied to any case of fulminating vasculitis. O'Duffy et al. subsequently reported the clinical and autopsy findings in 11 cases of hypersensitivity angiitis as defined by Zeek.[67] The average duration of illness was 3.7 months. These cases were also selected from autopsy records. Forty-five per cent of the individuals in this study had cutaneous lesions.

The duration and severity of illness are the sole differences between Zeek's hypersensitivity angiitis and the cutaneous-systemic angiitis complex under discussion; the histopathology and morphology of the cutaneous lesions, as well as the other clinical features of the two entities, are identical. The brief case reports of 30 patients with necrotizing vasculitis reported by McCombs in 1956 also illustrate the spectrum of illness encountered in cutaneous-systemic angiitis.[71]

A few case histories from McCombs' article are cited. One patient developed cutaneous and renal angiitis following a reaction to penicillin and died of uremia six weeks later (Case 6). A second patient also developed angiitis in the skin, gut, lungs, and kidney, following penicillin therapy. Although a moderate degree of uremia ensued, this patient recovered after several weeks of conservative therapy (Case 7). A third patient suffered from vasculitis of the skin and kidneys for 16 months before she died of renal failure. Etiology was not determined (Case 9). A fourth patient had migratory arthralgias and erythematous skin nodules that appeared intermittently for four years. A biopsy of a nodule showed necrotizing angiitis. Pulmonary, gastrointestinal, and renal involvement then developed, and the patient died of uremia two years later (Case 29). A fifth patient was still living after a seven-year history of idiopathic angiitis involving the skin, kidney, and bladder (Case 8).

In 1965 McCombs reported 72 cases of necrotizing angiitis, which he labeled *systemic "allergic" vasculitis.*[66] Drugs induced the disease in some of the patients. McCombs made the following comments:

> All of Zeek's patients who had hypersensitivity angiitis died within a few weeks of onset. Our cases of drug-induced vasculitis certainly fit into Zeek's category of hypersensitivity angiitis except that most of our patients recovered. We would agree that periarteritis nodosa deserves to be considered in a special category because of its poor prognosis. There are, however, many other cases in our series that fit neither of these groups and they may be designated as cases of *idiopathic "systemic" vasculitis* or because of the implications of allergy we have chosen to use the term *systemic "allergic" vasculitis.*

In spite of the identical histopathology in all his cases of small vessel angiitis, McCombs still diagnosed his patient's disorders as hypersensitivity angiitis if the illnesses were drug-induced and ran a fulminant course. However, in three of Zeek's ten cases, there was no history of preceding drug ingestion, and the etiology was never determined.[2]

The varied manifestations and unpredictable clinical course of cutaneous-systemic angiitis can be illustrated by four of our own patients.

The first patient was a 39-year-old woman who developed crops of lesions in association with fever and arthralgias over a three-year period. Plate 24*A* shows the eruption: hemorrhagic bullae, purpuric wheals, and scarring. Oral steroids controlled the cutaneous angiitis. During the three years, neither an underlying illness nor an etiology could be uncovered. Extracutaneous involvement did not seem to be present. The nephrotic syndrome arose abruptly, and the skin lesions became less prominent and manifested themselves only as small spots of purpura. Percutaneous biopsy of the kidney showed a moderately severe glomerulonephritis with glomerular changes compatible with LE. However, no other evidence of LE was present. The patient died of renal insufficiency seven and one-half years after the onset of her illness. The first three years of her angiitic syndrome conformed to the cutaneous vasculitides described by the dermatologists, whereas the last four and one-half years conformed to the systemic syndromes described by the internists and pathologists.

The second case was that of a 16-year-old boy who developed a fever and recurrent episodes of pain and swelling in his calf muscles. After eight months, a muscle biopsy was taken, and a diagnosis of leukocytoclastic angiitis was made. Oral steroid therapy suppressed signs and symptoms of the disease, but when the medicine was tapered, an ulceration developed over one ankle (Plate 24*B*). The ulcer promptly healed when the dose of prednisone was increased and indomethacin was added to the regimen. The disease entered a remission within a few months, and the patient remained well without medication for four years. No follow-up observations have been made. Etiology was never determined in the case.

The third patient was a 50-year-old woman with pemphigus vulgaris that was being treated with oral steroids. Because of fluid retention, she was given chlorothiazide to induce diuresis. Three days later she developed fever; purpuric wheals on her arms, legs, and trunk; a migrating pulmonary infiltrate; and eosinophilia. The diagnosis of leukocytoclastic angiitis in the skin was established by biopsy. Discontinuation of the diuretic was followed by prompt defervescence and remission of her cutaneous and visceral angiitis.

The fourth case was that of a 24-year-old woman whose illness began at age 15, three weeks after she had had a severe sore throat. She was confined to bed for over one week. The organism was not identified. Her illness was characterized by sharp pains in the shoulders, elbows, and knees; the pains occurred each morning and lasted for several hours. Erythematous nodules appeared intermittently on the palms and the palmar surfaces of the fingers. Recurrent purpuric ulcerations developed on the buttocks and legs, and cutaneous infections frequently resulted in deep ulcerations. On one occasion an extensive ulceration resembling pyoderma gangrenosum developed on her lower abdomen, and skin grafts were required. The diagnosis of leukocytoclastic angiitis was made four years after the onset of the illness. It was at this time that mild proteinuria, cylindruria, and hematuria were first noted. Seven years after her illness had begun, she still had an abnormal urinalysis, but her BUN was normal. She continued to require oral steroids and antibiotics intermittently for control of the cutaneous vasculitis and infections. During the succeeding two years she was relatively asymptomatic and was not on steroid therapy. In the ninth year of her illness, severe menorrhagia and a flare of her cutaneous vasculitis brought her back to the hospital where she was noted to have diffuse purpura, anemia, and a BUN of 189 mg per 100 ml. However, she did not exhibit any of the usual signs and symptoms of uremia. A renal biopsy showed three hyalinized glomeruli and one with a crescent formation, and her creatinine clearance was 4 ml/min. Kidney transplantation was performed two months later, but the patient died one and one half months after the surgery. Etiology was not determined in this patient.

The history of an upper respiratory illness preceding the onset of vasculitis, as in this last patient, is not an unusual finding in many cases of necrotizing angiitis. Also, our patient probably received antibiotics for her pharyngitis. Renal function did not deteriorate until the last two years of her nine-year illness, and during the first four years, there was no evidence of renal disease. While renal insufficiency was progressing in the last two years, the cutaneous vasculitis, arthralgias, and infections appeared to be in remission. This unpredictability makes prognosis and evaluation of therapy exceedingly difficult for this disorder.

Winkelmann and Ditto,[4] McCombs,[66] Wilkinson,[68] and Ramsay and Fry[69] have presented a realistic view of leukocytoclastic angiitis that is based on the study of living patients rather than on autopsies. Only four of 36 patients in Winkelmann's series died as a result of the vasculitis. Renal failure occurred in all four patients after intervals of four months, six months, 20 months, and seven years. In two patients, vascular lesions that were in muscular arteries and that were compatible with periarteritis nodosa were said to have been present at autopsy in addition to cutaneous leukocytoclastic angiitis. The colon and kidney were affected in one patient; the jejunum and colon were affected in the other patient. Both of these patients had pulmonary involvement during the course of illness. The duration of illness was at least seven years in some of the remaining 32 patients, but exact statistics were not provided.

McCombs presented similar data on prognosis in 55 patients with leukocytoclastic angiitis. Thirty-eight were still alive one to eleven years after the diagnosis of angiitis had been made, and 13 died of the disease. (Follow-up information was inadequate in four patients.) Fifteen patients entered a remission and the rest continued to show varying degrees of activity in their disease.

In Wilkinson's series, 5 of 23 patients died, but in Ramsay and Fry's group, all the patients had had a benign course at the time of the report.

In contrast, classic periarteritis nodosa is usually a rapidly fatal disease. Knowles et al. observed that their 14 patients died 5 to 52 weeks after the periarteritis had begun[2]; Rose and Spencer reported that 85 per cent of their patients did not survive for more than one year.[9] In O'Duffy's series, the mean duration of periarteritis was five and one-half months.[67] More recent studies by Frohnert and Sheps indicate that the survival rate in untreated periarteritis nodosa would not be expected to exceed 30 ± 10 per cent at two years.[11] In McCombs' series, 12 of 17 patients with periarteritis died soon after the onset; but 5 were alive 2 to 11 years later, and 2 of these patients were in apparent remission.[66] The differentiation of *microscopic* periarteritis (leukocytoclastic angiitis) from *classic* periarteritis nodosa is of more than academic interest.

EED, which was discussed earlier, is a chronic indolent form of leukocytoclastic angiitis. Serious systemic involvement is not usually a feature of EED, and until recently there has not been much emphasis on its associated signs and symptoms. However, recent reports have pointed out that fever, chills, malaise, and arthralgias often accompany acute exacerbations of this disorder.[56, 57] In the series of Katz et al., streptococcal infections caused the disease to flare and oral antibiotics were useful in controlling the disorder.[56] The role of the streptococci was further emphasized by the response to intradermal injections of streptokinase-streptodornase. Skin tests became positive at four hours and showed the histological features of an Arthus reaction, and in one patient the EED flared and was accompanied by the development of new lesions within 24 hours.[56] In the report by Winkelmann and Ditto, Case 11 had urticarial papules and vesicles of acute leukocytoclastic angiitis, as well as the chronic plaques of EED. This patient also had proteinuria, hematuria, and a positive test for rheumatoid factor.[4] This chronic form of leukocytoclastic angiitis is also unusual in that it responds dramatically to sulfones, unlike the acute form.[56]

The evolution of leukocytoclastic angiitis to EED is demonstrated by one of our patients.

A 21-year-old woman with juvenile diabetes mellitus developed recurrent crops of purpura with ulceration on her legs. Biopsy showed leukocytoclastic vasculitis. Oral steoids in small doses completely suppressed her disease. There was no evidence of systemic involvement, any associated underlying disease, or

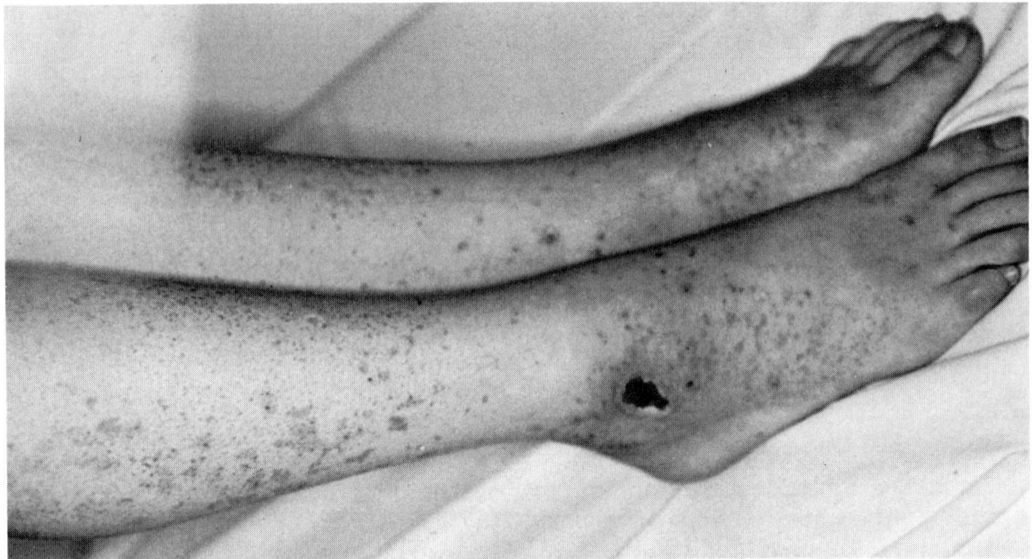

Figure 8–32. Leukocytoclastic vasculitis with ulceration on legs of patient who had lesions of EED on elbows and knees. Patient illustrated in Figures 8–27 and 8–28.

relationship to her medications, including insulin. Approximately five and one-half years later, her vasculitis recurred on the legs and buttocks and was not controlled by increasing doses of prednisone (Figs. 8–32 and 8–33). In addition, she began to develop reddish-brown papules and plaques on her knees and elbows (Figs. 8–27 and 8–34). Biopsies showed leukocytoclastic vasculitis in the purpuric lesions on the buttocks and legs and EED in the plaques and papules. The

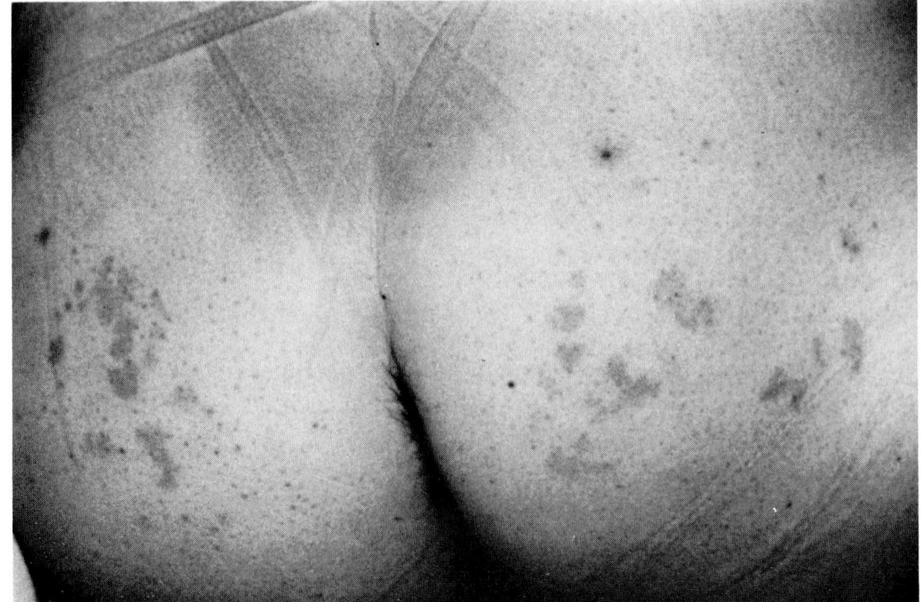

Figure 8–33. Leukocytoclastic vasculitis on buttocks of patient shown in Figure 8–32.

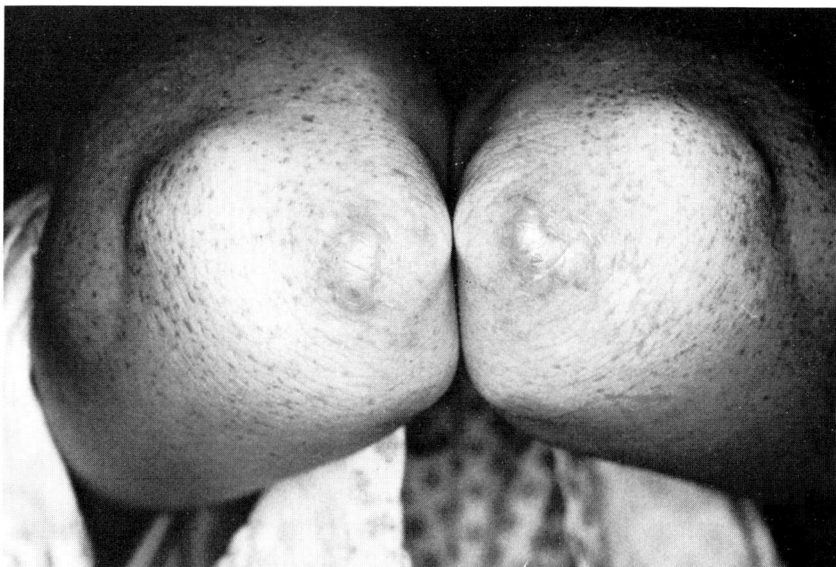

Figure 8–34. Plaques of EED over elbows of patient shown in Figure 8–32.

institution of sulfone therapy was followed by the prompt disappearance of both purpura and the lesions of EED. Her disease remains completely suppressed by the sulfone (dapsone) therapy.

Pathogenesis

Current clinical and experimental evidence indicates that leukocytoclastic angiitis and periarteritis nodosa are immune complex diseases. With the exception of thrombosis and the size of the affected vessels, both entities display similar histologic features, which are identical to the Arthus reaction and experimental serum sickness produced in animals by single or multiple injections of a foreign protein.[72] In both experimental models, a necrotizing angiitis is produced by antigen-antibody complexes that have been trapped within the vessel walls. In experimental serum sickness, circulating immune complexes also accumulate in the glomeruli to produce nephritis. Antigen, host antibody, and complement can be identified in these vascular lesions by immunofluorescent techniques. The physical size of complexes, rather than the specificity of the antibody, is responsible for the trapping and the subsequent tissue damage. Both complement and neutrophils are required for producing the tissue damage. Cochrane has shown that complexes with a sedimentation rate of greater than 19S are necessary for producing vasculitis in serum sickness.[73-75] Smaller complexes do not lodge in the vessels.

The mechanism is believed to operate as follows. Antigen-antibody complexes formed in antigen excess are soluble and larger than 19S. After gaining access to the vascular wall, they become lodged and trapped in the basement membrane material between the endothelial cells and the pericytes because of their larger size. The antigen-antibody aggregates fix complement and activate the complement system with the elaboration of C5a and the trimolecular complex C5-6-7, both chemotactic factors for neutrophils. The neutrophils move into the vascular wall to phagocytize and catabolize the immune complexes, and during the process of phagocytosis they release lysosomal proteolytic enzymes that can damage the vascular wall.[76] Janoff and Scherer[77] and Lazarus et al.[78] have isolated a collagenase and elastase from human granulocytes that can function at physiologic pH to attack the basement membrane and internal elastic lamina of the blood vessel, the sites of damage in experimental serum sickness. These events produce vascular permeability, inflammation, and hemorrhage. In human skin, these factors produce *palpable purpura*.

Vasoactive amines are required for the immune complexes to gain entrance to the vascular wall. The mechanism that has been elucidated in a rabbit model most likely is also operative in man.[79] The antigen responsible for initiating the eventual production of vasculitis produces an IgE antibody that coats circulating basophils. On reexposure to the antigen, basophils sensitized with IgE antibody degranulate and release both preformed histamine and platelet-activating factor. The latter causes nearby platelets to aggregate and to release a vasoactive amine, which in the rabbit is histamine. In man, platelets contain the vasoactive amine serotonin. Both serotonin and histamine, when injected into the skin of man and animals, cause endothelial cells in the postcapillary venules to reversibly separate from one another.[80] The endothelial cell gaps persist for up to 30 minutes, thereby allowing the circulating complexes to gain entrance to the vascular wall and initiate the neutrophil-complement–mediated tissue injury.

Many observations in clinical medicine support an immune complex mechanism for both leukocytoclastic vasculitis and periarteritis nodosa. Glomerulonephritis is frequently associated with necrotizing vasculitis (see Table 8–1). Stringa et al. and Schroeter et al. have demonstrated immunoglobulins and complement in the cutaneous lesions of leukocytoclastic angiitis by immunofluorescent methods.[81, 82] Gary et al. described two patients with small vessel vasculitis whose renal function declined and spontaneously recovered in association with acute exacerbations and subsequent remissions of their cutaneous vasculitis.[83] Circulating immune complexes have been demonstrated in serum directly as cryoproteins (cryoglobulins),[55, 84-86] indirectly by assays that detect C1q precipitins,[87] by material that binds to receptors on human lymphocytoid (Raji) cells,[88] and by inference from depressed levels of serum complement during disease activity. Immune complexes have been visualized as electron-dense bodies by electron microscopy in cutaneous lesions less than 24 hours old.[89] In both periarteritis nodosa and leukocytoclastic vasculitis, hepatitis B antigen-antibody complexes have been detected in both the serum and the vascular lesions of individual patients. Immunoglobulins and complement have been present with hepatitis B antigen in the vascular lesions.[12, 90] Hepatitis B antigen-antibody complexes have been found during active phases of periarteritis, but not during quiescent or improving phases.[13] Hepatitis B antigen-antibody complexes have been detected in the serum and in the vasculitic cutaneous lesions along with immune reactants during the prodromal serum sickness phase of acute viral hepatitis type B.[91]

It is difficult to demonstrate immune reactants by immunofluorescence in vasculitic lesions older than 24 hours because they have been removed by the neutrophils.[92] Electron microscopic studies of such lesions show only fibrin deposition and disintegrating neutrophils and no evidence of electron-dense material characteristic of immune complexes. In order to remove these obstacles in our studies of leukocytoclastic angiitis, we resorted to an artifice. Histamine was injected intradermally into the clinically normal-appearing forearm skin of individuals who had active vasculitis. A wheal with endothelial cell gaps was produced, which permitted circulating immune complexes to be trapped in the vessel walls. The area was biopsied three to four hours later and examined for the presence of immune complexes by electron microscopy and direct immunofluorescent techniques.[89] The results of our studies confirmed by others[93-95] showed that immune complexes were trapped and could be identified by electron microscopy and immunofluorescence (Figs. 8–35 and 8–36); the histologic appearance of the Arthus reaction or serum sickness could be reproduced; the fibrinoid deposition of light microscopy is fibrin; fibrin deposition was minimal compared to spontaneous lesions in which it is massive; normal-appearing nonmanipulated skin contained immune deposits in vascular walls, in the absence of inflammatory cells indicating that they are present before the purpuric lesions develop, and are not deposited secondary to inflammation; the complexes were deposited almost exclusively in postcapillary venules and rarely in arterial capillaries; examination of spontaneous vasculitic lesions less than 24 hours old revealed that electron-dense deposits were present both in the vascular wall and within cytoplasmic vacuoles of neutrophils; and the relative absence of fibrin in histamine-induced lesions indicates that fibrin is not a major factor in the production of the vasculitic lesion, as had been previously believed.[96] The "necrosis" of vessels (smudged images) seen by light microscopy appears to be an illusion produced by the massive deposition of fibrin between the cellular elements of the vascular wall. We found no evidence of necrosis morphologically in endothelial cells or pericytes by electron microscopy in either spontaneous or artificially induced lesions.

Although there is evidence that a low-grade DIC occurs in some patients with leukocytoclastic angiitis,[97] the rarity of thromboses in such lesions suggests that DIC is a parallel phenomenon that does not directly participate in the genesis of the vasculitic lesions. In addition, since the major deposition of fibrin is in the vascular wall and surrounding tissues, it seems likely that leakage of fibrinogen secondary to vascular permeability has occurred with the conversion to fibrin developing in these extravascular locations.

There is a seeming paradox between the absence of immune reactants in lesions older than 24 hours and the persistence of the diagnostic features of leukocytoclasis and fibrinoid degeneration for several days. This discrepancy may be explained by the fact that human neutrophils contain a lysosomal enzyme capable of cleaving C5 to C5a.[98] The presence of immune complexes in the vasculitic lesions would set the stage for phagocytosis by neutrophils with release of C5-cleaving enzyme and subsequent production of C5a that would then attract more neutrophils. Additional cleaving enzyme would be released as the cells disintegrated. A cycle would thus be established for several days. Since plasma proteins readily pass through inflamed vessels, it is likely that the

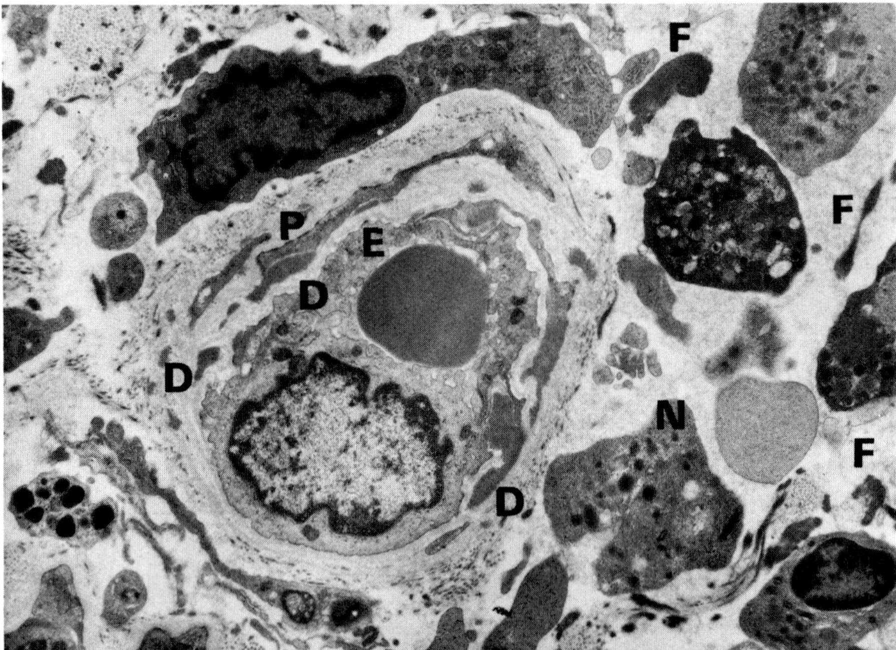

Figure 8–35. Histamine wheal. Electron-dense deposits (D) are present in vessel wall between endothelial cell (E) and pericytes (P). Clumps of fibrin (F) are present in perivascular area. Neutrophil (N). × 6840. (From Braverman, I. M., and Yen, A.: Demonstration of immune complexes in spontaneous and histamine-induced lesions and in normal skin of patients with leukocytoclastic angiitis. J. Invest. Dermatol., *64*:105, 1975.)

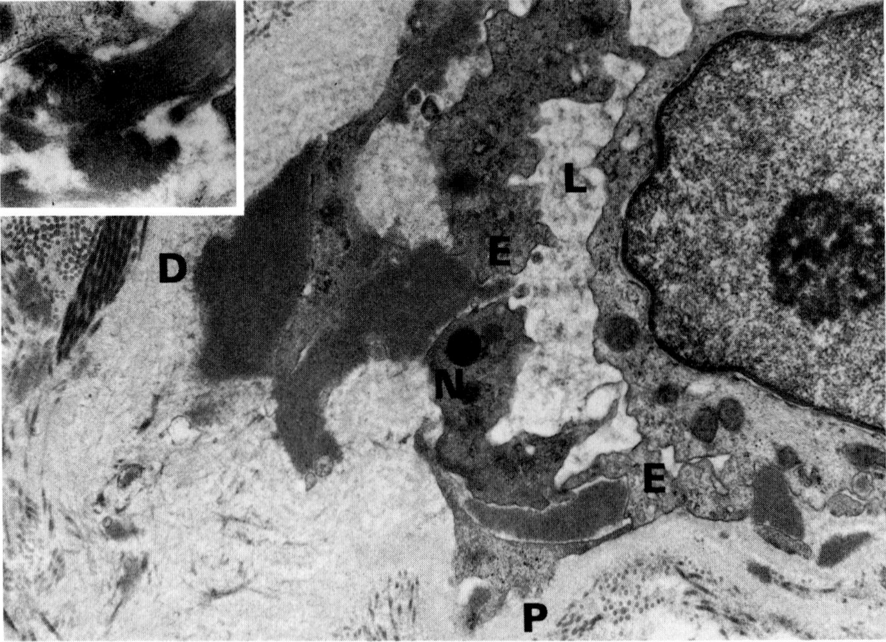

Figure 8–36. Histamine wheal. Electron-dense deposits (D) are present in endothelial cell gap (E-E) along with portion of neutrophil (N) identified by its granule. Deposit is dense and amorphous. Lumen (L), pericyte (P). × 14,630. Inset shows fibrillar nature of fibrin. × 21,500. (From Braverman, I. M., and Yen, A.: Demonstration of immune complexes in spontaneous and histamine-induced lesions and in normal skin of patients with leukocytoclastic angiitis. J. Invest. Dermatol., *64*:105, 1975.)

substrate C5 is being continually delivered into the perivascular space for a time. A similar scenario is believed to be responsible for the perpetuation of articular inflammation in rheumatoid joints.[99]

Although the release of C5-cleaving enzyme is usually associated with phagocytosis, it may also accompany the disintegration of neutrophils. Tick bites are an example of a nonimmunologically induced tissue injury mediated through complement and neutrophils.[100] C5a is initially generated by the action of tick salivary gland extract on C5, but subsequently production is related to C5-cleaving enzyme derived from the chemotactically attracted neutrophils.

Although almost all the available evidence indicates that leukocytoclastic vasculitis is primarily an immune complex disease, Soter et al. have suggested that in some patients a delayed hypersensitivity mechanism may be important.[10] In their series of patients with leukocytoclastic vasculitis, two groups were found: those with hypocomplementemia and those with normocomplementemia. In the former group, the perivascular infiltrate was composed primarily of neutrophils, while in the latter, lymphocytes were prominent. Gower et al. were unable to confirm these observations.[93] They noted that in their patients with vasculitis and normal levels of serum complement, virtually all the lesions contained both neutrophils and mononuclear cells. The relative proportions varied not only from patient to patient, but also in the same patient. The variety of histologic patterns encountered probably reflects the age of the evolving vasculitic process and other as-yet-unknown factors.

The postcapillary venules are almost exclusively involved in leukocytoclastic angiitis. In our studies arterial capillaries were only rarely affected. The postcapillary venular segment has important physiologic functions not present in other parts of the microcirculation.[102] A gradient of permeability, which begins in the arterioles, reaches a peak in the postcapillary venule and then decreases gradually along the veins; diapedesis of white cells occurs here in response to a variety of stimuli; and histamine, serotonin, and bradykinin act on this segment to produce endothelial cell contraction and gap formation, resulting in increased vascular permeability. These are some of the physiologic factors that influence the deposition of immune complexes in the postcapillary venules. This segment of the microcirculation comprises the majority of vessels in the upper dermis, where the histologic findings of leukocytoclastic angiitis are most prominent.

Clinical observations suggest that stasis and dependency may be predisposing factors for the development of vasculitic lesions. They most frequently arise on the legs and feet in ambulatory patients and can be found over the sacrum, back, and elbows in individuals confined to bed (Figs. 8–37 and 8–38).

Since the cutaneous postcapillary venule is the major site of involvement in small vessel angiitis, the term *cutaneous necrotizing venulitis* may be a more appropriate term than *leukocytoclastic angiitis*.

A major breakthrough in our understanding of immune complex disorders has been the recognition that circulating antigen-antibody aggregrates often behave as cryoglobulins.[86, 103-107] The cryoglobulins are usually of the mixed variety (Types II and III of Brouet) in which monoclonal (Type II) or polyclonal (Type III) IgM rheumatoid factors are combined with polyclonal IgG (see p. 226). Rarely, IgG or IgA may

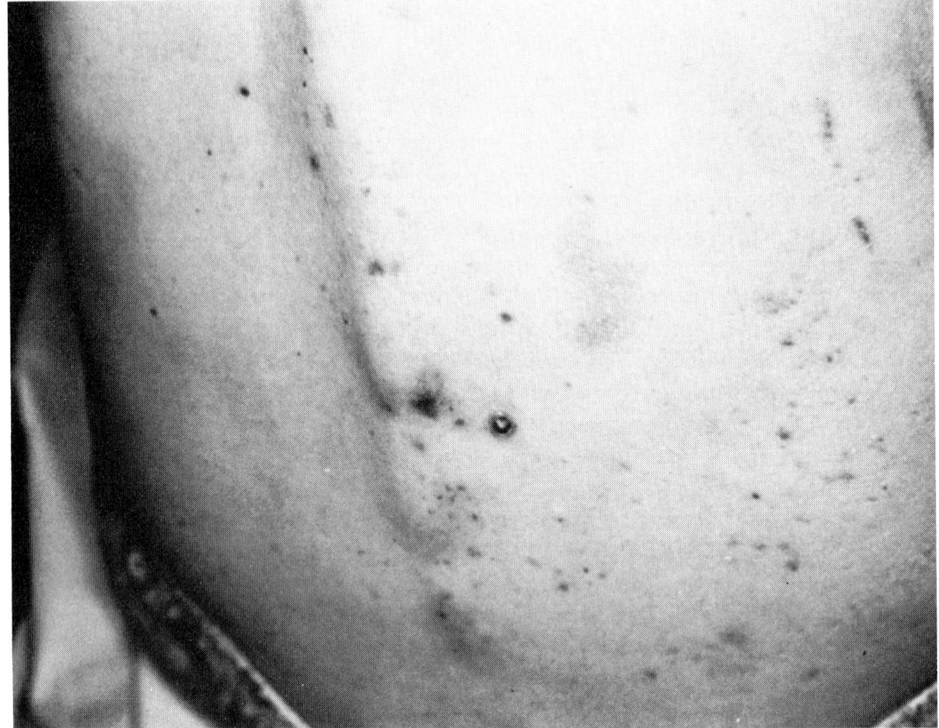

Figure 8–37. Leukocytoclastic vasculitis arising in dependent area of back in patient confined to bed.

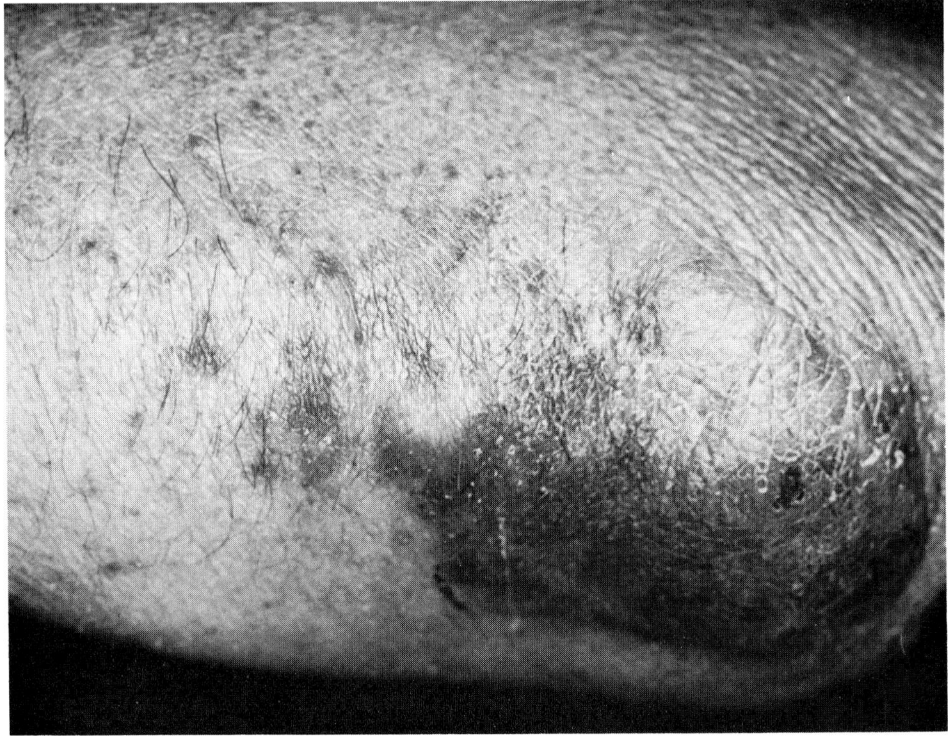

Figure 8–38. Leukocytoclastic vasculitis arising over the elbows of a bedridden patient.

develop rheumatoid factor activity and produce Type II cryoglobulins of the IgG-IgG or IgA-IgG types.[107] IgA, C3, C1q, and beta-lipoprotein are occasionally found as components of the cryoglobulins. In systemic LE, the cryoglobulins may be composed solely of IgM and C1q, or IgM, IgG, and C1q. In the latter instance, the IgM is a minor component.[108] Although the physicochemical basis for cryoprecipitation is not fully understood, it has been established that the IgM rheumatoid factor is responsible for this phenomenon in Type II cryglobulins; and C1q, in the Type III cryoglobulins containing this component in LE.

LoSpalluto et al.[109] and Meltzer et al.[85, 110] were responsible for bringing the association of mixed cryoglobulinemia with vasculitis to the attention of clinicians. Their patients had the typical features of cutaneous-systemic angiitis: palpable purpura, arthralgias, hypocomplementemia, and glomerulonephritis. Since their initial reports many patients with this syndrome have been recognized. Mixed cryoglobulins are found primarily in association with connective tissue disorders, chronic bacterial, viral, and parasitic infections, and chronic liver disease. The level of Type II cryoglobulins is usually high (> 1 mg/ml), whereas that of Type III is characteristically low (< 1 mg/ml).[107] Cryoglobulins may be found in normal individuals in small amounts in the absence of clinical illness.[86]

However, analysis of these cryoglobulins has shown that the polyclonal IgG, to which the IgM rheumatoid factor is reactive, *usually* displays no antibody activity against agents presumed to be responsible for the clinical disorder. This was an unexpected observation, because it was assumed that the cryoglobulins were identical to the antigen-antibody complexes believed to be causing the disease. The complexes should have contained the responsible antigen, as exemplified by bovine serum albumin in experimental serum sickness. Hurwitz et al. found that serum antibodies to the offending bacterial organisms in patients with chronic bacterial endocarditis were not preferentially concentrated in the cryoglobulins.[105] Although DNA–anti-DNA complexes are believed to be a major pathogenetic factor in lupus nephritis, DNA is not concentrated in the cryoglobulins of patients with LE.[107, 108] In other studies, antibacterial, antiviral, anticardiolipid, antinuclear, or red cell antibody activities found in the sera of patients with corresponding diseases were not concentrated in their cryoglobulins.[107] The major exception to this observation thus far is mixed cryoglobulinemia associated with hepatitis B antigenemia.[111]

In most instances, therefore, the mixed cryoglobulins that are capable of producing vasculitic syndromes do not contain the antigen that presumably initiated their formation. Bacterial, drug, or other antigens may be capable of altering IgG so that it becomes antigenic for IgM with subsequent formation of an immunoglobulin–anti-immunoglobulin immune complex (cryoglobulin) that produces a vasculitic syndrome. Alternatively, the cryoglobulin may be formed by IgM interacting with IgG molecules bound to an unknown and unsuspected antigen.

However, specific antibody activity *can* sometimes be detected in cryoglobulins, as in the case of a man with pulmonary coccidioidomycosis associated with purpura, arthralgias, glomerulonephritis, and Type II cryoglobulinemia.[112] In this unusual case, anticoccidioidin activity was found in the polyclonal IgG component of an IgA-IgG cryoglobulin. Although at present such an example is considered unusual, additional cases will undoubtedly be uncovered as cryoglobulins from individual patients in the future are more exhaustively studied. At present, there are at least two seemingly unrelated groups of circulating immune complexes that are capable of causing disease — those displaying the property of cryoprecipitation, and those that do not, as exemplified by DNA–anti-DNA aggregates.

The initiation of vasculitis is frequently attributed to drug reactions or infections. Yet it is only in a minority of cases that discontinuation of the suspected drug is followed by remission of the disease.[4, 66] McCombs had suggested that drugs may be one of the triggers that set off the pathogenetic mechanism responsible for the vasculitic disorder. That mechanism might be drug-induced alteration of IgG so that it becomes antigenic for IgM. In addition, if the immune system itself were abnormal in certain individuals, the production of these cryoglobulins could become self-perpetuating.

Recent studies of patients with Schönlein-Henoch purpura have demonstrated mixed cryoglobulinemia in patients with acute disease and in those with chronic nephritis but not in individuals who have recovered from this illness.[113] One third of the cryoglobulins tested have contained IgA, C1q, C3, and properdin in addition to the expected IgM and IgG. Direct immunofluorescent examination of affected kidneys and skin lesions has demonstrated IgA and C3 in renal glomeruli and cutaneous blood vessels.[63, 113, 114] Electron-dense deposits have been identified in the renal glomeruli by electron microscopy.[115] In one series, elevated serum levels of IgA were found in the presence of normal levels of IgG and IgM.[64] These observations suggest that the respiratory tract or gastrointestinal mucosa may be the initial site of contact with the agents, infectious or otherwise, responsible for initiating anaphylactoid purpura.

At present, in 1981, no one would dispute the fact that a wide spectrum of cutaneous and visceral syndromes are associated with leukocytoclastic angiitis (cutaneous necrotizing venulitis). A single organ can be involved initially with eventual spread of the angiitis to other organs; multiple systems may be affected at the onset of the disease; the illness may remain chronic and indolent or suddenly become more active and progressive; exacerbations and periods of relative inactivity are characteristic; and the joints, skin, and kidneys are the organs most frequently involved.

However, recent advances in our understanding of the mechanisms and etiologies underlying immune complex disorders do permit one to place some of the syndromes into clinically recognizable groups. These subsets are set down below in a *provisional* listing that may be useful in determining natural history and prognosis, and in devising effective therapy in future studies dealing with these syndromes.

I. Schönlein-Henoch Purpura. A characteristic entity observed in children following an infectious prodrome, probably viral in nature, but occasionally related to beta-streptococcal disease. It is distinct from the other vasculitic syndromes because it affects primarily children and young adults; it involves the skin, joints, gut, and kidney, but tends to spare the nervous system, lungs, and heart; it is usually benign and of relatively short duration; and it is not associated with drug reactions and connective tissue disorders.

II. Hepatitis B Infections. Hepatitis B antigen-antibody complexes have been the etiologic factor in the serum sickness prodrome of acute hepatitis type B,[90] and in some cases of leukocytoclastic angiitis.[91]

III. (Essential) Mixed Cryoglobulinemia (LoSpalluto-Meltzer-Franklin). Originally the entity was placed in the idiopathic category and was even considered to be a possible harbinger of lymphoproliferative disorders because the IgM rheumatoid factor component was often monoclonal. However, it has been demonstrated that 74 per cent of the mixed cryoglobulins studied in one series contained hepatitis B antigen.[111] The clinical syndrome of essential mixed cryoglobulinemia (purpura, arthralgias, nephritis) is distinctive enough to warrant a separate line in a classification, even though it may be shown that most instances of this syndrome represent a response to infection, especially with hepatitis B virus, as is currently suspected.

IV. Syndrome of Urticaria, Arthralgias, Hypocomplementemia, and Mild Glomerulonephritis (commonly called urticarial vasculitis). This clinical subset occurs primarily in women and is associated with an elevated sedimentation rate. Angioedema is sometimes present in addition to the characteristic urticarial eruption produced by leukocytoclastic angiitis (Fig 8–14).[54, 116] In some patients the eruption resembles erythema multiforme or bullous erythema multiforme.[117] The syndrome is considered to be unrelated to systemic LE or essential mixed cryoglobulinemia. Etiology is unknown.

V. Cutaneous-systemic Angiitis. The main clinical features of this subset are the cutaneous lesions of leukocytoclastic angiitis in association with a wide spectrum of visceral involvement that is unpredictable in behavior. This subset may be associated with the following disorders:

a. Manifestation of an underlying connective tissue disease such as systemic LE, Sjögren's syndrome, or rheumatoid arthritis (Fig. 8–39).
b. Sequel to beta-streptococcal infections as in EED and in some cases of livedo reticularis with intradermal nodules.[118]
c. Manifestation of a drug reaction.
d. Associated with lymphomas, leukemias, and carcinoma.[97] Figure 3–3 demonstrates purpuric papules in an untreated eight-month-old male infant with acute lymphatic leukemia. The upper dermis showed leukocytoclastic vasculitis and the lower dermis, a leukemic infiltrate.
e. Manifestation of chronic bacterial infections, e.g., subacute bacterial endocarditis, infected ventriculoatrial shunts, and infections in prosthetic valves and aortic grafts. Typical palpable purpuric lesions may occur in subacute bacterial endocarditis.[119] The classic peripheral signs of bacterial endocarditis, Osler nodes, Janeway lesions, Roth spots, subungual hemorrhages, and even petechiae are now considered to be manifestations of vasculitis rather than emboli from vegetations on the valves.[120] Figure 18–55 shows an erythematous papule on the palm of a 55-year-old man who developed a subacute bacterial endocarditis–like syndrome secondary to a staphylococcal infection around the base of his aortic valve graft. The lesion was biopsied 12 to 18 hours after it appeared. Culture of the biopsy for bacteria was sterile. Light microscopy showed a leukocytoclastic angiitis, immunofluorescent studies

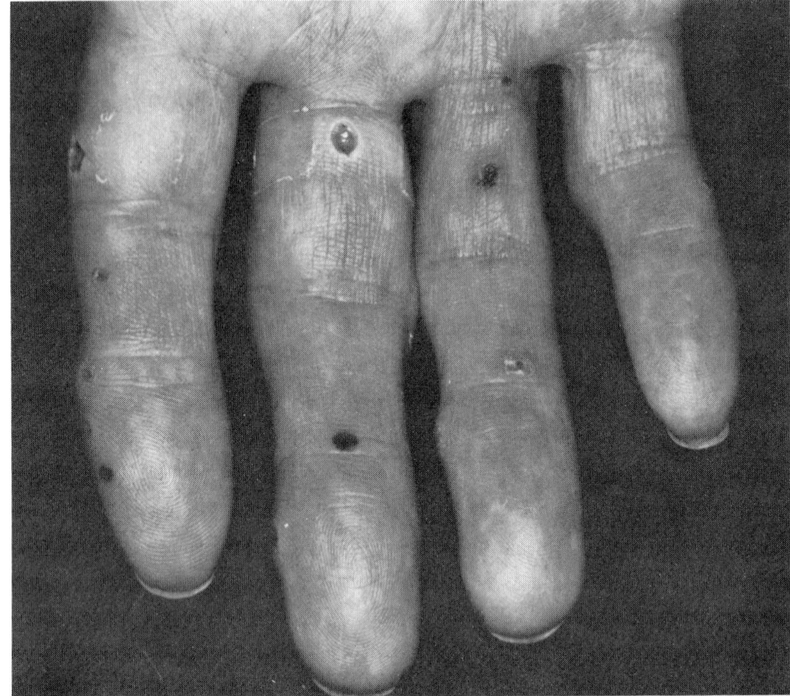

Figure 8–39. Leukocytoclastic angiitis. Ulcerated papules on fingers of man with rheumatoid arthritis. (Ulcer on proximal phalanx of second finger is a biopsy site.)

revealed IgG and C3 in the vascular walls, and electron microscopy demonstrated electron-dense deposits in the same sites.

f. Histologic basis for erythema nodosum in lepromatous leprosy, which is often precipitated by chemotherapeutic agents.
g. Manifestation of the serum sickness–like phase of infectious mononucleosis (arthralgias and an urticarial eruption).[121]
h. Sequel to intestinal bypass surgery for extreme obesity with urticarial, vesicular, and erythema nodosum–like lesions and arthralgias. A bacterial antigen, presumably related to bacterial overgrowth in the bypassed intestinal segment, has been suggested as the stimulus for the formation of immune complexes.[122]
i. Frequently idiopathic, with no obvious relationship to any of the potential antigens mentioned above: drugs, infectious agents, or abnormal cells or serum proteins in lymphoproliferative disorders.

In summary, leukocytoclastic angiitis (cutaneous necrotizing venulitis) can be diagnosed easily because of the characteristic skin lesions and diagnostic histopathology. However, it is a syndrome associated with several recognized diseases and with many etiologies, almost all of which are still unknown. The inciting agents and associated diseases need to be sought, since if they are eliminated or corrected, the vasculitis may remit. Usually, however, the disease does not remit and therapy with corticosteroids is indicated. The prognosis is good, compared to periarteritis nodosa, although the vasculitic process is completely unpredictable. One cannot determine in which patient the illness will remain stable and in which one it will become progressively more active. A significant number of individuals with leukocytoclastic angiitis remit either spontaneously or following therapy.

A point made earlier, related to the classification of vasculitis, needs to be reemphasized. There are patients with vasculitic syndromes in whom both visceral muscular arteries and cutaneous postcapillary venules are affected. These overlap syndromes of periarteritis nodosa and leukocytoclastic angiitis occur idiopathically as well as following serous otitis media and some hepatitis B infections. Fauci et al. have called these syndromes "systemic necrotizing vasculitis" and include them under the category of periarteritis nodosa. In many of their patients they were able to demonstrate aneurysms, vessel irregularities, and infarcts in viscera by angiography.[5] This is a severe, often fatal, form of systemic vasculitis if untreated, and behaves differently from the systemic syndromes associated with leukocytoclastic vasculitis in which postcapillary venules in the skin and viscera are affected.[3] This distinction cannot be overemphasized. The systemic syndromes of leukocytoclastic vasculitis have a much better prognosis than the overlap syndromes that are the equivalent of classic periarteritis nodosa. Since therapy with immunosuppressive drugs may be indicated in the overlap syndromes[123] but not in the leukocytoclastic syndromes, it is important that an effort be made to distinguish between the two by biopsies of organs that are reasonably accessible and by angiography of those that are not. The distinction between the two systemic vasculitic syndromes cannot always be made reliably on clinical grounds alone.

It is likely that after appropriate antigenic stimulation certain predisposed individuals produce soluble antigen-antibody complexes just large enough to be trapped in vessels and glomeruli. The physical size of the complex, rather than the specificity of the antibody, is a major factor responsible for the tissue localization and the initiation of the subsequent tissue damage. The inability of the reticuloendothelial system to effectively remove these complexes in order to prevent tissue damage has been ascribed to solubility of the complexes, because immune complexes formed at equivalence or in antibody excess are insoluble and easily removed. However, two recent studies in patients with systemic LE and cutaneous vasculitis indicate that there is a defect in the ability of their reticuloendothelial system to remove complexes containing IgG.[124, 125] The macrophages appear to be defective in receptor function for the Fc portion of the IgG molecule. This defect is correlated with disease activity and the amount of circulating soluble immune complexes. Plasma exchange is able to correct this defect. It is not clear whether the inability to remove complexes from the circulation is caused by a primary defect in Fc receptor function or simply because of receptor saturation by other circulating complexes. The slow clearance of immune complexes by the reticuloendothelial system would contribute to tissue deposition and damage.

It is likely that the pathogenetic mechanism for forming soluble circulating complexes that produce tissue damage is latent in a portion of the population and is activated by a variety of unrelated antigens. This possibility would explain in part why some patients develop urticarial drug reactions characterized by nonspecific perivascular lymphocytic cuffing, whereas others develop necrotizing arteritis and venulitis in response to the same medication. Experimental serum sickness cannot be produced in all rabbits. Only those animals that produce just enough antibody to make soluble complexes of appropriate size develop arteritis and glomerulonephritis; the same type of immunologic reactivity may apply to individuals with leukocytoclastic angiitis.

Although the etiology and pathogenesis of Wegener's granulomatosis and allergic granulomatosis are unknown, the small vessel arteritic phase of both disorders might be produced by circulating immune complexes that are related to the necrotizing respiratory granulomas and asthma, respectively, which are the major as well as the initial features of these diseases.

CRANIAL ARTERITIS (GIANT CELL ARTERITIS)

The carotid artery system is the site of an unusual necrotizing panarteritis that is characterized by granulomas and giant cells. The arterial divisions primarily affected are the superficial temporal and occipital and the branches of the internal ophthalmic, which supplies the optic nerve and retina. The angiitis occurs in a spotty fashion, so that it may be necessary to examine multiple sections over the length of the biopsy specimen in order to find the characteristic histologic changes. Synonyms for this disorder are temporal or giant cell arteritis. However, the angiitis is not limited to the carotid system; the subclavian, coronary, renal, mesenteric, pulmonary, and cutaneous muscular arteries can also be involved. The extracranial vascular involvement is frequently asymptomatic and discovered only at necropsy.

Cranial arteritis occurs almost exclusively in white men and women past the age of 55, but it may occur in the fourth and fifth decades.[126] Women are affected twice as often as men. The disease can be divided into prodromal, acute, and chronic phases. During the prodrome, which can last from a few weeks to three years, the patient may complain of fever, weight loss, and muscular pain mimicking polymyalgia rheumatica. Most clinicians believe this latter entity to be one of the manifestations of cranial arteritis.[127-129] Although a very rapid sedimentation rate is found in most individuals with temporal arteritis, it may be normal. The finding of a normal sedimentation rate should not be used to exclude this diagnosis in an otherwise typical case.[130]

The acute phase is classically ushered in with a severe and often unilateral headache that is accompanied by exquisite tenderness in the scalp over the temporal and occipital arteries. A common symptom is pain in the area of the temporomandibular joint during chewing or opening the mouth; this has been attributed to ischemia of the muscles of mastication. The affected arteries are tender, prominent, tortuous, and nodular; and the overlying skin is erythematous. The vessels pulsate less vigorously than normal; it is unusual for the pulse to disappear completely. Thrombosis of the superficial temporal or occipital arteries, which has been caused by the severe necrotizing inflammation in the vessel wall, can result in unilateral or bilateral gangrene of the scalp. Lingual artery involvement produces a red sore tongue that may develop gangrene.

In 50 per cent of patients with cranial arteritis, the eyes are affected at any time from a few days to two months after the acute attack has begun; the longest interval is six months and the average interval is one month. The ocular complications include ophthalmoplegia and a loss of vision secondary to retinal artery occlusion. Ophthalmoplegia is five to six times less frequent than blindness and is reversible; however, ophthalmoplegia may be followed by loss of vision in the affected eye. In most cases, blindness develops in only one eye, but the other may be affected a few weeks later. Unfortunately, the visual loss is almost always permanent; and ironically, the ocular complications frequently develop when the headache improves or ceases.

The chronic phase, which follows the headache and visual loss, can persist from six months to three years. During this period, patients may continue to have pains in the joints and muscles. An elevated sedimentation rate indicates that the disease is still active. Eventually most patients are restored to normal health, although their loss of vision persists. In one series, a second attack of headache, arteritis, and renewed ocular symptoms developed in 4 of 53 patients.

In some individuals extracranial arteritis has produced purpura, mesenteric thrombosis, renal insufficiency, peripheral neuropathy, pericarditis, myocardial infarction, and gastrointestinal hemorrhage.[131] When the aorta and its major branches are involved, intermittent claudication of extremities, Raynaud's phenomenon, aortic valve incompetence, and dissecting aneurysm and rupture of the aorta often develop.[132]

Although headache and scalp tenderness are invariable features of temporal arteritis, a patient with all the classic manifestations of the syndrome, but without pain, has been described.[133] Cranial arteritis needs to be considered in an elderly individual with the characteristic neurological and ocular signs and symptoms even in the absence of pain.

DIFFERENTIAL DIAGNOSIS

The differential diagnosis of the cutaneous lesions found in the necrotizing angiitides include those illnesses associated with purpura. Purpuric diseases can be subdivided into two groups based on whether or not vascular inflammation plays a significant role in the cutaneous bleeding.

Although purpura is the commonest skin sign in the necrotizing angiitides, it occurs in a variety of other disorders. The morphology of purpura can provide a clue to the correct diagnosis. Purpura may take the form of petechiae or larger spots and patches up to 5 cm. Larger areas of involvement are best called ecchymoses. Purpura may be oval and round, or irregularly outlined; it may be flat, or elevated because of edema and induration. Bullae and ulcerations can develop in any of the lesions larger than petechiae. The organization of the cutaneous microcirculation determines in great part the morphology of purpura (Fig. 8–40).

The microcirculation in the skin forms a horizontal plexus of capillary size vessels in the upper third of the dermis from which the capillary loops of the dermal papillae arise, and another horizontal plexus of larger vessels, arterioles and venules, at the dermal-subcutaneous junction. The lower plexus is derived from arteries and veins in the fat and underlying muscle. Petechiae and oval or round purpuric lesions are produced by involvement of the superficial plexus, and irregularly outlined (infarctive) patches are produced by involvement of the lower plexus and vessels in the subcutis. The pathogenetic mechanisms underlying purpura must operate through this vascular organization. Diseases with purpura as a major manifestation can be divided into two groups based on whether or

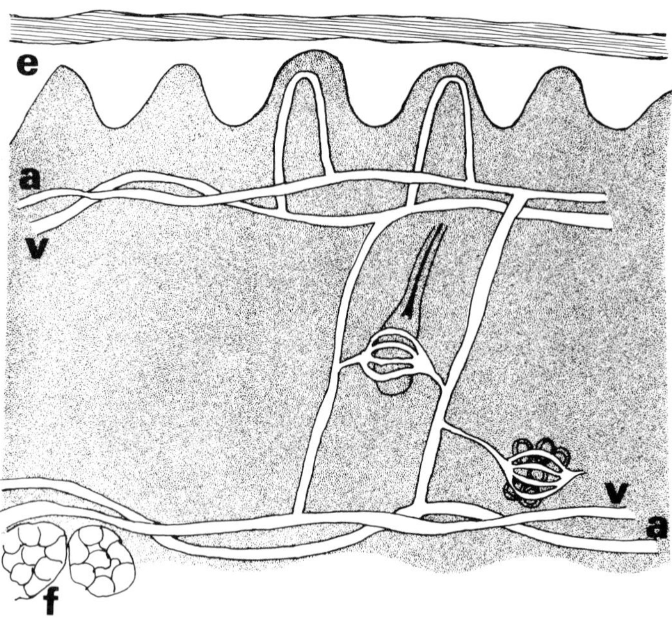

Figure 8–40. Organization of cutaneous microcirculation: e = epidermis, a = arterioles, v = venules, f = fat.

not vascular inflammation plays a significant role in the cutaneous bleeding.

Noninflammatory purpura includes those disorders associated with thrombocytopenia: the leukemias, the lymphomas, drug reactions, LE, thrombotic thrombocytopenic purpura, and rarely infections such as varicella, measles, and streptococcal disease. Petechiae and flat purpuric spots are characteristic of these diseases. The vessels in the dermal papillae and upper horizontal plexus are the source of the red cell extravasation. Scurvy (Fig. 8–41), uremia, and amyloidosis also produce flat noninflammatory purpuric spots but through mechanisms unrelated to thrombocytopenia. Common varieties of cutaneous bleeding include petechiae in areas of stasis dermatitis secondary to venous insufficiency, and large purpuric splotches (ecchymoses) that follow minor trauma to sun-aged skin (Fig. 8–42) or to the skin of individuals with hypercorticism. In both of these instances, bleeding probably results from poor vascular support provided by altered collagen and elastin in the dermis. Disseminated intravascular coagulation (purpura fulminans) can produce extensive flat hemorrhagic areas (Fig. 8–43) as one of its manifestations. The flat purpuric spots and petechiae characteristic of the above disorders are rarely observed in the necrotizing angiitides.

The cutaneous lesions in the necrotizing angiitides are produced by inflammation with its attendant increased vascular permeability and leakage of erythrocytes. However, two major differences exist between the small (leukocytoclastic) and large (periarteritis nodosa) vessel varieties. The upper vascular plexus is affected in leukocytoclastic vasculitis and the lower plexus and subcutaneous vessels are involved in periarteritis nodosa. In addition, thrombosis is usually a characteristic accompanying feature of inflammation in large vessel disease but is almost never observed in small vessel vasculitis. Thus, increased vascular permeability

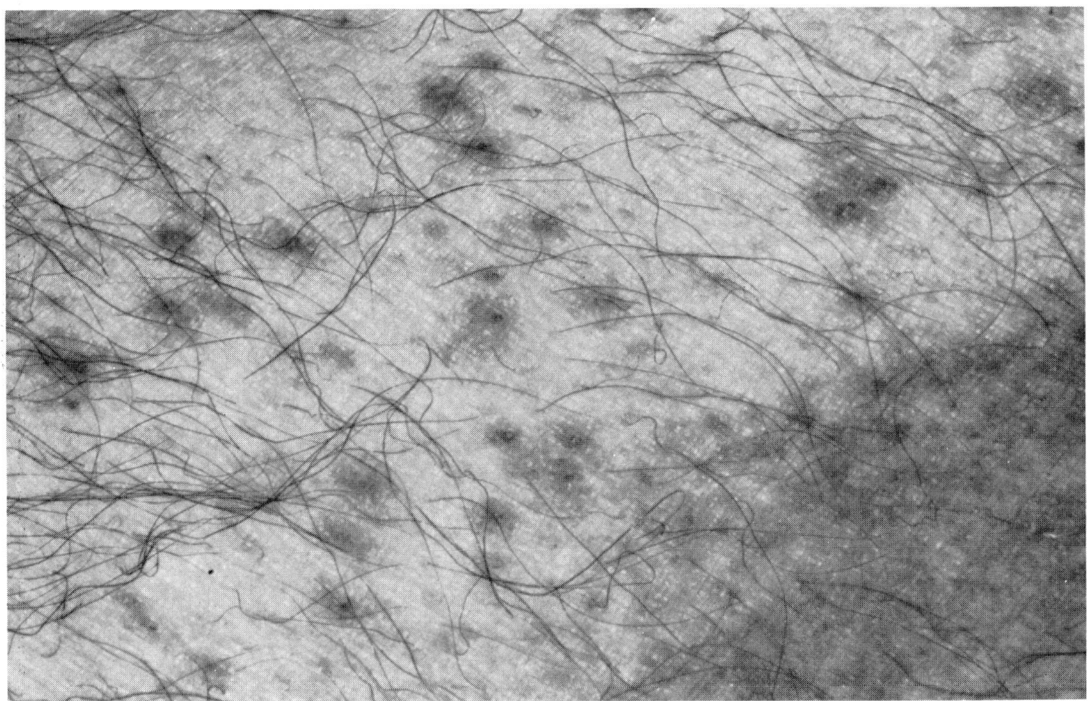

Figure 8–41. Scurvy. Perifollicular purpura. Corkscrew hairs are present in the center of many of these spots.

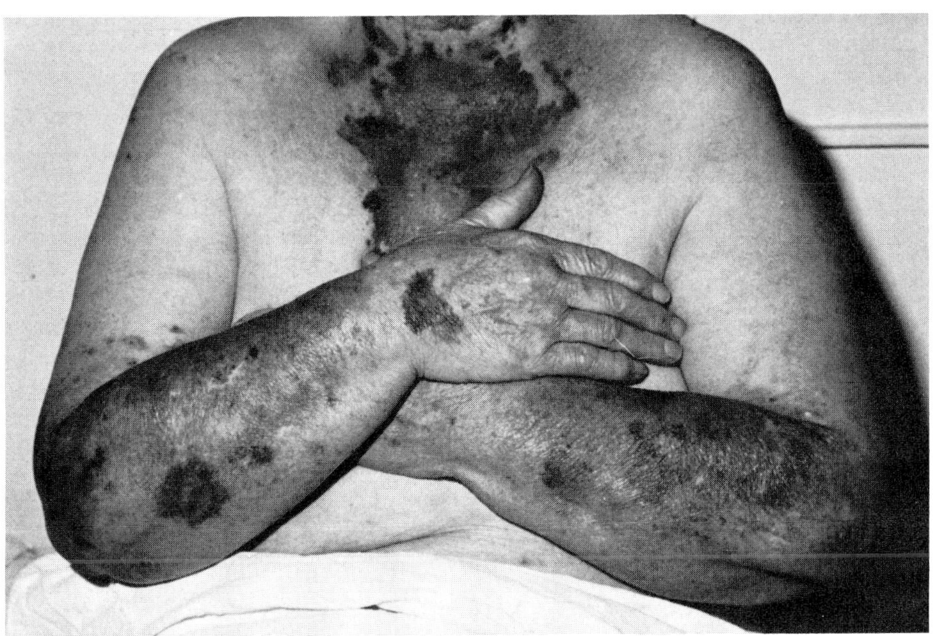

Figure 8–42. Purpura in actinically damaged skin.

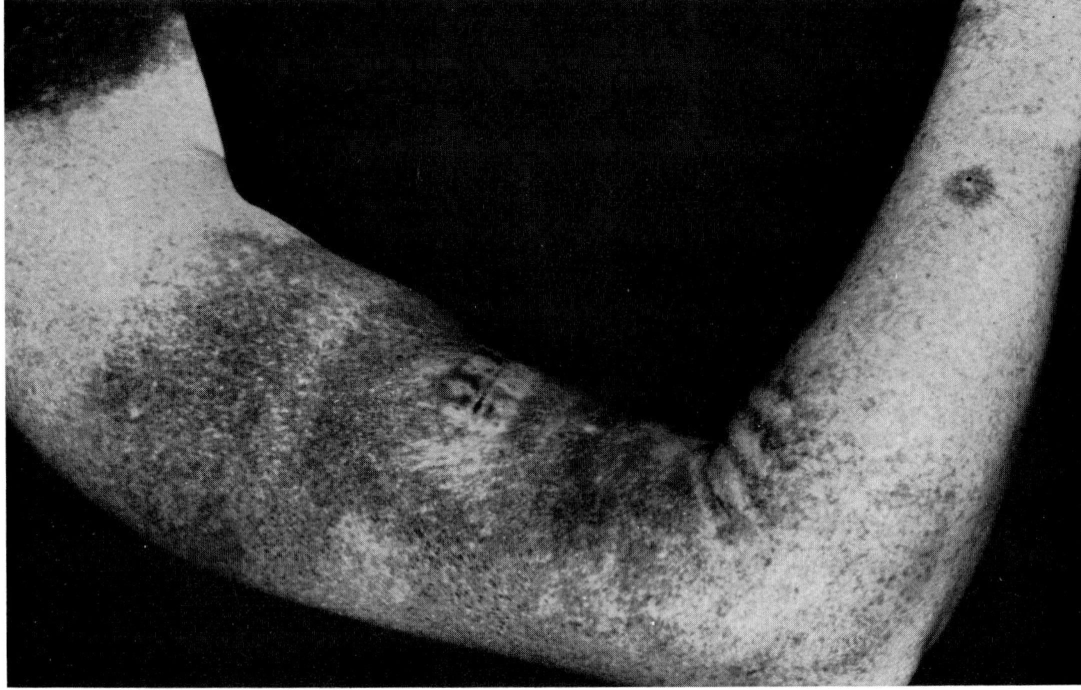

Figure 8–43. Purpura fulminans occurring postpartum. (Courtesy of Dr. Gerard Burrow.)

coupled with leakage of red cells from the upper plexus produces by radial diffusion *oval* or *round* urticarial wheals that become purpuric; inflammation and thrombosis of the deep dermal and subcutaneous vessels results in irregularly outlined areas of hemorrhagic infarction.

Other diseases can produce cutaneous hemorrhagic infarction. The most important illness in this group is acute meningococcemia. The cutaneous hemorrhage is usually slate-grey, indurated, deep, and irregular in outline (Fig. 8–44; Plate 24*C*). This purpuric exanthem is usually generalized and ranges from spots of 1 mm to infarctive plaques of several centimeters. The lesions in acute meningococcemia are most likely caused by a combination of direct bacterial injury to the vessels and disseminated intravascular coagulation. The meningococcus can be isolated from the eruption. Sometimes viral meningitis, caused by ECHO virus type 9 and Coxsackie virus, group A, type 9, may be accompanied by petechiae that mimic the shower of flat petechiae observed in meningococcemia. Rocky Mountain spotted fever is characterized by erythematous and purpuric macules, papules, and vesicles that begin on the distal parts of the extremities and spread centripetally. Disseminated intravascular coagulation also produces infarctive hemorrhagic and bullous plaques, but they are usually much larger and fewer in number than those seen in meningococcemia or vasculitis (Figs. 18–13 to 18–15). However, all of these individuals are critically ill and toxic, whereas individuals with localized or even widespread cutaneous vasculitis appear relatively healthy at the onset of the angiitis.

Acute gonococcemia is associated with small numbers of cutaneous lesions, primarily on the hands and fingers, accompanied by fever, chills, arthralgias, tenosynovitis, and myalgias. The eruption is characterized by

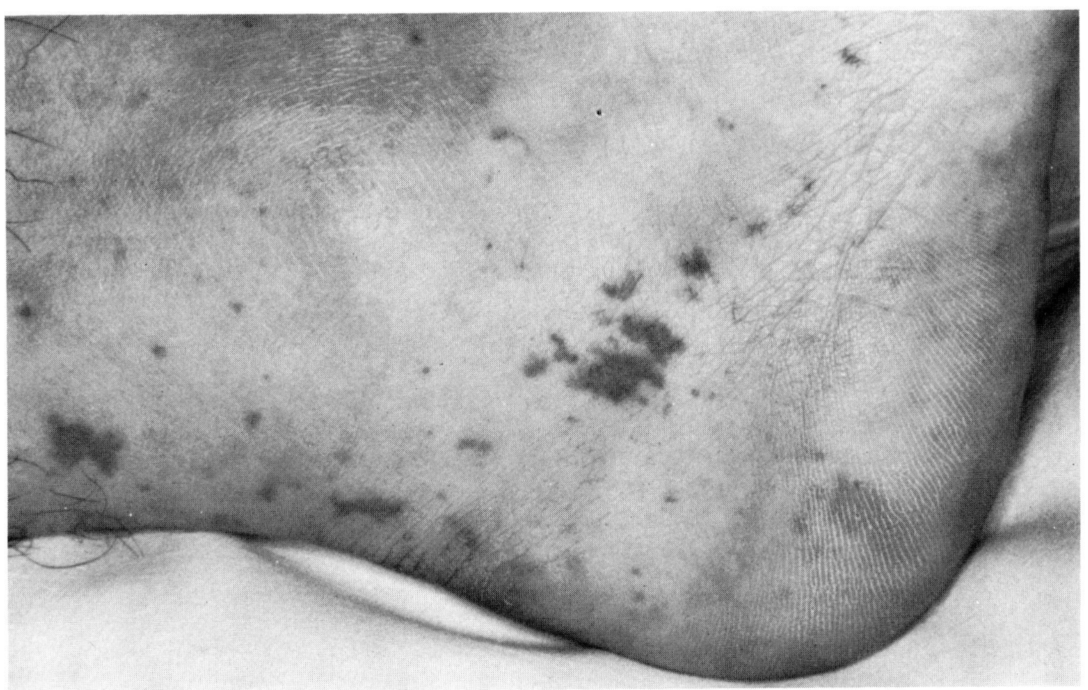

Figure 8–44. Meningococcemia. Purpuric lesions are irregular in outline, indurated, and often "gun-metal" gray.

hemorrhagic vesicopustules, or erythematous macules and papules that develop purpura limited to the central portion of the lesion (Plate 40*D*), in contrast to the erythematous wheals of leukocytoclastic angiitis which becomes uniformly purpuric (Fig. 8–12). The gonococcus can be identified in the skin lesions by smears and immunofluorescent techniques, but it is not easily cultured.[134, 135]

Chronic meningococcemia is usually characterized by a morbilliform eruption in association with fever, joint pain, and bacteremia. However, in a minority of cases, lesions indistinguishable from those of acute gonococcemia appear during the febrile episodes. The erythematous macules and papules may develop purpuric centers and ulcerate, but the organism is rarely isolated from the lesions.[136]

Although erythema multiforme is characterized by urticarial lesions that become purpuric, the quality of the cutaneous hemorrhage distinguishes this disease from the vasculitides. In erythema multiforme, the purpura is frequently petechial and requires a magnifying lens to be seen; homogeneous heavy bleeding within a wheal is not observed. The purpuric urticarial lesions of leukocytoclastic angiitis may ulcerate with or without preceding blister formation. In erythema multiforme, the bullae are rarely hemorrhagic, and the wheals never ulcerate in the absence of blisters. Cutaneous necrosis is an important sign of vasculitis, but it is infrequent in erythema multiforme. If iris lesions are present, the diagnosis of erythema multiforme can be established. Histologic examination of a cutaneous lesion will also differentiate the two disorders.

Schamberg's disease is a common benign capillaritis that also should not be confused with the vasculitides (Figs. 8–45 and 8–46; Plate 24*D*). Collections of lymphocytes are found around the dermal capillaries; neutrophils, nuclear dust, and fibrinoid necrosis are not present. Variants

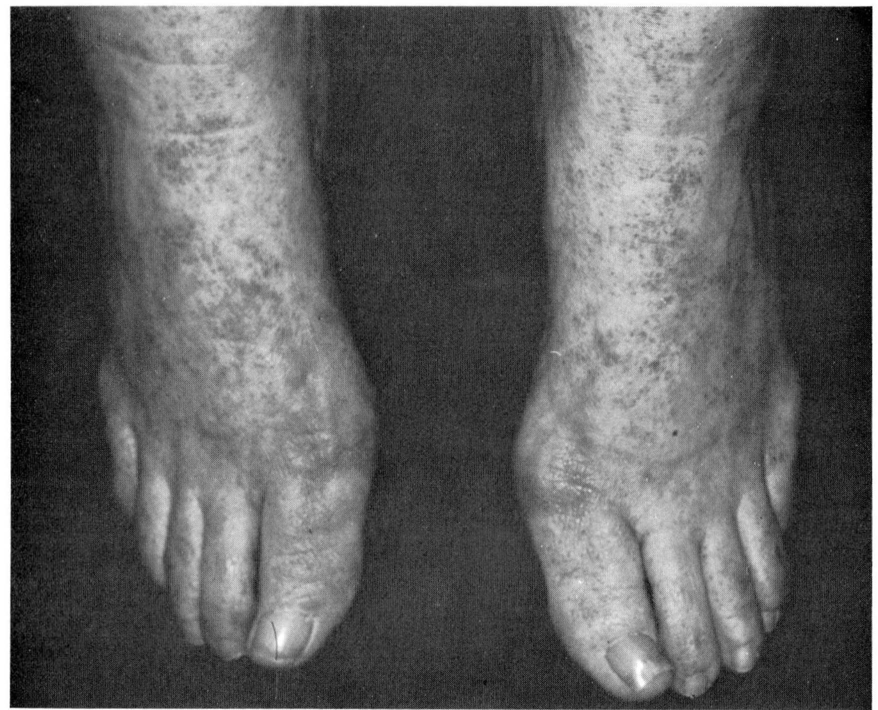

Figure 8–45. Schamberg's disease (benign capillaritis).

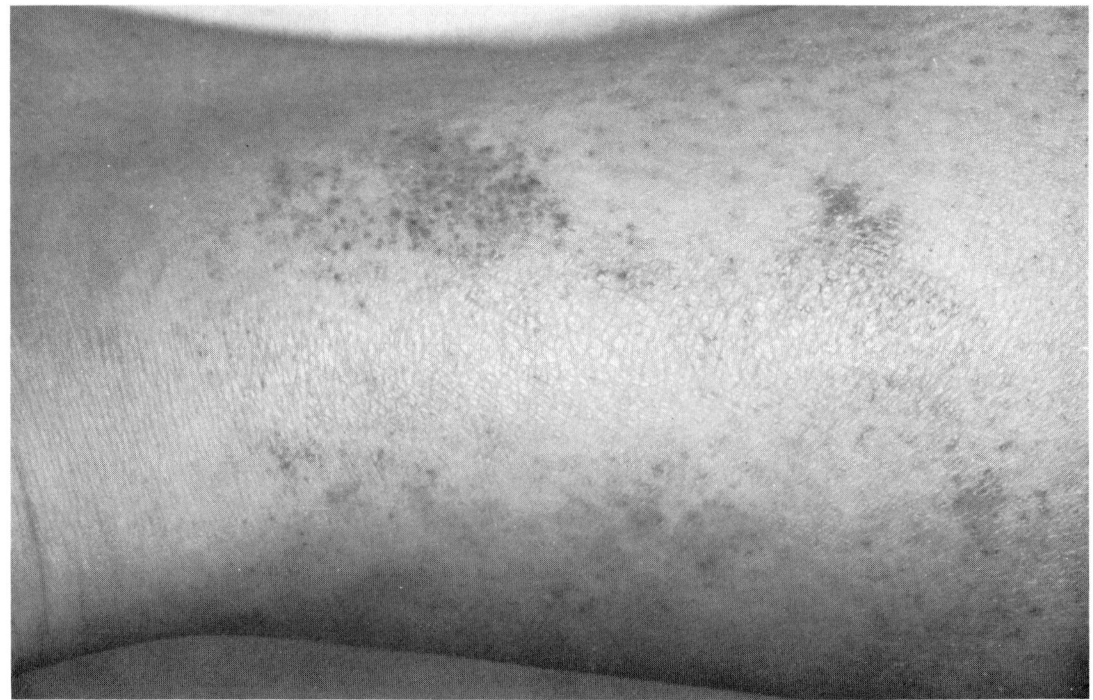

Figure 8–46. Schamberg's disease. Note the fine petechiae on a background of hemosiderin characteristic of capillaritis.

of this disease are Majocchi's purpura annularis telangiectodes and the pigmented purpuric lichenoid dermatosis of Gougerot and Blum.[137] The typical lesions are discrete brown or yellow-brown patches sprinkled with red or reddish-brown spots the size of pinpoints, representing freshly extravasated red cells and hemosiderin, respectively. Schamberg's disease begins on the lower legs and may spread to involve the entire limb. Extension to the trunk and upper limbs is rare. Pruritus is uncommon.

Itching purpura is the name given to a rare entity that clinically and histologically seems to represent a generalized Schamberg's disease. In one of our patients, typical Schamberg's disease was present on the legs for one year before the generalized capillaritis developed. The pruritus appeared with dissemination of the lesions. In two other individuals, lesions began on the legs and spread to involve the body within several weeks (Fig. 8–47 and 8–48). In our patients, this disorder remitted after one to three years.[138, 139]

Waldenström's hyperglobulinemic purpura is distinguished from Schamberg's disease by the absence of the brown or yellow-brown patches in which the fine petechiae appear; in Waldenström's disease the petechiae are larger and occur over the legs in a generalized, rather than a spotty, fashion (Plate 14*A*).

Purpura, petechiae, and hemorrhagic gangrene involving the tips of the fingers and toes can be a manifestation of vasculitis affecting the large and small digital vessels (Fig. 8–49). However, in the majority of such presentations, it is more likely that one of the following processes is responsible: DIC typically produces hemorrhagic gangrene of the fingers and toes (Fig. 8–50); persistent vasospasm of brachial and femoral arteries can produce a similar picture (Figs. 7–32 and 7–33); a prolonged decrease in cardiac output for any reason can be followed by gangrene of the digits because of inadequate perfusion of the terminal microcirculatory vessels (Figs. 8–51 and 8–52); and emboli from atrial myxoma[140] and from fungal vegetations on cardiac valves can produce petechial lesions on the digits as well as on other areas of the skin surface (Figs. 18–56 and 18–57). Cholesterol emboli from atheromata can produce not only acral petechiae, but also cutaneous ulcerations and subcutaneous nodules secondary to fat necrosis. A livedo pattern frequently develops in association with the ulceration and subcutaneous nodules, simulating periarteritis nodosa (Fig. 8–53). Biopsy of a subcutaneous nodule will show cholesterol clefts and atheromatous debris, but multiple step sections are often necessary to find these diagnostic features.[141] Primary hyperparathyroidism or secondary hyperparathyroidism caused by chronic renal insufficiency can result in vascular calcification leading to digital gangrene because of decreased perfusion (Plate 30*D*). Infection and birth control pills may precipitate small thromboses leading to persistent digital cyanosis or gangrene of the fingers in individuals with preexisting vascular anomalies of the hands and fingers.[142] Hypertensive patients being treated with beta-blockers often develop Raynaud's phenomenon and when stressed by cold weather may in addition develop pain and cutaneous necrosis of the feet and toes.[143, 144] The anticoagulant bishydroxycoumarin and its congeners can produce gangrene of the toes and feet as well as areas of hemorrhagic infarction elsewhere on the skin surface. These events typically appear within the third to tenth day after initiating anticoagulant therapy, and almost exclusively in women.[145] Histologically

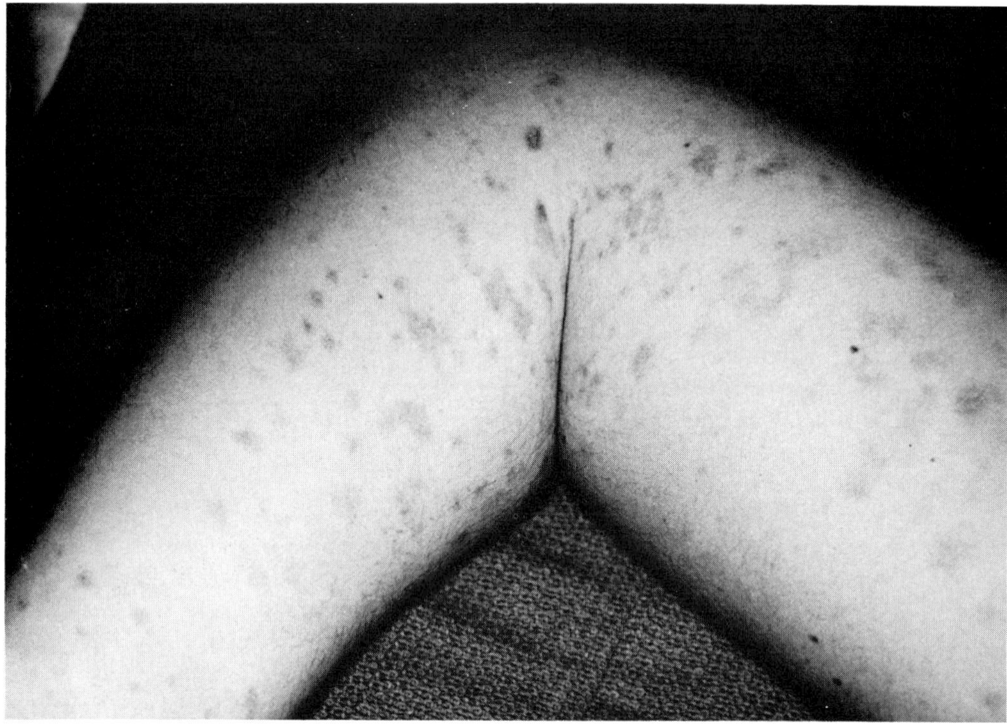

Figure 8–47. Itching purpura. Lesions were generalized over limbs and trunk.

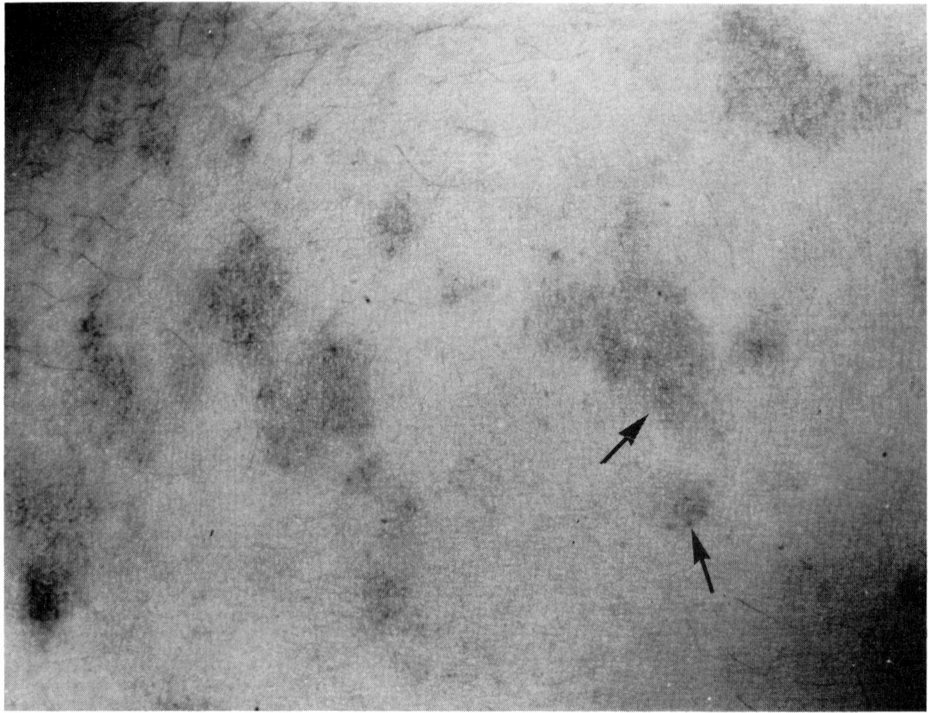

Figure 8–48. Itching purpura. Close-up of individual lesions depicted in Figure 8–47, showing flat brown patches of hemosiderin containing petechiae (arrows).

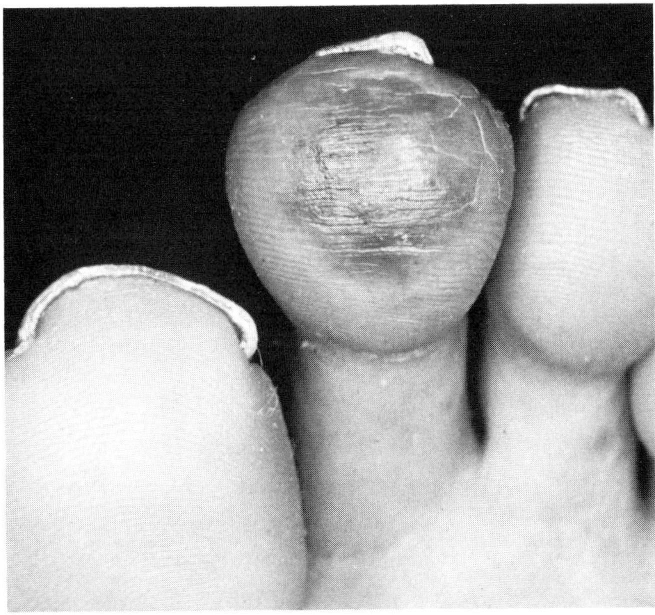

Figure 8–49. Leukocytoclastic vasculitis affecting toe of patient with rheumatoid arthritis.

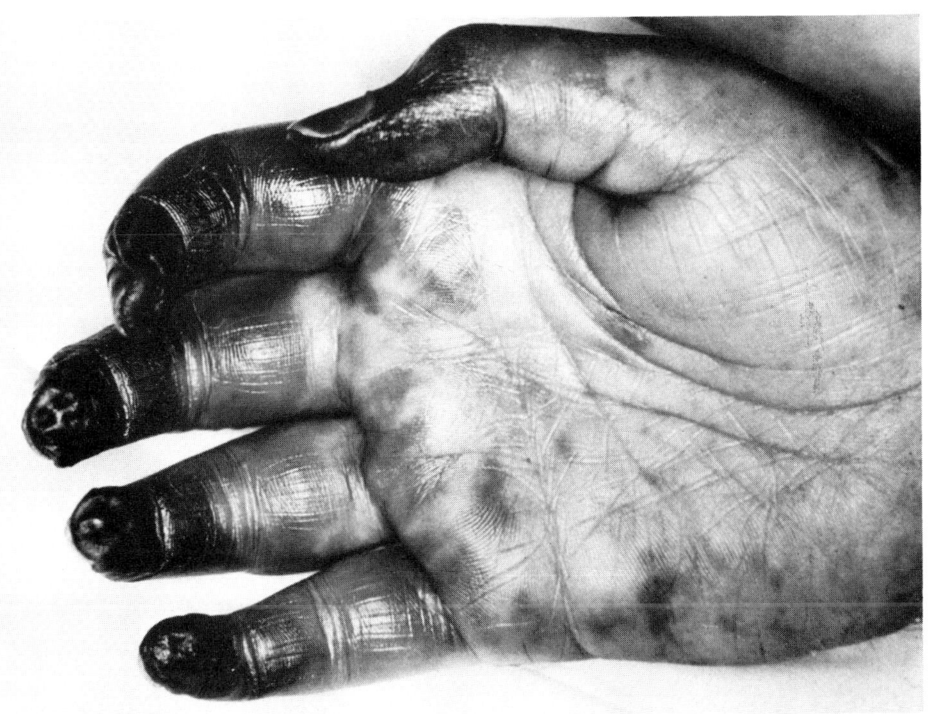

Figure 8–50. Disseminated intravascular coagulation producing hemorrhage and gangrene of fingers in patient with septicemia.

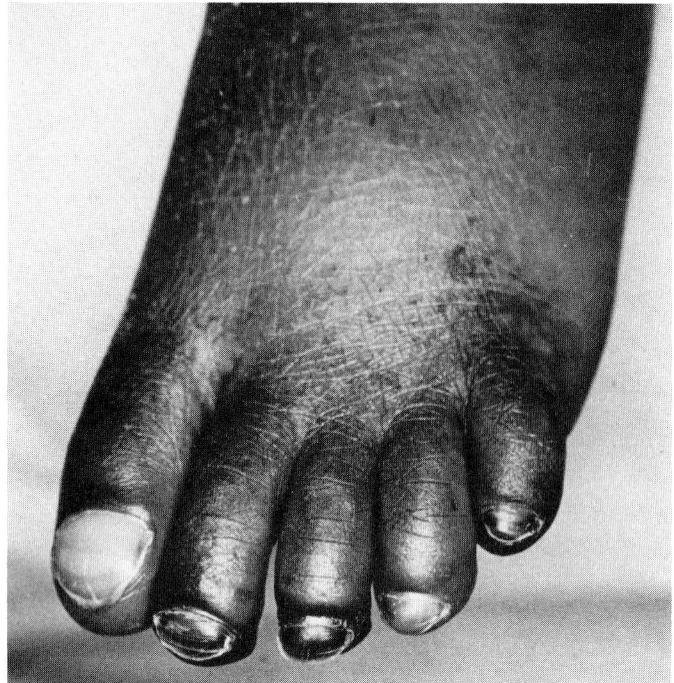

Figure 8–51. Digital gangrene produced by prolonged decrease in cardiac output in nine-year-old girl following open heart surgery.

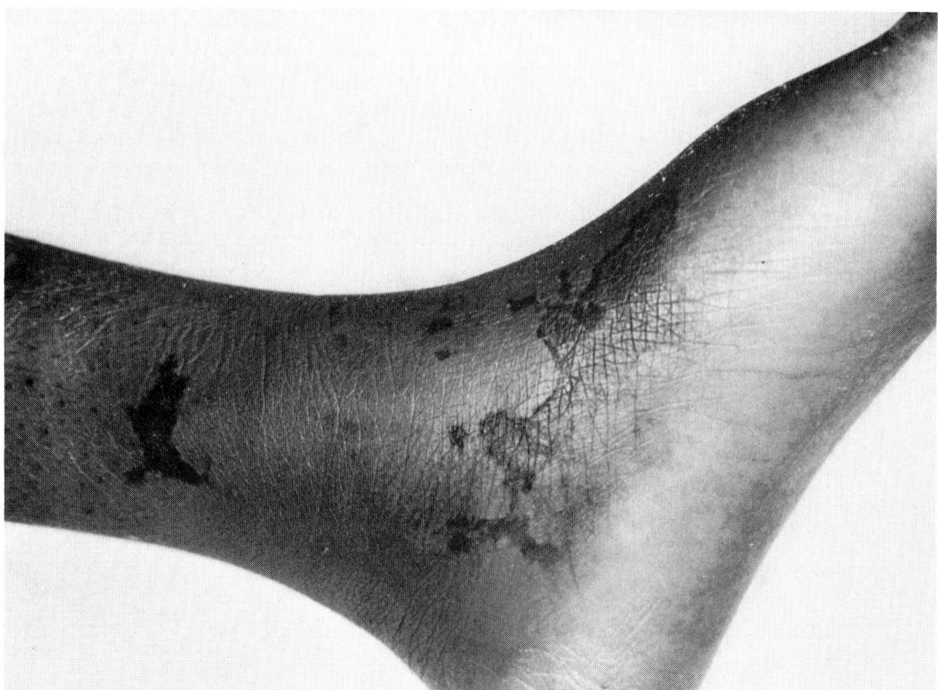

Figure 8–52. Hemorrhagic infarction of feet and legs in patient shown in Figure 8–51.

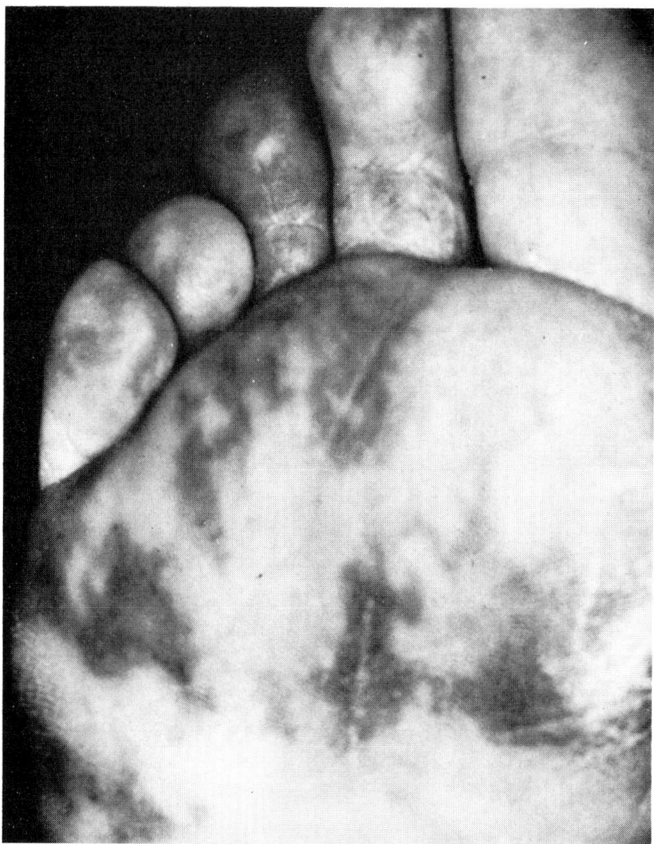

Figure 8–53. Cholesterol emboli from atheromatous plaques producing a dusky to purpuric livedo pattern.

one finds thromboses in the capillaries and venules in the skin and subcutaneous fat. There is no evidence of vasculitis. The reasons for this toxic localized intravascular coagulation are not known. Digital gangrene can also be a manifestation of polycythemia vera, one of whose major complications is arterial and venous thromboses.

Chilblain or pernio is characterized by patches of cyanosis or reddish-blue nodules on the fingers and toes (Figs. 8–54 to 8–59; Plate 24*E*, *F*). The lower parts of the legs and heels can also be affected. Ulceration occurs uncommonly. Chilblain represents chronic vasospasm of dermal arterioles in response to prolonged exposure to a cold, damp environment. The lesions persist during the winter months and disappear in the summer, only to recur the following fall or winter. The clinical course and histologic findings readily distinguish chilblain from necrotizing vasculitis. The histologic changes of chronic chilbain are those of an obliterative endarteritis affecting arterioles that is indistinguishable from that seen in chronic livedo reticularis with ulceration, to be described shortly.[146]

In the differential diagnosis of necrotizing angiitis, two other manifestations must be considered: cutaneous nodules and livedo reticularis. The cutaneous and subcutaneous nodules of necrotizing angiitis can resemble those of erythema nodosum, thrombophlebitis, lymphoma, sarcoidosis, and panniculitis. This manifestation of vasculitis is much less common than palpable purpura, and the correct diagnosis can be established by biopsy.

Livedo reticularis is a reddish-purple blotchy or reticulated pattern that is found chiefly on the trunk and extremities (Figs. 8–60 and 8–61). It

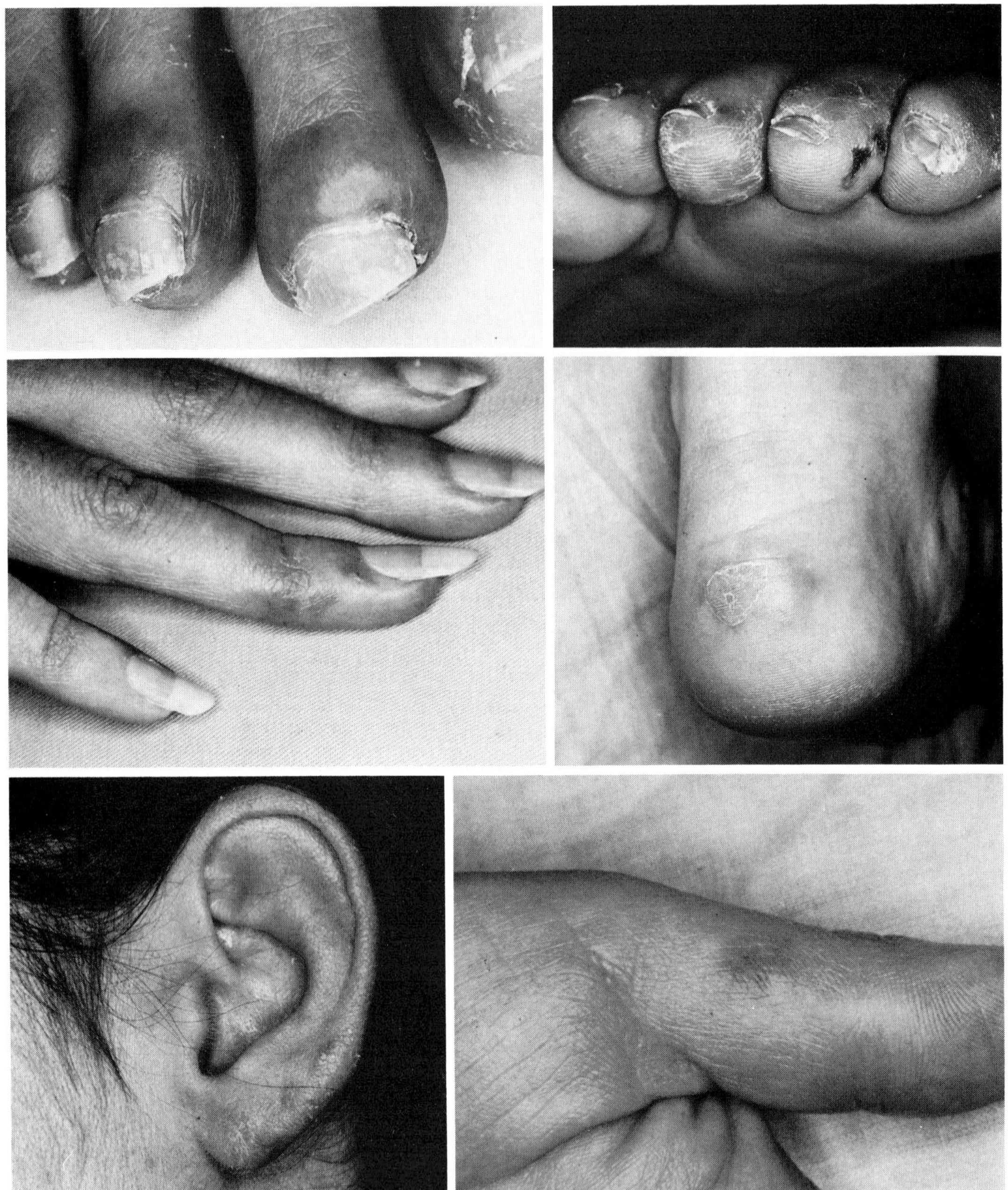

Figure 8-54. Top left. Chilblain. Reddish-blue painful nodules on toes.

Figure 8-55. Top right. Chilblain of second, third and fourth toes with ulceration of the fourth toe.

Figure 8-56. Center left. Chilblain on fourth finger.

Figure 8-57. Center right. Chilblain on heel.

Figure 8-58. Bottom left. Chilblain on inferior border of ear lobe. Induration, erythema and scaling are present.

Figure 8-59. Bottom right. Chilblaim on thumb.

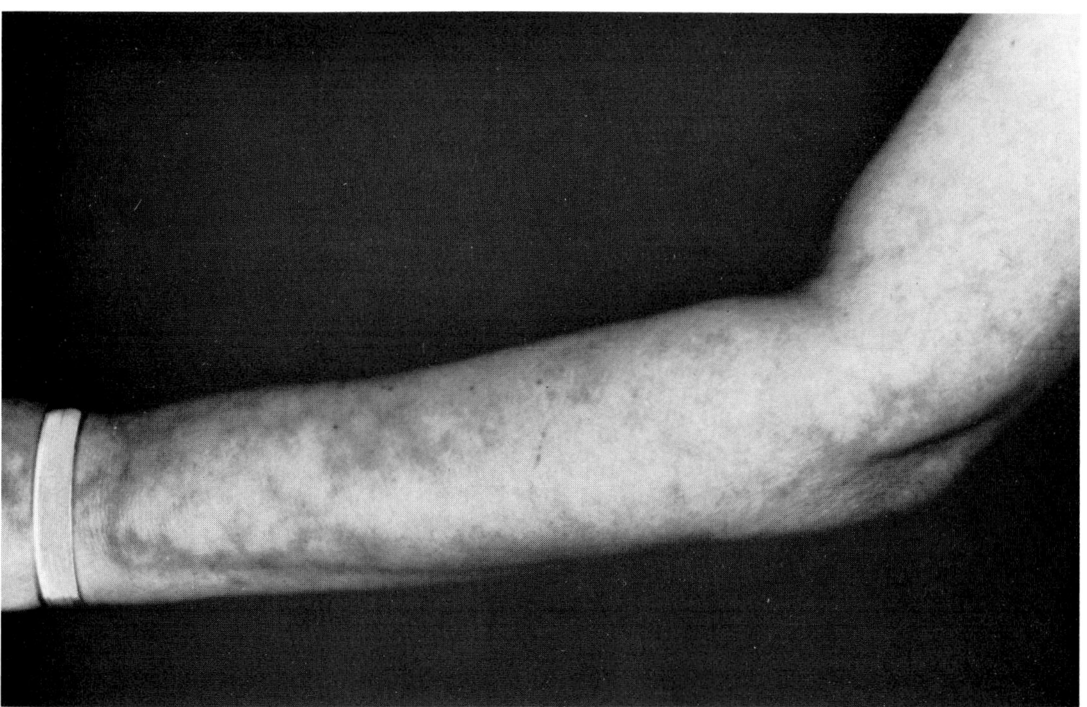

Figure 8–60. Livedo reticularis in patient with thrombotic thrombocytopenic purpura.

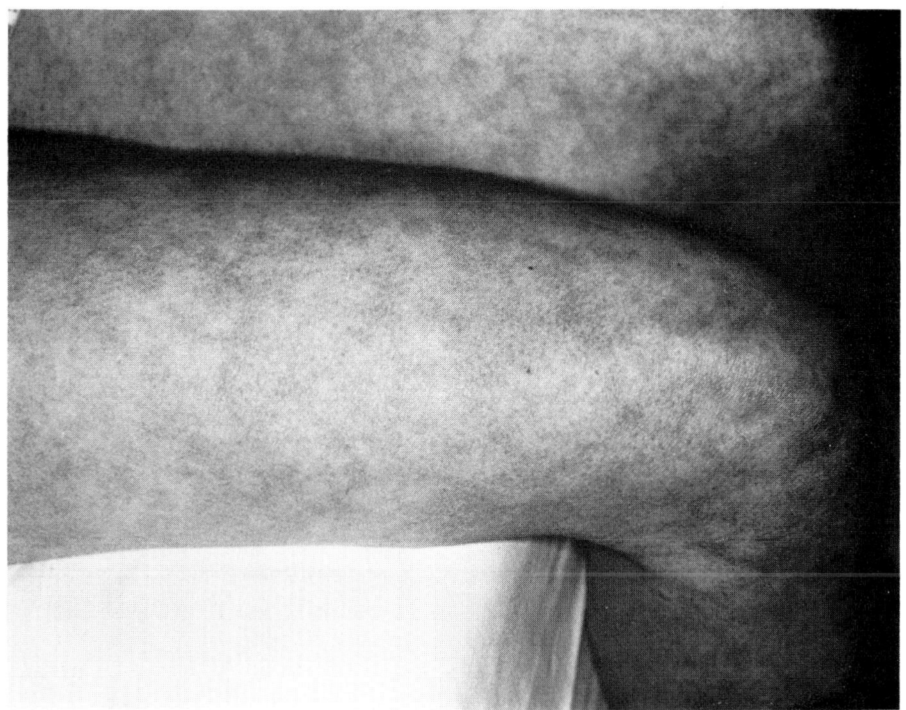

Figure 8–61. Livedo reticularis in patient with lupus erythematosus.

can involve the entire trunk and limb or it may be present in these sites as discontinuous patches. The discoloration persists even after the skin has been warmed, in contrast to the physiologic livid mottling of skin (cutis marmorata) produced by cold in infants and young children.

Although the blood flow through the purplish network, which corresponds to the superficial horizontal vascular plexus, is slower than through the intervening normal skin, the livedo pattern is thought to be caused by vasospasm of the deeper arterioles that supply this plexus.[147, 148] A biopsy shows arteriolar intimal thickening with narrowing of the lumen in patients who have had the disorder for several years. Sympathectomy and raising the skin temperature are sometimes helpful in alleviating the livedo pattern.[149] Whether venules are involved is still a controversial point. Leukocytoclastic vasculitis is not present in the livedo itself.

Livedo reticularis that develops in a blotchy interrupted configuration is usually a sign of a systemic illness. A continuous reticulated pattern that affects the entire trunk or limbs may also be indicative of an underlying disorder, but it is less likely. Livedo reticularis can be a manifestation of rheumatoid arthritis, rheumatic fever, idiopathic thrombocythemia, LE, scleroderma, thrombotic thrombocytopenic purpura, cryoglobulinemia, and periarteritis nodosa.[118, 148]

Livedo reticularis, accompanied by cutaneous nodules and ulcerations on the lower legs, can also be a manifestation of an underlying connective tissue disease. They may be the only manifestations of such a disorder for several years, before the other features of the disease reveal themselves. The nodules or ulcerations represent necrotizing vasculitis; the livedo pattern, arteriolar vasospasm. One of our patients had recurrent malleolar ulcerations in association with livedo reticularis for six years before the typical features of systemic LE appeared.

In some individuals the livedo pattern may become very intense in spots, producing irregular stellate-shaped deeply cyanotic papules and patches or deeply cyanotic puncta, 1 to 2 mm in diameter. (Figs. 8–62 to 8–69). These spots break down to form painful ulcers with black eschars, chiefly on the lower legs and ankles. This form of the disease has been called livedo vasculitis, livedoid vasculitis, and livedo reticularis with summer or winter ulceration depending upon the season in which ulceration developed.[150-154] Histologic examination shows hyalinization of the vascular wall with marked intimal thickening. The lumen is narrowed or occluded with or without fibrin thrombi. There is a surprising lack of inflammatory cells in and around the vascular walls in both livedoid vasculitis and chronic livedo reticularis. (Cutaneous periarteritis [Diaz-Perez and Winkelmann] can produce lesions that resemble the ulcerations found in livedoid vasculitis, but a biopsy would be able to distinguish between them.) Immunoglobulins and C3 have been detected in the vascular walls of livedoid vasculitis, but without any accompanying inflammatory cells.[155] A few patients with livedoid vasculitis have developed systemic LE, periarteritis nodosa, Raynaud's phenomenon, and peripheral neuropathy, but the majority have not had any associated significant illnesses.[154] One of our patients developed an IgA monoclonal gammopathy, and another, lymphomatoid granulomatosis, four years after the onset of their diseases.

When one reviews the literature on this subject, it becomes apparent that there is a spectrum of disease that begins with livedo reticularis and

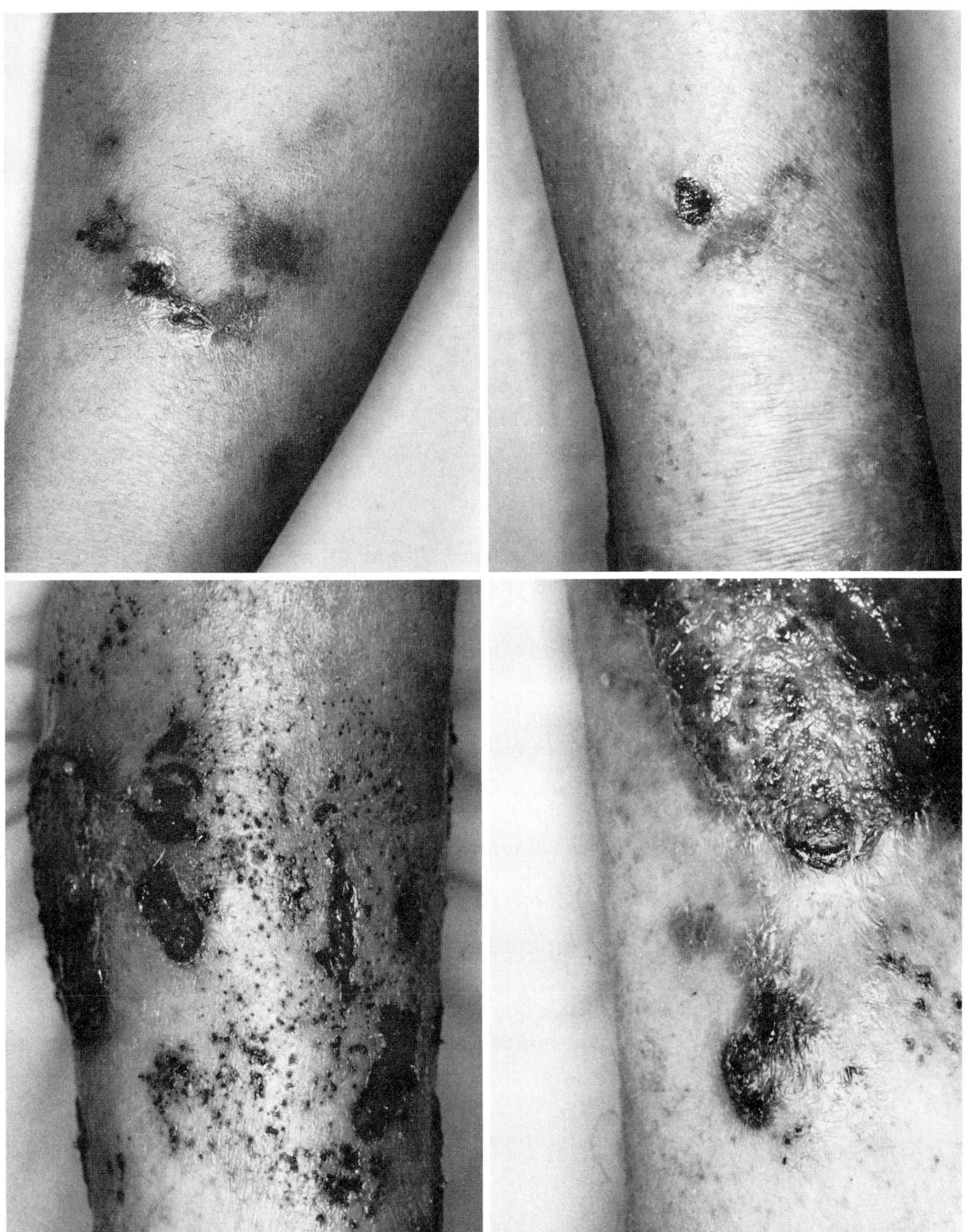

Figure 8–62. Top left. Livedoid vasculitis. Livedo pattern develops irregularly shaped dusky areas that become purpuric and ulcerate over the course of days to weeks.

Figure 8–63. Top right. Livedoid vasculitis.

Figure 8–64. Bottom left. Livedoid vasculitis. Punctate areas of necrosis are present in addition to large ulcers.

Figure 8–65. Bottom right. Livedoid vasculitis. Purpuric area undergoing necrosis.

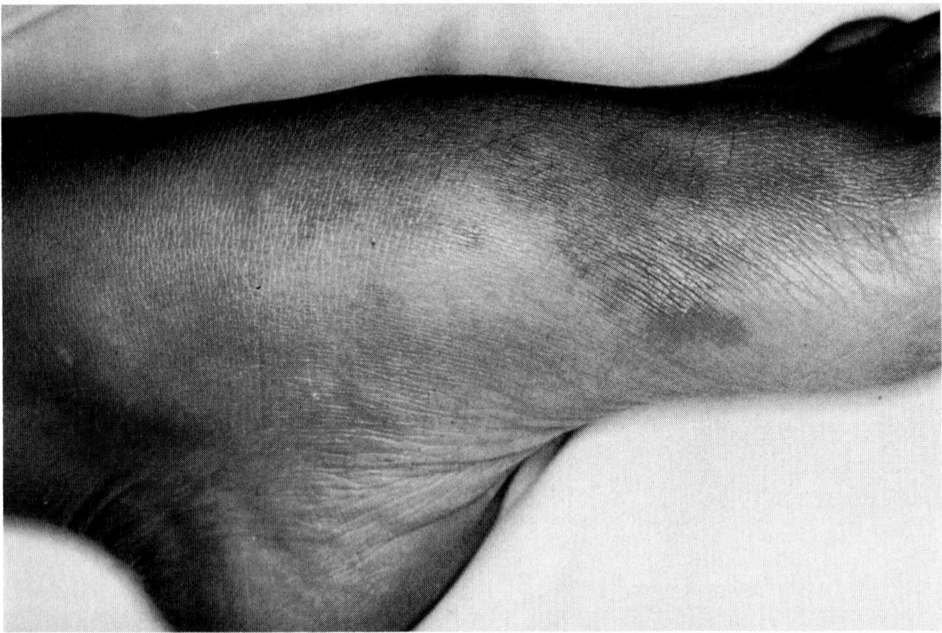

Figure 8–66. Livedoid vasculitis. In this patient, the livedo pattern was accompanied by the development of tender red nodules that showed the histologic features of livedoid vasculitis — an unusual manifestation. Same patient shown in Figure 8–62.

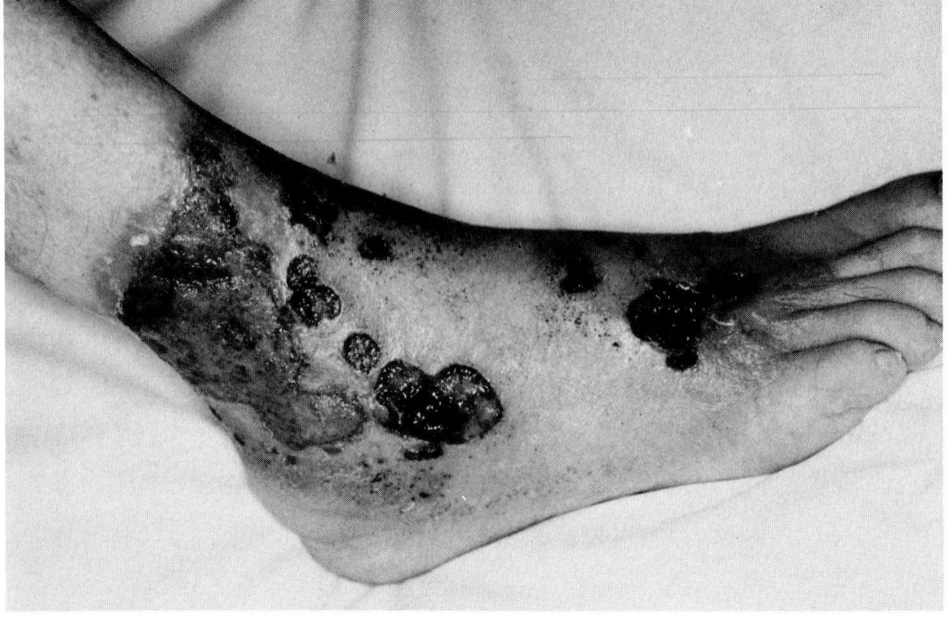

Figure 8–67. Livedoid vasculitis.

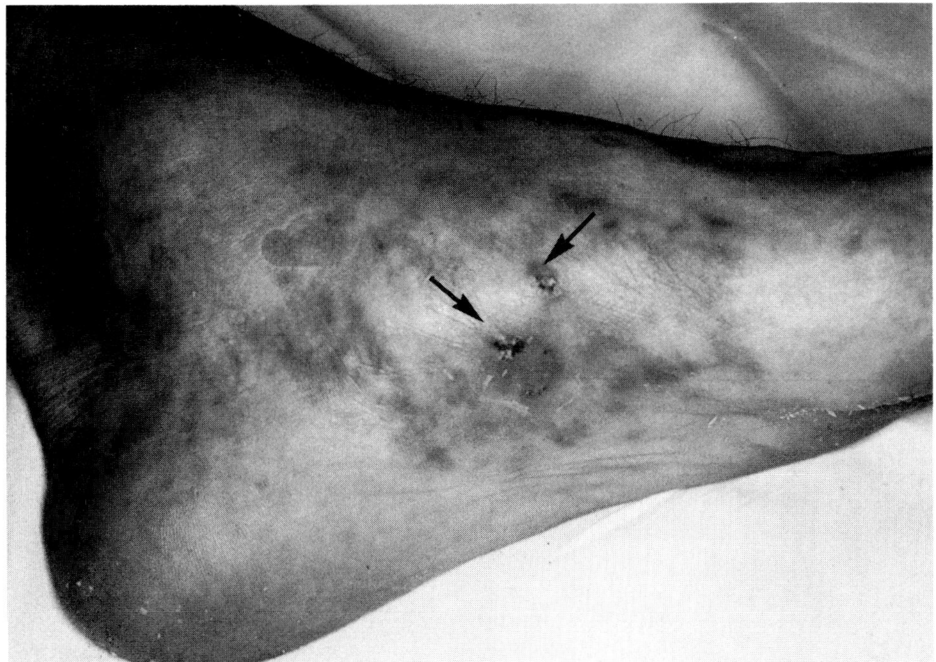

Figure 8–68. Livedoid vasculitis. Livedo pattern becoming intense and undergoing focal necrosis (arrows).

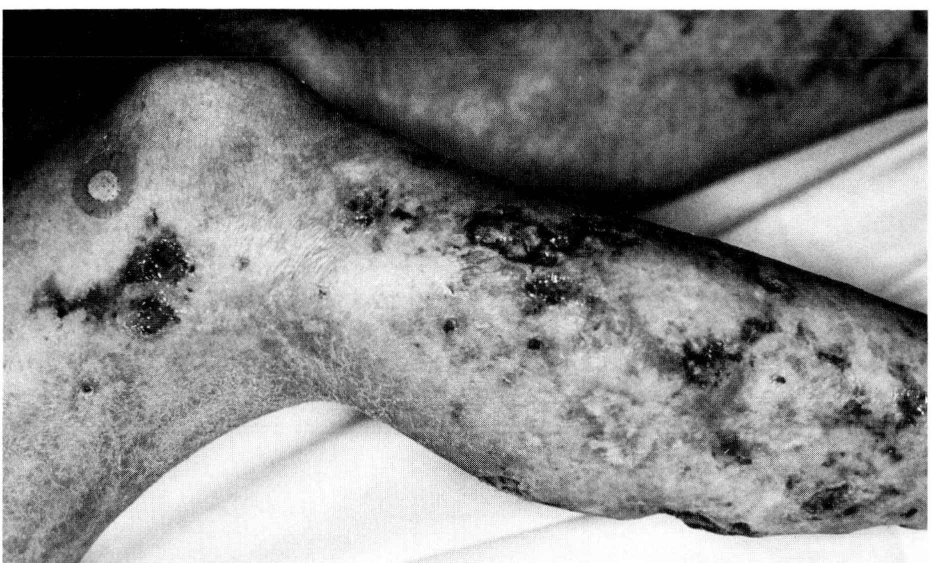

Figure 8–69. Livedoid vasculitis.

ends with livedoid vasculitis. Some cases originally diagnosed as livedo reticularis with ulcers have been later rediagnosed as livedoid vasculitis.[154] The histology of livedo reticularis and livedoid vasculitis differs only in the intensity of the endarteritis and is similar to the endarteritic changes found in Raynaud's phenomenon, chilblain, and the vascular lesions of scleroderma. A few patients with livedoid vasculitis have Raynaud's phenomenon, and their cutaneous lesions have been made worse by exposure to cold and emotional stress.[154] Cold weather has induced lesions on the arms, legs, and feet in one of our patients each winter for the past seven years (Fig. 8–66). I believe that livedo reticularis and livedoid vasculitis are merely two more clinical expressions of a basic underlying vasospastic process that also includes Raynaud's phenomenon, acrocyanosis, and chilblain. Vasospasm is a characteristic of connective tissue disease, and all of the phenomena mentioned above, except for acrocyanosis, have been associated with them. Careful long-term observations of patients with livedo reticularis and livedoid vasculitis may disclose that a larger percentage of them than we currently appreciate develop connective tissue disorders.

The presence of immune reactants without inflammation in livedoid vasculitis does not establish this disorder as an immune complex disease. Circulating immune complexes can be deposited and trapped in vessels made permeable by a variety of nonspecific stimuli such as intradermal injections of histamine, cutaneous application of ice, and dermographism.[89, 156] Chronic vasospasm produces endothelial cell damage that would also permit trapping of circulating complexes. Since circulating complexes can be detected in normal individuals as well as in those with serious diseases, the presence of immune reactants in livedoid vasculitis may not necessarily be significant. Long-term observation of these particular patients will be important in attempting to relate livedoid vasculitis to connective tissue disorders.

When the ulcers of livedoid vasculitis heal, they produce a characteristic ivory-white plaque that is studded with telangiectases and ringed with a hyperpigmented border. The term *atrophie blanche* has been applied to such scars (Fig. 8–70).[157, 158] Atrophie blanche is the end result of a variety of vascular diseases whose common feature is partial or complete occlusion of dermal blood vessels.

Sneddon described six patients with cerebrovascular accidents in association with livedo reticularis. In three persons the livedo and neurologic disturbances appeared simultaneously, and in the others the livedo had been present for many years. Angiitis was not found in the areas of livedo, and the cause of the strokes was not determined.[159]

Erythema ab igne, or fire stains, should not be confused with livedo reticularis (Fig. 8–71). This entity represents a reticulated postinflammatory hyperpigmentation that develops over the shins and abdomen as a result of prolonged exposure to heat from radiators, hot water bags, and fireplaces.

MUCHA-HABERMANN DISEASE

All of the necrotizing angiitides that have been discussed in this chapter are characterized by neutrophilic infiltration and nuclear dust.

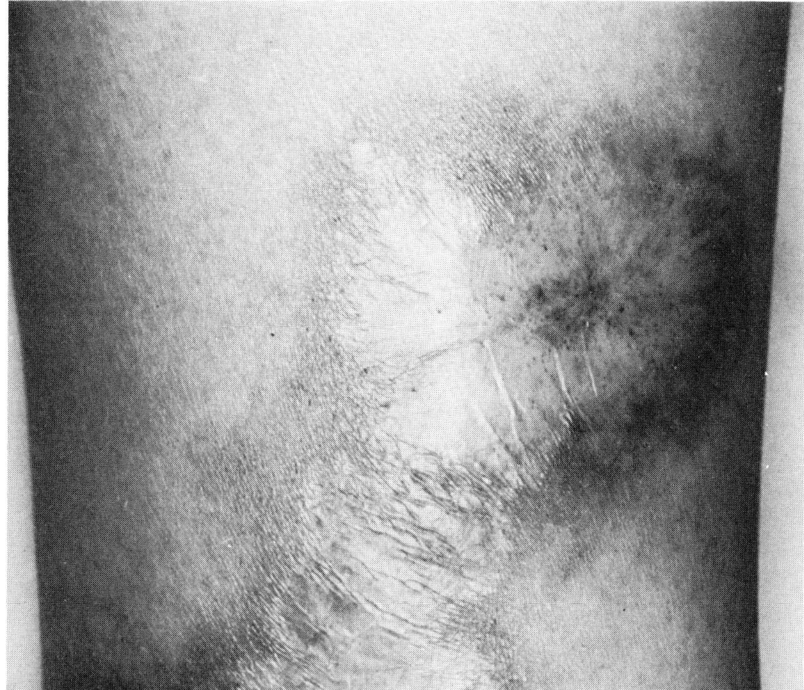

Figure 8–70. Atrophie blanche. End stage of a variety of vascular diseases but characteristic of livedoid vasculitis. Ivory-white scar studded with telangiectases and ringed by a hyperpigmented border.

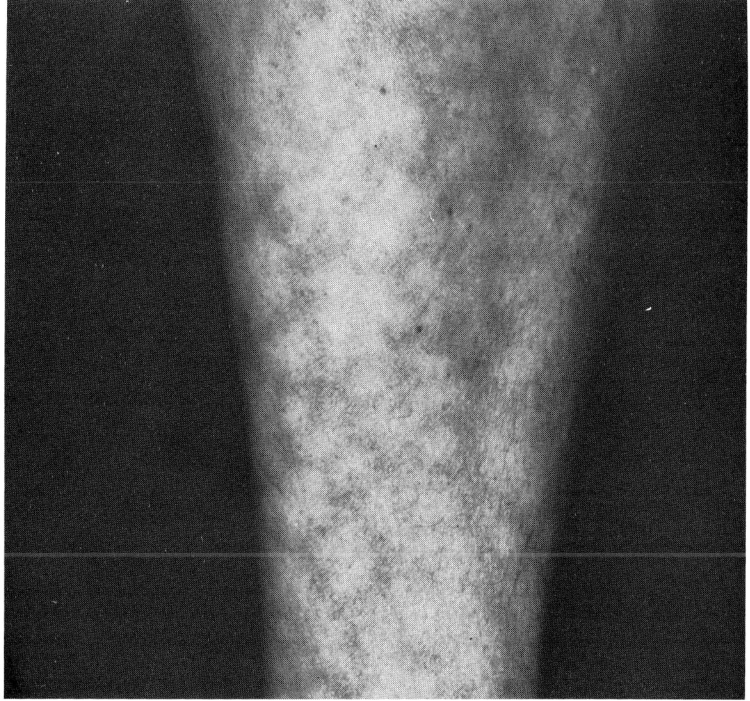

Figure 8–71. Erythema ab igne (fire stains).

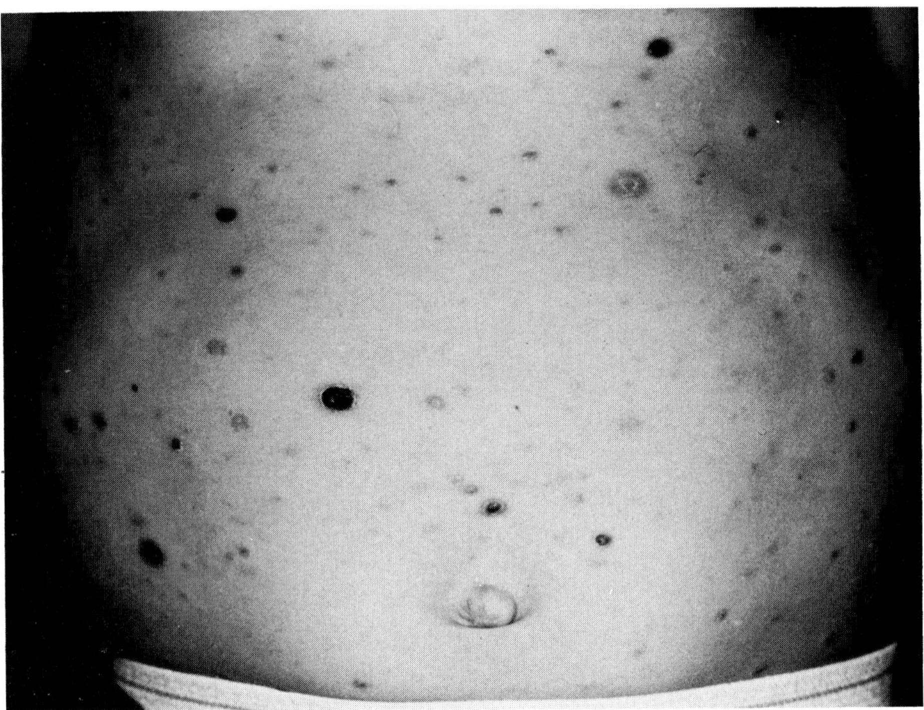

Figure 8–72. Mucha-Habermann disease. Crops of papules and papulovesicles in various stages from an acute eruption to necrosis and healing.

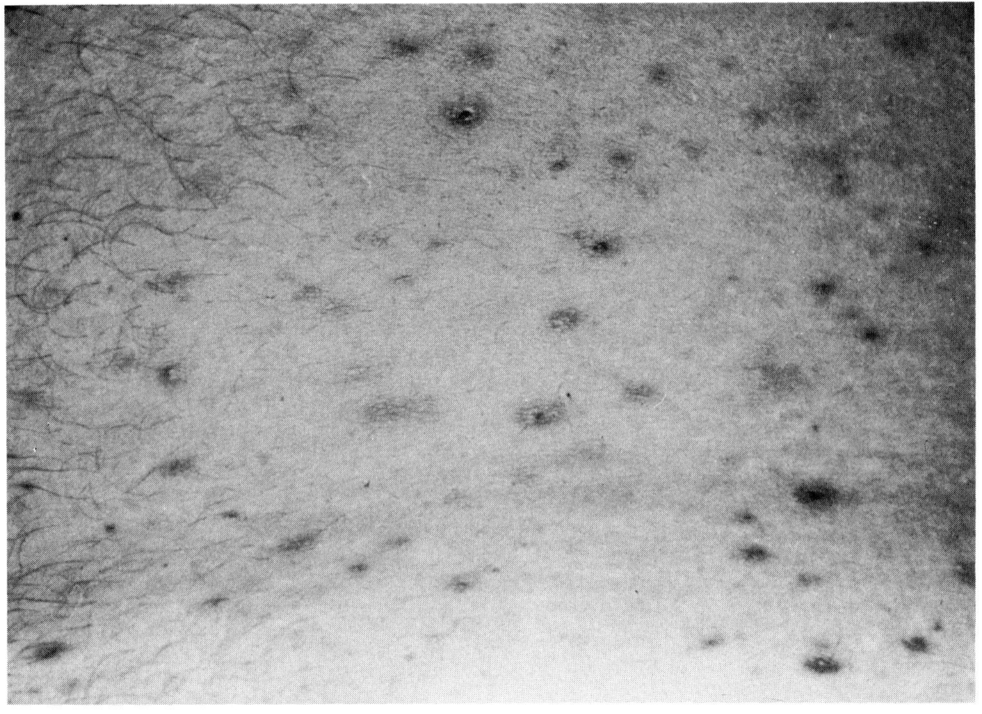

Figure 8–73. Mucha-Habermann disease. Close-up of the papules and papulovesicles.

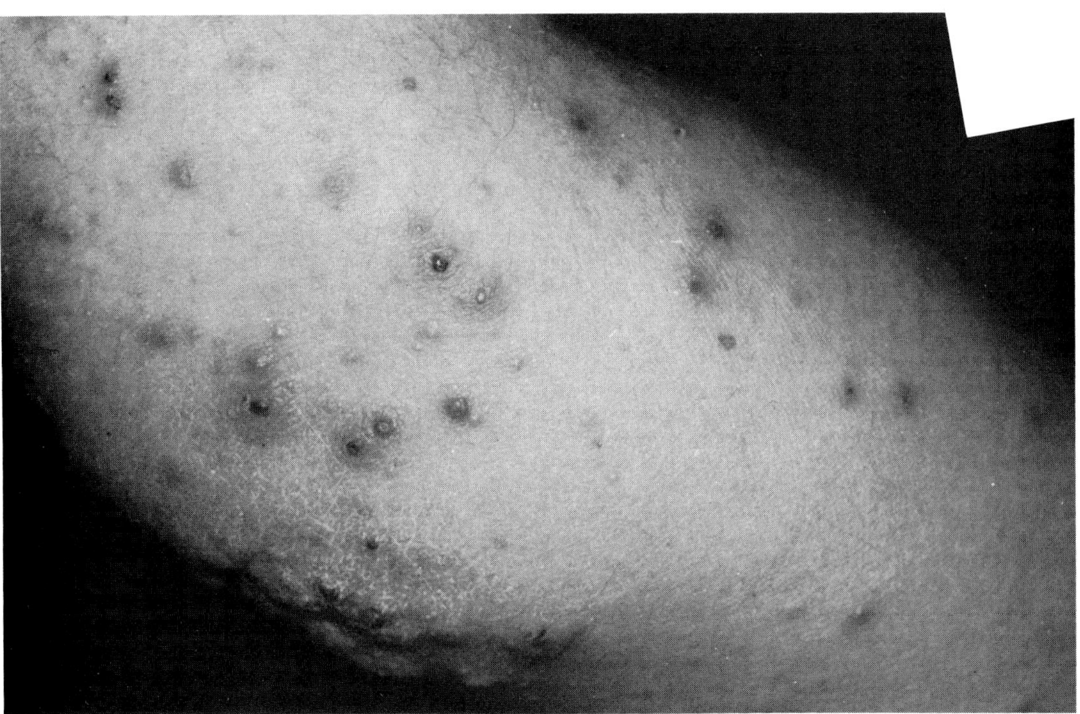

Figure 8–74. Mucha-Habermann disease. The eruption is composed of papules and papulovesicles, many of which exhibit superficial necrosis (crusts or mild ulceration).

Another cutaneous necrotizing vasculitis is recognized in which the predominant cell is the lymphocyte. *Acute parapsoriasis, Mucha-Habermann disease,* and *acute pityriasis lichenoides et varioliformis* are synonyms for this disorder, which is not known to be associated with any underlying disease and which follows a self-limiting course that lasts from a few weeks to two or three years.[160] Some dermatologists believe that this disorder represents the acute phase of chronic guttate parapsoriasis. The lesions appear in crops, persist from one to two weeks, and heal with or without varioliform scarring depending upon the severity of the necrotizing inflammation (Figs. 8–72 to 8–74). Fever and malaise may accompany severe attacks, but most patients with this disorder are asymptomatic. The lesions are papules or papulovesicles, 2 to 4 mm in size, that develop central necrosis with crusts soon after they arise. The cause of this disease is not known. It can be differentiated from leukocytoclastic angiitis by the pattern of papules and papulovesicles with central crusting and by the generalized distribution of lesions at the onset of the disease. Mucha-Habermann disease is more common in children and young adults than in older people, and it is frequently diagnosed as chronic chickenpox by physicians who have not had previous experience with this disorder.

Studies by Clayton and Haffenden demonstrated IgM and C3 in the dermal vessels of 72 per cent of 27 patients with Mucha-Habermann disease.[161] If confirmed, this would suggest that pityriasis lichenoides may be an immune complex disease.

REFERENCES

1. Zeek, P. M.: Periarteritis nodosa: a critical review. Am. J. Clin. Pathol., *22*:777, 1952.
2. Knowles, H. C., Jr., Zeek, P. M., and Blankenhorn, M. A.: Studies on necrotizing angiitis IV. Periarteritis nodosa and hypersensitivity angiitis. Arch. Intern. Med., *92*:789, 1953.
3. Zeek, P. M.: Periarteritis nodosa and other forms of necrotizing angiitis. N. Engl. J. Med., *248*:764, 1953.
4. Winkelmann, R. K., and Ditto, W. B.: Cutaneous and visceral syndromes of necrotizing or "allergic" angiitis: a study of 38 cases. Medicine (Balt.), *43*:59, 1964.
5. Fauci, A. S., Haynes, B. F., and Katz, P.: The spectrum of vasculitis. Clinical, pathologic, immunologic, and therapeutic considerations. Ann. Intern. Med., *89*:660, 1978.
6. Kussmaul, A., and Maier, R.: Über eine bisher nicht beschriebene eigenthumliche Arterienerkrankung (Periarteritis nodosa). Deutsch. Arch. Klin. Med., *1*:484, 1866.
7. Magilavy, D. B., Petty, R. E., Cassidy, J. T., and Sullivan, D. B.: A syndrome of childhood polyarteritis. J. Pediatr., *91*:25, 1977.
8. Blau, E. B., Morris, R. F., and Yunis, E. J.: Polyarteritis nodosa in older children. Pediatrics, *60*:227, 1977.
9. Rose, G. A., and Spencer, H.: Polyarteritis nodosa. Q. J. Med., *27*:43, 1957.
10. Sack, M., Cassidy, J. T., and Bole, G. G.: Prognostic factors in polyarteritis. J. Rheumatol., *2*:411, 1975.
11. Frohnert, P. P., and Sheps, S. G.: Long term followup study of periarteritis nodosa. Am. J. Med., *43*:8, 1967.
12. Gocke, D. J., Hsu, K., Morgan, C., Bombardieri, S., Lockshin, M., and Christian, C. L.: Vasculitis in association with Australia antigen. J. Exp. Med., *134*:330, 1971.
13. Trepo, C. G., Zuckerman, A. J., Bird, R. C., and Prince, A. M.: The role of circulating hepatitis B antigen/antibody immune complexes in the pathogenesis of vascular and hepatic manifestations in polyarteritis nodosa. J. Clin. Pathol., *27*:863, 1974.
14. Belasario, J. C.: Cutaneous manifestations in polyarteritis (periarteritis) nodosa. Arch. Dermatol., *82*:526, 1960.
15. Lyell, A., and Church, R.: The cutaneous manifestations of polyarteritis nodosa. Br. J. Dermatol., *66*:335, 1954.
16. Lindgren, I., and Lundmark, C.: Periarteritis nodosa as a skin disease. Acta Dermatovenerol., *36*:343, 1956.
17. Guequierre, J. P., and Greenbaum, S. G.: Periarteritis nodosa. Arch. Dermatol. Syph., *46*:566, 1942.
18. Oliver, E. A.: Panarteritis. Arch. Dermatol. Syph., *58*:530, 1948.
19. Carol, W. L. L., and Prakken, J. R.: Die kutane Form der Periarteritis nodosa. Acta Dermatovenereol., *18*:102, 1937.
20. Slinger, W. N., and Starck, V.: Cutaneous form of polyarteritis nodosa. Arch. Dermatol. Syph., *63*:461, 1951.
21. Kimberly, L. W.: A case for diagnosis (periarteritis nodosa). Arch. Dermatol. Syph., *54*:233, 1946.
22. Citron, B. P., Halperin, M., McCarron, M., Lundberg, G. D., McCormick, R., Pincus, I. J., Tatter, D., and Haverback, B. J.: Necrotizing angiitis associated with drug abuse. N. Engl. J. Med., *283*:1003, 1970.
23. Glass, D., Soter, N. A., and Schur, P. H.: Rheumatoid vasculitis. Arthritis Rheum., *19*:950, 1976.
24. Schimmer, H. M., and Bloch, K. J.: Mixed IgM-IgG cryoglobulinemia terminating in polyarteritis nodosa. J. Rheumatol., *2*:241, 1975.
25. Sergent, J. S., Lockshin, M. D., Christian, C. L., and Gocke, D. J.: Vasculitis with hepatitis B antigenemia: long term observations in nine patients. Medicine, *55*:1, 1976.
26. Ingelfinger, J. R., McCluskey, R. T., Schneeberger, E. E., and Grupe, W. E.: Necrotizing arteritis in acute poststreptococcal glomerulonephritis. Report of a recovered case. J. Pediatrics, *91*:228, 1977.
27. Diaz-Perez, J. L., and Winkelmann, R. K.: Cutaneous periarteritis nodosa. Arch. Dermatol., *110*:407, 1974.
28. Sergent, J. S., and Christian, C. L.: Necrotizing vasculitis after acute serous otitis media. Ann. Intern. Med., *81*:195, 1974.

28a. Verbov, J., and Stansfeld, A. G.: Cutaneous polyarteritis nodosa and Crohn's disease. Trans. St. Johns Hosp. Dermatol. Soc., *58*:261, 1972.

28b. Solley, G. O., Winkelmann, R. K., and Rovelstad, R. A.: Correlation between regional enterocolitis and cutaneous polyarteritis nodosa. Gastroenterology, *69*:235, 1975.

28c. Feurle, G. E.: Regional enteritis and polyarteritis nodosa. Gastroenterology, *72*: 560, 1977.

29. Cheson, B. D., Bluming, A. Z., and Alroy, J.: Cogan's syndrome; a systemic vasculitis. Am. J. Med., *60*:549, 1976.
30. Kawasaki, T., Kosaki, F., Okawa, S., Shigematsu, I., and Yanagawa, H.: A new infantile acute febrile mucocutaneous lymph node syndrome (MLNS) prevailing in Japan. Pediatrics, *54*:271, 1974.
31. Melish, M. C., Hicks, P. M., and Larson, E. J.: Mucocutaneous lymph node syndrome in the United States. Am. J. Dis. Child., *130*:599, 1976.
32. Landing, B. H., and Larson, E. J.: Are infantile periarteritis nodosa with coronary artery involvement and fatal mucocutaneous lymph node syndrome the same? Comparison of 20 patients from North

America with patients from Hawaii and Japan. Pediatrics, *59*:651, 1977.
33. Churg, J., and Strauss, L.: Allergic granulomatosis, allergic angiitis, and periarteritis nodosa. Am. J. Pathol., *27*:277, 1951.
34. Varriale, P., Minogue, W. F., and Alfenito, J. C.: Allergic granulomatosis; case report and review of the literature. Arch. Intern. Med., *113*:235, 1964.
35. Sokolov, R. A., Rachmaninoff, N., and Kaine, H. D.: Allergic granulomatosis. Am. J. Med., *32*:131, 1962.
36. Cooper, B. J., Bacal, E., and Patterson, R.: Allergic angiitis and granulomatosis. Prolonged remission induced by combined prednisone-azathioprine therapy. Arch. Intern. Med., *138*:367, 1978.
37. Godman, G. C., and Churg, J.: Wegener's granulomatosis; pathology and review of the literature. Arch. Pathol., *58*:533, 1954.
38. Reed, W. B., Jensen, A. K., Konwaler, B. E., and Hunter, D.: The cutaneous manifestations in Wegener's granulomatosis. Acta Dermatovenereol., *43*:250, 1963.
39. Fauci, A. S., and Wolff, S. M.: Wegener's granulomatosis: studies in eighteen patients and a review of the literature. Medicine, *52*:535, 1973.
40. Hu, C-H., O'Loughlin, S., and Winkelmann, R. K.: Cutaneous manifestations of Wegener granulomatosis. Arch. Dermatol., *113*:175, 1977.
41. Kraus, Z., Vortel, V., Fingerland, A., Salavec, M., and Krch, V.: Unusual cutaneous manifestations in Wegener's granulomatosis. Acta Dermatovenereol., *45*:288, 1965.
42. Haynes, B. F., Fishman, M. L., Fauci, A. S., and Wolff, S. M.: The ocular manifestations of Wegener's granulomatosis. Fifteen years experience and review of the literature. Am. J. Med., *63*:131, 1977.
43. Reza, M. J., Dornfeld, L., Goldberg, L. S., Bluestone, R., and Pearson, C. M.: Wegener's granulomatosis. Long term follow-up of patients treated with cyclophosphamide. Arthritis Rheum., *18*:501, 1975.
44. Carrington, C. B., and Liebow, A. A.: Limited forms of angiitis and granulomatosis of Wegener's type. Am. J. Med., *41*:497, 1966.
45. Fechner, R. E., and Lamppin, D. W.: Midline malignant reticulosis. A clinicopathologic entity. Arch. Otolaryngol., *95*:467, 1972.
46. Spear, G. S., and Walker, W. G., Jr.: Lethal midline granuloma (granuloma gangraenescens) at autopsy. Bull. Hopkins Hosp., *99*:313, 1956.
47. Fauci, A. S., Johnson, R. E., and Wolff, S. M.: Radiation therapy of midline granuloma. Ann. Intern. Med., *84*:140, 1976.
48. Fauci, A. S.: Granulomatous vasculitides: distinct but related. Ann. Intern. Med., *87*:782, 1977.
49. Liebow, A. S., Carrington, C. R. B., and Friedman, P. J.: Lymphomatoid granulomatosis. Hum. Pathol., *3*:457, 1972.
50. Israel, H., Patchefsky, A. S., and Saldana, M. J.: Wegener's granulomatosis, lymphomatoid granulomatosis, and benign lymphocytic angiitis and granulomatosis of lung. Recognition and treatment. Ann. Intern. Med., *87*:691, 1977.
51. DeRemee, R. A., McDonald, T. J., Harrison, E. G., Jr., and Coles, D. T.: Wegener's granulomatosis. Anatomic correlates, a proposed classification. Mayo Clin. Proc., *51*:777, 1976.
52. Kay, S., Fu, Y.-S., Minars, N., and Brady, J. W.: Lymphomatoid granulomatosis of the skin: light microscopic and ultrastructural studies. Cancer, *34*:1675, 1974.
53. Yockey, C. C., Leighter, S. B., and Hampton, J. R., III: Lymphomatoid granulomatosis presenting as fever of unknown origin. J.A.M.A., *237*:2633, 1977.
54. Soter, N. A., Austen, K. F., and Gigli, I.: Urticaria and arthralgias as manifestations of necrotizing angiitis (vasculitis). J. Invest. Dermatol., *63*:485, 1974.
55. Mraz, J. P., and Newcomer, V. D.: Erythema elevatum diutinum. Arch. Dermatol., *96*:235, 1967.
56. Katz, S. I., Gallin, J. I., Hertz, K. C., Fauci, A. S., and Lawley, T. J.: Erythema elevatum diutinum: skin and systemic manifestations, immunologic studies, and successful treatment with dapsone. Medicine, *56*:443, 1977.
57. Fort, S. L., and Rodman, O. G.: Erythema elevatum diutinum. Arch. Dermatol., *113*:819, 1977.
58. Gairdner, D.: The Schönlein-Henoch syndrome (anaphylactoid purpura). Q. J. Med., *17*:95, 1948.
59. Michaelsson, G., Pettersson, L., and Juhlin, L.: Purpura caused by food and drug additives. Arch. Dermatol., *109*:49, 1974.
60. Allen, D. M., Diamond, L. K., and Howell, D. A.: Anaphylactoid purpura in children (Schönlein-Henoch syndrome). Am. J. Dis. Child., *99*:833, 1960.
61. Emery, H., Larter, W., and Schaller, J. G.: Henoch-Schönlein vasculitis. Arthritis Rheum., *20*:385, 1977.
62. Norkin, S., and Wiener, J.: Henoch-Schönlein syndrome. Review of pathology and report of two cases. Am. J. Clin. Pathol., *33*:55, 1960.
63. Henoch-Schönlein purpura. Br. Med. J., *1*:190, 1977.
64. Trygstad, C. W., and Stiehm, E. R.: Elevated serum IgA globulin in anaphylactoid purpura. Pediatrics, *47*:1023, 1971.
65. Ayoub, E. M., and Hoyer, J.: Anaphylactoid purpura: Streptococcal antibody titers and β_1C globulin levels. J. Pediatr., *75*:193, 1969.
66. McCombs, R. P.: Systemic "allergic" vasculitis. J.A.M.A., *194*:1059, 1965.
67. O'Duffy, J. D., Scherbel, A. L., Reidbord, H. E., and McCormack, L. J.: Necrotizing angiitis: I. A clinical review of twenty-

seven autopsied cases. Cleveland Clin. Q., *32*:87, 1965.

68. Wilkinson, D. S.: Some clinical manifestations and associations of "allergic" vasculitis. Br. J. Dermatol., *77*:186, 1965.
69. Ramsay, C., and Fry, L.: Allergic vasculitis. Clinical and histologic features and incidence of renal involvement. Br. J. Dermatol., *81*:96, 1969.
70. Gougerot, H., and Duperrat, B.: The nodular dermal allergides of Gougerot. Br. J. Dermatol., *66*:283, 1954.
71. McCombs, R. P., Patterson, J. F., and MacMahon, H. E.: Syndromes associated with "allergic" vasculitis. N. Engl. J. Med., *255*:251, 1956.
72. Weigle, W. L.: Fate and biologic action of antigen-antibody complexes. *In* Advances in Immunology, vol. 1. Academic Press, New York, 1961, p. 283.
73. Cochrane, C. G.: Studies on the localization of circulating antigen-antibody complexes and other macromolecules in vessels. I. Structural studies. J. Exp. Med., *118*:489, 1963.
74. Cochrane, C. G.: Studies on the localization of circulating antigen-antibody complexes and other macromolecules in vessels. II. Pathogenetic and pharmacodynamic studies. J. Exp. Med., *118*:503, 1963.
75. Cochrane, C. G., and Hawkins, D.: Studies on circulating immune complexes. III. Factors governing the ability of circulating complexes to localize in blood vessels. J. Exp. Med., *127*:137, 1968.
76. Cochrane, C. G.: Immunologic tissue injury mediated by neutrophilic leukocytes. *In* Advances in Immunology, vol. 9. Academic Press, New York, 1968, p. 97.
77. Janoff, A., and Scherer, J.: Mediators of inflammation in leucocyte lysosomes. IX. Elastolytic activity in granules of human polymorphonuclear leucocytes. J. Exp. Med., *128*:1137, 1968.
78. Lazarus, G. S., Brown, R. S., Daniels, J. R., and Fullmer, H. M.: Human granulocyte collagenase. Science, *159*:1483, 1968.
79. Beneveniste, J., Henson, P. M., and Cochrane, C. G.: Leukocyte-dependent histamine release from rabbit platelets. The role of IgE, basophils, and a platelet-activating factor. J. Exp. Med., *136*:1356, 1972.
80. Majno, G., and Palade, G. E: Studies on inflammation. I. The effect of histamine and serotonin on vascular permeability: an electron microscopic study. J. Biophys. Biochem. Cytol., *11*:571, 1961.
81. Stringa, S. G., Bianchi, C., Casala, A. M., and Bianchi, O.: Allergic vasculitis (Gougerot-Ruiter syndrome). Arch. Dermatol., *95*:23, 1967.
82. Schroeter, A. L., Copeman, P. W. M., Jordan, R. E., Sams, W. M., Jr., and Winkelmann, R. K.: Immunofluorescence of cutaneous vasculitis. J. Clin. Invest., *48*:75a, 1969.
83. Gary, N. E., Mazzara, J. T., and Holfelder, L.: The Schönlein-Henoch syndrome. Report of two patients with recurrent impairment of renal function. Ann. Intern. Med., *72*:229, 1970.
84. Soter, N. A., Austen, K. F., and Gigli, I.: The complement system in necrotizing angiitis of the skin: analysis of complement component activities in serum of patients with concomitant collagen-vascular disease. J. Invest. Dermatol., *63*:219, 1974.
85. Meltzer, M., and Franklin, E. C.: Cryoglobulinemia — a study of twenty-nine patients. I. IgG and IgM cryoglobulins and factors affecting cryoprecipitability. Am. J. Med., *40*:828, 1966.
86. Weisman, M., and Zvaifler, N.: Cryoimmunoglobulinemia in rheumatoid arthritis. Significance in serum of patients with rheumatoid vasculitis. J. Clin. Invest., *56*:725, 1975.
87. Asghar, S. S., Faber, W. R., and Cormane, R. H.: C1q precipitin in the sera of patients with allergic vasculitis (Gougerot-Ruiter syndrome). J. Invest. Dermatol., *64*:113, 1975.
88. Theofilopoulos, A. N., Wilson, C. B., and Dixon, F. J.: The Raji cell radioimmune assay for detecting immune complexes in human sera. J. Clin. Invest., *57*:169, 1976.
89. Braverman, I. M., and Yen, A.: Demonstration of immune complexes in spontaneous and histamine-induced lesions and in normal skin of patients with leukocytoclastic angiitis. J. Invest. Dermatol., *64*:105, 1975.
90. Gower, R. G., Sausker, W. F., Kohler, P. F., Thorne, G. E., and McIntosh, R. M.: Small vessel vasculitis caused by hepatitis B virus immune complexes. Small vessel vasculitis and HBsAg. J. Allergy Clin. Immunol., *62*:222, 1978.
91. Dienstag, J. L., Rhodes, A. R., Bhan, A. K., Dvorak, A. M., Mihm, M. C., Jr., and Wands, J. R.: Urticaria associated with acute viral hepatitis type B. Ann. Intern. Med., *89*:34, 1978.
92. Cream, J. J., Bryceson, A. D. M., and Ryder, G.: Disappearance of immunoglobulin and complement from the Arthus reaction and its relevance to the studies of vasculitis in man. Br. J. Dermatol., *84*:106, 1971.
93. Gower, R. G., Sams, W. M., Jr., Thorne, E. G., Kohler, P. F., and Claman, H. N.: Leukocytoclastic vasculitis: sequential appearance of immunoreactants and cellular changes in serial biopsies. J. Invest. Dermatol., *69*:477, 1977.
94. Wolff, H. H., Maciejewski, W., Scherer, R., and Braun-Falco, O.: Immunoelectronmicroscopic examination of early lesions in histamine induced immune complex vasculitis in man. Br. J. Dermatol., *99*:13, 1978.
95. Sams, W. M., Jr., Claman, H. N., Kohler, P. F., McIntosh, R. M., Small, P., and Mass, M. F.: Human necrotizing vasculi-

tis: immunoglobulins and complement in vessel walls of cutaneous lesions and normal skin. J. Invest. Dermatol., *64*:441, 1975.

96. Cunliffe, W. J., and Menon, I. S.: The association between cutaneous vasculitis and decreased blood fibrinolytic activity. Br. J. Dermatol., *84*:99, 1971.
97. Handell, D. W., Roenigk, H. H., Jr., Shainoff, J., and Deodhar, S.: Necrotizing vasculitis. Etiologic aspects of immunology and coagulopathy. Arch. Dermatol., *111*:847, 1975.
98. Ward, P. A., and Zvaifler, N. J.: Complement-derived leukotactic factors in inflammatory synovial fluids of humans. J. Clin. Invest., *50*:606, 1971.
99. Zvaifler, N. J.: Immunoreactants in rheumatoid synovial effusions. J. Exp. Med., *134*:276S, 1971.
100. Benerberg, J. L., Ward, P. A., and Sonenshine, D. E.: Tick-bite injury: mediation by complement-derived chemotactic factor. J. Immunol., *109*:451, 1972.
101. Soter, N. A., Mihm, M. A., Jr., Gigli, I., Dvorak, H. F., and Austen, K. F.: Two distinct cellular patterns in cutaneous necrotizing angiitis. J. Invest. Dermatol., *66*:344, 1976.
102. Yen, A., and Braverman, I. M.: Ultrastructure of the human dermal microcirculation: the horizontal plexus of the papillary dermis. J. Invest. Dermatol., *66*:131, 1976.
103. Cream, J. J.: Clinical and immunological aspects of cutaneous vasculitis. Q. J. Med., *45*:255, 1976.
104. MacKechnie, H. L., Ogryzlo, M. A., and Pruzanski, W.: Heterogeneity of IgM/IgG cryocomplexes: immunological-clinical correlation. J. Rheumatol., *2*:225, 1975.
105. Hurwitz, D., Quismorio, F. P., and Friou, G. J.: Cryoglobulinaemia in patients with infectious endocarditis. Clin. Exp. Immunol., *19*:131, 1975.
106. Grey, H. M., and Kohler, P. F.: Cryoimmunoglobulins. Sem. Hematol., *10*:87, 1973.
107. Brouet, J.-C., Clauvel, J.-P., Danon, F., Klein, M., and Seligmann, M.: Biologic and clinical significance of cryoglobulins. A report of 86 cases. Am. J. Med., *57*:775, 1974.
108. Stastny, P., and Ziff, M.: Cold-insoluble complexes and complement levels in systemic lupus erythematosus. N. Engl. J. Med., *280*:1376, 1969.
109. LoSpalluto, J., Dorward, B., Miller, W., Jr., and Ziff, M.: Cryoglobulinemia based on interaction between a gamma macroglobulin and 7S gamma globulin. Am. J. Med., *32*:142, 1962.
110. Meltzer, M., Franklin, E. C., Elias, K., McCluskey, R. T., and Cooper, N.: Cryoglobulinemia — a clinical and laboratory study. II. Cryoglobulins with rheumatoid factor activity. Am. J. Med., *40*:837, 1966.
111. Levo, Y., Gorevic, P. D., Kassab, H. J., Zucker-Franklin, D., and Franklin, E. C.: Association between hepatitis B virus and essential mixed cryoglobulinemia. N. Engl. J. Med., *296*:1501, 1977.
112. Gamble, C. N., and Ruggles, S. W.: The immunopathogenesis of glomerulonephritis associated with mixed cryoglobulinemia. N. Engl. J. Med., *299*:81, 1978.
113. Garcia-Fuentes, M., Chantler, C., and Williams, D. G.: Cryoglobulinemia in Henoch-Schönlein purpura. Br. Med. J., *2*:163, 1977.
114. Zuckner, J., Tsai, C., Giangiacomo, J., Baldassare, A. R., and Auclair, R.: IgA deposition in normal and purpuric skin of patients with Henoch-Schönlein purpura. Arthritis Rheum., *20*:395, 1977.
115. Urizar, R. E., Michael, A., Sisson, S., and Vernier, R. L.: Anaphylactoid purpura. II. Immunofluorescent and electron microscopic studies of the glomerular lesions. Lab. Invest., *19*:437, 1968.
116. McDuffie, F. C., Sams, W. M., Jr., Maldonado, J. E., Andreini, P. H., Conn, D. L., and Samayoa, E. A.: Hypocomplementemia with cutaneous vasculitis and arthritis. Possible immune complex syndrome. Mayo Clin. Proc., *48*:340, 1973.
117. Gammon, W. R., and Wheeler, C. E., Jr.: Urticarial vasculitis. Arch. Dermatol., *115*:76, 1979.
118. Bradford, W. D., Cook, C. D., and Vawter, G. F.: Livedo reticularis: a form of allergic vasculitis. J. Pediatr., *60*:266, 1962.
119. Rubenfeld, S., and Min, K.-W.: Leukocytoclastic angiitis in subacute bacterial endocarditis. Arch. Dermatol., *113*:1073, 1977.
120. Farrior, J. B., III, and Silverman, M. E.: A consideration of the differences between a Janeway's lesion and an Osler's node in infectious endocarditis. Chest, *70*:239, 1976.
121. Wands, J. R., Perrotto, J. L., and Isselbacher, K. J.: Circulating immune complexes and complement sequence activation in infectious mononucleosis. Am. J. Med., *60*:269, 1976.
122. Goldman, J. A., Casey, H. L., Davidson, E. D., Hersh, T., and Pirozzi, D.: Vasculitis associated with intestinal bypass surgery. Arch. Dermatol., *115*:725, 1979.
123. Fauci, A. S., Katz, P., Haynes, B. F., and Wolff, S. M.: Cyclophosphamide therapy of severe systemic necrotizing vasculitis. N. Engl. J. Med., *309*:235, 1979.
124. Frank, M. M., Hamburger, M. I., Lawley, T. J., Kimberley, R. P., and Plotz, P. H.: Defective reticuloendothelial system Fc-receptor function in systemic lupus erythematosus. N. Engl. J. Med., *300*:518, 1979.
125. Lockwood, C. M., Worlledge, S., Nicholas, A., Cotton, C., and Peters, D. K.: Reversal of impaired splenic function in patients with nephritis or vasculitis (or both) by plasma exchange. N. Engl. J. Med., *300*:524, 1979.
126. deFaire, U., Millstedt, H., and Norden-

stam, H.: Granulomatous giant cell arteritis (temporal arteritis) in a young female. Acta Med. Scand., *201*:215, 1977.

127. Russell, R. W. R.: Giant-cell arteritis. A review of 35 cases. Q. J. Med., *28*:471, 1959.
128. Kinmont, P. D. C., and McCallum, D. I.: The aetiology, pathology and course of giant-cell arteritis. The possible role of light sensitivity. Br. J. Dermatol., *77*:193, 1965.
129. Ettlinger, R. E., Hunder, G. G., and Ward, L. E.: Polymyalgia rheumatica and giant cell arteritis. Annu. Rev. Med., *29*:15, 1978.
130. Kansu, T., Corbett, J. J., Savino, P., and Schatz, N. J.: Giant cell arteritis with normal sedimentation rate. Arch. Neurol., *34*:624, 1977.
131. Balmforth, G. V.: Temporal arteritis and renal failure. Arch. Intern. Med., *113*:230, 1964.
132. Klein, R. G., Hunder, G. G., Stanson, A. W., and Sheps, S. G.: Large artery involvement in giant cell (temporal) arteritis. Ann. Intern. Med., *83*:806, 1975.
133. Barot, A. J., Finton, C. K., Brannon, W. L., Jr., and Riley, R. L.: Temporal arteritis without pain. J.A.M.A., *243*:61, 1980.
134. Ackerman, A. B., Miller, R. C., and Shapiro, L.: Gonococcemia and its cutaneous manifestations. Arch. Dermatol., *91*:227, 1965.
135. Kahn, G., and Danielsson, D.: Septic gonococcal dermatitis. Arch. Dermatol., *99*:421, 1969.
136. Ognibene, A. J., and Dito, W. R.: Chronic meningococcemia. Further comments on the pathogenesis of associated skin lesions. Arch. Intern. Med., *114*:29, 1964.
137. Randall, A. J., Kierland, R. R., and Montgomery, H. Pigmented purpuric eruptions. Arch. Dermatol., *64*:177, 1951.
138. Mosto, S. J., and Casala, A. M.: Disseminated pruriginous angiodermatitis (itching purpura). Br. J. Dermatol., *91*:351, 1965.
139. Loewenthal, L. J. A.: Itching purpura. Br. J. Dermatol., *66*:95, 1954.
140. Huston, K. A., Combs, J. J., Jr., Lie, J. T., and Giuliani, E. R.: Left atrial myxoma simulating peripheral vasculitis. Mayo Clin. Proc., *53*:752, 1978.
141. Reed, W. B., Anderson, R., Weiss, L., and Harris, R.: Atheromatous embolism (with cutaneous manifestations resembling polyarteritis nodosa). Cutis, *16*:264, 1975.
142. Rowell, N.: Digital ischemia due to vascular anomalies. Br. J. Dermatol., *96*:615, 1977.
143. Marshall, A. J., Roberts, C. J. C., and Barritt, D. W.: Raynaud's phenomenon as side effect of beta-blockers in hypertension. Br. Med. J., *1*:1498, 1976.
144. Gokal, R., Dornan, T. L., and Ledingham, J. G. G.: Peripheral skin necrosis complicating beta-blockade. Br. Med. J., *1*:721, 1979.
145. Nalbandian, R. M., Mader, I. J., Barrett, J. L., Pearce, J. F., and Rupp, E. C.: Petechiae, ecchymoses, and necrosis of skin induced by coumarin congeners. Rare, occasionally lethal complications of anticoagulant therapy. J.A.M.A., *192*:107, 1965.
146. Spittell, J. A., Jr.: Diseases of the vascular system related to environmental temperature. *In* Peripheral Vascular Diseases, 4th ed., edited by J. F. Fairbairn, II, J. L. Juergens, and J. A. Spittell, Jr. W. B. Saunders Company, Philadelphia, 1972, p. 421.
147. Lewis, T.: The Blood Vessels of the Human Skin and Their Responses. Shaw, London, 1927, pp. 189, 259.
148. Champion, R. H.: Livedo reticularis. A review. Br. J. Dermatol., *77*:167, 1965.
149. Barker, N. W., Hines, E. A., and Craig, W. McK.: Livedo reticularis: a peripheral arteriolar disease. Am. Heart J., *21*:592, 1941.
150. Ebert, M. H.: Livedo reticularis. Arch. Dermatol. Syph., *16*:426, 1927.
151. Barker, N. W., and Baker, T. W.: Proliferative intimitis of small arteries and veins associated with peripheral neuritis, livedo reticularis, and recurring necrotic ulcers of the skin. Ann. Intern. Med., *9*:1134, 1936.
152. Feldaker, M., Hines, E. A., Jr., and Kierland, R. R.: Livedo reticularis with ulcerations. Circulation, *13*:196, 1956.
153. Bard, J. W., and Winkelmann, R. K.: Livedo vasculitis. Segmental hyalinizing vasculitis of the dermis. Arch. Dermatol., *96*:489, 1967.
154. Winkelmann, R. K., Schroeter, A. L., Kierland, R. R., and Ryan, T. M.: Clinical studies of livedoid vasculitis (segmental hyalinizing vasculitis). Mayo Clin. Proc., *49*:745, 1974.
155. Schroeter, A. L., Diaz-Perez, J. L., Winkelmann, R. K., and Jordan, R. E.: Livedo vasculitis. (The vasculitis of atrophie blanche.) Immunohistopathologic study. Arch. Dermatol., *111*:188, 1975.
156. Soter, N. A., Mihm, M. C., Jr., Dvorak, H. F., and Austen, K. F.: Cutaneous necrotizing venulitis: a sequential analysis of the morphological alterations occurring after mast cell degranulation in a patient with a unique syndrome. Clin. Exp. Immunol., *32*:46, 1978.
157. Stevanovic, D. V.: Atrophie blanche. A sign of dermal blood occlusion. Arch. Dermatol., *109*:858, 1974.
158. Gilliam, J. N., Herndon, J. H., and Prystowsky, S. D.: Fibrinolytic therapy for vasculitis of atrophie blanche. Arch. Dermatol., *109*:664, 1974.
159. Sneddon, I. B.: Cerebro-vascular lesions and livedo reticularis. Br. J. Dermatol. *77*:180, 1965.
160. Szymanski, F. J.: Pityriasis lichenoides et varioliformis acuta: histopathologic evidence that it is an entity distinct from parapsoriasis. Arch. Dermatol., *79*:7, 1959.
161. Clayton, R., and Haffenden, G.: An immunofluorescence study of pityriasis lichenoides. Br. J. Dermatol., *99*:491, 1978.

9

Hypersensitivity Syndromes

The important dermatologic disorders of hypersensitivity are urticaria, erythema nodosum, and erythema multiforme. They are usually referred to as "the erythemas" in medical textbooks. Diagnosis of these disorders is easy, but difficulties arise in determining their etiologies because each entity is associated with an incredible number of underlying factors. Occasionally combinations of the three appear together in one person: for example, erythema multiforme with erytherma nodosum or erythema multiforme with urticaria. Also included in this chapter are several disorders that may be confused with urticaria and erythema multiforme.

URTICARIA

Urticaria is common. Acute self-limited eruptions of hives usually represent reactions to drugs, serum injections, food, insect bites, inhalant or contact allergens, or psychogenic factors. Often the etiology of an acute episode of urticaria can be determined, but the factors responsible for chronic urticaria are usually not uncovered. Urticaria is considered to be chronic when it has been present continually or intermittently for more than six to eight weeks. Chronic urticaria may persist for months or years.[1, 2]

Several groups of systemic diseases in which acute and chronic urticaria are important clues will be discussed in this section. However, urticaria is one of the least common markers of internal disease, and intensive investigations of patients with acute and chronic hives will disclose relatively few associated systemic disorders.

Hives are transient erythematous or white swellings in the skin and are produced by localized edema. They may be oval, round, or polycyclic when confluent, and occasionally appear as incomplete rings (Figs. 9–1 and 9–2). Wheals are minimally or markedly elevated and are often surrounded by an erythematous halo. They change in size and shape with time and usually are present for only a few hours, although they may persist for one or two days. The lesions are frequently pruritic.

Histamine has been shown to be the final chemical mediator in most varieties of urticaria.[3, 4] The mast cells that are distributed along the course of the dermal blood vessels contain granules that are the source of histamine and other mediators influencing vascular permeability and inflammation. Mast cells can be activated to release their granules and contents by antigen interacting with IgE (reagin) on their cell surface; by

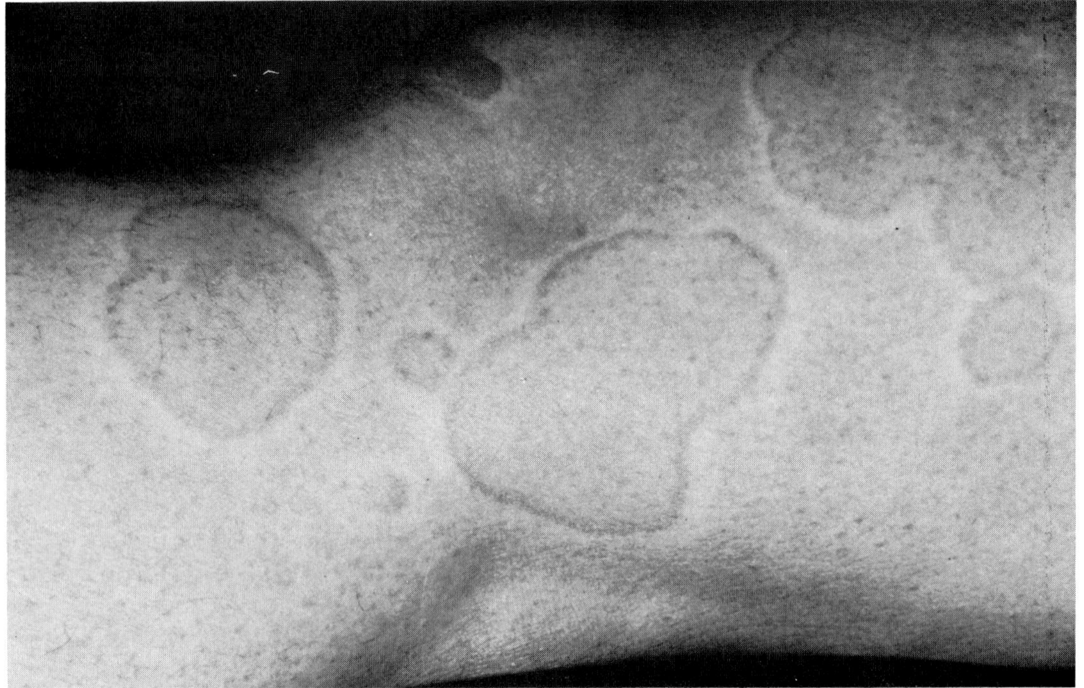

Figure 9–1. Urticaria.

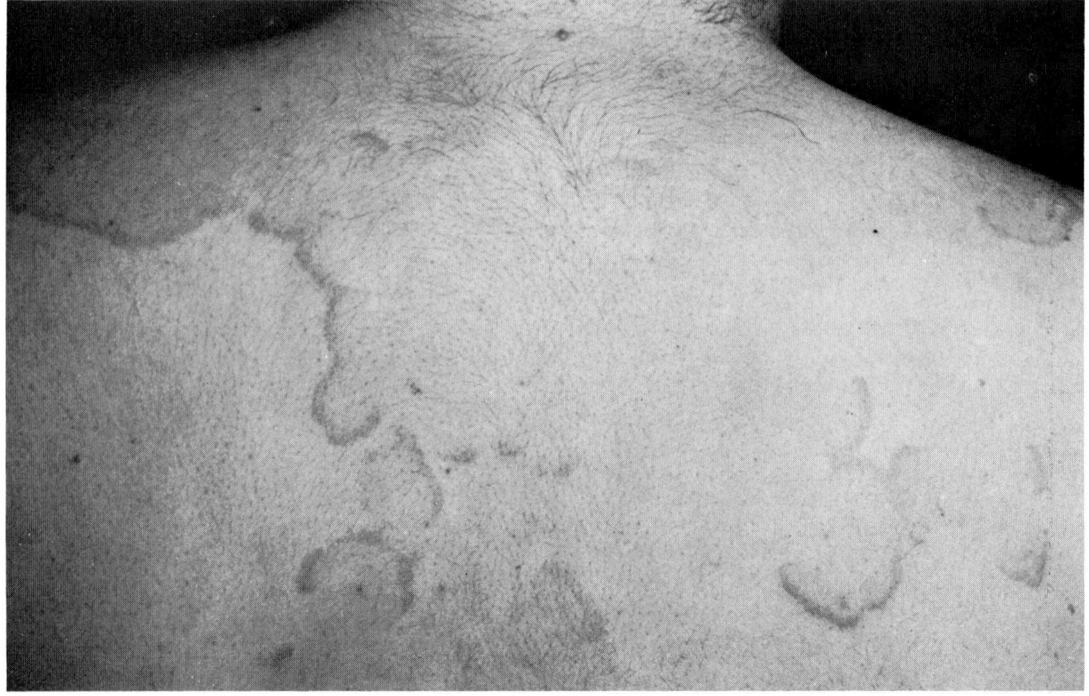

Figure 9–2. Urticaria in annular formations.

anaphylotoxins C3a and C5a generated from classic and alternative complement pathways through both immunologic and nonimmunologic mechanisms; and by direct action of agents such as codeine, morphine, polymyxin B, ethanol, and toxins found in various bacteria, invertebrates, and vertebrates. Thus, hives represent the morphologic expression of an intense, localized, increased vascular permeability produced by any of several immunologic and nonimmunologic mechanisms.

Virtually all agents capable of stimulating mast cells to release these granules do so by altering the intracellular levels of the cyclic nucleotides AMP and GMP. The release of histamine is inhibited by agents that raise the level of cyclic AMP and facilitated by those that increase the levels of cyclic GMP.[3] The actual mechanism of granule release proceeds through a process in which the membrane of the cell fuses with the membrane surrounding the granule, following which an opening to the exterior milieu develops.[5]

The granules are composed of a heparin-protein matrix to which the histamine is bound by ionic bonding. When the granule is exposed to the exterior, sodium ions exchange for histamine molecules in a cation exchange. Heparin is subsequently released into the tissues as well.[6] Other mediators released along with histamine and heparin include eosinophilic chemotactic factor of anaphylaxis (ECF-A) and neutrophil chemotactic factor of anaphylaxis (NCF-A). Slow-reacting substance of anaphylaxis (SRS-A) also appears in the tissues, but it is believed to be formed in the mast cell only after immunologic activation and immediately before its release, whereas ECF-A and NCF-A are stored as preformed molecules in the granules.[7, 8]

Histamine produces its various effects through receptors on cell membranes. Two different receptors have been discovered: H_1 (blocked by classic antihistamines) and H_2 (blocked by cimetidine).[3] Blood vessels contain both H_1 and H_2 receptors.[9] These discoveries concerning the mechanisms underlying mast cell activation and histamine-receptor interaction permit the rational development of therapy for histamine-mediated inflammatory responses.

Histologic examination of the early phase of urticaria shows only dermal edema. Hives that have been present for several hours may show a mild perivascular infiltrate of lymphocytes and eosinophils, the latter presumably attracted by the secretion of ECF-A. Neutrophils, however, are not present in significant numbers in spite of the release of NCF-A by mast cells. Center et al. have proposed that deactivation of the chemotactic mechanism for neutrophils develops *in vivo* as part of a regulatory mechanism.[10] They proposed that histamine or ECF-A may be the deactivators that limit the influx into the tissues of neutrophils with their potentially injurious lysosomal enzymes. An abnormality in such a mechanism could result in the accumulation of neutrophils in the dermis—a phenomenon seen in Sweet's syndrome (p. 753), the erysipelas-like reaction in familial Mediterranean fever (p. 578), and in two varieties of urticaria described later in this chapter.

Traditionally, urticaria is diagnosed on the basis of morphology and duration. On this basis, urticaria has been diagnosed in about 10 per cent of cases of acute rheumatic fever,[11] as a component of the serum sickness prodrome of serum (B) hepatitis, and as a chronic ailment in systemic LE. However, in the hepatitis B syndrome and in systemic LE, histologic examination of the urticaria has revealed a leukocytoclastic vasculitis and not true urticaria.[12, 13] The exact nature of the urticaria in acute rheumatic fever needs to be determined. It may represent true urticaria, but it could also be a variant of the figurate erythemas (see below). Therefore, in cases of apparent urticaria, especially in the chronic variety in which the cause is not readily established, a biopsy is indicated to distinguish between true urticaria and those entities that are mimics.

Urticaria is idiopathic in about 80 per cent of individuals with hives. The rest have well-defined genetic or acquired syndromes, most of which can be classified as physical urticarias. Before making a diagnosis of chronic true urticaria and seeking a possible underlying systemic disorder, urticaria produced by physical stimuli need to be excluded.

Urticaria develops in some people when they are exposed to a sudden drop in air temperature or when they swim in cold water. In the highly sensitive individual, massive transudation of fluid into the skin during swimming may produce hypotension and syncope,with dire consequences. Swelling of the lips, tongue, and pharynx may follow the drinking of cold liquid. This type of cold urticaria is an acquired disorder that often begins in adolescence and frequently is self-limited. Cases following viral infections, immunizations, drug reactions, and psychogenic stress have been reported. Ice applied to the skin will produce a local hive (Fig. 9–3). Cold urticaria can be transferred by the Prausnitz-Küstner technique, indicating that it is mediated by IgE (reaginic antibody).[14]

Patients with cryoglobulinemia (Type I, Brouet) may exhibit cold urticaria; but usually purpura, cutaneous ulceration, and Raynaud's phenomenon are also present. Cold urticaria as the sole manifestation of

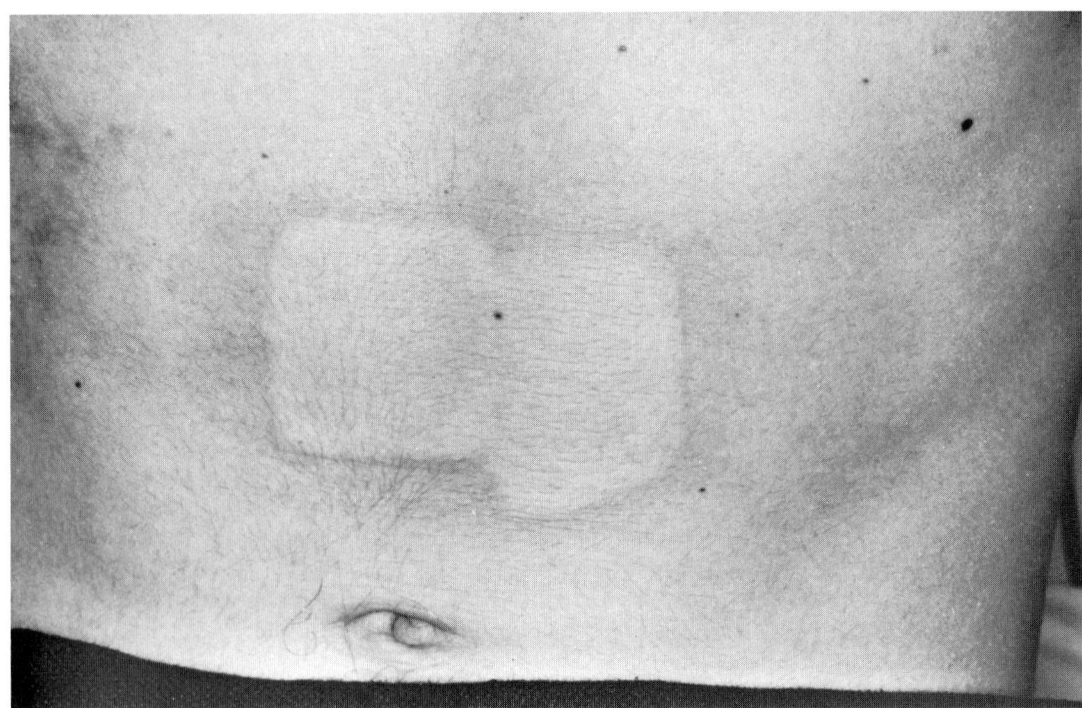

Figure 9–3. Cold urticaria. Positive test following application of two ice cubes to skin.

cryoglobulinemia is rare. Syphilitic paroxysmal cold hemoglobinuria is characterized by cold urticaria followed by hemoglobinuria when the chilled patient is warmed. Red blood cell hemolysins are responsible for the hemoglobinuria. Cold urticaria does not develop in nonsyphilitic hemoglobinuria, which is caused by cold hemagglutinins.

Familial cold urticaria is a life-long autosomal dominantly transmitted illness that begins in infancy.[15-17] Cooling of the skin by exposure to cold air, but not by direct contact with cold substances, produces urticaria-like lesions on exposed parts after one-half hour to several hours. If the exposure is severe, lesions develop on covered parts of the body in association with chills, fever, headache, arthralgias, swelling of hands and feet, nausea, and malaise. These manifestations may persist for several days, depending upon the severity of the exposure. The lesions begin as erythematous macules that become slightly palpable before resolving. They range in size from 0.5 to 15 cm. Petechiae may develop. Sensations of burning and itching are common. In severe exposures, leukocytosis up to 34,000 has been observed as the initial response preceding the appearance of the skin lesions.[16] Histologic examination of the hivelike lesions reveals a marked perivascular infiltrate of neutrophils with leukocytoclasia. However, there is no histologic evidence of necrotizing vasculitis. The mediator is unknown, the disease cannot be passively transferred by the Prausnitz-Küstner technique, and the illness has not been associated with any systemic disease.

Delayed cold-induced urticaria is a rare dominantly transmitted disorder.[18] Instead of developing a localized hive *immediately* after contact with a cold object, affected individuals develop red tender edematous areas 9 to 24 hours later. Soter et al. described a family with this entity. The propositus was a 10-year-old black boy who would develop erythema and swelling of his hands, feet, and legs 9 to 18 hours after playing in the snow. The lesions were mildly pruritic. Biopsy of an urticarial lesion showed a perivascular accumulation of mononuclear cells. They found no evidence for histamine release or participation by mast cells. However, the generation of a tissue factor was suspected, because intradermal injection of a supernatant made from skin prechallenged with cold produced an erythematous reaction.

Solar urticaria develops in susceptible individuals after exposure to the sun for only a few minutes and is rarely associated with an underlying disorder. Two broad-action spectra have been identified: 310 to 370 nm and 400 to 500 nm. The urticarial response to sunlight can be passively transferred by serum from patients who react to the first ultraviolet spectrum but not from those who react to the second. The possibility of an underlying connective tissue disease, drug-induced photosensitivity reaction, or abnormalities of porphyrin metabolism should be ruled out in all cases of solar urticaria, since this disorder has been described in one case of erythropoietic protoporphyria and in three cases of porphyria cutanea tarda.[19, 20]

Cholinergic (generalized heat) urticaria occurs primarily in young adults after exercise; the ingestion of hot food or drink, sweating, and emotional stress.[4] Classically, a small hive with a large red flare appears (Plate 25*D*; Fig. 9–4). The common factor is believed to be a rise in the temperature of the blood, which triggers a neural reflex that releases acetylcholine at nerve endings. Acetylcholine activates mast cells to

PLATE 25

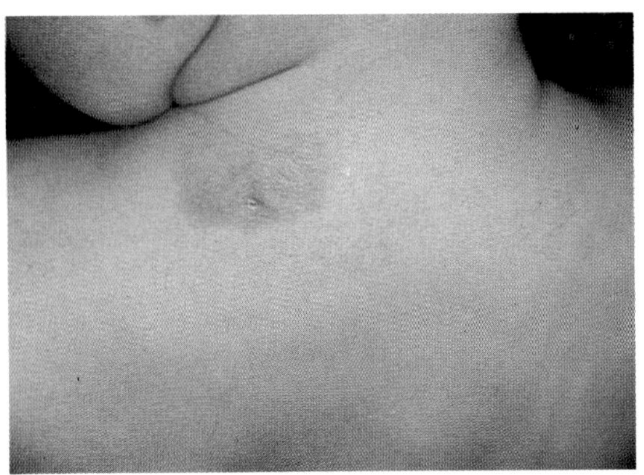

A, Urticaria pigmentosa occurring as a solitary lesion in a child.

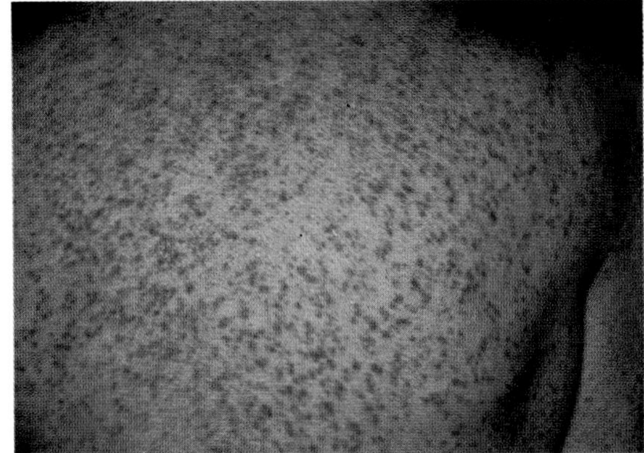

B, Urticaria pigmentosa in an adult. Red-brown freckle-like lesions are characteristic of the adult form of this disease.

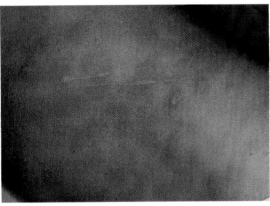

C, Urticaria pigmentosa. Many red-brown macules are present. Localized urticaria. (Darier's sign) and beaded dermographism have resulted from rubbing the macules.

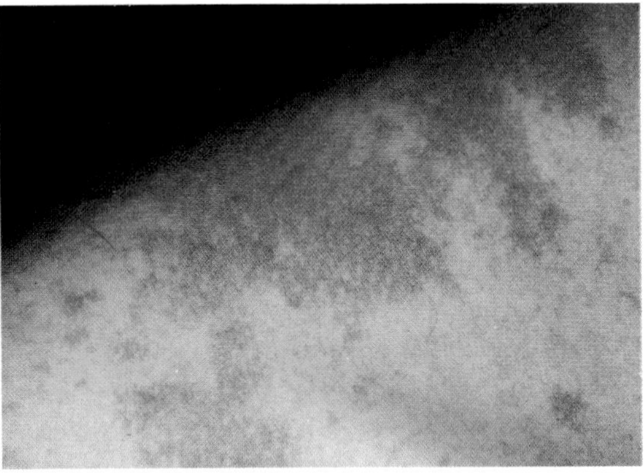

D, Cholinergic urticaria. Small wheals with large red flares.

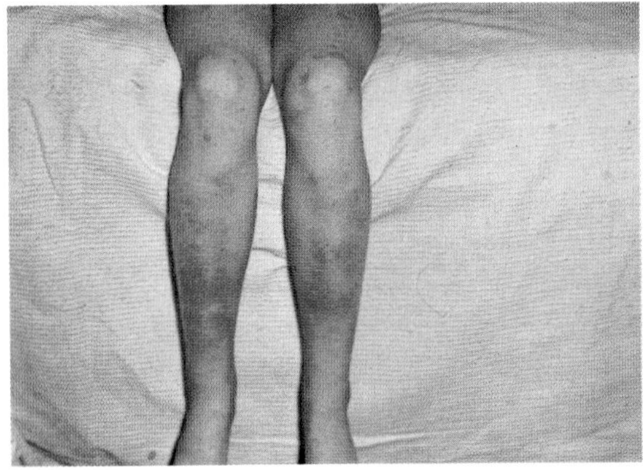

E, Erythema nodosum. Confluent lesions on the shins.

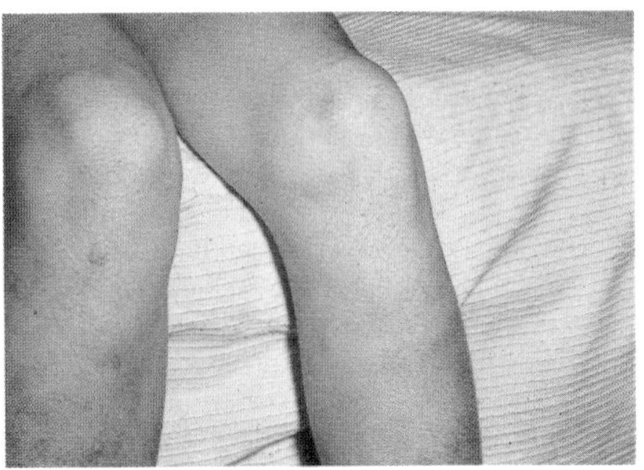

F, Erythema nodosum. Discrete nodules around the left knee.

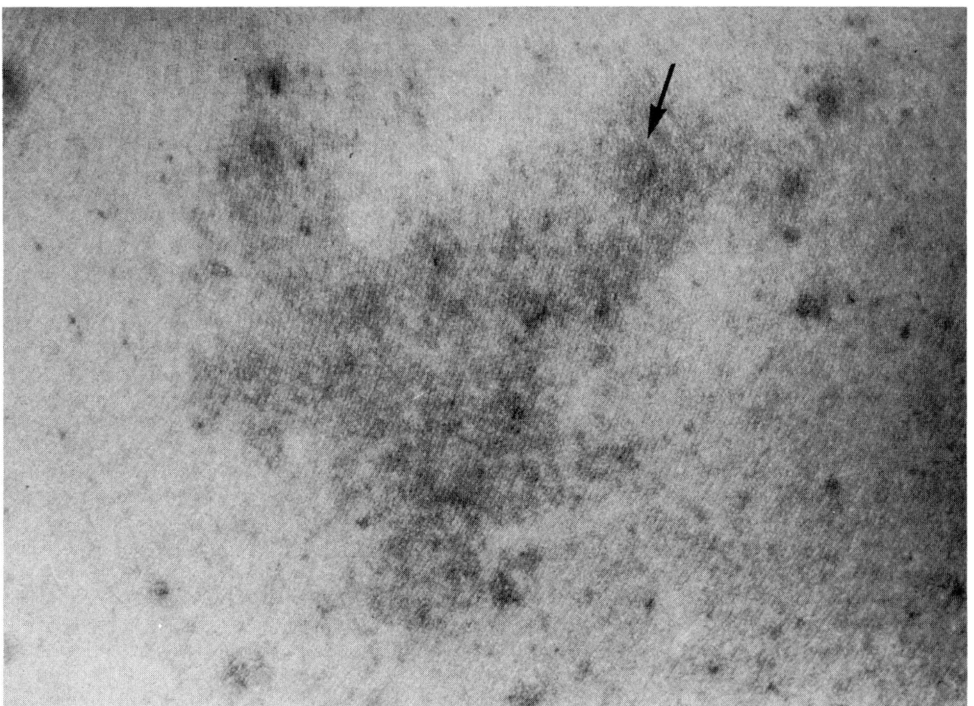

Figure 9–4. Cholinergic urticaria. Small wheal (arrow) with large flare.

release histamine by raising the intracellular level of cyclic GMP. Patients with cholinergic urticaria appear to have an increased sensitivity to the action of acetylcholine. Intradermal injection of acetylcholine or mecholyl in these patients produces urticaria with satellite lesions. Cholinergic (generalized heat) urticaria is considered a physical allergy and not a sign of a systemic disease. In some patients, passive transfer of the disease with serum has been accomplished.

Local heat urticaria is a variant of cholinergic urticaria. Localized hives appear after the application of warm objects.[21, 22]

Muckle and Wells,[23] Kennedy et al.,[24] and Black[25] have described an autosomal dominantly transmitted urticarial disorder that appears for the first time in adolescence. Bouts of urticaria and sometimes angioneurotic edema are brought on by heat and emotion. Chills and malaise may accompany bouts of urticaria. Progressive nerve deafness and amyloidosis of the kidney develop after a variable period. The urticaria in this syndrome behaves like cholinergic urticaria in many ways.[24]

Dermographism (factitious urticaria) represents the development of a wheal and flare in response to a stretching action on the skin, as produced by a scratch or a stroke (Fig. 9–5). It is a common condition. Although dermographism has been passively transferred with serum in some cases, histamine release has not yet been demonstrated. In the common variety of dermographism, there has been no evidence that mast cells are increased in number in the skin or that an underlying systemic disease is present.[26]

Pressure urticaria is a related disorder in which local pressure produced by clothing, jewelry, or weight bearing is followed immediately or after a several-hour delay by hives or a deeper swelling simulating

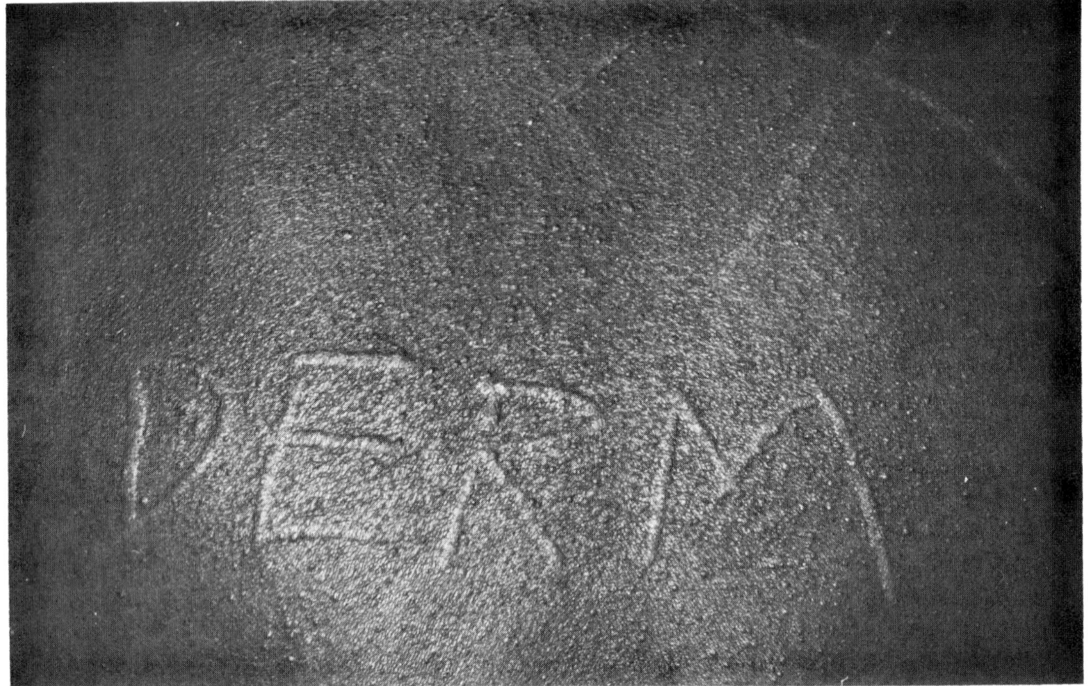

Figure 9–5. Dermographism.

angioedema.[26] Because of the delayed appearance of the hives, patients may not realize that they were provoked by pressure. Both dermographism and pressure urticaria may be confused with chronic urticaria if the relationship to trauma is not appreciated. Many individuals with chronic urticaria exhibit mild dermographism. This probably represents a nonspecific sensitivity of the skin to trauma.

Another syndrome closely related to factitious urticaria is vibratory angioedema, a dominantly transmitted disorder.[27] Localized swellings develop within a few minutes after the skin has been rubbed or subjected to vibratory motion. Headache and facial or generalized flushing may develop if the rubbing is severe enough.[28] These patients do not exhibit dermographism. Histamine release has been demonstrated in these cases.[27, 29]

We have seen an unusual type of physical urticaria. A 45-year-old man had a 10-year history of immediate pressure urticaria that would develop only following a warm shower, exercise, or sweating. The lesions were intensely pruritic and persisted for one to two hours.

Aquagenic urticaria is a rare form of hives that is produced by prolonged contact with water. It has been proposed that the water combines with sebum to produce a histamine-releasing factor that is subsequently absorbed and acts upon the perifollicular mast cells.[30] I have seen an 18-year-old woman who has had this entity since age 14. The hives are provoked by showering, but the temperature of the water does not appear to play a role in the production of her hives.

It seems likely that physical stimuli of various types impinging on the skin release an antigen to which the individual develops an IgE-mediated allergic response. Elevated levels of histamine, ECF-A, and NCF-A have been detected in the sera of patients with various forms of physical urticaria subjected to appropriate stimulation.[4, 7, 8] This combination implicates the mast cell as the source of histamine in these responses. Histamine release has been demonstrated in acquired cold urticaria, cholinergic urticaria, solar urticaria, local heat urticaria, immediate and delayed pressure urticarias, and vibratory angioedema.[4] Dermographism has not yet been shown to be associated with significant histamine release, but passive transfer experiments have been successful in a few patients, suggesting that this should be the case.[26]

Although chronic idiopathic urticaria has always been assumed to be histamine mediated, it has only recently been demonstrated that this actually may be the case. Preliminary observations by Kaplan et al. indicate that in some patients the levels of histamine in the lesions of chronic urticaria are higher than in the normal skin while in others, both the normal skin and hives show elevated levels.[31] Kern and Lichtenstein proposed that there may be defective histamine release in chronic urticaria based on their studies of the response of basophils in this disorder.[32]

Chronic urticaria is frequently attributed to longstanding infections of the sinuses, teeth, gallbladder, and urinary tract; however, extremely few cases are actually proved to be associated with such infections. Foods are rare causes, but diets rich in dairy products containing small amounts of penicillin may cause hives in penicillin-sensitive individuals. Urticaria can be caused by parasitic infections such as intestinal worms, African trypanosomiasis, and malaria.[33]

In the past, etiologies of chronic urticaria were not commonly uncovered, after physical urticarias and parasitic infections had been excluded. However, in the past 10 years, several authors have pointed out that 30 to 70 per cent of patients with chronic urticaria may have exacerbations of their hives when they ingest salicylates, including aspirin; benzoates; azo dyes such as tartrazine and New Coccine; paracetamol; and indomethacin.[33-35] Provocative tests with these agents may induce urticaria or angioedema to appear during quiescent periods. Less often they may induce a scarlet flush that begins on the scalp and spreads to the shoulders and chest. Diets eliminating these agents have been reported to be associated with improvement or remission in up to 80 per cent of individuals who have adhered to them.[33-35] In some patients, cross reactions may occur between salicylates, benzoates, and the azo dyes. Patients with cholinergic and pressure urticaria may also be sensitive to these agents. There is no evidence that allergic mechanisms are involved in these drug sensitivities. Doeglas has speculated that mechanisms involving prostaglandins may be involved because aspirin, indomethacin, sodium salicylate, and paracetamol have in common an effect on the synthesis of these molecules.[34]

Chronic idiopathic urticaria has been reported to be the presenting feature, as well as an indicator of disease activity, in about 7 per cent of patients with systemic LE. However, O'Loughlin et al. have demonstrated that the urticaria in their patients actually was a manifestation of leukocytoclastic angiitis.[13] Whether or not chronic idiopathic urticaria occurs in LE with increased frequency remains to be determined.

Chronic urticaria can be a feature of hyperthryoidism.[36]

After Soter et al. pointed out that leukocytoclastic angiitis could produce nonpurpuric wheals resembling urticaria that often persisted for

48 to 72 hours,[37] clinicians have begun to biopsy lesions of chronic idiopathic urticaria to detect this syndrome. Phanuphak et al. reported in an abstract that in 26 consecutive cases of chronic urticaria, 50 per cent showed histologic evidence of vasculitis.[38] The diagnosis was apparently based solely on the presence of inflammatory cells within the vessel walls; fibrinoid deposition and vascular wall necrosis were not mentioned. In five cases, the inflammatory cells were chiefly neutrophils; in two, mononuclear; and in six, a mixture of both. Three of the specimens showed IgM deposition in the vascular walls by immunofluorescence, but the character of the accompanying infiltrate was not described. After 1 to 12 months of follow-up they found no evidence of any systemic disease, not were they able to distinguish on clinical grounds between patients who had "vasculitis" and those who did not. It needs to be emphasized that the histologic diagnosis of vasculitis cannot be made solely on the basis of finding inflammatory cells in the vascular wall without other accompanying evidence of tissue damage. It does not matter whether the cells are neutrophils or mononuclear cells.

We have studied three women who have exhibited an unusual finding in association with their chronic idiopathic urticaria. The first patient is a 28-year-old white woman who has had almost continual episodes of urticaria for two years. She has complained of arthralgias of the knees with the most severe flares, but never has had fever, an elevated sedimentation rate, or signs of any underlying disease. The unusual aspect to her otherwise typical hives has been petechiae that appeared as the hives resolved (Fig. 9–6). Biopsies revealed a marked perivascular infiltrate of neutrophils with leukocytoclasis but without fibrinoid degen-

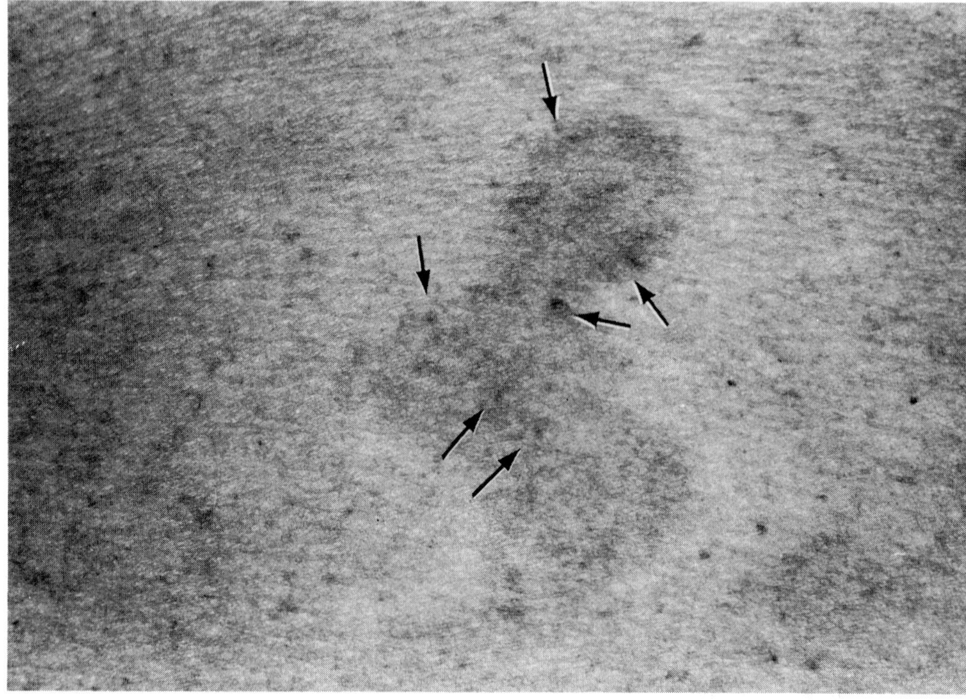

Figure 9–6. Resolving urticaria with prominent petechiae (arrows).

eration or signs of vascular wall necrosis. Direct examination of urticarial lesions less than 24 hours old by immunofluorescent techniques failed to demonstrate immunoglobulins or complement. It was not possible to detect circulating immune complexes by trapping them in dermal vessels with the histamine technique described earlier (see p. 417). The other two women were both 62 years old and had had their chronic urticaria for one year. The clinical and histologic features were identical to those of the first woman except for the absence of arthralgias. None of the women has developed any evidence of vasculitis or an underlying disease after three to five years of follow-up.

It is possible that the patients reported by Phanuphak et al. are similar to these three. Since clinicians have only recently begun to biopsy the lesions of chronic urticaria, it is not yet known how often urticaria may show a neutrophilic response. It is possible that such cases of chronic urticaria may be related to the NCF-A of mast cells: abnormal or prolonged release or failure of deactivation of chemotaxis. The petechiae most likely result from markedly increased vascular permeability. Familial cold urticaria, familial Mediterranean fever, and Sweet's disease exhibit similar neutrophilic responses in their associated skin lesions.

Chronic urticaria may be associated with an underlying malignancy but it is uncommon.[39] Acne urticata, which consists of small urticarial papules surmounted by a vesicle or excoriation, is one of the rare manifestations of polycythemia vera. A characteristic feature of acute necrotizing angiitis, primarily of the Schönlein-Henoch type, are urticarial lesions that quickly become purpuric and ulcerated because of fluid loss and leakage of red blood cells through the damaged vessel wall (see Chapter 8).

Urticaria is a diagnostic marker of juvenile rheumatoid arthritis (Still's disease).[40,41] Still's disease often begins as a fever of unknown origin that persists for weeks to years before arthritis develops. However, it may also begin with monoarticular or polyarticular arthritis. The characteristic rash is found in 9 to 48 per cent of patients. It is almost always present when the illness begins as a fever of unknown origin and is less common in the arthritic presentation. The rash consists of discrete pink to red macules or slightly elevated (edematous) papules that usually range in size from 5 to 10 mm. They may coalesce into larger macules and plaques. The eruption appears mainly on the trunk and extremities and is most intense at the peak of fever in the late afternoon. The lesions last for only a few hours and return in new areas when the fever recurs on the following day. The spots do not migrate or change in shape and almost never itch (Figs. 9–7 to 9–9). The eruption exhibits the Koebner phenomenon. The behavior of the rash in relation to the fever is close to that of cholinergic urticaria; however, the morphology is different. Histologic examination reveals dermal edema and a mild perivascular infiltrate of lymphocytes. A few neutrophils may be present. The histology is most consistent with mild urticaria. Isdale and Bywaters noted that neutrophils rather than mononuclear cells were the principal perivascular cells in their four patients.[42]

In the series of patients reported by Calabro and Marchesano, patients who presented with a fever of unknown origin had their eruptions persist for one week to nine years before the arthritis developed (average time, two years; median, six months). In those individuals whose illness

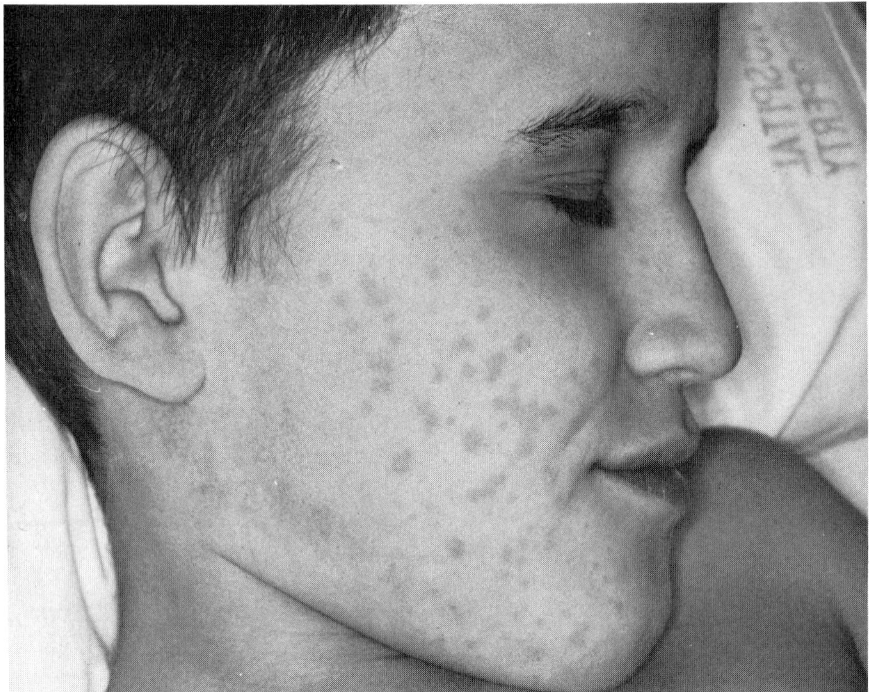

Figure 9–7. Characteristic rash of juvenile rheumatoid arthritis.

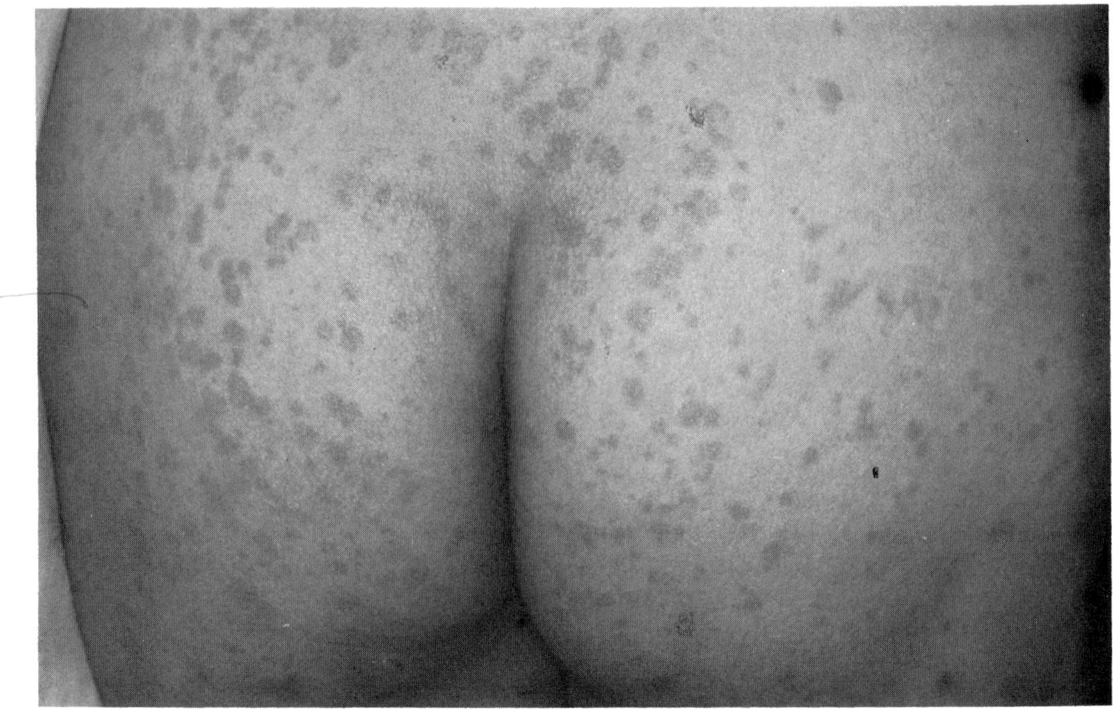

Figure 9–8. Characteristic rash of juvenile rheumatoid arthritis.

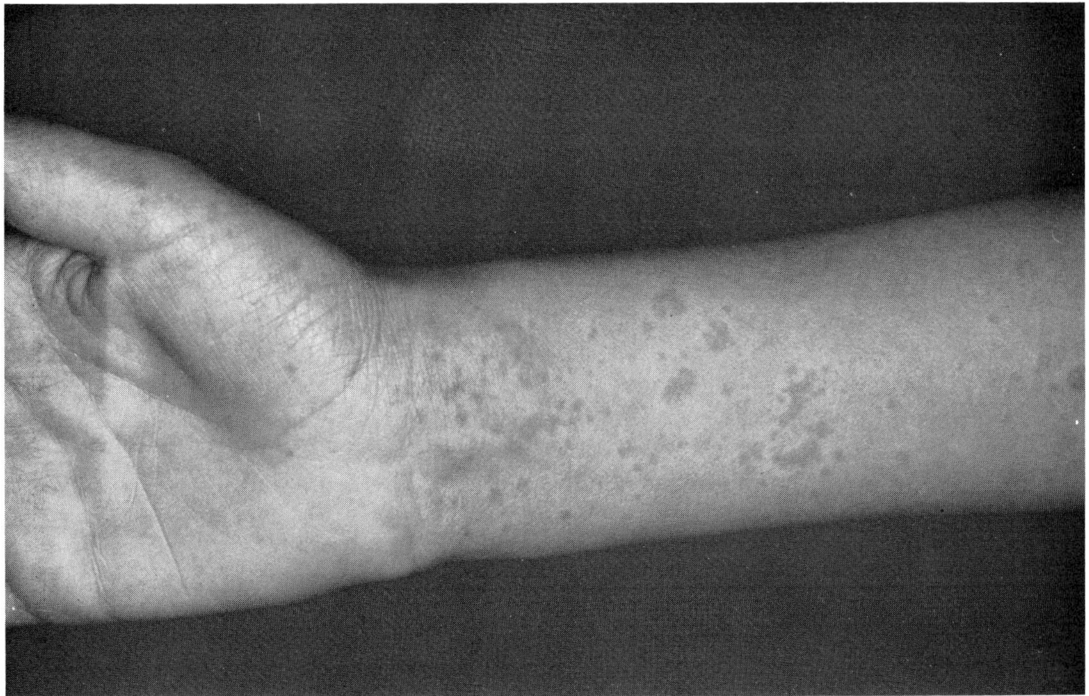

Figure 9–9. Characteristic rash of juvenile rheumatoid arthritis.

began with arthritis, the rash either preceded joint involvement by one to two weeks, or developed five months to 11 years later. In some patients the rash persisted for as long as 12.5 years. Often the eruption appeared or disappeared without any relationship to the course or treatment of the disease. Injections, surgery, emotional upsets, or any type of febrile illness could trigger a recurrence of the rash. Such exacerbations usually lasted for only a few days. The rash in Still's disease has not been found to be useful for prognosis. Still's disease is not limited to children; it occasionally occurs in adults with identical manifestations.

Patients with urticaria pigmentosa (cutaneous or systemic mastocytosis) seek medical attention because of urticaria. The itchy hives often develop following a hot bath, vigorous rubbing with a towel, or pressure against the skin. Close inspection reveals brown to reddish-brown macules on an urticarial base. The lesions are composed of increased numbers of mast cells in the dermis underlying a hyperpigmented epidermis. When stroked or subjected to heat, the mast cells degranulate and release histamine, thereby producing localized urticaria and pruritus (Darier's sign).

Urticaria pigmentosa in children is almost always a purely cutaneous disease and usually resolves spontaneously. The eruption in children is composed of brown or red-brown macules and papules, but large mast cell nodules can be yellow-brown (Plate 25*A*). Solitary mastocytomas as large as 6 cm may develop in children. Bullae or vesicles may arise from solitary or multiple mast cell tumors in children under three years of age. Rarely, the bullae may be hemorrhagic, and petechiae or purpura may appear in cutaneous lesions. Diffuse erythroderma with lichenification is an extremely rare manifestation of childhood mastocytosis. In the adult form of the disease, red-brown freckle-like spots are characteristic (Plate

25B; Fig. 9–10). (This type of lesion can also develop in childhood mastocytosis but is very uncommon.) Adults with urticaria pigmentosa may also have another unique lesion: telangiectasia macularis eruptiva perstans. This is characterized by red to reddish-brown macules with superimposed fine threadlike telangiectases (Figs. 9–11 to 9–13). They do not urticate as well as the more common types of mast cell lesions.

Thirty to 50 per cent of adult patients with urticaria pigmentosa have some evidence of systemic involvement.[4] Collections of mast cells may be found in the bones, gastrointestinal tract, lungs, liver, spleen, and bone marrow. Involvement of the gastrointestinal tract can be detected by barium studies. The liver and spleen may become enlarged. The accumulation of mast cells in the bones may produce either osteosclerotic or osteolytic shadows on radiographs. Degranulation of this enormous pool of mast cells can be produced in some patients by ingestion of codeine or alcohol or by injection of polymyxin B, with the resultant symptoms of headache, flushing, palpitations, diarrhea, and pruritus. Dermographia can often be demonstrated; it sometimes occurs only over each mast cell aggregation and results in a beaded line (Plate 25*C*). Usually, however, the normal-appearing skin also participates so that an uninterrupted line forms. Dermographia by itself is rarely a sign of urticaria pigmentosa, and usually no underlying disorder is found (Fig. 9–5). For a comprehensive presentation of mastocytosis, the reader is referred to the classic work of Sagher and Even-Paz.[44]

Angioneurotic edema is an extreme form of urticaria marked by massive transudation of fluid in the tissues. The face, tongue, lips, larynx, and gastrointestinal tract are the sites of predilection. Typical urticaria also may be present elsewhere. The causes of *allergic* angioneurotic

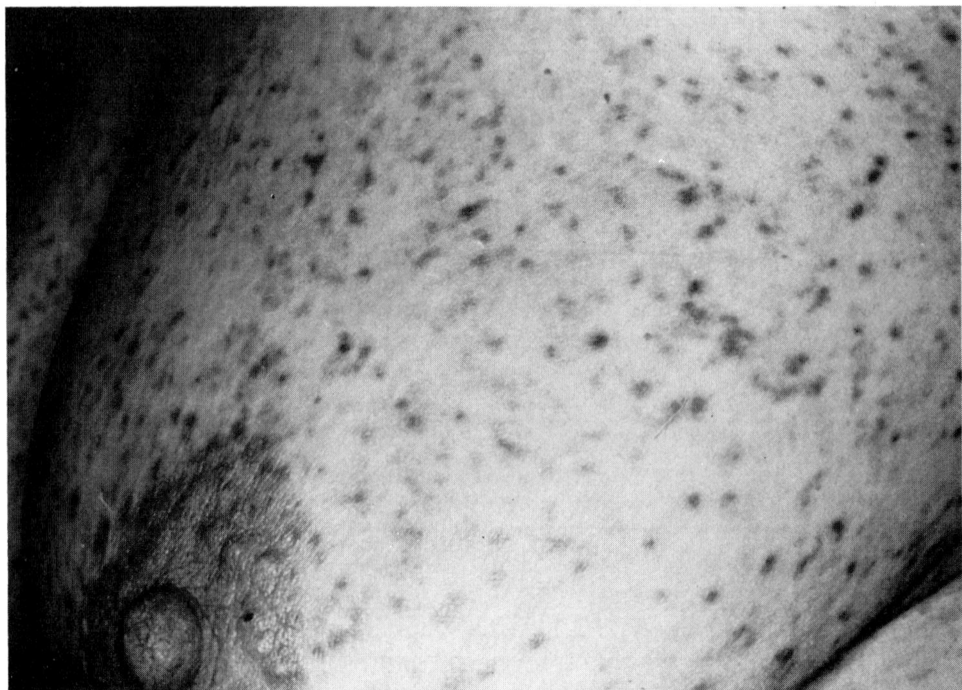

Figure 9–10. Urticaria pigmentosa. Adult form. Red-brown macules.

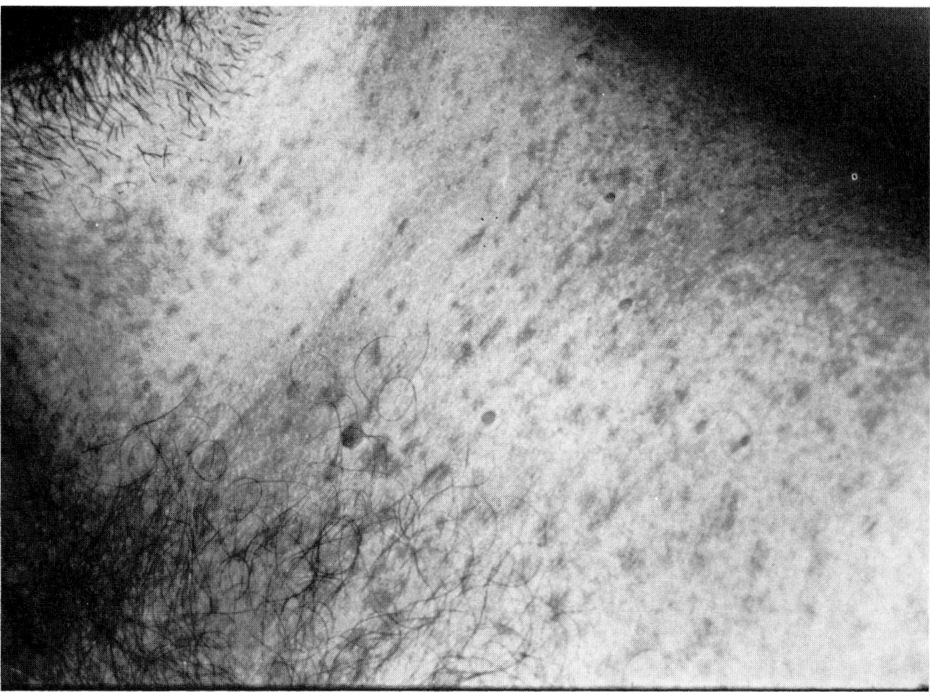

Figure 9–11. Urticaria pigmentosa. Adult form. Telangiectasia macularis eruptiva perstans. Red to reddish-brown macules with superimposed fine threadlike telangiectases.

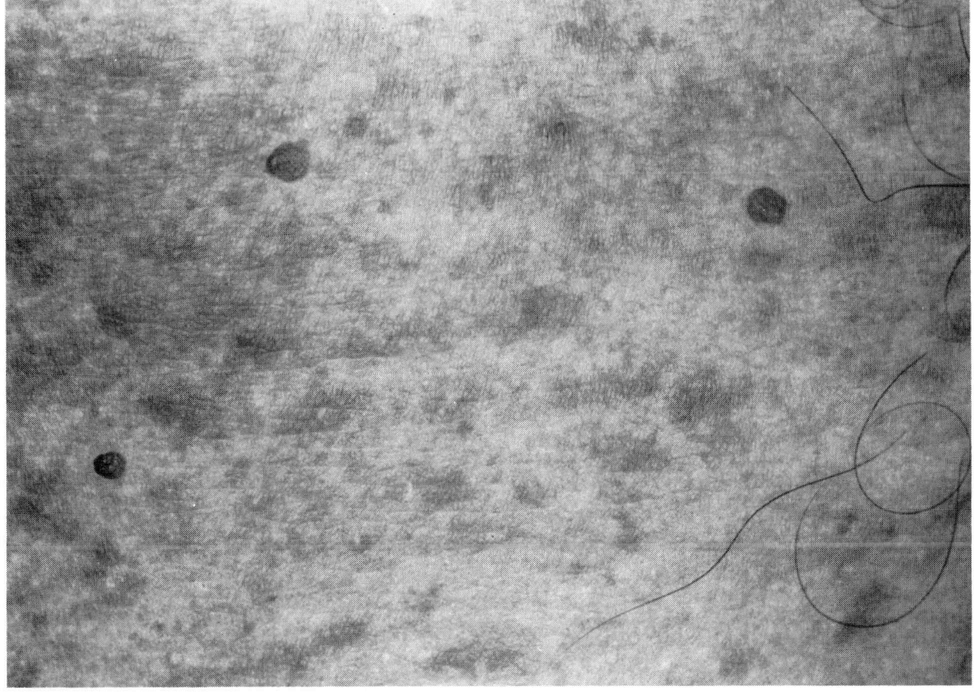

Figure 9–12. Urticaria pigmentosa. Close-up of lesions shown in Figure 9–11.

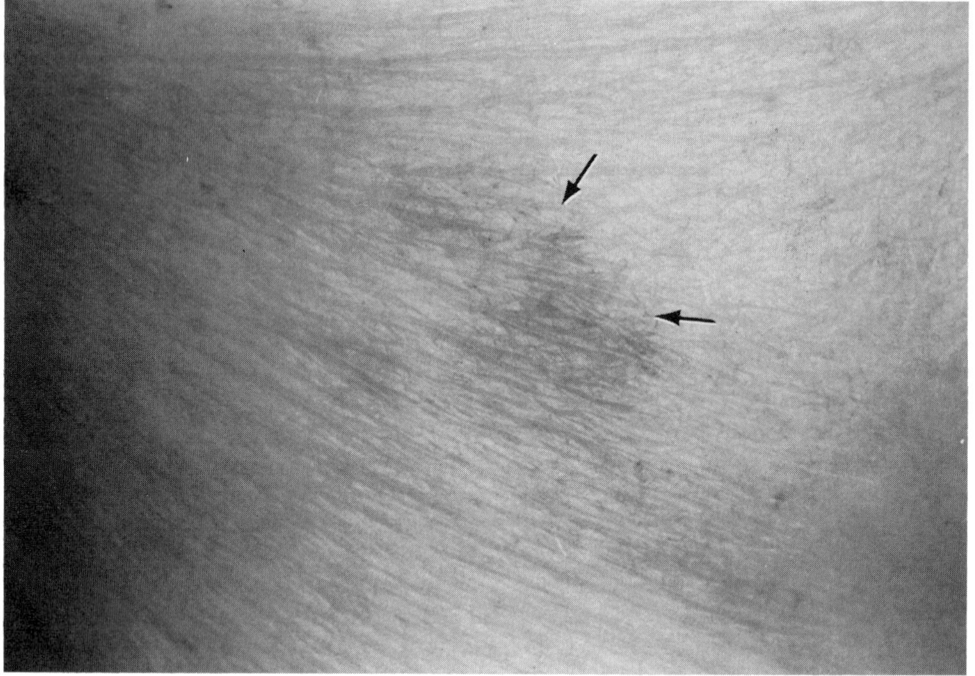

Figure 9–13. Urticaria pigmentosa. Close-up of lesions shown in Figure 9–11. Fine telangiectases (arrows) on red-brown macules.

edema are the same as those of acute urticaria. Angioneurotic edema is an uncommon clinical feature of lupus erythematosus.

Familial angioneurotic edema is a *nonallergic* dominantly transmitted disorder.[11] Usually the edema begins in infancy, though at times it appears as late as the forties. Swelling may develop anywhere, but the skin, gastrointestinal tract, and larynx are the most common sites. Fatal laryngeal edema occurs in 25 per cent of the patients. Acute attacks of abdominal pain and vomiting are common and last two or three days. The episodes of edema are precipitated by trauma, strenuous exercise, emotional excitement, and anxiety. The basis for the disorder is the lack of a serum inhibitor directed against the activated form of C1 (C1 esterase). Eighty-five per cent of patients with this disorder lack the inhibitor; 15 per cent have the inhibitor present as a nonfunctional molecule. The inhibitor is present in individuals with *allergic* angioneurotic edema.

The lack of inhibitor permits unrestricted interaction of activated C1 with its natural substrates C4 and C2 to produce a kinin-like protein from C2. This C2-kinin is subsequently cleaved by fibrinolysin to produce a molecule that enhances the permeability of postcapillary venules resulting in angioedema.[46] The serum levels of C4 are low during asymptomatic periods and fall to zero during an attack. The levels of C2 also decrease during the acute episodes. Measurement of serum levels of C4 is a good screening test for this disorder. Any event that can activate C1 will trigger an attack in these patients.[4]

Acute attacks can be successfully treated with fresh frozen plasma[47] or fibrinolytic inhibitors such as ε-aminocaproic acid and tranexamic acid.[48] Currently danazol, a nonvirilizing androgenic steroid, is being used as a prophylactic and therapeutic agent.[49] It restores the levels of both C4 and C1-esterase inhibitor to normal. This steroid stimulates the synthesis of the C1 inhibitor. Fresh frozen plasma and fibrinolytic inhibitors will still be used in young children and pregnant women for whom danazol is currently contraindicated.[48]

Acquired forms of this type of angioedema have developed in patients with lymphosarcoma, leukemia, and adenocarcinoma of the colon.[50] Individuals with this variant have a complement profile different from those with the hereditary form of the disease. There is a reduction in the serum level of C1, as well as C2, C4, and C1 inhibitor. The reasons for the complement abnormalities in these malignancies are not known.

In summary, urticaria is not as compelling a marker for the investigation of internal disease as Raynaud's phenomenon, erythema nodosum, xanthomas, and purpura. A detailed history, complete physical examination, and relatively simple laboratory tests will usually establish whether or not systemic disease is present. Fever and urticaria should suggest the possibility of juvenile rheumatoid arthritis or the prodrome of serum (B) hepatitis. However, in my experience, chronic idiopathic urticaria has rarely been associated with an internal disease. Those cases in which a cause is uncovered can usually be attributed to one of the following: drugs, including penicillin in dairy products; food and inhalant allergens; physical urticarias; dermographism; emotional stress; hyperthyroidism; and rarely dental infections.[1, 51, 52] The majority of cases, however, will prove to be idiopathic. A significant number may be provoked by salicylates, benzoates, and azo dyes through as-yet-undetermined mechanisms.

Related Disorders

The figurate erythemas are a group of disorders which begin as red macules or papules that spread centrifugally, producing rings with pale or clear centers. Although they are edematous and have an urticarial appearance, they persist for days to months, moving outward at variable rates. Biopsy shows a moderate to intense infiltrate of lymphocytes sharply localized to the perivascular zone — unlike the histologic pattern of ordinary urticaria. The figurate erythemas probably are a manifestation of cell-mediated hypersensitivity. These disorders can be divided into three basic types: erythema annulare centrifugum (EAC), erythema chronicum migrans (ECM), and erythema gyratum repens (EGR).[53]

EAC is the most common variety encountered. As the edematous border moves outward, it often carries a desquamating scale on its trailing edge. The lesions may be so edematous that vesicles or bullae arise on the advancing edge or in the center (Figs. 9–14 to 9–20). Pruritus is sometimes present. Synonyms for EAC include gyrate erythema and erythema perstans. The latter term is used when the figurate erythema arises as an erythematous plaque that persists for weeks to months without developing centrifugal spread. Erythema marginatum is a form of EAC that occurs in rheumatic fever. It differs from the more common varieties of EAC by being a transient eruption.

Most cases of EAC are idiopathic and characterized by a chronic recurrent course with unpredictable periods of remission. In a minority of instances, the eruption has been related to cutaneous infections with

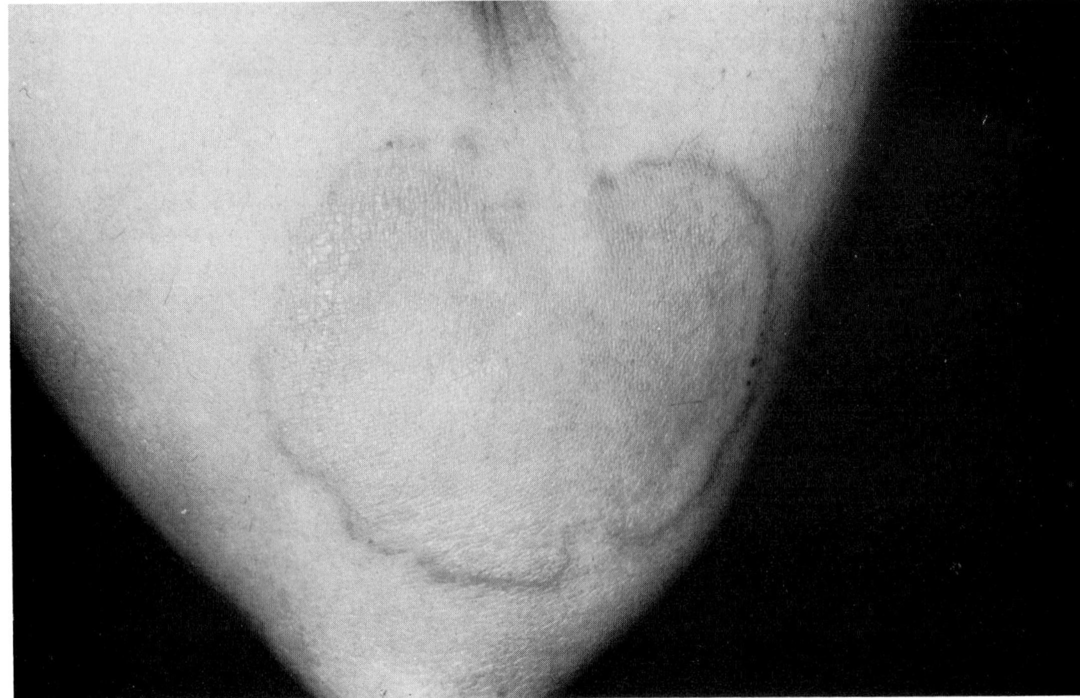

Figure 9–14. Erythema annulare centrifugum of unknown etiology.

dermatophytes and *Candida albicans;* cheese fungi; chloroquine therapy; virginal breast hypertrophy; and benign and malignant tumors.[53] Leimert et al. reported a patient in whom the activity of EAC was related to activity of Hodgkin's disease.[54] In one of our patients, a 13-year-old white girl, EAC developed in association with poststreptococcal glomerulonephritis. One of our patients had an associated benign ovarian tumor (see p. 45).

EAC has also been reported as a genetic disorder. Beare et al. reported an Irish family in which EAC was dominantly transmitted.[55] Four persons in three generations were affected. The eruption appeared shortly after birth. In one person the tongue was involved.

We saw a 55-year-old woman with erythema perstans that had been present recurrently for two years. The individual lesions would persist for approximately three months before fading. The trunk, extremities, and face were affected (Figs. 9–21 and 9–22). Pruritus was mild. One year after the eruption appeared she was found to have desquamative interstitial pneumonitis. However, 25 years earlier, during each of two pregnancies, she had lesions resembling erythema perstans limited to her palms. Both infants developed similar lesions on their faces when they were four to five months old. The erythematous patches spontaneously disappeared one to two months later and have not recurred. This patient had a 25-year remission from her figurate erythema.

Erythema chronicum migrans (ECM) is a well-known entity in Europe, Scandinavia, and Russia.[56, 57] Weeks or months following a tick bite, and in some areas probably a mosquito bite, the individual develops a red papule that slowly expands, producing a ring with a clear center. The rings may attain diameters of 50 cm. The border of the expanding

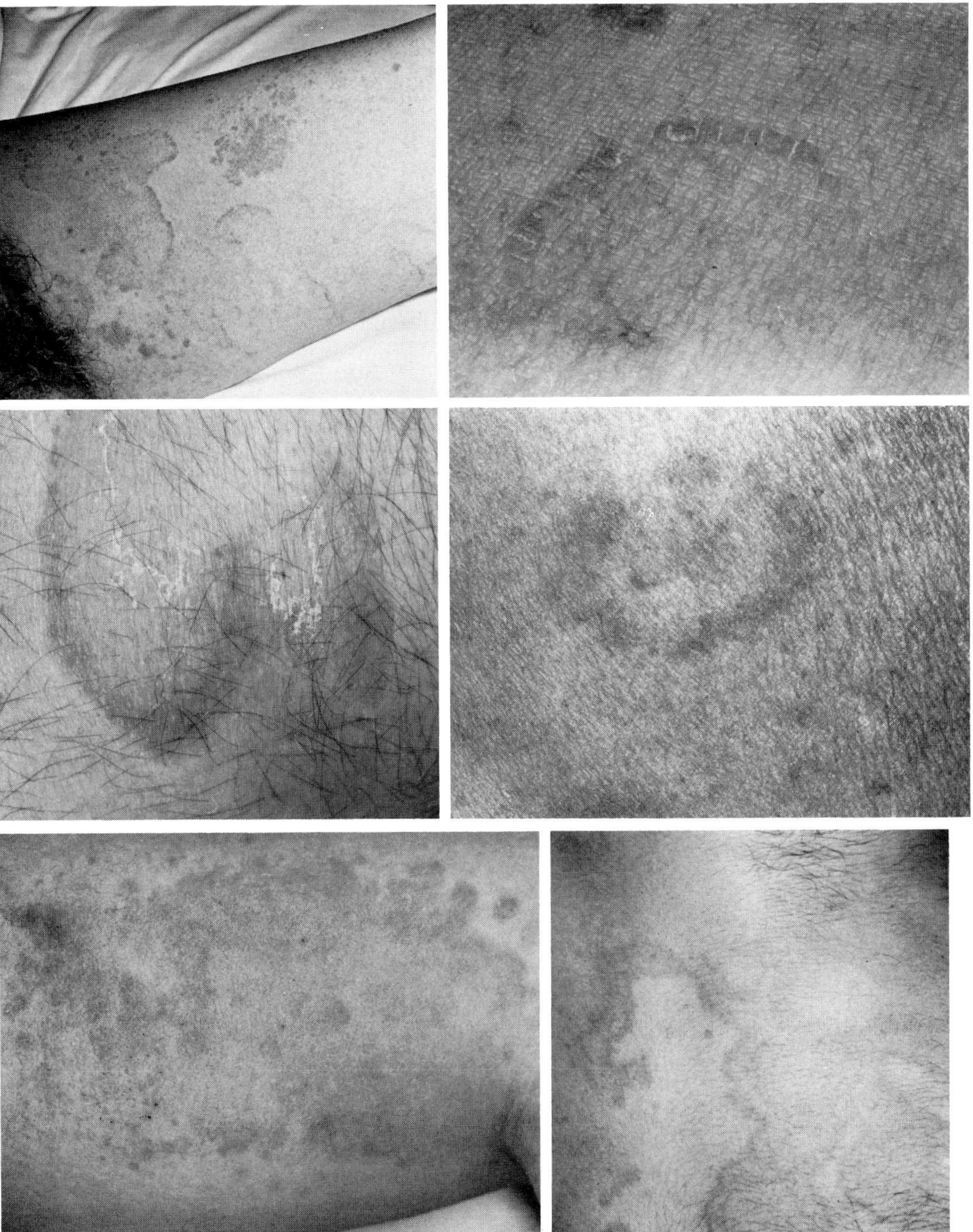

Figure 9–15. Top left. Erythema annulare centrifugum simulating tinea cruris. Ringed lesions with edematous, slightly scaly borders.

Figure 9–16. Top right. Erythema annulare centrifugum. Close-up of lesions in Figure 9–15.

Figure 9–17. Center left. Erythema annulare centrifugum. Edematous border with trailing edge of desquamating scale.

Figure 9–18. Center right. Erythema annulare centrifugum. Advancing border with relatively clear center.

Figure 9–19. Bottom left. Erythema annulare centrifugum. Coalescence of many individual lesions.

Figure 9–20. Bottom right. Erythema annulare centrifugum. Coalescence of large lesions to produce serpiginous pattern.

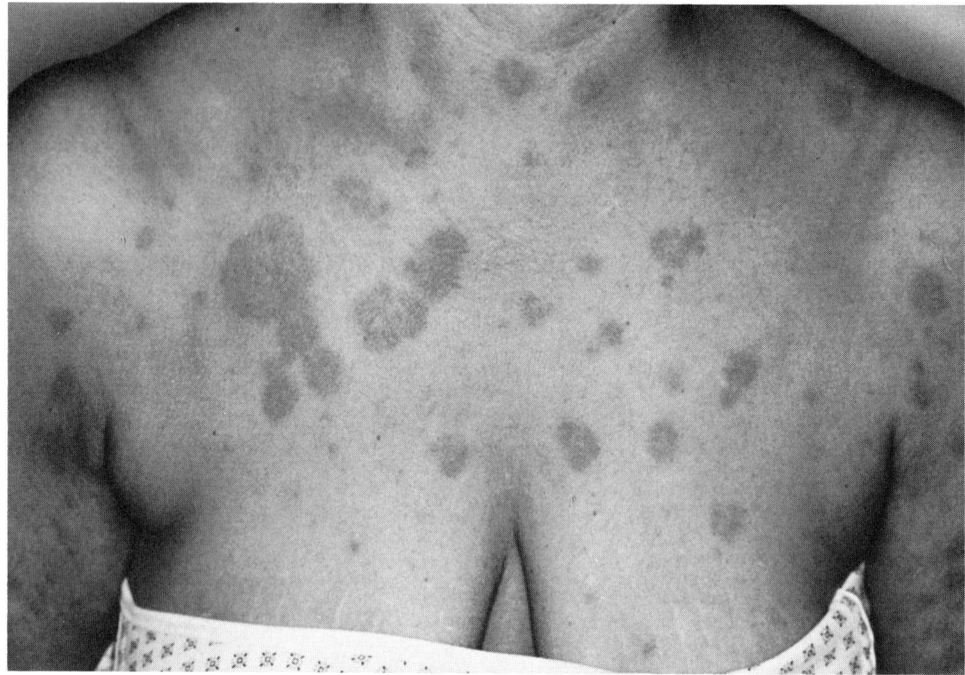

Figure 9–21. Persistent figurate erythema of three months' duration.

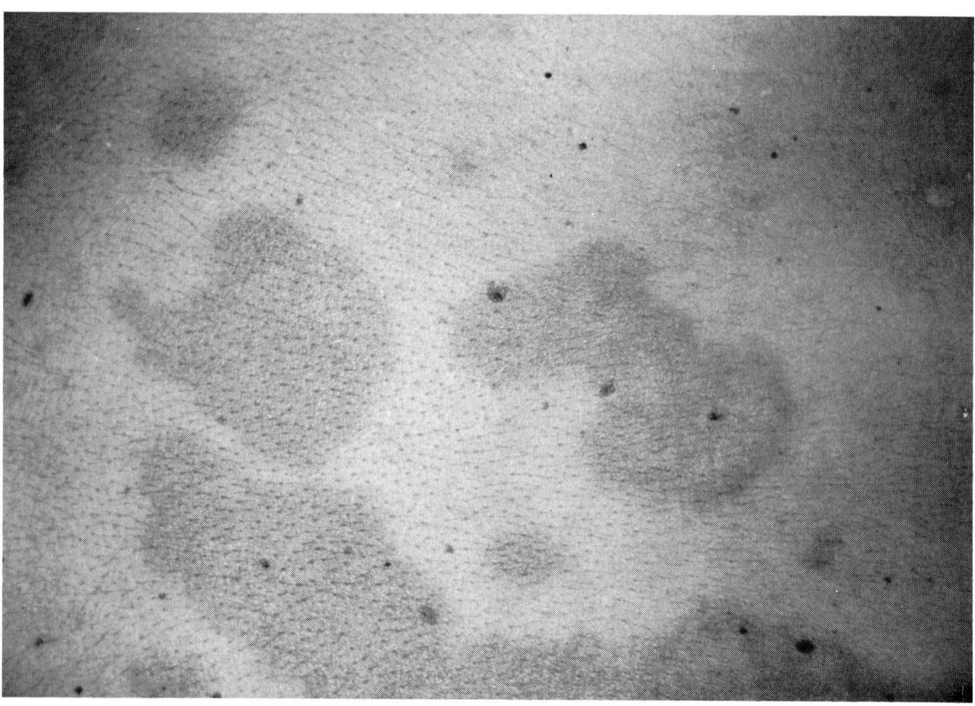

Figure 9–22. Close-up of lesions in Figure 9–21.

lesion is generally smooth without scale, and it is unusual for a person to develop more than one ring. These circular lesions may continue to expand for as long as one and one-half years before spontaneously resolving in untreated cases. Penicillin and tetracycline are said to be effective in producing prompt resolution of the eruption. Both spirochetes and rickettsiae have been implicated as etiologic agents, but neither has been isolated. Undoubtedly there is an infectious etiologic agent in ECM because the disease has been transmitted to unaffected individuals by intradermal inoculation of the ECM tissue. In some individuals, chronic lymphocytic meningitis, peripheral and cranial nerve palsies, and neuropathies have developed as complications of ECM. Prognosis for recovery has been good even though these signs and symptoms may persist for at least three months.

ECM was virtually unseen in the United States until 1972 when an endemic focus appeared in Southeastern Connecticut in the community of Lyme.[58] The illness, initially called Lyme arthritis, but now designated Lyme disease, presented as an unusual inflammatory arthritis that frequently developed after an episode of ECM. Since 1972, 135 patients have been identified and studied by Steere, Malawista, and associates at Yale. ECM developed 4 to 20 days after a tick bite in those who remembered the event. The illness began with a single lesion in all patients, although some later developed multiple rings (4 to 20) (Figs. 9–23 and 9–24). On the average, the ECM spontaneously disappeared in three weeks (range 0.3 week to 8 weeks). Secondary rings formed within the original one in some individuals. In those with multiple lesions, some rings disappeared before others. The rings of Lyme disease are identical to the European form of ECM: they lack a scale on the trailing border; are associated chiefly with sensations of burning, although rarely pain or itching have been described; and they disappear without leaving residual scarring or hyperpigmentation.

In 19 of 32 patients followed prospectively, asymmetric mono-, oligo-, or migratory polyarthritis appeared four days to five months after the development of ECM. The attack of arthritis usually affected only a single joint at a time and lasted for a few days (median eight days, range 1 to 90 days). The knees and other large joints and the temporomandibular joints were most commonly affected. The small joints of the fingers and toes were less frequently involved. The joints were often hot and swollen, but rarely red. In four patients, Baker's cysts formed and ruptured after the onset of the arthritis. At least half of the patients with ECM had malaise, fatigue, chills, fever, headache, stiff neck, and less commonly lymphadenopathy either a few days before or at the time of the skin lesion.

Most patients had recurrent attacks of arthritis lasting about eight days (range 1 to 90) usually separated by periods of remission measured in weeks (average 4 weeks, range 1 to 9). The severity and duration of the attacks and the intervals between them were highly variable and therefore unpredictable. During these recurrent attacks about half the patients reexperienced the initial symptoms of the disease and in a few the original skin lesion or lesions became faintly visible. In some, there was an exacerbation of the lymphadenopathy.

As in the European form of the disease, 4 of 19 patients with Lyme disease followed prospectively developed cranial nerve palsy (Bell's

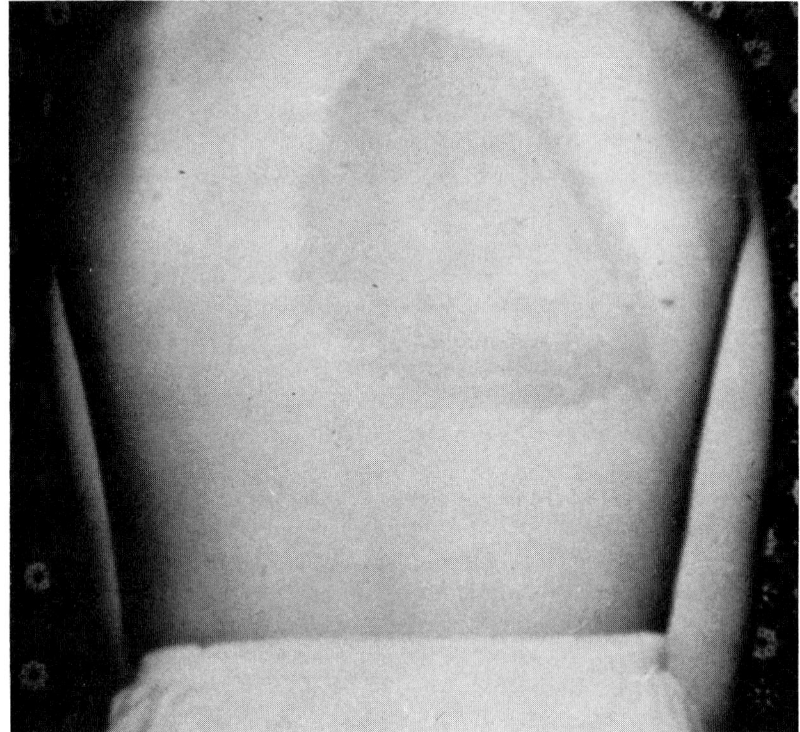

Figure 9–23. Erythema chronicum migrans. (From Steere, A. C., Malawista, S. E., Hardin, J. A., Ruddy, S., Askenase, P. W., and Andiman, W. A.: Erythema chronicum migrans and Lyme arthritis. The enlarging clinical spectrum. Ann. Intern. Med., *86*:685, 1977.)

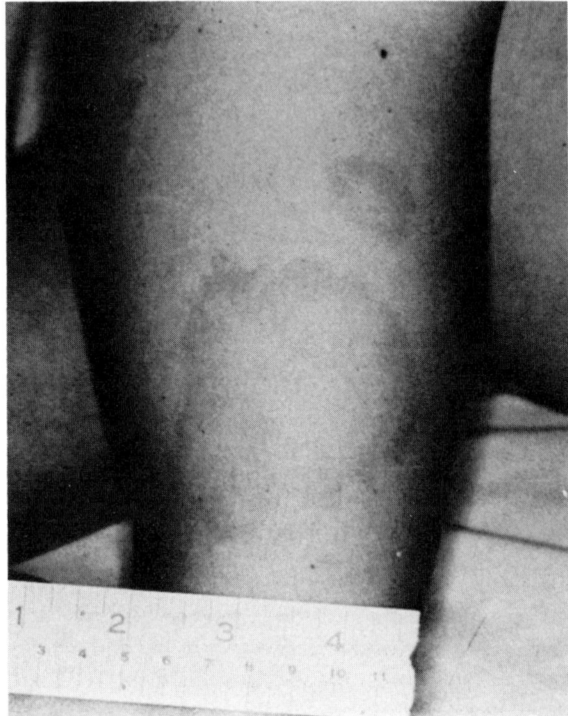

Figure 9–24. Erythema chronicum migrans. (From Steere, A. C., Malawista, S. E., Hardin, J. A., Ruddy, S., Askenase, P. W., and Andiman, W. A.: Erythema chronicum migrans and Lyme arthritis. The enlarging clinical spectrum. Ann. Intern. Med., *86*:685, 1977.)

palsy), asymmetric sensory radiculopathy, and cutaneous paresthesias. In addition, two patients developed fluctuating degrees of atrioventricular block, and one showed alternating left and right bundle branch block. Thirteen of 32 patients who developed ECM did not develop arthritis. Of 78 patients studied, 59 per cent developed arthritis, 23 per cent only ECM, and 18 per cent neurologic and cardiac abnormalities. All the patients in this last category also developed arthritis.

Although the vector in Connecticut has been identified as the tick *Ixodes dammini*, the presumed infectious agent has not been identified. Lyme disease is described here in considerable detail because it is likely that it is not limited to Southeastern Connecticut. It is beginning to appear in other areas of the United States where the tick species *I. dammini* and *I. pacificus* abound. Cases have been found in other areas of Connecticut, Massachusetts, Rhode Island, Long Island (New York), and Wisconsin. Naversen and Gardner reported a case of ECM from Sonoma County, California, secondary to a tick bite.[61] This particular individual showed no sequelae after one year of follow-up.

Steere, Hardin, and Malawista found cryoglobulins composed primarily of IgM in those with ECM, and mixed cryoglobulins (IgM-IgG) in those with active arthritis, implicating a pathogenetic role for circulating immune complexes in Lyme disease. Those who did *not* have cryoglobulins in association with ECM were at a greatly reduced risk for developing arthritis and the other complications of the disease. Subsequent studies by these workers showed that the cryoglobulins were composed of two moieties that coprecipitated in the cold: circulating immune complexes detected by C1q binding and Raji cell assays and an independently generated nonimmunoglobulin cold-precipitable protein.[60] Only 60 per cent of the sera exhibiting abnormal C1q binding contained cryoprecipitates. The circulating immune complexes were present in virtually all patients during the first two weeks after the development of ECM but tended to decline markedly in those with ECM only, or with arthritis. The C1q binding activity in the blood remained abnormally elevated in those who developed cardiac and neurologic complications. The inflamed joints, however, contained abnormal C1q binding activity as well as cryoprecipitates. Although cryoprecipitation is not a property of the circulating immune complexes, the detection of cryoprecipitates containing immunoglobulins is a simple and reliable screening test for the presence of immune complexes in this disorder. In cases in which cryoglobulins are not found, the C1q binding assay becomes both the screening and definitive test.

Currently, the following sequence of events has been proposed for the pathogenesis of Lyme disease. A causative agent is introduced into the skin by a tick bite. Four days to three weeks later, ECM develops at the site in some patients, accompanied by the generation of circulating immune complexes. If the agent is not eradicated in the prearticular phase of the disease, or if the immune system continues to generate immune complexes for other reasons, Lyme disease occurs. If the immune complexes remain disseminated, neurologic and cardiac dysfunction develops; if their production is limited to the synovium, as in rheumatoid arthritis, inflammatory arthritis ensues.[60]

In the absence of skin lesions, brief but recurrent attacks of inflammatory oligoarticular arthritis, particularly if cryoglobulins are present, is suggestive but not diagnostic of Lyme disease. A patient with peripheral neuropathy (particularly cranial nerve palsies), sensory radiculopathy, lymphocytic meningitis, atrioventricular node blocks, or myopericarditis may also have this same illness.[58] The most recent report by Steere et al. suggests that penicillin therapy shortens the duration of ECM and may prevent or attenuate subsequent arthritis.[61a] Penicillin therapy does not decrease the frequency of neurologic and cardiac abnormalities.

In EGR, the thin elevated borders of erythema annulare are replaced by constantly changing broad polycyclic edematous bands that cover the body and resemble the grain pattern of wood (Fig. 1–26). Gyrate erythema has occurred most often in patients with carcinoma.[62] Shelley published the case report of a young woman with massive breast hypertrophy and gyrate erythema. Antibodies to her breast tissue and positive tests for lupus erythematosus cells were found[63] (see p. 44).

ERYTHEMA NODOSUM

Erythema nodosum has been recognized as an entity ever since it was first described by Willan in 1798. In 1866 Hebra added a few other observations. Their clinical descriptions have not been improved upon and are worth repeating.

Willan stated:

> In the erythema nodosum, many of the red patches are large and rounded. The central parts of them are very gradually elevated and on the 6th or 7th day form hard and painful protuberances, which are often taken for impothumes (abscesses), but from the 7th to the 10th they constantly soften and subside without ulceration. On the 8th or 9th day the red colour changes to bluish or livid and the affected limb appears as if it had been severely bruised. This appearance remains for a week or ten days, when the cuticle begins to separate in scurf. The erythema nodosum usually affects the foreparts of the legs. I have only seen it in females, most of whom were servants. It is preceded by irregular shiverings, nausea, headache and fretfulness with a quick unequal pulse and a whitish fur on the tongue. These symptoms continue for a week or more but they usually abate on the appearance of the erythema, so that in the latter stages of the disease, the only sensations of uneasiness are languor, thirst and disrelish for food.[64]

Hebra added the following information:

> In other cases, a second or even a third eruption of these tumors takes place, affecting each time parts previously free from them so that the thighs, forearms and upper arms, the trunk and even the face are in succession covered with them. The duration of the disease as a whole is of course prolonged by the occurrence of these repeated attacks; and the sympathy of the system generally is likewise shown by the fact that paroxysms of fever of more or less severity precede each fresh outbreak. However, none of the more important organs of the body are ever especially attacked; and the extent to which the skin is affected is surely in itself sufficient to account for the febrile symptoms.
>
> Whether this form of erythema is partial or diffused over all parts of the body it always terminates within from two weeks to a month. In particular these tumors never suppurate or break down into abscesses. . . . Lastly the redness of the individual tubercles never spreads to the skin around them; a character which distinguishes the erythema nodosum essentially from furuncular affections, erysipelas and urticaria as well as from the other varieties of erythema already

PLATE 26

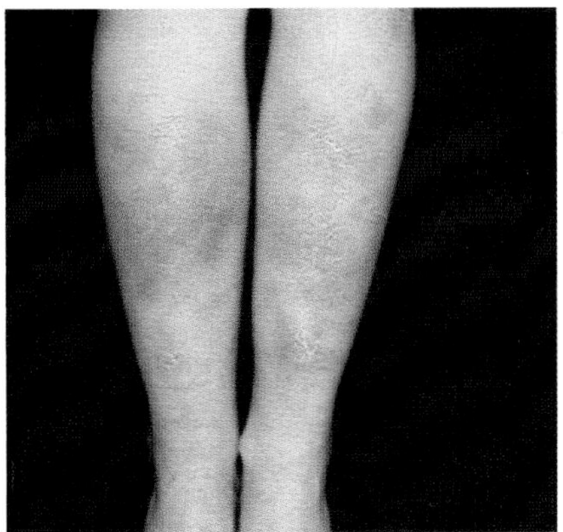

A, Erythema nodosum.

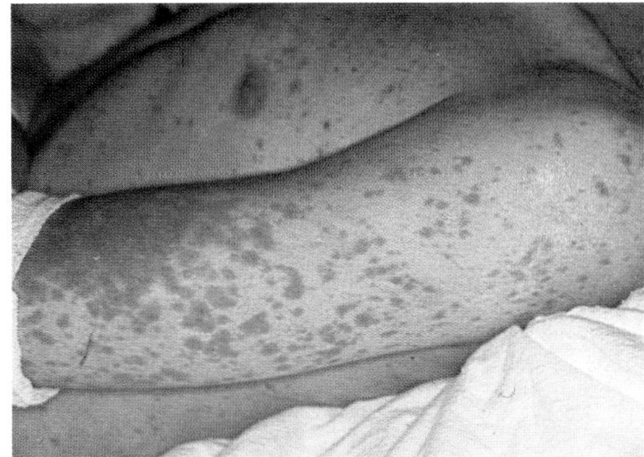

B, Erythema multiforme. Urticarial macules are faintly purpuric. Some have a central petechial punctum.

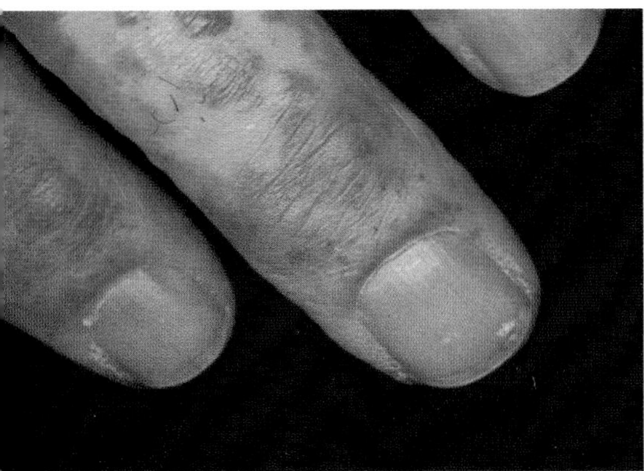

C, Erythema multiforme. Petechiae are evident in the urticarial-bullous lesions.

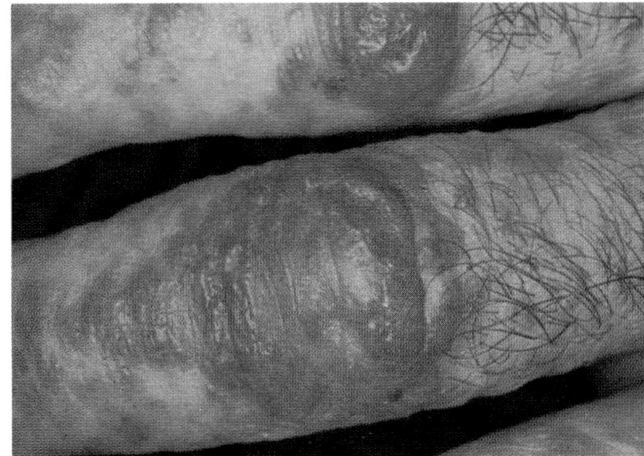

D, Erythema multiforme. Urticarial-bullous lesions with mild purpura.

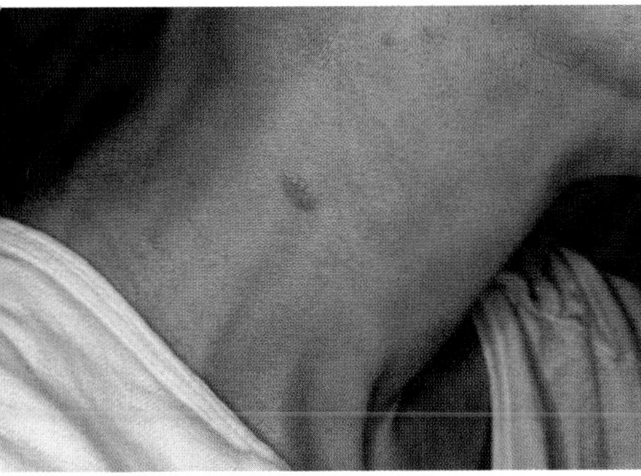

E, Sarcoid. This violaceous nodule on the neck was the sole cutaneous sign in this patient with endobronchial sarcoidosis.

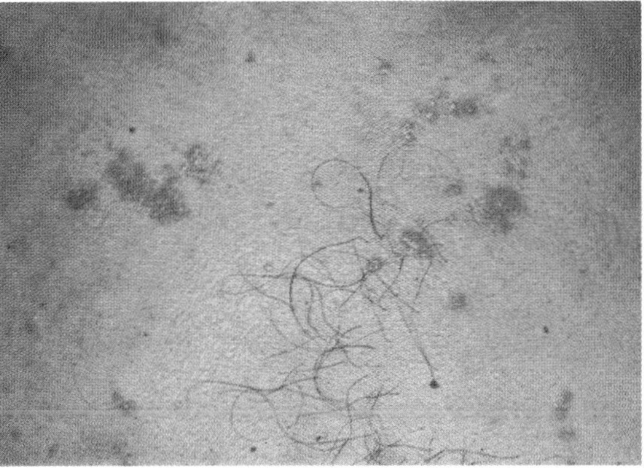

F, Sarcoid. Characteristic violaceous translucent papules.

> mentioned. . . . As I have already stated, all these forms of erythema come to an end spontaneously within a definite period and leave behind them no ill effects. Moreover they invariably terminate in recovery.[65]

Hebra also commented that erythema nodosum was more frequent in women than in men and coined the term *dermatitis contusiformis* as an alternate name.

These clinical descriptions must be amended only to a minor degree. Although the lesions of erythema nodosum are usually deep nodules, they also may develop as superficial, mildly edematous, warm, red, tender areas (Plates 25*E*, *F* and 26*A*). They can form a confluent patch that covers the entire shin and resembles erysipelas. The lesions do not always evolve in a spectrum of colors resembling a bruise; sometimes the bright erythema fades directly into the normal color of skin. The absence of color changes does not exclude a diagnosis of erythema nodosum. Although the usual duration is from three to six weeks, erythema nodosum may persist for six to ten months. Bäfverstedt describes a less common manifestation that he calls erythema nodosum migrans. The individual lesions divide and extend peripherally as they evolve (Fig. 9–25).[66, 67]

Two features of erythema nodosum need to be emphasized: lesions can arise anywhere in the skin where subcutaneous fat is present, and recurrent attacks separated by months or years are not unusual.

Episcleral nodules also may appear in association with erythema nodosum and follow the same course as the skin lesions. The nodules usually develop in the palpebral fissure near the insertion of the medial rectus muscle. They are bilateral and more superficial than other types of episcleral nodules. Their histopathology resembles Aschoff bodies and the subcutaneous nodules of rheumatic fever. Granulomas are not present.[68, 69]

Kerbel observed a unique manifestation in one of his patients with erythema nodosum. A 33-year-old Scottish woman had three attacks of erythema nodosum during a five-year period. With the third episode, which followed a cold and sore throat, she also developed tender red nodules in the depths of old scars from an appendectomy and from a surgical repair of the median nerve in the forearm. A biopsy of the shin lesions revealed the characteristic histopathology of erythema nodosum. There was no evidence of sarcoidosis clinically or on radiographic examination of the chest, and it is likely that subcutaneous fat adjacent to the scars developed lesions of erythema nodosum.[70]

Erythema nodosum often begins with fever, chills, and malaise.[71] The temperature may reach 105° F. Leukocytosis with a shift to less mature granulocytes on the differential blood count is not unusual.

Articular involvement may accompany the febrile phase or may precede it by two to six weeks. About 60 to 70 per cent of patients with erythema nodosum have associated arthropathy. The most commonly affected joints are the knees, ankles, wrists, fingers, shoulders, elbows, and hips. The arthropathy appears in a number of ways. Patients may complain only of morning stiffness or of pain and stiffness; but more often erythema, swelling, and tenderness are found over the joints and may be associated with effusions. Fortunately, crippling arthritis does not develop. The arthropathy frequently persists after the lesions of erythema nodosum have resolved. Truelove observed that in his series of 41

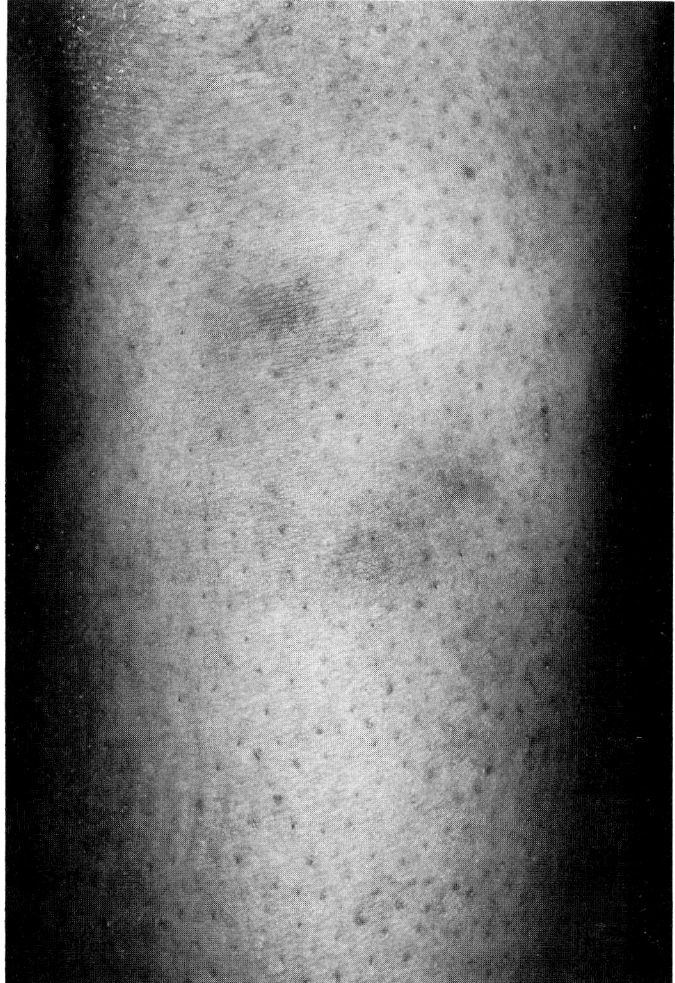

Figure 9–25. Erythema nodosum migrans. Erythematous nodule formed two separate lesions as it extended peripherally and cleared in the center.

patients, about 40 per cent had joint complaints for less than six weeks and 30 per cent had joint complaints for six weeks to six months. Two years after the attack, 30 per cent still had some complaints, mainly of pain and stiffness.[72]

Erythema nodosum can be diagnosed easily when the typical nodules are present on the shins. However, difficulty arises when lesions over the joints occur not as discrete nodules but as red, superficial, slightly edematous patches. It is not unusual for erythema nodosum to begin this way; and the tenderness of the skin may be misinterpreted as a painful joint and diagnosed as acute arthritis instead of erythema nodosum.

Bilateral or unilateral pulmonary hilar adenopathy is an integral feature of erythema nodosum, although it does not occur in every case. The incidence of hilar node enlargement depends upon the particular patients comprising the series of erythema nodosum; consequently a meaningful figure cannot be given. It is clear, however, that hilar adenopathy develops as part of the erythema nodosum reaction. Hilar adenopathy occurs in cases of erythema nodosum associated with tuberculosis, upper respiratory infections, coccidioidomycosis, histoplasmosis, and streptococcal disease, as well as with sarcoidosis.[73] Therefore, bilateral hilar adenopathy in association with erythema nodosum is not an *unequivocal* diagnostic sign of sarcoidosis. It is not known if hilar adenopathy also occurs in erythema nodosum that is caused by drugs.

Erythema nodosum displays a seasonal incidence — spring and late fall through the winter — as well as appearing all year. During childhood, girls are affected slightly more than boys, but in adult life women develop the disorder three to four times as often as men. The peak incidence in women occurs at 20 to 35 years. After the age of 50, erythema nodosum is not common.

On the basis of my review of the medical literature, it seems that erythema nodosum has been more prevalent in the British Isles and Scandinavian countries than in the United States. During the past twenty years this disorder has become less common all over the world.

Erythema nodosum belongs to the panniculitis group of diseases and is a delayed hypersensitivity response to a number of bacterial, fungal, and viral agents. In most cases the pathologic features are those of inflammation of veins in the fibrous septa of the fat. The septal collagen is markedly edematous and infiltrated by mononuclear cells and neutrophils.[74] Necrotizing angiitis is not present. Hemorrhage in the septa is a characteristic finding and accounts for the color changes responsible for the name "contusiformis." Dilatation of the vessels in the overlying dermis contributes to the erythema and warmth of the lesions. However, Winkelmann and Förström have pointed out that there is a spectrum of histologic changes in clinically typical erythema nodosum.[75] There may be acute inflammation with neutrophils and necrosis in the septa and, by extension, into the periphery of the fat lobules. In a few cases, they found acute neutrophilic inflammation involving the entire fat lobule. Even less commonly there may be granulomatous inflammation affecting the septa and fat lobules. However, these granulomatous and acute inflammatory changes must make up only a minor portion of the clinical lesion, because erythema nodosum resolves without scarring — a major distinction from the rest of the panniculitides. These recent studies emphasize  two practical clinical points: an excisional biopsy is necessary for the proper evaluation of tender nodose lesions on the legs, and correlation of clinical features with histologic findings is required for arriving at the correct diagnosis. Reliance on histologic findings alone may lead to erroneous conclusions. This spectrum of histologic changes in erythema nodosum, which has not been sufficiently appreciated in the past, is most likely the result of variations in the intensity of the delayed hypersensitivity response. In the other panniculitides described elsewhere (Chapter 14), fat necrosis and granulomatous inflammation with subsequent clinically recognizable scarring are the major histologic and clinical features that distinguish these disorders from erythema nodosum.

Since its delineation in the eighteenth and nineteenth centuries, erythema nodosum has been associated both with "rheumatism," because of the articular symptoms, and with tuberculosis. However, within the past 30 years the true nature of the disorder with its multiple etiologies has been uncovered. Thirty years ago the underlying factors varied throughout the world; but today, with certain minor exceptions, the etiologies are similar.

Erythema nodosum develops as a delayed hypersensitivity reaction to a previous β-streptococcal infection such as pharyngitis, tonsillitis, or scarlet fever. Intradermal skin testing with extracts from the streptococcus will produce a tuberculin type reaction, as well as exacerbate or induce the lesions of erythema nodosum, in susceptible persons.[76]

Erythema nodosum also follows the development of primary tuberculosis, coccidioidomycosis, histoplasmosis, North American blastomycosis, psittacosis, lymphogranuloma venereum, and cat-scratch disease. The development of erythema nodosum correlates with the individual's temporal conversion from a negative to a positive reactor to (e.g.) tuberculin, histoplasmin, and coccidioidin.[77, 78] Here as well, a positive skin test may exacerbate or induce lesions of erythema nodosum. In a few cases of histoplasmosis, coccidioidomycosis, and psittacosis, erythema multiforme has accompanied the erythema nodosum. Other infections associated with erythema nodosum include dental abscesses, tinea capitis with kerion formation, nonstreptococcal acute bronchitis or upper respiratory diseases, toxoplasmosis, and leptospirosis. In France and Scandinavia, especially Finland, infection with Yersinia bacilli is a common cause of erythema nodosum.[79, 80] The Yersinia bacilli (enterocolitica and pseudotuberculosis) that belong to the Pasteurella group cause acute diarrhea and abdominal pain simulating acute appendicitis, secondary to mesenteric lymphadenitis or terminal ileitis. In a few patients, erythema multiforme has accompanied the erythema nodosum reaction.

Noninfectious illnesses of importance that are associated with erythema nodosum include ulcerative colitis and regional enteritis, especially when there is a marked activity of the inflammatory bowel disease. I have seen erythema nodosum in a patient with sinus tracts in the abdominal wall that were caused by retained sutures that were being discharged intermittently. Rheumatic fever, surprisingly, is only rarely associated with erythema nodosum, even though both represent hypersensitivity reactions to the streptococcus. Much of the early confusion on this point stemmed from assumptions that the arthralgia of erythema nodosum represented rheumatic fever.

Drug reactions are not a common cause of nodose lesions, but medications most frequently implicated are the sulfonamides, iodides and bromides, and most recently, the oral contraceptives.[81] Pregnancy can also be a cause of erythema nodosum. Bombardieri et al. reported the case of a woman who developed erythema nodosum in each of four pregnancies and while on birth control pills.[82] The erythema nodosum appeared during the second month of pregnancy and remitted by the fifth month each time. I have also seen women with erythema nodosum in whom pregnancy was assumed to be the etiologic factor after all other known causes had been excluded. Sarcoidosis is a very important associated disease and is discussed in more detail later in this chapter and in Chapter 10.

During the period from 1956 to 1966, 38 patients with erythema nodosum were hospitalized at the Yale-New Haven Hospital. The etiologic factors are listed in Table 9–1. Streptococcal infections were the cause in 38 per cent of children and 25 per cent of adults. Sarcoidosis was present in 16 per cent of adults. In about 25 per cent of cases of erythema nodosum, including some with hilar adenopathy, no etiology was es-

Table 9–1. ANALYSIS OF ETIOLOGIC FACTORS IN 38 PATIENTS WITH ERYTHEMA NODOSUM

	Female	Male	Total
Children	3	3	6
Adults	26	6	32
Children:			
Streptococcal infection	0	2	2
Ulcerative colitis	1	1	2
Unknown etiology	2	0	2
Adults:			
Streptococcal infection	7	1	8
Ulcerative colitis	4	1	5
Sarcoidosis	4	1	5
Rheumatic fever	1	0	1
Drug reaction*	1	1	2
Tuberculosis	0	2	2
Unknown	9	0	9

*Furadantin, bromides.

tablished. Comparable data were obtained by James et al., who analyzed several series from 1960 to 1974 totalling 1043 patients:[83] streptococcal infections were present in 22 per cent; sarcoid, in 37 per cent; and no cause was discovered in 24 per cent.

It has been customary in various reviews on erythema nodosum to include other associated disorders. However, upon studying some of these cited references, I have found that the diagnoses were based on insufficient information or on a misinterpretation of clinical and histologic findings.

The misinterpreted associated disorders include the lepra reaction of lepromatous leprosy, which actually represents a leukocytoclastic angiitis[84]; meningococcemia, gonococcal disease, and measles, for which the reports are not documented well enough to be certain what the cutaneous lesions represent[85]; and various kinds of acute leukemia for which neither histologic proof nor studies to exclude other causes of erythema nodosum were performed.[86] However, we have seen one patient with granulocytic leukemia who had two biopsy-proven episodes of erythema nodosum one year apart. No specific cause other than leukemia could be determined.

Twenty to 30 years ago in the United States, especially in New England, streptococcal infection and bronchitis accounted for about 80 per cent of the cases of erythema nodosum.[76] Tuberculosis, sarcoidosis, and other disorders were responsible for the rest. In the southwest United States and in the Ohio Valley, coccidioidomycosis and histoplasmosis, respectively, were the main causes. In Great Britain and Scandinavia, primary tuberculosis and streptococcal disease were the most important; sarcoidosis was implicated in only about 10 per cent of the cases.

With the advent of antituberculous therapy and penicillin, the incidence of erythema nodosum caused by tubercle bacilli and streptococci has decreased greatly. In fact, today erythema nodosum is becoming uncommon. The incidence has decreased exclusively in children, among whom tubercle bacilli and streptococci used to be the chief culprits. There has not been a similar decrease in the number of adult cases of erythema nodosum because primary tuberculosis and streptococcal infections are much less common in adults. Löfgren's data show that the incidence of primary tuberculosis associated with erythema nodosum decreased from 58 per cent in 1944 to 17 per cent in 1949 and to 12 per cent in 1966. The incidence of sarcoidosis rose from 9 per cent in 1944 to 40 per cent in 1949. In 1966, 88 per cent of the cases were nontuberculous in origin, and no children with erythema nodosum were seen in Löfgren's clinic in Sweden.[87] Similar decreases in erythema nodosum associated with tuberculosis have been reported in England and in Finland.[88, 89]

Currently, the causes of erythema nodosum are relatively uniform over the world with the exception of endemic foci of coccidioidomycosis, histoplasmosis and yersiniosis. In children, streptococcal or upper respiratory infections are the most common etiologies, and primary tuberculosis is the next most frequent cause. Any child under five years of age who develops erythema nodosum in association with a positive tuberculin test and without evidence of a β-streptococcal infection or other respiratory illness should be considered to have tuberculosis. Tuberculosis is more prevalent in some areas of the world than it is in others.

Sarcoidosis accounts for a proportion of the adult cases of idiopathic erythema nodosum. The exact percentage will not be known until more cases are studied via biopsies of the liver or of mediastinal and scalene nodes. Bilateral hilar adenopathy together with erythema nodosum does not establish the diagnosis of sarcoidosis, since hilar node enlargement also occurs in erythema nodosum produced by streptococcal infection, tuberculosis, histoplasmosis, coccidioidomycosis, and viral upper respiratory diseases. It is likely that the development of hilar adenopathy in all these disorders is related to the portal of entry of the infectious agents.

Milliken and Tattersall in Northern Ireland published data indicating that sarcoidosis is a frequent cause of adult idiopathic erythema nodosum.[90] Over a five-year period, they examined 47 patients with this disease: 36 women and 11 men, 17 to 76 years old, comprised the study group. Except for hilar adenopathy in some, no signs or symptoms of sarcoidosis were present. Biopsies of scalene nodes were performed in 43 patients. Twenty-three of the 43 patients had hilar adenopathy, and the scalene node biopsies revealed sarcoid granulomas; 4 had hilar node enlargement, but their scalene biopsies showed normal histology; 3 had normal chest x-rays, but the scalene nodes revealed granulomas; and the remaining 3 had normal chest roentgenograms and normal scalene biopsies. Forty per cent of the patients with sarcoid granulomas reacted to tuberculin; this is the percentage found in most series on sarcoidosis.

Subsequently, the same investigators studied an additional 24 patients using a reliable Kveim antigen. Eleven of the 24 patients with hilar adenopathy had a positive Kveim test; one person with hilar node enlargement did not react to the Kveim antigen; 5 persons with normal chest radiographs developed Kveim positivity; and 7 with normal chest films did not.

In this last group, 63 per cent of the patients with erythema nodosum and hilar adenopathy presented histologic or serologic evidence of sarcoidosis. The remaining cases were ascribed to streptococcal infection, viral upper respiratory disease, and possibly, tuberculosis. These studies also indicate that hilar adenopathy does not always accompany sarcoidal erythema nodosum.

Textbooks and articles have created the impression that sarcoidosis always runs a benign, self-limited course when erythema nodosum is its initial manifestation.[91, 92] However, we have now observed five patients who have developed progressive sarcoidosis involving liver, lung, and skin after such an onset.

Hormonal factors may be important in sarcoidosis manifesting itself as erythema nodosum. The majority of the patients are women in their reproductive prime, 20 to 35 years old. Sarcoidosis can improve with pregnancy only to relapse when pregnancy ends. Löfgren noted that 30 per cent of his female patients developed sarcoidosis with the resumption of menstruation during the puerperium.

In summary, an adult patient with erythema nodosum today most likely has one of the following underlying disorders; streptococcal or other upper respiratory illness or sarcoidosis. The less common causes — coccidioidomycosis, histoplasmosis, primary tuberculosis, drug reactions, ulcerative colitis, regional enteritis, lymphogranuloma venereum, and psittacosis — should be excluded.

A child with erythema nodosum probably has a streptococcal or other upper respiratory infection or primary tuberculosis. Sarcoidosis with erythema nodosum is rare in children. The other associated disorders should be ruled out by appropriate tests.

Erythema nodosum behaves as a recurrent disorder in 10 per cent of the patients. In such cases, it is assumed that the individual has been reexposed to the same antigen(s), which in most instances is the streptococcus.

Racial factors also may be important in the pathogenesis of erythema nodosum, since not all people with (e.g.) streptococcal disease and tuberculosis develop nodose lesions. James stated that erythema nodosum occurred most frequently in Irish women living in London, and Siltzbach said that the Puerto Rican immigrants in New York City were especially susceptible to the disease.[93]

The differential diagnosis of erythema nodosum includes superficial and deep thrombophlebitis, erysipelas, angiitis, and the fat-destructive panniculitides. Palpable linear cords are diagnostic clues for thrombophlebitis; unilateral lesions with sharply demarcated and advancing elevated borders are the features of erysipelas; and a hyperpigmented depression in the skin, following resolution of a nodose lesion, is a sign of panniculitis with fat necrosis. The clinical diagnosis of erythema nodosum can be confirmed by biopsy.

ERYTHEMA MULTIFORME

Erythema multiforme has been a confusing entity for many physicians, partly because of terminology. It seems to me that the adjective *multiforme* permits one to consider any erythematous eruption occurring in an acutely ill person as an example of this disorder. (Other synonyms include erythema multiforme exudativum or bullosum, ectodermosis erosiva pluriorificialis, and Stevens-Johnson syndrome.)

The adjective *multiforme* was first introduced by Hebra probably to indicate that a variety of cutaneous lesions occur. Although a single type of lesion might predominate during a particular attack, different kinds might appear either in the eruption associated with a single attack or during subsequent recurrences. A polymorphous appearance could also be produced by crops of lesions at different stages of development.

Basically, erythema multiforme consists of only two kinds of lesions: macular-urticarial and vesiculobullous; the clinical diagnosis can be made readily if they are kept in mind.

The eruption has a predilection for the backs of the hands, palms, soles, and the extensor surfaces of the limbs. The lesions may develop initially at these sites and then spread to the rest of the body, or they may be generalized from the beginning. In 25 per cent of patients, the mucous membranes are affected, and such involvement can be the sole manifestation of erythema multiforme. Pruritus may be present. Resolution of cutaneous lesions takes place without scarring, but hyperpigmentation often develops and persists at these sites for many months before spontaneously fading away. The evolution and resolution of individual lesions lasts about a week, but the efflorescence may continue to appear in crops for as long as two to three weeks. The latter feature contributes to the multiforme appearance.

Histologically erythema multiforme is characterized by the development of subepidermal edema that produces urticarial lesions when moderate and bullae when severe. Intercellular edema of epidermal cells frequently accompanies the subepidermal lesion. In addition, necrosis of epidermal cells may be present in the basal cell layer or may be generalized in the entire epidermis, simulating the histologic picture of toxic epidermal necrolysis. Focal epidermal changes are common in the macular-urticarial lesions, and generalized necrosis in the bullous and iris lesions. Curiously, the stratum corneum is unaffected despite intense inflammation in the papillary dermis composed by lymphocytes and a few neutrophils. However, the features of necrotizing angiitis are not present.

The macular lesions are bright red and well circumscribed; and they frequently become urticarial within a few hours as the dermal edema accumulates. Mild purpura ensues and produces a livid, cyanotic, or violaceous color in the majority of lesions. It is rare for the macules not to undergo any change (Plate 26*B, C*).

Iris lesions are urticarial patches with dusky centers and bright red active borders (Figs. 9–26 and 9–27). They can undergo renewed activity by developing red urticarial centers and enlarging centrifugally. It is not unusual to see targets of concentric circles whose bright red rings alternate with cyanotic or violaceous ones. Sometimes iris lesions link up to produce colorful polycyclic and gyrate festooning. Target lesions are found only in erythema multiforme. Careful inspection of the eruption in erythema multiforme discloses fine petechiae, which is the clinical feature that distinguishes erythema multiforme from annular urticaria (Plate 26*D*).

Massive exudation in the upper dermis lifts the epidermis and produces a vesicle or bulla located most commonly in the center of urticarial or iris lesions (Figs. 9–28 and 9–29). Sometimes small vesicles stud the active red border of the iris lesion. The blisters can be grossly bloody, but this is extremely unusual. In some patients the blisters seem to arise from normal skin or minimally edematous and erythematous patches. Such a bullous efflorescence may be the sole manifestation of the disorder.

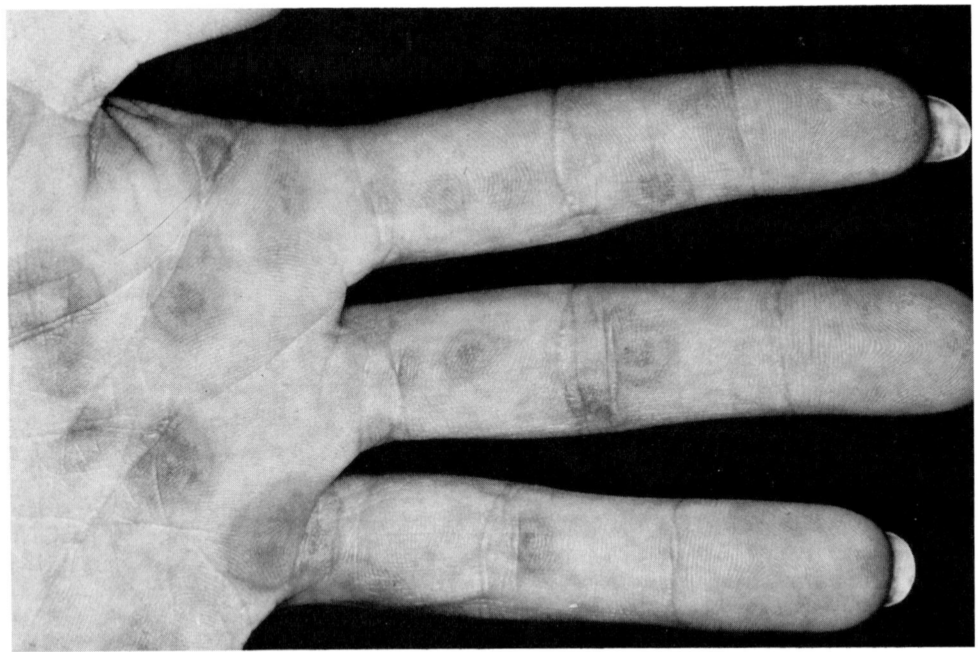

Figure 9–26. Erythema multiforme. Iris (target, bull's-eye) lesions on palm.

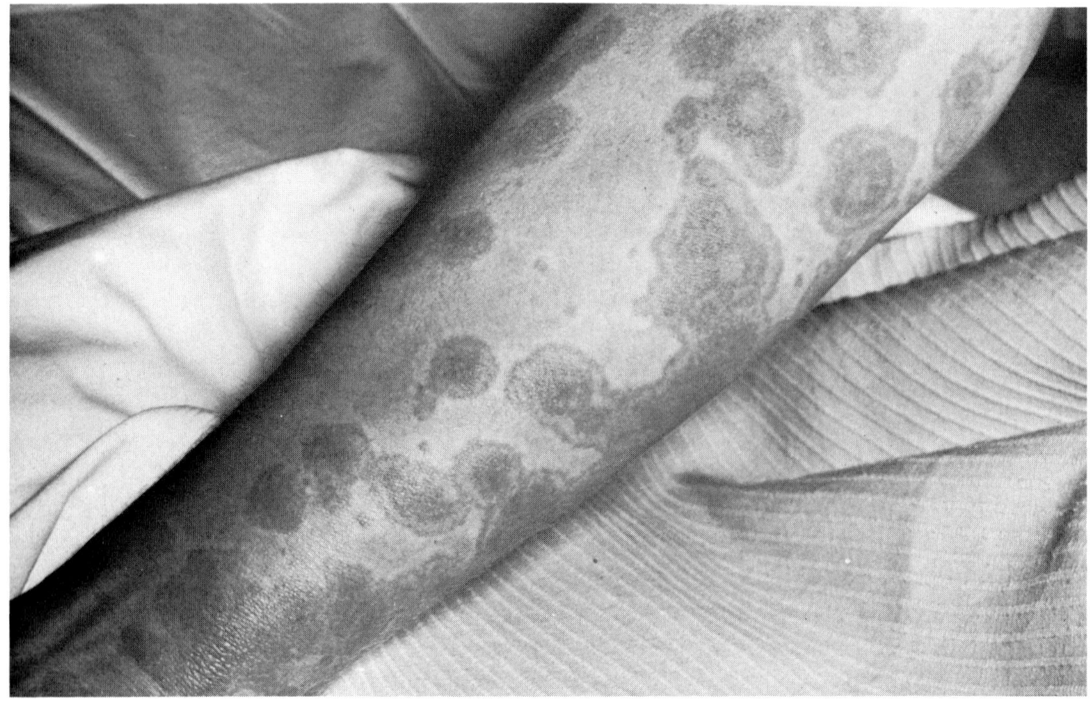

Figure 9–27. Erythema multiforme. Iris (target, bull's-eye) lesions.

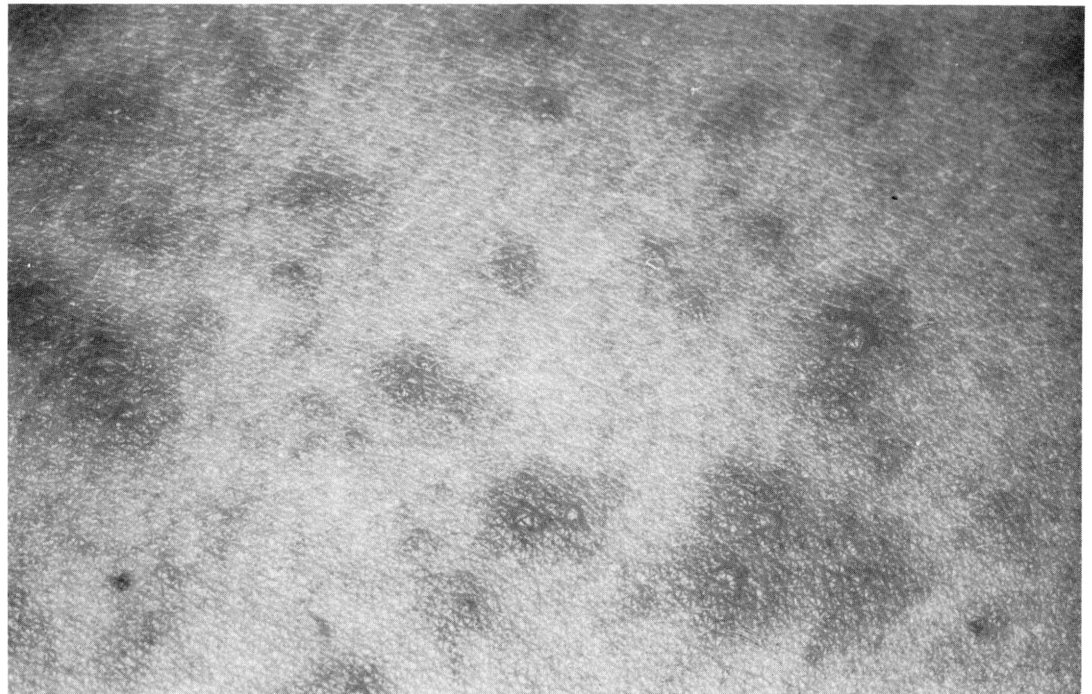

Figure 9–28. Erythema multiforme. Erythematous macules with blister formation.

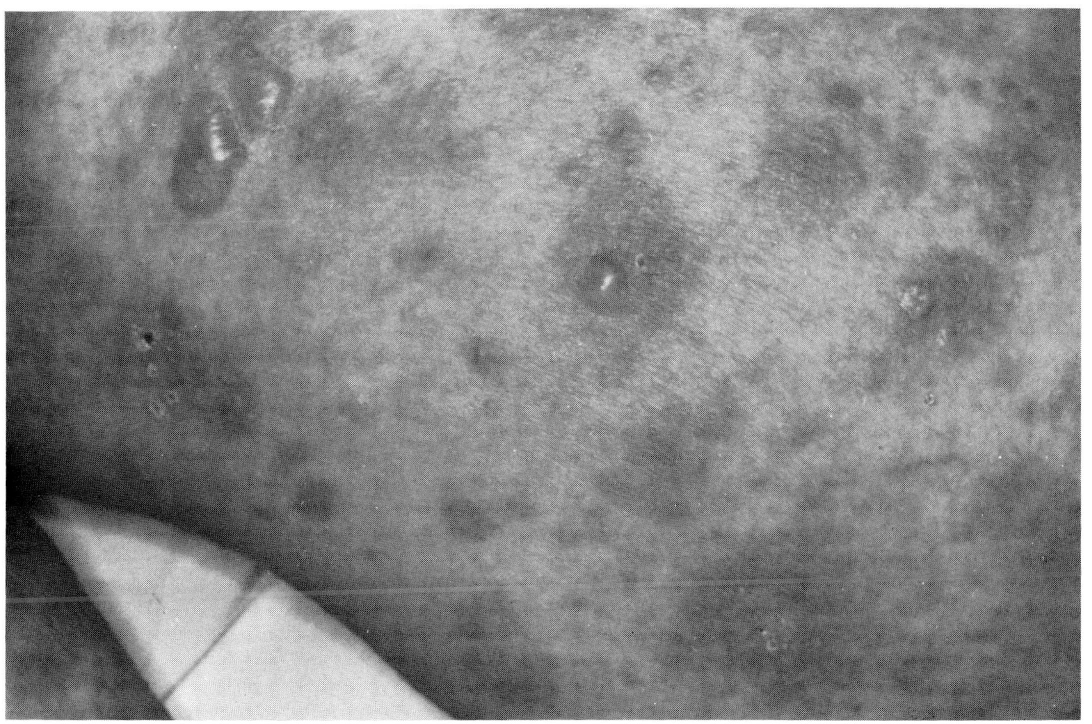

Figure 9–29. Erythema multiforme. Bullae are filled with clear serum.

Mucosal involvement occurs alone or in conjunction with cutaneous lesions (Figs. 9–30 to 9–35). The lips, buccal mucosa, palate, conjunctivae, urethra, and vagina are the areas most frequently involved. In severe cases, the pharyngeal, tracheobronchial, and esophageal lining can also be affected. The anal and nasal mucosae are less common sites.

Mucosal involvement begins with bullae that break very soon after formation and leave denuded areas that undergo a variety of changes. There may be simply a grayish surface membrane that persists until healing occurs, or extensive bloody crusts may form. Patients are unable to eat because of painful stomatitis. They are also susceptible to secondary bacterial infection of the conjunctivae. Surprisingly, healing of mucosal lesions takes place without scarring, unless there has been severe secondary bacterial infection.[95]

Erythema multiforme is seen in all age groups, although the causes in children and young adults tend to be different from those found in older persons. A seasonal incidence in the fall and spring is characteristic; and the disease generally lasts from two to four weeks, though it may continue for two months. The prodromal symptoms range from almost no constitutional complaints to severe toxic manifestations. This variance is most likely due to the etiology of the particular episode; for instance, drug reactions and visceral carcinoma tend to produce fewer symptoms than does an infection. The general pattern is one of fever, sore throat, cough, and malaise, which are followed by mucosal and cutaneous lesions. However, in addition to the constitutional symptoms, mucosal or skin involvement may be the only manifestations in any given attack. The fever may be short-lived or it may continue for two to three weeks. The upper respiratory symptoms may be present a few days to two weeks before the mucosal and skin lesions appear. Unfortunately, the very severe cases with mucocutaneous involvement have been labeled Stevens-Johnson disease, which incorrectly implies a separate entity.[96]

Although erythema multiforme is generally considered to be acute and self-limiting, recent observations indicate that it behaves as a chronic,

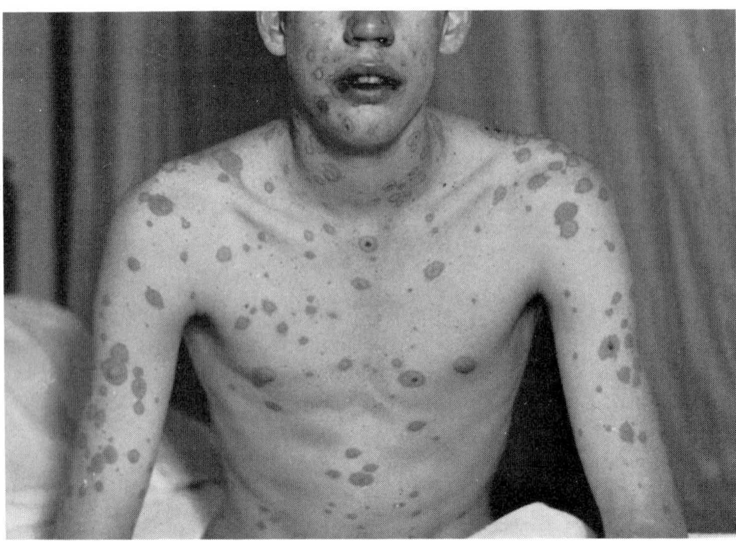

Figure 9–30. Erythema multiforme. Mucocutaneous syndrome.

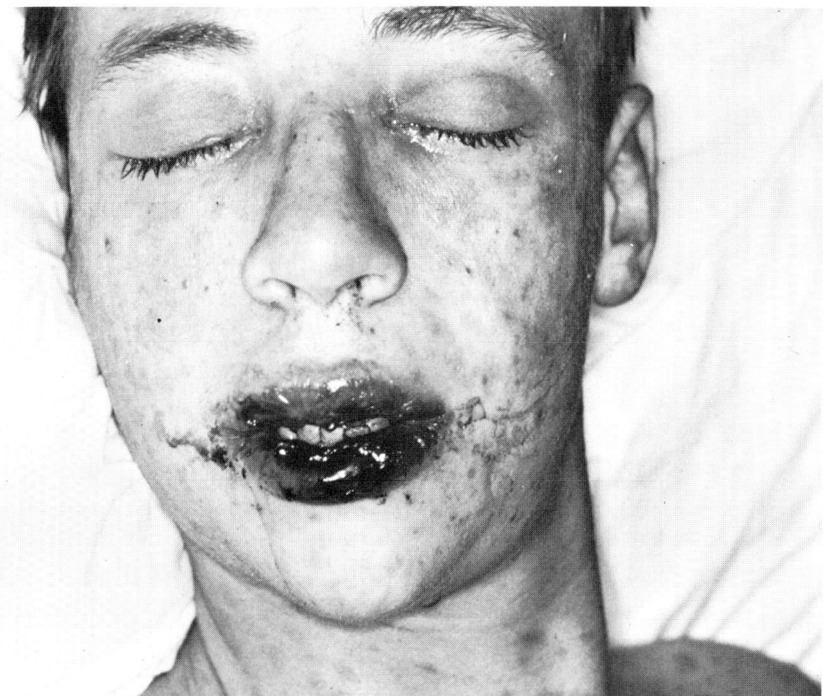

Figure 9–31. Erythema multiforme. Mucocutaneous syndrome. Bleeding and crusting of lips are typically seen in this syndrome.

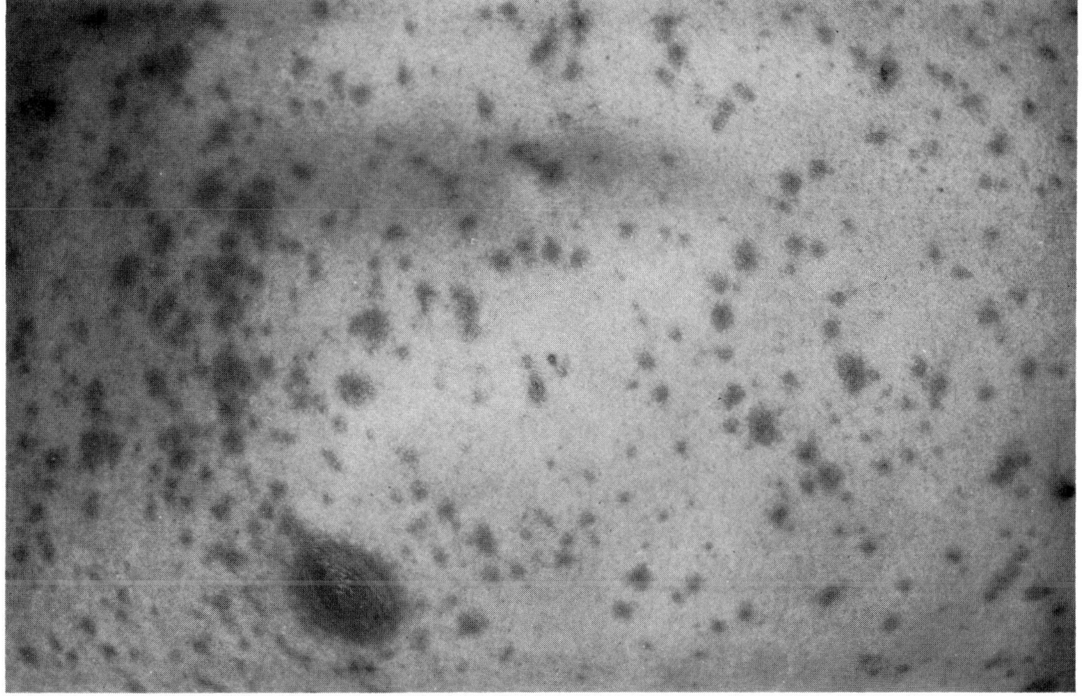

Figure 9–32. Erythema multiforme. Same patient shown in Figure 9–31. Macules are faintly purpuric and are becoming urticarial and bullous.

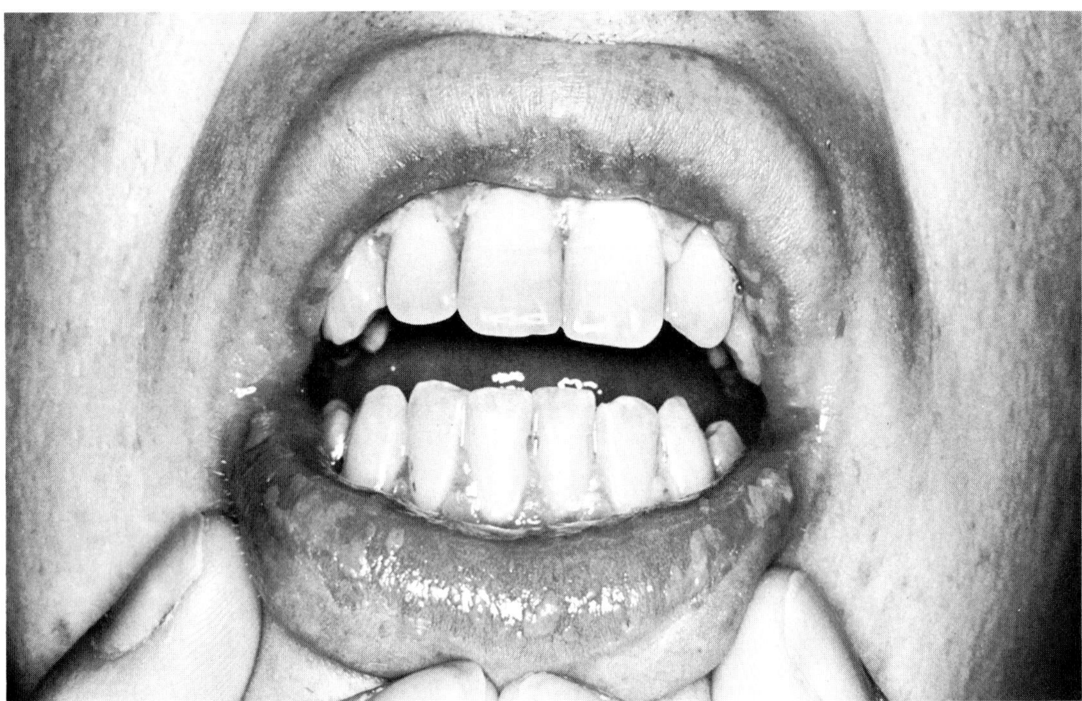

Figure 9–33. Erythema multiforme. Stomatitis was the sole manifestation in this patient who had mycoplasma pneumonitis.

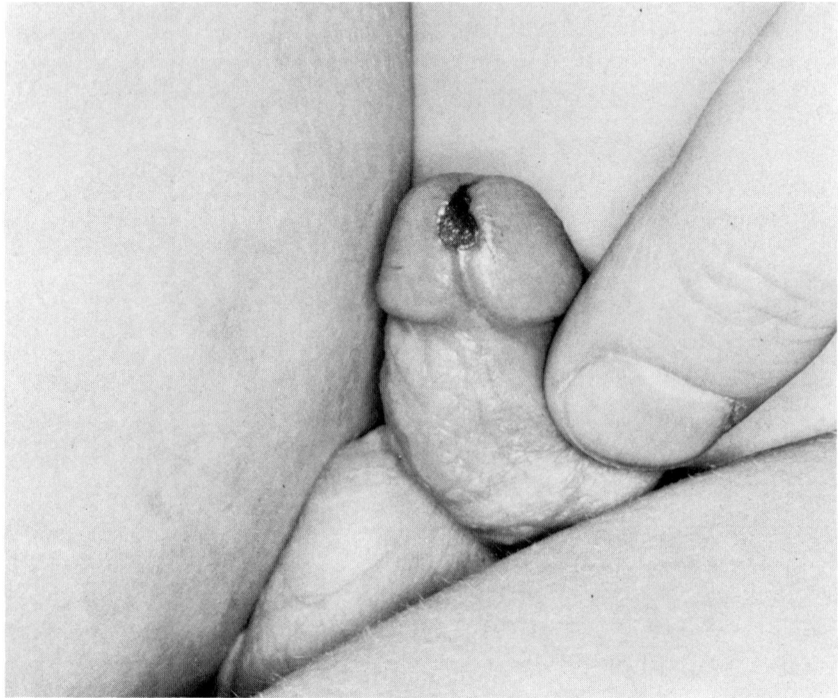

Figure 9–34. Erythema multiforme: Urethral mucosa is involved.

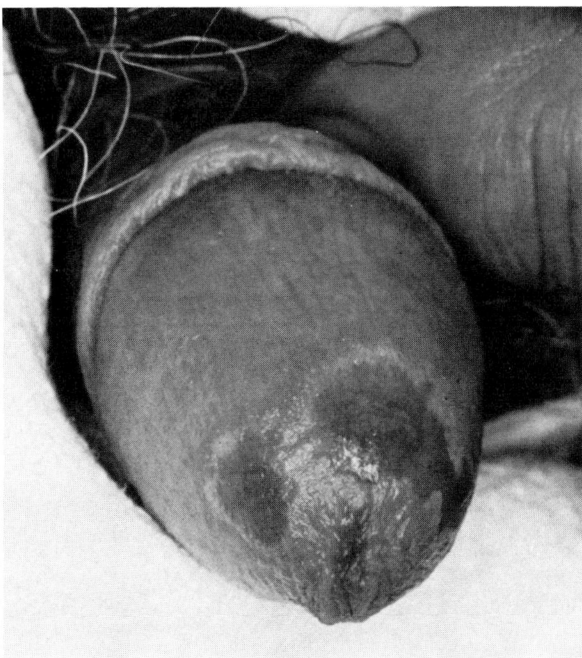

Figure 9–35. Erythema multiforme. Iris lesions on glans penis.

recurrent disorder in a significant number of individuals. In a recent review of 50 consecutive patients with erythema multiforme examined at a dental clinic, only 20 per cent were found to have self-limited disease.[95a] In the other patients the disorder recurred at irregular intervals, or cycled every 12 to 24 weeks over the course of 1 to 21 years, or had been present almost continually without any significant period of remission. The mucous membranes or skin or both can be involved in the chronic form of the disease (Figs. 9–36 and 9–37). Although patients who have had two or three episodes are assumed to have been reexposed to the same stimuli, the causes of the chronic form of the disease are unknown. Medical centers ought to review their experience with erythema multiforme to determine the percentage of patients in this category. In the past 10 years, we have seen two men and three women in whom the disease has been chronic with irregularly occurring episodes of acute activity. The total duration of their illnesses has ranged from 10 to 30 years. Etiology was not determined in any of these patients. In contrast to patients with the acute form of erythema multiforme, these individuals had marked scarring of the buccal and lingual mucosae.

Erythema multiforme, like erythema nodosum, has multiple etiologies. Herpes simplex infections, usually of the lip or genitals, may be followed in seven to ten days by erythema multiforme. Shelley estimated that 15 per cent of cases of recurrent erythema multiforme were due to recurrent herpes simplex. Lozada and Silverman found the same percentage in their series.[95] Shelley showed that the intradermal injection of formalin-inactivated herpes vaccine into a patient with erythema multiforme secondary to herpes simplex not only produced a bullous lesion at the site of injection but also, 48 hours later, produced identical lesions over the rest of the body. Two patients with erythema multiforme, which

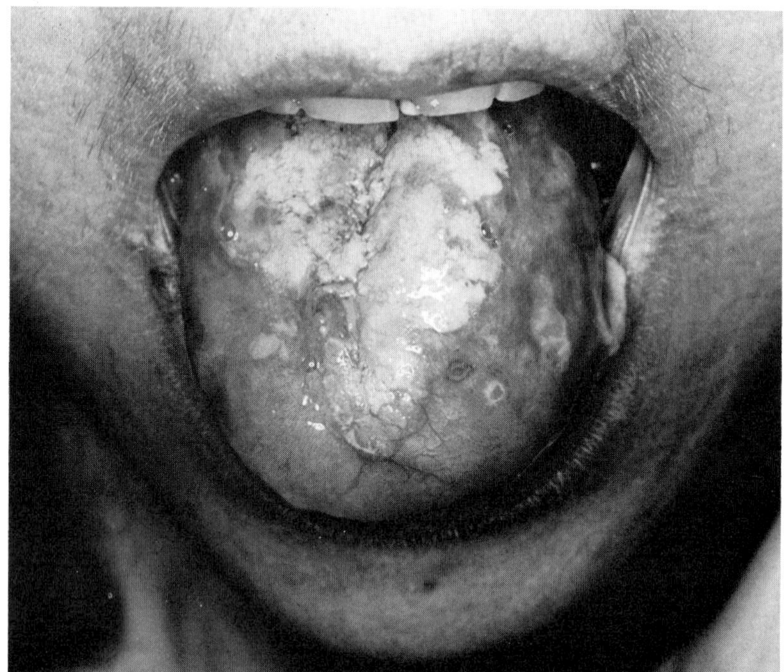

Figure 9–36. Chronic erythema multiforme producing ulceration and scarring of tongue.

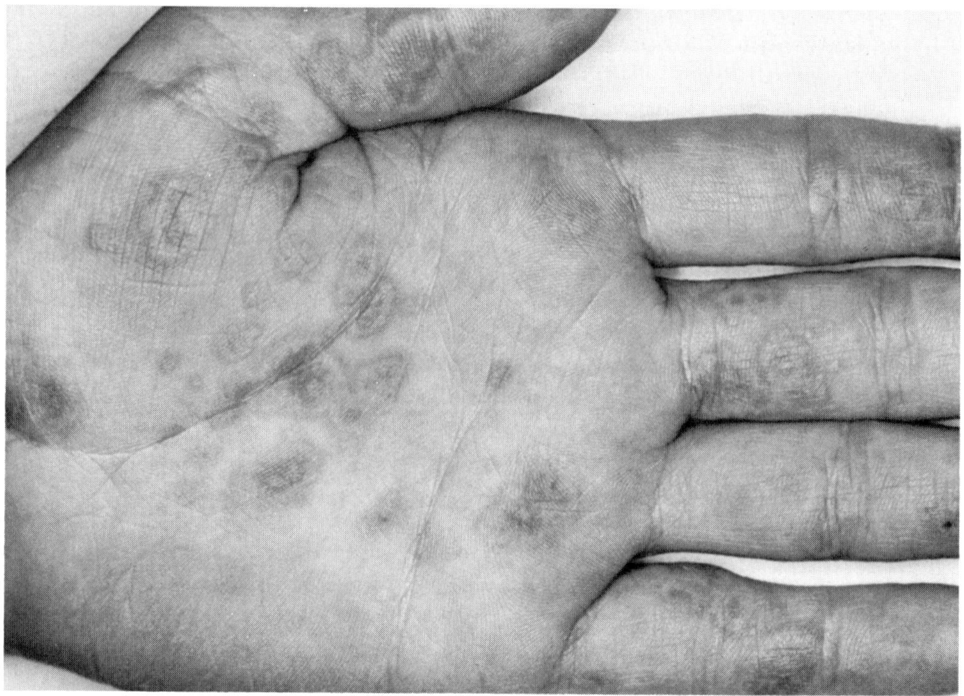

Figure 9–37. Chronic erythema multiforme affecting palms.

in one case was related to cancer and in the other to a drug reaction, did not react in this fashion to the skin test; nor did patients who had only herpes simplex infections.[97] Shelley was also able to produce local and generalized target lesions with intradermal injections of five different heat-killed enteric gram-negative bacteria and bacterial endotoxin, respectively, in another patient. These studies suggest that erythema multiforme may arise in true association with respiratory, gastrointestinal, and urinary tract infections.[98]

Infection with *Mycoplasma pneumoniae* (Eaton agent) can be followed by erythema multiforme. The association between atypical pneumonia and erythema multiforme has been known since 1945, but the etiologic agent was first demonstrated by cultural and serologic techniques 20 years later.[98-100] Other etiologic infectious agents are Coxsackie B-5, influenza type A, and ECHO viruses.[101] In one case, the agent appeared to be Trichomonas.[102] Persons with psittacosis, histoplasmosis, coccidioidomycosis, and yersiniosis can develop erythema multiforme together with erythema nodosum. Although erythema multiforme has been reported along with Pseudomonas and meningococcal infections, review of the publications reveals that urticaria, not erythema multiforme, was the more probable diagnosis. Vaccination with BCG, vaccinia, and poliomyelitis viruses has resulted in erythema multiforme. Söltz-Szöts reported a patient who developed erythema multiforme after receiving herpes simplex vaccine for the therapy of recurrent herpes simplex.[103]

Erythema multiforme can also be a hypersensitivity reaction to drugs or foods, and all cases should be investigated with this possibility in mind. The mucocutaneous features are identical to those occurring in response to known infectious agents. Probably any drug is capable of producing erythema multiforme, but the most common ones are penicillin, phenolphthalein (found in laxatives), sulfonamides, and barbiturates. Arsenicals, bromides, iodides, sulfa-related compounds (chlorothiazide, tolbutamide), gold salts, mercurials, salicylates, and hydantoins are less common offenders. DeFeo reported an epidemic of erythema multiforme among college chemistry students exposed to 9-bromofluorene.[104] A nationwide epidemic occurred in Holland in 1960 and was due to the addition of a modified triglyceride to a new commercial margarine.[105] Shellfish ingestion can cause erythema multiforme in some persons.

Erythema multiforme is one of the manifestations of autoimmune progesterone dermatitis (see p. 774). It appears regularly five to ten days before the menstrual cycle and spontaneously resolves after menstruation. Hypersensitivity to progesterone is believed to be the underlying cause. Herpes gestationis is a bullous disease peculiar to pregnancy which in the past has been difficult to distinguish from erythema multiforme because of their similar clinical and histologic features. However, they can now be distinguished on the basis of immunoglobulin and complement deposition in the skin of patients with herpes gestationis. Prospective studies employing these diagnostic aids should be able to determine the prevalence of erythema multiforme in pregnancy.

Although not a common etiology, internal malignancy should be considered a possibility in adults in whom no other cause of erythema multiforme can be found. Deep x-radiation therapy may produce erythema multiforme that is most likely a reaction to necrotic tumor tissue.[106]

Erythema multiforme can be an indicator of disease activity in ulcerative colitis and Crohn's disease.[107]

Infectious diseases are the important causes of erythema multiforme in children and young adults, whereas drug reactions and malignancy are the important factors in older persons.

As techniques in virology continue to advance and as our appreciation for and detection of environmental toxins improve, the number of idiopathic cases of erythema multiforme should decrease. All of the various etiologies noted above apply to the acute self-limited form of the disease. The causes of the chronically persistent variety are still unknown.

Internal organ involvement directly related to erythema multiforme is rare. The mucosal lesions of the esophagus, pharynx, and tracheobronchial tree merely are a serious extension of those in the mouth, and the pneumonitis is related to the Eaton agent.

Renal lesions have been documented in only a few cases of erythema multiforme, but they may be more frequent.[108] There are many reports of albuminuria and hematuria with erythema multiforme, but the urinary findings have been attributed to the associated fever. Cardiac arrhythmias accompanied nephritis in one patient with erythema multiforme.[109] The incidence of renal disease in erythema multiforme needs further study, and investigations to determine whether the erythema multiforme and nephritis have a common etiology should be conducted.

Erythema multiforme is considered to be a hypersensitivity response to a variety of agents because of its association with erythema nodosum, mycoplasma infections, recurrences following attacks of herpes simplex, and its development following reactions to drugs, foods, and injections. The mechanism has been assumed to be on the basis of humoral rather than cell-mediated hypersensitivity. In two cases associated with Eaton agent, and in several associated with herpes simplex, the mycoplasma and virus, respectively, have been isolated from intact skin blisters.[110-113] The significance of such isolations has been unclear, since the histology of erythema multiforme is that of subepidermal blisters without histologic evidence of viral infection.

Wuepper et al. proposed that erythema multiforme is a disorder produced by circulating immune complexes. They demonstrated IgM and C3 in the vessels of the papillary dermis by direct immunofluorescence in early lesions of erythema multiforme. Circulating immune complexes were assumed to be present because of increased binding of immunoglobulins by the Raji cell radioimmunoassay and by demonstration of IgM in the dermal blood vessels of the patients' normal skin that had been made permeable by the earlier injection of histamine.[114] Other workers have detected circulating immune complexes in serum specimens by C1q binding and monoclonal rheumatoid factor inhibition assays.[114a, 114b] Safai et al. studied the blister fluids of two patients with erythema multiforme. They demonstrated complement activation and the presence of immune complexes by C1q binding in the blisters. However, complement activation and circulating immune complexes could not be demonstrated in the serum.[115] These observations are preliminary, and further work is necessary before a pathogenetic mechanism for circulating immune complexes can be established in this disorder.

The clinical and laboratory observations in erythema multiforme suggest another hypothesis. If it is demonstrated that *local* complement activation and immune complex formation in the blisters are the major pathogenetic events in erythema multiforme, analogous to the findings in rheumatoid joints, then the isolation of mycoplasma and herpes simplex from the skin lesions and the induction of erythema multiforme by intradermal and subcutaneous injections of herpes simplex vaccine become highly significant. If erythema multiforme caused by mycoplasma or herpes simplex were associated with hematogenous dissemination of the organisms, the widespread deposition of the infectious agents in the skin reacting with circulating antibodies in and around the blood vessels could produce an Arthus reaction. Complement activation and immune complex formation would be present and detectable. The studies of Safai et al. support such an hypothesis.[115] In addition, the generalized nature of the eruption in such cases of erythema multiforme could be accounted for.

Unfortunately, the histologic finding in erythema multiforme is not that of an Arthus response but rather a lymphohistiocytic reaction with only a few neutrophils present. Kazmierowski and Wuepper were also concerned about the lack of neutrophilic response in relation to their hypothesis that erythema multiforme is an immune complex disorder. They suggested that differences in membrane receptors for immunoglobulins and complement on inflammatory cells might account for the different histologic patterns in leukocytoclastic angiitis and mononuclear cell vasculitis such as Mucha-Habermann disease. Neutrophils have membrane receptors for the Fc fragment of IgG, and C3b, but not IgM or C3d. Monocytes and B lymphocytes have receptors for the Fc fragment of IgG, C3b, and C3d, but not IgM. If relatively large amounts of C3d were incorporated into the lattice structure of IgM containing immune complexes, monocytes and lymphocytes rather than neutrophils might be preferentially attracted to such immune aggregates when they were deposited in the tissues. Thus, the presence or lack of a C3d receptor on inflammatory cells might account for different histologic findings in various types of immune complex vasculitis.[114] Clayton et al. reported that they identified IgM and C3 in the vessels of the cutaneous lesions of Mucha-Habermann disease.[116] In eight of their ten patients circulating immune complexes were detected by polyethylene glycol precipitation.

Cultures of the blister fluid for herpes simplex and mycoplasma organisms in appropriate cases of erythema multiforme, coupled with measurements of complement components and immune complexes in both blisters and serum, should establish whether some of these hypotheses are correct.

Differential Diagnosis

A number of disorders superficially resemble erythema multiforme. Urticaria may develop into circinate and polycyclic forms, and erythema annulare centrifugum may evolve into similar configurations that resemble the iris and urticarial lesions of erythema multiforme. However, fine petechiae or mild purpura are never present in true urticaria or erythema annulare. If clinical differentiation is impossible, histologic examination of the lesions will reveal the correct diagnosis.

Bullous pemphigoid can be far more troublesome. *Tense* clear bullae arise on erythematous, slightly edematous bases or, occasionally, on normal-appearing skin (Figs. 9–38 to 9–41). The blisters erupt in crops,

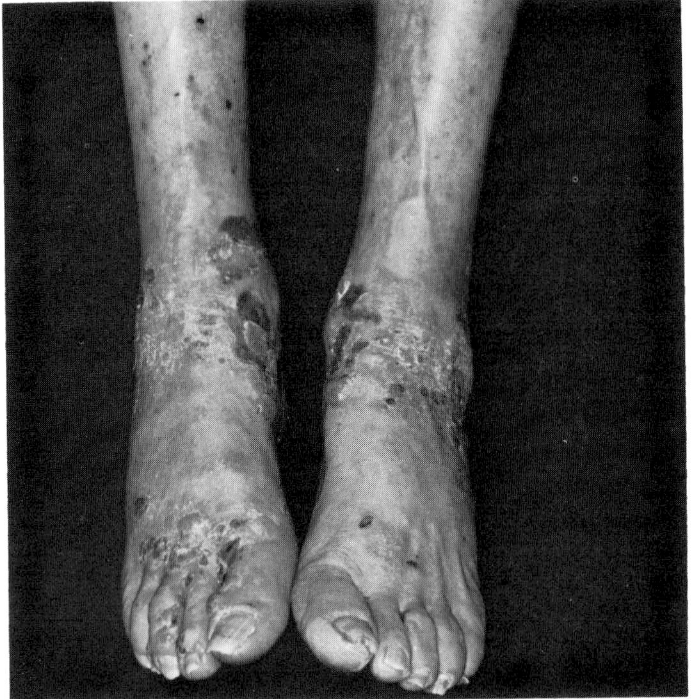

Figure 9–38. Pemphigoid. Cause not determined.

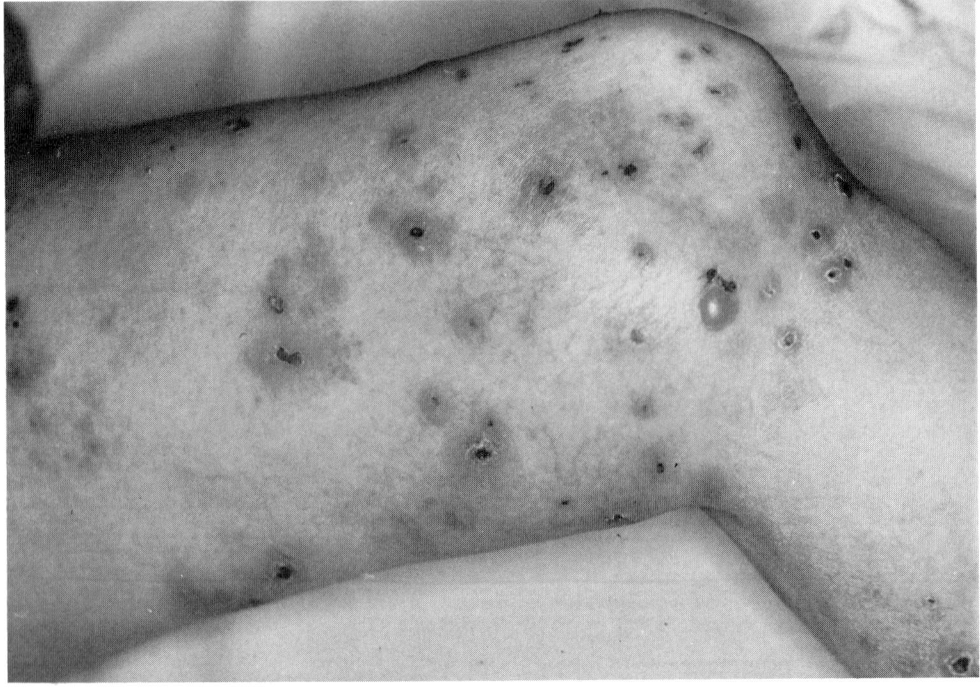

Figure 9–39. Bullous pemphigoid. Tense blisters arising from relatively normal skin or urticarial bases.

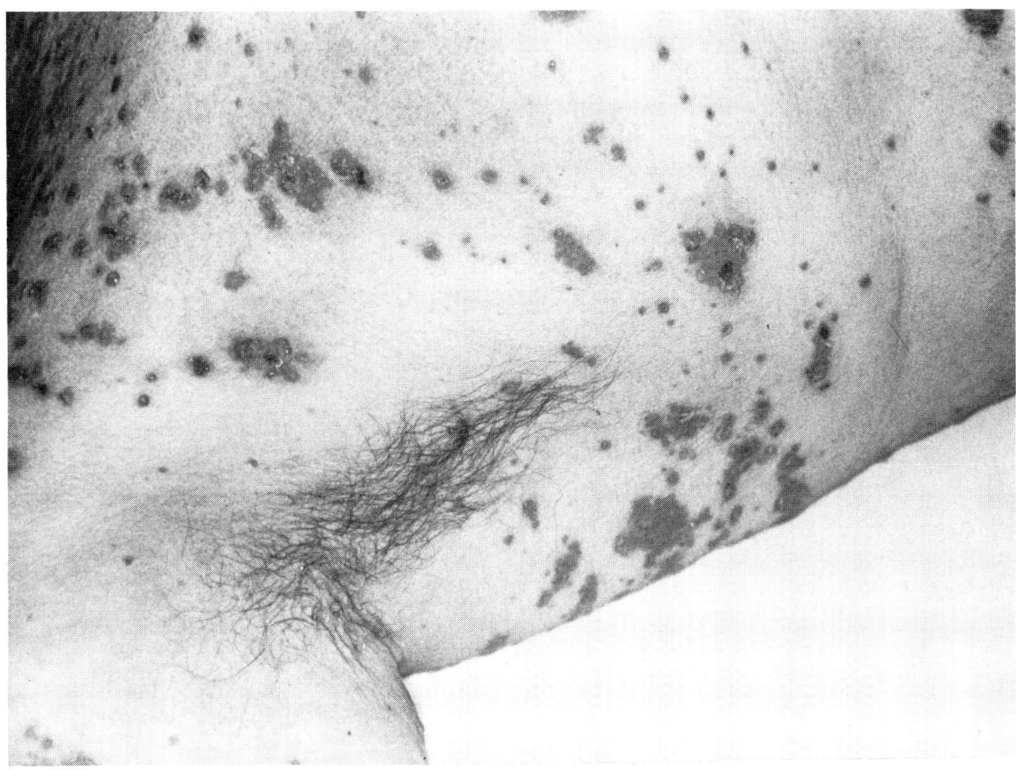

Figure 9–40. Bullous pemphigoid.

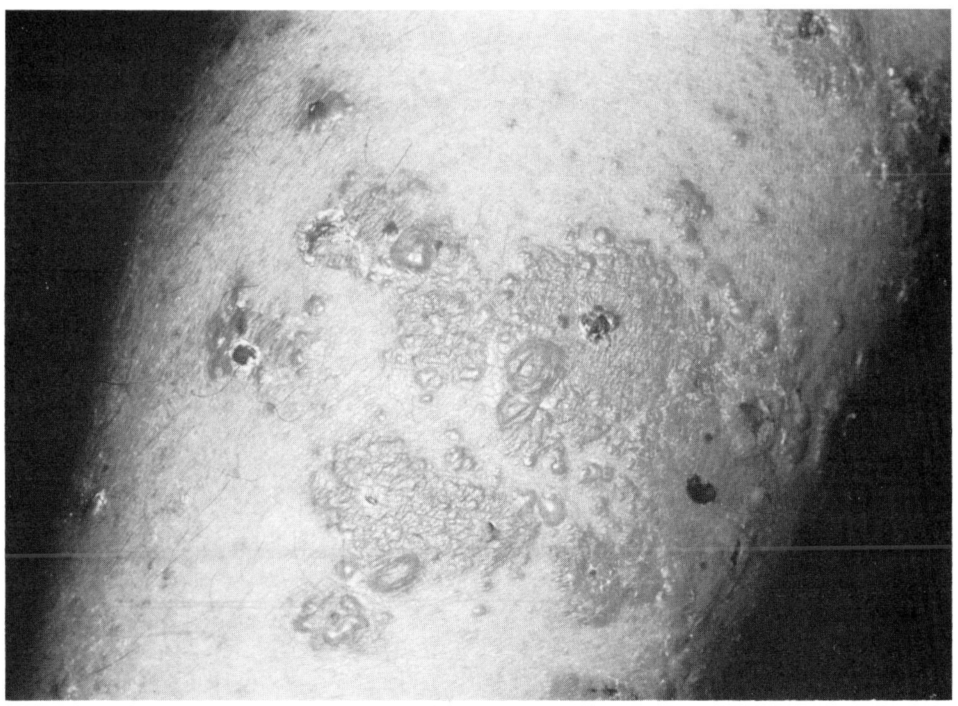

Figure 9–41. Bullous pemphigoid. Bullae arising from urticarial bases.

vary greatly in size — they may be as large as 10 cm. in diameter — and often have an irregular outline. They may be generalized or localized, and the localized blisters may precede a generalized spread. There is a limited form of the disease that involves primarily the extremities and scalp. In one of our patients, pemphigoid developed under a cast applied for a fractured ankle. The skin from the mid-shin to the ankle was affected, and no other areas of the body were involved. Pruritus is often present and may be severe, unlike the mild pruritus seen in erythema multiforme.

In about one third of the cases, the buccal mucosa is also the site of blisters. The blisters tend to be small, and the extent of involvement is mild; consequently, the severe stomatitis of erythema multiforme does not result. Hemorrhagic crusted lips are not a feature of pemphigoid.

Bullous pemphigoid occurs primarily in children and in adults over 60 years old (Fig. 9–42). Young adults rarely develop the illness. Several series of patients have been reported which confirm Lever's original assessment of the disease: a relatively benign, self-limited illness in most instances.[117, 118] In at least half the patients, the disease remitted in less than six years. In a few it persisted for as long as 15 to 22 years.[119-121] In some patients, the course is characterized by remissions and exacerbations that occur over a period of months.

In the past some clinicians believed that pemphigoid was a chronic form of erythema multiforme because of similarities in histology and clinical appearance. However, immunofluorescent studies have shown that they are not related. Patients with pemphigoid have circulating antibodies against the basement membrane zone of the epidermis. Direct immunofluorescent examination of the blisters and immediately adjacent

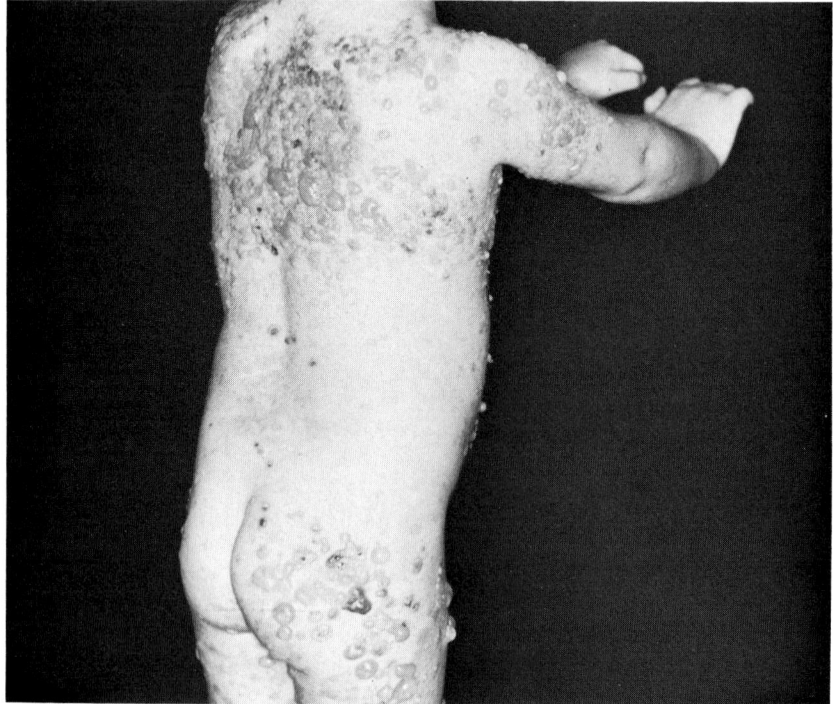

Figure 9–42. Pemphigoid of childhood.

skin will reveal immunoglobulin and complement deposition at this site.[118, 122] Erythema multiforme lacks these findings.

Ocasionally pemphigoid can be a reactive expression of an underlying carcinoma, as illustrated in Figure 1–25. However, there is no increased prevalence of malignancy in this disorder.

Psoriasis and immunologically proven pemphigoid have occurred together.[123, 124] In some patients the pemphigoid has been generalized and in others, limited to the legs. We have seen two patients in the first category and one in the second. In the latter, discontinuation of tar and ultraviolet therapy was followed by prompt disappearance of the bullae with no relapse during two years of follow-up. Cram and Fukuyama have shown that ultraviolet irradiation of the normal-appearing skin of patients with pemphigoid can produce fresh lesions that exhibit the typical histologic and immunofluorescent changes of this disorder.[125]

Pemphigus can be differentiated from bullous pemphigoid on the basis of clinical features and histopathologic and immunofluorescent studies. The bullae are flaccid, arise from normal-appearing skin, break easily, and produce large denuded areas of skin. The blister forms within the epidermis, rather than subepidermally, by acantholysis. Finally, sera of patients with pemphigus contain antibodies that fix to the intercellular epidermal spaces but not to the basement membrane of the epidermis.[122] Direct immunofluorescent examination of spontaneous lesions shows immunoglobulin and complement deposition in the same intercellular epidermal spaces. There is convincing evidence presented by Schiltz and Michel and confirmed by others that the pemphigus antibody is capable of inducing acantholysis in human epidermis grown in organ culture in the absence of complement.[126, 127]

Since erythema multiforme can pursue a chronic course involving only the oral mucosa, three mimicking disorders need to be distinguished. Pemphigus often begins with oral ulcerations that may be the sole manifestation of the disease for as long as six months before diagnostic skin lesions develop. In this early phase, biopsy of fresh oral lesions for examination by light microscopy and direct immunofluorescence, coupled with a search for circulating antiepithelial antibodies in the serum, will establish the correct diagnosis.

Cicatricial pemphigoid (benign mucous membrane pemphigoid) is an uncommon *subepidermal* blistering disorder that primarily affects mucosal epithelium.[128, 129] Other synonyms for this entity have included chronic pemphigus, ocular pemphigus, and essential shrinkage of the conjunctiva. In contrast to bullous pemphigoid, spontaneous remissions are uncommon. Cicatricial pemphigoid can produce recurrent blistering in the mucosa of the mouth, nose, eyes, upper respiratory tract, esophagus, and genitals. The skin is much less often affected. The repeated blistering is followed by scarring that produces laryngeal and esophageal strictures. Permanent tracheostomy and repeated dilatations of the esophagus may be necessary. Ocular involvement may be manifested only as conjunctivitis, but it frequently progresses to conjunctival ulcerations that result in scarring between the bulbar and palpebral conjunctivae. The lids become fixed and the palpebral opening narrowed (symblepharon), leading to corneal ulcers and pannus formation which often produce blindness (Figs. 9–43 to 9–45). In one of our patients, the major manifestations of the disease were fusion of the labia minora with obstruction to the urethral

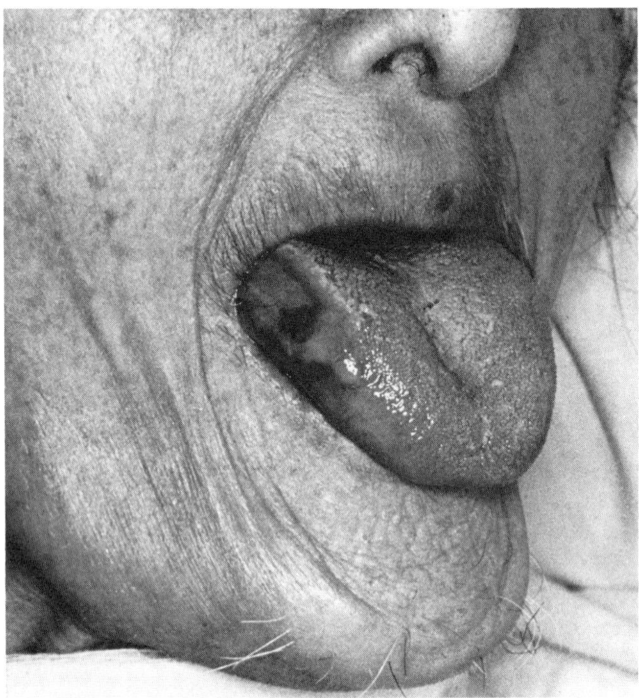

Figure 9–43. Cicatricial pemphigoid. Ulcer on tongue.

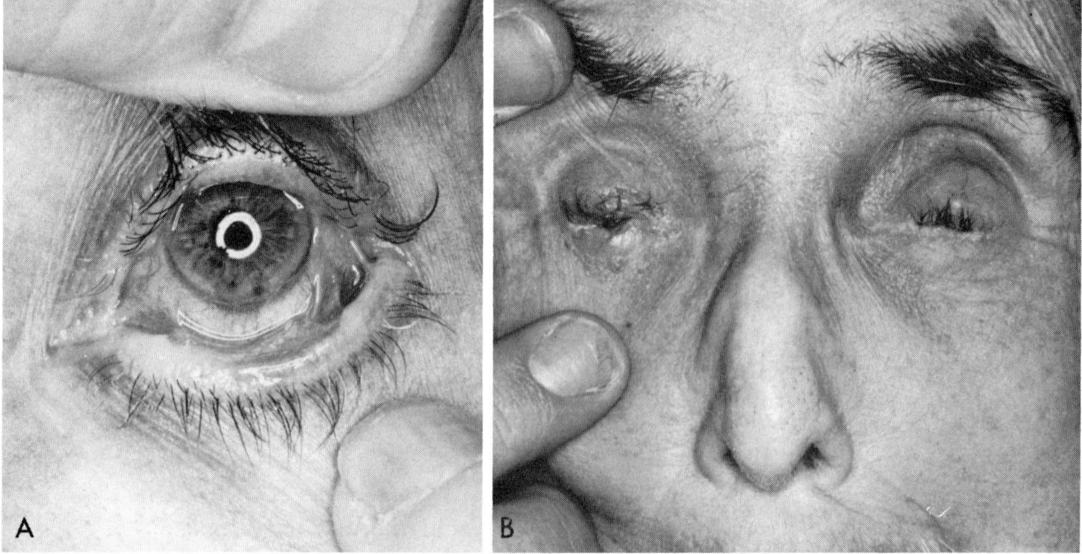

Figure 9–44. *A*, Cicatricial pemphigoid. Conjunctival ulcerations with scarring between palpebral and bulbar conjunctivae. *B*, Advanced stage. Symblepharon formation and blindness.

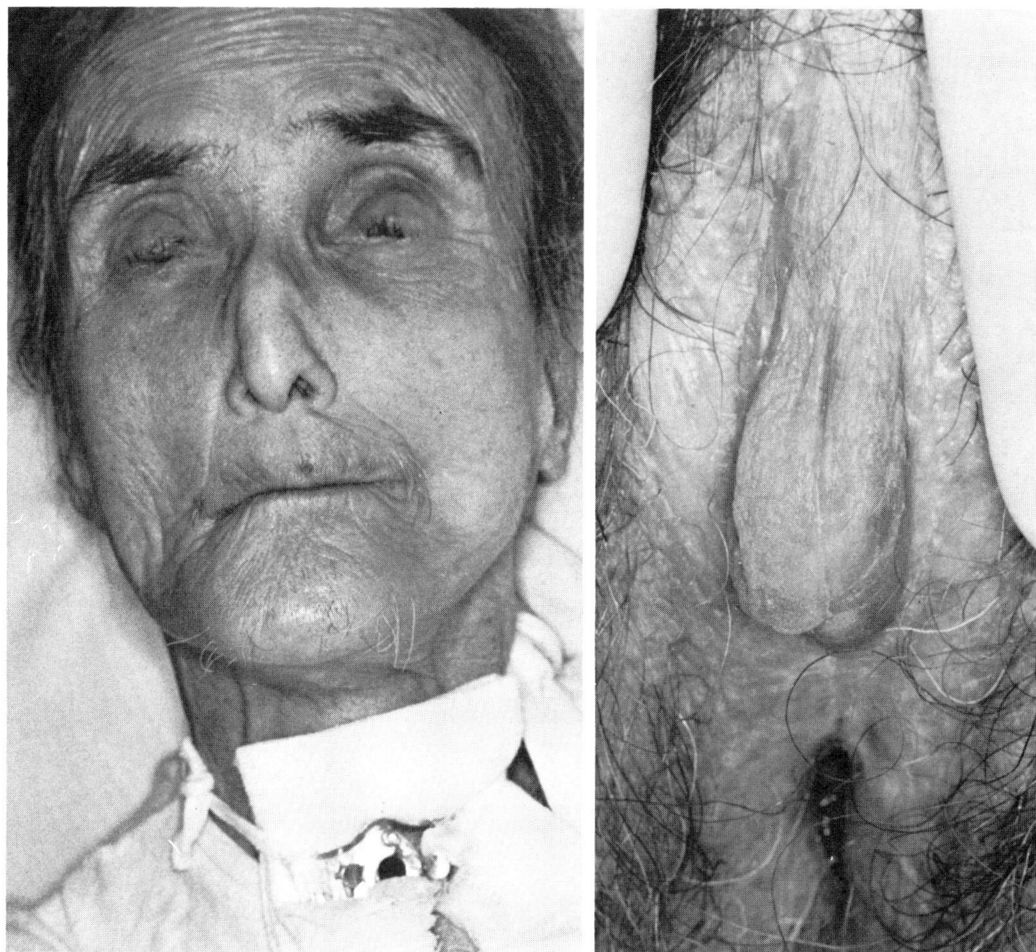

Figure 9–45. Cicatricial pemphigoid. Laryngeal stricture required tracheostomy.

Figure 9–46. Cicatricial pemphigoid. Fusion of labia minora, obstruction of urethral meatus, and narrowing of vaginal introitus.

opening, and narrowing of the vaginal introitus, which required periodic surgical lysis (Fig. 9–46). She had dysphagia secondary to esophageal scarring, but her eyes and mouth were never involved. In another patient, chronic ulcers in the mouth and nose and on the gingivae were followed in three months by dysphagia produced by scarring from esophageal ulcerations (Figs. 9-47 and 9-48). A biopsy of the esophagus showed subepithelial cleavage. The eyes have not been affected in this individual.

An uncommon variety of this syndrome, known as the Brunsting-Perry type, is characterized by skin lesions without mucosal involvement. Red macules with recurrent crops of blisters develop chiefly on the head and neck — rarely on the chest and back — to produce atrophic scarring.[130]

Direct immunofluorescent examination of the oral and cutaneous blisters shows IgG and complement localized to the basement membrane zone of the epithelium as in bullous pemphigoid. However, only an occasional patient has circulating antibasement membrane antibodies — mostly in those with extensive disease.[128, 129]

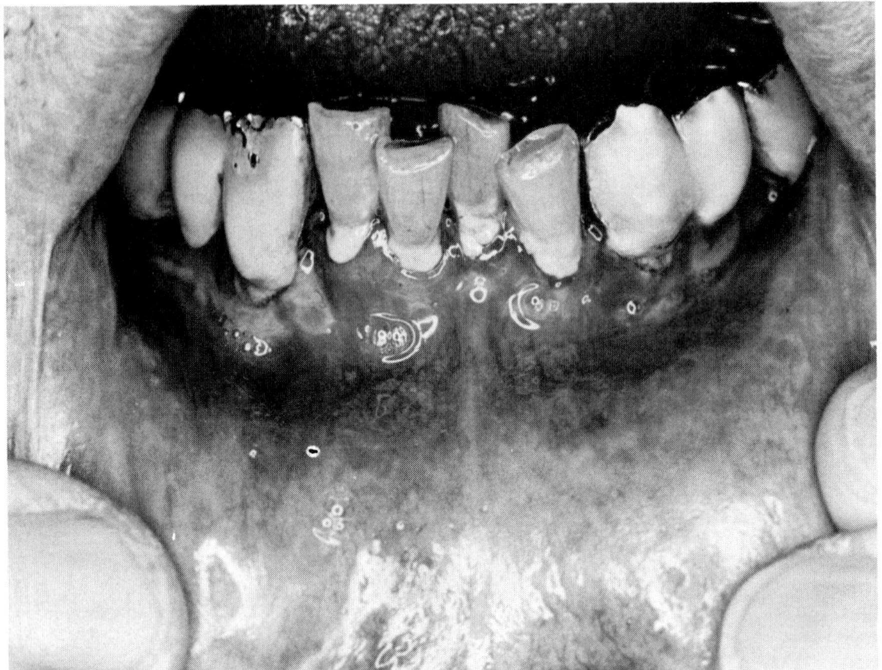

Figure 9–47. Cicatricial pemphigoid. Gingival blistering and ulceration, which had been mistaken for periodontal disease.

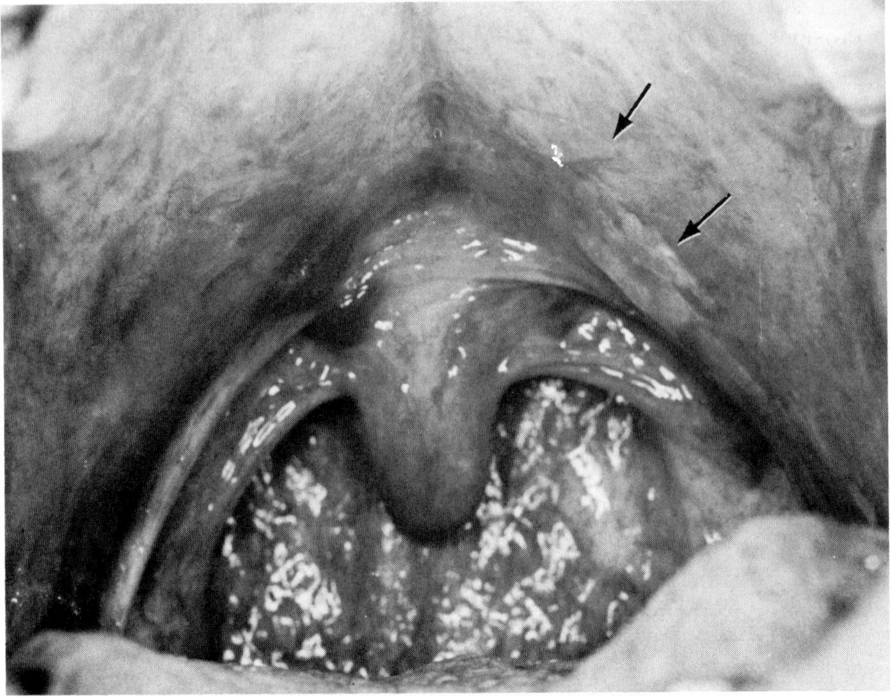

Figure 9–48. Cicatricial pemphigoid. Blisters on palate (arrows). Same patient as in Figure 9–47.

Desquamative gingivitis is an uncommon entity that was originally believed to be primarily dental in origin.[129, 131] In its mildest form, desquamative gingivitis displays a painless diffuse erythema of the marginal, interdental, and attached gingivae. Moderate involvement is characterized by sensations of burning. The epithelial surface is red, glistening smooth, and peels away with ease. The gingivae are edematous and pit with pressure. The adjacent oral mucosa may also be red and edematous. Severe involvement is characterized by pain and burning sensations in the gums. The gingivae show red and edematous patches that contain areas of denudation. Intact vesicles and bullae may be seen. The adjacent oral mucosa is red and edematous. In all forms of desquamative gingivitis the lingual surfaces of the gingivae are less involved than the buccolabial.

The term *desquamative gingivitis* encompasses several disorders. It is currently believed that in most patients desquamative gingivitis represents a variant of cicatricial pemphigoid. Some cases have evolved into the clinical syndrome of cicatricial pemphigoid and, in a few, direct immunofluorescent examination of the gingival tissue has shown the same pattern as observed in cicatricial pemphigoid and bullous pemphigoid.[129] Lichen planus, pemphigus vulgaris, and bullous pemphigoid, as well as periodontal disease, can also produce the clinical picture of desquamative gingivitis. Immunoflourescent studies of involved tissues and serum would assist in differentiating these entities from cicatricial pemphigoid.

Mucocutaneous lymph node syndrome (Kawasaki's disease) might be confused with erythema multiforme on superficial inspection because of the constellation of fever, conjunctival injection, oral mucosal involvement, and a polymorphous skin eruption that may be scarlatiniform, morbilliform, urticarial, vesicular, or iris-like.[132] The distinguishing features of Kawasaki's disease based on morphology alone include a diffuse erythema of the lips that is followed by dryness, fissuring, and superficial erosions rather than bloody crusted lips; a diffusely red oropharynx; diffuse erythema and prominent lingual papillae simulating a "strawberry" tongue; and indurated edema and erythema of the hands and feet (see Chapter 18).

Toxic epidermal necrolysis (TEN) has also been confused with erythema multiforme. TEN begins abruptly with patches of red tender skin. Within 24 to 72 hours, the skin begins to be shed in large sheets (Fig. 9–49). Histologically there is widespread necrosis of the epidermis in the absence of significant dermal inflammation. Flaccid bullae may appear before the slough occurs because of fluid accumulation in the developing dermal-epidermal space (Fig. 9–50). However TEN is not a bullous disorder. In some patients the oral mucosa may slough as well (Fig. 9–51). TEN can develop as a reaction to drugs, as a complication of pustular psoriasis of Von Zumbusch, or on an idiopathic basis.[133, 134] Rarely, features of erythema multiforme and TEN have occurred in the same patient. This is most likely a manifestation of two separate pathogenetic processes developing in response to the inciting agent, as can be seen in patients with combinations of erythema nodosum and erythema multiforme or erythema multiforme and urticaria. A similar-appearing entity follows staphylococcal infections in children, in whom it is currently referred to as "*staphylococcal scalded skin syndrome*" (SSSS) (Figs. 9–52 and 9–53). SSSS has an excellent prognosis in children, while TEN is

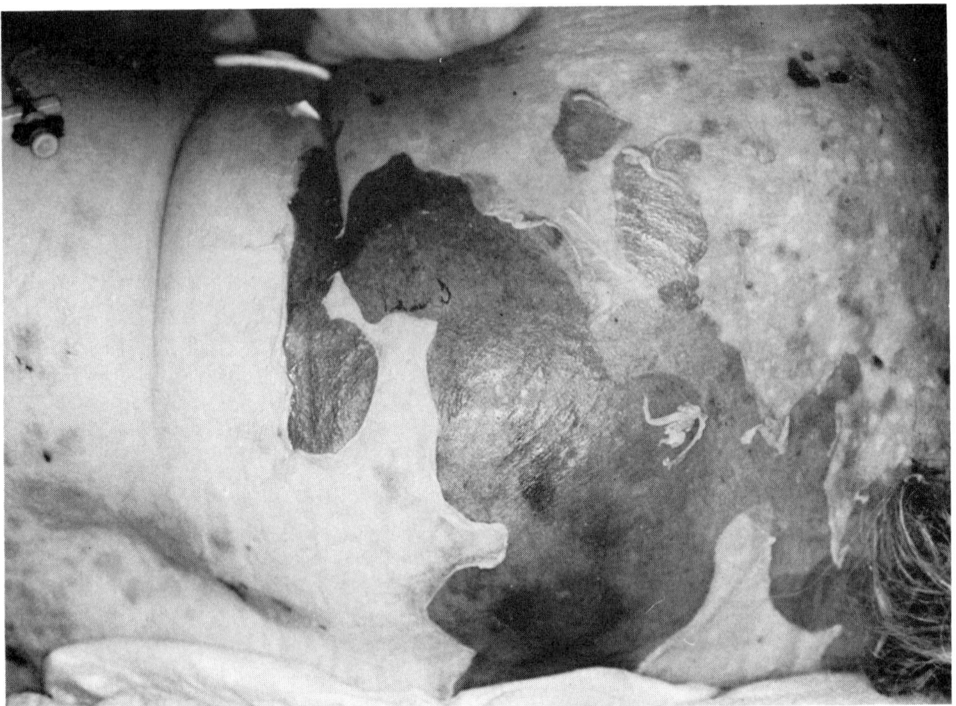

Figure 9–49. Toxic epidermal necrolysis. Widespread denudation of skin.

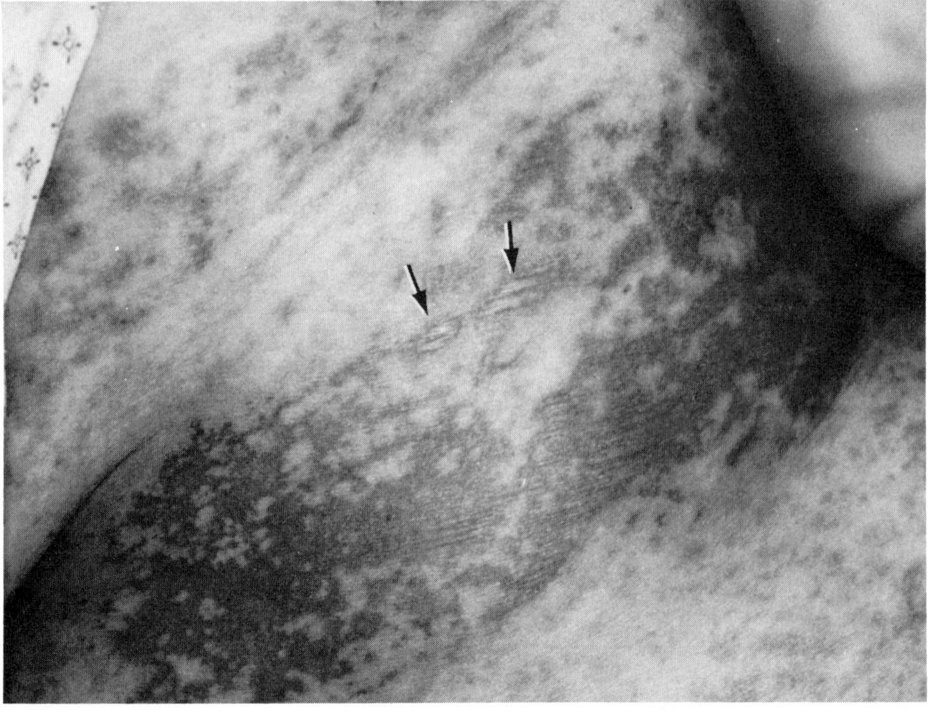

Figure 9–50. Toxic epidermal necrolysis. Flaccid bullae (arrows) developing in areas of tender red skin before there is cutaneous shedding.

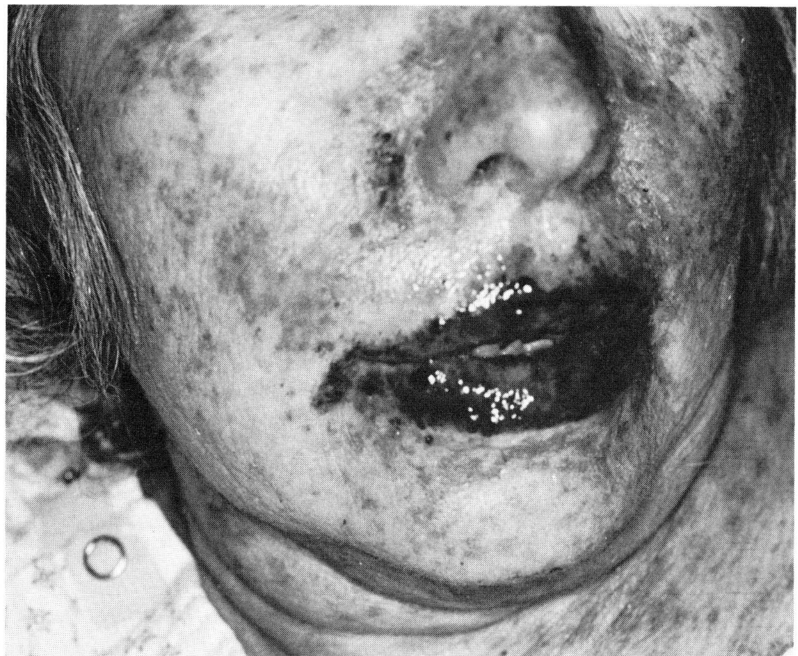

Figure 9–51. Toxic epidermal necrolysis. Involvement of the oral mucosa.

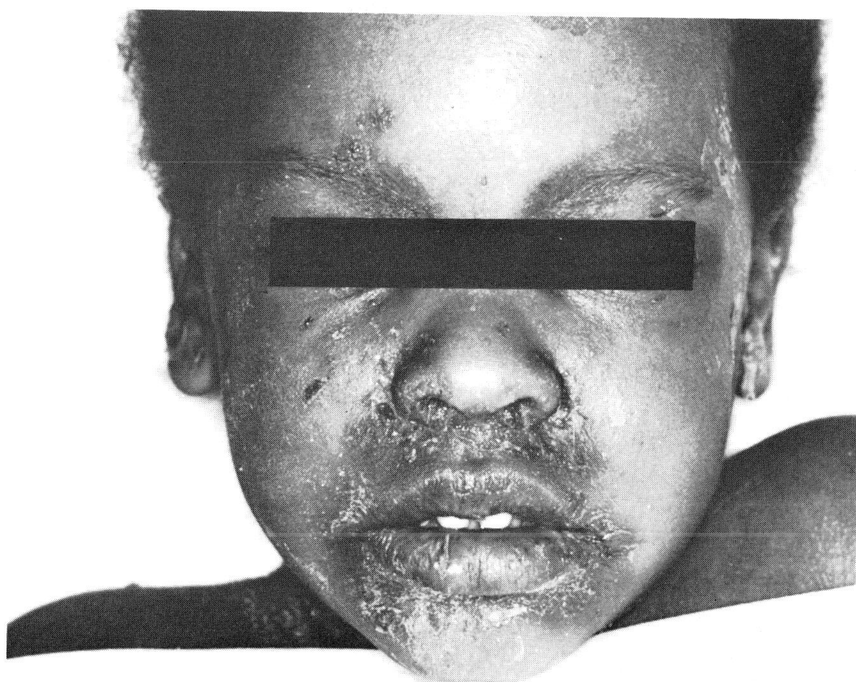

Figure 9–52. Staphylococcal scalded skin syndrome. Periorificial eruption.

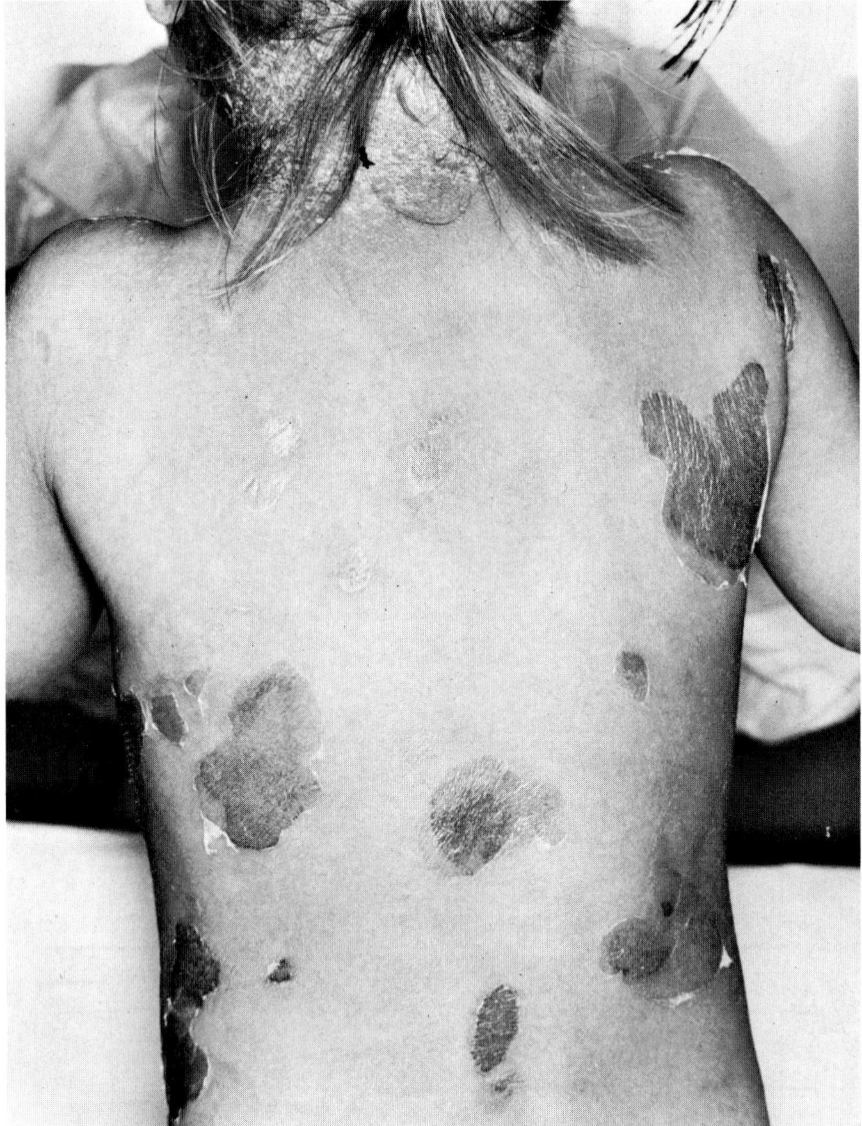

Figure 9–53. Staphylococcal scalded skin syndrome. Characteristic appearance of denuded skin.

associated with high mortality in adults. SSSS differs from TEN in both pathogenesis and pathology (see Chapter 18).

Leukocytoclastic angiitis produces lesions that might be confused with erythema multiforme, but histologic examination will always differentiate the two. In this type of angiitis there are hemorrhagic bullae, which rarely occur in erythema multiforme, and urticarial plaques and papules that rapidly become purpuric and sometimes ulcerate. Ulceration without a preceding blister is not a feature of erythema multiforme, and the degree of purpura in the lesions of erythema multiforme is mild in comparison with that seen in necrotizing angiitis.

Behçet's disease is another chronic mucocutaneous disorder that should not be confused with erythema multiforme. Although most prevalent in Great Britain, Japan, and in the Middle East, Behçet's disease has been reported from all over the world.[135, 136]

The disorder is defined by the triad of oral and genital ulcerations and inflammatory disease of the eyes (Fig. 9–54). Behçet's disease is said to be twice as common in men, but if the milder forms are included — that is, those with only oral and genital ulceration — the predominance of men is not as striking. Women have fewer ocular lesions than men.

Behçet's disease is punctuated by attacks that last from a few days to a month and may occur several times a year or less frequently. The typical episode begins with aphthous stomatitis and ulcers on the scrotum or labia in association with fever, malaise, and arthralgia. (The penis, vagina, cervix, and perineum are less frequently ulcerated). Ocular involvement may be present in the initial episodes but usually does not develop until later, sometimes after an interval of 10 years. Dowling found lesions of the eye in 80 per cent of 124 cases collected from the literature.[137] but Haim found eye involvement in only 22 per cent of his 23 cases,[138] and Chamberlain found 25 per cent in her 35 cases.[139]

The ulcers in Behçet's disease are of three types: superficial greyish erosions indistinguishable from ordinary aphthae (canker sores); deeply punched-out erosions that resemble periadenitis mucosa necrotica recurrens (Sutton); and, rarely, superficial punctate erosions described as herpetiform. The usual sites affected are the lips, gums, cheeks, and tongue. In severe cases the pharynx and palate may be affected. Ulcerations may develop in the esophagus, stomach, intestine, and anus followed by perforations. Intestinal involvement produces recurrent colitis or mimics regional enteritis. The genital ulcers may produce

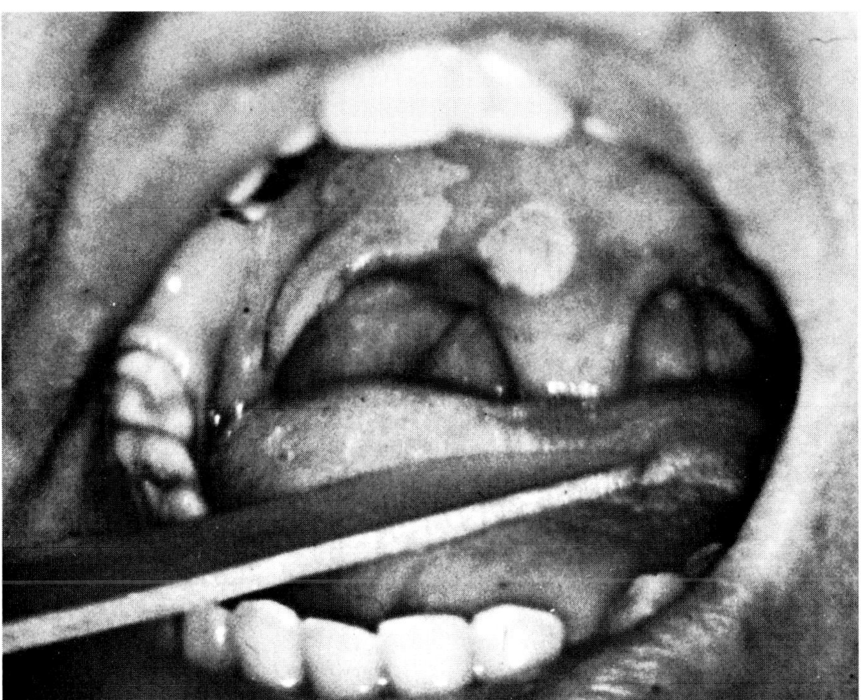

Figure 9–54. Behçet's syndrome. Severe oral aphthae. (Courtesy of Dr. Helen Curth.)

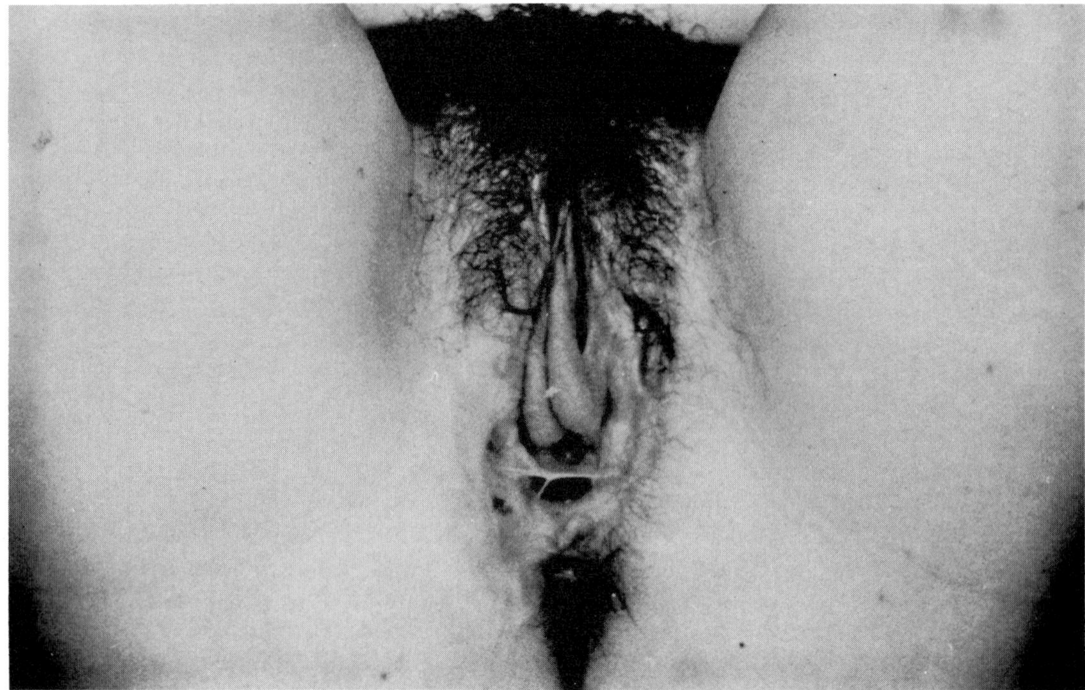

Figure 9–55. Behçet's syndrome. Perforation of labia secondary to severe genital aphthae. (Courtesy of Dr. Helen Curth.)

perforation of the labia minora (Fig. 9–55). Patients often are unable to eat during attacks because of a painful mouth. The aphthous lesions, whether of the mouth or genitalia, begin as vesicles or pustules and tend to heal with scar formation, a phenomenon not seen in erythema multiforme. The deep ulcerations begin as submucosal or dermal nodules and always heal with scarring. Individual ulcers may persist for as long as a month before they heal.[140]

Ocular attacks occur with iritis or uveitis and hypopyon. Initially there may be only unilateral involvement, but eventually the process becomes bilateral and blindness follows. Secondary glaucoma with enucleation may be the end result.

Other features that accompany the acute episodes or that appear in between attacks are arthralgias, synovitis, or noninflammatory joint effusions involving primarily large joints in an asymmetric fashion; superficial and deep thrombophlebitis; phlebitis of retinal veins, dural sinuses, and the superior and inferior venae cavae; gastrointestinal ulceration; orchitis and epididymitis; pyoderma; furunculosis; and nodose lesions of the legs. Although the last sign has been called erythema nodosum, it actually represents an angiitis.[141] Benign pericarditis and aortic aneurysms also are features of Behçet's disease.[142, 143] In many cases, a pustule or red papule develops at a cutaneous site that has been punctured by a needle or injected intradermally with distilled water.

The currently acceptable diagnostic criteria for the diagnosis of Behçet's disease are listed in Table 9–2.

Neurologic involvement is the only poor prognostic sign. It develops in 15 to 20 per cent of patients on an average of two to five years after the

Table 9–2. CURRENTLY ACCEPTABLE DIAGNOSTIC CRITERIA FOR BEHÇET'S DISEASE*

Recurrent aphthous stomatitis
Recurrent genital ulcers
Uveitis, both anterior and posterior
Vasculitis of either cutaneous or large vessels
Arthritis
Meningoencephalitis
Cutaneous hyperreactivity to minor trauma

*Compiled from O'Duffy, J. D.: Summary of international symposium on Behçet's disease. J. Rheumatol., *5*:229, 1978, and Pallis, C. A.: Behçet's disease and the nervous system. Trans. St. John Hosp. Dermatol. Soc., *52*:201, 1966.

Combinations of three or more (one being recurrent aphthae) are considered diagnostic of Behçet's disease. Incomplete form: two criteria are present, one being recurrent aphthae. Exclusions: diagnosis of inflammatory bowel disease, SLE, Reiter's syndrome, and herpetic infections.

disease has begun. Fifty per cent of the patients die within one year. The neurologic manifestations have been divided into three types: brain stem lesions, meningoencephalitis, and organic confusional states.[145] The clinical features have included hemiparesis, quadriparesis, cerebellar ataxia, pseudobulbar palsies, and transient ocular palsies.[145, 146]

Renal involvement is an uncommon complication of Behcet's disease. Three types of renal lesions have been described: amyloidosis, acute glomerulonephritis, and proteinuria with hematuria. Renal involvement may lead to renal failure.[147, 148]

Currently, it is believed that aberrations in humoral and cellular immunity play a role in the pathogenesis of Behçet's disease. Circulating antimucosal antibodies can be found in the patient's sera,[149] and in some, but not all, patients circulating immune complexes can be correlated with disease activity, but not with duration or specific organ involvement.[150] Cell-mediated hypersensitivity has been linked to the aphthous ulcer component of Behçet's disease. The histopathologic appearance of early aphthous lesions is compatible with cell-mediated hypersensitivity.[151, 152] Lehner demonstrated lymphocyte transformation in response to extracts of oral mucosa in five of nine patients with Behçet's syndrome.[153] Rogers et al. demonstrated that the circulating lymphocytes of patients with Behçet's disease and those with ordinary aphthous stomatitis are cytotoxic for suspensions of oral epithelium held in culture for 18 hours. Cell viability was defined by exclusion of trypan blue dye.[154] Cytotoxicity was less active in normal patients whose aphthae were in remission. Cytotoxicity was not found in control patients composed of normal healthy individuals; in patients with active oral erosive disease (bullous and cicatricial pemphigoids, erythema multiforme, herpes simplex, lichen planus, and leukoplakia); or in other patients with active skin disease but without oral lesions (psoriasis, atopic dermatitis, pyoderma gangrenosum, Sézary syndrome, and bullous pemphigoid).

Israeli, Turkish, and Japanese investigators have found that HLA-B5 is significantly increased among their patients, but this has not been found in American and British cases.[155] Familial cases occur but are uncommon.[156]

Curth believes that the combination of oral and genital ulceration should be accepted as sufficient evidence to support a diagnosis of Behçet's disease, and perhaps her view is correct.[157] It remains to be determined whether or not Lipschütz's acute vulvar ulceration and Sutton's periadenitis mucosa necrotica recurrens represent monosymptomatic forms of Behçet's disease.

RHEUMATIC FEVER

Various erythemas occur in 10 per cent of patients with rheumatic fever.[11] Among them are included ordinary urticaria and the figurate erythemas.

The most common variety of erythema is erythema annulare, which usually is labeled erythema marginatum when found in rheumatic fever. Erythema annulare is characterized by red macules or urticarial papules that slowly expand peripherally, leaving clear centers and producing complete or incomplete rings (Fig. 9–56). Sometimes these lesions meet in polycyclic patterns. The borders can be either *flat* or *elevated* and are various shades of red. The lesions may persist for a few hours or for two to three days, and they characteristically develop in crops. Although they are usually present during the active stages of rheumatic fever and tend to be associated with carditis, they may arise for the first time after the disease seems to be inactive. In some patients, erythema marginatum has been present continuously for two years without evidence of rheumatic activity.

Erythema papulatum is the designation for another variety of erythema encountered in rheumatic fever. It consists of small red macules and urticarial papules that arise on the elbows, knees, arms, and buttocks. These lesions also develop in crops and persist for a length of time similar

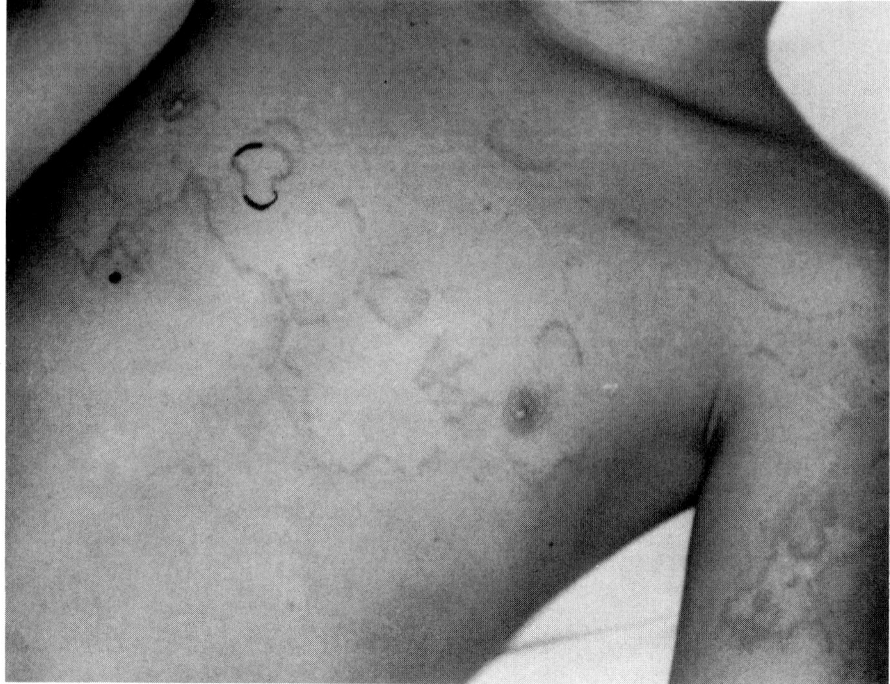

Figure 9–56. Erythema marginatum. Note annular and serpiginous patterns.

to that of erythema marginatum. However, they do not form rings. Both erythema marginatum and erythema papulatum are asymptomatic.

Subcutaneous nodules of rheumatic fever are also associated with carditis and can coexist with erythema marginatum. The nodules in rheumatic fever are smaller than those in rheumatoid arthritis and last for shorter periods of time, usually less than one month. The histopathology is similar in the two diseases. The nodules are located over bony surfaces or prominences or in proximity to tendons; they also develop in crops. It is unusual to have rheumatic nodules without carditis.

An unusual variety of subcutaneous nodules was described by Rosenberg in 1934 and by Burns et al. in 1964. Instead of developing in the subcutaneous layer, the nodules arose within the dermis over the back and abdomen and were red and yellow-red. In Burns' patient, the lesions remained for two years and were accompanied by erythema marginatum during that period.[158]

As noted previously, erythema nodosum is an unusual manifestation of rheumatic fever. In the past, the arthralgias of erythema nodosum were probably misinterpreted as a sign of rheumatic fever.

REFERENCES

1. Warin, R. P., and Champion, R. H.: Urticaria. W. B. Saunders, Philadelphia, 1974, p. 173.
2. Monroe, E. W., and Jones, H. E.: Urticaria. An updated review. Arch. Dermatol., *113*:80, 1977.
3. Beaven, M. A.: Histamine. N. Engl. J. Med., *294*:301, 320, 1976.
4. Kaplan, A. P.: Mediators of urticaria and angioedema. J. Allergy. Clin. Immunol., *60*:324, 1977.
5. Lagunoff, D., and Chi, E. Y.: Mast cell secretion: membrane events. J. Invest. Dermatol., *71*:81, 1978.
6. Uvnäs, B.: Chemistry and storage function of mast cell granules. J. Invest. Dermatol., *71*:76, 1978.
7. Soter, N. A., and Austen, K. F.: The diversity of mast cell-derived mediators: implications for acute, subacute and chronic cutaneous inflammatory disorders. J. Invest. Dermatol., *67*:313, 1976.
8. Wasserman, S. I., Soter, N. A., Center, D. M., and Austen, K. F.: Cold urticaria. Recognition and characterization of a neutrophil chemotactic factor which appears in serum during experimental cold challenge. J. Clin. Invest., *60*:189, 1977.
9. Greaves, M., Marks, R., and Robertson, I.: Receptors for histamine in human skin blood vessels: a review. Br. J. Dermatol. *97*:225, 1977.
10. Center, D. M., Soter, N. A., Wasserman, S. I., and Austen, K. F.: Inhibition of neutrophil chemotaxis in association with experimental angioedema in patients with cold urticaria; a model of chemotactic deactivation in vivo. Clin. Exp. Immunol., *35*:112, 1979.
11. Keil, H.: The rheumatic erythemas; a critical survey. Ann. Intern. Med., *11*:2223, 1938.
12. Dienstag, J. L., Rhodes, A. R., Bhan, A. K., Dvorak, A. M., Mihm, M. C., Jr., and Wands, J. R.: Urticaria associated with acute viral hepatitis type B. Ann. Intern. Med., *89*:34, 1978.
13. O'Loughlin, S., Schroeter, A. L., and Jordon, R. E.: Chronic urticaria-like lesions in systemic lupus erythematosus. Arch. Dermatol., *114*:879, 1978.
14. Warin, R. P., and Champion, R. H.: *op. cit.*, p. 146.
15. Kile, R. I., and Rusk, H. A.: A case of cold urticaria with an unusual family history. J.A.M.A., *114*:1067, 1940.
16. Tindall, J. P., Beeker, S. K., and Rosse, W. F.: Familial cold urticaria: a generalized reaction involving leukocytosis. Arch. Intern. Med., *124*:129, 1969.
17. Doeglas, H. M. G., and Bleumink, E.: Familial cold urticaria. Clinical findings. Arch. Dermatol., *110*:382, 1974.
18. Soter, N. A., Joshi, N. P., Twarog, F. J., Zeiger, R. S., Rothman, P., and Colten, H. R.: Delayed cold-induced urticaria: a dominantly inherited disorder. J. Allergy Clin. Immunol., *59*:294, 1977.
19. Ive, H., Lloyd, J., and Magnus, I. A.: Action spectra in idiopathic solar urticaria. Br. J. Dermatol. *77*:229, 1965.
20. Epstein, J. H.: Solar urticaria. Int. J. Dermatol., *16*:388, 1977.
21. Warin, R. P., and Champion, R. H.: *op. cit.*, p. 154.
22. Daman, L., Lieberman, P., Gauier, M., and Hashimoto, K.: Localized heat urticaria. J. Allergy Clin. Immunol., *61*:273, 1978.
23. Muckle, T. J., and Wells, M.: Urticaria, deafness and amyloidosis. A new heredo-

familial syndromes. Q. J. Med., *31*:235, 1962.

24. Kennedy, D. D., Rosenthal, F. D., and Sneddon, I. B.: Amyloidosis presenting as urticaria. Br. Med. J., *1*:31, 1966.
25. Black, J. T.: Amyloidosis, deafness, urticaria and limb pains. A hereditary syndrome. Ann. Intern. Med., *70*:989, 1969.
26. Warin, R. P., and Champion, R. H.: *op. cit.*, p. 120.
27. Patterson, R., Mellies, C. J., Blankenship, M. L., and Pruzansky, J. J.: Vibratory angioedema: A hereditary type of physical hypersensitivity. J. Allergy Clin. Immunol., *50*:174, 1972.
28. Metzger, W. J., Kaplan, A. P., Beaven, M. A., Irons, J., and Patterson, R.: Hereditary vibratory angioedema: Confirmation of histamine release in a type of physical hypersensitivitiy. J. Allergy Clin. Immunol., *57*:605, 1976.
29. Kaplan, A. P., and Beaven, M. A.: In vivo studies of the pathogenesis of cold urticaria, cholinergic urticaria, and vibration induced swelling. J. Invest. Dermatol., *67*:327, 1976.
30. Shelley, W. B., and Rawnsley, H. M.: Aquagenic urticaria. Contact sensitivity reaction to water. J.A.M.A., *189*:895, 1964.
31. Kaplan, A. P., Horakova, Z., and Katz, S. I.: Assessment of tissue histamine levels in patients with urticaria. J. Allergy Clin. Immunol., *61*:350, 1978.
32. Kern. F., and Lichtenstein, L. M.: Defective histamine release in chronic urticaria. J. Clin. Invest., *57*:1369, 1976.
33. Juhlin, L.: Recurrent urticaria. Int. J. Dermatol., *15*:271, 1976.
34. Doeglas, H. M. G.: Reactions to aspirin and food additives in patients with chronic urticaria, including the physical urticarias. Br. J. Dermatol., *93*:135, 1975.
35. Fisherman, E. W., and Cohen, G. W.: Recurring and chronic urticaria: identification of etiologies. Ann. Allergy, *36*:400, 1976.
36. Pace, J. L., and Garretts, M.: Urticaria and hyperthyroidism. Br. J. Dermatol., *93*:97, 1975.
37. Soter, N. A., Austen, K. F., and Gigli, I.: Urticaria and arthralgias as manifestations of necrotizing angiitis (vasculitis). J. Invest. Dermatol., *63*:485, 1974.
38. Phanuphak, D., Kohler, P. F., Stanford, R. E., Carr, R. I., Thorne, G. E., and Claman, H. N. Vasculitis in chronic urticaria. J. Allergy Clin. Immunol., *61*:181, 1978.
39. Urbach, E.: Endogenous allergy. Arch. Dermatol., *45*:697, 1942.
40. Calabro, J. J., and Marchesano, J. M.: Rash associated with juvenile rheumatoid arthritis. J. Pediatrics, *72*:611, 1968.
41. Schlesinger, B.: Still's disease. *In* Copeman, W. S. C. (ed.): Textbook of the Rheumatic Diseases. E. & S. Livingstone, Edinburgh, 1964, p. 240.
42. Isdaile, I. C., and Bywaters, E. G. L.: The rash of rheumatoid arthritis and Still's disease. Q. J. Med., *25*:377, 1956.
43. Demis, D. J.: The mastocytosis syndrome: clinical and biological studies. Ann. Intern. Med., *59*:194, 1963.
44. Sagher, F., and Even-Paz, Z.: Mastocytosis and the Mast Cell. Year Book Medical Publishers, Chicago, 1967, pp. 427.
45. Donaldson, V. H., and Evans, R. R.: A biochemical abnormality in hereditary angioneurotic edema. Am. J. Med., *35*:37, 1963.
46. Donaldson, V. H., Ratnoff, O. D., DaSilva, W. D., and Rosen, F. S.: Permeability — increasing activity in hereditary angioneurotic edema plasma. II. Mechanism of formation and partial characterization. J. Clin. Invest., *48*:642, 1969.
47. Pickering, R. J., Good, R. A., Kelly, J. R., and Gewurz, H.: Replacement therapy in hereditary angioedema. Successful treatment of two patients with fresh frozen plasma. Lancet, *1*:326, 1969.
48. Rosen, F. S., and Austen, K. F.: Androgen therapy in hereditary angioneurotic edema. N. Engl. J. Med., *295*:1476, 1976.
49. Gelfand, J. A., Sherins, R. J., Alling, O. W., and Frank, M. M.: Treatment of hereditary angioedema with danazol. Reversal of clinical and biochemical abnormalities. N. Engl. J. Med., *295*:1444, 1976.
50. Cohen, S. H., Koethe, S. M., Kozin, F., Rodey, G., Arkins, J. A., and Fink, J. N.: Acquired angioedema associated with rectal carcinoma and its response to danazol. J. Allergy Clin. Immunol., *62*:217, 1978.
51. Tas, J.: Chronic urticaria. A survey of 100 hospitalized cases. Dermatologica, *135*:90, 1967.
52. Miller, D. A., Freeman, G. L., and Akers, W. A.: Chronic urticaria. A clinical study of fifty patients. Am. J. Med., *44*:68, 1968.
53. Shelley, W. B.: Erythema annulare centrifugum. A case due to hypersensitivity to blue cheese Penicillium. Arch. Dermatol., *90*:54, 1964.
54. Leimert, J. T., Corder, M. P., Skibba, C. A., and Gingrich, R. D.: Erythema annulare centrifugum and Hodgkin's disease. Association with disease activity. Arch. Intern. Med., *139*:486, 1979.
55. Beare, J. M., Froggatt, P., Jones, J. A., and Neill, D. W.: Familial annular erythema — an apparently new dominant mutation. Br. J. Dermatol. *78*:59, 1966.
56. Hellerstrom, S.: Erythema chronicum migrans Afzelii. Acta Dermatol. Venereol., *11*:315, 1930.
57. Goette, D. K., and Odom, R. B.: Erythema chronicum migrans in three soldiers. Int. J. Dermatol., *17*:732, 1978.
58. Steere, A. C., Malawista, S. E., Hardin, J. A., Ruddy, S., Askenase, P. W., and Andiman, W. A.: Erythema chronicum migrans and Lyme arthritis. The enlarging clinical spectrum. Ann. Intern. Med., *86*:685, 1977.
59. Steere, A. C., Hardin, J. A., and Malawista, S. E.: Erythema chronicum migrans arthritis: cryoimmunoglobulins and clinical

activity of skin and joints. Science, *196*:1121, 1977.

60. Hardin, J. A., Steere, A. C., and Malawista, S. E.: Immune complexes and the evolution of Lyme arthritis. Dissemination and localization of abnormal Clq binding activity. N. Engl. J. Med., *301*:1358, 1979.
61. Naversen, D. N., and Gardner, L. W.: Erythema chronicum migrans in America. Arch. Dermatol., *114*:253, 1978.
61a. Steere, A. C., Malawista, S. E., Newman, J. H., Spieler, P. N., and Bartenhagen, N. H.: Antibiotic therapy in Lyme disease. Ann. Intern. Med., *93*:1, 1980.
62. Gammel, J. A.: Erythema gyratum repens. Arch. Dermatol., *66*:494, 1952.
63. Shelley, W. B., and Hurley, H. J.: An unusual autoimmune syndrome. Arch. Dermatol., *81*:889, 1960.
64. Willan, R.: On Cutaneous Diseases. vol. 1. Kimber and Conrad, Philadelphia, 1809, p. 369.
65. Hebra, F.: Diseases of the Skin. vol. 1. C. Hilton Fagge, tr. New Sydenham Society, London, 1866, p. 289.
66. Bäfverstedt, B.: Erythema nodosum migrans. Acta Dermatovenereol., *34*:1, 1954.
67. Bäfverstedt, B.: Erythema nodosum migrans. Acta Dermatovenereol., *48*:381, 1968.
68. McCarthy, J. L.: Episcleral nodules and erythema nodosum. Report of a case with the pathologic findings. Am. J. Ophthalmol., *51*:60, 1961.
69. Bluefarb, S. M.: Erythema nodosum with conjunctival nodules. Q. Bull. Northwestern Univ. Med. School, *34*:194, 1960.
70. Kerbel, N. C.: An unusual case of erythema nodosum. Can. Med. Assoc. J., *83*:820, 1960.
71. James, D. G.: Erythema nodosum. Br. Med. J., *1*:853, 1961.
72. Truelove, L. H.: Articular manifestations of erythema nodosum. Ann. Rheum. Dis., *19*:174, 1960.
73. Löfgren, S.: Erythema nodosum. Studies on etiology and pathogenesis in 185 adult cases. Acta Med. Scand., *124*: (Suppl. 174):1946.
74. Löfgren, S., and Wahlgren, F.: On the histopathology of erythema nodosum. Acta Dermatovenereol., *29*:1, 1949.
75. Winkelmann, R. K., and Forstrom, L.: New observations in the histopathology of erythema nodosum. J. Invest. Dermatol., *65*:441, 1975.
76. Favour, C. B., and Sosman, M. C.: Erythema nodosum. Arch. Intern. Med., *80*:435, 1947.
77. Beerman, H.: Erythema nodosum. Am. J. Med. Sci., *223*:433, 1952.
78. Saslaw, S., and Beman, F.: Erythema nodosum as a manifestation of histoplasmosis. J.A.M.A., *170*:1178, 1959.
79. Debois, J., Vandepitte, J., and Degreef, H.: Yersinia enterocolitica as a cause of erythema nodosum. Dermatologica, *156*:65, 1978.
80. Hannuksela, M.: Human Yersiniosis: a common cause of erythematous skin eruptions. Int. J. Dermatol., *16*:665, 1977.
81. Baden, H. P., and Holcomb, F. D.: Erythema nodosum from oral contraceptives. Arch. Dermatol., *98*:634, 1968.
82. Bombardieri, S., DiMunno, O., DiPunzio, C., and Pasero, G.: Erythema nodosum associated with pregnancy and oral contraceptives. Br. Med. J., *1*:1509, 1977.
83. James, D. G., Neville, E., and Carstairs, L. S.: Bone and joint sarcoidosis. Sem. Arthritis. Rheum., *6*:53, 1976.
84. Canizares, O., Costello, M., and Gigli, I.: Erythema nodosum type of lepra reaction. Arch. Dermatol., *85*:29, 1962.
85. See references 15, 22, 55, 72 and 84*d* cited by Beerman, H.: Erythema nodosum. Am. J. Med. Sci., *223*:433, 1952.
86. Bluefarb, S. M., Wallk, S., and Gecht, M. L.: Acute monocytic leukemia with erythema nodosum. Arch. Dermatol., *75*:596, 1957.
87. Löfgren, S.: The concept of erythema nodosum revised. Scand. J. Resp. Dis., *48*:348, 1967.
88. Similä, S., and Pietilä, J.: The changing etiology of erythema nodosum in children. Acta. Tuberc. Scand., *46*:159, 1965.
89. Aetiology of erythema nodosum in children. A study by a group of pediatricians. Lancet, *2*:14, 1961.
90. Milliken, T. G., and Tattersall, P. E. R.: Scalene node biopsy in cases of erythema nodosum. Acta Med. Scand., *176*(Suppl. 425):248, 1964.
91. James, D. G.: Dermatological aspects of sarcoidosis. Q. J. Med., *28*:109, 1959.
92. Sharma, O. P.: Cutaneous sarcoidosis: clinical features and management. Chest, *61*:320, 1972.
93. Erythema nodosum. Lancet, *1*:256, 1962.
94. Bedi, T. R., and Pinkus, H.: Histopathological spectrum of erythema multiforme. Br. J. Dermatol., *95*:243, 1976.
95. Lozada, F., and Silverman, S., Jr.: Erythema multiforme. Clinical characteristics and natural history in fifty patients. Oral Surg., *46*:628, 1978.
95a. Wooten, J. W., Katz, H. I., Hoffman, S., and Fink, J.: Development of oral lesions in erythema multiforme exudativum. Oral Surg., *24*:808, 1967.
96. Keil, H.: Erythema multiforme exudativum (Hebra): a clinical entity associated with systemic features. Ann. Intern. Med., *14*:449, 1940.
97. Shelley, W. B.: Herpes simplex virus as a cause of erythema multiforme. J.A.M.A., *201*:153, 1967.
98. Shelley, W. B.: Bacterial endotoxin (lipopolysaccharide) as a cause of erythema multiforme. J.A.M.A., *243*:58, 1980.
99. Sontheimer, R. D., Garibaldi, R. A., and Krueger, G. G.: Stevens-Johnson syndrome associated with Mycoplasma pneumoniae infections. Arch. Dermatol., *114*:241, 1978.
100. Ludlam, G. B., Bridges, J. B., and Benn, E. C.: Association of Stevens-Johnson syn-

drome with antibody for Mycoplasma pneumoniae. Lancet, *1*:958, 1964.
101. Wasserman, E., and Glass, W.: Stevens-Johnson syndrome. Arch. Intern. Med., *104*:787, 1959.
102. March, C. H.: Erythema multiforme bullosum associated with trichomonas infection. Arch. Dermatol., *92*:674, 1965.
103. Söltz-Szöts, J.: Nachweis des Herpes Simplex-Virus aus Effloreszenzen eines Falles von Erythema exudativum multiforme. A Haut Geschlechtskr., *34*:25, 1963.
104. DeFeo, C., Jr.: Erythema multiforme bullosum caused by 9-Bromofluorene. Arch. Dermatol., *94*:545, 1966.
105. Mali, J. W. H., and Malten, K. E.: The epidemic of polymorph toxic erythema in the Netherlands in 1960. Acta Dermato-venereol., *46*:123, 1966.
106. Nawalkha, P. L., Mathor, N., Malholtra, Y., and Saksena, H.: Severe erythema multiforme (Stevens-Johnson syndrome) following telecobalt therapy. Br. J. Radiol., *45*:768, 1972.
107. Chapman, R. S., Forsyth, A., and MacQueen, A.: Erythema multiforme in association with acute ulcerative colitis and Crohn's disease. Dermatologica, *154*:32, 1977.
108. Comaish, J. S., and Kerr, D. N. S.: Erythema multiforme and nephritis. Br. Med. J., *2*:84, 1961.
109. Bloom, A., and Lovel, T. W. I.: Erythema multiforme with renal and myocardial injury. Proc. R. Soc. Med., *57*:175, 1964.
110. Foerster, D. W., and Scott, L. V.: Isolation of herpes simplex virus from a patient with erythema multiforme exudativum (Stevens-Johnson syndrome). N. Engl. J. Med., *259*:473, 1958.
111. Lyell, A., Gordon, A. M., Dick, H. M., and Somerville, R. G.: Mycoplasmas and erythema multiforme. Lancet, *2*:1116, 1967.
112. Major, P. P., Morisette, R., Kurstak, C., and Kurstak, E.: Isolation of herpes simplex virus type 1 from lesions of erythema multiforme. Can. Med. Assoc. J., *8*:821, 1978.
113. MacDonald, A., and Feinwel, M.: Isolation of herpes virus from erythema multiforme. Br. Med. J., *2*:570, 1972
114. Wuepper, K. D., Watson, P. A., and Kazmierowski, J. A.: Immune complexes in erythema multiforme and the Stevens-Johnson syndrome. J. Invest. Dermatol., *74*:368, 1980.
114a. Bushkell, L. L., Mackel, S. E., and Jordon, R. E.: Erythema multiforme: direct immunofluorescence studies and detection of circulating immune complexes. J. Invest. Dermatol., *74*:372, 1980.
114b. Huff, J. C., Weston, W. L., and Carr, R. I.: Mixed cryoglobulinemia, ^{125}I Clq binding and skin immunofluorescence in erythema multiforme. J. Invest. Dermatol., *74*:375, 1980.
115. Safai, B., Good, R. A., and Day, N. K.: Erythema multiforme: report of two cases and speculation on immune mechanisms involved in pathogenesis. Clin. Immunol. Immunopathol., *7*:379, 1977.
116. Clayton, R., and Haffenden, G.: An immunofluorescence study of pityriasis lichenoides. Br. J. Dermatol., *99*:491, 1978.
117. Lever, W. F.: Pemphigus and Pemphigoid. Charles C Thomas, Springfield, 1965, p. 75.
118. Lever, W. F.: Pemphigus and pemphigoid. A review of the advances made since 1964. J. Am. Acad. Dermatol., *1*:2, 1979.
119. Person, J. R., and Rogers, R. S., III: Bullous and cicatricial pemphigoid. Clinical, histopathologic, and immunopathologic correlations. Mayo Clin. Proc., *52*:54, 1977.
120. Kim, R., and Winkelmann, R. K.: Dermatitis herpetiformis in children. Relationship to bullous pemphigoid. Arch. Dermatol., *83*:895, 1961.
121. Ahmed, A. R., Maize, J. C., and Provost, T. T.: Bullous pemphigoid. Clinical and immunologic follow-up after successful therapy. Arch. Dermatol., *113*:1043, 1977.
122. Beutner, E. H., Jordan, R. E., and Chorzelski, T. P.: The immunopathology of pemphigus and bullous pemphigoid. J. Invest. Dermatol., *51*:63, 1968.
123. Person, J. R., and Rogers, R. S., III: Bullous pemphigoid and psoriasis: does subclinical bullous pemphigoid exist? Br. J. Dermatol., *95*:535, 1976.
124. Koerber, W. A., Jr., Price, N. M., and Watson, W.: Coexistent psoriasis and bullous pemphigoid. Arch. Dermatol., *114*:1643, 1978.
125. Cram, D. L., and Fukuyama, K.: Immunohistochemistry of ultraviolet-induced pemphigus and pemphigoid lesions. Arch. Dermatol., *106*:819, 1972.
126. Schiltz, J., and Michel, G.: Production of epidermal acantholysis in normal human skin in vitro by the IgG fraction from pemphigus serum. J. Invest. Dermatol., *67*:254, 1976.
127. Deng, J.-S., Beutner, E. H., Shu, S., and Chorzelski, T. P.: Pemphigus antibody action on skin explants. Arch. Dermatol., *113*:923, 1977.
128. Tagami, H., and Imamura, S.: Benign mucous membrane pemphigoid. Demonstration of circulating and tissue-bound membrane antibodies. Arch. Dermatol., *109*:711, 1974.
129. Rogers, R. S., III, Sheridan, P. J., and Jordon, R. E.: Desquamative gingivitis. Clinical, histopathologic and immunopathologic investigations. Oral Surg., *42*:316, 1976.
130. Brunsting, L. A., and Perry, H. O.: Benign pemphigoid. A report of seven cases with chronic scarring, herpetiform plaques about the head and neck. Arch. Dermatol., *75*:489, 1957.
131. Rogers, R. S., III: Recent advances in erosive, ulcerative, and bullous diseases of

the oral mucosa. Prog. Dermatol., *12*:1, 5, 1978.
132. Kahn, G.: Mucocutaneous lymph node syndrome (Kawasaki's disease). A new disease remaking its debut. Arch. Dermatol., *114*:948, 1978.
133. Lyell, A.: A review of toxic epidermal necrolysis in Britain. Br. J. Dermatol. *79*:662, 1967.
134. Lyell, A., Dick, H. M., and Alexander, J. O'D.: Outbreak of toxic epidermal necrolysis associated with staphylococci. Lancet, *1*:787, 1969.
135. Mamo, J. G., and Baghdassarian, A.: Behçet's disease. A report of 28 cases. Arch. Ophthalmol. *71*:4, 1964.
136. Haim, S., and Sherf, K.: Behçet's disease. Presentation of 11 cases and evaluation of treatment. Isr. J. Med. Sci., *2*:69, 1966.
137. Dowling, G. B.: Behçet's disease. Proc. R. Soc. Med., *54*:101, 1961.
138. Haim, S.: Contribution of ocular symptoms in the diagnosis of Behçet's disease. Study of 23 cases. Arch. Dermatol., *98*:478, 1968.
139. Chamberlain, M. A.: Behçet's syndrome in 32 patients in Yorkshire. Ann. Rheum. Dis., *36*:491, 1977.
140. France, R., Buchanan, R. N., Wilson, M. W., and Sheldon, M. B., Jr.: Relapsing iritis with recurrent ulcers of the mouth and genitalia (Behçet's syndrome). Medicine (Balt.), *30*:335, 1951.
141. Forman, L.: Behçet's disease. Br. J. Dermatol., *63*:417, 1951.
142. Sigel, N., and Larson, R.: Behçet's syndrome. A case with benign pericarditis and recurrent neurologic involvement treated with adrenal steroids. Arch. Intern. Med., *115*:203, 1965.
143. Hills, E. A.: Behçet's syndrome with aortic aneurysms. Br. Med. J., *4*:152, 1967.
144. O'Duffy, J. D.: Summary of international symposium on Behçet's disease. J. Rheumatol., *5*:229, 1978.
145. Pallis, C. A.: Behçet's disease and the nervous system. Trans. St. John. Hosp. Dermatol. Soc., *52*:201, 1966.
146. O'Duffy, J. D., and Goldstein, N. P.: Neurologic involvement in seven patients with Behçet's disease. Am. J. Med., *61*:170, 1976.
147. Orsson, P. J.: Behçet's syndrome. N. Engl. J. Med., *302*:407, 1980.
148. Bach, C. D., and Rubin, R. J.: Behçet's syndrome. N. Engl. J. Med., *302*:408, 1980.
149. Lehner, T.: Behçet's syndrome and autoimmunity. Br. Med. J., *1*:465, 1967.
150. Gupta, R. C., O'Duffy, J. D., McDuffie, F. C., Meurer, M., and Jordon, R. E.: Circulating immune complexes in active Behçet's disease. Clin. Exp. Immunol., *34*:213, 1978.
151. Lehner, T.: Pathology of recurrent oral ulceration and oral ulceration in Behçet's syndrome: Light, electron and fluorescence microscopy. J. Pathol., *97*:481, 1969.
152. Graykowski, E. A., Barile, M. F., Lee, W. B., and Stanley, H. R., Jr.: Recurrent aphthous stomatitis — clinical, therapeutic, histopathologic and hypersensitivity aspects. J.A.M.A., *196*:637, 1966.
153. Lehner, T.: Stimulation of lymphocyte transformation by tissue homogenates in recurrent oral ulceration. Immunology, *13*:159, 1967.
154. Rogers, R. S., III, Sams, W. M., Jr., and Shorter, R. G.: Lymphocytotoxicity in recurrent aphthous stomatitis. Lymphocytotoxicity for oral epithelial cells in recurrent aphthous stomatitis and Behçet syndrome. Arch. Dermatol., *109*:361, 1974.
155. Yazici, H., Akokan, G., Yalcin, B., and Müftüoğlu, A.: The high prevalence of HLA-B5 in Behçet's disease. Clin. Exp. Immunol., *30*:256, 1977.
156. Nahir, M., Scharf, Y., Gidoni, O., Barzilai, A., Friedman-Birnbaum, R., and Haim, S.: HL-A antigens in Behçet's disease. A family study. Dermatologica, *156*:205, 1978.
157. Curth, H. O.: Recurrent genito-oral aphthosis and uveitis with hypopyon (Behçet's syndrome). Report of two cases. Arch. Dermatol. Syph., *54*:179, 1946.
158. Burns, R. E., Boyer, P., and Fine, G.: Cutaneous papules heralding rheumatcc carditis (Rosenberg). Arch. Dermatol., *89*:334, 1964.

10

Sarcoidosis

Boeck's sarcoid is a systemic granulomatous disorder of unknown etiology. Rather than a single entity, it is probably a syndrome produced by diverse stimuli. The granulomatous reaction is composed of *naked* tubercles — collections of epithelioid cells with a thin rim of lymphocytes. Giant cells are often present. Necrosis does not occur. Sometimes the collar of lymphocytes is absent. The lungs, liver, lymph nodes, spleen, eyes, joints, muscles, exocrine glands, and nervous system are frequently involved in an identical granulomatous response. Skin lesions occur in 10 per cent to 100 per cent of the cases, depending upon whether the internist or dermatologist is the observer. In four representative series[1-4] composed of adults, cutaneous lesions histologically specific for sarcoid occurred in 16 to 36 per cent of the patients. The prevalence of skin lesions in children is the same.[5]

The skin markers of sarcoid, as in other disorders, are both specific and nonspecific. The gross appearance of the specific eruption encompasses papules, nodules, plaques, subcutaneous tumors, and scaly erythematous and atrophic flat lesions. Although the lesions do not have a pathognomonic clinical morphology, they do exhibit highly characteristic features that should strongly suggest the presence of the disease. Sarcoidosis can be diagnosed almost with certainty by histologic examination of specific lesions, thereby eliminating the need to biopsy lymph nodes, liver, muscle, or bronchial mucosa solely for diagnostic purposes. In James' series, the cutaneous manifestations of sarcoidosis occurred four times more often in women than in men.[1]

SPECIFIC LESIONS

The lesions of sarcoidosis are usually red or purple, but they can also have a reddish-brown or yellowish-brown hue (Plates 26*E*, *F* and 27*A*, *B*). If the erythema is pressed out with a glass slide (diascopy), one can often see tiny yellow-brown nodules produced by the granulomas; these nodules are similar to those seen in lupus vulgaris, the common form of cutaneous tuberculosis. Sarcoid lesions characteristically have a waxy translucent appearance. They are almost never pruritic or painful.

Papules of sarcoidosis can arise anywhere on the body, but they are found most often on the face, periorbitally, and in the nasolabial folds (Figs. 10–1 to 10–3). These small elevated lesions are usually flat-topped, translucent, red or brown, and from 2 to 5 mm in diameter. Initially, papular lesions might be confused with flat warts or acne vulgaris; but on

PLATE 27

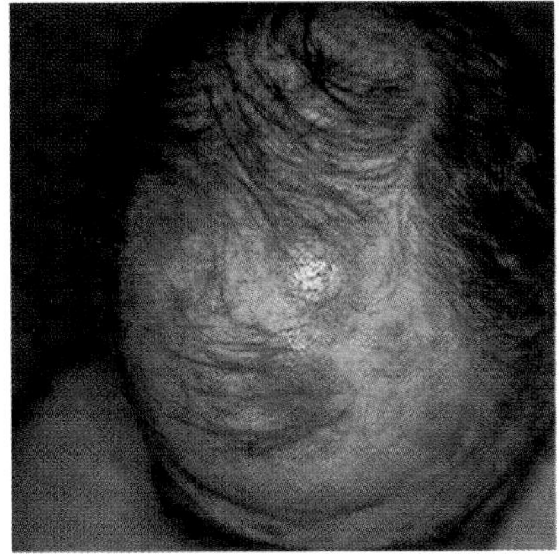

A, Sarcoid. Red translucent plaques on scalp.

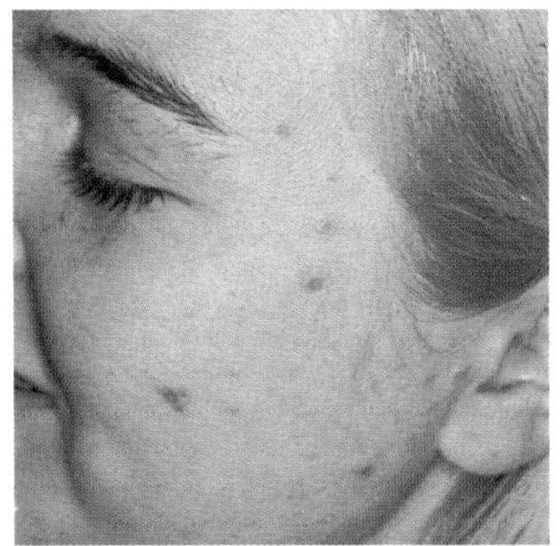

B, Sarcoid. Red translucent papules on face which are sometimes misdiagnosed as acne.

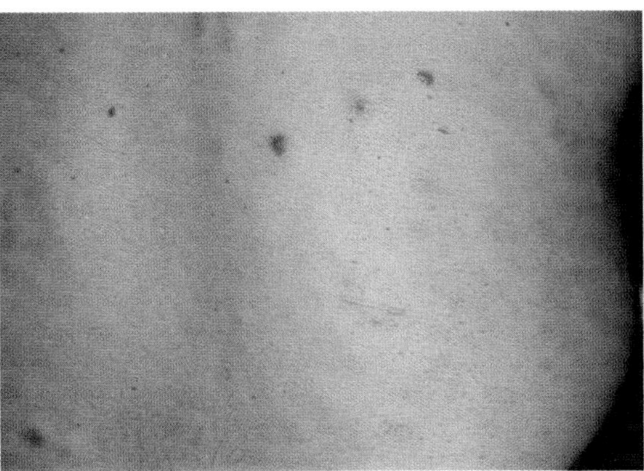

C, Sarcoid. Deep subcutaneous nodules which are often purple in color.

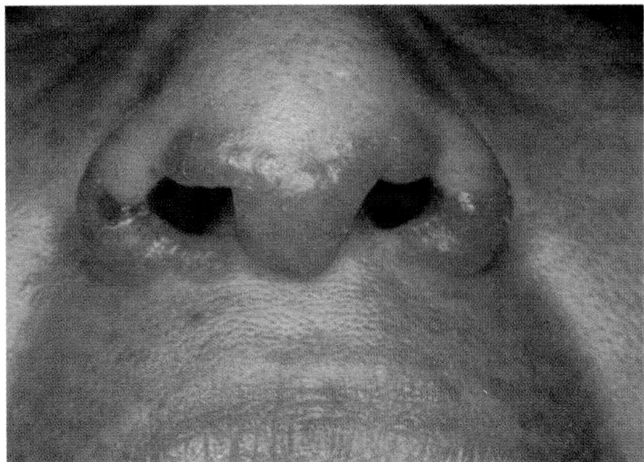

D, Sarcoid. Lupus pernio of the nose.

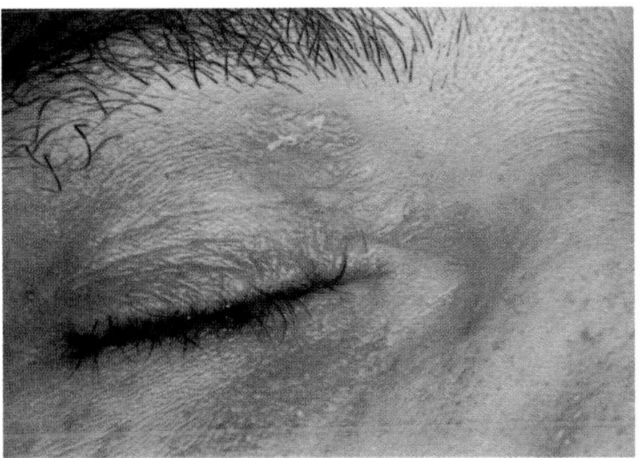

E, Sarcoid. Characteristic scaly yellow-brown plaques.

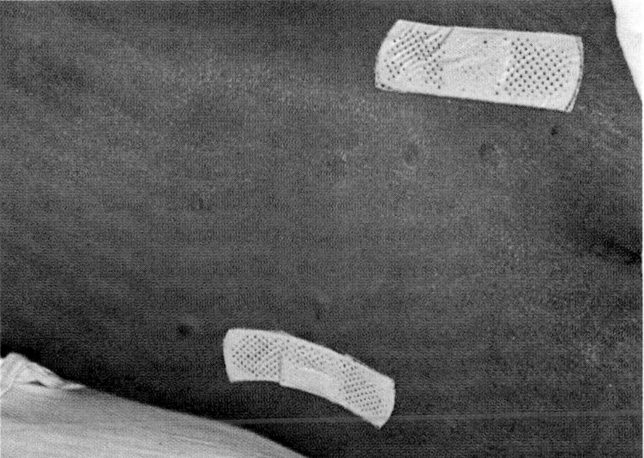

F, Sarcoid. Moderately scaly nodules on the back of this patient proved to be composed of noncaseating naked tubercles characteristic of sarcoidosis.

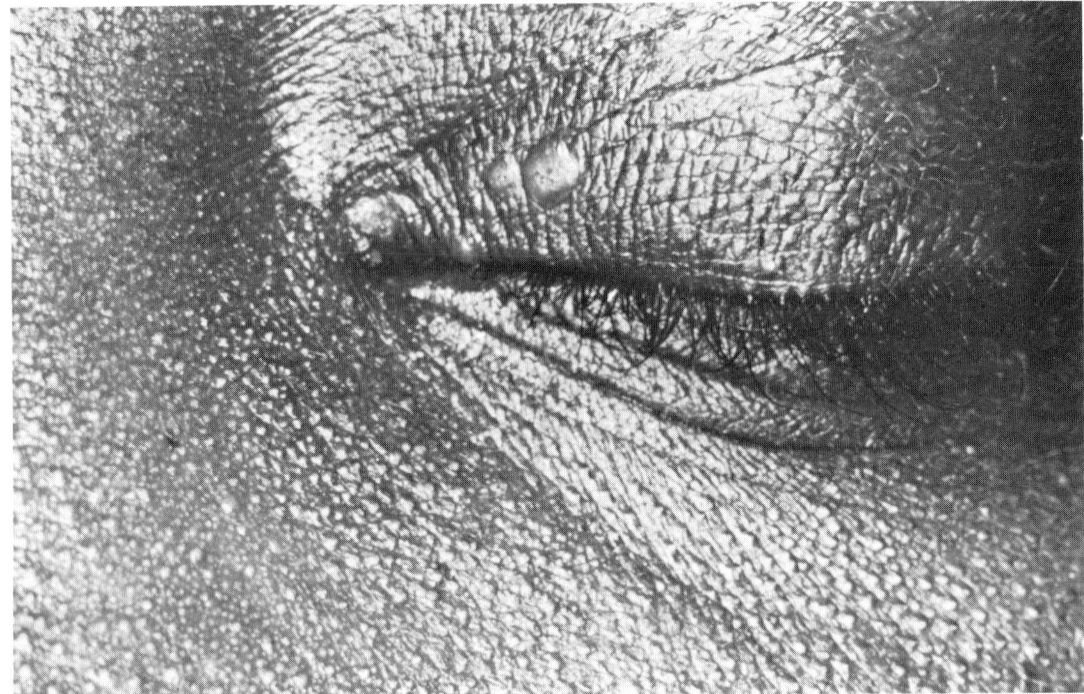

Figure 10–1. Sarcoid. Characteristic flat-topped papules are present on the upper eyelid.

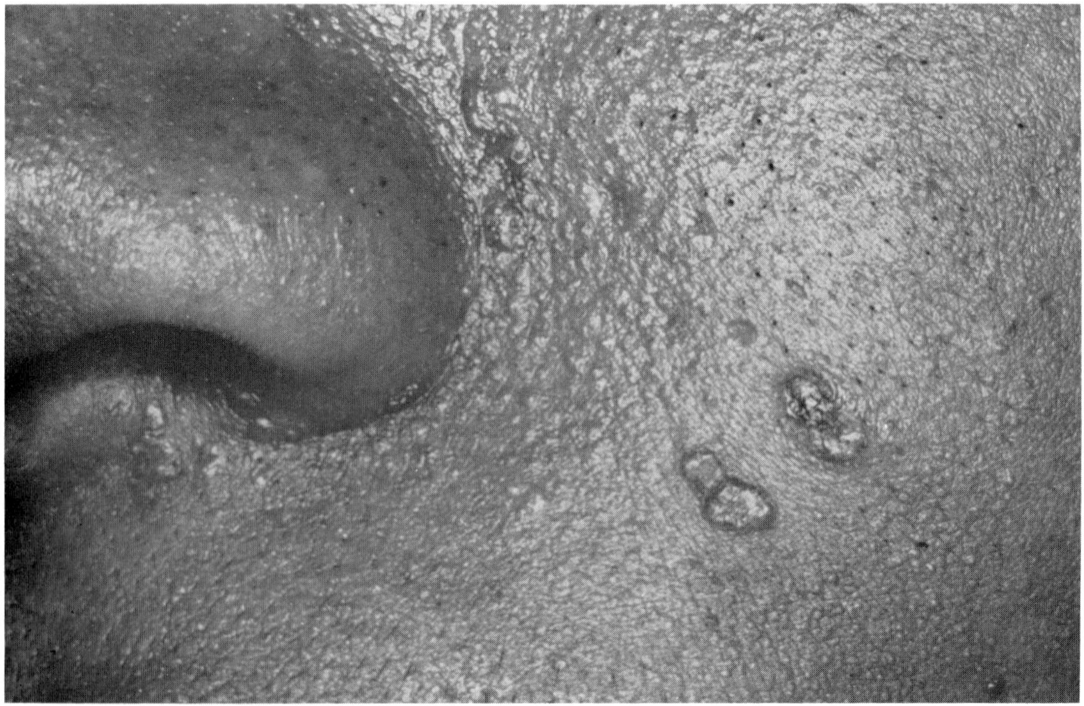

Figure 10–2. Sarcoid. Characteristic flat-topped papules are present at nostril, ala nasi, and nasolabial fold.

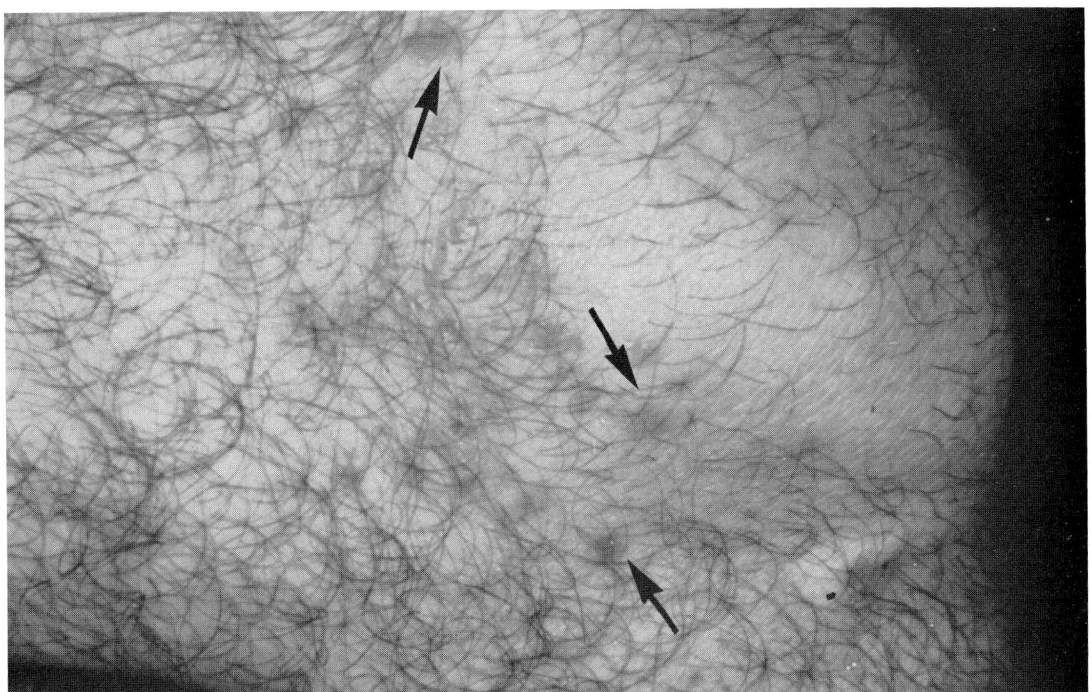

Figure 10–3. Sarcoid. Papules (arrows) about the knee.

careful inspection, one can detect their characteristic translucence and color. James uses the term *maculopapular* to describe these small papules.[1]

Papules can form a ring simulating the banal disorder, granuloma annulare (Fig. 10–4). However, the color and translucent quality of the lesions in sarcoid distinguish them from those of granuloma annulare; the borders of the latter are made up of *skin-colored* papules. Annular lesions of sarcoid begin as papules that slowly expand peripherally and usually leave an atrophic and sometimes scaly center (Figs. 10–5 to 10–7). In granuloma annulare, the center is neither scaly nor atrophic. Annular lesions also can be produced by plaques that undergo central atrophy. If the annular lesions have a yellow-brown color, as they sometimes can, it may be difficult to distinguish them clinically, but not histologically, from necrobiosis lipoidica.[6] Ring lesions seem to occur most frequently in American blacks.

Nodules show a predilection for the extremities and trunk (Plate 27*C*). Translucency is not characteristic, but the red and purple colors are. The nodules arise in the deep dermis and subcutaneous layer. Calcification is a rare development in subcutaneous nodules.[8] Although deep nodules of sarcoidosis are often called Darier-Roussy sarcoid, the eponym is not correct. *Darier-Roussy sarcoid* is a term used by dermatologists to describe several nonspecific inflammatory disorders that involve the subcutaneous fat.[7]

Plaques of sarcoidosis are almost always violaceous and translucent with ill-defined borders (Plate 27*D*). Large telangiectatic vessels can be present on the surface, and some authors call these plaques angiolupoid lesions. However, when such extensive plaque formation arises on the ear lobes, nose, fingers, and toes, the term *lupus pernio* has been used.

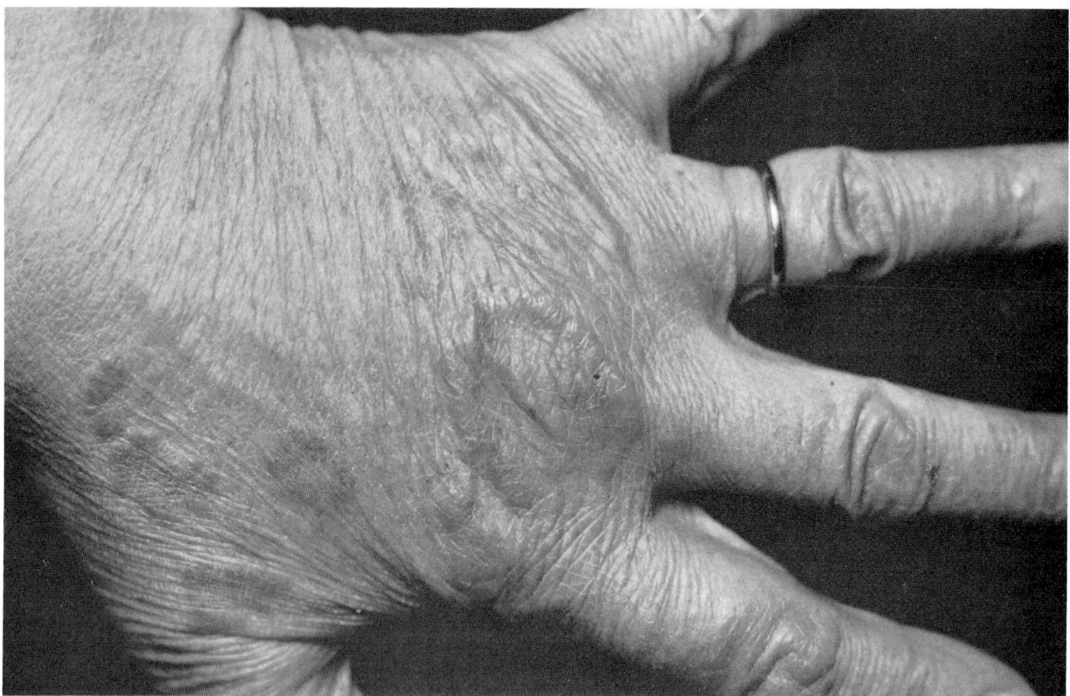

Figure 10–4. Granuloma annulare. Several lesions are present. Border of lesion is made up of discrete, but joined, papules. Center is normal skin.

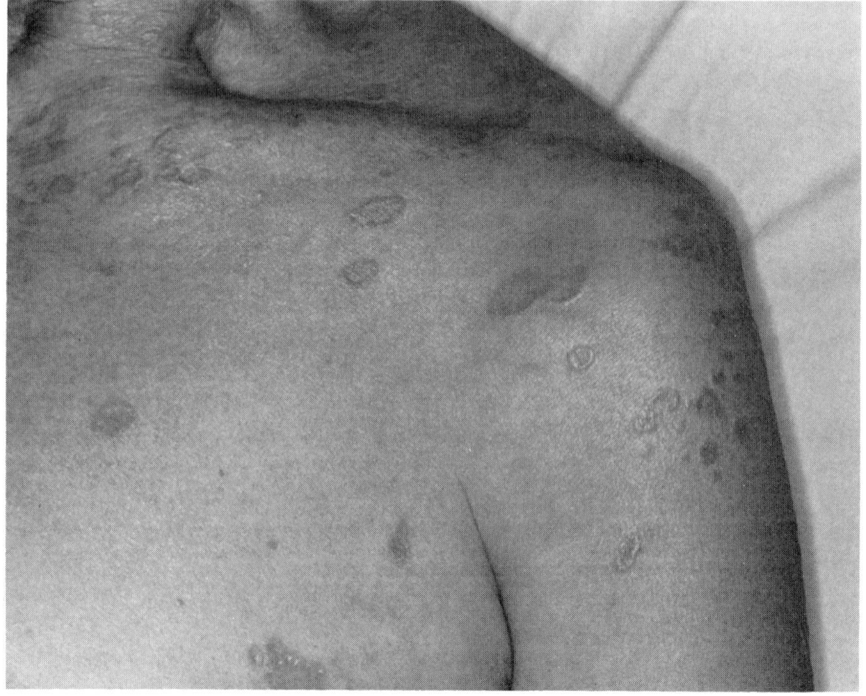

Figure 10–5. Sarcoid. Granuloma annulare–like lesions.

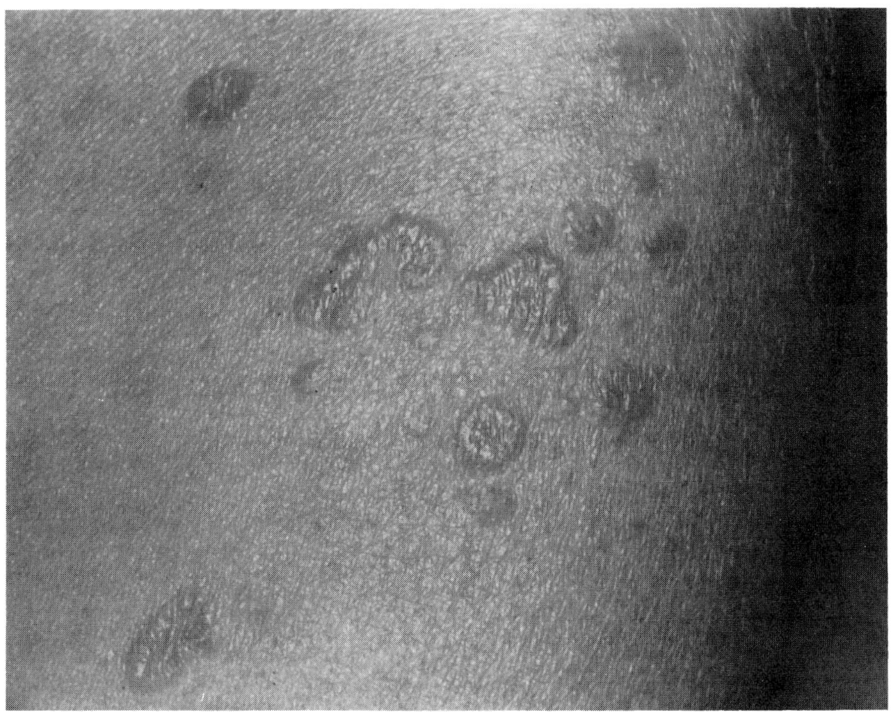

Figure 10–6. Sarcoid. Granuloma annulare–like lesions.

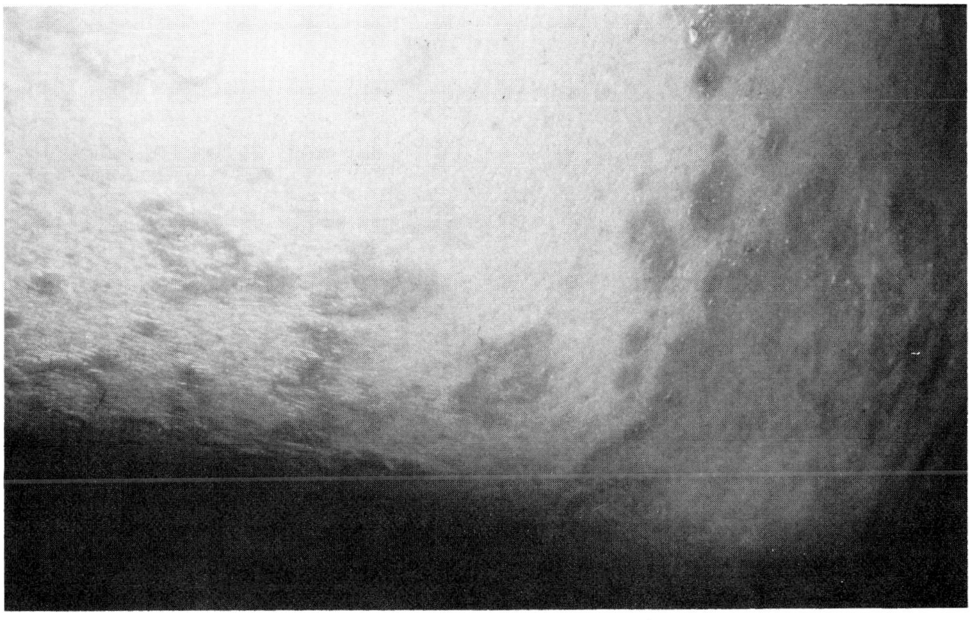

Figure 10–7. Sarcoid. Granuloma annulare–like lesions.

Lupus pernio of the fingers and toes produces bulbous and sausage-shaped digits and is almost always associated with lytic lesions in the underlying phalanges (Figs. 10–8 and 10–9). When the tip of the nose is involved by lupus pernio, the nasal bones may show osteoporosis and cystic lesions. The nasal mucosa may also be affected, producing purulent catarrh and obstructive symptoms. Bone involvement is present in 10 to 20 per cent of patients with sarcoidosis. Although the bones most frequently involved are those of the hands and feet, occasionally the skull, long bones, vertebrae, and ribs show identical lytic lesions. However, James emphasizes that radiographic examination of the hands and feet of patients with sarcoid is worthwhile only if they have lupus pernio or chronic skin lesions elsewhere.[1, 9] Bone involvement may also portend a poorer prognosis. The mortality rate of such patients was 21 per cent in James' series, four times greater than the overall rate.[9]

Sarcoidal lesions can also take the form of red, violaceous, yellowish-brown, or reddish-brown scaly macules or patches (Plate 27*E*, *F*). These eruptions tend to involute spontaneously and produce cutaneous atrophy. The scale varies from thin and scant to heavy and thick. When the scalp is affected by such sarcoidal lesions, alopecia frequently results, and the clinical appearance of lupus erythematosus is mimicked. On the trunk and extremities the picture of psoriasis can be simulated; and on the palms, the appearance of secondary syphilis is duplicated. The psoriasiform lesion is said to be characteristic of sarcoid in American blacks.

In a few patients, this type of scaling eruption covered the legs, buttocks, and trunk and has been called "erythrodermic" sarcoidosis. In

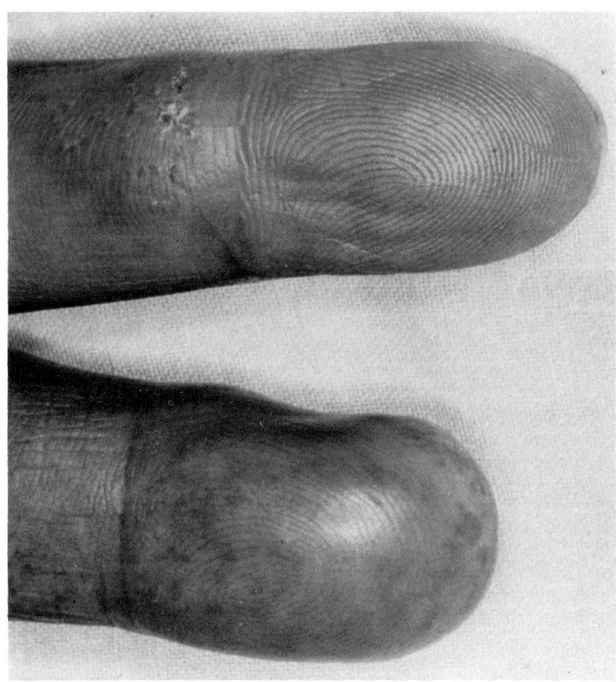

Figure 10–8. Sarcoid. Bulbous and sausage-shaped fingers with underlying lytic lesions in the bone (lupus pernio).

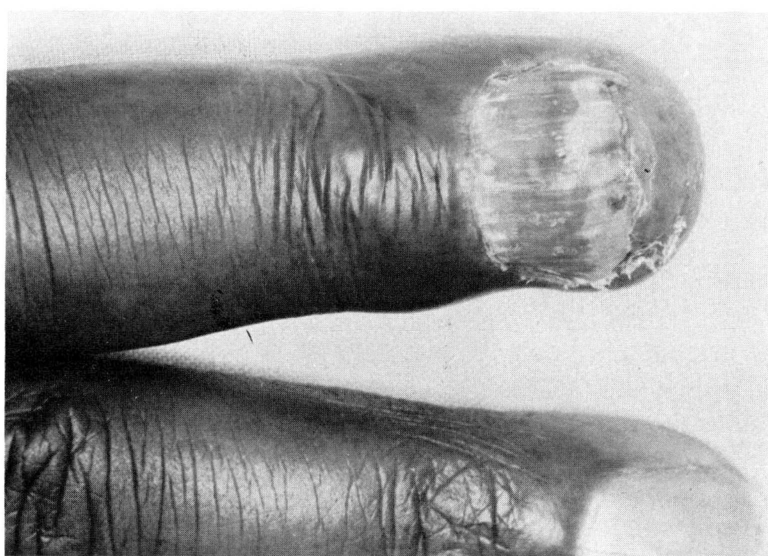

Figure 10–9. Sarcoid. Lupus pernio.

three persons, generalized skin involvement developed, simulating an exfoliative dermatitis.[10, 11]

A brief history of one of our patients is illustrative. A 40-year-old white woman developed several red to purple papules on the cheeks and the sides of the neck and an atrophic red scaling area with alopecia on the scalp. Biopsy of lesions from the face and scalp showed the *naked* tubercles of sarcoidosis. Radiographs of the chest disclosed the typical pulmonary findings of sarcoid. The cutaneous lesions regressed spontaneously during the following six months. The patient returned to the clinic after a seven year absence and displayed a noninflammatory scarring alopecia that was indistinguishable from pseudopelade of Brocq (Fig. 10–10). Biopsy disclosed neither sarcoidosis nor inflammation.

Ulceration may be a complication of lupus pernio on the nose and ears. Rarely, cutaneous plaques and deep cutaneous and subcutaneous nodules may ulcerate.[12, 13] Moser et al. reported a patient with generalized perifollicular papules and pustules as the specific cutaneous markers of sarcoidosis.[14] Fong and Sharma reported the case of a 41-year-old white man who had a severely pruritic and generalized eruption of small papules for 20 years that had been diagnosed as neurodermatitis. He was treated with topical corticosteroids, but the rash never cleared completely. Repeated exacerbations resulted in frequent hospitalizations. A skin biopsy finally established the diagnosis of sarcoidosis. His only other positive findings were enlarged supraclavicular and inguinal lymph nodes. A scalene node biopsy showed noncaseating granulomas. The skin lesions and pruritus disappeared following oral steroid therapy.[15]

An ichthyosis-like picture developed six months before the diagnosis of sarcoid in one of our patients illustrated in Figures 10–11 and 10–12. Only the ichthyotic areas showed the histopathology of sarcoidosis. Additional examples of this ichthyosiform manifestation have been reported in the literature.[16, 17]

Hypopigmentation is an uncommon manifestation.[4, 18, 19] It may develop over papules and nodules or it may exist as patches that feel

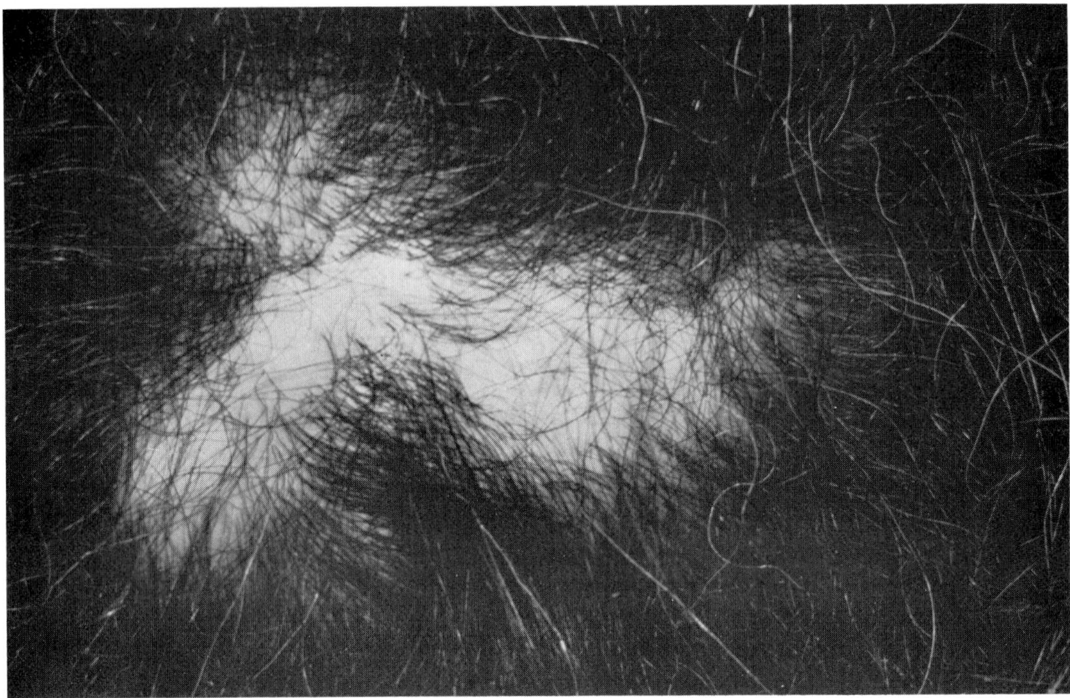

Figure 10–10. Sarcoid. Alopecia simulating pseudopelade. Sarcoid lesions had been present in this area several years before.

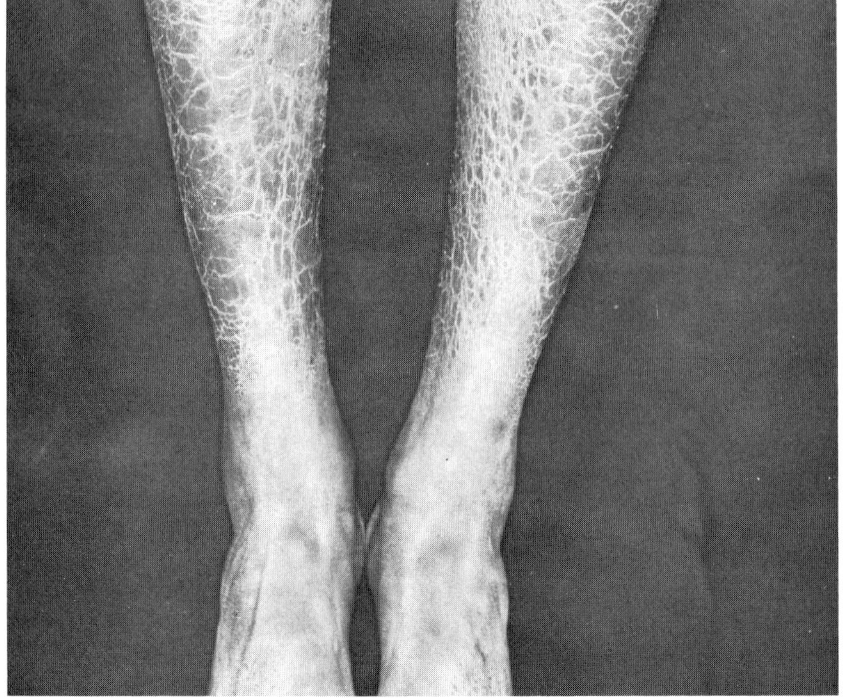

Figure 10–11. Sarcoid. Ichthyosis-like lesions.

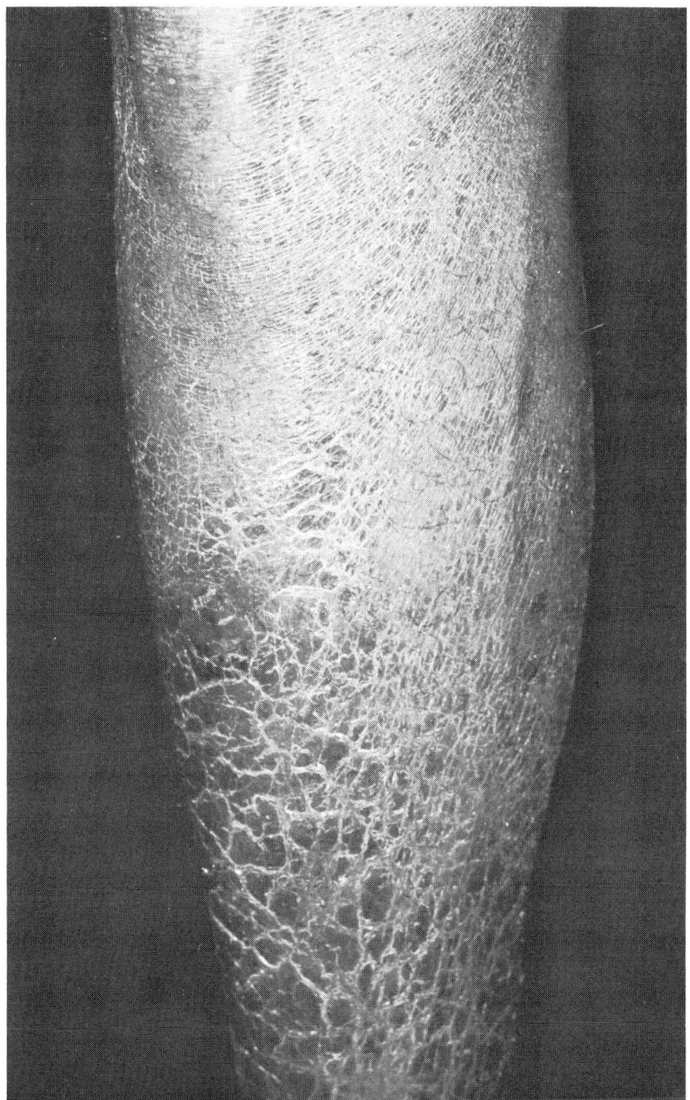

Figure 10–12. Sarcoid. Closer view of ichthyosis-like lesions shown in Figure 10–11.

normal or slightly indurated. Papules and nodules usually develop later from the hypopigmented macules. Biopsies have shown sarcoid granulomas in the macules, papules, and nodules. All of the patients have been black where that information has been reported.[18, 19] The hypopigmentation appears to be related to decreased melanization of the overlying epidermal cells. The melanocyte count was normal, and there was no evidence for postinflammatory hypopigmentation in the study by Cornelius et al.[18]

Nathan et al. described a patient with chronic lymphedema and ulcerations of the legs that were present for 11 years before uveitis, inguinal node enlargement, and cutaneous papules and nodules developed. Biopsy of a node and skin lesion showed sarcoidosis. Both the lymphedema and skin lesions disappeared following steroid therapy.[20]

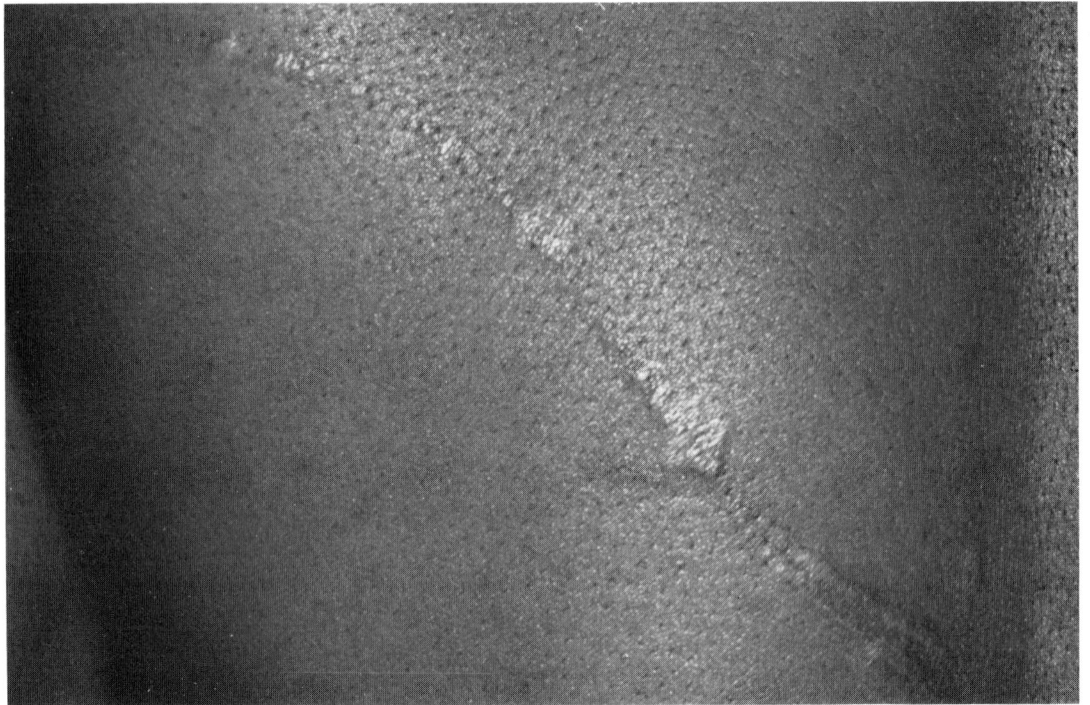

Figure 10–13. Sarcoid lesions arising in scar.

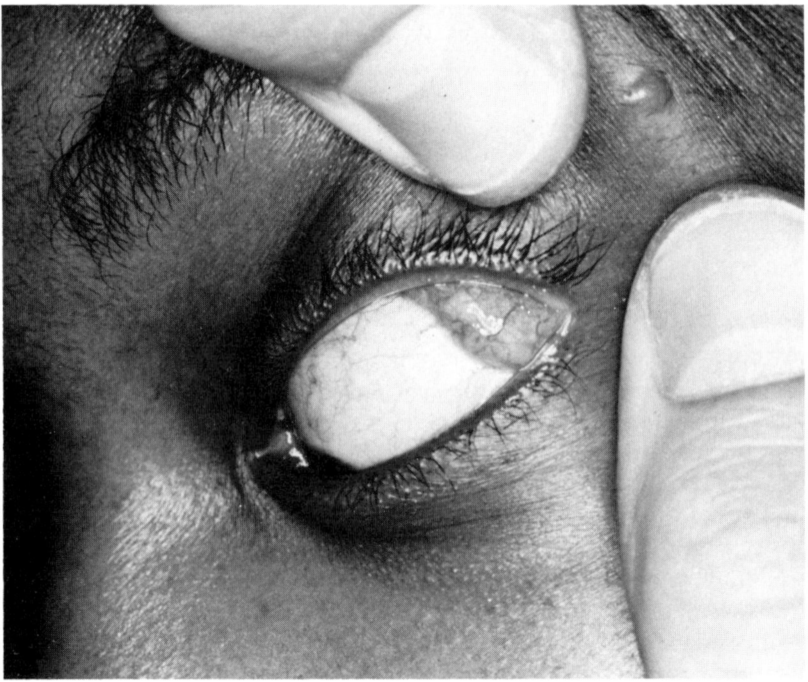

Figure 10–14. Sarcoid. Enlarged lacrimal gland.

Shumes et al. described a patient with sarcoid in whom the papules and nodules had a verrucous surface.[21]

It is worthwhile to take a biopsy of any lesion, no matter how trivial, in a patient suspected of having sarcoidosis. We have seen two patients in whom granulomas typical of sarcoid developed at sites of an earlier folliculitis. Clinically, the lesions looked like small scars. A biopsy of the banal marks established the diagnosis of sarcoidosis in these two patients, both of whom also had radiographic findings characteristic of pulmonary sarcoidosis. Surgical scars are favorite sites for the development of cutaneous sarcoid. Even scars many years old suddenly can become affected by the granulomatous reaction (Fig. 10–13).

Occasionally, the oral mucosa and palpebral conjunctivae are involved with granulomas. Enlarged lacrimal and parotid glands, uveitis, and fever (uveoparotid fever) are characteristic features of sarcoidosis. Enlargement of only the lacrimal glands is also observed (Fig. 10–14).

The differential diagnosis of specific papules and nodules includes cutaneous amyloidosis, lichen planus, flat warts, syringoma, trichoepithelioma, lupus erythematosus, lymphoma cutis, and xanthoma. The plaques resemble those seen in lupus erythematosus, lymphoma, and photosensitivity reactions. In addition, the deep nodules could be confused with those of malignant lymphoma. However, all of these entities can be distinguished easily from one another and from sarcoidosis by histologic examination.

NONSPECIFIC MANIFESTATIONS

Erythema nodosum is a striking but nonspecific sign of sarcoidosis. The clinical features of this fascinating hypersensitivity syndrome are detailed in Chapter 9. Erythema nodosum with hilar adenopathy, arthralgia, fever, and chills is frequently the initial manifestation of sarcoidosis as well as a sign of previous streptococcal infection, primary tuberculosis, or deep fungal diseases. When erythema nodosum occurs in sarcoid, the latter usually behaves as a benign self-limited disorder.[9] This manifestation of sarcoid occurs most frequently in women 20 to 35 years old. However, I have seen five patients in whom sarcoid began in this manner but did not resolve; progressive sarcoidosis involving lung and liver ensued. Siltzbach and Greenberg observed erythema nodosum in only one out of 18 children with sarcoidosis. Their ages ranged from 9 to 15 years.[23]

Several large series from different countries compiled from 1960 to 1974 indicate that sarcoidosis is the cause of erythema nodosum in 37 per cent of the cases (range 11 to 74 per cent).[9] The prevalence of erythema nodosum in sarcoidosis ranges from 4 to 35 per cent (average 17 per cent).[2, 9, 24, 25] In our experience, sarcoid has accounted for 16 per cent of the cases of erythema nodosum, and erythema nodosum has occurred in 10 per cent of patients with sarcoidosis.[25]

Whether or not cutaneous sarcoidosis indicates a poor prognosis is controversial, but the limited data suggest that involvement of the skin has no influence on the course of the disease.[2] However, information concerning the outcome of the various types of skin lesions is available.[26] Erythema nodosum always disappears without scarring. James[26] observed that the associated hilar adenopathy cleared within one year, although Sones and Israel[27] reported that in their patients erythema nodosum and hilar adenopathy cleared less quickly and less often. (However, the latter authors supplied no data that would indicate how many failed to clear and the nature of the clinical course in those patients.) Unlike most reported series, they had only six cases of erythema nodosum in their patient population of 211.[27] The papules and nodules of sarcoidosis tend to disappear with or without scarring, but the plaques — angiolupoid and lupus pernio — usually persist, especially in patients over 30 years old. It should be stressed that the number of specific cutaneous lesions bears no relation to the extent of visceral involvement.

ETIOLOGY AND PATHOGENESIS

The pathogenesis of sarcoidosis is still unclear. Although anergy to various skin tests, such as tuberculin, mumps, Candida, and trichophytin is present in two thirds of patients, it can be overcome by strong antigenic challenge. The anergy is relative and not absolute as in Hodgkin's disease. Whether there is a basic defect in the suppressor T cell population itself, or whether there is a serum inhibitor acting in conjunction with suppressor T cells to produce depression of cell-mediated hypersensitivity has not been settled.[28-31] Overactivity of B cells as manifested by elevated serum levels of immunoglobulins can be found in up to 80 per cent of patients with *active* sarcoidosis, but there is *no* correlation of immunoglobulin elevation with the degree of disease activity or depression of delayed hypersensitivity.[31] Circulating immune complexes have been found in a few patients with erythema nodosum.[32-34] Although their presence has been correlated with the course of the erythema nodosum, they probably represent a parallel immunologic event and are not causally related. Only a minority of patients with erythema nodosum and sarcoidosis have been shown to have circulating immune complexes.

Granulomatous inflammation is a characteristic response to a number of mycotic and bacterial agents and minerals. The histology of granulomas ranges from the pure epithelioid cell granuloma without inflammation or necrosis to tubercles composed of multiple cell types accompanied by necrosis. The discovery of *naked* tubercles is presumptive evidence of sarcoidosis; but the diagnosis cannot be made unequivocally, nor should it be made unless correlated with the clinical findings. Sometimes tuberculosis, histoplasmosis, brucellosis, syphilis, leprosy, and toxoplasmosis produce similar granulomas; but usually these diseases are associated with inflammatory granulomas exhibiting necrosis. All granulomas should be examined both with polarizing lenses to detect foreign bodies and after selective staining to uncover microorganisms.

Fifty to 60 per cent of patients with active sarcoidosis have elevated serum levels of angiotensin-converting enzyme (ACE), whose main source is the granuloma.[35-37] The serum level may reflect the magnitude of the body mass of granulomas because an involved lymph node can show elevated amounts of ACE in the presence of a normal concentration in the serum. ACE levels parallel the serum levels of lysozyme. Ten per cent of the elevated serum levels of ACE are false positives. Nevertheless, it is a useful test when positive, because it decreases in remission or following steroid therapy and increases during relapse. If it does not decrease following adequate steroid therapy, it may indicate progressive disease with a poorer prognosis.[37]

The Kveim-Siltzbach test is positive in 54 to 92 per cent (average 78 per cent) of patients with sarcoid.[31] This skin test is particularly useful when histologic confirmation of sarcoidosis is lacking or equivocal. It is useful in the differential diagnosis of diffuse pulmonary mottling, uveitis, or erythema nodosum. The combination of the Kveim-Siltzbach test and determination of ACE levels should be especially helpful in such circumstances.

For many years attention has been focused on tuberculosis as the major cause of sarcoidosis because of the similar histopathology of the two entities and the increased incidence of tuberculosis in some patients with sarcoid. Scadding has described English patients in whom tuberculosis preceded the development of sarcoidosis. In one instance, sarcoidosis developed after the successful treatment of pulmonary tuberculosis but disappeared when the tuberculosis became active again. Scadding also described five cases of sarcoidosis that evolved into tuberculosis. In three of the five patients, the typical cutaneous and pulmonary radiographic findings of sarcoidosis disappeared when the transition to active tuberculosis occurred.[38]

Although tuberculosis is not believed to play an important role in the etiology of most cases of sarcoidosis, it nevertheless cannot be entirely excluded. James has pointed out that wherever tuberculosis is rampant, sarcoid is rarely seen, but as tuberculosis is brought under control, sarcoid becomes more frequent.[31] This phenomenon has been observed among the Bantus in South Africa and the population in Uruguay. Some of the Bantu patients with sarcoid were found in leprosaria, just as many English patients had been discovered in sanitaria. Sarcoid is common in the West Indian population living in Britain and in the natives of Martinique living in France. James suggests that sarcoid may appear not only in the wake of tuberculosis, but also following the eradication of leprosy.[31]

Most likely sarcoid has multiple etiologies that vary in different parts of the world. In the United States, sarcoid is most common in the black American. Although hypersensitivity to the lipids of pine pollen, which also react positively with acid-fast stains, is no longer considered to be an important cause of sarcoidosis in the United States, the most promising clues to the nature of sarcoid still involve acid-fast bacilli.[39]

Mankiewicz has presented data suggesting that atypical mycobacteria are important etiologic agents in sarcoidosis.[40, 41] She found that patients with tuberculosis and sarcoidosis are infected with mycobacteriophages. However, individuals with sarcoidosis do not develop neutralizing antibodies to these phages, whereas those with tuberculosis do. Mankiewicz has suggested that sarcoidosis may develop in the following way: tubercle bacilli in the presence of unneutralized mycobacteriophage may be altered to an unrecognizable form that elicits only a noncaseating granulomatous reaction. Mycobacteria resembling the atypical varieties have appeared in cultures of virulent tubercle bacilli injected with mycobacteriophage-neutralizing rabbit sera.

Mankiewicz and colleagues also showed that blast transformation of human leukocytes induced by the mitogen phytohemagglutinin is significantly reduced when mycobacteriophage is added to the *in vitro* system.[42] Mankiewicz has postulated that the absence of pathogenicity of the mycobacteriophage and of the saprophytic mycobacteria does not preclude the possibility that their presence as particulate material or antigens interferes with *in vivo* and *in vitro* immune reactions. This interesting theory requires further study.

DIFFERENTIAL DIAGNOSIS

The differential diagnosis of cutaneous sarcoidosis includes granulomas produced by zirconium, beryllium, silica, and other foreign bodies.[43, 44] In some persons, deodorants and topical poison ivy remedies containing zirconium can produce a sarcoidal eruption by delayed hypersensitivity. Systemic involvement is not known to be a feature in these cases. Cutaneous zirconium granulomas are clinically and histologically indistinguishable from those of sarcoidosis; beryllium, silica, and other foreign bodies produce similar, but not identical, granulomas.

Other granulomatous diseases to be considered in the differential diagnosis include tuberculoid leprosy, lupus vulgaris, tertiary syphilis, the deep mycoses, and swimming pool granuloma caused by *Mycobacterium marinum (balnei).*

M. marinum, an atypical mycobacterium, is found primarily in poorly chlorinated rough-walled swimming pools and in tropical fish aquaria. Trauma to the skin followed by inoculation of the organism results in a focal granulomatous reaction that produces papules or ulcers. Lymphangitic spread producing a picture indistinguishable from sporotrichosis is common. A tuberculin-negative individual becomes a positive reactor after infection with *M. marinum.* The histopathology resembles tuberculosis more than sarcoidosis.[45]

REFERENCES

1. James, D. G.: Dermatological aspects of sarcoidosis. Q. J. Med., *28*:109, 1959.
2. Labow, T. A., Atwood, W. G., and Nelson, C. T.: Sarcoidosis in the American Negro. Arch. Dermatol., *89*:682, 1964.
3. Sharma, O. P.: Cutaneous sarcoidosis: clinical features and management. Chest, *61*:320, 1972.
4. Mayock, R. L., Bertrand, P., Morrison, C. E., and Scott, J. H.: Manifestations of sarcoidosis. Analysis of 145 patients, with a review of nine series selected from the literature. Am. J. Med., *35*:67, 1963.
5. Kendig, E. L., Jr.: The clinical picture of sarcoidosis in children. Pediatrics, *54*:289, 1974.
6. Rudolph, R. I., and Goldschmidt, H.: Annular sarcoidosis of the face. Cutis, *16*:1025, 1975.
7. Irgang, S.: Darier-Roussy's sarcoid. Report of a case and a discussion of the histopathologic features. Dermatologica, *118*:145, 1959.
8. Kroll, J. J., Shapiro, L., Koplon, B. S., and Feldman, F.: Subcutaneous sarcoidosis with calcification. Arch. Dermatol., *106*:894, 1972.
9. James, D. G., Neville, E., and Carstairs, L. S.: Bone and joint sarcoidosis. Sem. Arthritis Rheum., *6*:53, 1976.
10. Schaumann, J.: Benign lymphogranuloma and its cutaneous manifestations. Brit. J. Dermatol., *36*:515, 1924.
11. Wigley, J. E. M., and Musso, L. A.: A case of sarcoidosis with erythrodermic lesions. Treatment with calciferol. Br. J. Dermatol., *63*:398, 1951.
12. Schiffner, J., and Sharma, O. P.: Ulcerative sarcoidosis. Report of an unusual case. Arch. Dermatol., *113*:676, 1977.
13. Meyers, M., and Barsky, S.: Ulcerative sarcoidosis. Arch. Dermatol., *114*:447, 1978.

14. Moser, H. S., Solowey, C. M., and Leider, M.: An unusual form of cutaneous sarcoidosis. N. Y. J. Med., *62*:1859, 1962.
15. Fong, Y. W., and Sharma, O. P.: Pruritic maculopapular skin lesions in sarcoidosis. An unusual clinical presentation. Arch. Dermatol., *111*:362, 1975.
16. Kauh, Y. C., Goody, H. E., and Luscombe, H. A.: Ichthyosiform sarcoidosis. Arch. Dermatol., *114*:100, 1978.
17. Kelly, A. P.: Ichthyosiform sarcoid. Arch. Dermatol., *114*:1551, 1978.
18. Cornelius, C. E., III, Stein, K. M., Hanshaw, W. J., and Spott, D. A.: Hypopigmentation and sarcoidosis. Arch. Dermatol., *108*:249, 1973.
19. Hubler, W. R., Jr.: Hypomelanotic canopy of sarcoidosis. Cutis, *19*:86, 1977.
20. Nathan, M. P. R., Pinsker, R., Chase, P. H., and Elguezabel, A.: Sarcoidosis presenting as lymphedema. Arch. Dermatol., *109*:543, 1974.
21. Shmunes, E., Lantis, L. R., and Hurley, H. J.: Verrucose sarcoidosis. Arch. Dermatol., *102*:665, 1970.
22. Scadding, J. G.: Sarcoidosis. Eyre and Spottiswoode. London, 1967, p. 55.
23. Siltzbach, L. E., and Greenberg, G. M.: Childhood sarcoidosis — a study of 18 patients. N. Engl. J. Med., *279*:1239, 1968.
24. Löfgren, S., and Stavenow, S.: Course and prognosis of sarcoidosis: Stockholm. Am. Rev. Resp. Dis., *84*(part 2):71, 1961.
25. Sulavik, S.: Personal communication.
26. James, D. G.: Course and prognosis of sarcoidosis: London. Am. Rev. Resp. Dis., *84*(part 2):66, 1961.
27. Sones, M., and Israel, H. L.: Course and prognosis of sarcoidosis: Philadelphia. Am. Rev. Resp. Dis., *84*(part 2):60, 1961.
28. Kantor, F. S., Dwyer, J. M., and Mangi, R. J.: Sarcoid. J. Invest. Dermatol., *67*:470, 1976.
29. Daniele, R. P., and Rowlands, D. T.: Antibodies to T cells in sarcoidosis. In Siltzbach, L. E. (ed.): Proceedings of the VII International Conference on Sarcoidosis. Ann. N.Y. Acad. Sci., *278*:88, 1976.
30. Israel, H. L.: Some controversial aspects of sarcoidosis. Ann. Allergy, *38*:112, 1977.
31. James, D. G., Neville, E., and Walker, A. N.: Immunology of sarcoidosis. Am. J. Med., *59*:388, 1975.
32. James, D. G., and Neville, E.: Pathobiology of sarcoidosis. Pathobiol. Annual, *7*:31, 1977.
33. Hedfors, E., and Norberg, R.: Evidence for circulating immune complexes in sarcoidosis. Clin. Exp. Immunol., *16*:493, 1974.
34. Vernier-Jones, J., Cumming, R. H., Asplin, C. M., Lazlo, G., and White, R. J.: Circulating immune complexes in erythema nodosum and early sarcoidosis. Lancet, *1*:153, 1976.
35. Studdy, P., Bird, R., and James, D. G.: Serum angiotensin-converting enzyme (SACE) in sarcoidosis and other granulomatous disorders. Lancet, *2*:1331, 1978.
36. Silverstein, E., Friedland, J., Kitt, M., and Lyons, H. A.: Increased serum angiotensin converting enzyme in sarcoidosis. Isr. J. Med. Sci., *13*:995, 1977.
37. Silverstein, E., Friedland, J., and Lyons, H. A.: Serum angiotensin converting enzyme in sarcoidosis: clinical significance. Isr. J. Med. Sci., *13*:1001, 1977.
38. Scadding, J. G.: Mycobacterium tuberculosis in the etiology of sarcoidosis. Br. Med. J., *2*:1617, 1960.
39. Scadding, J. G.: Sarcoidosis. *op. cit.*, p. 470.
40. Mankiewicz, E.: The relationship of sarcoidosis of anonymous bacteria. Acta Med. Scand., Suppl. *425*:68, 1964.
41. Mankiewicz, E., and Walbeck, M. Van: Mycobacteriophages: their role in tuberculosis and sarcoidosis. Arch. Environ. Health, *5*:122, 1962.
42. Mankiewicz, E., Kurti, V., and Adominis, H.: The effect of mycobacteriophage particles on cell mediated immune reactions. Can. J. Microbiol., *20*:1209, 1974.
43. Shelley, W. B., and Hurley, H. J.: The allergic origin of zirconium granulomas. Br. J. Dermatol., *70*:75, 1958.
44. Epstein, W. L.: Contribution to the pathogenesis of zirconium granulomas in man. J. Invest. Dermatol., *34*:183, 1960.
45. Philpott, J. A., Jr., Woodburne, A. R., Philpott, O. S., Schaefer, W. B., and Mollohan, C. S.: Swimming pool granuloma: a study of 290 cases. Arch. Dermatol., *88*:158, 1963.

11

Blood Vessels

The circulatory system provides important clues to the presence of systemic disease. Some of them are among the first signs taught to medical students who are beginning to learn the principles of physical examination. These signs include the pallor of anemia; the plethora of polycythemia; the cherry red color of carbon monoxide poisoning; the cyanosis of cardiopulmonary disorders; erythema produced by fever, drug reactions, and histamine release in mastocytosis; the cyanotic suffusion of the head and neck in the superior vena caval syndrome; and the vasopastic signs of Raynaud's phenomenon.

These changes are well known and need not be discussed further. Instead, this chapter is concerned with focal derangements of blood vessels — telangiectasia, vascular malformations, and neoplastic vascular disorders — and how they serve as markers of systemic disease.

TELANGIECTASIA

Telangiectasia consists of dilated venules, capillaries, or arterioles in the skin; they vary in appearance from fine wires to heavy cords of 0.5 mm in diameter. Although such vascular changes can usually be detected without magnification, a hand lens is sometimes required.

Dilated blood vessels in the skin usually are considered a cosmetic problem and of no medical significance. One purpose of this chapter is to discuss the varieties and features of the most common types of telangiectasia and to distinguish them from the telangiectatic syndromes indicating systemic disease. If the distribution and morphology of telangiectasia were observed as carefully as those of other lesions, such as erythema nodosum and secondary syphilis, the telangiectatic syndromes associated with systemic disease would be easily recognized.

Perhaps the most common example of telangiectasia is that found in actinically damaged skin. The affected individual is often of Anglo-Saxon origin, has blue eyes, freckles, and does not tan well. Mottled hyperpigmentation and ruddiness appear on the face, the V of the neck and chest, and other exposed parts after many years of exposure to sunlight. Fine and coarse telangiectatic vessels, scattered randomly like separate twigs in the sun-damaged skin, contribute to the ruddy complexion.

In rosacea, broad elongated bluish venules traverse the cheeks and nose over a background of erythema and pustules. The telangiectasia of rosacea is distinct from that of actinically damaged skin and resembles the facial vascular changes found in hypercorticism and polycythemia vera.

In fact, polycythemia vera with facial rubor and telangiectasia is often misdiagnosed as acne rosacea. Chronic flushing in the carcinoid syndrome produces identical changes (Plate 2*B*).

The hallmarks of radiodermatitis are short coarse telangiectatic vessels developing in atrophic hyperpigmented and hypopigmented skin. Without telangiectasia, a diagnosis of radiodermatitis cannot be made.

The spider angioma is the best known type of telangiectasia. It consists of a central pulsating punctum, often slightly elevated, with symmetrically radiating legs (Figs. 11–1 and 11–2; Plate 28*A–C*). When the central point is compressed, the legs disappear. In its earliest stage, the spider is merely a tiny red spot with a pale halo. The surrounding pallor probably is due to the shift of blood from the periphery to the center, because when the punctum is compressed, the skin returns to its normal pink color, and when central pressure is released and the punctum re-forms, the ring of pallor reappears. In its most highly developed state, when the arterioles feeding the center proliferate and produce an elevated mass, the spider angioma looks like a strawberry hemangioma and can measure up to 2 cm in diameter.

Spiders develop most frequently on the face, trunk, arms, hands, and fingers and rarely below the umbilicus. Although spiders are associated most commonly with cirrhosis and pregnancy, they occur idiopathically in children and young adults. Some patients with metastatic carcinoma of the liver may show the cutaneous signs associated with cirrhosis, including spider angiomas.

In two thirds of the patients with connective tissue disease, specific patterns of telangiectasia develop. These patterns have the same diagnos-

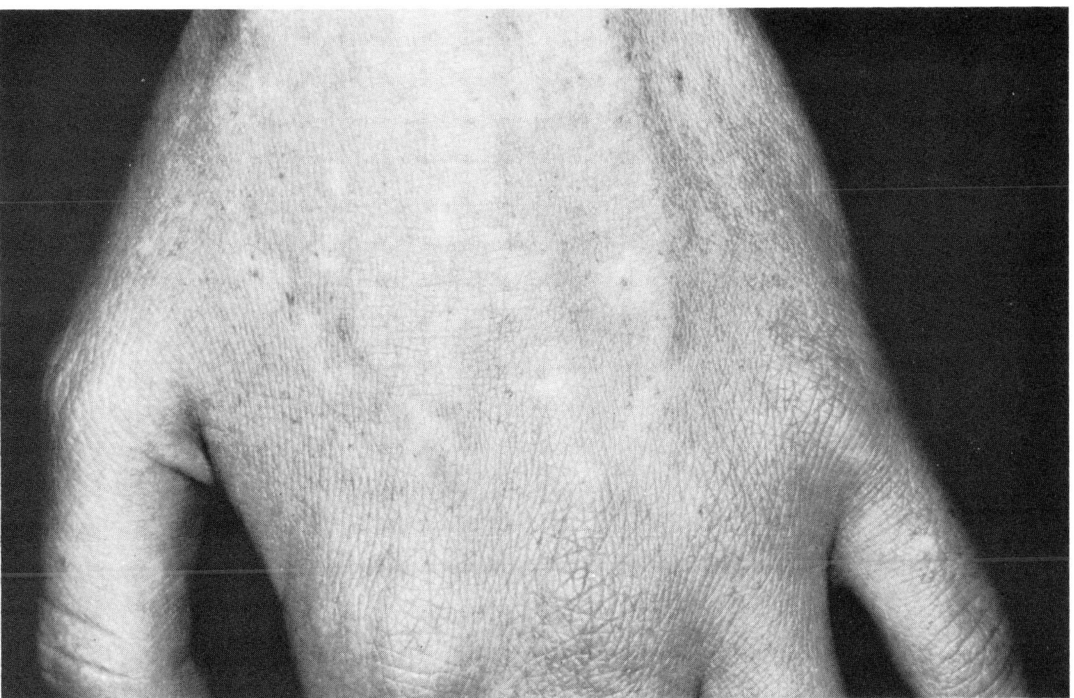

Figure 11–1. Spider angioma. Earliest stage with pale halo around central feeding vessel.

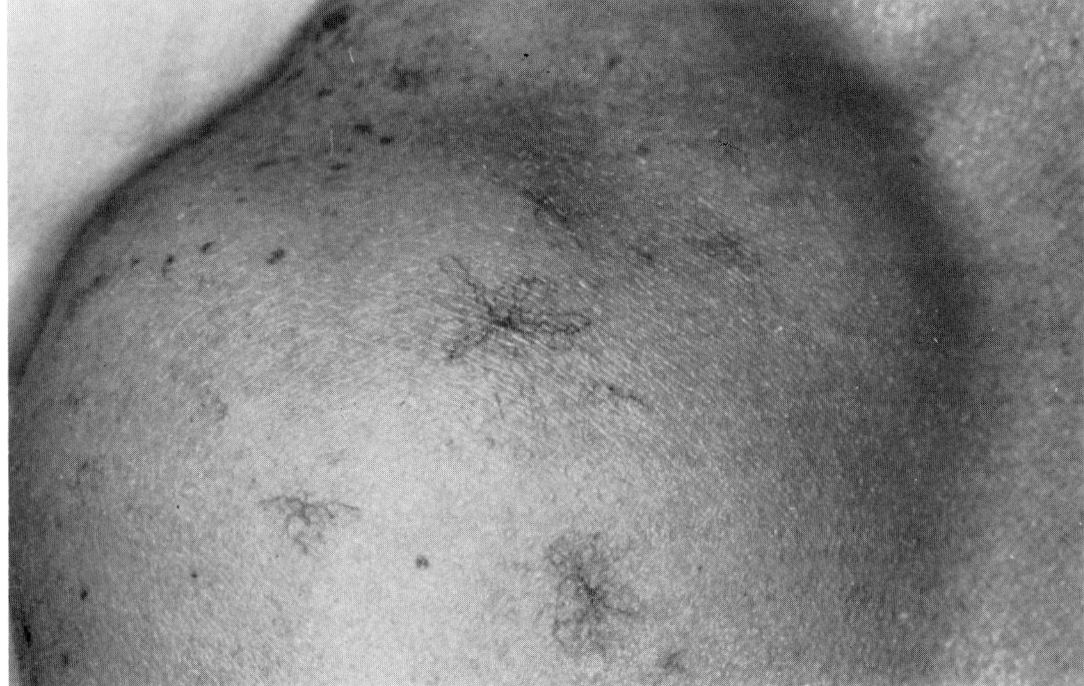

Figure 11–2. Spider angioma. More advanced stage with central feeder and radiating legs.

tic significance as the other cutaneous signs of these kinds of disorders, and at times they are the only cutaneous stigmata.

A pathognomonic sign of connective tissue disease, such as lupus erythematosus, dermatomyositis, and scleroderma, is cuticular telangiectasia (Plate 18*C*). Linear wiry vessels that are perpendicular to the base of the nail overlie the posterior nailfold. They are usually bright red, but they appear black if thrombosed. In lupus erythematosus and dermatomyositis there is usually an associated periungual erythema, but in scleroderma the dilated vessels develop on normally colored skin. Although these dilated vessels have been studied extensively by capillary microscopy, neither their easy detection with the naked eye nor their clinical significance has been sufficiently emphasized. Cuticular telangiectasia occurs in at least two thirds of the patients with one of the three connective tissue diseases, in 5 per cent of the patients with rheumatoid arthritis,[1] and in an occasional patient with leukocytoclastic angiitis. Only twice have I found such lesions in a healthy person without evidence of an underlying disorder.

Large numbers of telangiectatic vessels may develop on the periungual tissue of every nail, or only a few may appear at the base of one or two nails; however, the significance is the same. This sign is particularly helpful in diagnosing connective tissue diseases in their early phases before the other diagnostic features of lupus erythematosus, dermatomyositis, and scleroderma develop.

Palmar-digital telangiectasia is a pattern seen almost exclusively in lupus erythematosus (Plate 18*D*). Red to violaceous, discrete, elevated, oval spots appear on the palms and palmar aspects of the fingers. They are distinguished from the palmar erythema of pregnancy and cirrhosis by

PLATE 28

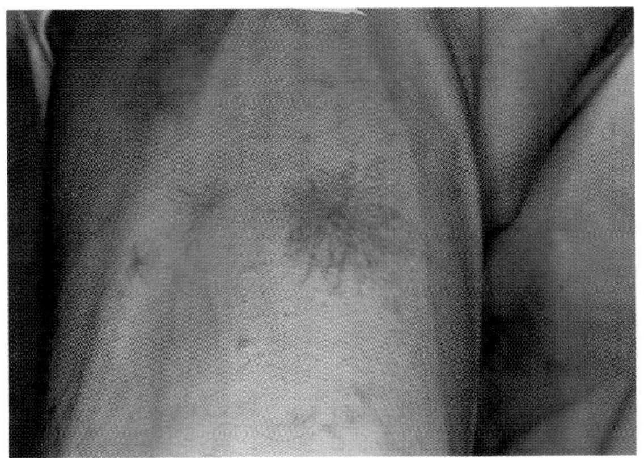

A, Spider angioma.

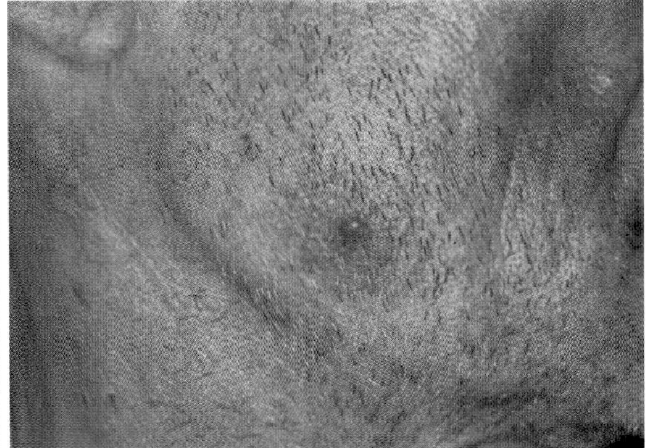

B, Spider angioma. Central feeder has enlarged considerably.

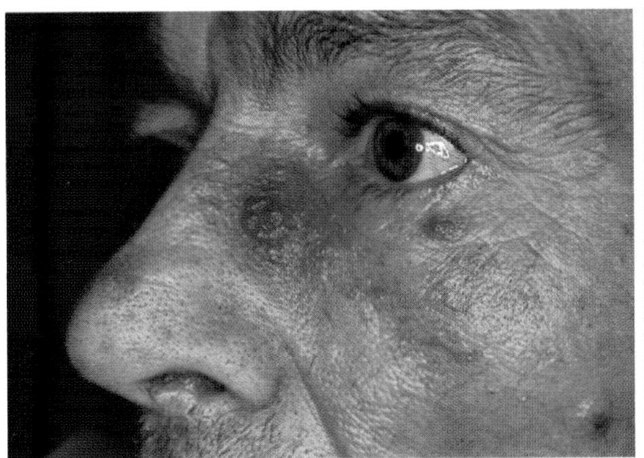

C, Spider angioma has developed into a large hemangiomatous lesion.

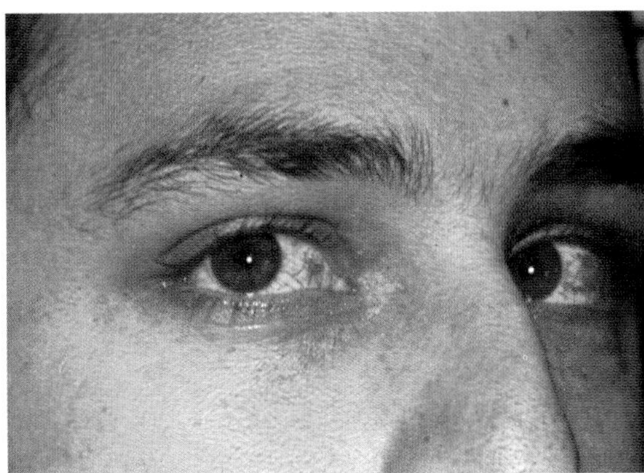

D, Ataxia-telangiectasia. Scleral telangiectases. (Courtesy of Dr. Byron Waksman.)

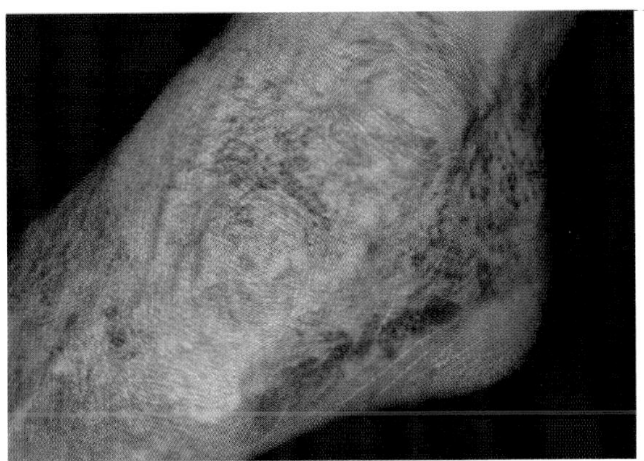

E, Essential telangiectasia. Venous stars.

F, Essential telangiectasia. Fine wiry closely-packed telangiectases on the thigh of one of our patients.

their discreteness, elevation, and extension onto the fingers all the way to the fingertips. The individual lesion blanches easily. This sign is not common and has been described only in lupus erythematosus. We have not seen such lesions in dermatomyositis and scleroderma.

Violaceous flat-topped papules develop over the dorsal interphalangeal joints in about one third of the patients with dermatomyositis. The papules evolve into atrophic hypopigmented macules; and the fine wiry telangiectasia, which may have been difficult to see in the papules, becomes obvious. These early and late lesions, designated Gottron's sign, are pathognomonic of dermatomyositis (Fig. 7–46; Plate 20*B*).

In scleroderma, two other kinds of telangiectasia are found in at least 50 per cent of the patients. The most common is a pink-to-red well-marginated macule that ranges in size from 1 to 6 mm and occurs most often on the face, palms, and dorsa of the hands (Plate 21). These lesions can also be found on the lips, tongue, palate, and buccal mucosa. The distinctive feature of these spots is their square, rectangular, polyangular, oval, or arciform shape. They may look like flattened cherry angiomas. Closely packed fine vessels can sometimes be seen in these macules. These vascular macules are called telangiectatic mats.

This pattern of telangiectasia is seen almost exclusively in scleroderma. However, I have seen them in one case of sclerodermatomyositis, and only on the fingertips in two patients with systemic LE.

The second type of telangiectasia, which is found less often in scleroderma, is indistinguishable from the lesions of hereditary hemorrhagic telangiectasia (Rendu-Osler-Weber disease) in both its appearance and its distribution. This less common variety of vascular ectasia is also a salient feature of the CRST syndrome (see p. 335). However, most of the reported patients with this latter entity, as well as those I have examined at clinical dermatologic meetings, have had telangiectatic mats rather than the lesions of Rendu-Osler-Weber disease. I have found telangiectasia that is indistinguishable from that observed in Osler's disease in only 2 of 20 patients with the CRST syndrome.

Both of these varieties of telangiectasia may be the only cutaneous signs of scleroderma. We have seen patients with extensive sclerotic involvement of the gastrointestinal tract and lungs in whom these telangiectases were the only cutaneous abnormalities.

The development of Raynaud's phenomenon always raises the possibility of an underlying connective tissue disease. If patients with Raynaud's syndrome are examined carefully, many will be found to have cuticular telangiectasia, polyangular telangiectatic mats, or hereditary telangiectasia-like lesions, all of which indicate the presence of scleroderma.

The telangiectasia of scleroderma usually arises in skin that is clinically and histologically normal. The relationship between the vascular abnormalities and the other pathologic findings in systemic sclerosis is not understood. However, an hypothesis attempting to integrate the pathologic findings in scleroderma, including telangiectasia, has been presented earlier in this book (see p. 357).

In Rendu-Osler-Weber disease, the vascular lesions develop primarily on the lips, nasal mucosa, tongue, palms, and palate; but they also can be found under the nails (Fig. 11–3), on the soles of the feet, and even on the tympanic membrane. The true lesion of Osler's disease tends to be

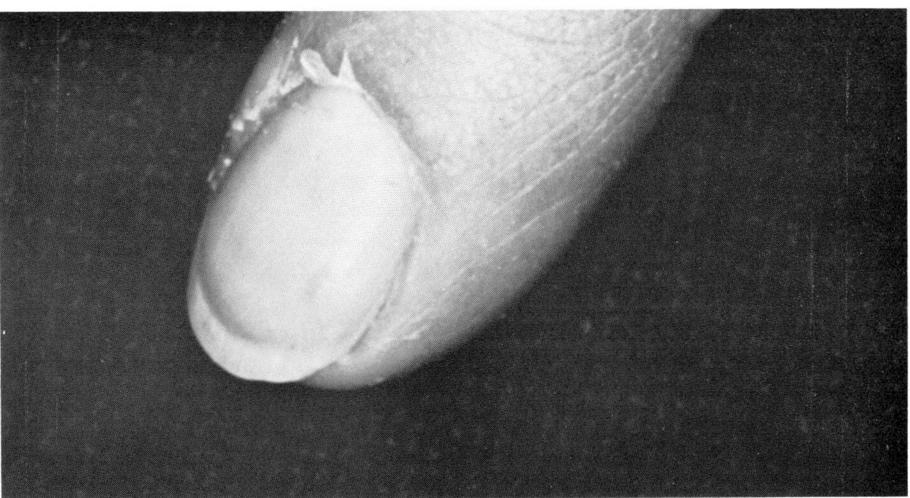

Figure 11–3. Rendu-Osler-Weber disease. Telangiectasis under fingernail.

slightly elevated with an ill-defined border and one or more legs radiating from an eccentrically placed punctum (Plate 29; Fig. 11–4). This is easily demonstrated by stretching the lip. The color is usually dark red, resembling a ruby. Although some lesions in Osler's disease can be flat with sharp borders, the majority conform to the above description. Stress is placed on these fine distinctions between the telangiectases of scleroderma and those of Osler's disease because of their extremely important diagnostic significance. When the red telangiectatic mat of scleroderma is stretched, it becomes fainter and pink; radiating legs are not present.

Melena and epistaxes are the most frequent complications of Rendu-Osler-Weber disease because of telangiectasia in the gastrointestinal tract and nasal mucosa. If the patient is very anemic, the cutaneous telangiectasia will be invisible. With adequate blood replacement the dilated vessels will be refilled, and the diagnosis of Rendu-Osler-Weber disease can be made.

Arteriovenous fistulae may develop in the lung and produce coin lesions on chest radiographs. Clubbing, cyanosis, and polycythemia can be associated with extensive fistula formation; and these features may be the major manifestations of Osler's disease in an individual.[2] Less frequently, one may encounter arteriovenous fistulae in the splenic, intracerebral, retinal, and mesenteric arteries. Vascular malformations may be present in the colon and stomach. Aortic aneurysms are a rare development. In the liver, the vascular malformations are surrounded by broad fibrous septa, a picture which has been interpreted as an unusual form of cirrhosis by some investigators.[3]

Conlon et al. described two families in whom hereditary telangiectasia and von Willebrand's disease coexisted.[4] In one family, the bleeding was nasal and oral, while in the other, it was both nasal and gastrointestinal. The authors cite three individuals in two other families who may have had the same combination. These studies suggest that persons with von Willebrand's disease who have recurrent bleeding, especially from the gastrointestinal tract, ought to be examined for the presence of telangiectases.

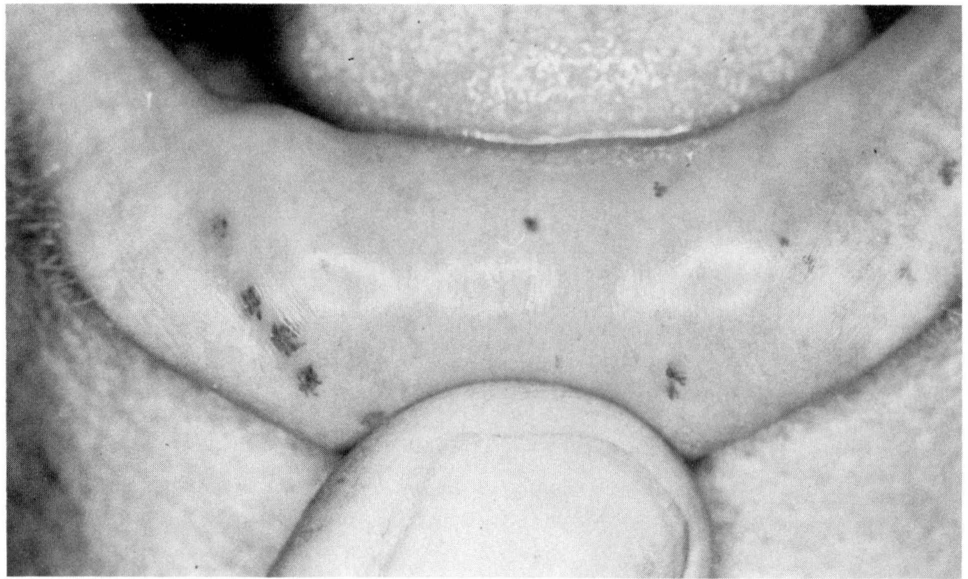

Figure 11–4. Rendu-Osler-Weber disease. Stretching lips demonstrates branching vessels in telangiectases.

Osler's disease is inherited as an autosomal dominant, and the telangiectasia appears during the second and third decades.[5]

Telangiectasia is also the diagnostic cutaneous sign of the Louis-Bar syndrome, or ataxia-telangiectasia, which appears as cerebellar ataxia in children shortly after they begin to walk. Sinopulmonary infections are frequent, immunoglobulin synthesis is impaired, and many of the patients develop malignant lymphomas if they survive into their late teens and early twenties. The diagnosis can be established at about 3 years of age when telangiectasia appears. Fine wiry elongated vessels course over the pinnae and bulbar conjunctivae, and short stubby vessels appear in the antecubital and popliteal spaces and on the sides of the neck (Figs. 11–5 and 11–6; Plate 28*D*). Such vascular lesions can also appear on the butterfly area of the face and on the palate.[6]

In addition to being a diagnostic sign of systemic diseases, telangiectasia is also an important component of several other disorders. Basal cell tumors are very common and can be diagnosed early if one looks for the characteristic telangiectasis (Fig. 11–7). Basal cell tumors are translucent papules or nodules that tend to expand with an elevated pearly border, meanwhile leaving behind a necrotic center. Many fine wiry vessels can be found on the raised margin. In its earliest stage, when the tumor is no more than 1 to 2 mm in diameter, a wiry vessel running from the base to the apex can almost always be found. Such telangiectasia is not a feature of epidermoid cancer.

Degos' disease, malignant atrophic papulosis, is a rare disorder in which the vascular lumina undergo gradual obliteration. When the dermal vessels are affected, a wedged-shaped area of acellular homogeneous-appearing collagen with an overlying atrophic epidermis results. Involvement of other organs, such as the gastrointestinal tract, brain, and eye, results in analogous tissue changes so that the gross appearance of the lesion is remarkably similar to that seen in the skin.[7] Clinically the lesions are discrete porcelain-white spots with wiry telangiectases palisading on

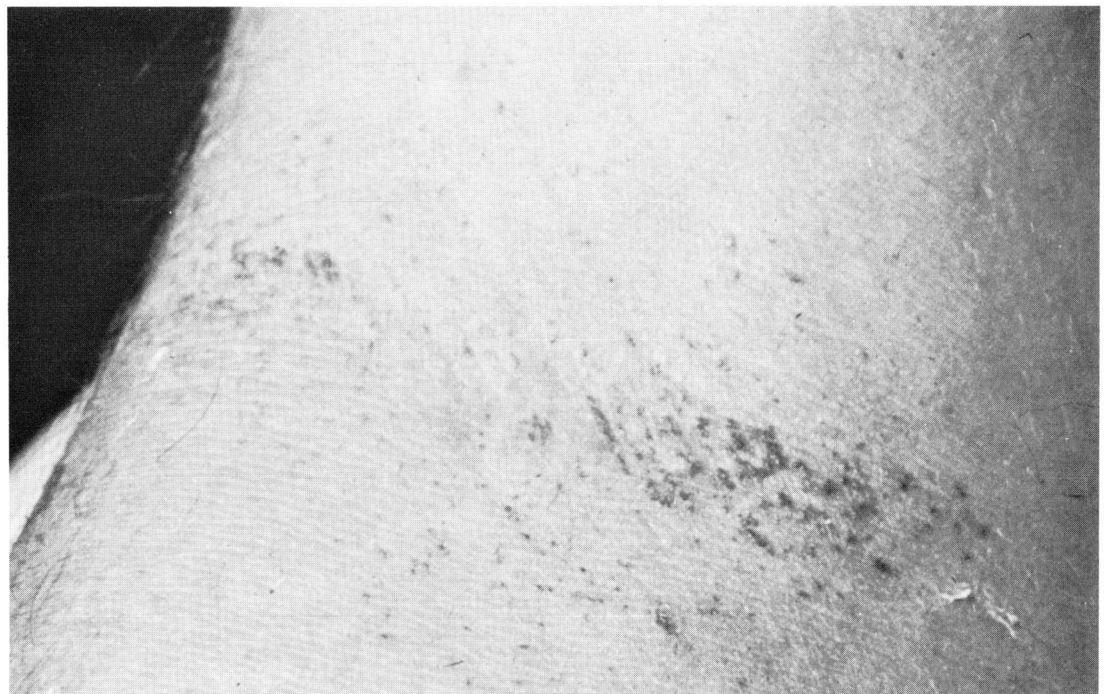

Figure 11–5. Ataxia-telangiectasia. Telangiectases in cubital space. (Courtesy of Dr. William Epstein.)

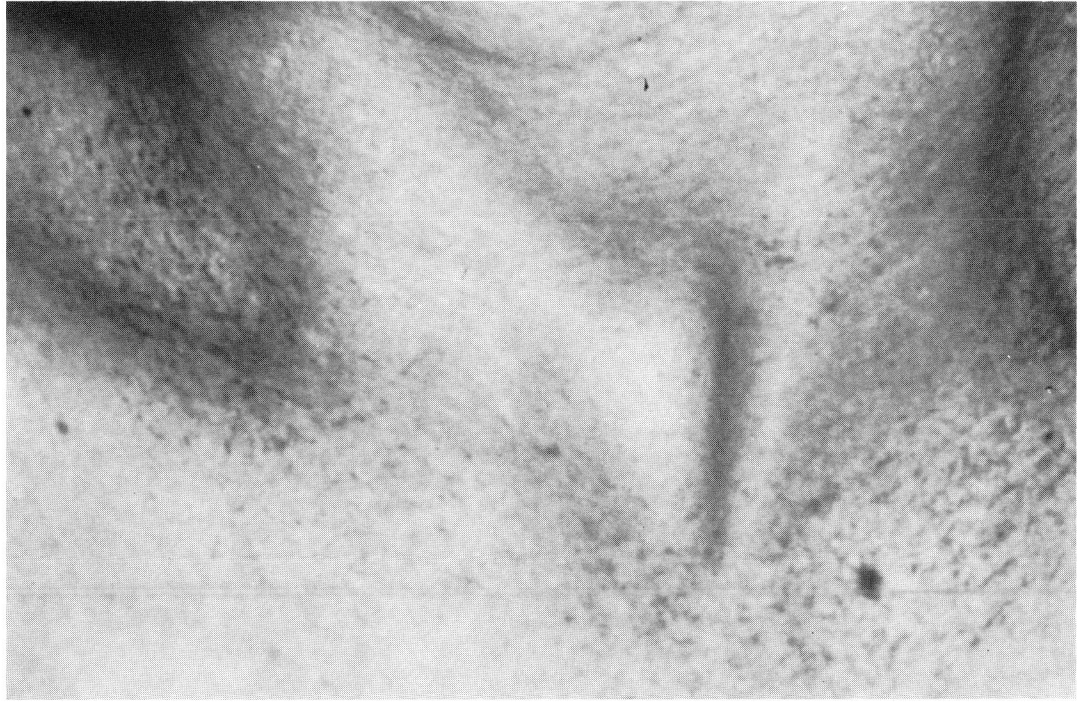

Figure 11–6. Ataxia-telangiectasia. Telangiectases on upper chest and neck. (Courtesy of Dr. Byron Waksman.)

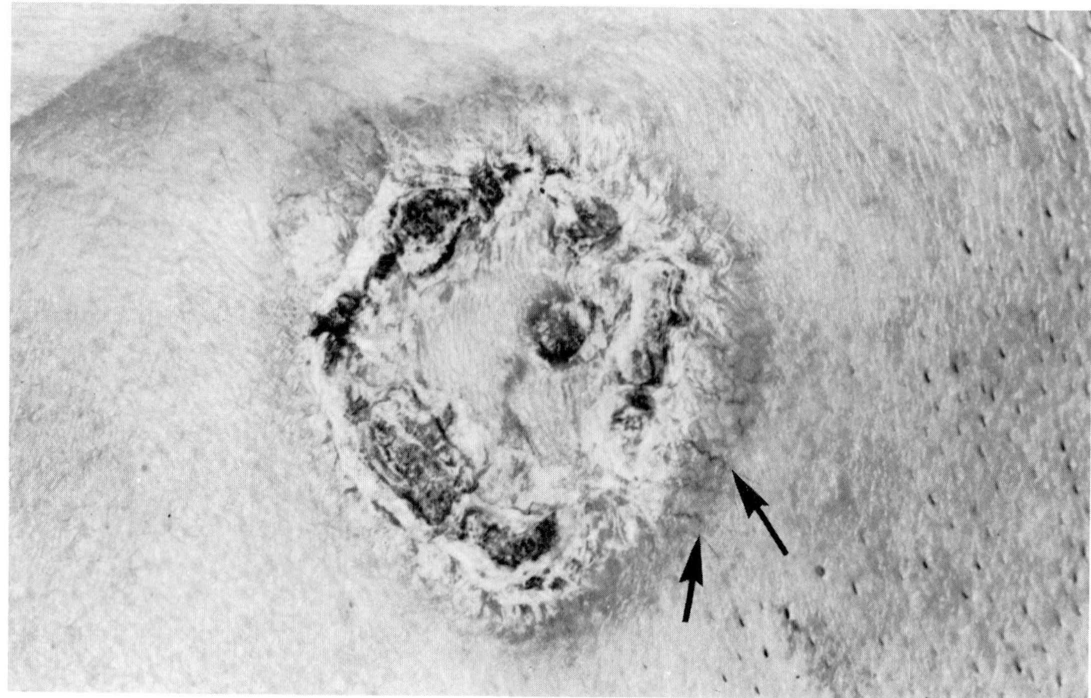

Figure 11–7. Basal cell tumor with characteristic telangiectasia (arrows) on rolled border.

the periphery. Identical lesions are found in the cerebral cortex, sclerae, and gastrointestinal tract. Post-traumatic scarring does not mimic this unique lesion. The most common cause of death in Degos' disease is intestinal perforation through the atrophic spots and attendant secondary peritonitis.

In sarcoidosis and the malignant lymphomas, red and purplish plaques and tumors may have large dilated venules running over their surfaces. This telangiectasia, made up of large vessels, differs strikingly from the fine short telangiectases found in the skin lesions of lupus erythematosus.

The term *poikiloderma* is applied to skin affected with mottled hyperpigmentation and hypopigmentation, atrophy, and fine telangiectases that impart an over-all erythematous color to the affected area. Poikilodermatous change is found most often on the light-exposed areas of the body during the chronic phases of dermatomyositis and lupus erythematosus.

In poikiloderma vasculare atrophicans, the erythema is replaced by a red-brown color, and the lesions develop as large patches over the lower back, buttocks, and thighs. It is a precursor of mycosis fungoides (see p. 139).

In xeroderma pigmentosum the skin rapidly deteriorates on exposure to sunlight, simulating generalized radiodermatitis. By three or four years of age, the patients have multiple skin cancers: epidermoid and basal cell tumors and melanomas.

Telangiectasia is the striking feature of necrobiosis lipoidica, which is usually a sign of diabetes mellitus or the prediabetic state.

Not all widespread telangiectasia indicates systemic disease. Gener-

PLATE 29

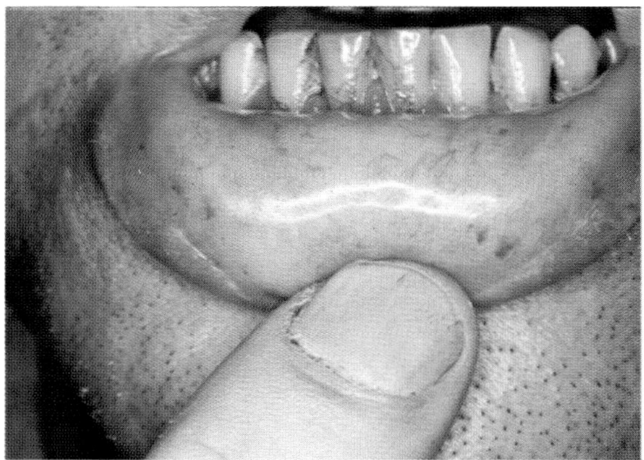

A, Rendu-Osler-Weber disease. Eccentrically placed punctum with radiating legs is the characteristic feature of the telangiectases in this disease.

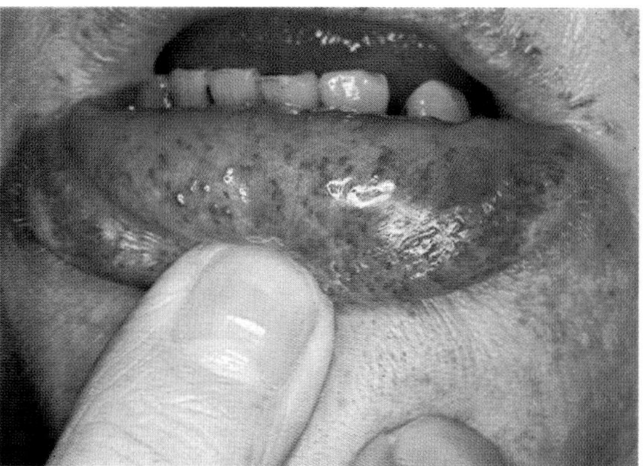

B, Telangiectasia in Rendu-Osler-Weber disease.

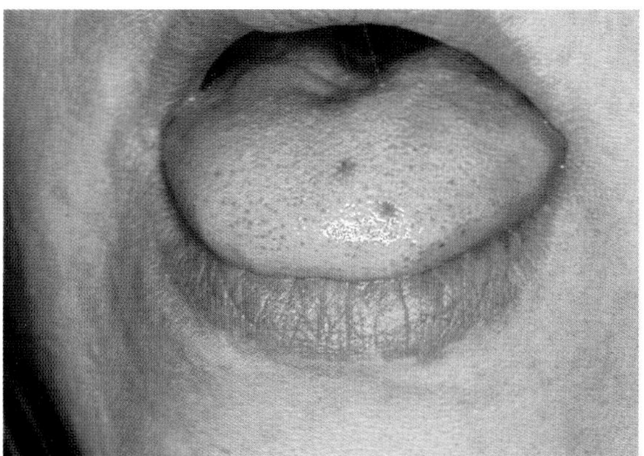

C, Telangiectasia on the tongue in Rendu-Osler-Weber disease.

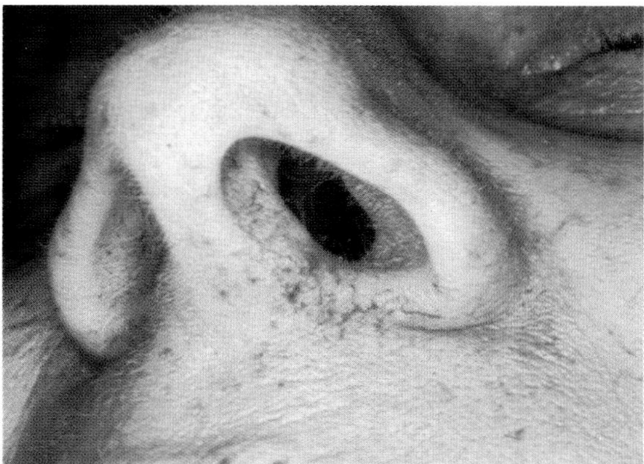

D, Telangiectasia in Rendu-Osler-Weber disease.

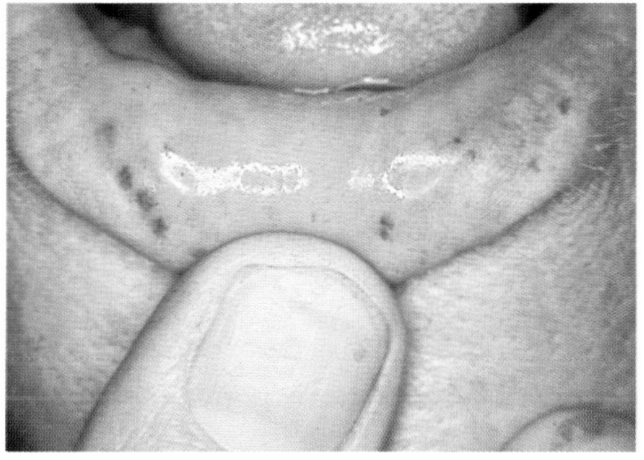

E, Telangiectasia in Rendu-Osler-Weber disease. Stretching the lip reveals the eccentric punctum with radiating legs.

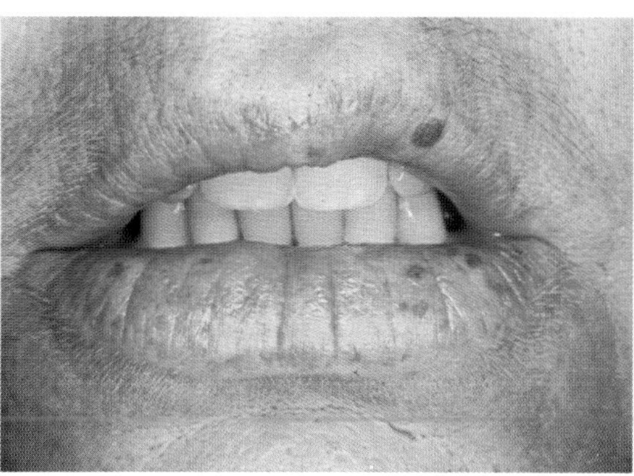

F, Scleroderma (CRST syndrome). Telangiectasis is a polyangular mat without a punctum and radiating legs.

PLATE 30

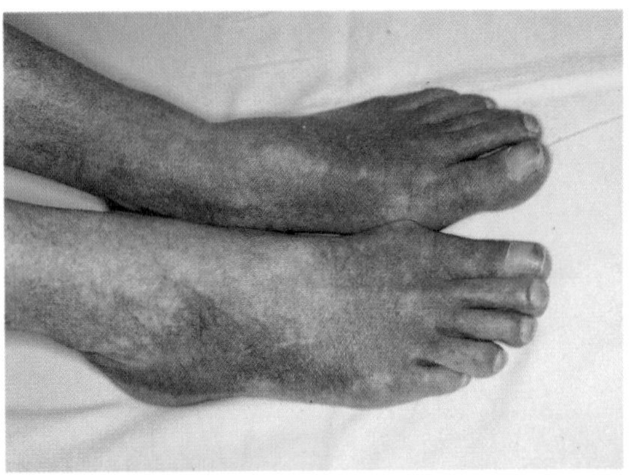

A, Generalized essential telangiectasia. Fine wiry telangiectatic vessels produces purplish color of feet.

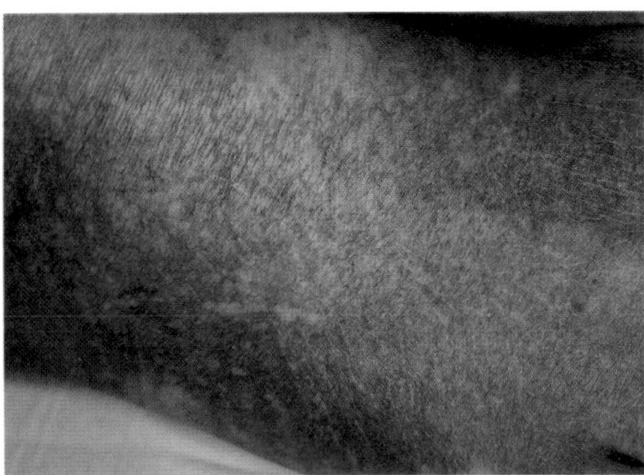

B, Close-up of fine wiry telangiectasia in *A*.

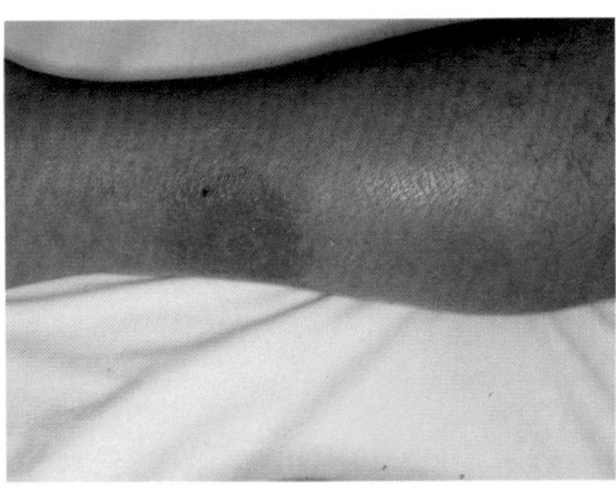

C, Pretibial myxedema. The skin of the posterior and lateral calf is erythematous and warm, mimicking cellulitis. The more intensely inflamed area above the ankle is a contact dermatitis.

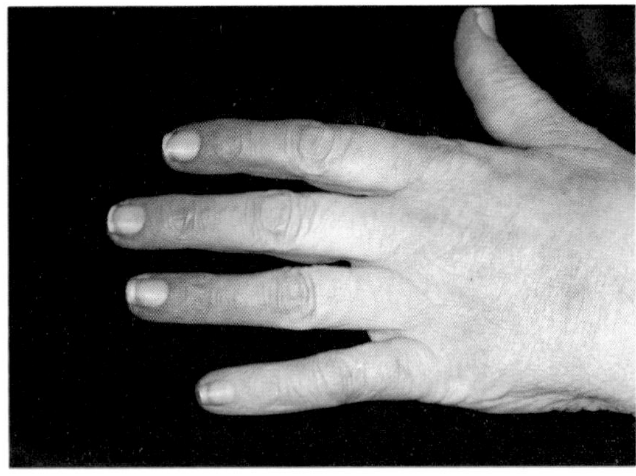

D, Cyanosis of finger tips as a result of decreased perfusion from vascular calcification. The calcification was produced by secondary hyperparathyroidism of chronic renal disease.

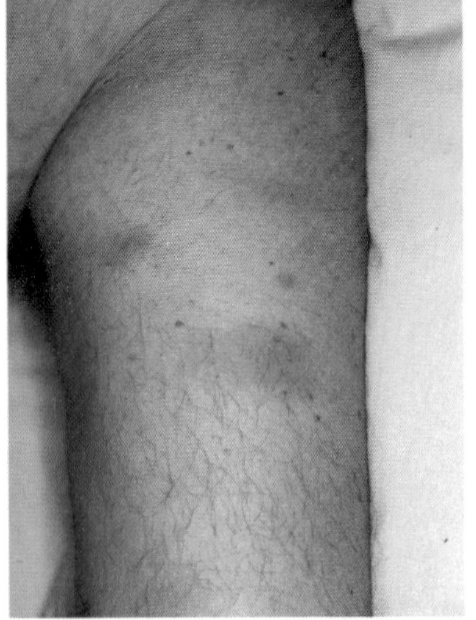

E, Sweet's syndrome. Erythematous plaques and pustules on upper arm.

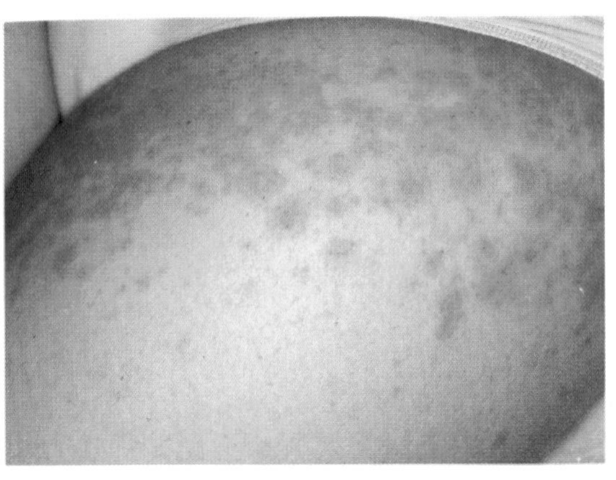

F, Pruritic urticarial papules and plaques of pregnancy (PUPPP syndrome). Erythematous papules on the thigh, some with more intensely red centers, simulating the lesions of erythema multiforme.

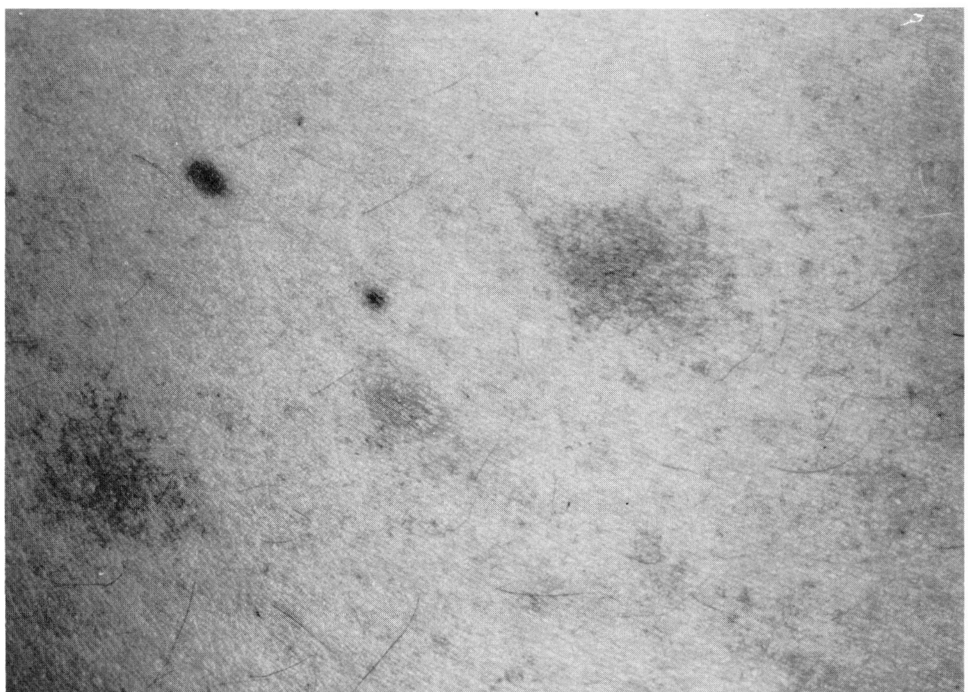

Figure 11–8. Generalized essential telangiectasia. Clusters of wiry vessels forming fairly discrete patches.

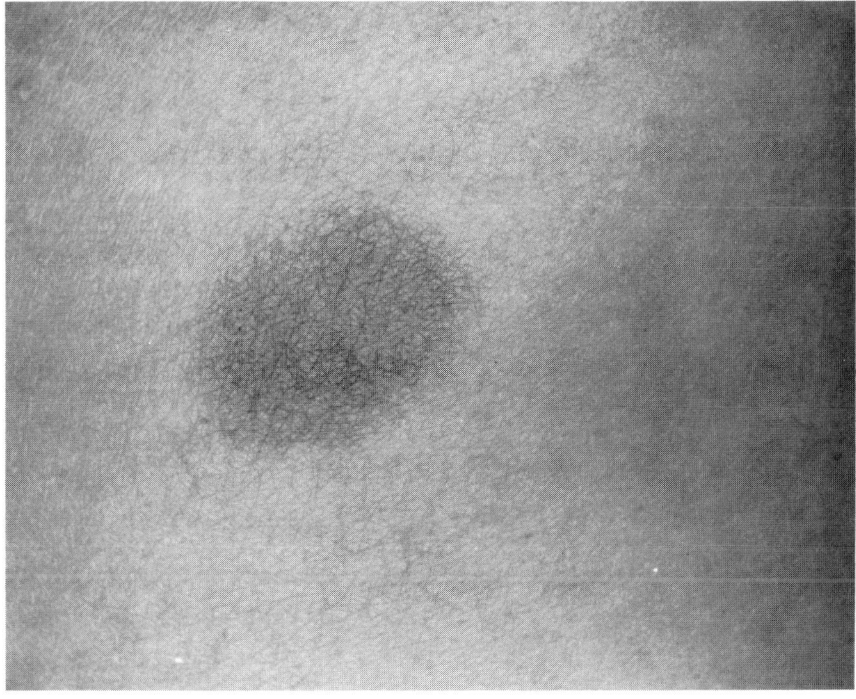

Figure 11–9. Generalized essential telangiectasia. Telangiectases may form large oval lesions.

alized essential telangiectasia is a spectacular but benign cutaneous entity that develops most commonly in women in the fourth and fifth decades. In some instances this telangiectasia is familial. The disorder begins on the legs and slowly spreads to involve the thighs, lower abdomen, and occasionally the arms. Three varieites of telangiectases are present: large venous stars consisting of superficial varicosities on the lower legs; bright red blotchy erythema produced by many wiry vessels on the feet, legs, and thighs; and a few discrete red macules measuring 0.5 to 1.0 cm on the thighs, lower abdomen, or arm (Plates 28*E*, *F* and 30*A*, *B*; Figs. 11–8 and 11–9). Spontaneous regression is rare, but it developed in one of our patients after the disorder had been present for four to five years. Although this syndrome presents a serious cosmetic problem for some patients, it is not a manifestation of an underlying systemic disorder.[8]

Spider angiomas, as well as clusters of dilated vessels, can appear in a segmental distribution shortly after birth or in early childhood. They are uncommon, not associated with systemic involvement, and represent a vascular birthmark.

The morphologic and distributional patterns of the telangiectases are many, but careful examination allows one to separate the banal from the significant. In the process, systemic disease can be uncovered.

HAMARTOMAS AND HEMANGIOMAS

By tradition, benign vascular tumors of any size are called hemangiomas, whereas malignant varieties are termed angiosarcomas. The vast majority of vascular tumors encountered in medical practice, however, have a benign cytology and clinical course and should be referred to as hamartomas, that is, developmental rather than neoplastic tumors. Although these vascular malformations arise most commonly in children, they also develop in adults. Lymphatic vascular elements participate in variable degrees in the formation of these hamartomas.

Vascular tumors are common, but fortunately they ordinarily do not present serious problems from the medical viewpoint. In this section the vascular tumors of diagnostic import, as well as those of lesser significance, will be discussed.

Common Trivial Lesions

Cherry angiomas, venous lakes, and caviar spots are banal vascular lesions of cosmetic significance only.

The cherry angiomas (de Morgan's spot) is a ruby-red papule that arises primarily on the trunk (Fig. 11–10). Originating as pinpoint red marks, they increase in size and number with age. Some spots may be 4 mm in diameter. The cherry angiomas do not blanch with pressure, and histologically they are composed of increased numbers of dilated capillaries.

Venous lakes develop most frequently on exposed areas: the ears, face, lips, and less often on the neck and other parts of the body (Plate 31*A*). These vascular marks are dark blue. Some resemble blood blisters, and others appear to be focal collections of superficial dilated veins.

Caviar spots arise on the undersurface of the tongue as spherical

PLATE 31

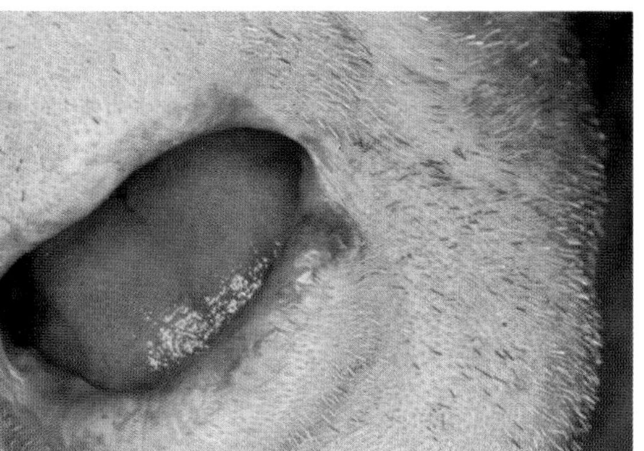

A, Venous lake.

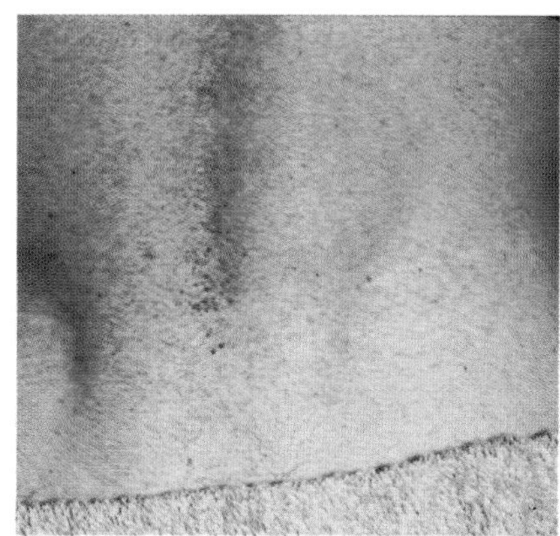

B, Angiokeratomas of Fabry's disease. (Courtesy of Dr. Andrew Simone.)

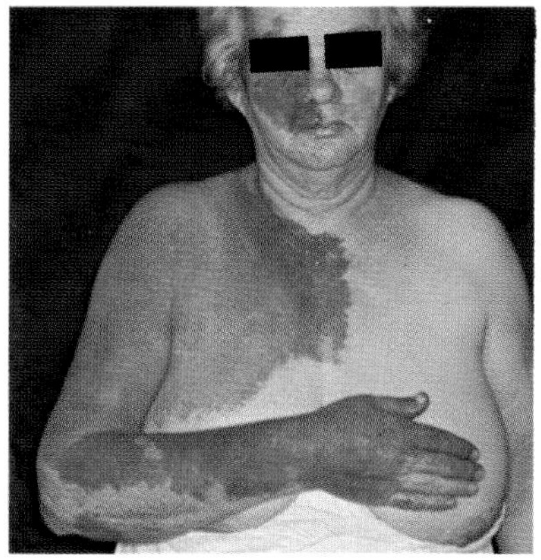

C, Port-wine stain (nevus flammeus).

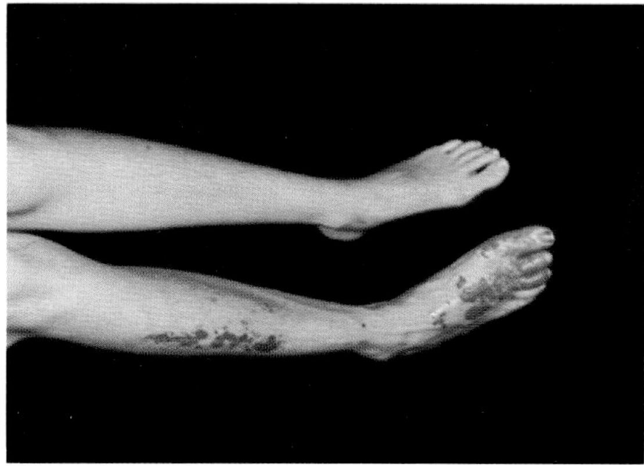

D, Klippel-Trenaunay-Parkes-Weber syndrome. Hypertrophy of tissue affected by diffuse hemangiomatosis.

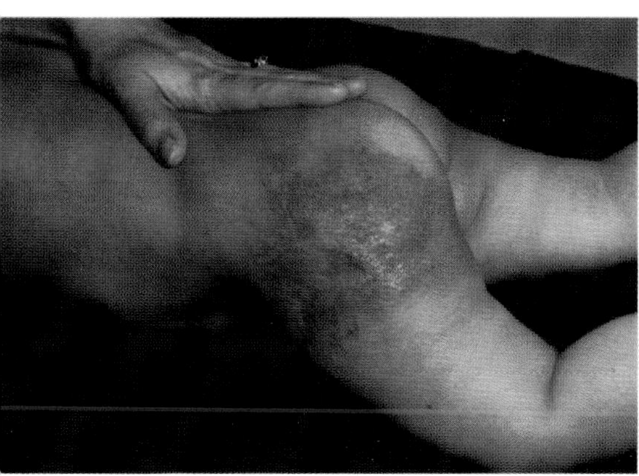

E, Cavernous hemangioma associated with thrombocytopenia.

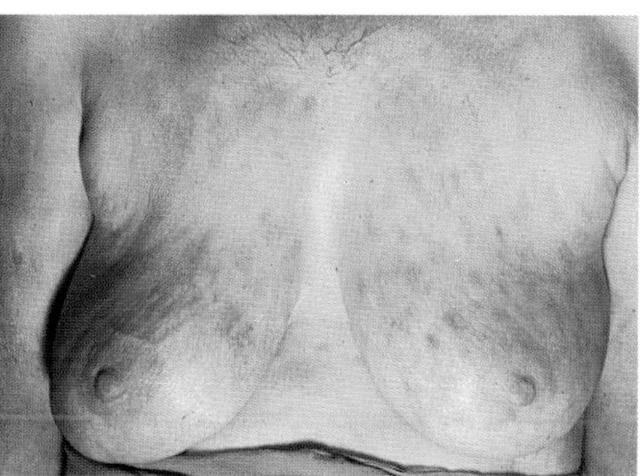

F, Malignant endotheliomatosis. Bluish patches were slightly infiltrated. Fine tortuous vessels were present on the surface. (From Arch. Dermatol., *84*:22, 1961. Case of Braverman and Lerner.)

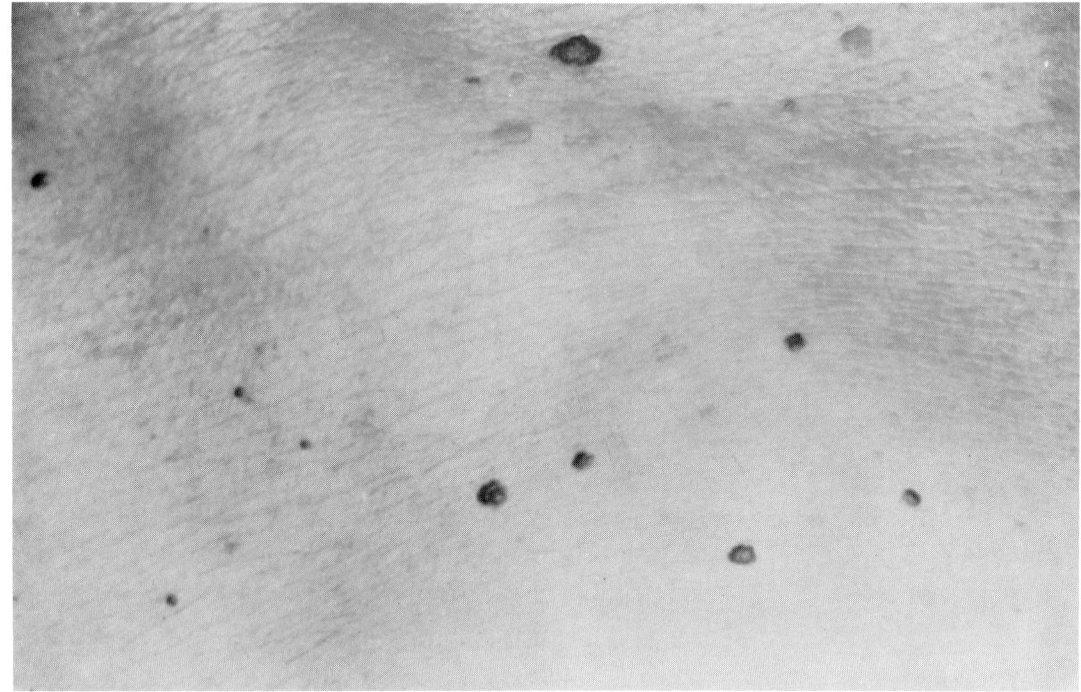

Figure 11–10. Cherry angiomas.

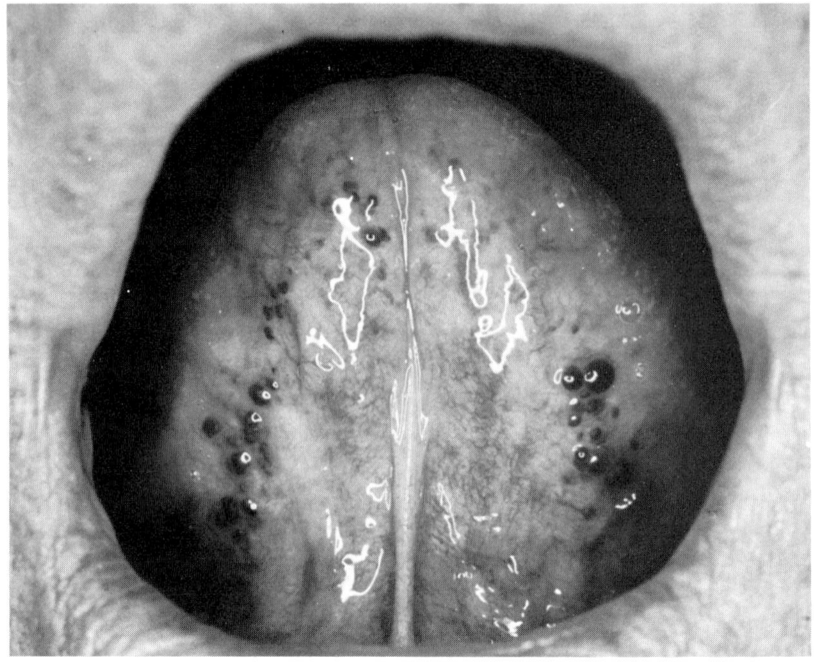

Figure 11–11. Caviar spots. Varicose lingual veins.

varicose enlargements along the collecting lingual veins (Fig. 11–11). Their appearance has been likened to buckshot. Twenty per cent of persons over age 40 have caviar spots, and by age 80, the incidence is 70 per cent.[9]

Spontaneous bleeding is not a feature of any of these three vascular marks.

Lesions and Syndromes of Indeterminate Significance

Miller and Akers reported the fourth case of an individual suffering from melena as a result of multiple phlebectasias of the jejunum associated with caviar spots and scrotal angiokeratomas (Fordyce lesions). Since caviar spots and Fordyce lesions are common, it is difficult to be sure whether or not this association was fortuitous.[10]

On the other hand, Guis et al. described three kinds of vascular lesions that were statistically associated with the presence of peptic ulcer: the microcherry mark, which is a circumscribed red spot less than 1 mm in size; the glomerulus-like lesion, composed of several convoluted vessels that could be as large as 2 mm; and venous lakes. The three types of lesions were found most often on the inner surface of the lower lip and on the vermilion border of the upper lip. All three occurred in greater numbers and at an earlier age in individuals with peptic ulcer disease than in those without ulcers.[11] The significance of this association is not understood.

Significant Vascular Tumors

Angiokeratoma. Angiokeratoma is a horny vascular papule, black or blue in color and no larger than 4 to 5 mm in diameter. Histologically it is composed of markedly dilated vessels within the dermal papillae. Sometimes the vessels appear to be surrounded by the epidermis. The amount of scale present on the surface of the papule varies from one keratoma to another, being absent in some and prominent in others.[12]

Three forms of angiokeratomas are recognized. The first two represent cosmetic problems only. The Mibelli variety arises primarily on the dorsa of the hands and feet, including the fingers and toes; but other exposed parts of the body may also be involved. Lesions occur singly or in clusters (Fig. 11–12). The Fordyce type is found principally on the scrotum in older men (Fig. 11–13). When traumatized, the angiokeratomas bleed readily.

The angiokeratoma of importance is that occurring in Fabry's disease (angiokeratoma corporis diffusum).[13] These spots vary greatly in size and color from pinpoint flat black spots without scale to bluish-black papules that have a fine scale and measure up to 3 and 4 mm. These spots are concentrated between the umbilicus and knees and may number in the thousands (Fig. 11–14 and 11–15; Plate 31*B*). The lesions tend to cluster, and they vary in size within each group. The lower back, buttocks, scrotum, and penis are the sites of predilection. The angiokeratomas also aggregate about the elbows and on the lips, buccal mucosa, uvula, and palate. Grouping around the nails is also characteristic. The only areas spared seem to be the face, scalp, and ears. Because angiokeratomas vary in size, the afflicted patient has been said to resemble an individual

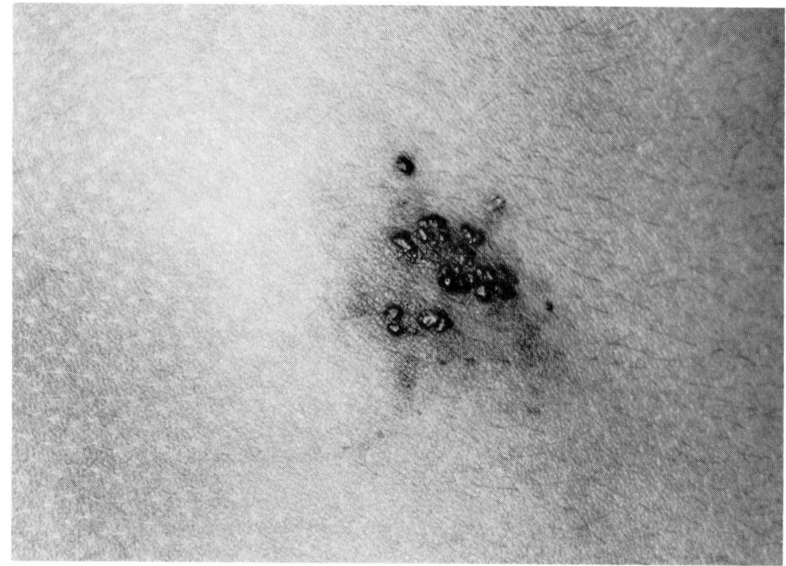

Figure 11–12. Angiokeratoma of Mibelli on back of 12-year-old boy.

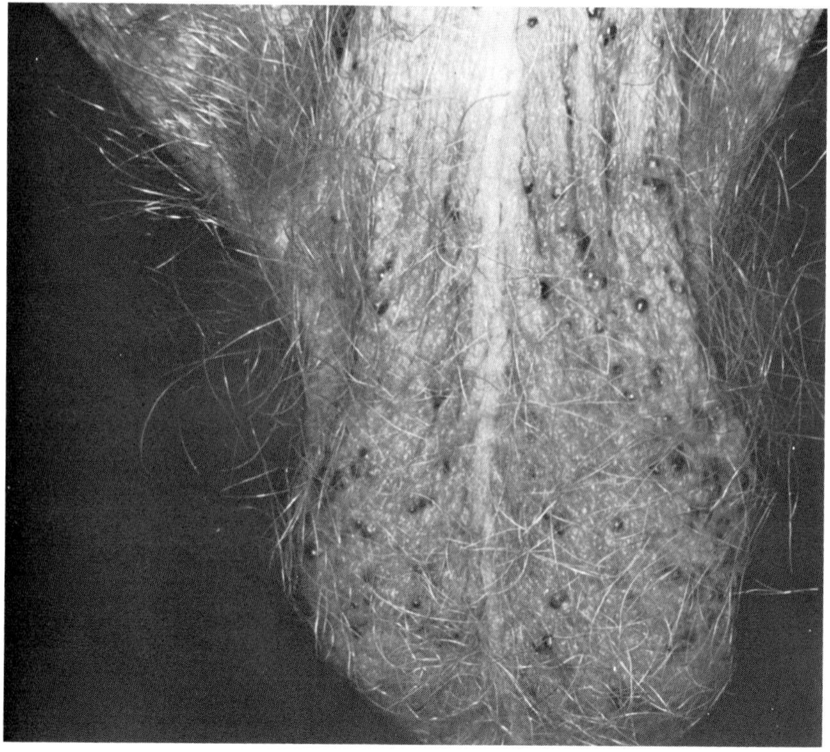

Figure 11–13. Angiokeratomas on scrotum (Fordyce).

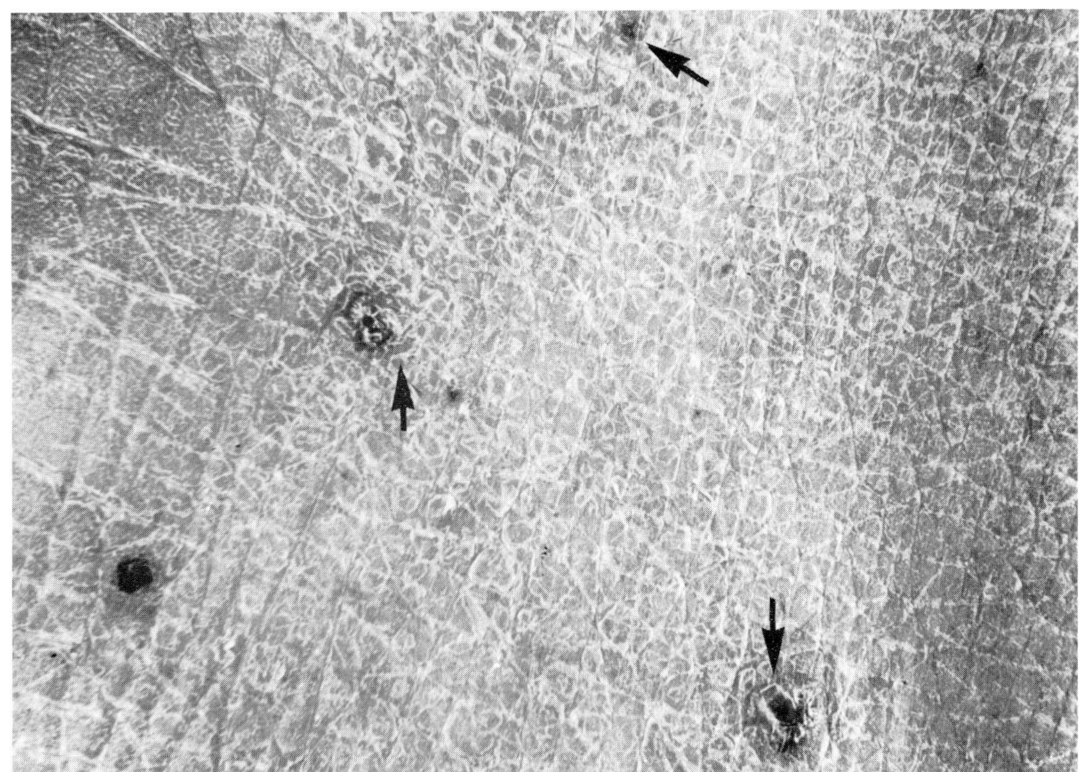

Figure 11–14. Fabry's disease. These angiokeratomas (arrows) characteristically vary in size. (Courtesy of Dr. Richard Sagebiel.)

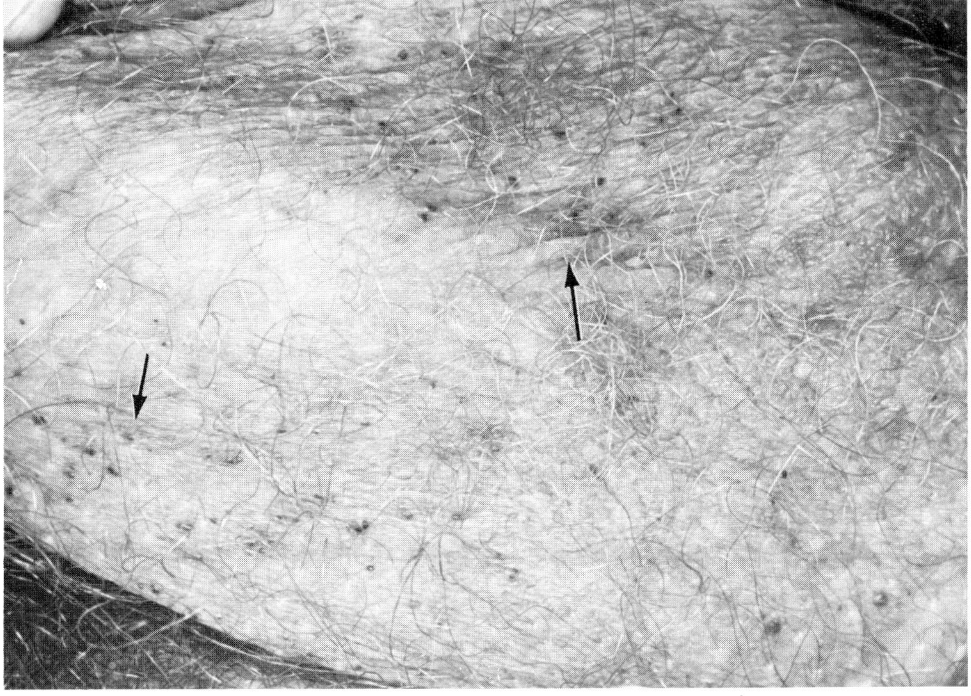

Figure 11–15. Fabry's disease. Angiokeratomas on scrotum (arrows).

peppered with buckshot. Some patients have coarse telangiectases over the shoulders and trunk and in the axilla.[14]

Fabry's disease is a sex-linked disorder in which two neutral glycolipids are abnormally stored in many different types of cells: vascular endothelium; dermal histiocytes; neurons; smooth, striated, and cardiac muscle fibers; and renal glomeruli and tubules. The two glycolipids, trihexosylceramide (galactosylgalactosylglucosylceramide) and diagalactosylceramide, are also excreted in elevated amounts in the urine. The enzyme α-galactosidase A (formerly called ceramidetrihexosidase) is absent in hemizygous males, but present in intermediate amounts in heterozygous females. Males develop the complete clinical picture, but in heterozygous females the course of the disease is less severe and the clinical features are milder or absent.[15, 16] The enzyme α-galactosidase A catalyzes the cleavage of the terminal α-galactose from trihexosylceramide and digalactosylceramide. This enzyme is present in the plasma, white cells, hair roots, and tears, which facilitates measurement for the detection of heterozygous females and suspected cases.[17, 18] The abnormal storage of these glycolipids is believed responsible for the signs and symptoms of the disorder.

The diagnostic skin lesions appear at 7 to 13 years of age, a time much too early for the onset of Fordyce lesions. A case of biochemically proved Fabry's disease with only scrotal lesions has been observed, but this must be an extremely rare event.[14] Although angiokeratomas are usually present in patients with Fabry's disease, two patients exhibited proteinuria as the only manifestation of the illness, and a third, proteinuria plus burning sensations in the hands and feet.[19, 20] The vascular ectasias also have been seen in the gastrointestinal, respiratory, and genitourinary tracts.

The clinical features are as striking as the skin lesions: incapacitating pain in the fingers, toes, and occasionally in the entire extremity may be brought on by fever, heat, cold, or exertion. The pain may affect the glans penis. Attacks of abdominal and flank pain simulate appendicitis or renal colic. Although the pain usually arises in crises, it may also be present as a constant nagging discomfort in the hands and feet. The pain also takes the form of burning sensations and paresthesias. The pain may be the earliest manifestation of the illness, preceding the appearance of skin lesions by months or years.[21] Other features include chronic edema of the feet when serum proteins are normal and cardiac and renal diseases are not detectable; central nervous system signs and symptoms, such as paresis, aphasia, tremor, sensory disturbances, loss of consciousness, and decreased visual acuity — all of which are often transient; heat intolerance because of poor sweating; intermittent nonbloody diarrhea and proctocolitis with the rare complication of bowel perforation[22, 23]; a peculiar arthritis of the distal interphalangeal joints with some loss of motion; limitation of movement of the temporomandibular joints and other large joints; and vascular necrosis of the head of the femur.

The ocular changes are distinctive and can be diagnostic.[24] They range from a diffuse haziness of the epithelial layer of the cornea to corneal opacities characterized by whorled streaks extending from a central point to the periphery of the cornea. (Chloroquine toxicity can produce an identical pattern.) Posterior capsular cataracts with spoke formation can develop. The retinal and conjunctival vessels may show mild to marked tortuosity and angulation. There may be aneurysmal and segmental sausage-like dilations. Fortunately, none of these abnormalities results in impairment of vision.

Most of the affected men have died in their thirties of renal failure with uremia and hypertension. Some have succumbed to congestive heart failure and cerebrovascular accidents. The oldest known living male is 56 years of age. The affected heterozygous women tend to have skin lesions, cataracts, and a benign and milder clinical course than hemizygous men. However, some women become more symptomatic with age and die from the disease.[16] Renal biopsies from heterozygous women demonstrate that the characteristic deposits of trihexosylceramide may be absent, or present in lesser amounts, then in men. When present, the glycolipid is irregularly deposited throughout the kidney in contrast to the uniform generalized deposition in men.[25]

Examination of angiokeratomas with lipid and PAS stains discloses the abnormally deposited glycolipid in the endothelial cells.[26] Identical glycolipid deposits can also be found in the normal-appearing skin of affected individuals.[27] Electron microscopy shows that these inclusions have a characteristic appearance that is diagnostic for the disorder: concentric, lamellar, myelin-like profiles (Figs. 11–16 and 11–17). The urine sediment contains cells with birefringent inclusions, which can be helpful in diagnosis. Demonstration of glycolipid in the endothelial cells is a useful method for distinguishing Fordyce lesions from those of Fabry's disease in a confusing case.

The accumulation of trihexosylceramide in endothelial cells results in swelling of the cells with a concomitant narrowing of the vascular lumen. This narrowing is believed to produce most of the clinical features of the disease through vascular occlusion and ischemia.[15, 28] The major source of the accumulated glycolipid is thought to be senescent erythrocytes, because the endothelial cells are primarily affected. Johnson and Desnick have proposed that since the trihexosylceramide and digalactosylceramide are transported by low- and high-density lipoproteins in the blood, their entry into the endothelium may result from receptor-mediated uptake of circulating lipoproteins saturated with these glycolipids.[15] Their accumulation then results from the lack of α-galactosidase A activity in the endothelial cell.

Attempts have been made to correct the enzymatic defect in patients by infusion of plasma from healthy individuals, and of purified enzyme from human placenta. These attempts produced only short-term beneficial responses. Renal transplantation has also been employed. This technique was designed to supply a continuous source of the missing enzyme or to be a sink into which the circulating trihexosylceramide would pass and be metabolized. However, many of these transplants have failed to produce a beneficial response.[29]

A phenocopy of Fabry's disease has recently been discovered in another inborn lysosomal disease—fucosidosis. In this disorder there is an absence or profound deficiency of α-L-fucosidase, which results in a widespread tissue accumulation of fucose-containing glycosphingolipids and oligo- and polysaccharides, in association with an increased urinary excretion of fucosides.[30-34] The initial family with this disease traces its origin to Calabria in Southern Italy. Two clinical forms exist. The *severe* form is characterized by progressive psychomotor retardation; moderate

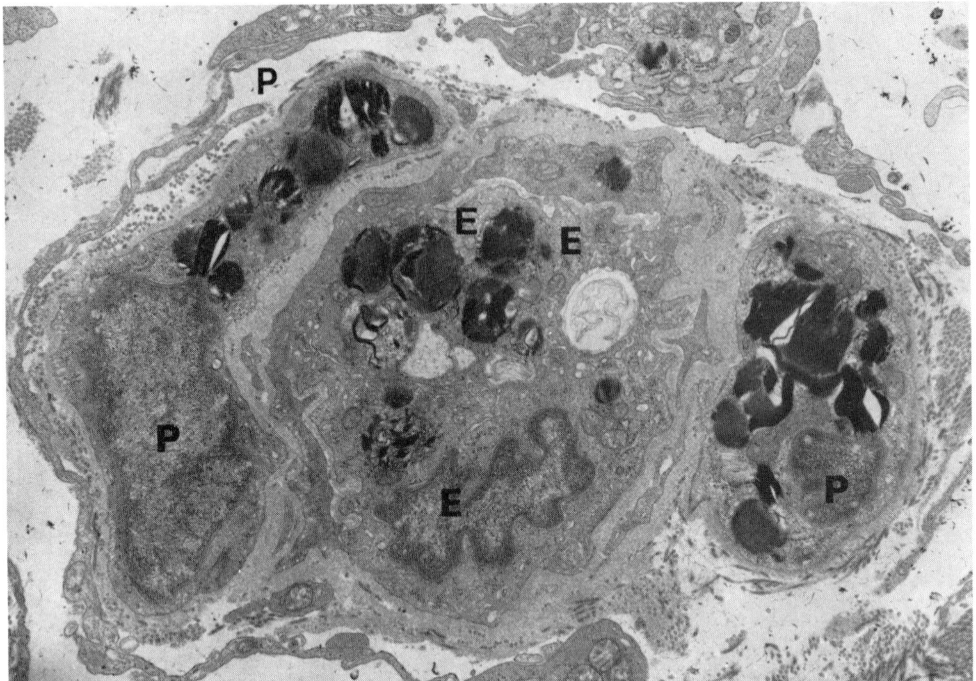

Figure 11–16. Fabry's disease. Characteristic inclusions in this disease are found in endothelial cells (E) and pericytes (P) of vessels as well as in other tissue cells. Electron microscopy is a diagnostic procedure in this disorder. × 10,000.

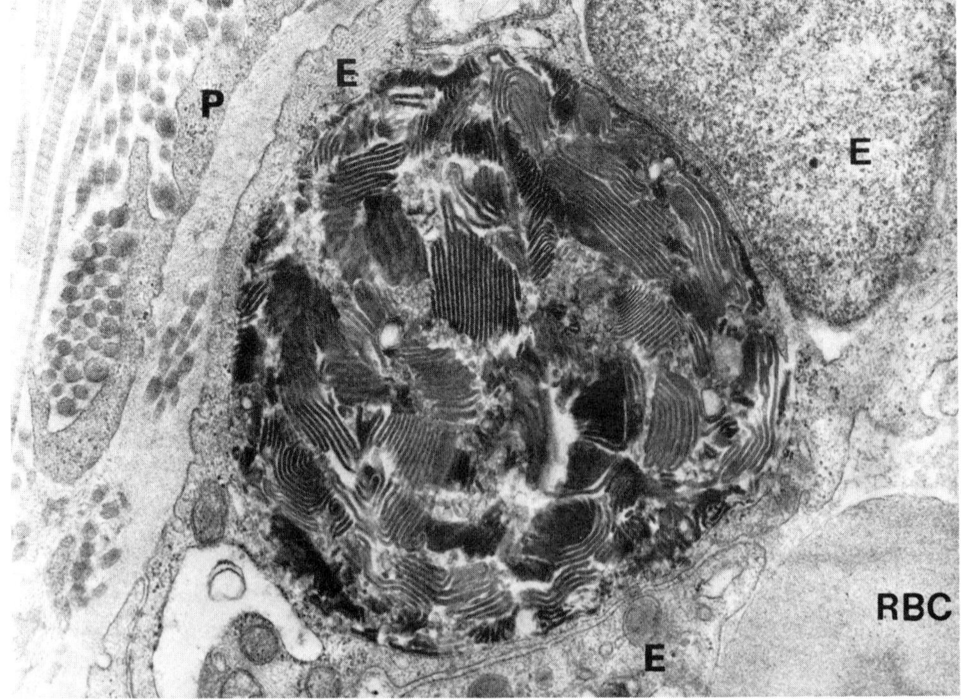

Figure 11–17. Fabry's disease. Close-up of inclusions shows their lamellar myelin-like profiles. × 28,000.

chondrodystrophy similar to that found in the mucopolysaccharidoses; coarse facial features, thick lips, and macroglossia; hepatosplenomegaly; cloudy corneas; lumbar hyperlordosis; and protuberant abdomen and umbilical hernia. Life expectancy is less than three to five years. The *mild* variety has angiokeratomas, and tortuous vessels on the retina and conjunctivae indistinguishable from those of Fabry's disease. These children have survived into adolescence and beyond. They exhibit milder psychomotor retardation but have many of the other features seen in the severe form. The inclusions in the cells have a different electron microscopic appearance from those of Fabry's disease. The disease can be detected by measuring the enzyme level in tears or white blood cells.[30] Screening for the disease by measuring plasma levels of the enzyme can be misleading because there are normal individuals whose enzyme levels are low in the plasma but normal in leukocytes. Therefore, both white cells and plasma need to be measured. The endothelial cells in the angiokeratomas of fucosidosis do not stain for fat as they do in Fabry's disease.[35] The disease may be more common than is realized and may not be limited to individuals of Italian origin. The first case of non-Italian background was recently diagnosed in Great Britain.[36]

An additional phenocopy resembling Fabry's disease was reported by Pelletier et al. Thus far, this is the only case. The patient had angiokeratomas, lens opacities, and a moderately depressed creatinine clearance. However, he had neither fucosidosis nor Fabry's disease according to the measurements of the appropriate enzymes. Electron microscopy of the skin and kidneys showed inclusions in cells that were unlike those of either Fabry's disease or fucosidosis.[37]

Hemangioma. The hemangiomas are classified into three groups: port-wine stain, cavernous hemangioma, and strawberry hemangioma.

The port-wine stain (nevus flammeus, mature capillary hemangioma) is flat and bluish-red. It is present at birth and increases only as the affected part grows. Occasionally hypertrophic vascular nodules arise from the flat hemangioma in adult life.

The cavernous hemangiomas are deep vascular tumors that involve the dermis and subcutaneous tissue. Histologic examination reveals dilated vascular spaces lined by a single layer of endothelial cells and surrounded by a fibrous wall. Cavernous lesions are present at birth and grow with the involved area. They appear as smooth, bluish intradermal or subcutaneous masses. If very deep, they are of a flesh color. The term cavernous hemangioma is sometimes incorrectly applied to vascular malformations composed of large vessels arranged in cerebriform and plexiform configurations, especially when these hamartomas have a deep cutaneous component. Both arteries and veins participate in the hamartomas, and arteriovenous communications are common. Lymphatic vascular elements often are admixed with these bizarre vascular tumors.

The strawberry hemangioma (capillary hemangioma), present at birth or appearing within the first few weeks of life, is appropriately named. This vascular lesion often grows rapidly for about six to eight months and then spontaneously ceases its expansion and begins to involute spontaneously in most cases. Histologic examination of such a lesion discloses sheets and clumps of endothelial cells forming vascular channels. Although the rapid growth and increase in size fulfill one definition of neoplasia, the cytologic characteristics of the endothelial cells are benign. Strawberry angiomas are bright red with a pebbly surface. Although these angiomas are usually localized to the upper dermis, they can extend deeply, even into the subcutaneous layer. Also, it is not unusual for a strawberry angioma to overlie a cavernous hemangioma. The strawberry hemangioma need not be treated unless a vital organ — such as the eyes, lips, pharynx, or larynx — is affected.

These three types of hemangiomas usually do not signify the presence of internal disease; they are simply cosmetic problems. However, they can be the major sign of some important medical disorders, as discussed below.

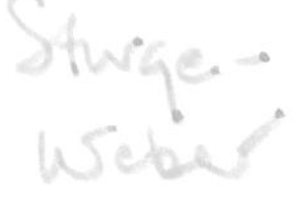

The Sturge-Weber syndrome (encephalotrigeminal angiomatosis) is characterized by a port-wine stain in the trigeminal distribution in association with a vascular malformation involving the ipsilateral meninges and cerebral cortex.[38] Epilepsy, mental retardation, ocular defects, and contralateral hemiplegia are the associated functional disturbances. Ocular abnormalities include exophthalmos, choroidal atrophy, glaucoma, and megalocornea. The intracranial angiomatosis can often be visualized by x-ray because of intralesional calcification. The port-wine stain is not always limited to the face in this syndrome; it may also involve the extremities and trunk either unilaterally or bilaterally (Plate 31*C*). In addition, cavernous hemangiomas may also be present elsewhere on the skin. The occurrence of a port-wine stain on a limb or the trunk may be accompanied by hypertrophy of the soft tissues and bones underneath the vascular lesion. In such cases, a deep vascular malformation is present that results in an increased blood flow through the soft tissue and bone with an attendant increase in the size and volume of the affected parts.

Cavernous hemangiomas and other bizarre vascular malformations can also be associated with hypertrophy of limbs and other parts of the body in the absence of the Sturge-Weber syndrome. The eponym applied to these states of hemihypertrophy is the Klippel-Trenaunay-Parkes-Weber syndrome (Plate 31*D*).

Allied to the Sturge-Weber syndrome are three other entities which have congenital hemangiomas involving the skin and central nervous system. The Cobb syndrome combines primarily a nevus flammeus or cavernous hemangioma in a dermatomal distribution with an angioma in the spinal cord that corresponds to the cutaneous distribution within one or two segments.[39, 40] The neurological deficit does not appear until late childhood or adolescence. Bonnet-Dechaume-Blanc syndrome is characterized by a nevus flammeus of the face, retinal angiomatosis, and intracranial angiomas in the region of the thalamus and mesencephalon. Wyburn-Mason syndrome combines an arteriovenous aneurysm of the mid-brain with a malformation of the retinal vessels unilaterally. A nevus flammeus is present in the skin in the region of the affected eye.[40]

The strawberry angioma is not associated with these two latter syndromes; but it can produce disastrous effects when vital areas are affected: laryngeal lesions cause respiratory embarrassment, angiomas of the pharynx and lips interfere with sucking and eating, and involvement of the eyelids produces amblyopia through disuse.

Hemangiomatosis of the gut is well known to the gastroenterologist, but in only a few cases has the skin been similarly affected.[41, 42] Conversely, the gastrointestinal tract is rarely affected in cases of hemangiomatosis of the skin. Nevertheless the presence of cavernous hemangiomas in the skin should alert one to possible gastrointestinal lesions; and the skin of any person having melena for obscure reasons should be examined carefully for the presence of hemangiomas.

In most cases of hemangiomatosis of the skin and gut, the cutaneous angiomas have been of the ordinary cavernous type — smooth bluish cutaneous masses — and the submucosal gastrointestinal component has had a similar appearance.[43, 44] The angiomas of the gut not only bleed but also can produce perforation of the bowel.

In several cases of angiomatosis of the skin and gut, the cutaneous cavernous angioma has had an unusual appearance, being nipple- or bladder-like, soft, and easily compressible. It slowly refills with blood when the pressure is released. The angiomas have been pedunculated as well as sessile. These unusual vascular lesions are the hallmark of the *blue rubber-bleb nevus syndrome*.[45-48]

A 15-year-old boy was reported to have these typical bladder-like angiomas in the skin, but no lesions had been found in the gastrointestinal tract.[47] Rice and Fischer described the blue rubber-bleb nevus syndrome in a young woman who not only had extensive skin and gut involvement but also had angiomas in the mouth, lungs, and muscles. A medulloblastoma was a complicating disorder in this individual.[48] A number of authors have noted that spontaneous pain associated with sweating can be a feature of this kind of angioma; and histologically, sweat glands and smooth muscle were intimately associated with the vascular tissue.[47, 49]

Although the blue rubber-bleb character of the cavernous hemangioma is distinctive and should direct one's attention to the possible involvement of other organs, especially the gut, the ordinary cavernous hemangioma is *more* frequently found in skin-gut angiomatosis.

Cavernous hemangiomas are also a feature of Maffucci's syndrome, a mesodermal dysplasia characterized by enchondromas, dyschondroplasia, and bony abnormalities produced by unequal and irregular development of the osseous tissue.[50] The vascular hamartomas develop independently, in both time and location, of the bony and cartilaginous abnormalities. Pathologic fractures are common, and malignant degeneration of both cartilage and vascular angiomas is a serious complication of Maffucci's syndrome. A case of blue rubber-bleb nevus syndrome and Maffucci's disease was described by Sakurane, Sugai, and Saito.[49]

Thrombocytopenia, caused by platelet sequestration and destruction, in giant cavernous hemangiomas — the Kasabach-Merritt syndrome — produces local and widespread purpura (Plate 31*E*). This syndrome has been associated primarily with cavernous hemangiomas, occasionally with hemangiosarcomas, but never with strawberry angiomas or port-wine stains. Some hemangiomas have been present for many months before the platelet sequestration and purpura develop.[51] The number of platelets increases to normal when the vascular tumor shrinks following irradiation or corticosteroid therapy. Although in most cases the hemangiomas have been very large and deep, some vascular tumors have measured only 10 by 15 cm.[52]

Vascular hamartomas can be extraordinarily extensive and pervasive in an individual and can affect such diverse structures as bone, serosal surfaces, lungs, and other viscera in addition to the skin. In some instances lymphatic vascular elements also contribute to the hamartoma, and it can be difficult separating blood vascular from lymphatic vascular elements in such malformations. Koblenzer and Bukowski reported the case of a 3.5-year-old girl who developed a large cavernous hemangioma over the left side of the chest at one year of age. Histologically, the vascular tumor showed benign cytologic features, but it invaded the underlying ribs and communicated with the pleural spaces to produce recurrent bloody pleural effusions. The hamartomatous process became multicentric so that by age 3.5 years, when the child died, there were osteolytic lesions of the right parietal bone, clavicle, scapula, ribs, pelvis, vertebral bodies, and long bones of the upper and lower extremities. At autopsy, angiomatosis was found in all these areas, and the cytologic characteristics still were benign. Some of the elements were believed to be lymphatic in origin, and extensive lymphatic venous communications were thought to be present. The authors called this entity hamartomatous hem-lymphangiomatosis and culled seven other similar cases from the literature.[53] The clinical features of these cases depended upon the sites of involvement: bone, lungs, liver, spleen, kidneys, bladder, gut, heart, and pleurae, in addition to the skin. Visceromegaly was present in some cases. Massive effusions — chylous, bloody, or both — were common, depending upon the origin of the vascular elements within the hamartoma.

In some cases, bone has been involved almost exclusively. The occurrence of massive osteolysis has been called "disappearing bone disease," or Gorham's disease. The disorder has begun in childhood in most cases and has been progressive. In a few instances the onset was in adult life, and the disease became stationary after a time.[54]

MALIGNANT VASCULAR TUMORS

The most import malignant vascular tumors are of two types: the lymphangiosarcoma of Stewart-Treves, which originates in chronic lymphedematous limbs (see Chapter 1), and the hemangiosarcomas that arise as solitary tumors in normal skin and metastasize widely to liver, lungs, and other viscera (Fig. 11–18). The hemangiosarcomas of skin often resemble the ordinary deep cavernous hemangiomas and can be diagnosed as malignant disorders only by histologic examination. They are divided into hemangioendothelioma and hemangiopericytoma, depending upon whether the malignant cell is an endothelial one or a pericyte.

Multicentric neoplastic proliferation of vascular endothelium is a newly discovered entity reported by Tappeiner and Pfleger in 1959 and by Braverman and Lerner in 1961. Gross tumors as seen in hemangiosarcoma do not develop, nor do metastases. Several terms have been applied to this entity: diffuse malignant proliferation of vascular endothelium, systemic endotheliomatosis, and endotheliomatosis proliferans systemisata. As of 1970, eight additional cases had been reported: six satisfy the histologic criteria of this entity; and two are possible, but not proved, cases.

As the descriptive titles indicate, there is a malignant neoplastic proliferation of endothelial cells throughout the body without concomitant changes in any of the other cellular or structural elements in blood vessels. The signs and symptoms in this disease are related to vascular obstruction produced in the affected organs. Only rarely do the malignant

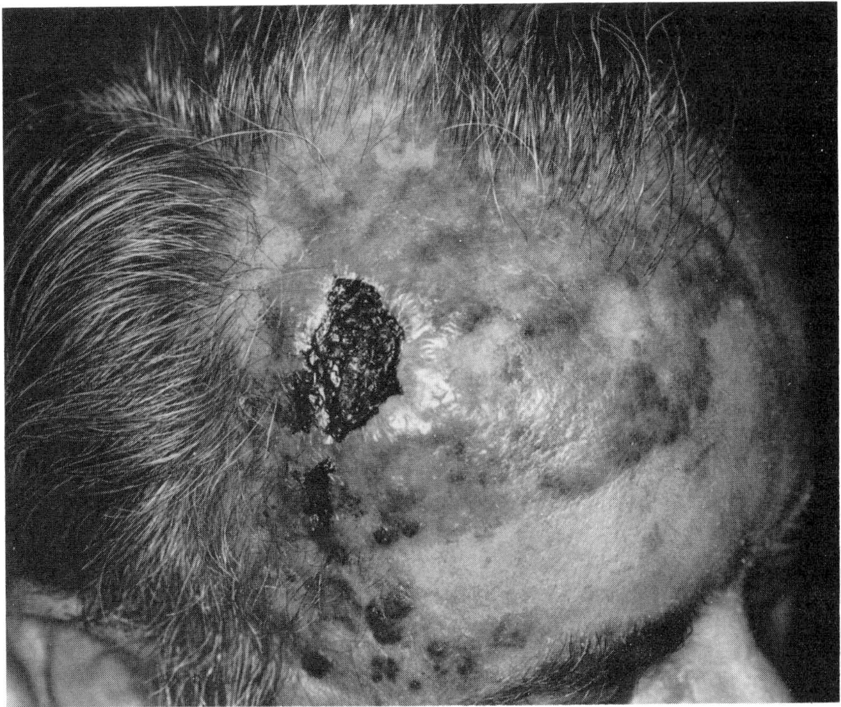

Figure 11–18. Hemangiosarcoma.

cells break out of the vascular lumina and invade the surrounding parenchyma.

The cutaneous markers have been different in all reported cases, and the disease can be identified only by its unique histopathology. Histologic examination of cutaneous and visceral lesions reveals dilated thin-walled vessels arranged in clusters resembling renal glomeruli (Figs. 11–19 to 11–21). Within the lumina of the dilated vessels, the cells lining the endothelium proliferate and detach, forming clumps. In some vessels, thrombi may be associated with the groups of tumor cells. The vascular walls are normal and without evidence of necrosis or inflammation. The pathologic process is not that of a necrotizing angiitis.[55-57]

Some of the reported cases have had a benign course, whereas others have been fatal. The spectrum of this disorder is best illustrated by summarizing each case.

The first patient, described by Tappeiner and Pfleger, was a 31-year-old Greek nurse whose illness was characterized by recurrent episodes of fever, chills, and a cutaneous eruption.[55, 56] The latter consisted, for the most part, of slightly raised infiltrated red annular lesions ranging in size from that of a fingernail to that of a palm (Fig. 11–22). They had a markedly red border. A minor part of the eruption was made up of homogeneous red blotches. During the first six years of the patient's illness, her skin was free of lesions between acute attacks, but thereafter the eruption became persistent. Remission eventually was induced in the seventh year by treatment with penicillin and oral corticosteroids, but the patient was lost to follow-up. On the basis of the histopathology, Tappeiner and Pfleger diagnosed their case as an unclassified unusually high-grade endothelial proliferation, which might best be called a nonmalignant hemangioendothelioma.

Braverman and Lerner reported the second case, a 66-year-old woman who lived for only eight months.[57] The cutaneous findings were 1- to 4-cm slightly tender

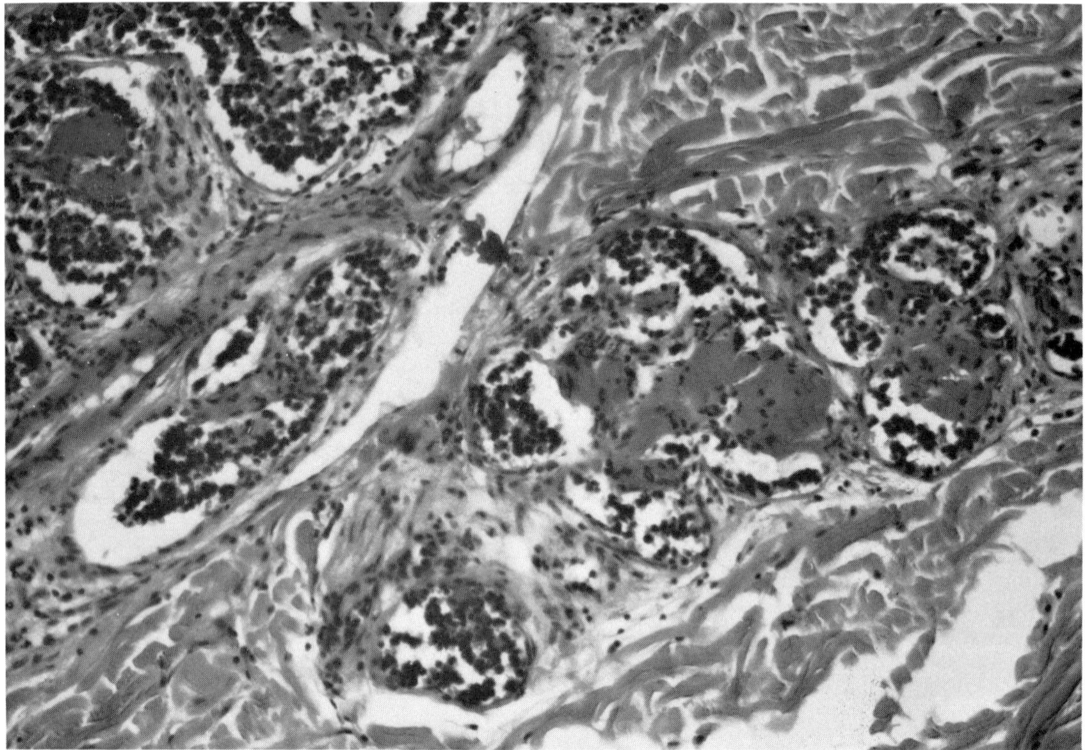

Figure 11–19. Malignant endotheliomatosis. Clusters of vessels are filled with tumor cells arising from the endothelium. Fibrin thrombi also present. Hematoxylin and eosin. × 100.

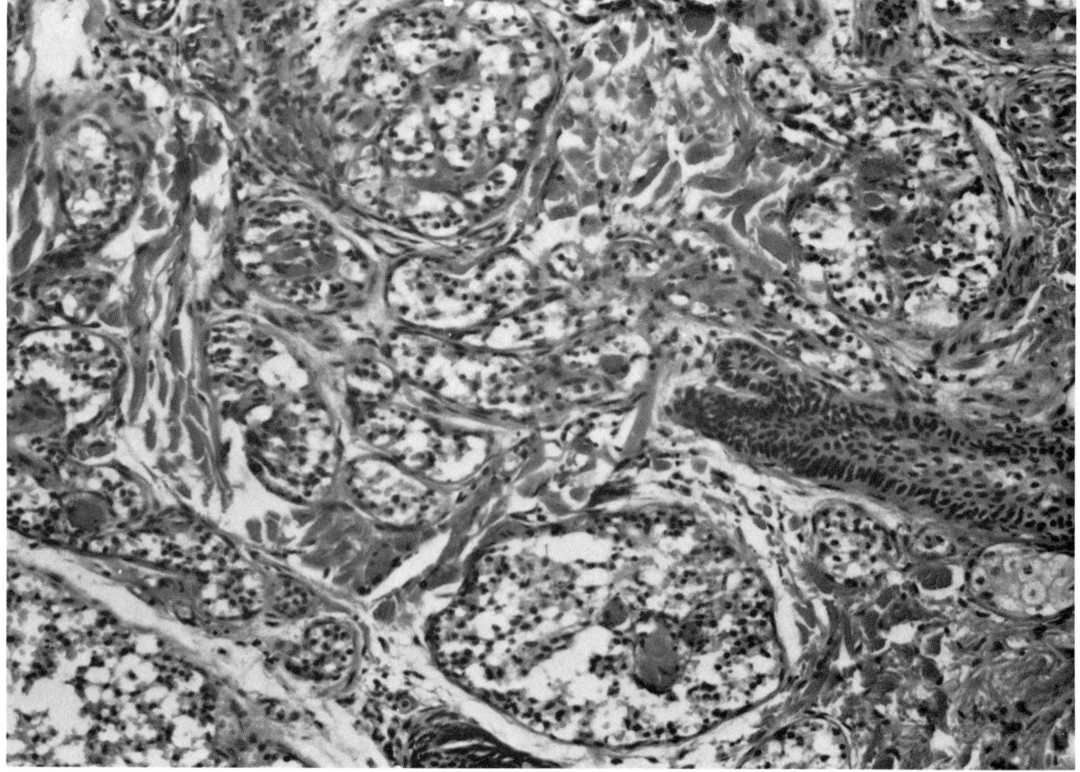

Figure 11–20. Malignant endotheliomatosis. Histopathology. Hematoxylin and eosin. × 100.

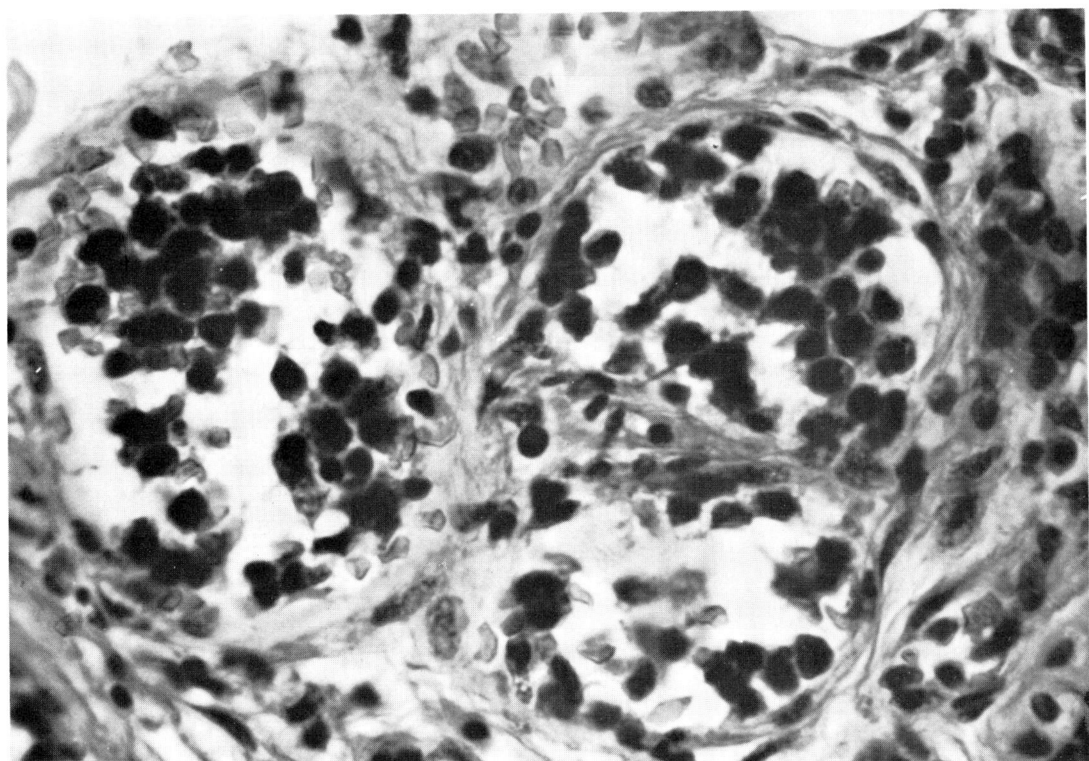

Figure 11–21. Malignant endotheliomatosis. Tumor cells can be seen arising from the endothelium. Hematoxylin and eosin. × 400.

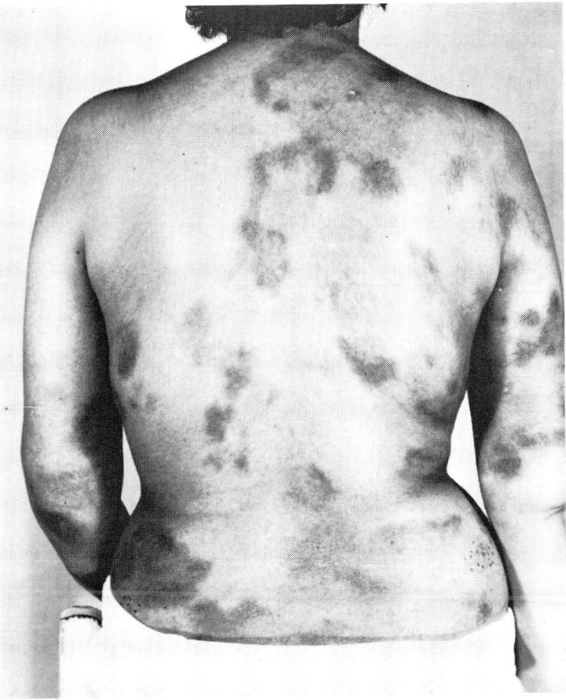

Figure 11–22. Malignant endotheliomatosis. Eruption in patient reported by Tappeiner and Pfleger. (Courtesy of Dr. Josef Tappeiner.)

bluish patches, some of which were minimally infiltrated (Plate 31*F*). Tortuous fine vessels coursed over the surface of the lesions. The patient's main complaints were progressive loss of vision and hearing, malaise, and weakness. Fever and chills did not occur. Serial biopsies of the skin during the course of the illness showed at first a benign endothelial proliferation, but it gradually assumed a frankly malignant appearance. The cells were confined to the vascular channels. One month before death, tissue invasion occurred, manifesting itself as red subcutaneous nodules on the trunk and extremities. Our clinical diagnosis was atypical reticulum cell sarcoma. Autopsy disclosed that the vessels in all organs were similarly affected: proliferating malignant-appearing endothelial cells occluded the lumina. Tissue invasion occurred in a patchy fashion in the heart, thyroid, and skin. The parenchyma of the spleen, liver, and lymph nodes was not involved; but the vessels of these structures were full of malignant cells. Deafness was produced by infiltration of the petrous portion of the temporal bone, and blindness was caused by invasion of the uveal tract and vitreous humor of the eye.

Dr. Walter Lever called our attention to Tappeiner and Pfleger's case, the tissues of which he had examined. It was obvious that we were dealing with a new entity — a multicentric proliferation of vascular endothelium. In our patient it was possible to observe the transition from a benign to a malignant phase. The tissue invasion, where present, was mild, considering that all the vessels examined at autopsy showed endothelial changes.

This entity differs from the recognized forms of angiosarcoma in that neither new vascular channels nor sheets and clusters of cells resembling an undifferentiated sarcoma were present. The tumor cells apparently arose from the endothelium of the vessels and merely filled the lumina.

These first two examples are the prototypes of the eight additional patients that have since been reported. Tappeiner and Pfleger's case exhibited crops of lesions, in association with fever, that disappeared between attacks; it had a benign course for at least seven years; and as far as is known it remained a benign disorder. Our patient steadily deteriorated and the disease behaved like a malignant disorder.

Haber et al. reported the third instance, a 46-year-old woman who died of a stroke one year after her illness began.[58] The cutaneous lesions were plum-colored subcutaneous nodules that arose on the legs and spread to the buttocks and trunk. The histopathology was identical to the previous cases. Although an autopsy was not performed, this patient most likely had lesions in the blood vessels of the brain similar to those we had found in our own patient.

Strouth et al. described additional examples of this disorder in two men, 42 and 63 years old.[59] Both had bizarre neurologic signs and symptoms culminating in dementia that was ultimately shown to have been produced by ischemic necrosis secondary to lesions in the cerebral vessels. The skin was not involved.

Ruiter and Mandema[60] and Gottron and Nikolowski[61] each described the disease in two women 55 and 52 years old, respectively. Both suffered from a febrile illness with features suggesting subacute bacterial endocarditis. However, no organisms were isolated in either case. Both women had lesions on the cheeks; these lesions were described as firm brown-red patches with a smooth surface occasionally interrupted by pinpoint bluish-black papules and purpuric spots (Plate 32*A*). In Ruiter's patient the ear lobes were swollen and bluish-red, and on the forearms there were coalescent red patches studded with petechiae. Histologic examination of

PLATE 32

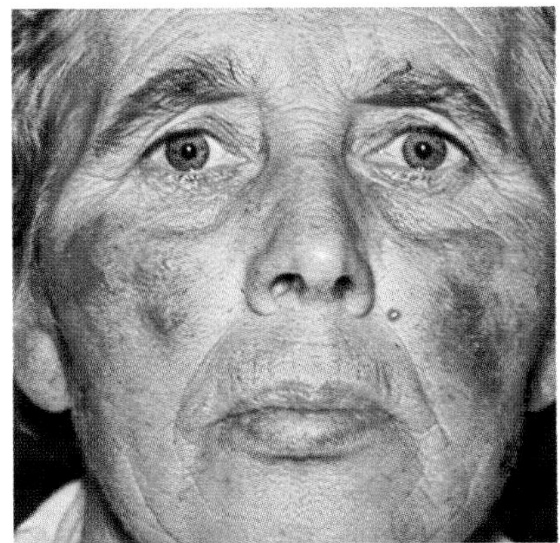

A, Malignant endotheliomatosis. Patient reported by Ruiter and Mandema. (From Arch. Intern. Med., *113*:283, 1964. Courtesy of Dr. M. Ruiter.)

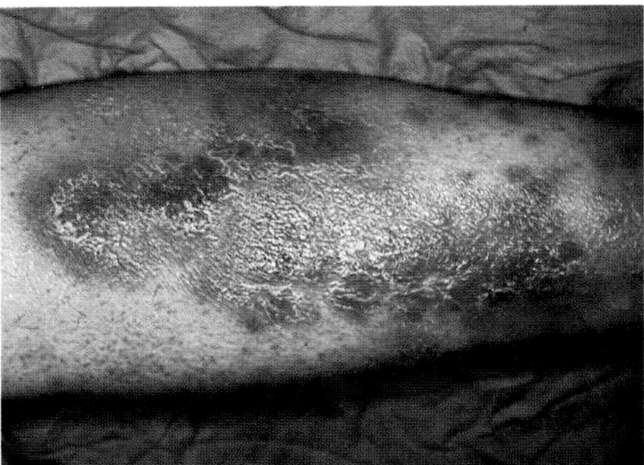

B, Malignant endotheliomatosis. Lesion on shin. Patient of Maibach. (Courtesy of Dr. Howard Maibach.)

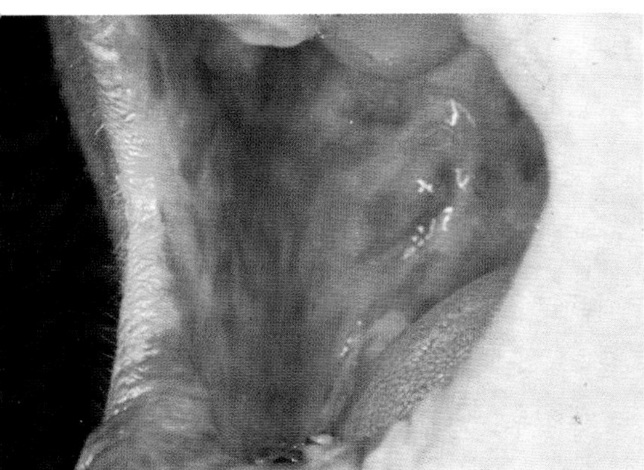

C, Peutz-Jeghers syndrome. Buccal pigmentation.

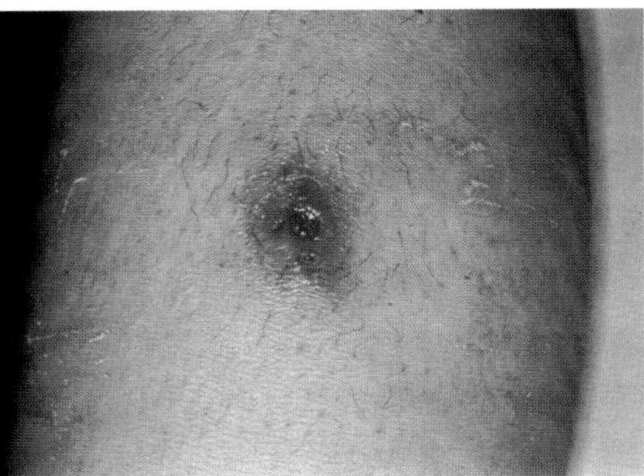

D, Pyoderma gangrenosum in a patient with ulcerative colitis.

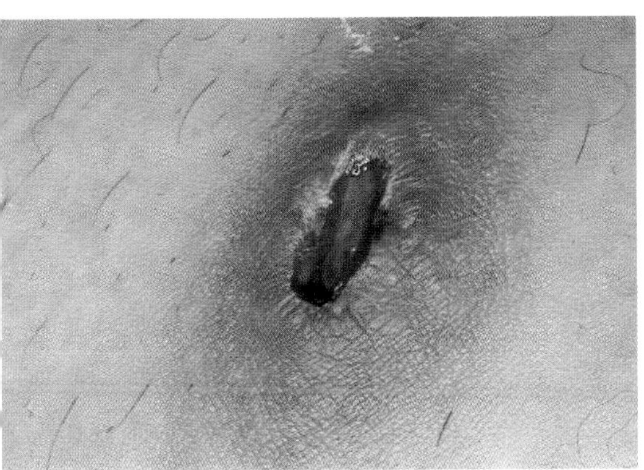

E, Pyoderma gangrenosum in a patient with ulcerative colitis. Note undermined necrotic bluish margins.

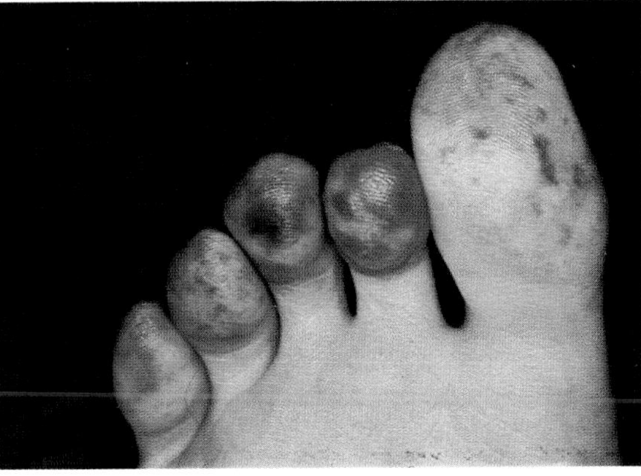

F, Gangrene produced by hypercoagulation syndrome in ulcerative colitis.

the lesions in both cases disclosed the pathognomonic features of systemic endotheliomatosis. Treatment with penicillin was followed by complete remission in both patients. In a personal communication, Ruiter reported that his patient was alive and well five years later but suffered cardiac decompensation secondary to mitral valve insufficiency. The skin lesions did not recur. Gottron's patient died of congestive heart failure two years after discharge from the hospital, but there was no evidence of active disease during that time. The relationship between the disease of the heart and the vascular endothelium is not known, if indeed they were related.

Maibach cared for a 68-year-old man with this disorder.[62] The patient had two lesions; a red plaque with an irregular surface on the right leg (Plate 32*B*) and an erythematous nodule on the abdomen. Neurologic signs and symptoms of increasing weakness of the legs with a wobbling gait, and decreased mental acuity with depression and difficulty in maintaining orderly thought processes developed 22 months after the beginning of his illness. Neurologic evaluation was consistent with a right-sided brain lesion of either vascular or neoplastic origin. His signs and symptoms initially improved followed irradiation to the cutaneous lesions and chemotherapy with vincristine and cyclophosphamide. However, his general condition later slowly deteriorated and he died one year later. No autopsy was performed. The course of his illness was 34 months.

Two other case reports probably are examples of this disorder, but we have not had the opportunity to review the histologic sections. Lund reported and illustrated a case of a man with disseminated carcinoma, primary site unknown.[63] The accompanying photomicrograph was labeled as representing tumor emboli in vessels, but in retrospect Lund thought this patient might be another example of this disorder.[64]

Midana and Ormea reported a 13-year-old girl who died after a four-month illness.[65] She abruptly developed nodules and tumors on the breast, below the eye, and generally, over her body. The larger ones ulcerated and resembled the mushroom tumors of mycosis fungoides. Although the photomicrographs in the article were consistent with this new entity, Wolff, who reviewed the biopsy material, believes that the girl suffered from a lymphoma rather than systemic endotheliosis.[66]

The eight proved cases fit into two categories: (1) a fatal disease and (2) a self-limited variety characterized by fever, chills, and the disappearance of skin lesions. Although the cutaneous lesions are not clinically diagnostic, the histopathology clearly is.

Since 1970, an additional 11 cases — six men and five women —have been diagnosed.[67-75] They continue to fit into the two categories of a neoplastic and an inflammatory process. One of the recent patients had an illness with features suggesting subacute bacterial endocarditis, although no organisms were isolated. Thus 3 of 17 cases have had an illness mimicking subacute bacterial endocarditis.[60, 61, 67] In one patient, a five-month-old boy, the disease ran a self-limited course of five months. The authors thought that he had a reticuloendothelial response to either multiple bacterial infections or the protein in cow's milk.[73] Hollander discovered an unsuspected case at autopsy. The patient was a 47-year-old woman who had had abdominal pain for three months. Diffuse radiographic changes suggested granulomatous enterocolitis. Small bowel obstruction and perforation of the transverse colon led to her demise. At autopsy there were mucosal ulcerations in the small intestine, mesenteric fat necrosis, and multiple foci of hepatic necrosis. Extensive intravascular proliferation of neoplastic cells was found in the intestine, pancreas, and liver, with multifocal ischemic infarcts. The extravascular component was minimal. Autopsy permission was limited to the abdomen, but full diagnostic work-up showed no primary malignancy. There was no clinical involvement of the central nervous system or skin.

This disorder behaves like a multicentric process, and tissue invasion is rare. The vessels proliferate or dilate to form clusters resembling renal glomeruli. Reticulum stains of these clustered vessels do not show anastomoses characteristic of hemangioendothelioma. Other examples of this entity undoubtedly exist and most likely are classified under the rubric of disseminated carcinomatosis with tumor emboli. The stimuli and mechanism underlying this endothelial proliferation are as yet unknown. Person suggested that a circulating angiogenic factor might be responsible for the proliferation, analogous to the tumor angiogenic factor of Folkmann.[76]

REFERENCES

1. Hamilton, E. B. D.: Nail studies in rheumatoid arthritis. Ann. Rheum. Dis., *19*:167, 1960.
2. Hodgson, C. H., Burchell, H. B., Good, C. A., and Clagett, O. T.: Hereditary hemorrhagic telangiectasia and pulmonary arteriovenous fistula. Survey of a large family. N. Engl. J. Med., *261*:625, 1959.
3. Trell, E., Johansson, B. W., Linell, F., and Ripa, J.: Familial pulmonary hypertension and multiple abnormalities of large systemic arteries in Osler's disease. Am. J. Med., *53*:50, 1972.
4. Conlon, C. L., Weinger, R. S., Cimio, P. L., Moake, J. L., and Olson, J. D.: Telangiectasia and von Willebrand's disease in two families. Ann. Intern. Med., *89*:921, 1978.
5. Bird, R. M., Hammarsten, J. F., Marshall, R. A., and Robinson, R. R.: A family reunion. A study of hereditary hemorrhagic telangiectasia. N. Engl. J. Med., *257*:105, 1957.
6. Reed, W. B., Epstein, W. L., Boder, E., and Sedgwick, R.: Cutaneous manifestations of ataxia telangiectasia. J.A.M.A., *195*:746, 1966.
7. Degos, R.: Malignant atrophic papulosis: a fatal cutaneo-intestinal syndrome. Br. J. Dermatol., *66*:304, 1954.
8. McGrae, J. D., and Winkelmann, R. K.: Generalized essential telangiectasia. Report of a clinical and histochemical study of 13 patients with acquired cutaneous lesions. J.A.M.A., *185*:909, 1963.
9. Bean, W. B.: Vascular Spiders and Related Lesions of the Skin. Charles C Thomas, Springfield, Ill., 1958, p. 255.
10. Miller, D. A., and Akers, W. A.: Multiple phlebectasia of the jejunum, oral cavity and scrotum. Arch. Intern. Med., *121*:180, 1968.
11. Guis, J. A., Boyle, D. E., Castle, D. D., and Congdon, R. H.: Vascular formations of the lip and peptic ulcer. J.A.M.A., *183*:725, 1963.
12. Imperial, R., and Helwig, E. B.: Angiokeratoma: a clinicopathological study. Arch. Dermatol., *95*:166, 1967.
13. Wise, D., Wallace, H. J., and Jellinek, E. H.: Angiokeratoma corporis diffusum. A clinical study of eight affected families. Q. J. Med., *31*:177, 1962.
14. Frost, P., Spaeth, G. L., and Tanaka, Y.: Fabry's disease: glycolipid lipidosis. Arch. Intern. Med., *117*:440, 1966.
15. Johnson, D. L., and Desnick, R. J.: Molecular pathology of Fabry's disease. Physical and kinetic properties of α-galactosidase A in cultured endothelial cells. Biochim. Biophys. Acta, *538*:195, 1978.
16. Burda, C. D., and Winda, P. R.: Angiokeratoma corporis diffusum universale (Fabry's disease) in female subjects. Am. J. Med., *42*:293, 1967.
17. Vermoken, A. J. M., Weterings, P. J. J. M., Spierenburg, G. Th., van Bennekom, C. A., Wirtz, P., de Bruyn, C. H. M. M., and Oei, T. L.: Fabry's disease: biochemical and histochemical studies on hair roots for carrier detection. Br. J. Dermatol., *98*:191, 1978.
18. Wadskov, S., Andersen, V., Kobayasi, T., Søndergaard, J., and Sørensen, S. A.: On the diagnosis of Fabry's disease. Acta Dermatovenereol., *55*:363, 1975.
19. Clarke, J. T. R., Knaack, J. H., Crawhall, J. C., and Wolfe, L. S.: Ceramide trihexosidosis (Fabry's disease) without skin lesions. N. Engl. J. Med., *284*:233, 1971.
20. Volk, B. W., Schneck, L., Clemmons, J. E., and Nicastri, A. D.: Fabry's disease in a black man without skin lesions. Neurology, *24*:991, 1974.
21. Taaffe, A.: Angiokeratoma corporis diffu-

sum: the evolution of a disease entity. Postgrad. Med. J., *53*:78, 1977.
22. Bryan, A., Knauft, R. F., and Burns, W. A.: Small bowel perforation in Fabry's disease. Ann. Intern. Med., *86*:315, 1977.
23. Rowe, J. W., Gilliam, J. I., and Warthin, T. A.: Intestinal manifestations of Fabry's disease. Ann. Intern. Med., *81*:628, 1974.
24. Spaeth, G. L., and Frost, P.: Eye lesions of Fabry's disease. Arch. Ophthalmol., *74*:760, 1965.
25. Gubler, M.-C., Lenoir, G., Grunfeld, J. P., Ulmann, A., Droz, D., and Habib, R.: Early renal changes in hemizygous and heterozygous patients with Fabry's disease. Kidney Int., *13*:223, 1978.
26. Frost, P., Tanaka, Y., and Spaeth, G. L.: Fabry's disease — glycolipid lipidosis. Am. J. Med., *40*:618, 1966.
27. Sagebiel, R. W., and Parker, F.: Cutaneous lesions of Fabry's disease: glycolipid lipidosis. J. Invest. Dermatol., *50*:208, 1968.
28. Desnick, R. J., Blieden, L. C., Sharp, H. L., Hofschire, P. J., and Moller, J. H.: Cardiac valvular anomalies in Fabry disease. Clinical morphologic and biochemical studies. Circulation, *54*:818, 1976.
29. Spence, M. W., MacKinnon, K. E., Burgess, J. M., d'Entremont, D. M., Beletsky, P., Lannon, S. G., and MacDonald, A. S.: Failure to correct the metabolic defect by renal allotransplantation in Fabry's disease. Ann. Intern. Med., *84*:13, 1976.
30. Libert, J., Van Hoof, F., and Tondeur, M.: Fucosidosis: ultrastructural study of conjunctiva and skin, and enzyme analysis of tears. Invest. Ophthalmol., *15*:626, 1976.
31. Gatti, R., Borrone, C., Trias, X., and Durand, P.: Genetic heterogeneity in fucosidosis. Lancet, *2*:1024, 1973.
32. Kousseff, B. G., Beratis, N. G., Danesino, C., and Hirschhorn, K.: Genetic heterogeneity in fucosidosis. Lancet, *2*:1387, 1973.
33. Kornfeld, M., Snyder, R. D., and Wenger, D. A.: Fucosidosis with angiokeratoma. Arch. Pathol. Lab. Med., *101*:478, 1977.
34. Epinette, W. W., Norins, A. L., Drew, A. L., Zeman, W., and Patel, V.: Angiokeratoma corporis diffusum with α-L-fucosidase deficiency. Arch. Dermatol., *107*:754, 1973.
35. Smith, E. B., Graham, J. L., Ledman, J. A., and Snyder, R. D.: Fucosidosis. Cutis, *19*:195, 1977.
36. MacPhee, G. B., Logan, R. W., and Primrose, D. A. A.: Fucosidosis: how many cases undetected? Lancet, *2*:462, 1975.
37. Pelletier, A., Herbeuval, E., Brondeau, M. T., Belleville, F., and Nabet, P.: Pseudoclinical Fabry's disease without alphagalactosidase deficiency. Biomedicine, *26*:194, 1977.
38. King, G., and Schwarz, G. A.: Sturge-Weber syndrome (encephalo-trigeminal angiomatosis). Arch. Intern. Med., *94*:743, 1954.
39. Cobb, S.: Haemangioma of the spinal cord associated with skin naevi of the same metamere. Ann. Surg., *62*:641, 1915.
40. Jessen, R. T., Thompson, S., and Smith, E. B.: Cobb syndrome. Arch. Dermatol., *113*:1587, 1977.
41. Kaijser, R.: Über Hämangiome des Tractus gastrointestinalis. Arch. Klin. Chir., *187*:351, 661, 1936.
42. Lazarus, J. A., and Marks, M. S.: Benign intestinal tumors of vascular origin. Surgery, *22*:766, 1947.
43. Shepherd, J. A.: Angiomatous conditions of the gastrointestinal tract. Br. J. Surg., *40*:409, 1953.
44. Heycock, J. B., and Dickinson, P. H.: Hemangiomata of the intestine. Br. Med. J., *1*:620, 1951.
45. Bean, W. B.: *op. cit.*, p. 178.
46. McClure, R. D., and Ellis, F. W.: Hemangiomatosis of the intestine. Am. J. Surg., *10*:241, 1930.
47. Fine, R. M., Derbes, V. J., and Clark, W. H.: Blue rubber bleb nevus. Arch. Dermatol., *84*:802, 1961.
48. Rice, J. S., and Fischer, D. S.: Blue rubberbleb nevus syndrome. Arch. Dermatol. *86*:503, 1962.
49. Sakurane, H. F., Sugai, T., and Saito, T.: The association of blue rubber bleb nevus and Maffucci's syndrome. Arch. Dermatol., *95*:28, 1967.
50. Bean, W. B.: Dyschondroplasia and hemangiomata (Maffucci's syndrome). II. Arch. Intern. Med., *102*:544, 1958.
51. Sutherland, D. A., and Clark, H.: Hemangiomas associated with thrombocytopenia. Am. J. Med., *33*:150, 1962.
52. Atkins, H. L., Wolff, J. A., and Sitarz, A.: Giant hemangioma in infancy with secondary thrombocytopenic purpura. Am. J. Roentgenol., *89*:1062, 1963.
53. Koblenzer, P. J., and Bukowski, M. J.: Angiomatosis (hamartomatous hemlymphangiomatosis). Pediatrics, *28*:65, 1961.
54. Gorham, L. W., Wright, A. W., Shultz, H. H., and Maxon, F. C., Jr.: Disappearing bones: a rare form of massive osteolysis. Am. J. Med., *17*:674, 1954.
55. Pfleger, L., and Tappeiner, J.: Zur Kenntnis der systemisierten Endotheliomatose der cutanen Blutgefasse (Reticuloendotheliose?) Hautarzt, *10*:359, 1959.
56. Tappeiner, J., and Pfleger, L.: Angioendotheliomatosis proliferans systemisata — ein klinisch und pathologisch neues Krankheitsbild. Hautarzt, *14*:67, 1963.
57. Braverman, I. M., and Lerner, A. B.: Diffuse malignant proliferation of vascular endothelium. Arch. Dermatol., *84*:72, 1961.
58. Haber, H., Harris-Jones, J. N., and Wells, A. L.: Intravascular endothelioma (endothelioma in situ, systemic endotheliomatosis). J. Clin. Pathol., *17*:608, 1964.
59. Strouth, J. C., Donahue, S., Ross, A., and Aldred, A.: Neoplastic angioendotheliosis. Neurology, *15*:644, 1965.
60. Ruiter, M., and Mandema, E.: New cutaneous syndrome in subacute bacterial endocarditis. Arch. Intern. Med., *113*:283, 1964.
61. Gottron, H. A., and Nikolowski, W.: Extrarenale Löhlein-Herdnephritis der Haut

bei Endocarditis. Arch. Klin. Exp. Dermatol., *207*:156, 1958.
62. Maibach, H. I.: Personal communication.
63. Lund, H. Z.: Tumors of the skin. *In* Atlas of Tumor Pathology. section I, fasc. 2, Armed Forces Institute of Pathology, Washington, 1957, p. 272 (accession no. 219474–268).
64. Lund, H. Z.: Personal communication.
65. Midana, A., and Ormea, F.: A propos d'un cas d'"angioendotheliomatosis proliferans systemisata" (de Tappeiner et Pfleger). Ann. Dermatol. Syph., *92*:129, 1965.
66. Wolff, K.: Personal communication.
67. Fievez, M., Fievez, C., and Hustin, J.: Proliferating systematized angioendotheliomatosis. Arch. Dermatol., *104*:320, 1971.
68. Shtern, R., and Likhachev, I. P.: Endotheliomatosis as a systemic neoplastic disease. Arkh. Pat., *25*:35, 1963. Cited by Fievez et al.[67]
69. Abulafia, J., Cigorraga, S., Saliva, S., et al.: Angioendotheliomatosis proliferates sistematica (Pfleger y Tappeiner). Derm. Ibero. Lat. Am., *11*:23, 1969. Cited by Fievez et al.[67]
70. Okagaki, T., and Richart, R. M.: Systemic proliferating angioendotheliomatosis. A case report. Obstet. Gynecol., *37*:377, 1971.
71. Madara, J., Shane, J., and Scarlata, M.: Systemic endotheliomatosis: a case report. J. Clin. Pathol., *28*:476, 1975.
72. Scott, P. W. B., Silvers, D. N., and Helwig, E. B.: Proliferating angioendotheliomatosis. Arch. Pathol., *99*:323, 1975.
73. Pasyk, K., and Depowski, M.: Proliferating systematized angioendotheliomatosis of a 5-month-old infant. Arch. Dermatol., *114*:1512, 1978.
74. Hollander, I. J.: Personal communication.
75. Kauh, Y. C., McFarland, J. P., Carnabuci, G. C., and Luscombe, H. A.: Malignant proliferating angioendotheliomatosis. Arch. Dermatol., *116*:803, 1980.
76. Person, J. R.: Systemic angioendotheliomatosis: a possible disorder of a circulating angiogenic factor. Br. J. Dermatol., *96*:329, 1977.

12

Diseases of the Gastrointestinal Tract

Many of the diseases with gastrointestinal and cutaneous manifestations that are included in this chapter have already been discussed extensively in other parts of this book. However, it is worthwhile to briefly review these diseases in relation to their major gastrointestinal features before considering the other important diseases of the gut, pancreas, and liver.

GASTROINTESTINAL HEMORRHAGE

Gastrointestinal bleeding is a common medical problem, and it is not unusual to encounter individuals in whom neither a diagnosis can be made nor the source of hemorrhage uncovered even after careful radiologic, endoscopic, and hematologic studies. In some of these patients, however, a diagnosis can be made by finding characteristic skin lesions, although the site of the bleeding may still not be pinpointed.

Hereditary hemorrhagic telangiectasia is perhaps the most well-known dermatologic entity associated with melena, but the diagnostic lesions may be missed if the patient is anemic. Hence, all patients with melena and anemia should be carefully examined for telangiectasia after adequate blood replacement. For instance, a 65-year-old black male had been admitted four times in four years to the Yale-New Haven Hospital for anemia and melena. During the fourth hospitalization, tiny red spots were seen on the patient's lips after he had been given a transfusion (Fig. 12–1). Gastroscopy revealed identical telangiectases on the gastric mucosa.

Cavernous hemangiomas in the bowel may be the source of bleeding. The correct diagnosis can be made if the skin is carefully scrutinized for the presence of similar angiomas. In some cases the cutaneous cavernous hemangiomas are blue, soft, and compressible and have been labeled blue rubber-bleb nevi.

The main complication of Kaposi's hemorrhagic sarcoma is gastrointestinal bleeding. Usually the cause of the melena is readily apparent because the cutaneous lesions are present. However, in the patient illustrated in Figures 12–2 and 12–3, gastrointestinal bleeding was present for one to two years before the pathognomonic skin lesions developed. The lesions of Kaposi's sarcoma can arise anywhere in the alimentary canal and can often be seen in the mouth (Plate 9*F*).

Necrotizing angiitis involves the gastrointestinal tract and produces

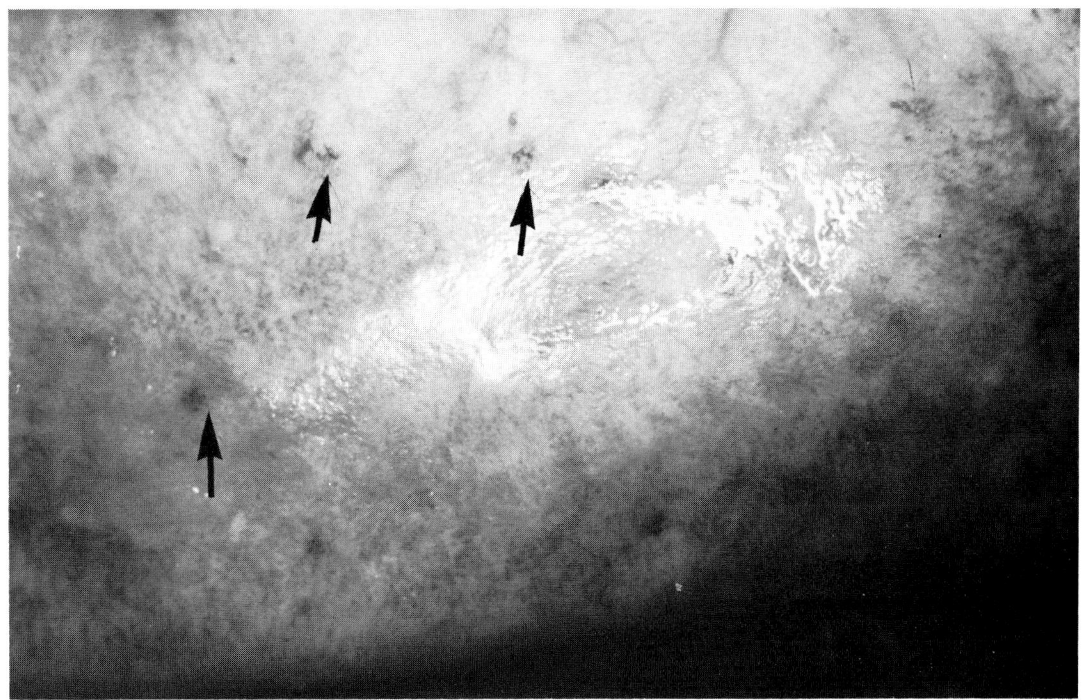

Figure 12–1. These minute telangiectases (arrows) present on the lips were also found by endoscopy on the gastric mucosa.

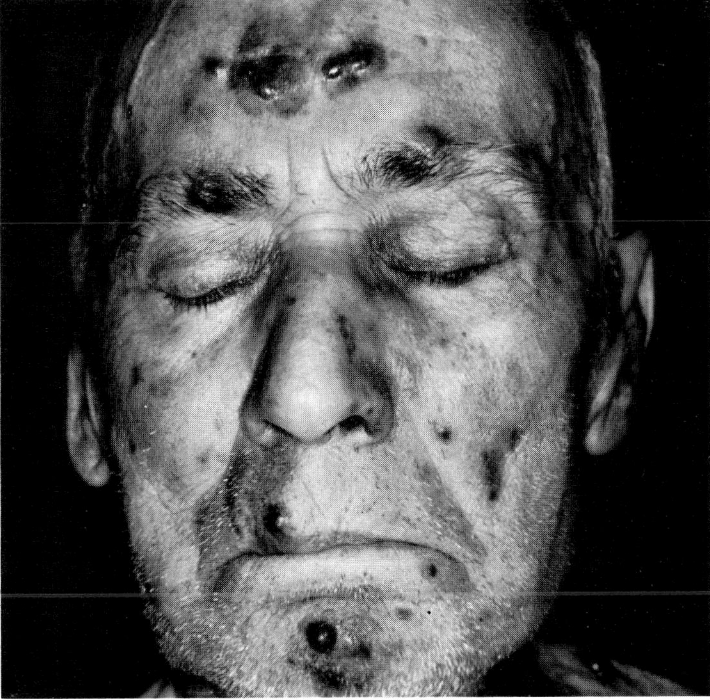

Figure 12–2. Kaposi's sarcoma. This patient had recurrent bouts of melena for almost two years before the cutaneous lesions of Kaposi's sarcoma developed.

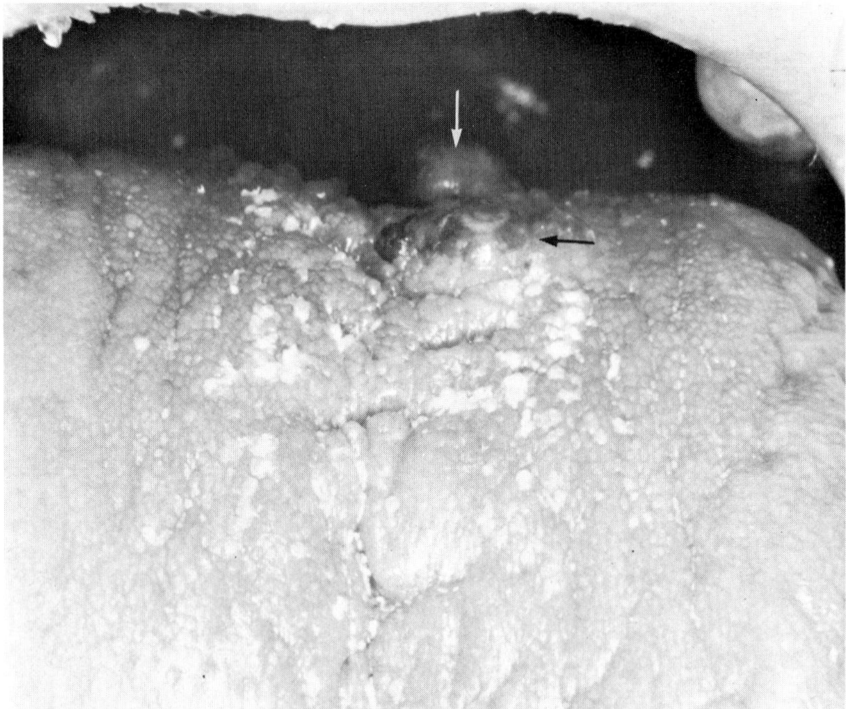

Figure 12–3. Kaposi's sarcoma. Arrows indicate lesions on the tongue of patient shown in Figure 12–2.

melena, diarrhea, cramps, and intussusception. The characteristic accompanying skin lesion is a palpable purpuric spot that may ulcerate. The eruption can be florid or subtle. Its severity cannot be correlated with the intensity of the visceral involvement.

Major gastrointestinal bleeding is also one of the most important complications of pseudoxanthoma elasticum. The diagnostic yellow papules are found on the neck and in the flexures. The abnormal proliferation of elastic tissue responsible for the cutaneous lesions also develops in the retina and produces angioid streaks. Hemorrhage occurs through mucosal vessels in which microaneurysms have formed secondary to abnormalities of the elastic tissue.

GASTROINTESTINAL POLYPOSIS

Intestinal polyposis can be a cause of melena. The polyps also may undergo malignant change, so early recognition of their presence is very important. Familial polyposis of the colon is a premalignant disorder requiring colectomy. There have been no skin markers for this entity except for the reticulated perineal hyperpigmentation observed in one of our patients (Plate 4*D*).

Gardner's syndrome is a dominantly transmitted disease characterized by premalignant colonic and rectal polyps and associated with cutaneous, osseous, and dental lesions.[1] The most frequent cutaneous signs are large disfiguring sebaceous cysts that are found primarily on the face; they may also appear on the trunk, scrotum, and extremities. Banal fibromas and desmoids, which are locally invasive fibrous tissue neoplasms that frequently develop in scars, are other frequent manifestations of this syndrome.

Osteomatosis of the cranium, maxilla, mandible, and sinuses may also produce disfiguring lumps in the skin; or osteomatosis may be detectable only by x-ray examination. The long bones are affected much less frequently. The dental abnormalities include odontomas, supernumerary and unerupted teeth, and dentigerous cysts.

The sebaceous cysts develop at birth or in early childhood. They do not continue to increase in size indefinitely. Fortunately the cysts are evident for many years before the polyps develop. It is unusual to find polyposis in children. However, half of the affected individuals have polyps by the age of 20, which is when malignant degeneration begins to develop. About 50 per cent of persons with this syndrome have developed carcinomatous polyps of the colon.[1] Duodenal, ileal, and gastric polyps may also develop in Gardner's syndrome. In a few patients, carcinomas have developed in polyps arising in the duodenum and in the area of the ampulla of Vater. In two instances carcinomas have arisen in the pancreas. Although colectomy or subtotal colectomy is the treatment of choice in Gardner's syndrome, as in familial polyposis, it may not be curative, because the small intestinal polyps appear to have a small but definite premalignant potential. Similarly, in familial polyposis, there are occasional occurrences of carcinomas of the small intestine and stomach.[2]

The combination of osteomas and sebaceous cysts occurs in no other entity. Multiple sebaceous cysts, osteomatosis, and colonic polyposis all occur as separate familial diseases. The association of multiple sebaceous cysts and premalignant polyposis of the colon — termed Oldfield's syndrome — is another recognized disorder.[3] Are all these entities variants of a single hereditary disease? Any patient with a family history of extensive facial sebaceous cysts should be studied for evidence of colonic polyposis.

Peutz-Jeghers syndrome is a dominantly transmitted disorder characterized by distinctive pigmentation and intestinal polyps.[4,5] In at least 90 per cent of the cases, the small intestine is involved; but in 50 per cent of the patients, the stomach, colon, and rectum are also affected. Polyposis of the nasal mucosa, bladder, bronchus, and appendix has been reported, though not very often. The pigmented spots, noted at birth or in early childhood, are flat and irregular and vary in size from 1 to 12 mm. They are black, brown, or blue; the intensity of the color may be light or dark. The sites of predilection are the vermilion borders of the lips and the oral mucosa (Fig. 12–4; Plate 32*C*); the perioral, perinasal, and periorbital skin; the dorsal aspects of the fingers and toes, especially over the joints; and the palms and soles. Pigmented spots may also develop on the elbows. The facial pigmentation can fade and eventually disappear with age; but the pigmentation on the buccal mucosa, tongue, and palate remain. This mucosal pigmentation is indistinguishable from that seen in black individuals and patients with adrenal insufficiency. In one patient pigmented papillomas were present on the buccal mucosa.[6] Less common sites of increased pigmentation are the palmar areas and the rectal mucosa. Dark linear bands on the nails, identical to those produced by

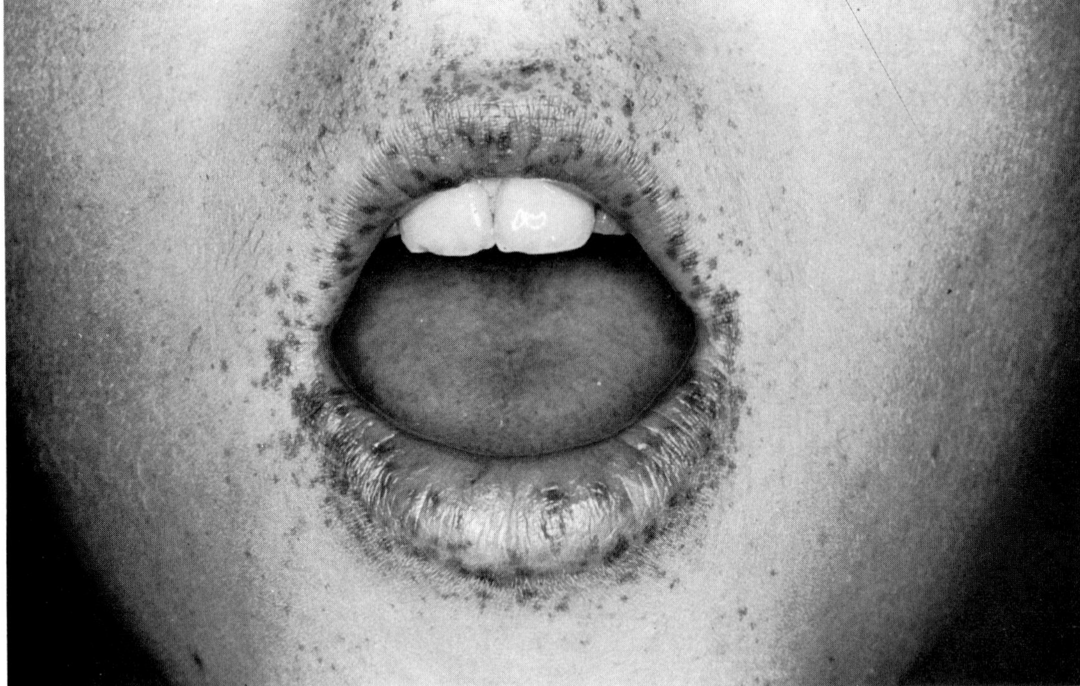

Figure 12–4. Peutz-Jeghers syndrome. Typical perioral pigmentation.

junctional nevi in the nail matrix, were found in two patients.[7, 8] Clubbing is a minor feature of the disease.

Melena and intussusception are the chief complications of the Peutz-Jeghers syndrome and usually develop in the second decade; sometimes, however, they appear in early childhood. The small bowel polyps are considered to be hamartomas, although in the initial reports of this disorder the histologic features of the polyps were misinterpreted as being those of carcinoma. There is controversy over the nature of the large bowel polyps — whether they are hamartomas, adenomas, or a mixture of both existing side by side.[9-11]

There have been case reports of 24 patients with Peutz-Jeghers syndrome who have developed gastrointestinal cancer. Approximately 6 per cent of patients with this disorder appear to be at risk (see p. 89).

The complete syndrome exhibits pigmentation and polyposis, but either feature can exist alone. The prevalence of patients with only pigmented spots is not known and probably varies from pedigree to pedigree. In one family, 10 individuals (half the family members) ranging in age from 8 to 46 years had only pigmented macules.[12] In comparison, all 21 patients in Dormandy's series had demonstrable polyps at the same ages.

Juvenile polyposis is another autosomal, dominantly transmitted disorder that can affect either the colon alone or the entire tract from stomach to colon.[13, 14] The polyps are considered to be hamartomas, although the histology is different from that in Peutz-Jeghers syndrome. Ninety to 95 per cent of them appear in the first decade. These polyps may produce acute or chronic gastrointestinal bleeding and repeated bouts of intussusception, but they are not premalignant. Gastrointestinal cancer and juvenile polyposis have been associated in one kindred. However, the cancers were not related to the polyps in location or in temporal sequence. Not every person with polyps developed a carcinoma, and vice versa.[14] There have been no cutaneous markers associated with juvenile polyposis which might clinically be mistaken for Peutz-Jeghers syndrome at first encounter.

Cronkhite and Canada[15] and Johnston et al.[16] described three middle-aged women who abruptly developed gastrointestinal symptoms and striking cutaneous abnormalities: diarrhea, cramps, weight loss, and sometimes melena, in association with alopecia of the scalp, eyebrows, and body and the loss of axillary and pubic hair. Pigmentation increased on the hands, arms, and face and became accentuated in body folds and palmar creases. One of the women developed buccal pigmentation. In some, the nails were shed; in others, dystrophic changes or onycholysis developed. Benign adenomatous polyposis of the stomach, ileum, colon, and rectum was present. Significant malabsorption could not be demonstrated by laboratory tests, and the patients died six to seventeen months after the onset of the symptoms. Jarnum and Jensen reported three additional cases, two women and one man.[17] The duration of the illness was six to eighteen months in four of the six patients. One woman entered a spontaneous remission even though no therapy was directed toward the polyps; the man recovered following hemicolectomy for intussusception. Protein-losing enteropathy was probably operative in these cases. The duration of the polyposis preceding the onset of the signs and symptoms in these patients is not known. Approximately 45 patients have been reported in the literature.[18, 19] The mortality rate from this disorder has been 75 per cent in women and 50 per cent in men. In four cases, malignant transformation of a polyp or an accompanying carcinoma arose in the colon and rectum.

DISTURBANCES IN GASTROINTESTINAL MOTILITY

Dysphagia is one of the main symptoms of scleroderma and is associated with disturbed esophageal motility. Radiographic examination of the esophagus and results of esophageal motility studies show decreased motility, atony, or loss of peristalsis in the majority of patients with scleroderma, even in the absence of symptoms. Other characteristic x-ray findings include a dilated atonic esophagus with narrowing at the esophageal gastric junction and a hiatus hernia. Esophageal stricture may develop as a consequence of esophagitis that is secondary to chronic gastric reflux. Radiographic examination of the small bowel may show puddling and retention of the barium meal. In the colon, square-shaped diverticula may be found.[20]

Hypomotility of the small intestine may result in stasis and bacterial overgrowth that in turn may produce a state of malabsorption similar to that seen with the blind loop syndrome. Oral broad-spectrum antibiotics are effective therapy for this disturbance.[21] Malabsorption was the first sign of scleroderma in one of our patients. Another patient developed multiple perforations in the descending colon. Prolonged constipation as a result of hypomotility produced pressure atrophy of the colon. The walls were tissue-paper thin.

Although visceral scleroderma occurs without cutaneous sclerosis, usually there are other telltale signs in the skin; cuticular telangiectasia, telangiectatic mats, and vascular spots resembling those of Osler's disease. The appearance of these telangiectases in association with Raynaud's phenomenon are as indicative of scleroderma as is sclerosis of the skin. These signs should be looked for in patients with unexplained dysphagia or malabsorption (Plates 18*C* and 21).

The Paterson-Brown-Kelly-Plummer-Vinson syndrome seems to be more prevalent in Great Britain than in the United States.[22-25] This disease almost exclusively affects women and is characterized by angular stomatitis, atrophic tongue, and brittle nails that are sometimes spoon shaped (koilonychia). Iron deficiency with or without anemia is present in most patients. From those who are normal, one can usually elicit a previous history of iron deficiency and anemia that has been corrected. Dysphagia completes the syndrome and is believed to be caused by spasm that is secondary to iron deficiency. Radiologically, a postcricoid esophageal web (a fold of normal mucosa) appears with swallowing. When the disorder continues for a long time, carcinoma may develop in the postcricoid area. Administration of iron relieves the dysphagia, causes the web to disappear, and cures the mucocutaneous lesions.

MISCELLANEOUS DISORDERS

Epidermolysis bullosa is a genetically determined group of bullous diseases in which minor trauma to the skin results in massive blisters (Figs. 12–5 and 12–6). The skin heals with scarring. In some children having this illness, the esophagus behaves in an identical way. Dysphagia secondary to strictures eventually results. The anal mucosa also may react to injury in the same fashion as the skin.[26] Twenty-one patients have developed squamous cell carcinomas, usually with metastases, in the areas of scarring. In five, the cancers arose on the tongue and in the pharynx, esophagus, stomach, or perianal area. In the rest, the carcinomas arose in areas of skin involvement.[27]

When urticaria pigmentosa involves the intestinal tract with submucosal nodules of mast cells, patients may experience spontaneous flushing, abdominal pain, cramps, and diarrhea. These symptoms of histamine release can also be induced by drinking alcohol and by eating.

Acanthosis nigricans, developing in a thin or muscular adult, almost always indicates the presence of an intra-abdominal cancer, usually of the stomach. Its development in children or in obese individuals is related to endocrine abnormalities or to other factors.

Intestinal bypass procedures for the treatment of morbid obesity have been followed by rheumatic syndromes in as many as 23 per cent of the cases.[28-30] Arthritis, arthalgias, and cutaneous lesions of leukocytoclastic vasculitis have developed. The latter consisted of erythematous papules, vesicopustules, and erythema nodosum–like lesions that arose on the extremities, trunk, and face. The antigenic stimulus for this immune complex syndrome is thought to be bacterial in origin, secondary to bacterial overgrowth in the excluded loop of bowel.

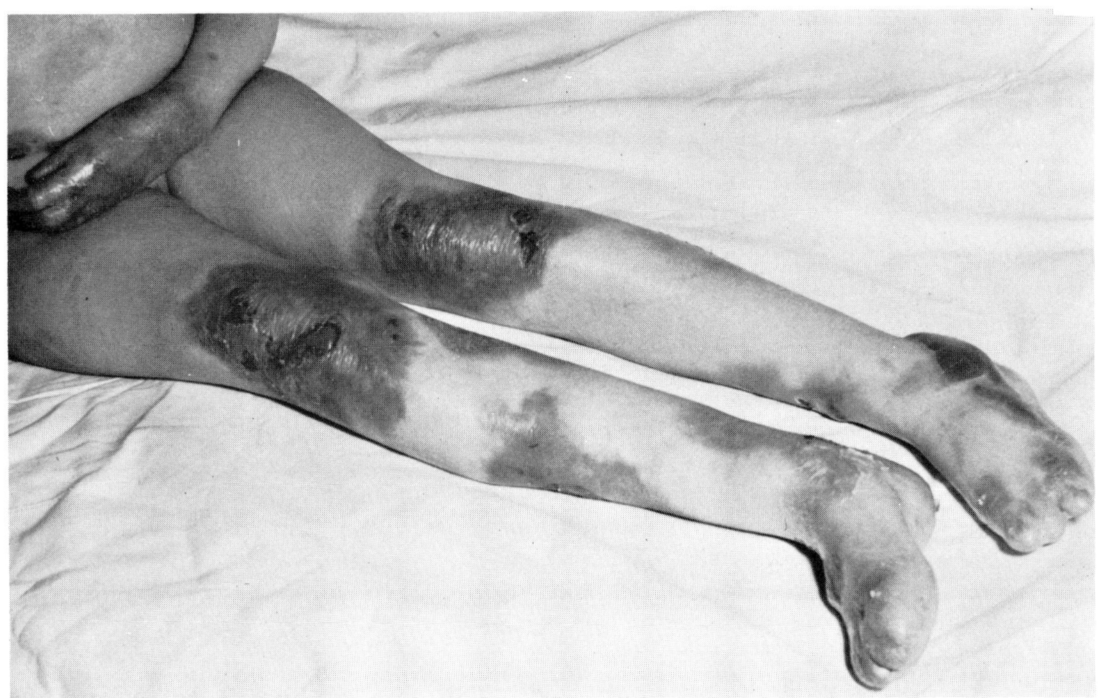

Figure 12–5. Epidermolysis bullosa.

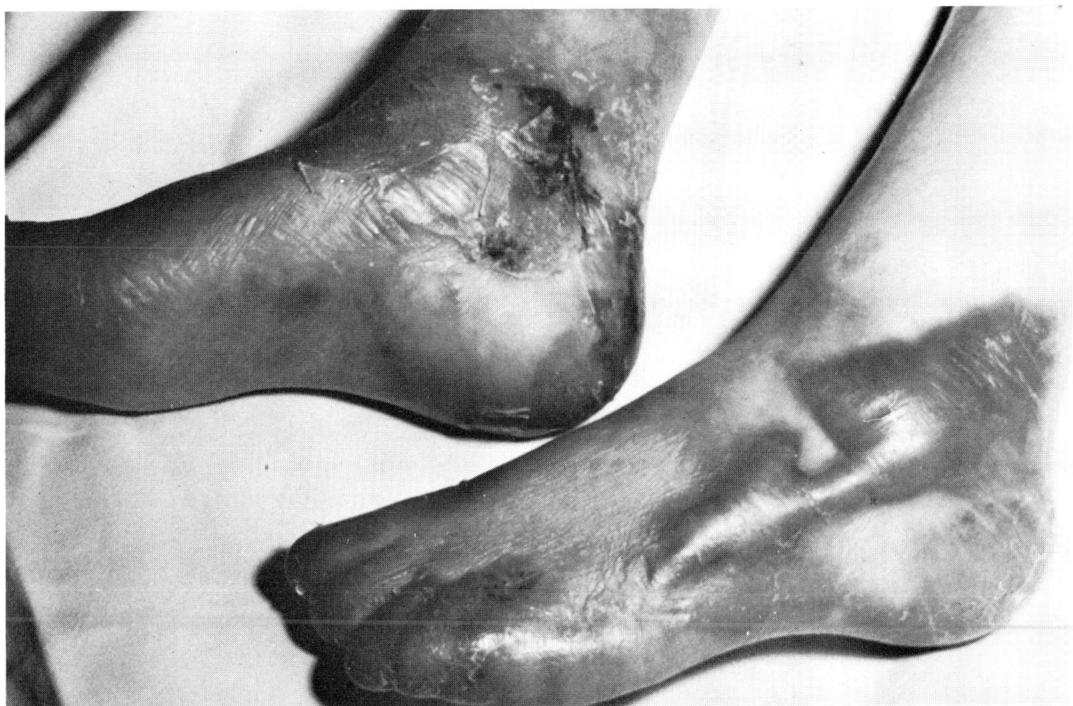

Figure 12–6. Epidermolysis bullosa. Bullae form in response to minimal trauma to the skin. In severe and longstanding instances of this disorder, the fingers and toes often become encased in a web of tissue.

DEGOS' DISEASE

Although Degos' disease (malignant atrophic papulosis) occurs rarely, its cutaneous features are so distinctive and unique that a single picture or verbal description should make the diagnosis of this disorder easy. In addition to the skin, the gastrointestinal tract is the system most frequently involved. The basic pathologic process is an endovasculitis characterized by endothelial cell swelling and proliferation, sometimes in association with fibrinoid necrosis within the intima. Fibrous tissue is deposited between the intima and internal elastic lamina, and thrombosis of the vessel eventually occurs. All these changes happen in the absence of significant inflammation or necrosis in the media or adventitia of the vessels.[31] These pathologic findings in no way resemble those of necrotizing angiitis.

The eruption of Degos' disease evolves as crops of erythematous papules that undergo umbilication and produce doughnut-shaped lesions with porcelain-white centers and slightly elevated red borders (Fig. 12–7, Plate 33*A–D*). Eventually they flatten out to produce brilliant white spots with a surrounding ring of erythema composed of fine palisading telangiectases. In our patient, evolution of the lesions occurred within a week. These spots can be as large as 10 mm, and it is not unusual for several lesions to coalesce and form a clover-leaf-like pattern. Individuals may have hundreds of these spots on the skin.

The histologic appearance of a fully evolved lesion is remarkable. The epidermis is only two or three cell layers thick, and it overlies a

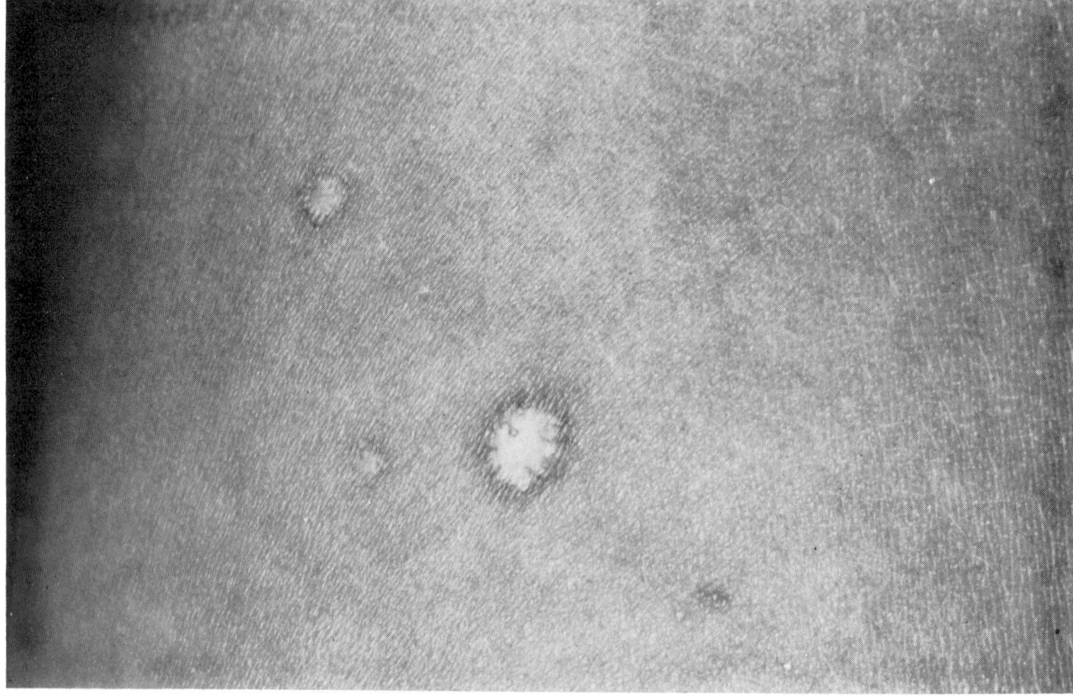

Figure 12–7. Degos' disease. Telangiectasia on periphery of porcelain-white skin spot.

PLATE 33

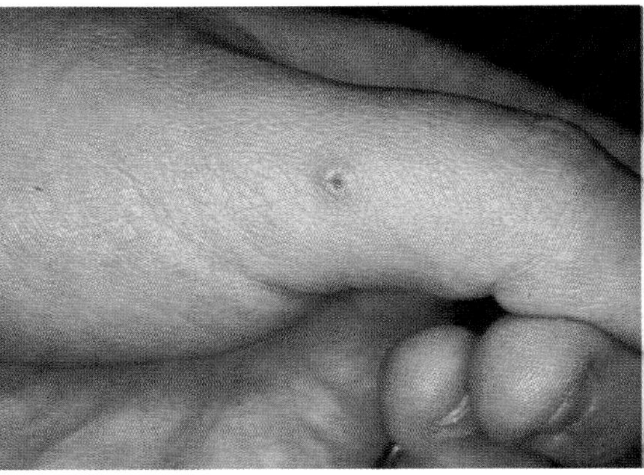

A, Degos' disease. Stages in the development of the diagnostic porcelain-white spot. The initial lesion is a papule.

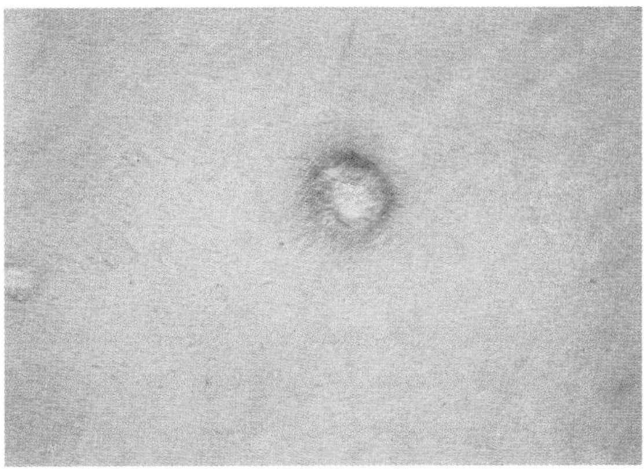

B, Degos' disease. Evolution of the papule into a "doughnut" form.

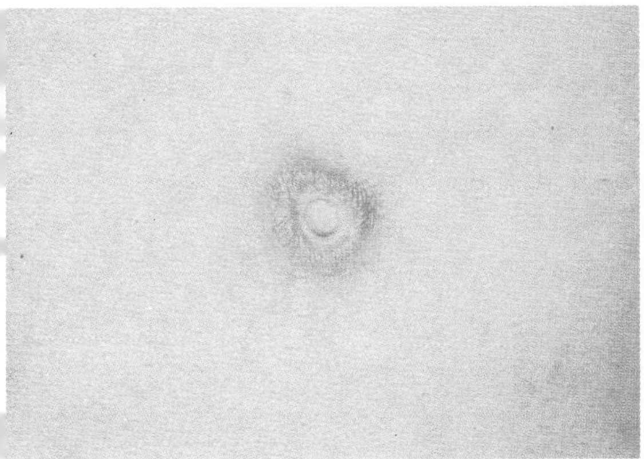

C, Degos' disease. Porcelain-white center developing.

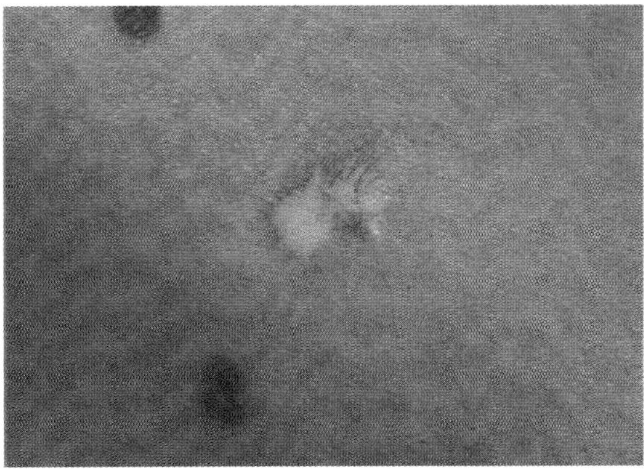

D, Degos' disease. Fully evolved white spot with palisading telangiectasia.

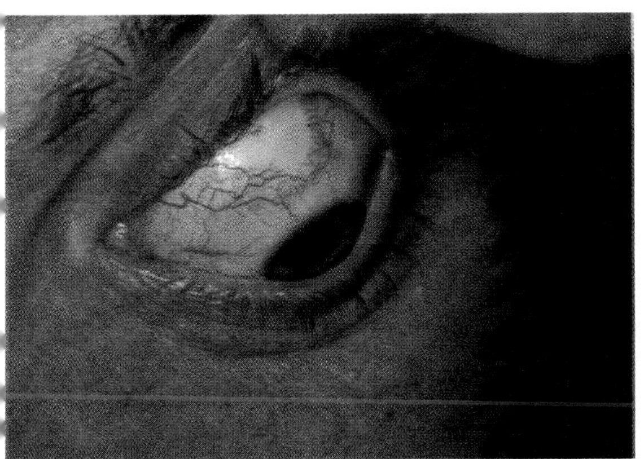

E, Degos' disease. Porcelain-white spot on sclera.

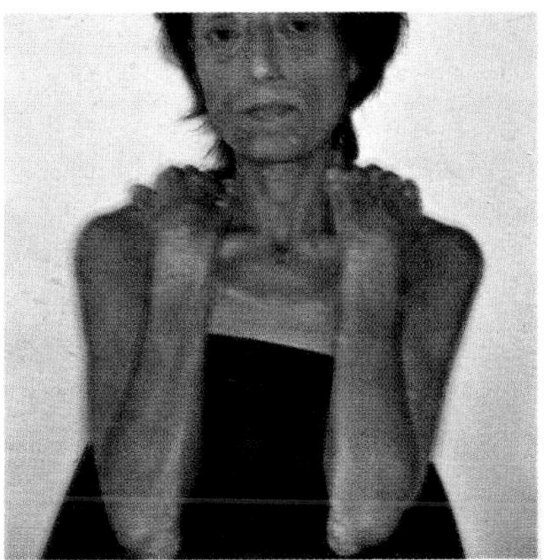

F, Biliary cirrhosis. Hyperpigmentation, jaundice, and pruritus are the important cutaneous signs and symptoms. This patient also had tuberous xanthomas on the elbows.

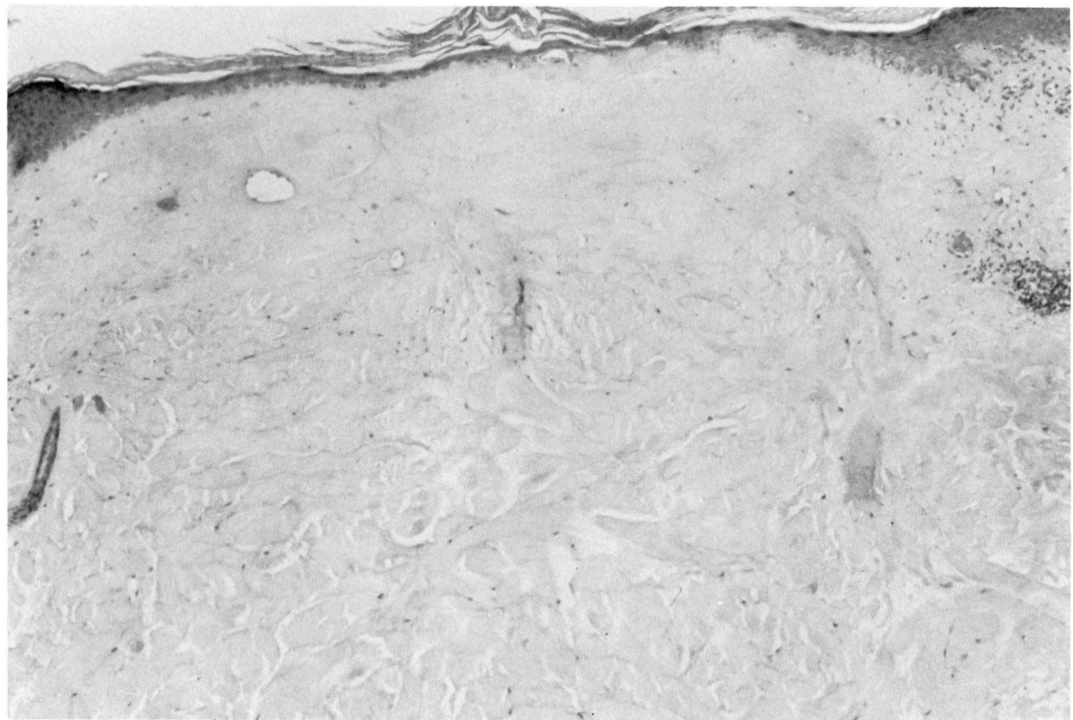

Figure 12–8. Degos' disease. Histopathology of cutaneous lesions. Homogeneous acellular collagen in upper dermis with atrophic epidermis above. Hematoxylin and eosin. × 40.

wedge-shaped area of acellular homogeneous-appearing collagen (Fig. 12–8). It is amazing that these lesions do not ulcerate.

Identical lesions frequently form in the walls of the gastrointestinal tract, and multiple minute perforations eventually develop and produce a fatal peritonitis. Fifteen of thirty patients have died in this fashion.[32-34] At the time these cases were reported, ten of the remaining patients were alive, and three of these had abdominal pain. Three patients have died from involvement of the central nervous system.

The gastrointestinal signs and symptoms include nausea, vomiting, ileus, melena, and severe pain in all areas of the abdomen. One patient had diarrhea with malabsorption. Neurological involvement produces dysphasia, headache, numbness of extremities, ataxia, and diplopia. The cerebral cortex has been involved by white plaques similar to those in the skin and gastrointestinal tract. The heart, kidneys, pericardium, bladder, conjunctivae, and oral and labial mucosae have also been affected in some patients.

Our patient, a 32-year-old woman whose case was reported by Howard et al., had Degos' disease for 11 years.[34] In addition to hundreds of skin lesions, she had retinal and scleral spots (Plate 33*E*). From 1964 to 1967, the skin and eye lesions were the only signs of her disease. In 1967 she began having recurrent pleural effusions that required repeated thoracenteses. In 1968 she complained of abdominal pain for the first time. X-ray studies showed submucosal edema in the duodenal bulb and an ulcerated mucosal lesion in the sigmoid colon. She never developed a perforation of her bowel. Her pleural effusions continued until 1975 when she was readmitted to the hospital because of congestive heart failure and increasing dyspnea. She was again found to have bilateral pleural effusions, but restrictive lung disease and constrictive pericarditis with marked calcification were also present. A pericardiectomy and decortication of the left lung were performed. However she died one month later from congestive heart failure and increasing respiratory insufficiency. At autopsy there was extensive calcification covering the entire epicardium. The lungs were adherent to the diaphragm and chest wall. Calcification was present over all the pleural surfaces. The white oval lesions characteristic of Degos' disease were present in the submucosa of the entire gastrointestinal tract. The brain was free of lesions. The patient of Strole et al. also had pleural effusions.[31]

May reported the case of a 26-year-old man with an acute fulminant illness which led to peritonitis.[33] He had all the general characteristics of Degos' disease, including the histopathologic features, except for one. Instead of following the pattern just described, the skin lesions began as papules that quickly developed black centers and ulcerated. The ulcers eventually healed and left depressed atrophic scars. The small bowel was involved in the fashion usual to Degos' disease. In this patient the cutaneous vascular insufficiency had developed more rapidly than usual, and consequently ulcers, rather than white spots, developed.

Degos' disease occurs about three times more frequently in men than in women. Individuals have lived for as long as nine years before succumbing, but the average duration of the disease is two years. In about three quarters of the cases, the disease has begun in patients 14 to 36 years old; the oldest patient was 57 years old. Some of the patients who were alive at the time of their case reports had had their illness for three to six years.

Approximately 50 patients with Degos' disease have been described since the initial reports by Köhlmeier and Degos et al. in 1941 and 1942.[35, 36] The etiology and pathogenesis are still unknown in spite of extensive histochemical, ultrastructural, immunologic, and coagulation studies in the past 10 years.[37-40]

FAMILIAL MEDITERRANEAN FEVER

Familial Mediterranean fever (FMF) is an inherited disease transmitted by an autosomal recessive gene. It occurs almost exclusively in Sephardic Jews, Armenians, and to a lesser degree, in Levantine Arabs. Sephardic Jews include those who have lived along the Mediterranean coast and as far inland as Iraq; Ashkenazic Jews come from central and eastern Europe. FMF has been described under a variety of names: benign or familial paroxysmal peritonitis, periodic disease, and familial paroxysmal polyserositis. The disease is one and one half times more frequent in men than in women and develops by the age of 20 in 60 to 90 per cent of the predisposed individuals.[41-45]

FMF is the most thoroughly studied variety of hereditofamilial amyloidosis. The amyloid is type AA, and therefore its formation is believed to be a consequence of this recurrent inflammatory disease. Two phenotypes of FMF exist. Type 1, the common variant, is characterized by attacks of fever and short self-limited episodes of peritonitis, pleuritis, arthritis, and erysipelas-like lesions. Renal amyloidosis, which manifests itself as the nephrotic syndrome, eventually develops in at least one quarter of the affected patients. Type 2, a rare variant, is characterized by amyloidosis as the initial or sole manifestation of the disease.[42] Epidemiologic data show that although FMF occurs among Ashkenazic Jews, Sephardic Jews, and Armenians; only the Sephardim run the risk of developing renal amyloidosis.[41, 42, 45]

The attacks of FMF last from twelve hours to two or three days and may recur every few days, weeks, or months without periodicity. Spontaneous remissions can occur, but they are unusual. The attack begins with pain in one of the characteristic sites and is followed by fever several hours later.

Abdominal pain, which occurs in 95 to 98 per cent of the patients, is the most common manifestation of the disorder. At first the pain is localized, but it soon spreads to involve the entire abdomen. The clinical signs and symptoms of peritonitis are exactly mimicked, and radiographic films of the abdomen show the findings characteristic of peritonitis. When a laparotomy is performed the surgeon may find a normal or hyperemic peritoneum and sometimes a small amount of cloudy fluid in the abdominal cavity. The fluid is sterile on bacteriologic culture and is composed chiefly of neutrophils. The abdominal pain subsides within one or two days after the fever has abated. Intestinal adhesions never develop.

When chest pain is a feature of the attack, pleurisy is simulated. A small pleural effusion, also composed of neutrophils, is often seen on chest x-ray. Within a day after the attack has subsided, the effusion disappears.

Joint involvement is usually manifested as an asymmetric monoarthritis. However, polyarthralgias and polyarthritis can occur. The knee, ankle, hip, and shoulder are most frequently affected. The arthritis is characterized by effusion, heat, tenderness, and loss of mobility. Usually the attack of arthritis abates within one week, but it sometimes persists for weeks or months. In spite of swelling and immobility for long periods, the joint returns to its normal state; chronic disability does not result. Histologic examination of the synovium during an attack shows the same acute inflammation seen in the histologic sections of the peritoneum: acute vasodilatation, edema, and perivascular collections of neutrophils.

Some of the cutaneous lesions associated with an attack are unique. Sharply demarcated red patches that are hot, tender, and edematous and that occur on the calves, around the ankles, and on the dorsa of the feet are the lesions seen most frequently. This eruption has been called erysipelas-like erythema. It may be the sole manifestation of an attack, or it may accompany the arthritis. Siguier et al. reported a case of a patient who developed intense back pain during an acute episode of FMF, and shortly thereafter a vast sheet of "cellulitis" appeared over the lower half of the back.[46] The attack terminated within a few hours. Sohar et al. noted that the erysipelas-like erythema and brief synovial attacks involving the legs are sometimes precipitated by prolonged standing, walking, or minor trauma to the extremity.[42]

Urticaria, rather than painful erythematous lesions, can arise during attacks of FMF. Subcutaneous nodules have also been observed in acute

Table 12–1. Ethnic Groups Affected by FMF

Series	New York City (Siegal)	Israel (Sohar et al.)	World (Sohar et al.)	Israel (Ehrenfeld et al.)	Lebanon (Reimann et al.)
Number of patients	50	470	345	55	72
Ethnic groups					
Ashkenazim	38	10	3	10	0
Sephardim	4	455	181	45	0
Armenians	7	0	87	0	49
Maltese	1	0	0	0	0
Arabs (Levantine)	0	5	36	0	23
Non-Jews	–	–	22*	–	–
Jews	–	–	16**	–	–

*Countries represented: France, Italy, Greece, Sweden, Spain, Turkey, Iran, and Holland.

**No information provided concerning origin or countries represented.

episodes, and histologic examination of these lumps is said to show only a nonspecific panniculitis. Azizi and Fisher have demonstrated that the histologic findings in the erysipelas-like erythema are identical to those found in peritoneal and synovial tissues biopsied during an attack: acute inflammation manifested by vasodilatation, edema, and perivascular collection of neutrophils.[47] The histologic basis of the urticaria is unknown. In some patients, purpura has been a manifestation during an attack.[43] The etiology and pathogenesis of the purpura are also unknown. The cutaneous manifestations of FMF need to be reevaluated histologically, especially with respect to the role of the neutrophil.

Sohar et al. noted that Schönlein-Henoch purpura occurred during childhood in 17 of 470 patients with FMF.[42] Rotem and Federgruen made similar observations.[48] The significance of this association, if any, has not been determined.

Table 12–1 summarizes the ethnic background of patients with FMF. Included in this table are cases culled from the literature by Sohar and associates.[42] The disease is far more common in Sephardim than in Ashkenazim in Israel, even though the Sephardic Jew and the Ashkenazic Jew are represented in approximately equal numbers in the overall Israeli population. The 22 cases of FMF among non-Jews are distributed among persons from Greece, Italy, France, Spain, Holland, Sweden, Turkey, and Iran. Only Levantine Arabs have been affected. Type 1 FMF has not been diagnosed among Iranian or Yemenite Jews, but type 2 was discovered in an Iranian. The Jews in the United States are predominantly Ashkenazim.

Some of the clinical features of FMF in the New York patients described by Siegal are different from those reported in Israelis by Sohar et al. (Table 12–2). Only 6 of the 50 patients in Siegal's series had cutaneous lesions, urticaria being the type of eruption seen.[41] The erysipelas-like erythema never appeared. However, in 45 per cent of Sohar's 470 patients, the cutaneous lesions were those of the erysipelas-like erythema, and urticaria did not occur. Joint involvement was more common in Sohar's patients. Splenomegaly occurred in 40 per cent of the patients in Sohar's series but in only 10 per cent of Siegal's patients.

Table 12–2. SIGNS AND SYMPTOMS IN FMF

Series	New York City (Siegal)	Israel (Sohar et al.)	Israel (Ehrenfeld et al.)
Number of patients	50	470	55
Signs and symptoms (in per cent)			
Peritonitis	98	95	98
Pleuritis	68	40	38
Arthritis	24	78	31
Skin lesions	12*	45**	8***
Splenomegaly	10	40	40
Renal amyloidosis	2	27	7

*Urticaria, only.
**Erysipelas-like erythema, only.
***Purpura, erythema, and subcutaneous nodules.

However, these latter patients were composed of Sephardic Jews, Armenians, and one Maltese.

The most important difference between the two series is the prevalence of renal amyloidosis, which is the cause of death in FMF. Only one patient in Siegal's series died of renal insufficiency, and he was a Sephardic Jew. The three other Sephardim in his series were 18, 30, and 38 years old at the time they were last studied. By contrast, in Sohar's series 27 per cent of the patients have thus far developed amyloidosis, and half of them succumbed to renal insufficiency by age 40. Only 10 per cent of Sohar's patients who died from renal amyloidosis lived past 40 years of age.

It seems that Ashkenazic Jews have a better prognosis with FMF because of the apparent freedom from renal amyloidosis. FMF behaves as a relatively benign disease in the United States, since the Sephardim constitute a minority of the Jewish population. Among the 100 Armenians with FMF living in California, eight exhibited erysipelas-like erythema, but none developed renal amyloidosis.[45]

ACRODERMATITIS ENTEROPATHICA

Acrodermatitis enteropathica is another uncommon disease, but it too has distinctive features that should make the diagnosis easy. As of 1965, about 180 cases had been reported in the literature.[49] This illness usually appears from two weeks to 20 months after birth, but at least three individuals have developed the disease as late as four and seven and one-half years. It often develops after weaning. Three individuals were not diagnosed until adulthood; however, careful inquiry revealed that the disease was present in a mild fashion in these latter three patients since early childhood. Boys and girls are equally affected by this disorder. In many instances, the disease was probably recessively transmitted, since siblings, never parents, were affected.[50, 51]

The cutaneous lesions involve the periorificial areas — mouth, nose, eyes, ears, and perineum — the extensor surfaces of the major joints, fingers, and toes; and the scalp (Figs. 12–9 and 12–10; Plate 34). The

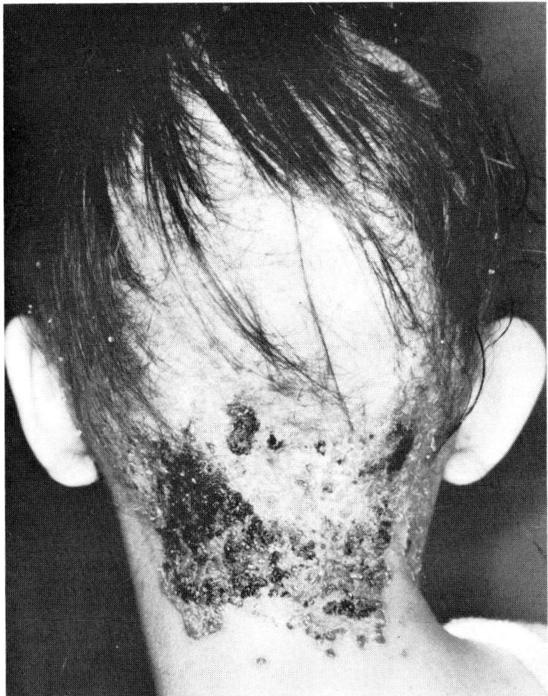

Figure 12–9. Acrodermatitis enteropathica. Alopecia with typical eruption.

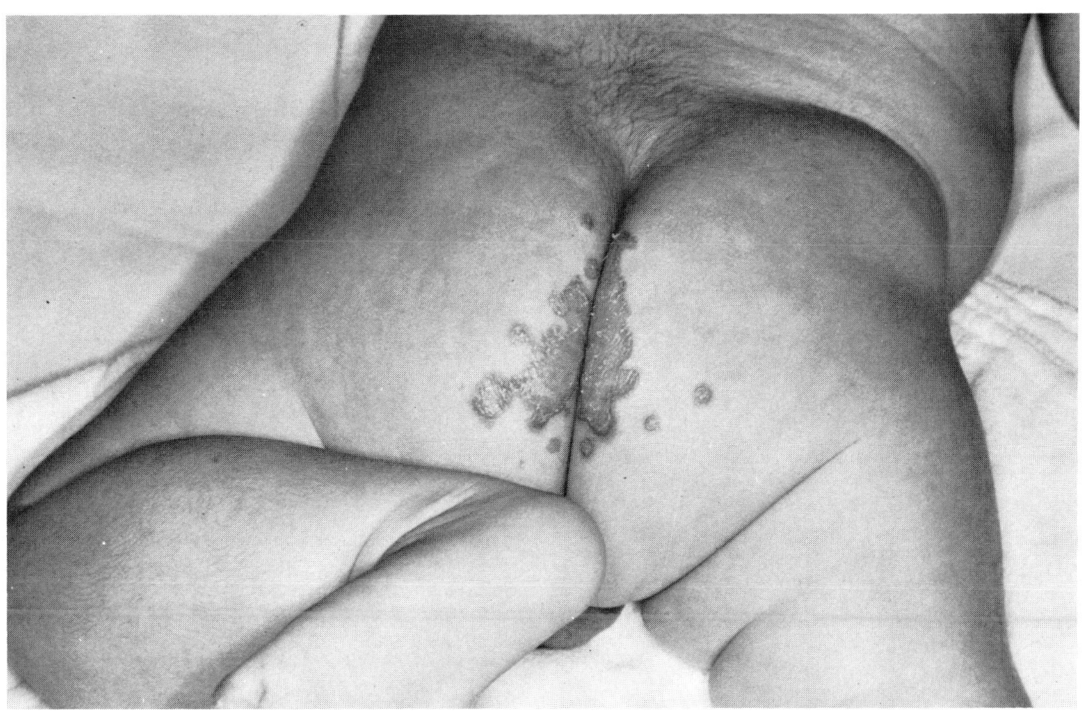

Figure 12–10. Acrodermatitis enteropathica. Characteristic perineal eruption.

PLATE 34

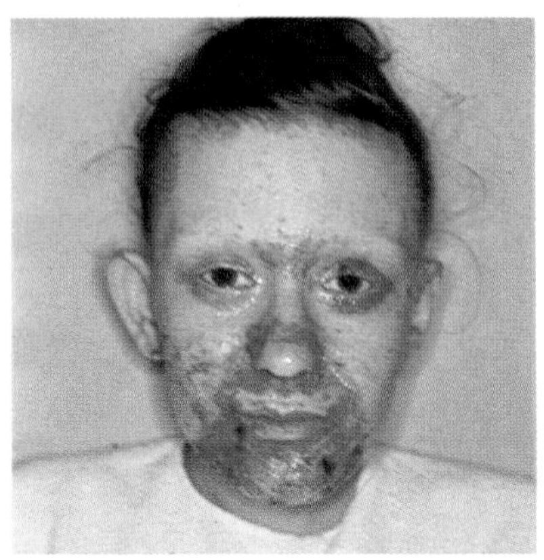

A, Acrodermatitis enteropathica. Typical periorificial eruption.

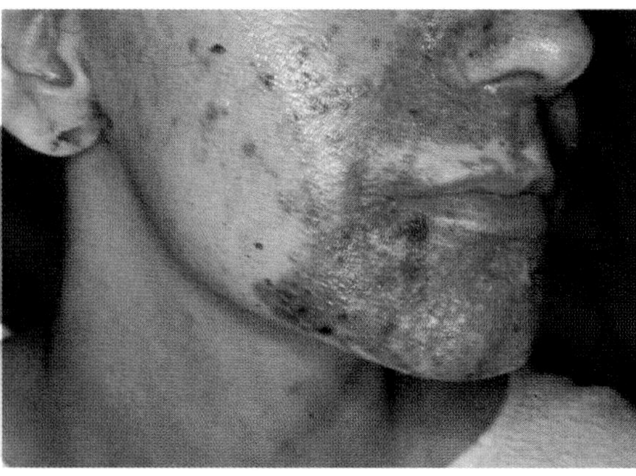

B, Acrodermatitis enteropathica. Close view of eruption in *A*.

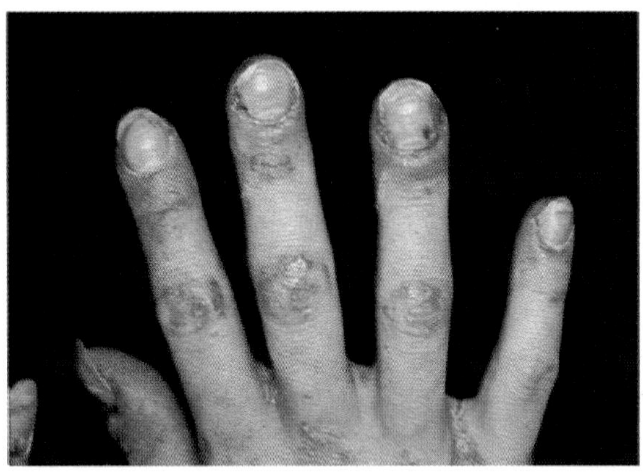

C, Acrodermatitis enteropathica. Involvement of fingers mimics candidiasis.

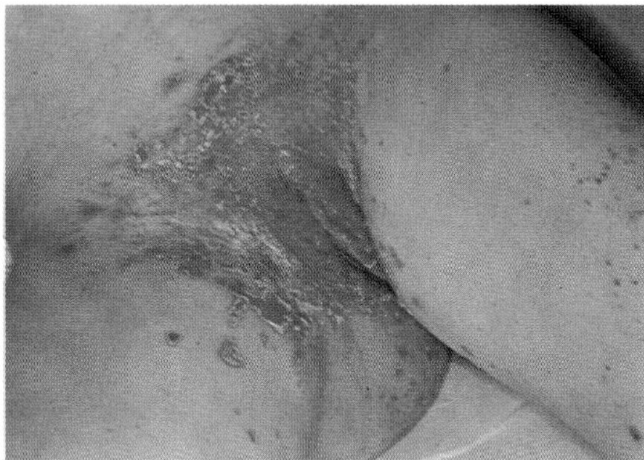

D, Acrodermatitis enteropathica. Perineal involvement also mimics candidiasis.

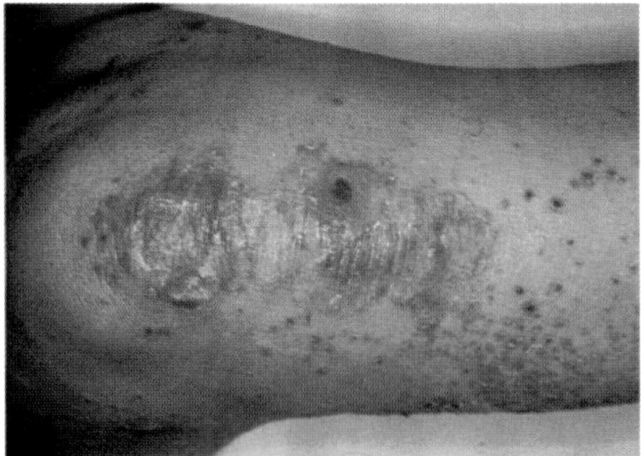

E, Acrodermatitis enteropathica. The initial lesions are erythematous macules and vesicles, which are shown here on the knees.

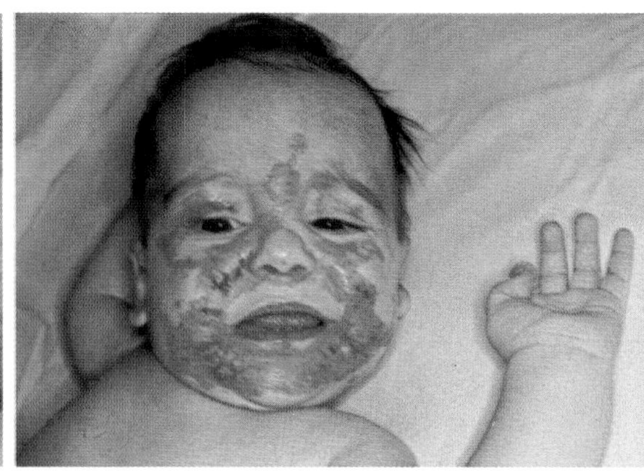

F, Acrodermatitis enteropathica in a 12-week-old male infant.

tongue and the buccal mucosa can also be affected. The basic lesion is a vesicobullous eruption arising from an erythematous base. The blisters quickly collapse, and discrete plaques with varying amounts of scale develop at these sites. Exudation sometimes is present. When the fingers and toes are involved there is marked erythema and swelling of the paronychial tissues, and the nails are transversely grooved and often lifted up by subungual thickening. The tongue and the buccal mucosa may be covered with white patches. Alopecia results when the scalp is involved.

The clinical picture is identical to that of either severe candidiasis or pustular psoriasis, depending upon the areas that are affected. *Candida albicans* has been isolated from the skin and mucosal lesions in 20 per cent of the cases, but this isolation is believed to represent a secondary infection and not a primary etiologic factor. Discrete bright red scaly plaques in the periorificial areas are markers of this disease.

Most children with this illness suffer from diarrhea, and in a few patients, the stools have resembled those of sprue. Before the advent of successful therapy with diiodohydroxyquin, human milk, and zinc, the weight loss and emaciation that accompanied the diarrhea predisposed the debilitated youngster to pneumonitis and death. Body growth is retarded, and personality changes develop. Depression, irritability, and slow cerebration are frequently observed in patients with acrodermatitis. These symptoms promptly disappear with diiodohydroxyquin and zinc therapy.[51, 53] Although the disease is usually lethal when untreated, eight cases have been reported in which untreated individuals survived into the fourth and fifth decades.[51] In some, the course was marked by permanent remission at puberty, and in others by fluctuation with long symptom-free intervals of months to years. In at least four patients, the disease flared with pregnancy and remitted post partum.[51, 54, 55] In one untreated woman, Parkinsonism developed prematurely at age 37, raising the possibility that prolonged zinc deficiency was responsible.[51]

Neither of our patients with acrodermatitis enteropathica has suffered from diarrhea. One patient is a 36-year-old woman who was first diagnosed at age 21, although the history revealed that she had had recurrent episodes of the eruption since early childhood. Major exacerbations occurred with her two pregnancies.

Our other patient is a 13-year-old boy whose disorder began at five weeks and was diagnosed at twelve weeks. His illness was well controlled with small doses of diiodohydroxyquin administered three or four days each month (Fig. 12–11). He is currently controlled by zinc sulfate taken twice a week. The mother was able to anticipate the monthly flare-up one or two days ahead because the youngster always became irritable and developed a foul breath, flatulence, increased salivation, and perianal erythema.

Before 1973, three pathogenetic mechanisms had been proposed for acrodermatitis: absorption of a dietary protein that had been rendered toxic by incomplete digestion; disordered metabolism of tryptophane; and defective interconversion of the unsaturated fatty acid linoleic acid to arachidonic acid.[56, 57] Modifications of this last hypothesis in conjunction with zinc deficiency currently best explain the pathogenesis of acroder-

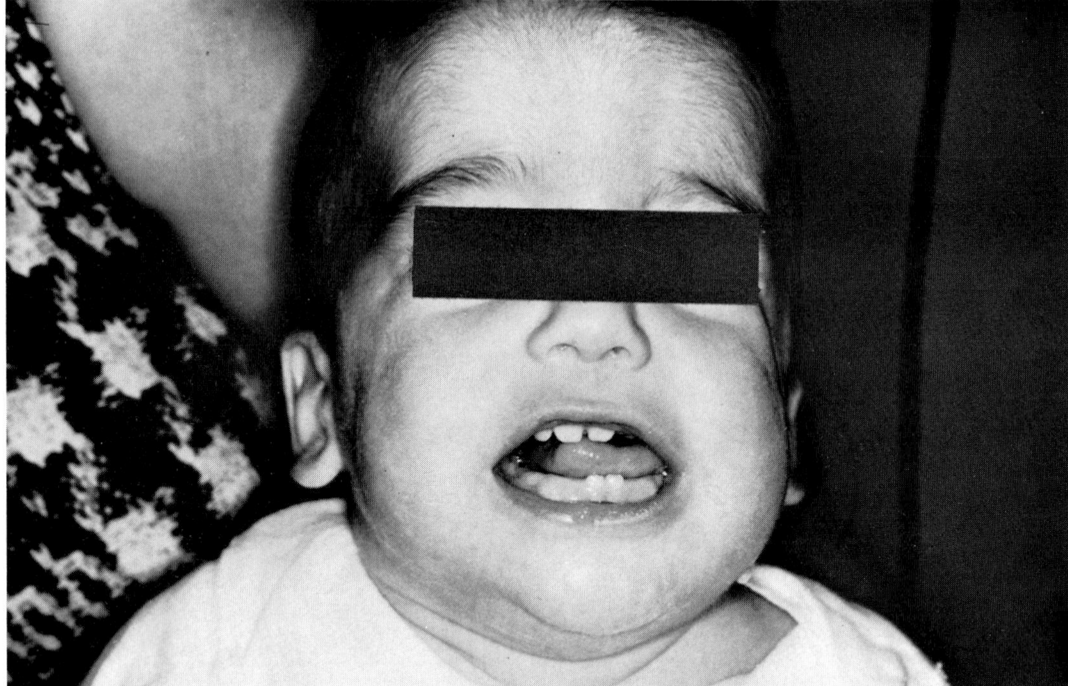

Figure 12–11. Acrodermatitis enteropathica. Same patient shown in Plate 34*F* two weeks after Diiodoquin therapy.

matitis. Linoleic acid deficiency appears to be important. In severe forms of the disease, the level of linoleic acid in the skin is low[58]; within 48 hours after intravenously administered linoleic acid, there is marked clinical improvement; orally administered arachidonic acid can restore abnormally low serum levels to normal, but produces no beneficial clinical response[56]; and successful treatment with diiodohydroxyquin restores the serum levels of linoleic acid to normal.[58] These data strongly suggest that linoleic acid is more important than arachidonic acid in the pathogenesis of the cutaneous eruption. However, the role, if any, of the defects in the metabolic interconversion of linoleic and linolenic acids to their more unsaturated forms in the pathogenesis of acrodermatitis has not been determined. Diiodohydroxyquin has been a specific remedy in almost every case. Although this chemical is poorly absorbed from the gut, it has a clear-cut therapeutic effect upon the skin, psyche, and gastrointestinal tract within seven to ten days (Fig. 12–11). Human milk is also effective therapy, but it is not helpful in every case and works more slowly.

In 1973, Moynahan and Barnes discovered that serum levels of zinc were markedly reduced in patients with acrodermatitis.[59] Small doses of zinc sulfate taken orally produced a dramatic response. Other workers have confirmed the observation that acrodermatitis is a syndrome related to zinc deficiency because of poor intestinal absorption.[60, 61] Evans and Johnson have proposed that the impaired absorption is related to inadequate levels of a zinc binding factor that is secreted by the pancreas.[62]

This zinc binding factor is present in *human* but not cow's milk and has been shown to be picolinic acid (pyridine-2-carboxylic acid).[63]

However, exceptional patients have been described in whom the serum levels of zinc were normal or borderline low.[63, 64] We have also seen a case of acrodermatitis with borderline low zinc levels. In all these instances the disease responded promptly to oral zinc therapy.

Diiodohydroxyquin produces a complete clinical response but does not restore the serum level of zinc to normal. The serum levels of zinc appear to remain at abnormally low levels in spite of the disappearance of intestinal and cutaneous symptoms, whether induced by the drug or occurring spontaneously as in the patient reported by Ølhom-Larsen.[51] Diiodohydroxyquin may enhance the absorption of zinc, but obviously not completely. But even following the institution of zinc therapy, complete clinical remissions occur before blood levels of zinc return to normal. The lag may be one to two weeks depending upon the therapeutic dose of zinc sulfate employed.[61] The slow return of zinc levels to normal may reflect slow saturation of body stores of zinc. The flare-up of acrodermatitis during pregnancy is undoubtedly a reflection of demands for zinc by the fetus that cannot be met by the mother.

Kelly et al. demonstrated histologic abnormalities of the duodenal mucosa that resembled those of sprue in three children: loss of villous architecture with flattening of villi accompanied by inflammatory cells in the lamina propria. Diiodohydroxyquin and human milk only partially reversed the bowel abnormalities; zinc restored them completely to normal.[65]

It is likely that the deficiencies in zinc and linoleic acid are intertwined because each produces a rapid clinical response. It is also possible that in some patients there may be an abnormal binding factor that facilitates the intestinal absorption of zinc at a low normal level but does not release it at the peripheral active tissue site. The abnormalities in the interconversion of linoleic to arachidonic acids with potential adverse effects on the subsequent biosynthetic steps to prostaglandins are at the present time of uncertain significance.[66]

Syndromes of zinc deficiency mimicking acrodermatitis enteropathica are now being seen in individuals receiving long-term parenteral nutrition (hyperalimentation) that typically does not contain zinc[67-70]; chronic alcoholics with poor nutrition[68, 70]; and in patients who have had small intestinal bypass procedures for treatment of obesity.[68] Zinc deficiency with the cutaneous manifestations of acrodermatitis can also develop as a complication of regional enteritis.[71] In addition to the typical cutaneous lesions found in acrodermatitis, several other types may be seen in zinc deficiency: generalized and localized eczema craquelè (Figs. 12–12 to 12–16); lesions resembling the migratory necrolytic erythema seen with glucagonoma; and angular stomatitis.[68] Apathy, depression, and irritability may accompany these cutaneous changes. Essential fatty acid deficiencies can produce a similar picture.[69] Histologic examination of the cutaneous lesions produced in these syndromes shows extensive necrosis of the mid-epidermis with production of microvesicles and some acantholysis as found in acrodermatitis enteropathica.[69]

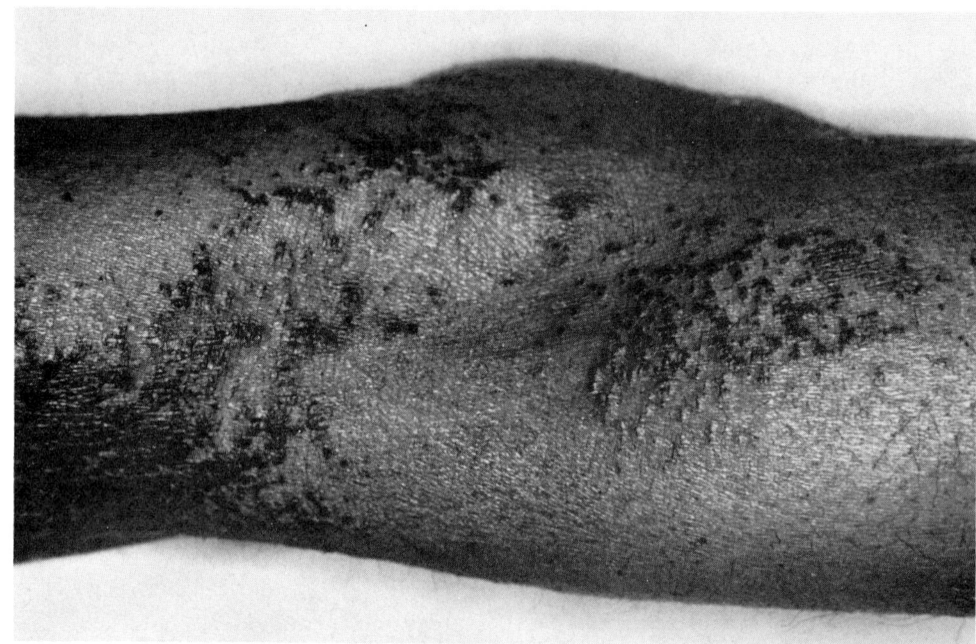

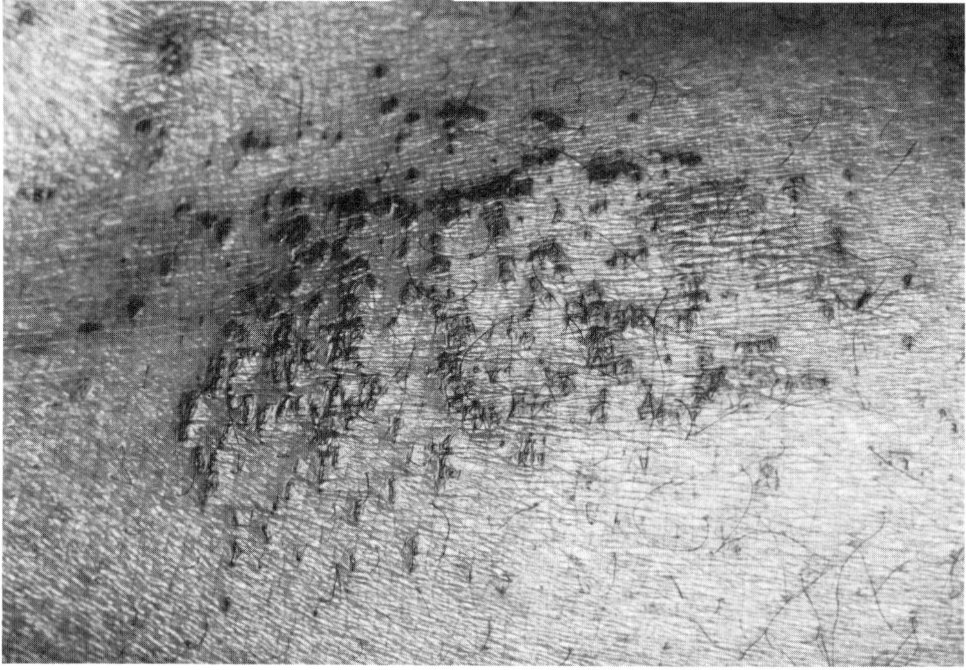

Figure 12–12. Top. Zinc deficiency occurring in patient receiving hyperalimentation. Figures 12–12 to 12–16 show spectrum of lesions in this patient.

Figure 12–13. Bottom. Close-up of lesions in Figure 12–12. Erythema with focal areas of fissuring and crusting.

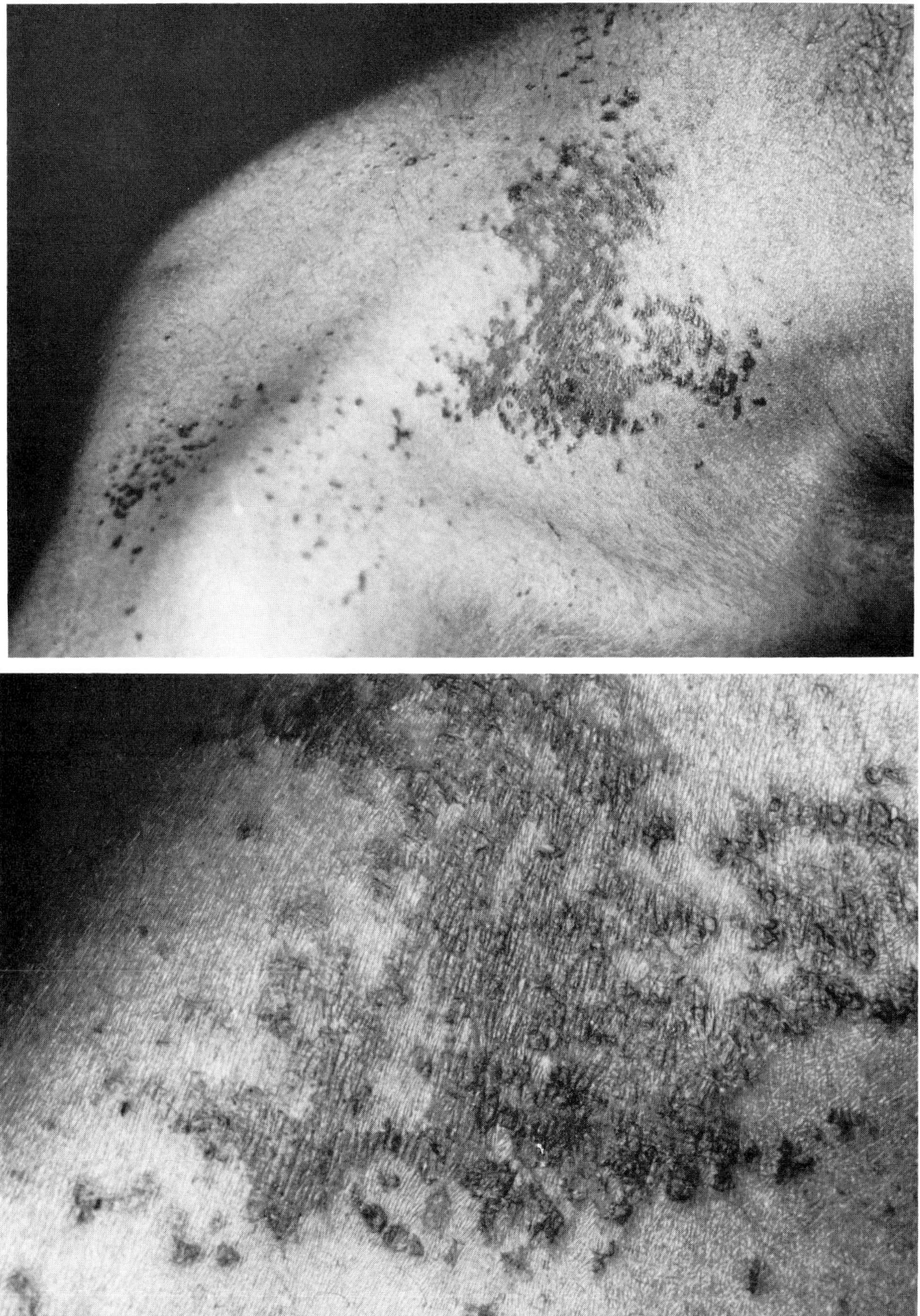

Figure 12–14. Top. Patches of erythema with superficial crusting on neck and shoulder.
Figure 12–15. Bottom. Close-up of Figure 12–14.

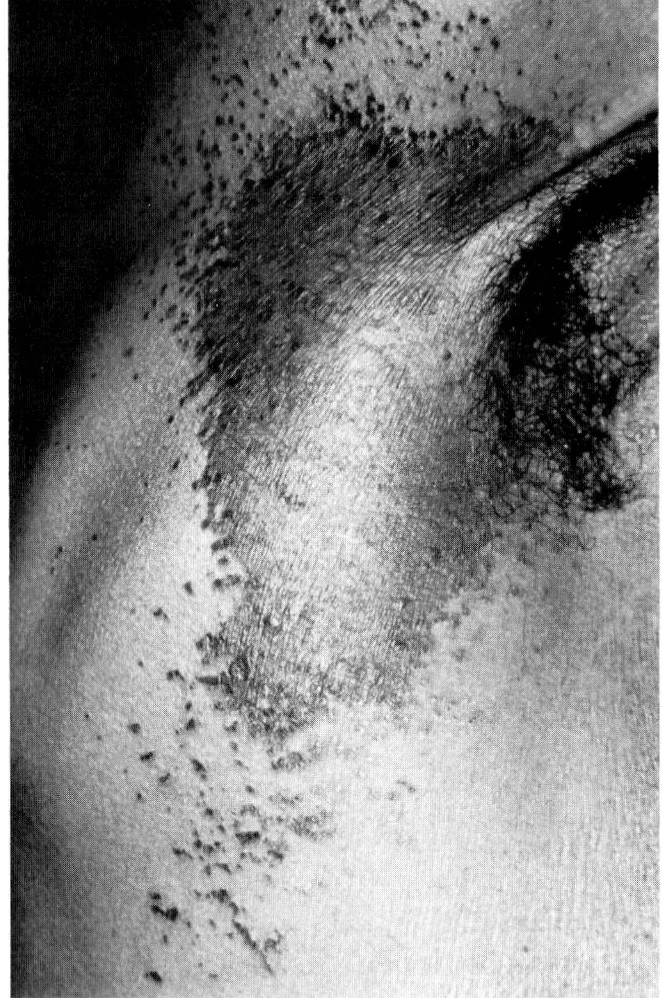

Figure 12–16. Involvement of axillary area.

INFLAMMATORY DISEASES OF THE BOWEL

Inflammatory diseases of the bowel can be divided into two main groups: ulcerative colitis and Crohn's disease. The latter is currently subdivided on the basis of the portion of the gastrointestinal tract that is affected: regional enteritis (ileitis) — small bowel; granulomatous colitis — colon; and ileocolitis — both large and small intestines. Ulcerative colitis is primarily an inflammatory disease of the mucosa and submucosa. In Crohn's disease the entire wall is affected. In 75 to 85 per cent of patients with Crohn's disease, one can find foci of granulomatous inflammation with giant cells in the bowel wall. This histologic picture is loosely referred to as a "sarcoid" reaction by some workers.

Ulcerative Colitis

Skin lesions are found in 6 to 34 per cent of patients with ulcerative colitis; the recorded prevalence depends upon the observer compiling the series.[72-75] One of the most common lesions is aphthous stomatitis (Fig. 12–17). Aphthous ulcers, indistinguishable from the ordinary variety, frequently develop with acute exacerbations of the illness. Erythema nodosum develops in 3 to 10 per cent of the cases and appears almost always during the acute phase of the disease.

Fernandez-Herlihy studied the significance of arthritis with ulcerative colitis in a series of 555 patients.[76] Typical rheumatoid arthritis and spondylitis developed in 46 patients, but in only 6 individuals did joint disease precede the onset of the bowel disorder. The development of rheumatoid arthritis is related to the chronicity of the underlying colitis and can be accompanied by iritis, uveitis, and episcleritis. On the other hand, arthralgias and acute toxic arthritis *are* related to the activity of the disease in the same way as erythema nodosum and pyoderma gangrenosum. Acute toxic arthritis is clinically different from ordinary rheumatoid arthritis. Swelling of large joints occurs with the initial attack of ulcerative colits and remits when the bowel disease remits. This type of joint disease does not remain active during the chronic and relatively quiescent phase of colitis.

Pyoderma gangrenosum, a term applied to ulcers having undermined necrotic bluish margins, occurs in 1 to 10 per cent of patients with active ulcerative colitis.[74, 75, 78] Pyoderma gangrenosum usually begins as a frank pustule, pustular nodule, or rarely as an erythematous nodule that quickly ulcerates and spreads to encompass areas as large as 9 to 12 inches (Plate 32*D, E*) (Fig. 12–18). Individual ulcerations also may coalesce to form larger lesions. No area of the body has been spared by this process.[78-80] In a few patients, pyoderma gangrenosum has developed before the ulcera-

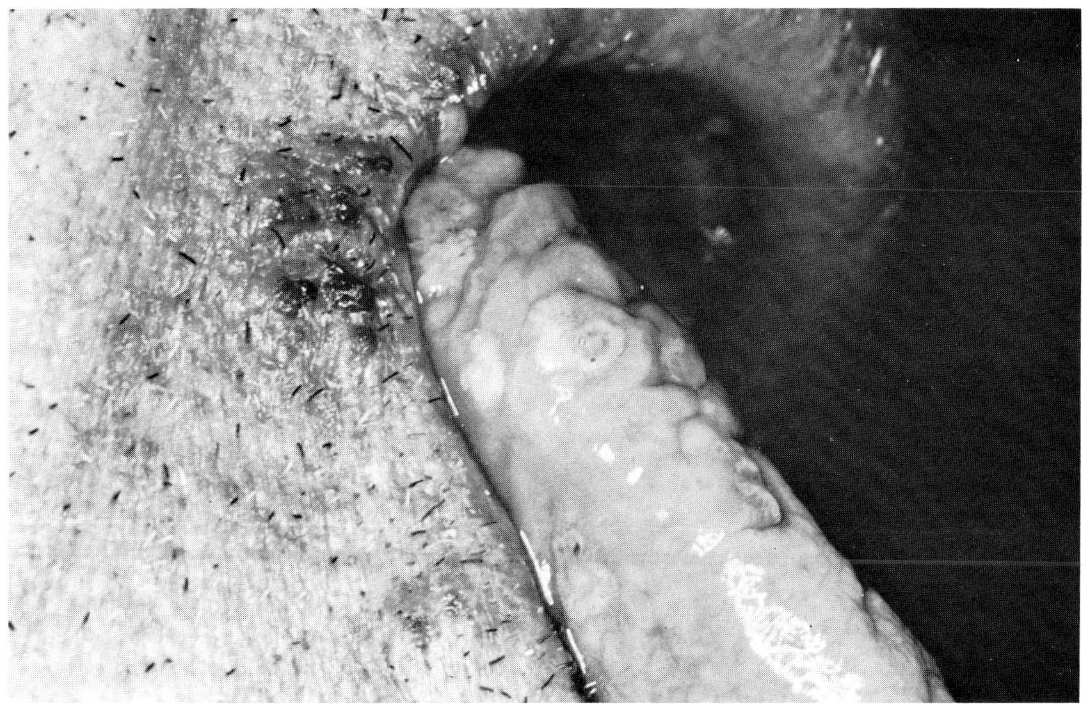

Figure 12–17. Ulcerative colitis. Aphthous ulcers of the tongue.

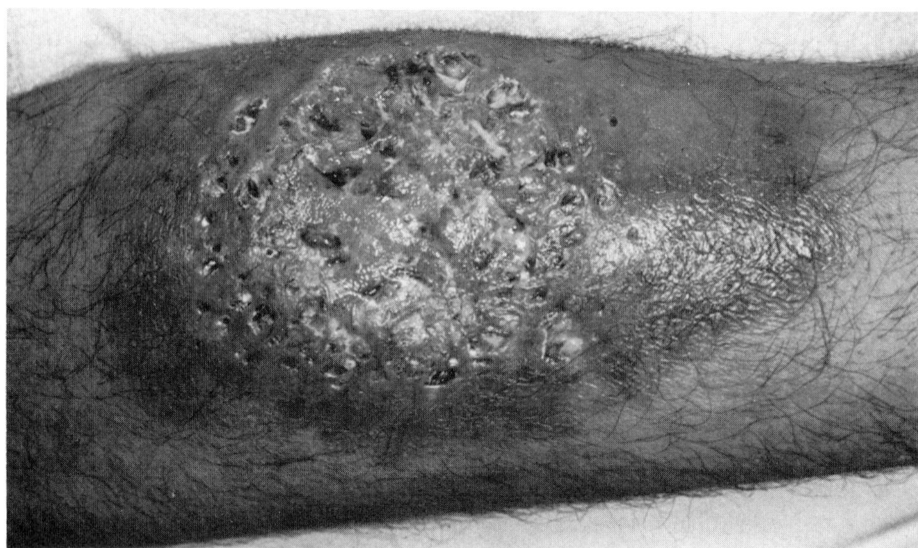

Figure 12–18. Pyoderma gangrenosum in 16-year-old boy with ulcerative colitis.

tive colitis has appeared. Although medical tradition has stated that pyoderma gangrenosum develops almost exclusively during periods of disease activity and can be used as an indication for colectomy, recent reviews have emphasized that pyoderma gangrenosum may arise during periods of remission, and even following colectomy by as long as 12 years.

Other types of pustular reactions can be seen in ulcerative colitis. They relate to disease activity as classic pyoderma gangrenosum does, but they do not always evolve into giant necrotic ulcerations. The inflammatory response in these reactions is probably less violent than in classic pyoderma gangrenosum and therefore less apt to produce extensive ulceration. The histology of these reactions when studied is indistinguishable from that found in pyoderma gangrenosum. A description of these pustular eruptions, which in my view represent variants of pyoderma gangrenosum, follows.

Ricketts et al. reported that in some of their patients with ulcerative colitis, erythematous and papulopustular nodules arose, but then resolved without undergoing ulceration. In some of the patients, vesicular eruptions on an erythematous base later appeared in the same sites, but these lesions also subsided without ulcerating.[81]

O'Loughlin and Perry described painful pustules involving the skin and oral mucosa in two patients in whom the colitis was flaring. The pustules on the skin displayed several patterns: some were in clusters; some arose from erythematous red plaques; and in others red papules appeared first, became pustular, and subsequently sloughed to form small ulcers. Crops of these pustules and papules arose during the time of disease activity and disappeared after colectomy. The histologic features were those of pyoderma gangrenosum.[82]

Basler and Dubin described discrete pustules that enlarged and coalesced into purulent necrotic plaques that later evolved into the typical lesions of pyoderma gangrenosum.[83]

Johnson and Wilson have described identical types of pustular lesions which they called "papulonecrotic lesions" and "ulcerating erythematous plaques." The papulonecrotic lesions began as scattered small red papules that became pustular and subsequently necrotic. The ulcers persisted for several weeks, leaving behind hyperpigmented scars after healing. The other lesions began as red plaques on the shins, which broke down in several places to produce noncoalescing small ulcers that eventually healed over the course of several weeks. Both types of lesions appeared during periods of disease activity, disease inactivity, and even two years after colectomy.[74]

Figures 12–19 to 12–24 show the sequence of these papulonecrotic lesions in a patient with ulcerative colitis. Some red nodules suppurated and became necrotic and others resolved with minor scar formation. This patient had several episodes of this eruption, always during periods of remission. They disappeared each time following a brief course of oral corticosteroids.

Fig. 12–25 shows the "ulcerating erythematous plaque" variety. This patient had a colectomy performed two years earlier. He developed this lesion twice, and each time it promptly disappeared after oral steroid

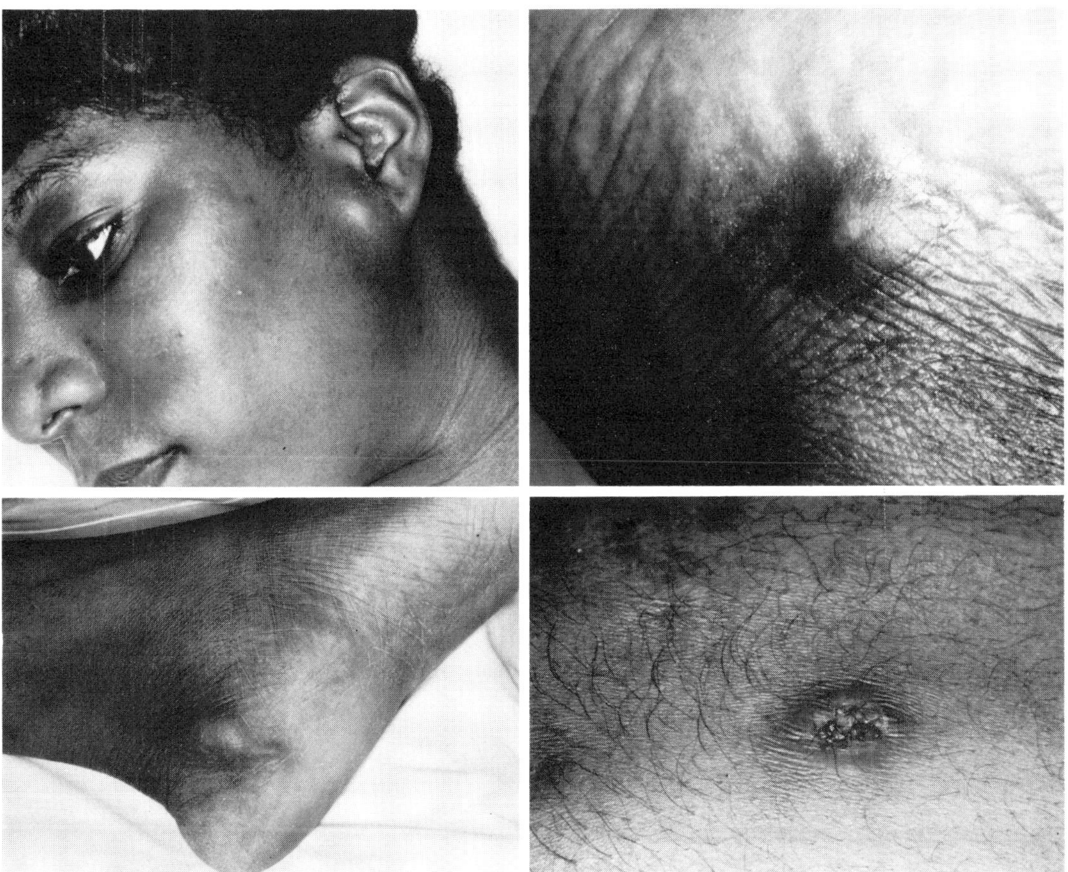

Figure 12–19. Top left. Ulcerative colitis. Figures 12–19 to 12–24 show sequence in development of "papulonecrotic lesions" and "ulcerating erythematous plaques." Erythematous nodule anterior to ear.
Figure 12–20. Top right. Erythematous nodule undergoing suppuration.
Figure 12–21. Bottom left. Erythematous nodule undergoing suppuration.
Figure 12–22. Bottom right. Nodule ulcerating after suppurative phase.

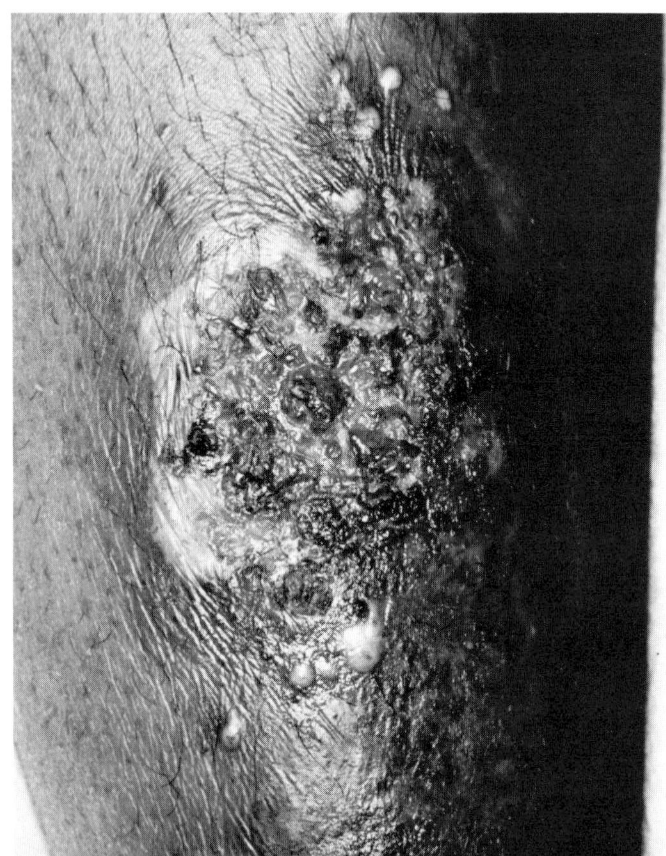

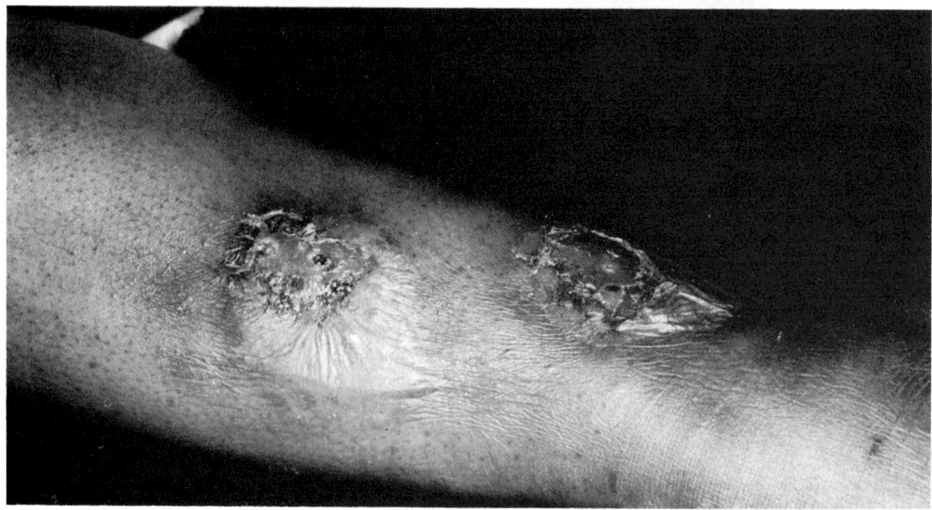

Figure 12–23. Top. Plaque ulcerating after suppurative phase.

Figure 12–24. Bottom. Plaques ulcerating after suppurative phase.

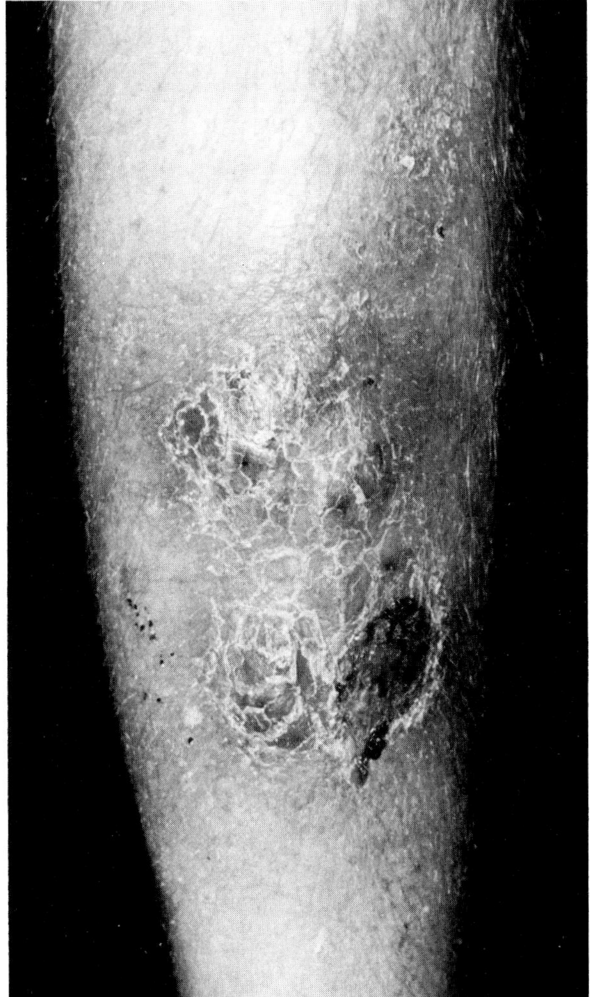

Figure 12–25. Ulcerative colitis. Ulcerating erythematous plaque.

therapy. The histology in both cases was characteristic of pyoderma gangrenosum. There was no evidence of necrotizing vasculitis.

Pyodermite végétante or pyoderma vegetans (Hallopeau) is most likely an exaggerated manifestation of the pustular lesions found in ulcerative colitis. These lesions have a predilection for the flexures, trunk, and upper thighs. They also can occur on the lip, in the mouth, on the palate, and on the palpebral conjunctivae. They begin as groups of pustules, rarely vesicles or clear bullae that break, resulting in the formation of a hyperplastic or vegetating epithelial surface over a boggy red base. The irregular surface of these lesions displays small pustular summits. Fresh pustules appear at the periphery of the vegetating plaques as they slowly expand. Extensive plaques can cover the trunk and abdomen. After months to years, the plaques stop forming pustules, become dry, and resolve, leaving behind hyperpigmented skin. Relapses may occur in the same sites. The conjunctivae show fine points of necrosis that may be followed by an area of velvety papillomatosis. The gums, hard and soft palates, buccal mucosa, and tongue may be similarly affected. The name *pyostomatitis vegetans* has been applied to the lesions when they affect the mouth.[84] One sees numerous closely set papillary projections that are red with small pockets of pus or ulcerations at their apices. In Forman's series, eight of 12 patients with pyoderma vegetans had ulcerative colitis that had developed one to 11 years earlier.[85] No underlying disease was discovered in the other four patients. The development of pyoderma vegetans was not always related to disease activity. In one patient the skin lesions persisted for 26 years. Bloom et al. described a case in association with hypogammaglobulinemia.[86] We have seen pyoderma vegetans develop in a patient with mycosis fungoides (see p. 146).

After reviewing the description and courses of these various pustular eruptions in ulcerative colitis, it appears that they are variations on a theme. They have many features in common, including histopathologic changes, not only among themselves, but also with pyoderma gangrenosum. These papers also emphasize that the pustular lesions can arise in response to disease activity as well as appear during periods of disease remission. They should be viewed as one of the extracolonic manifestations of ulcerative colitis.

The lesions of pyoderma gangrenosum frequently are sterile on bacteriologic culture. The histopathology of pyoderma gangrenosum is nonspecific — acute inflammation within the dermis and around vessels, with secondary ulceration of the epidermis. The bulk of the inflammatory cells are neutrophils. There is no evidence of a necrotizing angiitis. These histologic changes are those of the fully developed lesion complicated by epidermal ulceration. Histologic examination of the earliest phase of the lesion has not been well studied. Dantzig, however, was able to study two examples of pyoderma gangrenosum in its earliest phase.[87] Both showed a dense infiltrate of large and small lymphocytes and other mononuclear cells in the mid- and lower dermis. There was dermal necrosis and invasion and disruption of vascular walls by lymphocytes. This histology is characteristic of a cell-mediated hypersensitivity reaction. As the necrosis evolves and the epidermis ulcerates, neutrophils would be expected to invade the area.

Just as in Behçet's disease, the skin of patients with ulcerative colitis may develop pyoderma gangrenosum in response to trauma, especially that resulting from intradermal injections.

Erythema nodosum and acute toxic arthritis are invariably signs of disease activity and usually resolve after the diseased bowel has been successfully treated medically or surgically. Pyoderma gangrenosum is sometimes a sign of disease activity and in those instances it also disappears after successful therapy.

The term *pyoderma gangrenosum* is properly applied only to lesions that begin with pustules, or less commonly erythematous nodules, that break down to form spreading ulcers with necrotic undermined edges. In addition, the following diagnoses need to be excluded as a cause of the necrotic ulcer: necrotizing vasculitis, mixed bacterial infection producing Meleney's ulcer, iododerma or bromoderma, deep fungal infection, spider bites, and factitial ulceration. Although pyoderma gangrenosum was originally considered to be associated with ulcerative colitis in 50 per cent of cases, this may be a gross overestimate.[79, 88] Hickman and Lazarus found it to be associated with ulcerative colitis in only 1 of 15 patients at Duke University Medical Center.[89]

Previously, I had suggested that the term *pyoderma gangrenosum* be limited to necrotic ulcers in association with ulcerative colitis and the term *necrotic ulcers associated with disease X* be used in the other clinical settings. However, in view of the more recent histologic, clinical, and immunologic data, it is reasonable to view pyoderma gangrenosum as a possible expression of a severe cell-mediated hypersensitivity reaction that can be triggered by a variety of events.

Pyoderma gangrenosum has been reported in 0.5 to 20 per cent of cases of Crohn's disease[75, 89, 90]; chronic active hepatitis[91]; and seropositive rheumatoid arthritis without evidence of vasculitis.[89] It has been reported to precede the detection of acute and chronic granulocytic leukemia and polycythemia vera, as well as developing during the course of these disorders.[92, 93] Pyoderma gangrenosum associated with leukemia tends to be more superficial and less destructive. Bullae may develop on the margin of the lesion as it expands centrifugally. Pyoderma gangrenosum has also been associated with hypogammaglobulinemia and monoclonal gammopathy either secondary to myeloma or idiopathically.[86, 89]

Ayres and Ayres described four patients with pyoderma gangrenosum who had rheumatoid arthritis–like disease and a papulovesicular eruption. The eruption was polymorphous and consisted of grouped symmetrical pruritic flaccid vesicles, vesicopustules, and papules that occasionally were observed to develop into typical ulcers of pyoderma gangrenosum. A biopsy of a vesicle that had not yet ruptured exhibited histologic findings that lend further support to an underlying mechanism of cell-mediated hypersensitivity as suggested by Dantzig.[94] The unopened vesicle revealed a vesicopustule that was partially intraepidermal and partially subepidermal. It contained many neutrophils, lymphocytes, and considerable necrotic debris. There was a perivascular lymphocytic infiltrate throughout the cutis, adjacent to and beneath the vesicopustule.

The histology of pyoderma gangrenosum points to cell-mediated hypersensitivity complicated by a neutrophilic response to dermal necrosis. There has been no evidence for circulating immune complexes thus far.[89] Lazarus et al. demonstrated cutaneous anergy to skin testing in four patients.[95] However, these patients had only a partial deficiency in cell-mediated hypersensitivity because their lymphocytes could be stimulated by phytohemagglutinin and specific antigens to incorporate tritiated thymidine, but not to produce migration inhibitory factor (MIF). Two of these patients were restudied after their ulcers had healed and oral steroids had been discontinued.[89] Their lymphocytes were still unable to produce MIF after appropriate stimulation, suggesting that an abnormality in cell-mediated hypersensitivity might be a primary event in the disease. However, cutaneous anergy was present only in 3 of 11 patients recently studied by Lazarus et al.[89] In at least 50 per cent of patients with pyoderma gangrenosum, the disease is still idiopathic. A defect in cell-mediated hypersensitivity is the most attractive hypothesis offered thus far for pyoderma gangrenosum, and investigations along this line appear to offer the most promise for eventual understanding of this disorder.

Thrombophlebitis develops in 1 to 10 per cent of patients with ulcerative colitis, but in patients examined by autopsy, the prevalence of venous thromboses is 30 to 40 per cent.[96] Visceral venous thromboses are common. Studies by Lee et al. indicate that ulcerative colitis, like disseminated malignancy, is associated with the hypercoagulable state, one facet of disseminated intravascular coagulation (DIC). Lee found that increased Factor VIII activity, the most frequent abnormality in the 16 patients under study, appeared to be correlated with the acute stage of ulcerative colitis and to be responsible for the observed accelerated generation of thromboplastin.[97]

Morowitz and associates reported increased numbers of platelets — 500,000 to over 1,000,000 per cubic millimeter — in six patients with ulcerative colitis, granulomatous colitis, and regional enteritis. In three individuals the bowel disease was successfully treated, and the number of platelets returned to normal.[98] The thrombocytosis is also a manifestation of the hypercoagulable state.

Although the thromboses in ulcerative colitis occur chiefly in veins, Bargen and Barker described extensive arterial thromboses in one patient; and Kehoe and Newcomer reported the case of a young man who developed superficial gangrene of the glans penis during an acute episode of colitis.[99, 100] These latter authors also mention that brachial artery occlusions have been observed in other patients. The rare occurrence of arterial occlusion in ulcerative colitis prompts the inclusion of the following case reports of two of our patients that showed this phenomenon.

The first patient was a 15-year-old boy who developed an indolent ulcer over the right medial malleolus eight months before admission to the Yale-New Haven Hospital. The ulcer began as a "pimple" that broke down and spread. After several months of bedrest and antibiotic therapy, the ulcer healed. However, upon ambulation it recurred. Two weeks before admission to the hospital, the patient developed abdominal cramping and nonbloody diarrhea. The mallolar ulcer measured about 6 cm and was as large as it had been originally. A biopsy of the edge showed nonspecific inflammation; no evidence of necrotizing angiitis was found. Barium enema revealed right-sided ulcerative colitis. Treatment with oral prednisone was begun, and the patient was discharged from the hospital. Within one or two days after the steroid therapy had been started, the patient began to experience pain, pallor, and cyanosis in all of his toes. Over the next three weeks, definite peripheral gangrene appeared and slowly progessed (Plate 32*F*). His colitis also became worse. He was admitted to the hospital for the second time, and a bilateral sympathectomy was performed. Unfortunately, no benefit for the gangrene was realized, and his toes were amputated two months later. Because his colitis did not respond to oral steroid therapy, he underwent total colectomy one month after his toes had been removed. Sixteen days postoperatively, he died of septicemia. Autopsy gave no evidence of necrotizing angiitis in any organ, and no sign of thrombosis was present. Review of the surgically removed toes revealed arterial and venous occlusions in the absence of necrotizing angiitis.

The significance of this first case was not fully appreciated until the second patient came under our care eight years later.

The patient is a 52-year-old man who had developed ulcerative colitis 14 years previously. He was treated at another institution for three months with oral steroids, and his ulcerative colitis had remitted. During the course of the illness he developed gangrenous changes on his left great toe; these cleared spontaneously

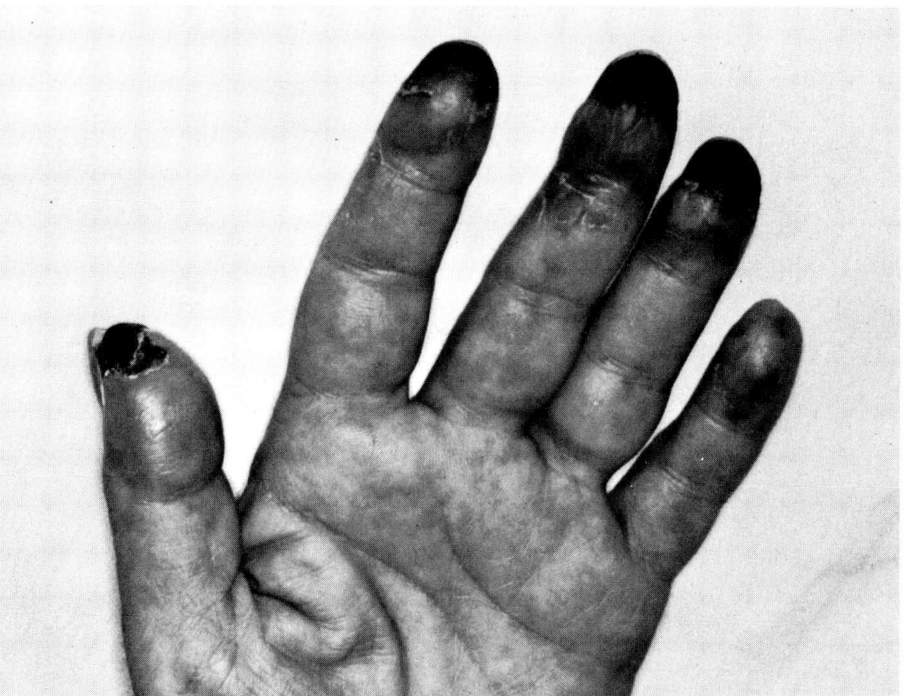

Figure 12–26. Ulcerative colitis. Digital gangrene caused by hypercoagulable state.

and required no surgical treatment. For the next 13½ years his ulcerative colitis remained in remission without steroid therapy. Four months before admission to our medical center, the ulcerative colitis flared. Treatment was begun with oral steroids, and two weeks later the patient noticed numbness and tingling of the fingers on his left hand. During the next few weeks, superficial gangrene of the distal phalanges developed (Fig. 12–26). The patient was admitted for a sympathectomy that proved to be beneficial. Two fingers were saved and the other three required surgical treatment.

Ball and Goldman described a 56-year-old man who developed gangrene of the fingers and toes and cutaneous infarction on the medial aspect of the left knee. Fibrin split products, a feature of DIC, were detected as cryofibrinogenemia in this patient.[101] A biopsy of the hemorrhagic infarction showed thrombosed vessels — the typical changes of DIC.

Crohn's Disease

Crohn's disease can affect the small bowel (regional enteritis), colon (granulomatous colitis), or small bowel and colon (ileocolitis). Perianal lesions, consisting of perianal and ischiorectal abscesses and sinuses, and fistulae-in-ano are found in 15 to 50 per cent of cases.[90, 102-104] *Painless anal* fissures can be found in 50 to 60 per cent.[104] It is not unusual for fistulae to be the first manifestation of Crohn's disease, even though the inflammatory bowel disease may have been mild or relatively asymptomatic. Fistulae have been noted to precede the bowel disease by an average of four years (range, 1 month to 22 years).[105] Although perianal abscesses and fistulae were believed to be an associated feature of ulcerative colitis in 10 to 20 per cent of cases, these observations were made before

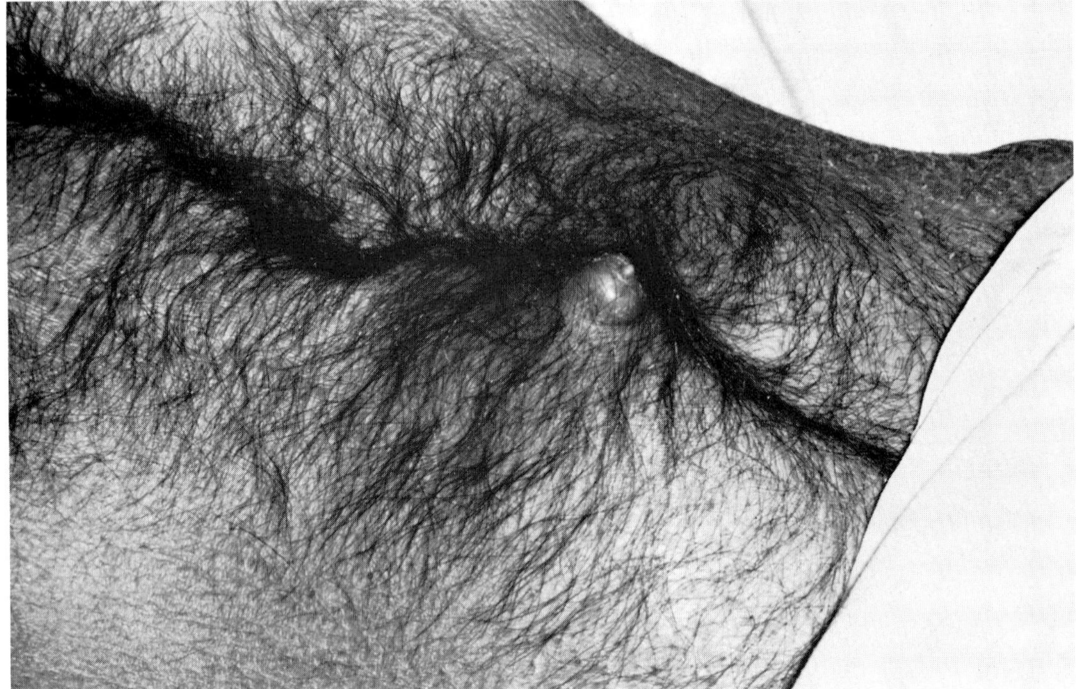

Figure 12–27. Regional ileitis. Fistula from small bowel to abdominal wall.

ulcerative colitis and granulomatous colitis were recognized to be separate entities.[105] Perianal lesions are not a manifestation of classic ulcerative colitis as it is currently defined. Abdominal wall fistulae develop in 20 per cent of patients with Crohn's disease — invariably postoperatively or in the scars from previous laparotomies (Fig. 12–27). Fistulae can also extend from the small bowel to the vagina, rectum, and bladder.

In one large series, arthralgias and rheumatoid arthritis developed in 9 to 23 per cent; conjunctivitis, episcleritis, and uveitis in 1 to 13 per cent; erythema nodosum in 4 to 15 per cent; and pyoderma gangrenosum in 1 to 1.6 per cent. The highest prevalence occurred in patients with granulomatous colitis and the lowest in those with regional enteritis.[75] Clubbing, palmar erythema, and phlebitis were found in 4 per cent of 183 patients studied by McCallum and Kinmont.[106]

Perianal lesions often begin with anal or perianal erythema that becomes edematous, producing a purplish-red discoloration. In more advanced cases, inflammation in the anal crypts of Morgagni produces red, swollen, fleshy anal tags (Fig. 12–28). These may progress to fissure-in-ano and abscesses. The latter can break down and extend to form large ulcers that cover the perineum, thighs, scrotum, base of the penis, vulva, and anterior abdominal wall. In most reported cases, the edges of the ulcers were clean and not undermined and showed the histologic "sarcoid" reaction of Crohn's disease on biopsy. In a minority of patients, the ulcers had the clinical appearance of pyoderma gangrenosum. The skin around colostomies can develop identical ulcers when the contiguous bowel is affected. However, in a few cases, there have been ulcerations under the breasts, at the base of the penis, in the groin, and behind the ears which have been unrelated to contiguous bowel involve-

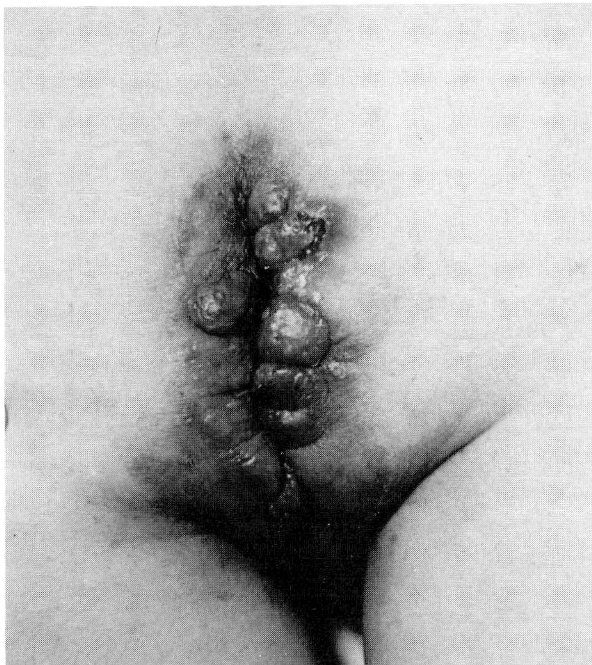

Figure 12–28. Crohn's disease. Red, swollen, fleshy nodules produced by inflammation in the anal crypts of Morgagni.

ment. These "metastatic" lesions showed the histologic "sarcoid" reaction.[102, 105-107]

In addition to aphthous ulcers, which are common, one may also find ulcerations of the buccal mucosa and lips, which show the same characteristic granulomatous changes. The ulcers develop hypertrophic granulation tissue which produces a cobblestone appearance. The granulomatous inflammation has produced swellings on the gingival margins and indurated polypoid tumors on the buccal mucosa.[102, 108-110]

Perianal lesions are more common in Crohn's colitis than in regional enteritis. Their development in regional enteritis is believed to be caused by retrograde lymph flow from the ileum to the perianal tissues.[104] The presence of such perianal lesions should make one consider the possibility of Crohn's disease even though bowel symptoms are absent or minimal. In the past, ischiorectal abscess was synonymous with tuberculosis, in part because of the granulomatous inflammation. However, currently it should be regarded as a sign of Crohn's disease until proven otherwise. Ileocecal tuberculosis, which is rare in the United States, ought to be considered when pulmonary tuberculosis is present, or in areas where milk borne tuberculosis is common. A negative skin test with tuberculin would exclude tuberculosis in such a differential diagnosis.

Cutaneous periarteritis nodosa as defined by Diaz-Perez and Winkelmann, has been reported as an associated syndrome in nine patients with Crohn's disease (see p. 383).

MALABSORPTION SYNDROME

The malabsorption syndrome is associated with several disorders. In the temperate climates the most common illness producing malabsorption is celiac sprue. The childhood phase, known as celiac disease, appears after the youngster has begun to eat cereals. The classic triad of this disorder is weight loss, a distended abdomen, and the bulky frothy stools of steatorrhea. After several years of spontaneous or therapeutically induced remission, celiac disease reappears in adult life. In some adults a history of preceding celiac disease cannot be obtained because of the mildness of the infantile form. Before it was realized that there were two phases of celiac sprue, the adult form of the disorder was called nontropical sprue or idiopathic steatorrhea. *Gluten-sensitive enteropathy* is a new term that is applied to both phases of the disease.

The severity of the malabsorption syndrome in adults varies from patient to patient. In addition to the defect in fat absorption, which is responsible for the presence of steatorrhea in almost every case, iron, folic acid, calcium, vitamin K, and the vitamin B complex may also be poorly absorbed. In some patients, protein-losing enteropathy also occurs and results in peripheral edema and signs of malnutrition. The histologic hallmark of celiac sprue is atrophy of the villi in the duodenal-jejunal mucosa. These changes are readily detected by peroral biopsy of the proximal small bowel. Gluten, a protein fraction of wheat, is believed to be responsible for producing the histologic and functional abnormalities of celiac sprue. Gluten instilled into the normal ileum of patients with celiac sprue produces the abnormal mucosal pattern characteristic of this disorder, whereas a gluten-free diet causes the signs and symptoms of celiac sprue to disappear and in most cases aids in correcting the abnormal small bowel pattern.

Malabsorption can also be produced by systemic disorders that affect the small bowel: Whipple's disease, lymphoma, amyloidosis, scleroderma, diabetes mellitus, and vascular insufficiency of the bowel. Steatorrhea can also be associated with cystic fibrosis of the pancreas and chronic pancreatitis; in these disorders, malabsorption of vitamins and minerals occurs less frequently than in celiac sprue.

Mucocutaneous abnormalities occur frequently in the malabsorption syndrome and have been the presenting features of the disease in a significant number of persons. In a series by Cooke et al., stomatitis developed in 90 per cent of the patients with malabsorption.[111] In the most severe cases the entire tongue and the buccal mucosa were bright red with multiple ulcers. When the disease was mild, the tips and edges of the tongue were smooth, red, and sore. In pernicious anemia the tongue is pale and smooth. Acute glossitis can develop within 48 hours in the malabsorption syndrome and can be accompanied by perianal soreness and dyspareunia. Folic acid and vitamin B complex deficiencies are believed to be responsible for the glossitis and stomatitis. Angular stomatitis was found in half of Cooke's patients.

Vitamin K deficiency is responsible for purpura, petechiae, melena, oral bleeding, hematuria, and even hemarthroses. Hemorrhage can be the first manifestation in some patients with malabsorption. Reversible clubbing occurred in 17 per cent of Cooke's patients. The findings in Cooke's series of 100 patients with sprue in Great Britain are comparable to those reported by Green and Wollaeger in 124 individuals with sprue in the United States.[112]

Dermatitis can also be the chief complaint of patients with malabsorption; it has been reported in 10 to 20 per cent of the cases.[113] The rash is an erythematous scaling eruption that has been said to resemble seborrheic dermatitis and psoriasis in some patients; in others it resembles eczema, asteatosis, and ichthyosis. The eczema often begins as solitary lichenified or weeping patches that become generalized and hyperpigmented. The dermatitis and hyperpigmentation promptly clear when the malabsorption has been successfully treated. Such cases need to be reevaluated with regard to possible zinc deficiency.

Increased pigmentation may also develop in the absence of dermatitis. The pigmentary patterns are of three types: melasmic (chloasmic) —a blotchy pigmentation on the face and neck; Addisonian — a distribution pattern, including buccal pigmentation, similar to that of adrenal insufficiency; and pellagroid — a purplish-brown color that occurs over the exposed parts and extensor areas of the limbs and that resembles pellagra but is not associated with cutaneous blisters or exudation. The pathogenesis of the Addisonian hyperpigmentation in malabsorption is not understood.

Purpura and hyperpigmentation are also characteristic features of Whipple's disease (intestinal lipodystrophy). The pattern of the increased pigmentation is Addisonian, but buccal involvement is said not to occur.

Hair and nail growth can be abnormal. The scalp and facial hair may be shed and remain sparse until malabsorption is corrected; the pubic and axillary hair are similarly affected. Koilonychia is not an unusual finding and responds to treatment with iron. The nails can also become brittle and crack along their free edges.

The precise factors responsible for the hair, nail, and cutaneous abnormalities in celiac sprue are difficult to delineate. Sometimes hypocalcemia appears to be the major deficiency, and when it is corrected, the cutaneous abnormalities disappear.[114-116] At other times identical dermatologic lesions occur in the presence of normal levels of serum calcium and remit following a gluten-free diet.[116]

Hypocalcemia *per se* appears to be important. Simpson[114] and Dent and Garetts[115] have reported patients with hypocalcemia secondary to hypoparathyroidism who have developed nail and hair abnormalities and extensive eczema identical to those conditions seen in celiac sprue. With acute hypocalcemia, the nails may be shed, or transverse grooves (Beau's lines) may develop in the nails with episodes of tetany (Fig. 12–29). In chronic hypocalcemia, the nails sometimes show longitudinal ridging and cracking. Not only is the scalp hair lost, but also the eyebrows, eyelashes, pubic hair, and axillary hair are shed. In addition, the skin may become dry, scaly, and hyperpigmented. All of these ectodermal changes can be corrected by restoring the level of serum calcium to normal.

On the basis of the preceding data, then, it seems clear that patients with intractable and hyperpigmented eczema should be studied for malabsorption and hypocalcemia.

Shuster and coworkers have emphasized two unsuspected relationships between skin and gut: one concerns dermatitis herpetiformis and celiac sprue; the other, termed dermatogenic enteropathy, is the effect of an extensive dermatitis on the small intestine.

Dermatitis herpetiformis is a chronic, extremely pruritic disease that is characterized by clusters of vesicles distributed symmetrically over the extensor surfaces of the knees and elbows, scalp, and back of the neck

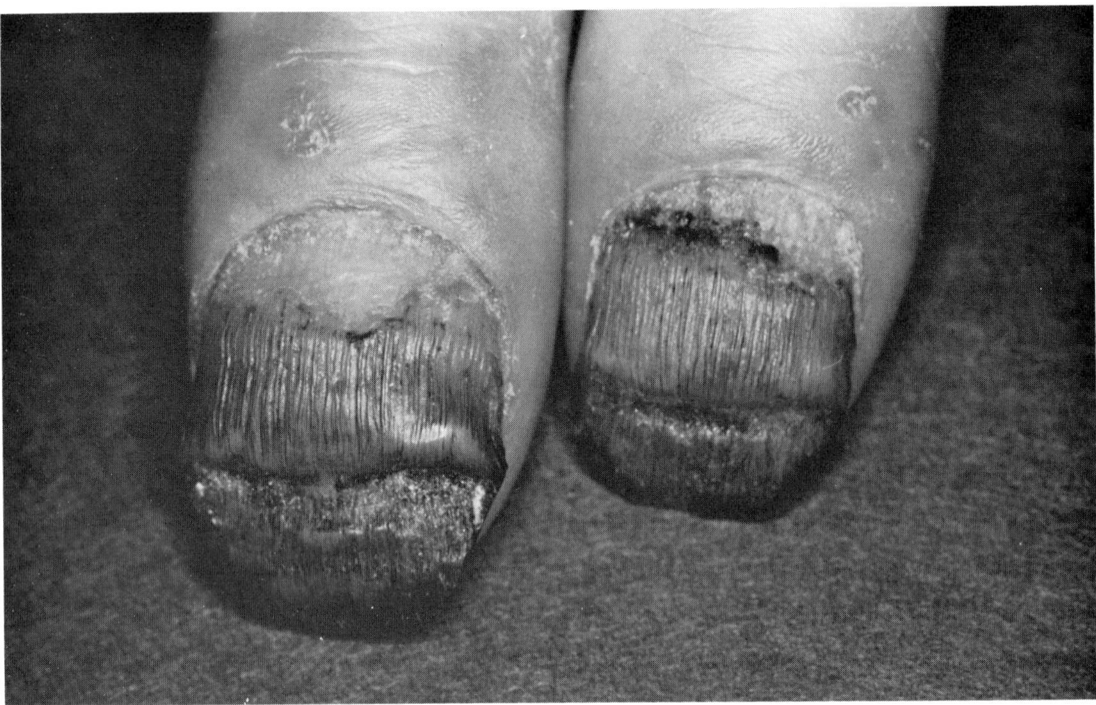

Figure 12–29. Beau's lines in a patient with psoriasis. These horizontal grooves develop as a nonspecific reaction to any stress that temporarily interrupts nail growth.

(Figs. 12–30 and 12–31). The face is infrequently affected and the oral mucosa only rarely. The disease responds dramatically to sulfones (e.g., dapsone) and sulfapyridine.

The illness may begin at any age, but it most frequently appears in the second to fourth decades. Although the disease appears to be lifelong in most individuals, it tends to become milder after it has been present for about 10 years. Spontaneous remissions persisting for several years or spontaneous cures have been recorded. In two series, spontaneous remissions of varying lengths and cures were observed in up to 35 per cent of patients, and milder courses developed in up to 70 per cent.[117, 118] These statistics, however, are derived from diagnoses made on the basis of clinical and histologic features and response to therapy — before the immunologic facets of the disease were discovered. Currently, it is believed that the diagnosis of dermatitis herpetiformis must be based upon immunofluorescent markers as well as upon the traditional features just mentioned. The natural history of the disease needs to be reevaluated in terms of these new criteria.

Dermatitis herpetiformis has been reported in association with an underlying carcinoma in a few instances. These reports were published before the immunofluorescent markers of the disease were discovered. This relationship needs reevaluation.

The histology of the skin lesions in their earliest phase is characterized by collections of neutrophils at the tips of the dermal papillae (microabscesses), often in association with separation of the papillary tips from overlying epidermis. As the lesions evolve, frank, subepidermal vesiculation develops that can be difficult to distinguish from the subepi-

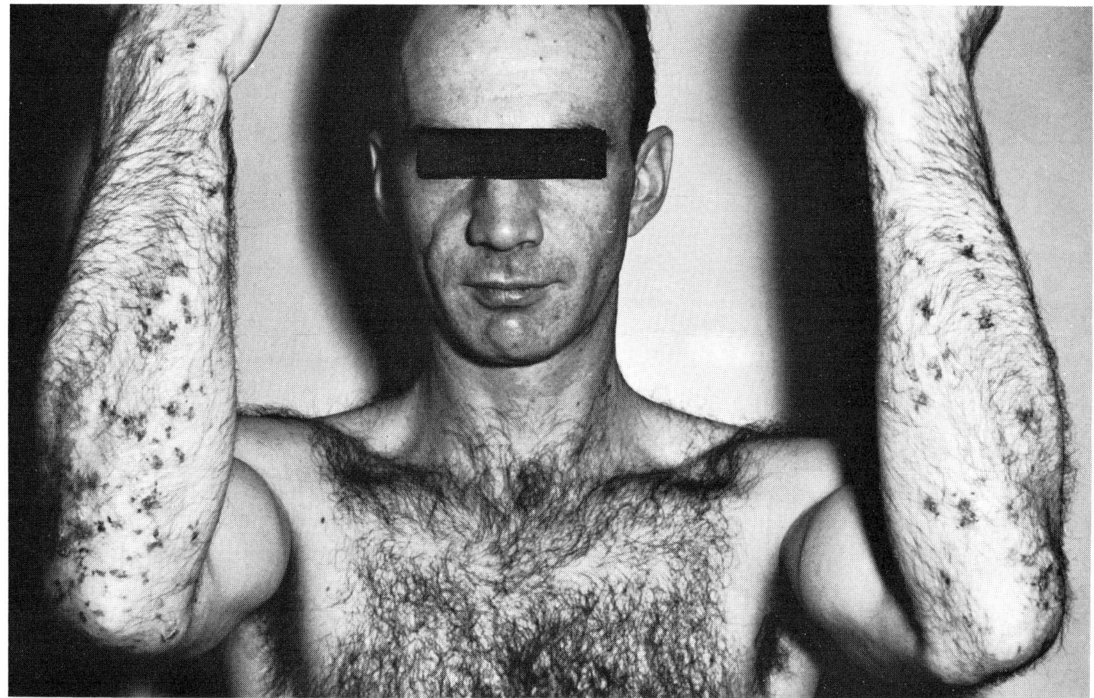

Figure 12–30. Dermatitis herpetiformis. Clusters of grouped vesicles occur symmetrically over the knees, elbows, buttocks, and scapulae and are associated with intense pruritus.

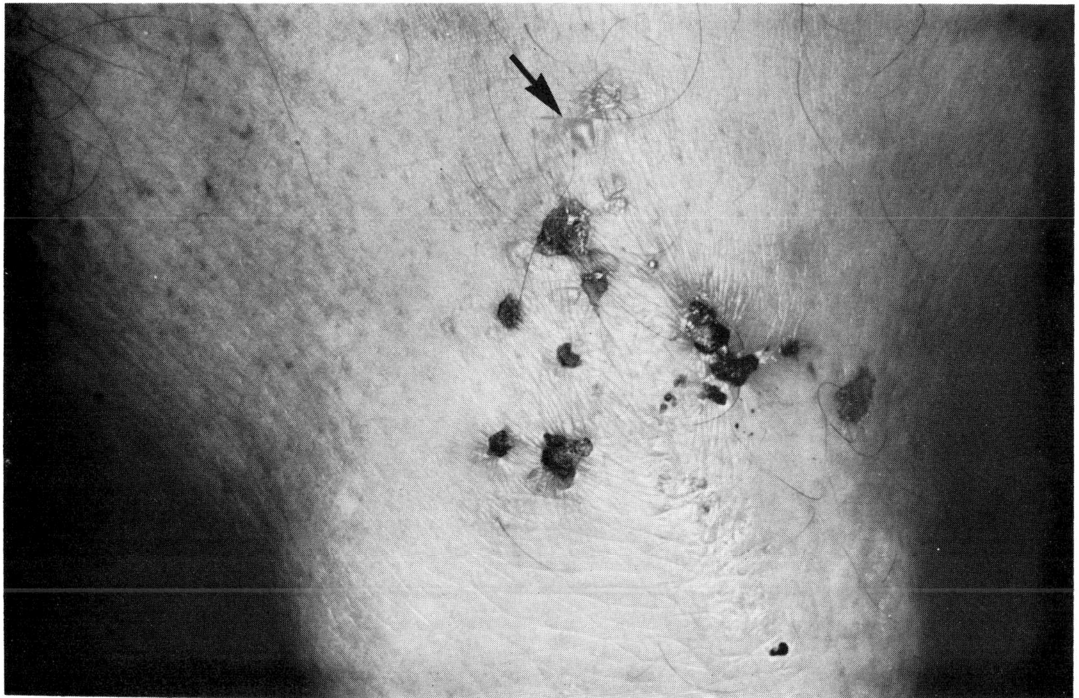

Figure 12–31. Dermatitis herpetiformis. Closer view of grouped vesicles. Arrow points to an intact vesicle. The rest of the small blisters have broken.

dermal blisters found in bullous pemphigoid, erythema multiforme, bullous drug eruptions, and herpes gestationis.

Most patients with dermatitis herpetiformis diagnosed on the basis of clinical and histologic features and their response to therapy have granular deposits of IgA identified by direct immunofluorescence in the dermal papillae of their cutaneous lesions, as well as in perilesional and normal skin. A minority of these patients have a linear deposit of IgA at the dermal-epidermal junction. C3 may be present as well in both sites. Other immunoglobulins in addition to IgA are found inconstantly in the dermal papillae, and only rarely at the dermal-epidermal junction.[119] In contrast, linear IgA deposits, which can be found at the basement membrane zone in bullous and cicatricial pemphigoids, are almost always accompanied by linear IgG deposits at this site.[119]

A few patients with a presumptive diagnosis of dermatitis herpetiformis based on classic criteria have lacked these immunologic markers. Fry and Seah have demonstrated that in 13 such individuals, the correct diagnoses proved to be pemphigus, subcorneal pustular dermatosis, vasculitis, juvenile dermatitis herpetiformis and eczema in six, and undiagnosed disorders in seven. In addition, intestinal biopsies in these 13 patients could be distinguished from those found in IgA-positive dermatitis herpetiformis on the basis of numbers of lymphocytes in the intestinal epithelium.[120] Immunofluorescent markers of IgA deposition appear to be necessary for the diagnosis of dermatitis herpetiformis. Dermatitis herpetiformis phenotypically appears to be a heterogeneous group of disorders. It needs to be emphasized, however, that multiple sections need to be studied before a conclusion can be reached that immunofluorescent studies are negative in an individual patient.[119]

Dermatitis herpetiformis is associated with mucosal changes in the small bowel that are indistinguishable from those of celiac sprue.[121-124] The atrophic villous pattern in dermatitis herpetiformis ranges from mild to severe. It is more prominent in the proximal small bowel than in the distal portion as observed in celiac sprue, but the atrophy occurs in a spotty fashion as opposed to more universal involvement in sprue. The differences in extent and degree of mucosal involvement in dermatitis herpetiformis have been proposed as the reasons for the rarity of clinical signs of malabsorption.[123] More recently, Scott and Losowsky have claimed that mucosal lesions in sprue are also patchy, but it is the intensity of the villous atrophy that is responsible for the clinical signs of malabsorption in sprue.[125]

Data from several series have shown that chemical evidence of steatorrhea was present in 22 of 69 patients, but in only six were there clinical signs and symptoms of malabsorption.[122, 126-129] Katz et al. found only 2 of 51 patients had symptoms of malabsorption.[119] Dermatitis herpetiformis preceded or followed malabsorption by as long as three to eight years. Ten to 33 per cent of patients have had abnormalities of D-xylose excretion, and anemia secondary to iron and folate deficiencies. Abnormalities in glucose, bicarbonate, and water absorption similar to those found in sprue have also been present.[119, 122, 126-129]

Sulfones produce remission in the skin lesions but have no effect on the enteropathy. However, a gluten-free diet in dermatitis herpetiformis will not only cause the intestinal lesion to revert to normal as in sprue, but in *most* patients it will induce a remission in the skin lesions or significantly reduce the dose of sulfones necessary to keep the skin clear.[130-132] It requires 6 to 12 months to achieve these cutaneous effects with a gluten-free diet. Return to a gluten-containing diet is followed by a relapse of skin disease in one to three weeks. Some patients with dermatitis herpetiformis do not respond to a gluten-free diet.[119, 124] Curiously, IgA and C3 can still be found in the normal skin of patients who have responded to a gluten-free diet.[119]

The pathogenesis of dermatitis herpetiformis is believed to involve the deposition of IgA at the dermal-epidermal junction of the skin with subsequent activation of complement by the alternative pathway. Neutrophils are attracted to the site and the histologic lesion is generated. However, the presence of IgA alone is insufficient to initiate the formation of the lesions, and other factors are necessary although they are still undefined. It has been established that patch tests with I^-, Cl^-, Br^-, F^-, and SCN^- will initiate local lesions within 24 to 48 hours. Oral potassium iodide can also induce lesions and exacerbate the disease. It is not understood how the halogens bring this about. The significance of IgA deposition in the skin is likewise unclear. It has been proposed that the IgA is directed against gluten protein or cross-reacting antigens, and that it originates in the gastrointestinal tract.[119] There is no evidence that circulating immune complexes, which are detectable in some patients,[132a] play a pathogenetic role in this disease.

Other evidence links dermatitis herpetiformis to sprue. Relatives of patients with dermatitis herpetiformis have been shown to have a high prevalence of villous atrophy assumed to be caused by celiac sprue.[126, 132] HLA-B8 and HLA-DRw3 are present with increased frequency in both sprue and dermatitis herpetiformis.[119]

Dermatitis herpetiformis associated with linear IgA deposits may be different pathophysiologically from the disorder associated with granular IgA deposits. Lawley et al. have studied 10 such individuals. The prevalence of HLA-B8 was not increased in these patients. Six of six individuals who were further evaluated had *normal* intestinal biopsies.[133] Circulating antibasement membrane zone antibodies of the IgA class can be found in patients with linear IgA deposits, but are rare in those with granular deposits.[119] Clearly, the phenotype called dermatitis herpetiformis is proving to be heterogeneous. The exact nosology of dermatitis herpetiformis with linear IgA deposits is uncertain. There is insufficient data at present to decide whether this syndrome, which is indistinguishable from dermatitis herpetiformis with granular deposits, is more likely to be a subtype of bullous pemphigoid than a subtype of dermatitis herpetiformis.

A single study of patients with rosacea revealed that 7 out of 60 patients had sprue-like patterns in the small bowel; 4 of these 7 patients also had celiac disease. The other three patients showed no evidence of malabsorption.[134]

Shuster and Marks have made a second important observation.[135] Exfoliative eczema or psoriasis is associated with increased fecal fat excretion, although the fat is not present in sufficient amount to produce symptomatic steatorrhea. When the dermatitis is successfully treated by topical therapy only, the chemical steatorrhea disappears. Three patients had relapses of their dermatitis and a concomitant return of the steatorrhea. When the skin was again successfully treated, the steatorrhea disappeared. The mucosal patterns of the small bowel were only mildly abnormal and did not resemble those of celiac sprue. The mechanism of dermatogenic enteropathy — extensive dermatitis that produces steatorrhea — is not understood.

Fry et al. and Doran et al. have reported that absorption studies with D-xylose and folic acid yield false positive results for malabsorption in patients with extensive eczema and psoriasis.[136, 137] The abnormal results from D-xylose testing have been attributed to decreased renal clearance, not malabsorption. The reason for decreased renal clearance has not been studied. Low serum folate levels are ascribed to increased utilization by the diseased epidermis rather than to faulty absorption. Serum folate and D-xylose levels, which are common screening tests for malabsorption, cannot be used for this purpose in patients with extensive skin disease. Correction of the serum folate levels has not benefited the eruptions in these patients.[138]

DISEASES OF THE PANCREAS

Most of the dermatologic signs of pancreatic disease have been covered in Chapter 1. Briefly, they include the syndrome of tender red cutaneous nodules, joint pain, fever, and eosinophilia, which are associated with acute and chronic pancreatitis and pancreatic carcinoma; and migratory superficial thrombophlebitis and migratory necrolytic erythema, which are associated with pancreatic cancer.

Acute hemorrhagic pancreatitis may be accompanied by purpura in the left flank (Grey-Turner's sign) or in the periumbilical area (Cullen's sign). Hematomas dissect along fascial planes from the retroperitoneal site of bleeding to the skin of the flank and periumbilical area.

DISEASES OF THE LIVER

In general, the cutaneous stigmata of liver disease are associated with the severity of the disorder. In acute liver disease, jaundice is a frequent sign, and pruritus can be a concomitant symptom if biliary obstruction is present. Serum hepatitis can have a serum sickness prodrome of urticaria, fever, and arthralgias, but these signs and symptoms have not been reported in cases of infectious hepatitis.[139]

Laennec's Cirrhosis

Laennec's cirrhosis is the most common type of chronic liver disease and displays a panorama of signs familiar to all physicians. Spider angiomas develop in at least three quarters of patients with cirrhosis. Spiders have been described previously (p. 533), and their spectrum is illustrated in Figures 11–1 and 11–2 and in Plate 28*A* to *C*. Although most spiders are planar, they can enlarge tremendously to form hemangioma-like masses. Spider nevi also occur in biliary cirrhosis, hemochromatosis, and postnecrotic cirrhosis following viral hepatitis. Spiders may even appear during the acute stage of viral hepatitis and disappear after recovery. The spider nevus, however, is not pathognomonic of liver disease; it is often seen in children, pregnant women, and otherwise normal young adults.

Spiders were observed in an unusual distribution in one of our female patients with advanced Laennec's cirrhosis. The telangiectatic lesions were distributed in a segmental fashion over the right side of the body and involved the forehead, face, upper back, chest, and arm. The lesions reached the midline but did not cross it. Spider nevi were found nowhere else on the body. Her only other cutaneous stigma of cirrhosis was bilateral palmar erythema.

American paper money skin describes the appearance of the integument of some patients with cirrhosis (Fig. 12–32). The thin wiry long vessels in the skin look like the fibers in our paper currency. This type of telangiectasia is not peculiar to cirrhotics; identical vascular patterns may be found in normal individuals of fair complexion.

Palmar erythema is a frequent accompaniment of spider nevi. A diffuse or blotchy erythema appears on the thenar and hypothenar eminences and on the tips of the fingers. Identical erythema can be found in persons during pregnancy and in those people with rheumatoid arthritis, thyrotoxicosis, and malnutrition. The diagnostic erythematous palmar spots of lupus erythematosus tend to be violaceous, papular, and more discrete than those of cirrhosis. Sometimes the distinction between lupus palms and liver palms cannot be made with certainty.

Although palmar erythema and spider nevi often occur in the clinical setting of presumed hyperestrogenism, the evidence that increased levels of estrogen are responsible for the pathogenesis of these lesions is only circumstantial.

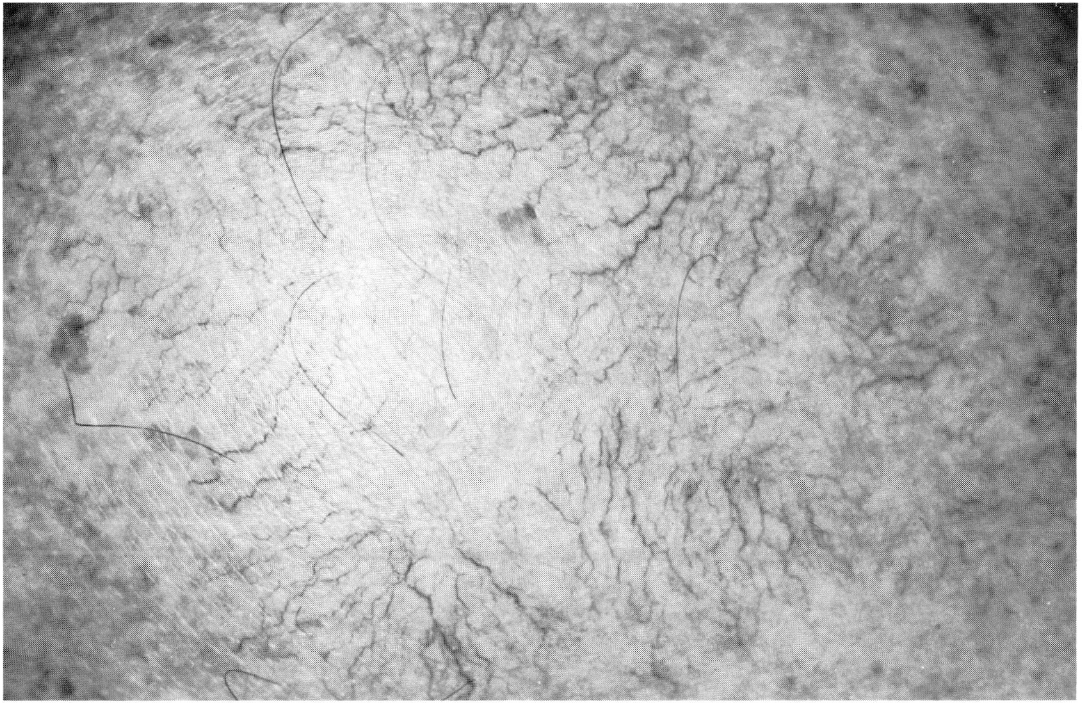

Figure 12–32. Laennec's cirrhosis. Wiry telangiectasia resembling fibers in American paper currency.

Men with cirrhosis tend to have sparse axillary, pubic, and pectoral hair; and they often are affected with loss of libido, gynecomastia, and testicular softening. The loss of hair has often been assumed to be a manifestation of feminization secondary to hyperestrogenism. However, both Spellberg and Klatskin have noted that according to the statements of many of their patients, sparse growth of axillary, pubic, and pectoral hair had been present for many years before cirrhosis developed.[140, 141] The possibility of a constitutional predisposition to cirrhosis is raised by these observations.

Gynecomastia is frequently associated with increasingly severe cirrhosis, but it may also occur when a severely malnourished patient begins to improve on a good diet. Jaundice develops as hepatic failure increases. It is characteristic for hyperpigmentation to develop primarily over the exposed areas, but the pathogenesis is not known. Similar hyperpigmentation can develop in any chronic debilitating disease. Clubbing has been observed in 5 to 18 per cent of patients with cirrhosis.[140] Dupuytren's contracture and parotid gland enlargement are also associated features of cirrhosis.

With advancing hepatic fibrosis and impaired hepatic function, prothrombin deficiency becomes a major problem that results in cutaneous purpura, epistaxis, and gingival bleeding. Hypoalbuminemia results in edema and ascites. When portal hypertension supervenes, collateral circulation between the portal and systemic systems develops in most patients and manifests itself as dilated superficial veins over the abdomen and chest. However, a marked enlargement of the periumbilical veins that produces a caput medusae is an uncommon finding in cirrhosis.

Pellagra can develop in alcoholics with severe nutritional deficiency.

Terry described the phenomenon of white nails in 82 of 100 persons affected by alcoholic, postnecrotic, and cholangiolitic cirrhosis.[142] Almost the entire nail was opaque white except for the distal portion, which retained its normal pink color (Fig. 12–33). Terry classified the abnormal nails into four groups. In group I the lunula was indistinguishable from the rest of the white nail. Only six patients had such nails. In group II the whiteness of the nail was less intense, and the lunula was just barely discernible. Twenty-three patients had this type of nail. In groups III and IV the lunula was readily visible, and the nails had only moderately or slightly increased whiteness; 53 patients were categorized under these last two groups. The white color was not within the nailplate but represented an opacification of the nailbed because the whiteness neither moved with nail growth nor altered when blood was forced into the subungual tissue by compression of digital vessels.

Terry also pointed out that white nails were not unique in patients with cirrhosis because they could also be found in children under four years old and in some normal women under 20 years of age. He also observed white nails of varying intensity in patients with congestive heart failure, diabetes mellitus, rheumatoid arthritis, and carcinoma. Bean reported finding white nails in 25 per cent of patients with cirrhosis and in 8 per cent of persons with other miscellaneous disorders.[143] Bean did not state whether the white nails were only of group I or of all the groups described by Terry. In our experience, about 5 per cent of cirrhotics were found to have white nails typical of group I. Morey and Burke reported the presence of white nails with absent lunulae in four patients with

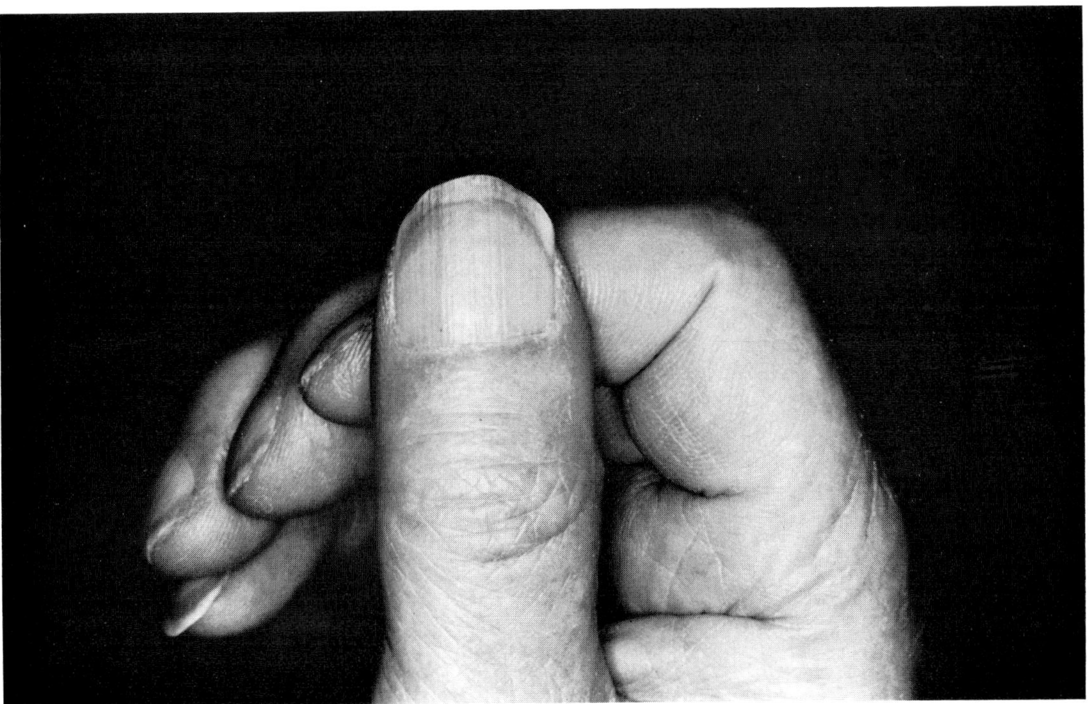

Figure 12–33. Laennec's cirrhosis. White nails. Lunula is absent.

cirrhosis.[144] The distal curved margin of the white area had a central or off-center peak.

These white nails are of interest even though they have a very limited diagnostic usefulness, since they may indicate an abnormal physiologic state. Muehrcke described a seemingly different kind of white nail in patients with *chronic* hypoalbuminemia (serum level of less than 2.2 gm/100 ml).[145] In these cases, two parallel white bands were present on the nail; and they were separated from each other, as well as from the lunula and free edge, by the normal pink color. These nail changes were found in many patients with chronic hypoalbuminemia of diverse etiologies, but not all patients with low levels of serum albumin developed these bands. The white lines were not present in the nailplate but represented an opacification in the nailbed. When the serum albumin was raised above 2.2 gm/100 ml, the lines disappeared; they returned when the hypoalbuminemia recurred. In one of Muehrcke's patients, the two white bands were replaced by a solid white opacity that produced the white nail, as described by Terry, for cirrhosis.

Although Terry did not publish any data correlating levels of serum albumin with white nails in cirrhosis, the four patients reported by Morey and Burke had levels of serum albumin of approximately 2.0 gm/100 ml. Only a single determination of the serum albumin was cited; consequently one cannot determine the duration of the hypoalbuminemia. However, it is known that the patients had signs and symptoms of cirrhosis for at least one year. The pathogenesis of the opacification in the nailbed that produces Terry's and Muehrcke's white nails is not known. However, anemia is not a factor.

Lewin has been able to study at autopsy the nails and nailbeds of over 80 individuals with a variety of systemic diseases, and his observations permit one to speculate on a possible mechanism for the production of these white nails.[146]

The lunula or half moon of the nail corresponds to the visible part of the nail matrix that is responsible for the production of the nailplate. The rest of the nail matrix extends proximally for about 3 mm under the cuticle. The epidermal cells of the nailbed, distal to the lunula, do not contribute to the formation of the nailplate under normal conditions. When a nail is removed, a white area corresponding to the lunula can be seen on its undersurface. This opacification is produced by the superficial layers of the nail matrix, which have remained attached to the nailplate. The nail matrix, corresponding to the lunula, is also pale white. Beneath the germinative epidermal cell layer of the lunula, the connective tissue is avascular and has a very loose texture. The connective tissue of the nailbed distal to the lunula is composed of compact collagen fibers and has a rich vascular supply. Lewin was also able to study normal nails that lacked a lunula, a relatively common finding. The connective tissue in the area where a lunula should have been was not loose but was dense with compact collagen. The white color of the lunula most likely results from the avascularity and loose stroma below the germinative epithelium.

It is possible, therefore, that hypoalbuminemia results in edema of the connective tissue just below the epidermal layer of the distal nailbed and converts a highly compact collagenous structure into a loosely knit one. In this way it simulates the organization of the lunula and produces a white color in the nail. The correlation of the presence or absence of white bands with the level of serum albumin is consistent with this hypothesis. Unfortunately, there are no data on the relationship between serum albumin levels and the white nails of cirrhosis except for the information reported by Morey and Burke concerning their four patients. Also, none of the 80 patients studied by Lewin had the white nails of cirrhosis. As a consequence, the histopathology of this condition is unknown.[147] Some nails normally lack a lunula; but the thumbs always have one, and it is they that should be examined for white nails.

The differential diagnosis of white nails includes leukonychia, a condition in which white spots are present within the nailplate and are most likely caused by focal abnormalities of keratinization. Leukonychia is manifested by spots, linear bands, and rarely, by total involvement of the nailplate. These white spots move as the nails grow.

Hemochromatosis

Hemochromatosis (bronzed diabetes) is inherited as an autosomal recessive disease with partial biochemical expression in the heterozygote.[148, 149] There is an abnormally increased absorption of iron which leads to deposition of this element in the skin, liver, heart, pancreas, and endocrine organs, including the pituitary. Hemochromatosis is 10 times more frequent in men than in women and usually becomes clinically apparent between 40 and 60 years of age.[150] Hyperpigmentation, cirrhosis, and diabetes mellitus constitute the triad of signs and symptoms of this disorder. Hyperpigmentation eventually develops in almost every patient and is the presenting sign in 25 to 40 per cent of affected individuals. The hyperpigmentation is generalized and accentuated over the exposed areas. The gums, palate, buccal mucosa, and sometimes the conjunctivae are affected in 15 to 20 per cent of patients.[140] The pigmentation can be brown or slate gray; these colors often occur together.

The increased pigmentation is produced by melanin and not by the deposition of iron in the skin. Perdrup and Poulsen demonstrated this point nicely in describing a patient who had both vitiligo and hemochromatosis. The white spots of vitiligo were typically dead white but contained as much histochemically demonstrated iron as did the hyperpigmented areas. The presence of the iron in the vitiliginous lesions, which were devoid of melanin, produced no hyperpigmentation.[151]

The skin of patients with hemochromatosis tends to be dry and scaly. The usual features of cirrhosis can also be found: gynecomastia, spider nevi, sparse body hair, and ecchymoses.

Biliary Cirrhosis

Biliary cirrhosis develops primarily in women. The combination of pruritus, hyperpigmentation, jaundice, and xanthomas occurs in no other disease and thus permits an easy clinical diagnosis (Plate 33*F*). The melanotic hyperpigmentation is brown, generalized, worse on exposed areas, and does not seem to affect the mucosal surfaces. In spite of these signs and symptoms, the patient appears relatively healthy, not wasted as one would expect of a person with Laennec's cirrhosis who had jaundice and hyperpigmentation.

Hyperlipidemia eventually develops in most patients with biliary cirrhosis and is responsible for the most spectacular xanthomatosis seen in medicine: xanthelasma, tuberous xanthomas over extensor and pressure areas, and flat or plane xanthomas in palmar creases and scars from acne or previous surgery. Tendon xanthomas are rare in biliary cirrhosis, but they were found in two of our patients.

The reasons for pruritus and hyperpigmentation in primary biliary cirrhosis are unknown, but Burton and Kirby have proposed a novel hypothesis.[152] Bile salts exhibit a nonspecific cytotoxicity, probably because of detergent action on lipid membranes. Bile salts produce itching when applied to the bases of cutaneous blisters produced in normal individuals. They proposed that the cytotoxic properties of the bile salts cause release of epidermal proteolytic enzymes, which are potent pruritogens. Proteolytic enzymes can also activate epidermal tyrosinase. Continued release of low concentrations of proteolytic enzymes in the skin secondary to the nonspecific cytotoxic effects of the bile salts could account for both the pigmentation and the pruritus of patients with biliary cirrhosis.

Fleming et al. reported an unusual manifestation in one patient with primary biliary cirrhosis who had high hepatic serum and urinary levels of copper.[153] Slit lamp biomicroscopy revealed pigmented corneal rings similar to Kayser-Fleischer rings. Wilson's disease was excluded in this patient on the basis of elevated serum levels of ceruloplasmin and copper, lack of neurologic disease, negative family history, and the typical clinical features of primary biliary cirrhosis.

An immunologic basis for biliary cirrhosis is suspected because of associated clinical and laboratory findings. Circulating antibodies to mitochondria are present in all patients, and rheumatic disorders are common accompanying features. In one series of 83 patients, 23 had a rheumatic disease. Fourteen of 23 had either various facets of CRST syndrome or mild scleroderma. Usually abnormalities were limited to disturbances in esophageal motility or decreased diffusion capacity in the lungs. Four of 83 had a destructive arthropathy of unknown type; nine had Sjögren's syndrome; and four had small joint polyarthritis of the hands and feet. Some patients had more than one rheumatic feature. The patients who had scleroderma had haplotypes HLA-A1, B8.[154]

Wilson's Disease

Hepatolenticular degeneration (Wilson's disease) is characterized by the triad of basal ganglia degeneration, cirrhosis of the liver, and a pathognomonic pigmentation of the corneal margins known as the Kayser-Fleischer ring. The disease usually begins in adolescence, but it may appear as early as the age of four or as late as age forty. In most cases the initial manifestation is related to the nervous system. In a few patients, signs of liver insufficiency are the first indications of the disease.[155, 156]

The most consistent sign of Wilson's disease is the Kayser-Fleischer ring: a golden brown or greenish-brown circle of pigment produced by the deposition of copper in Descemet's membrane at the periphery of the cornea.[140] The ring is best visualized with side lighting (Plate 35*A*). The Kayser-Fleischer ring disappears after successful therapy with *d*-penicillamine and thus serves as a useful monitor of therapy.

Blue lunulae have been reported in six patients with Wilson's disease.[155, 157] However, it has also been observed in a normal individual and in another person who had ingested phenolphthalein.[157] The copper content of the fingernails with blue lunulae in Wilson's disease does not differ significantly from the copper content of normal fingernails of patients with Wilson's disease or of individuals with ordinary cirrhosis.

Carotenemia

Carotenemia is a harmless but colorful disorder that is produced by an excessive dietary intake of carotene (which is found in leafy and yellow vegetables and fruits: carrots, spinach, squash, peaches, oranges, and apricots). Since carotene has an affinity for the horny layer of the skin, the palms and soles are the most strongly stained areas of the integument (Plate 35*B*). Carotenemia produces an orange-yellow color. Differentiation from jaundice is easy because the sclerae are not stained by carotene.

Carotenemia sometimes appears in individuals with hypothyroidism or diabetes mellitus. It is believed that carotene cannot be converted to vitamin A in the absence of thyroid hormone. In addition, myxedema may be accompanied by hyperbetalipoproteinemia and a Type II pattern which mimics that found in familial hypercholesterolemia. The level of carotene in the plasma is high because betalipoprotein is the major carrier of carotene in the blood.

In diabetes mellitus, carotenemia has been ascribed to both hyperlipemia and to a decrease in the capacity of the liver to convert carotene to vitamin A.[158, 159] Although it is stated that 10 per cent of patients with diabetes mellitus have carotenemia, this statement cannot be correct. This statistic must have been obtained many years ago when diabetics were treated by diets low in carbohydrates and high in yellow and leafy vegetables. Diabetics usually have hypertriglyceridemia rather than the hypercholesterolemia that is associated with increased blood levels of carotene. The prevalence and etiology of carotenemia in diabetes mellitus need to be reevaluated.

The skin can also be stained orange-yellow by carotenoids in lycopenemia. This disorder is produced by drinking large amounts of tomato juice for several months. Ninety per cent of the color in tomatoes is produced by carotenoids.

Hepatic Ductular Hypoplasia

Hepatic ductular hypoplasia is a disorder in which hypoplastic intrahepatic bile ducts are combined with patent extrahepatic bile ducts. In a series of 30 children with this entity, 15 were noted to form a clinically homogeneous and readily recognizable group. All had a characteristic facies. A mesosystolic murmur consistent with pulmonary artery hypoplasia or stenosis was present in 12; defects in fusion of vertebral arches in eight, sometimes accompanied by growth retardation; mental retardation (I.Q. 60 to 80) in nine; and hypogonadism in six.[160]

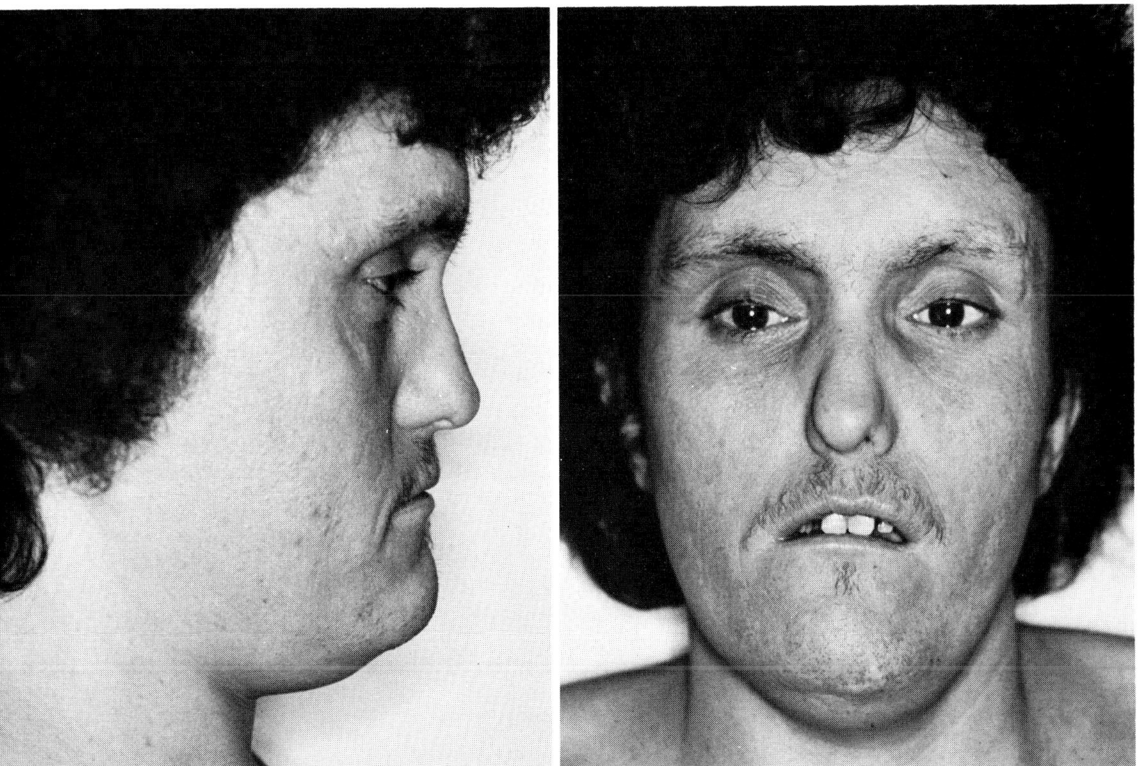

Figure 12–34. Left. Hepatic ductular hypoplasia. Typical facies.

Figure 12–35. Right. Hepatic ductular hypoplasia. Typical facies.

The earliest indication of the disease is persistent cholestasis, which appears during the first three months after birth, and intense pruritus with moderate elevations in serum bilirubin. Hepatosplenomegaly is a constant feature. Xanthomas are rare, but when present they are planar in type. During the second year, all the serum lipids become elevated. However, the disease is treatable. Thirteen of the 15 children no longer have pruritus, elevated lipids, or bilirubin following treatment with cholestyramine and fat-soluble vitamins. Those who were refractory to this therapy had a successful response to cholecystojejunostomy. The life expectancy in this disorder is not yet known.

The characteristic facies are present from the early months of life; all the patients resemble each other. The forehead is prominent and the eyes deeply set. There is mild hypertelorism, a straight nose, and a small pointed chin (Figs. 12–34 and 12–35). Hypogonadism is present in 40 per cent of affected persons. In 20 per cent of patients, there is a family history for neonatal cholestatic disorders in siblings. Thus, among the congenital disorders of bile duct hypoplasia, there appears to be a genetically transmitted form of the disease that has a better prognosis than other types of congenital intrahepatic cholestasis.

REFERENCES

1. Weary, P. E., Linthicum, A., Cawley, E. P., Coleman, C. C., Jr., and Graham, G. F.: Gardner's syndrome. Arch. Dermatol., *90*:20, 1964.
2. Coli, R. D., Moore, J. P., LaMarche, P. H., DeLuca, F. G., and Thayer, W. R., Jr.: Gardner's syndrome. A revisit to a previously described family. Am. J. Dig. Dis., *15*:551, 1970.
3. Oldfield, M. C.: Association of familial polyposis of colon with multiple sebaceous cysts. Br. J. Surg., *41*:534, 1954.
4. Dormandy, T. L.: Gastrointestinal polyposis with mucocutaneous pigmentation (Peutz-Jeghers syndrome). N. Engl. J. Med., *256*:1093, 1141, 1186, 1957.
5. Zegarelli, E. V., Kutscher, A. H., Mercadante, J. M., Kupferberg, N., and Piro, J. D.: Atlas of oral lesions observed in the syndrome of oral melanosis with associated intestinal polyposis (Peutz-Jeghers syndrome). Am. J. Dig. Dis., *4*:479, 1959.
6. Lowe, N. J.: Peutz-Jeghers syndrome with pigmented oral papillomas. Arch. Dermatol., *111*:503, 1975.
7. Kyle, J.: Peutz-Jeghers syndrome. Scot. Med. J., *6*:361, 1961.
8. Valero, A., and Sherf, K.: Pigmented nails in Peutz-Jeghers syndrome. Am. J. Gastroenterol., *43*:56, 1965.
9. Bartholomew, L. G., Dahlin, D. C., and Waugh, J. M.: Intestinal polyposis associated with mucocutaneous pigmentation (Peutz-Jeghers syndrome). Gastroenterology, *32*:434, 1957.
10. Dozois, R. R., Judd, E. S., Dahlin, D. C., and Bartholomew, L. G.: The Peutz-Jeghers syndrome. Is there a predisposition to the development of intestinal cancer? Arch. Surg., *98*:509, 1969.
11. Altemeier, W. A.: in discussion of ref. 10, p. 517.
12. Reid, J. D.: Duodenal cancer in the Peutz-Jeghers syndrome. Cancer, *18*:970, 1965.
13. Sachatello, C. R., Pickren, J. W., and Grace, J. T., Jr.: Generalized juvenile gastrointestinal polyposis. A hereditary syndrome. Gastroenterology, *58*:699, 1970.
14. Stemper, T. J., Kent, T. H., and Summers, R. W.: Juvenile polyposis and gastrointestinal carcinoma. A study of a kindred. Ann. Intern. Med., *83*:639, 1975.
15. Cronkhite, L. W., Jr., and Canada, W. J.: Generalized gastrointestinal polyposis. An unusual syndrome of polyposis pigmentation, alopecia and onychotrophia. N. Engl. J. Med., *252*:1011, 1955.
16. Johnson, M. M., Vosburgh, J. W., Wiens, A. T., and Walsh, G. C.: Gastrointestinal polyposis associated with alopecia, pigmentation and atrophy of the fingernails and toenails. Ann. Intern. Med., *56*:935, 1962.
17. Jarnum, S., and Jensen, H.: Diffuse gastrointestinal polyposis with ectodermal changes. Gastroenterology, *50*:107, 1966.
18. Chan, H. L., Ho, K. T., and Khoo, O. T.: Cronkhite-Canada syndrome in a Malay. Arch. Dermatol., *115*:98, 1979.
19. Tokuyasu, K., Takebayashi, S., Takahara, O., and Uchiyama, E.: An autopsy case of Cronkhite-Canada syndrome. Gastroenterol. Japon., *11*:215, 1976.

20. Fraser, G. M.: The radiological manifestations of scleroderma (diffuse systemic sclerosis). Br. J. Dermatol., *78*:1, 1966.
21. Cliff, I. S., Herber, R., and Demis, D. J.: Control of malabsorption in scleroderma. J. Invest. Dermatol., *47*:475, 1966.
22. Paterson-Brown-Kelly syndrome. Br. Med. J., *2*:258, 1967.
23. Crawfurd, M. D'A., Jacobs, A., Murphy, B., and Peters, D. K.: Paterson-Brown-Kelly syndrome in adolescence: a report of five cases. Br. Med. J., *1*:693, 1965.
24. Chisholm, M., and Wright, R.: Post-cricoid dysphagia and iron deficiency in men. Br. Med. J., *2*:281, 1967.
25. Schetman, D.: The Plummer-Vinson syndrome. Arch. Dermatol., *105*:720, 1972.
26. Katz, J., Gryboski, J. D., Rosenbaum, H. M., and Spiro, H. M.: Dysphagia in children with epidermolysis bullosa. Gastroenterology, *52*:259, 1967.
27. Reed, W. B., College, J., Jr., Francis, M. J. O., Zachariae, H., Mohs, F., Sher, M. A., and Sneddon, I. B.: Epidermolysis bullosa dystrophica with epidermal neoplasms. Arch. Dermatol., *110*:894, 1974.
28. Goldman, J. A., Casey, H. L., Davidson, E. D., Hersh, T., and Pirozzi, D.: Vasculitis associated with intestinal bypass surgery. Arch. Dermatol., *115*:725, 1979.
29. Dicken, C. H., and Seehafer, J. R.: Bowel bypass syndrome. Arch. Dermatol., *115*:837, 1979.
30. Utsinger, P. D., Shapiro, R. F., Ely, P. H., McLaughlin, G. E., and Wusner, K. B.: Clinical and immunologic study of the postintestinal bypass arthritis-dermatitis syndrome. Arth. Rheum., *21*:599, 1978.
31. Strole, W. E. Jr., Clark, W. H., Jr., and Isselbacher, K. J.: Progressive arterial occlusive disease (Köhlmeier-Degos). N. Engl. J. Med., *276*:195, 1967.
32. Roenigk, H. H., Jr., and Farmer, R. G.: Degos' disease (malignant papulosis). J. A. M. A., *206*:1508, 1968.
33. May, R. E.: Degos' syndrome. Br. Med. J., *1*:161, 1968.
34. Howard, R. O., Klaus, S. N., Savin, R. C., and Fenton, R.: Malignant atrophic papulosis (Degos' syndrome). Arch. Ophthalmol., *79*:262, 1968.
35. Kohlmeier, W.: Multiple Hautnekrosen bei Thrombangiitis Obliterans. Arch. Dermatol. Syph., *181*:783, 1941.
36. Degos, R., Delort, J., and Tricot, R.: Dermatite papulo-squameuse atrophiante. Bull. Soc. Fr. Dermatol. Syph., *49*:148, 1942.
37. Muller, S. A., and Landry, M.: Exchange autographs in malignant atrophic papulosis (Degos' disease). Mayo Clin. Proc., *49*:883, 1974.
38. Muller, S. A., and Landry, M.: Malignant atrophic papulosis (Degos' disease). A report of two cases with clinical and histologic studies. Arch. Dermatol., *112*:357, 1976.
39. Black, M. M.: Malignant atrophic papulosis (Degos' disease). Int. J. Dermatol., *15*:405, 1976.
40. Stahl, D., Thomsen, K., and Hou-Jensen, K.: Malignant atrophic papulosis. Treatment with aspirin and dipyridamole. Arch. Dermatol., *114*:1687, 1978.
41. Siegal, S.: Familial paroxysmal polyserositis. Am. J. Med., *36*:893, 1964.
42. Sohar, E., Gafni, J., Pras, M., and Heller, H.: Familial Mediterranean fever. A survey of 470 cases and review of the literature. Am. J. Med., *43*:227, 1967.
43. Ehrenfeld, E. N., Eliakim, M., and Rachmilewitz, M.: Recurrent polyserositis (familial Mediterranean fever; periodic disease). A report of 55 cases. Am. J. Med., *31*:107, 1961.
44. Reimann, H. A., Moadié, J., Semerdjian, S., and Sahyoun, P. F.: Periodic peritonitis — heredity and pathology. Report of 72 cases. J. A. M. A., *154*:1254, 1954.
45. Schwabe, A. D., and Peters, R. S.: Familial Mediterranean fever in Armenians. Analysis of 100 cases. Medicine, *53*:453, 1974.
46. Siguier, F.: Maladies vedettes. Maladies d'avenir. Maladies quotidiennes. Maladies d'exception. La maladie dite périodique. Paris, Masson et Cie, 1957, p. 295.
47. Azizi., E., and Fisher, B. K.: Cutaneous manifestations of familial Mediterranean fever. Arch. Dermatol., *112*:364, 1976.
48. Rotem, Y., and Federgruen, A.: Schoenlein-Henoch syndrome in familial Mediterranean fever. Harefuah, *62*:1, 1962.
49. Heite, H.-J., and Ody, R.: Die Acrodermatitis enteropathica im Lichte der Häufigkeitsanalyse. Hautarzt, *16*:529, 1965.
50. Wells, B. T., and Winkelmann, R. K.: Acrodermatitis enteropathica. Arch. Dermatol. *84*:40, 1961.
51. Ølholm-Larsen, P.: Untreated acrodermatitis enteropathica in adults. Dermatologica, *156*:155, 1978.
52. Deffner, N. F., and Perry, H. O.: Acrodermatitis enteropathica and failure to thrive. Arch. Dermatol., *108*:658, 1973.
53. Moynahan, E. J.: Zinc deficiency and disturbances of mood and visual behavior. Lancet, *1*:9, 1976.
54. Entwisle, B. R.: Acrodermatitis enteropathica. Aust. J. Dermatol., *8*:13, 1968.
55. Epstein, S., and Vedder, J. S.: Acrodermatitis enteropathica persisting into adulthood. Arch. Dermatol. *82*:135, 1960.
56. Cash, R., and Berger, C. K.: Acrodermatitis enteropathica: Defective metabolism of unsaturated fatty acids. J. Pediatr., *74*:717, 1969.
57. Nelder, K. H., Hagler, L., Wise, W. R., Stifel, F. B., Lufkin, E. G., and Herman, R. H.: Acrodermatitis enteropathica. A clinical and biochemical survey. Arch. Dermatol., *110*:711, 1974.
58. Ginsburg, R., Robertson, A., Jr., and Michel, B.: Acrodermatitis enteropathica. Abnormalities of fat metabolism and integumental ultrastructures in infants. Arch. Dermatol., *112*:653, 1976.
59. Moynahan, E. J., and Barnes, P. M.: Zinc deficiency and a synthetic diet for lactose intolerance. Lancet, *1*:675, 1973.

60. Lombeck, I., Schnippering, H. G., Ritzl, F., Feinendegen, L. H., and Bremer, H. J.: Absorption of zinc in acrodermatitis enteropathica. Lancet, *1*:855, 1975.
61. Neldner, K. H., and Hambridge, K. M.: Zinc therapy of acrodermatitis enteropathica. N. Engl. J. Med., *292*:879, 1975.
62. Evans, G. W., and Johnson, P. E.: Zinc binding factor in acrodermatitis enteropathica. Lancet, *2*:1310, 1976.
63. Kreiger, I., and Evans, G. W.: Acrodermatitis enteropathica without hypozincemia: therapeutic effect of a pancreatic enzyme preparation due to a zinc-binding ligand. J. Pediatr., *96*:32, 1980.
64. Garretts, M., and Molokhia, M.: Acrodermatitis enteropathica without hypozincemia. J. Pediatr., *91*:492, 1977.
65. Kelly, R., Davidson, G. P., Townley, R. R. W., and Campbell, P. E.: Reversible intestinal mucosal abnormality in acrodermatitis enteropathica. Arch. Dis. Child., *51*:219, 1976.
66. Evans, G. W., and Johnson, P. E.: Defective prostaglandin synthesis in acrodermatitis enteropathica. Lancet, *1*:52, 1977.
67. van Vloten, W. A., and Bos, L. P.: Skin lesions in acquired zinc deficiency due to parenteral nutrition. Dermatologica, *156*:175, 1978.
68. Weismann, K., Wadskov, S., Mikkelsen, H. I., Knudsen, L., Christensen, K. C., and Storgaard, L.: Acquired zinc deficiency dermatosis in man. Arch. Dermatol., *114*:1509, 1978.
69. Brazin, S. A., Johnson, W. T., and Abramson, L. J.: The acrodermatitis enteropathica-like syndrome. Arch. Dermatol., *115*:597, 1979.
70. Ecker, R. I., and Schroeter, A. L.: Acrodermatitis and acquired zinc deficiency. Arch. Dermatol., *114*:937, 1978.
71. McClain, C., Soutor, C., and Zieve, L.: Zinc deficiency: a complication of Crohn's disease. Gastroenterology, *78*:272, 1980.
72. Samitz, M. H., and Greenberg, M. S.: Skin lesions in association with ulcerative colitis. Gastroenterology, *19*:476, 1951.
73. Hightower, N. C., Broders, A. C., Haines, R. D., McKenney, J. F., and Sommers, A. W.: Chronic ulcerative colitis: diagnostic considerations, complications, treatment. Am. J. Dig. Dis., *3*:722, 861, 931, 1958.
74. Johnson, M. L., and Wilson, H. T. H.: Skin lesions in ulcerative colitis. Gut, *10*:255, 1969.
75. Greenstein, A. J., Janowitz, H. D., and Sachar, D. B.: The extraintestinal complications of Crohn's disease and ulcerative colitis: a study of 700 patients. Medicine, *55*:401, 1976.
76. Fernandez-Herlihy, L.: The articular manifestations of chronic ulcerative colitis. An analysis of 555 cases. N. Engl. J. Med., *261*:259, 1959.
77. Moschella, S. L.: Pyoderma gangrenosum. Arch. Dermatol., *95*:121, 1967.
78. Brunsting, L. A., Goeckerman, W. H., and O'Leary, P. A.: Pyoderma (ecthyma) gangrenosum: clinical and experimental observations in 5 cases occurring in adults. Arch. Dermatol. Syph., *22*:655, 1930.
79. Perry, H. O., and Brunsting, L. A.: Pyoderma gangrenosum. Arch. Dermatol., *75*:380, 1957.
80. Decherd, J. W., Leyden, J., and Holtzapple, P. G.: Facial pyoderma gangrenosum preceding ulcerative colitis. Cutis, *14*: 208, 1974.
81. Ricketts, W. E., Kirsner, J. B., and Rothman, S.: Pyoderma gangrenosum in chronic non-specific ulcerative colitis. Am. J. Med., *5*:69, 1948.
82. O'Loughlin, S., and Perry, H. O.: A diffuse pustular eruption associated with ulcerative colitis. Arch. Dermatol., *114*:1061, 1978.
83. Basler, R. S. W., and Dubin, H.: Ulcerative colitis and the skin. Arch. Dermatol., *112*:531, 1976.
84. McCarthy, P., and Shklar, G.: A syndrome of pyostomatitis vegetans and ulcerative colitis. Arch. Dermatol., *88*:913, 1963.
85. Forman, L.: The skin and the colon. Trans. St. John's Hosp. Derm. Soc., *52*:139, 1966.
86. Bloom, D., Fisher, D., and Dannenberg, M.: Pyoderma gangrenosum associated with hypogammaglobulinemia. Arch. Dermatol., *77*:412, 1958.
87. Dantzig, P. I.: Pyoderma gangrenosum. N. Engl. J. Med., *292*:47, 1975.
88. Perry, H. O.: Pyoderma gangrenosum. South. Med. J., *62*:899, 1969.
89. Hickman, J. G., and Lazarus, G. S.: Pyoderma gangrenosum: new concepts in etiology and treatment. *In* Moschella, S. L. (ed.): Dermatology Update. Reviews for Physicians. New York, Elsevier, 1979, p. 325.
90. McCallum, D. I., and Kinmont, P. D. C.: Dermatological manifestations of Crohn's disease. Br. J. Dermatol., *80*:1, 1968.
91. Byrne, J. P., Newitt, M., and Summerly, R.: Pyoderma gangrenosum associated with active chronic hepatitis. Arch. Dermatol., *112*:1297, 1976.
92. Callen, J. P., Dubin, H. V., and Gehrke, C. F.: Recurrent pyoderma gangrenosum and agnogenic myeloid metaplasia. Arch. Dermatol., *113*:1585, 1977.
93. Perry, H. O., and Winkelmann, R. K.: Bullous pyoderma gangrenosum and leukemia. Arch. Dermatol., *106*:901, 1972.
94. Ayres, S. A., Jr., and Ayres, S., III: Pyoderma gangrenosum with an unusual syndrome of ulcers, vesicles and arthritis. Arch. Dermatol., *77*:269, 1958.
95. Lazarus, G. S., Goldsmith, L. A., Rocklin, L. E., Pinals, R. S., deBuisseret, J. P., David, J. R., and Draper, W.: Pyoderma gangrenosum, altered delayed hypersensitivity and polyarthritis. Arch. Dermatol., *105*:46, 1972.
96. Graef, V., Baggenstoss, A. H., Sauer, W. G., and Spittell, J. A., Jr.: Venous thrombosis occurring in nonspecific ulcerative

colitis. Arch. Intern. Med., *117*:377, 1966.
97. Lee, J. C., Spittell, J. A., Jr., Sauer, W. G., Owen, C. A., Jr., and Thompson, J. H., Jr.: Hyper-coagulability associated with chronic ulcerative colitis: changes in blood coagulation factors. Gastroenterology, *54*:76, 1968.
98. Morowitz, D. A., Allen, L. W., and Kirsner, J. B.: Thrombosis in chronic inflammatory bowel disease. Ann. Intern. Med., *68*:1013, 1968.
99. Bargen, J. A., and Barker, N. W.: Extensive arterial and venous thromboses complicating chronic ulcerative colitis. Arch. Intern. Med., *58*:17, 1936.
100. Kehoe, E. L., and Newcomer, K. L.: Thromboembolic phenomena in ulcerative colitis. Arch. Intern. Med., *113*:711, 1964.
101. Ball, G. V., and Goldman, L. N.: Chronic ulcerative colitis, skin necrosis, and cryofibrinogenemia. Ann. Intern. Med., *85*:464, 1976.
102. Verbov, J. L.: The skin in patients with Crohn's disease and ulcerative colitis. Trans. St. John's Hosp. Derm. Soc., *59*:30, 1973.
103. Baker, W. N. W., and Milton-Thompson, G. J.: Management of anal fistulae in Crohn's disease. Proc. R. Soc. Med., *67*:58, 1974.
104. Fielding, J. F.: Perianal lesions in Crohn's disease. J. R. Coll. Surg., *17*:32, 1972.
105. Baker, W. N. W., and Milton-Thompson, G. J.: The anal lesion as the sole presenting symptom of intestinal Crohn's disease. Gut, *12*:865, 1971.
106. McCallum, D. I.: Personal communication.
107. Mountain, J. C.: Cutaneous ulceration in Crohn's disease. Gut, *11*:18, 1970.
108. Shiller, K. F. R., Golding, P. L., Peebles, R. A., and Whitehead, R.: Crohn's disease of the mouth and lips. Gut, *12*:864, 1971.
109. Stankler, L, Ewen, S. W. B., and Kerr, N. W.: Crohn's disease of the mouth. Br. J. Dermatol., *87*:501, 1972.
110. Verbov, J. L.: Crohn's disease with mouth and lip involvement. Br. J. Dermatol., *88*:517, 1973.
111. Cooke, W. T., Peeney, A. L. P., and Hawkins, C. F.: Symptoms, signs and diagnostic features of idiopathic steatorrhea. Q. J. Med., *22*:59, 1953.
112. Green, P. A., and Wollaeger, E. E.: The clinical behavior of sprue in the United States. Gastroenterology, *38*:399, 1960.
113. Wells, G. C.: Skin disorders in relation to malabsorption. Br. Med. J., *2*:937, 1962.
114. Simpson, J. A.: Dermatologic changes in hypocalcemia. Br. J. Dermatol., *66*:1, 1954.
115. Dent, C. E., and Garretts, M.: Skin changes in hypocalcemia. Lancet, *1*:142, 1960.
116. Friedman, M., and Hare, P. J.: Gluten sensitive enteropathy and eczema. Lancet, *1*:521, 1965.
117. Eyster, W. H., and Kierland, R. R.: Prognosis of dermatitis herpetiformis: treated and untreated. Arch. Dermatol., *64*:1, 1951.
118. Everall, J.: A clinical and followup study of 53 cases of dermatitis herpetiformis and electron microscopical examination in one case. Acta Dermato-Venereol., *34*:259, 1954.
119. Katz, S. I., and Strober, W.: The pathogenesis of dermatitis herpetiformis. J. Invest. Dermatol., *70*:63, 1978.
120. Fry, L., and Seah, P. P.: Criteria for the diagnosis of dermatitis herpetiformis. Proc. R. Soc. Med., *66*:749, 1973.
121. Brow, J. R., Parker, F., and Rubin, C. E.: Celiac sprue and the sprue-like lesion of dermatitis herpetiformis — separate or related entities? Gastroenterology, *54*:1223, 1968.
122. Fry, L., Keir, P., McMinn, R. M. H., Cowan, J. D., and Hoffbrand, A. V.: Small bowel structure and function and hematologic changes in dermatitis herpetiformis. Lancet, *2*:729, 1967.
123. Brow, J. R., Parker, F., Weinstein, M. W., and Rubin, C. E.: The small intestinal mucosa in dermatitis herpetiformis. I. Severity and distribution of the small intestinal lesions and associated malabsorption. Gastroenterology. *60*:355, 1971.
124. Weinstein, W. M., Brow, J. R., Parker, F., and Rubin, C. E.: The small intestinal mucosa in dermatitis herpetiformis. II. Relationship of the small intestinal lesion to gluten. Gastroenterology, *60*:362, 1 71.
125. Scott, B. B., and Losowsky, M. S.: Patchiness and mucosal abnormality in coeliac disease (CD) and dermatitis herpetiformis. Gut, *16*:393, 1975.
126. Shuster, S., Watson, A. J., and Marks, J.: Coeliac syndrome in dermatitis herpetiformis. Lancet, *1*:1101, 1968.
127. Bendl, B. J., and Williams, P. B.: Histopathological changes in the jejunal mucosa in dermatitis herpetiformis. Can. Med. Assoc. J., *98*:575, 1968.
128. Van Tongeren, J. H. M., Van der Staak, J. B. M., and Schillings, P. H. M.: Small bowel changes in dermatitis herpetiformis. Lancet, *1*:218, 1967.
129. Fraser, N. G., Murray, D., and Alexander, J. O'D.: Structure and function of the small intestine in dermatitis herpetiformis. Br. J. Dermatol., *79*:509, 1967.
130. Fry, L., Seah, P. P., Riches, D. J., and Hoffbrand, A. V.: Clearance of skin lesions in dermatitis herpetiformis after gluten withdrawal. Lancet, *1*:288, 1973.
131. Marks, R., and Whittle, M. W.: Results of treatment of dermatitis herpetiformis with a gluten-free diet after one year. Br. Med. J., *4*:772, 1969.
132. Marks, J., Birkett, D., Shuster, S., and Robert, D. F.: Small intestinal mucosal abnormalities in relatives of patients with dermatitis herpetiformis. Gut, *11*:493, 1970.

132a. Hall, R. P., Lawley, T. J., Heck, J. A., and Katz, S. I.: IgA-containing immune complexes in dermatitis herpetiformis, Henoch-Schönlein purpura, systemic lupus erythematosus and other diseases. Clin. Exp. Immunol., *40*:431, 1980.
133. Lawley, T. J., Strober, W., Yaoita, H., and Katz, S. I.: Small intestinal biopsies and HLA types in dermatitis herpetiformis patients with granular and linear IgA skin deposits. J. Invest. Dermatol., *74*:9, 1980.
134. Watson, W. C., Paton, E., and Murray, D.: Small bowel disease in rosacea. Lancet, *2*:47, 1965.
135. Shuster, S., and Marks, J.: Dermatogenic enteropathy. Lancet, *1*:1367, 1965.
136. Fry, L., Shuster, S., and McMinn, R. M. H.: D-xylose absorption in patients with eczema. Br. Med. J., *1*:967, 1965.
137. Doran, C. K., Everett, M. A., and Welsh, J D.: The D-xylose tolerance test. Arch. Dermatol., *94*:574, 1966.
138. Knowles, J. P., Shuster, S., and Wells, G. C.: Folic acid deficiency in patients with skin disease. Lancet, *1*:1138, 1963.
139. Mirick, G. S., and Shank, R. E.: An epidemic of serum hepatitis studied under controlled conditions. Trans. Am. Clin. Climat. Assoc., *71*:176, 1959.
140. Spellberg, M. A.: Disease of the Liver. New York, Grune and Stratton, Inc., 1954, p. 408.
141. Klatskin, G.: Personal communication.
142. Terry, R.: White nails in hepatic cirrhosis. Lancet, *1*:757, 1954.
143. Bean, W.: Vascular Spiders and Related Lesions of the Skin. Springfield, Charles C Thomas, 1958, p. 290.
144. Morey, D. A. J., and Burke, J. O.: Distinctive nail changes in advanced hepatic cirrhosis. Gastroenterology, *29*:258, 1955.
145. Muehrcke, R. C.: The finger nails in chronic hypoalbuminemia. A new physical sign. Br. Med. J., *1*:1327, 1956.
146. Lewin, K.: The normal finger nail. Br. J. Dermatol., *77*:421, 1965.
147. Lewin, K.: The finger nail in general disease. Br. J. Dermatol., *77*:431, 1965.
148. Cartwright, G. E., Edwards, C. Q., Kravitz, K., Skolnick, M., Amos, D. B., Johnson, A., and Buskjaer, L.: Hereditary hemochromatosis. Phenotypic expression of the disease. N. Engl. J. Med., *301*:175, 1979.
149. Kidd, K. K.: Genetic linkage and hemochromatosis. N. Engl. J. Med., *301*:209, 1979.
150. Sherlock, S.: Hemochromatosis: course and treatment. Ann. Rev. Med., *27*:143, 1976.
151. Perdrup, A., and Poulsen, H.: Hemochromatosis and vitiligo. Arch. Dermatol., *90*:34, 1964.
152. Burton, J. L., and Kirby, J.: Pigmentation and biliary cirrhosis. Lancet, *1*:458, 1975.
153. Fleming, C. R., Dickson, E. R., Hollenhorst, R. W., Goldstein, N. P., McCall, J. T., and Baggenstoss, A. H.: Pigmented corneal rings in patient with primary biliary cirrhosis. Gastroenterology, *69*:220, 1975.
154. Clarke, A. K., Galbraith, R. M., Hamilton, E. B. D., and Williams, R.: Rheumatic disorders in primary biliary cirrhosis. Ann. Rheum. Dis., *37*:42, 1978.
155. Dobyns, W. B., Goldstein, N. P., and Gordon, H.: Clinical spectrum of Wilson's disease (hepatolenticular degeneration). Mayo Clin. Proc., *54*:35, 1979.
156. Strickland, G. T., and Leu, M-L.: Wilson's disease. Clinical and laboratory manifestations in 40 patients. Medicine, *54*:113, 1975.
157. Leff, I. L.: Azure lunulae. Arch. Dermatol. *80*:224, 1959.
158. Emerson, K., Jr.: Disorders of pigment metabolism. *In* Harrison, T. R., Adams, R. D., Bennett, I. L., Resnik, W. H., Thorn, G. W., and Wintrobe, M. M. (eds.): Principles of Internal Medicine, 4th ed., New York, McGraw-Hill, Inc., 1962, p. 787.
159. Bondy, P. K.: Diabetes mellitus. *In* Beeson, P. B., and McDermott, W. (eds.): Cecil-Loeb Textbook of Medicine, 11th ed. Philadelphia, W. B. Saunders Company, 1963, p. 1305.
160. Alagille, D., Odièvre, M., Gautier, M., and Dommergues, J. P.: Hepatic ductular hypoplasia associated with characteristic facies, vertebral malformations, retarded physical, mental and sexual development, and cardiac murmur. J. Pediatr., *86*:63, 1975.

13

Endocrine and Metabolic Diseases

The major cutaneous manifestations of the endocrine and metabolic disorders are well known to clinicians and have been amply described in textbooks of medicine and endocrinology. I shall stress the less commonly appreciated signs and symptoms.

Two aspects of the dermatologic manifestations of these disorders need to be reevaluated; namely, skin texture and pruritus. Sweating, sebum production, and thickness all contribute to the texture of skin, but these factors cannot be accurately evaluated by clinical examination alone; they must also be measured by objective techniques. Coarseness and dryness of the skin may be caused by low humidity, too frequent bathing, excessive ultraviolet light exposure, topical medications, or genetically determined ichthyosis vulgaris. Dry skin is usually related to environmental or genetic factors rather than to the person's associated illness. Pruritus also has many etiologies that must be excluded before itching can be ascribed to the endocrine disorder which is present.

HYPOPITUITARISM

Pituitary insufficiency most often arises secondary to postpartum hemorrhage (Sheehan's syndrome) or to ablation of the gland by surgery or x-radiation for treatment of local tumors, visceral cancer, and diabetic retinopathy. Idiopathic hypopituitarism (Simmond's disease) is the least common variety of this endocrinopathy. The most obvious signs of pituitary insufficiency are pallor and a decreased ability to tan. These are the consequences of a decrease in melanin pigmentation secondary to diminished or absent secretion of a melanin-stimulating factor from the pituitary. In 1974, investigators discovered that the peptide sequence of beta–melanocyte-stimulating hormone (β-MSH) was part of the sequence of a larger pituitary peptide, β-lipotropin. β-MSH does not exist in nature but is split out from β-lipotropin during extraction procedures performed on pituitary glands. The peptide(s) responsible for melanin pigmentation in man need to be reevaluated. The role played by β-lipotropin or any of its degradation products in the physiologic control of human pigmentation remains to be defined (see p. 15).

The texture of the skin in hypopituitarism has been described both as smooth and as coarse with dryness and scaling. Fine wrinkling of the face and forehead is said to be characteristic. However, Sarver et al. described three patients, 16, 37, and 51 years old, with gigantism and fractional hypopituitarism.[1] The skin was smooth, and the patients had a youthful appearance even though two of the three persons were hypothyroid. I examined two patients with Sheehan's syndrome and found that their skin was smooth and "rubbery," similar to that of an infant.

Randall and Spong described a 49-year-old man who had had idiopathic hypopituitarism for 16 years.[2] This individual's skin was said to be thick, dry, and coarse over the distal arms and legs; also, the subcutaneous tissues over the entire body had a peculiar "doughy" feeling. The skin was pale and exhibited a diminished capacity to tan. The patient's PBI was 2.5 μg/100 ml and the BMR was minus 14 per cent. Dryness, coarseness, and scaling of the skin are said to be less pronounced in secondary myxedema than in primary myxedema. The texture of the skin in hypopituitarism needs to be reevaluated, especially in relation to the presence or absence of secondary hypothyroidism.

Secondary adrenal insufficiency is not accompanied by Addisonian pigmentation because of the lack of secretion of the pituitary peptide(s) responsible for pigmentation. Gonadal hypofunction produces a gradual loss of axillary, pubic, and body hair over a period of several years. Patients with chronic pituitary insufficiency remain in good nutritional status and do not develop the cachectic appearance of patients with anorexia nervosa. These latter individuals display some of the cutaneous features of hypopituitarism, but their endocrine glands function normally.

HYPERPITUITARISM

The excessive secretion of growth hormone by pituitary tumors produces gigantism in youngsters whose epiphyses have not yet closed; in adults whose normal bone growth has ceased, an excess of growth hormone produces acromegaly.

Growth hormone increases the mass of all the internal viscera as well as causes the obvious changes in the skin and bones. New periosteal bone is added, since the bones cannot grow in length. The skin thickens because of an increase in the dermal collagen. Over the face, neck, and scalp the excessive mass of skin may buckle and form burrows and ridges that resemble the gyri of the cerebral cortex (cutis verticis gyrata). The tongue is large and sometimes deeply furrowed. In its mildest form, the acromegalic facies resembles the coarse features of a myxedematous patient (Figs. 13–1 and 13–2). Thick lips, large nose, lantern jaw, and broad spadelike hands with squatty fingers are the striking findings in a person with advanced acromegaly (Fig. 13–3). Hyperpigmentation occurs in 40 per cent, and body hair is increased in about 50 per cent, of acromegalics.[3] The cause of the hirsutism is not understood, but the hyperpigmentation could be related to increased secretion of the pigment-promoting peptide(s).

The overgrowth of the soft tissues and of the facial and long bones occurs so slowly that the patient and close relatives rarely notice the presence or progression of the acromegaly. The affected individuals usually do not seek medical aid until the pituitary tumor — usually an eosinophilic adenoma — has enlarged sufficiently to produce headache or visual disturbances. Successful treatment of acromegaly by irradiation of

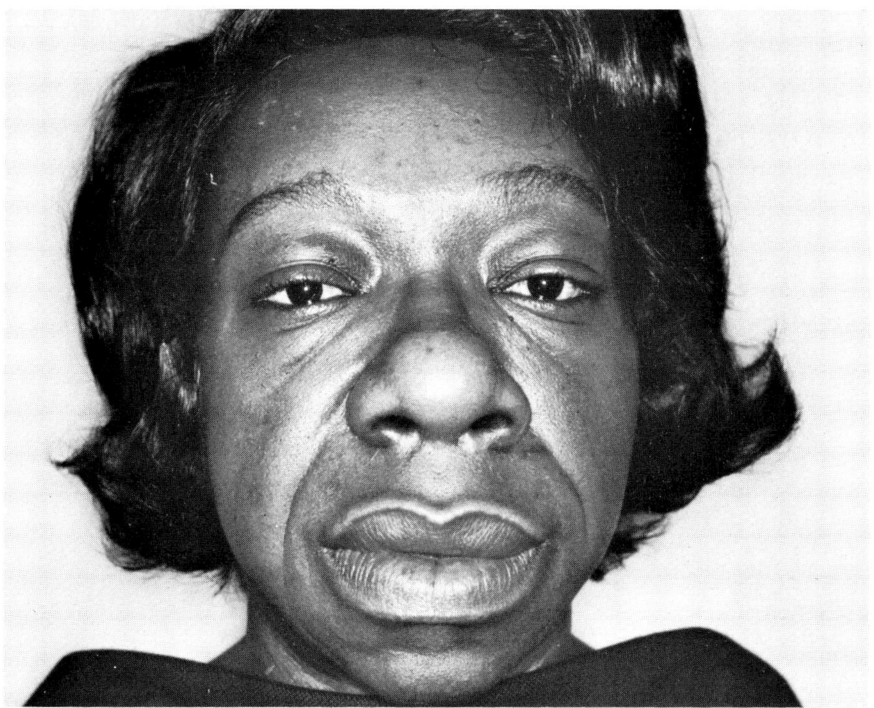

Figure 13–1. Acromegaly.

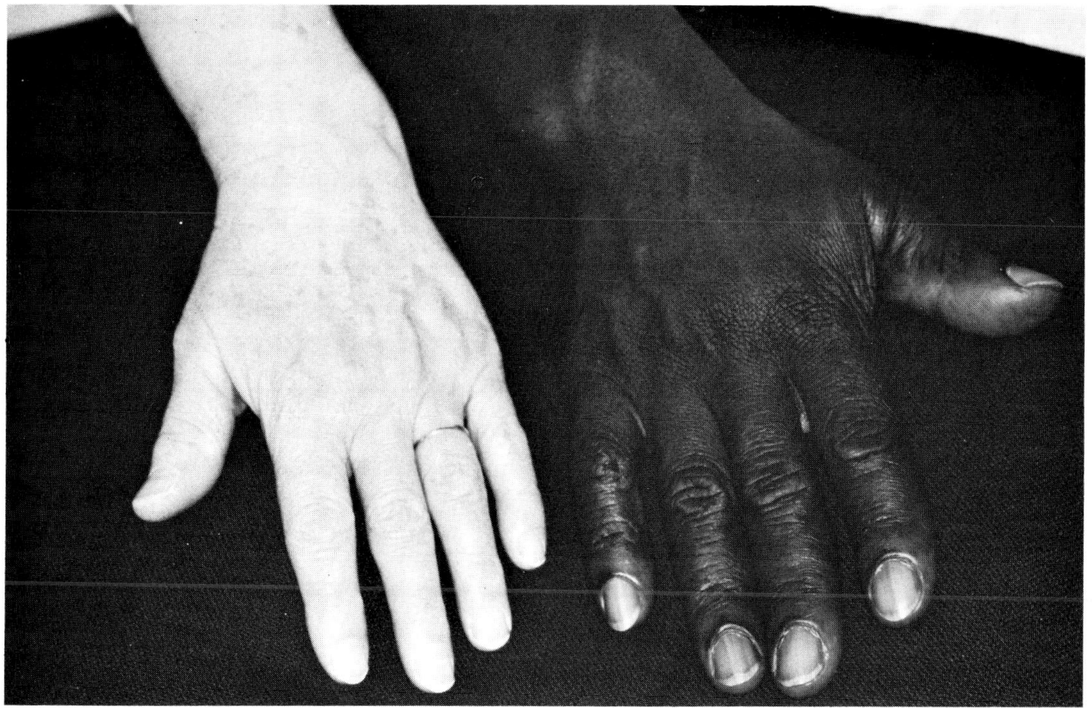

Figure 13–2. Acromegaly. Hand of the patient shown in Figure 13–1 compared with a normal-sized female hand.

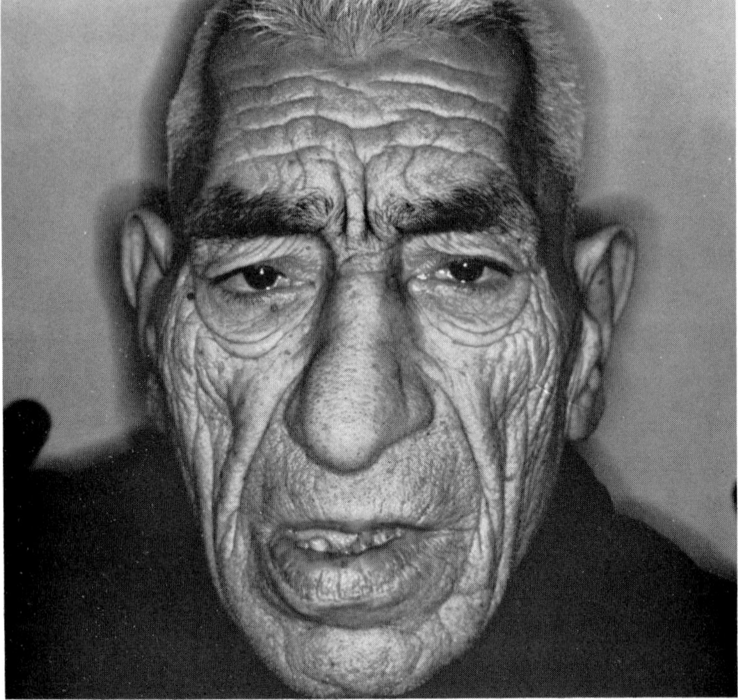

Figure 13–3. Acromegaly.

the pituitary is frequently accompanied by some improvement in the cutaneous and visceral abnormalities.

The clinical observation of cutaneous thickening in acromegalics has been substantiated by objective measurements.[4] However, the skin has also been described as being leathery with increased sweating and oiliness. Sweating and sebum production need to be objectively measured in order to determine whether or not growth hormone has a direct effect on sebaceous and exocrine sweat glands. Pochi has conducted preliminary studies on the effect of growth hormone on sebaceous gland function. He studied eight acromegalics, all of whom were women. Four were premenopausal, 22 to 32 years old, and the rest were postmenopausal, 50 to 58 years old. All of the postmenopausal acromegalics had normal sebum production, but three of the four younger women had moderately increased sebum secretion. The values were 3.3 to 3.6 mg (upper limit of normal: 2.8 mg). Pochi also found that adult pituitary dwarfs who lack growth hormone have normal sebaceous gland function.[5] These preliminary data suggest that sebaceous glands can function in the absence of growth hormone and that a moderate increase in sebaceous gland secretion occurs in some patients with acromegaly.

I have examined the skin of three patients with acromegaly. One man and one woman, both in their forties, had active untreated disease; and a third man, 70 years old, was in the inactive "burned-out" stage of the illness. The two patients with active disease had *smooth* rubbery skin that was hyperelastic, almost to the same extent as that observed in Ehlers-Danlos disease (Fig. 13–4). However, there was no evidence of hyperextensible joints or a family history of this disorder in either patient. The

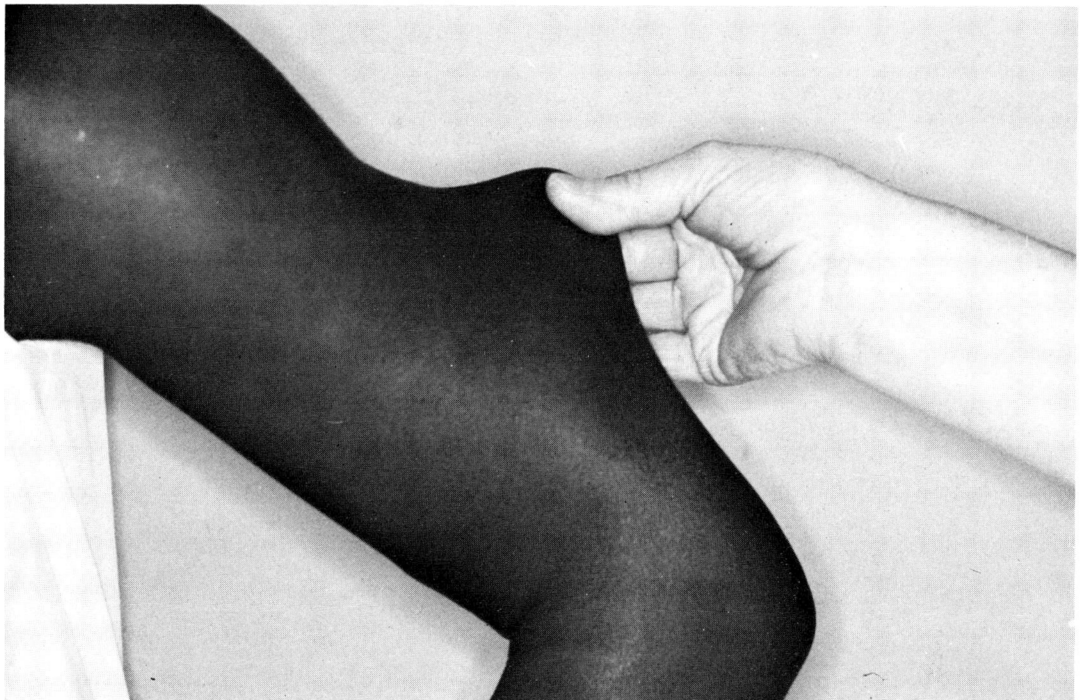

Figure 13–4. Acromegaly. Hyperelastic skin of the patient shown in Figure 13–1.

skin of the third patient was dry, rough, and did not feel thickened. The cutaneous findings were those of a 70-year-old man.

Hyperfunction of the pituitary gland is also responsible for most cases of Cushing's syndrome with bilateral adrenal hyperplasia. This disorder will be discussed later in this section.

Lerner reported the case of a 33-year-old Egyptian man who developed hyperpigmentation secondary to increased "MSH" secretion from a presumedly hyperplastic or hyperfunctioning pituitary gland.[6] There was no evidence of Cushing's syndrome or acromegaly, but the patient displayed the characteristic pattern of "MSH" hyperpigmentation on the face, neck, and genitalia and in the axillae, palmar creases, and recent scars. Increased "MSH" activity was detected in the patient's urine. Following treatment with 50 mg of cortisone daily, the hyperpigmentation faded somewhat, and abnormal urinary levels of "MSH" activity were no longer detected. X-ray examination showed that the sella turcica was not enlarged. Addison's disease was also excluded in this patient.

GRAVES' DISEASE

At present, Graves' or Basedow's disease is considered to be a syndrome with five components: hyperthyroidism or thyrotoxicosis associated with diffuse goiter; ophthalmopathy; pretibial myxedema; clubbing and subperiosteal new bone formation (acropachy); and the presence of long-acting thyroid stimulator (LATS) in the serum.[7] Each of these features may be present singly, in various combinations, or may follow one another in random sequence. For example, pretibial myxedema may precede or follow hyperthyroidism by months to years. Ophthalmopathy may exist in the absence of thyrotoxicosis, thus giving rise to the concept of euthyroid Graves' disease. Ophthalmopathy has even been described in patients with myxedema.[8] LATS is present in 40 to 60 per cent of individuals with hyperthyroidism and exophthalmos and in over 90 per cent of patients with pretibial myxedema.

Graves' disease is also believed to be closely related to Hashimoto's thyroiditis and myxedema because of common immunological abnormalities.[10, 11] Most instances of primary hypothyroidism and myxedema are now considered to be the consequence of preceding Hashimoto's thyroiditis, which may not have been clinically apparent. Circulating antibodies against thyroglobulin and thyroid microsomes, evidence of cell-mediated immunity against thyroid tissue and lymphocytic infiltration of the thyroid gland, are common features of these three disorders. In some families, thyroid antibodies including LATS have been detected in relatives of patients with Graves' disease and thyroiditis.[12] Relatives of patients with one of these three disorders often have an increased prevalence of one of the other two. Instances of myxedema or thyroiditis preceding thyrotoxicosis have been reported.[13]

LATS is a polyclonal IgG that behaves as an autoantibody against an as-yet-unidentified component of the thyroid cell membrane. LATS can stimulate the synthesis and release of thyroid hormone in animals, but not in man. LATS cannot be correlated with the severity of hyperthyroidism or pretibial myxedema, nor can it be directly implicated in the pathogenesis of the various components of Graves' disease. It is not present in *all* patients with hyperthyroidism or pretibial myxedema. However, the investigations centered about LATS led to the discovery by Adams and Kennedy[14] and Onaya et al.[15] of another IgG species, thyroid-stimulating immunoglobulin (TSI), that was important in thyrotoxicosis. TSI has four properties: it inhibits the binding of LATS to thyroid tissue extract (LATS protector); stimulates colloid droplet formation; activates cyclic AMP in human thyroid slices; and displaces thyrotropin (TSH) from its receptors on thyroid cells. TSI appears to behave as an antibody against TSH receptors on the plasma membrane of the thyroid follicular cell. TSI inhibits the binding of TSH to its receptors, while it simultaneously stimulates the thyroid cell to produce thyrotoxicosis.

Thus it is currently believed that the balance of interaction between TSI and cell-mediated immunity with its tissue destructive effects is the major determinant affecting the development of Graves' disease, thyroiditis, and hypothyroidism. TSI can be found in 15 per cent of patients with Hashimoto's thyroiditis. It has been suggested that the inflammatory tissue reaction in thyroiditis may limit the responsiveness of the gland to TSI, thereby explaining in part the phenomenon of euthyroid ophthalmopathy and euthyroid Graves' disease. Genetic factors also appear to be an important predisposing factor in the development of autoimmune thyroid disease.[12, 16, 17] Hyperthyroidism is an example of a newly described group of disorders known as antireceptor antibody diseases. Myasthenia gravis and the syndrome of diabetes mellitus, insulin resistance, and acanthosis nigricans are the other two entities that belong to this group. The antibodies in these latter two disorders inhibit, rather than stimulate, neuromuscular transmission and the action of insulin through the blocking of acetylcholine and insulin receptors, respectively.

The excess production and secretion of thyroid hormone responsible for the hyperthyroid component of Graves' disease produces characteristic cutaneous findings.

The skin is warm and moist because of an increase in cutaneous blood flow and sweating. Although the skin is frequently described as being fine, thereby implying thinness, radiographic studies show that the skin is of normal thickness. Palmar erythema and onycholysis (the separation of the distal nailplate from the nailbed) are present in some patients (Fig. 13–5; Plate 35*C*). However, neither sign is specific for hyperthyroidism. The scalp hair is said to be fine, friable, and not capable of retaining a wave. The scalp hair may be lost in a diffuse fashion during active hyperthyroidism, but it will regrow when the disease is brought under control.

Chronic active hyperthyroidism can be complicated by Addisonian hyperpigmentation, which is thought to be caused by increased "MSH" secretion from the pituitary. This feature occurs less frequently now, probably because patients with hyperthyroidism come to a physician for treatment earlier than they used to. Vitiligo develops in about 7 per cent of thyrotoxic individuals (Fig. 13–6).

Readett found that 33 per cent of 146 patients with hyperthyroidism suffered from atopic dermatitis.[18] Chronic urticaria and generalized pruritus are uncommon manifestations of this thyroid disorder.[19]

The ophthalmopathy varies from mild exophthalmos in which the eyes merely appear prominent to the more severe condition of proptosis. When the ophthalmopathy is mild, the sclera is visible on upward or downward gaze (lid lag); when more severe, the lids are edematous and

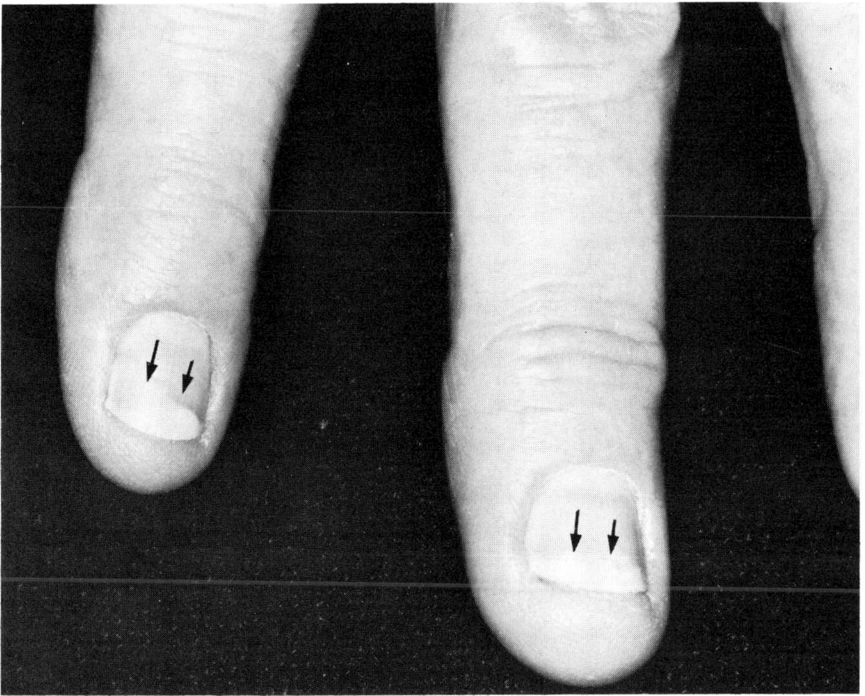

Figure 13–5. Onycholysis in hyperthyroidism. Arrows show extent of separation of nailplate from nailbed.

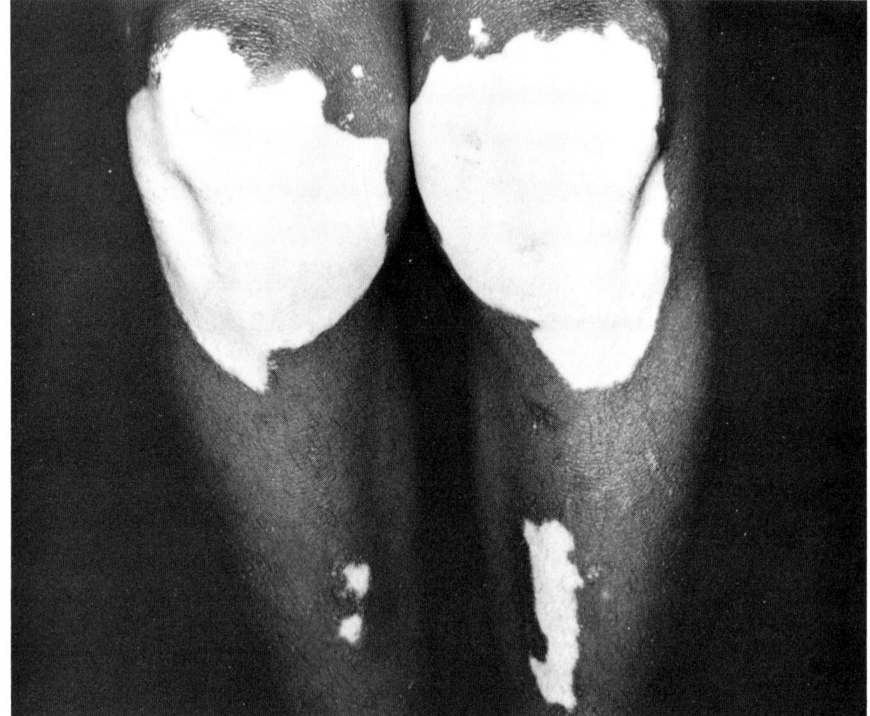

Figure 13–6. Vitiligo.

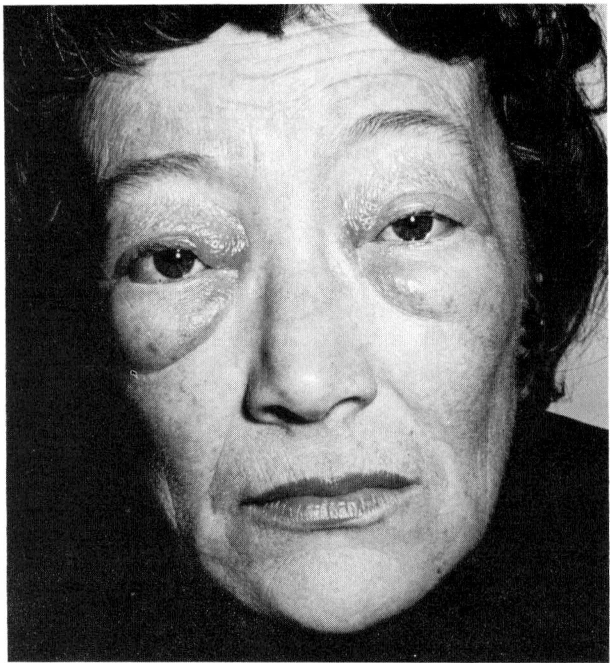

Figure 13–7. Graves' disease. Periorbital edema and chemosis.

PLATE 35

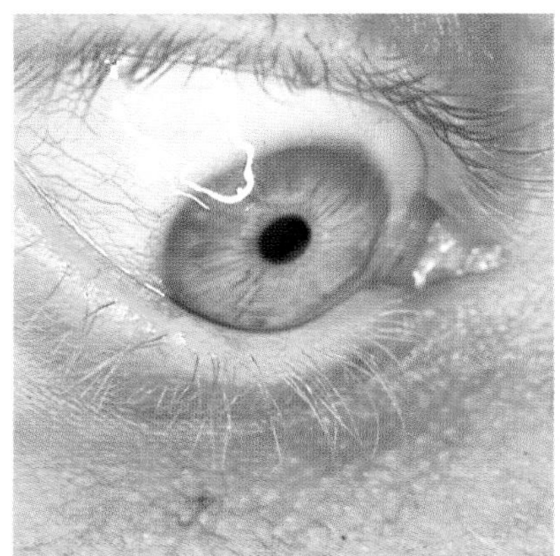

A, Kayser-Fleischer ring in Wilson's disease.

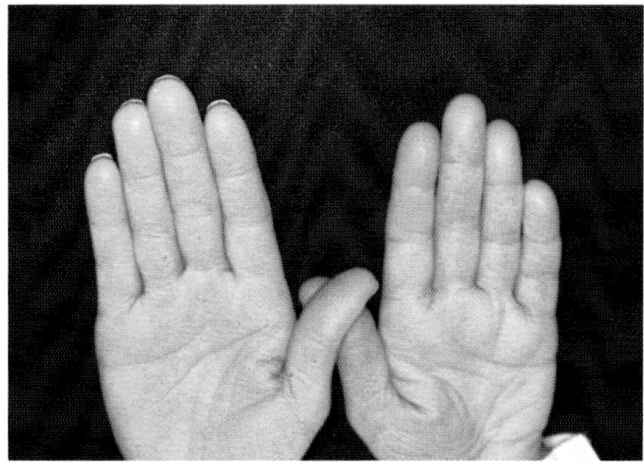

B, Carotenemia. The hand on the left belongs to patient; the hand on the right belongs to normal person.

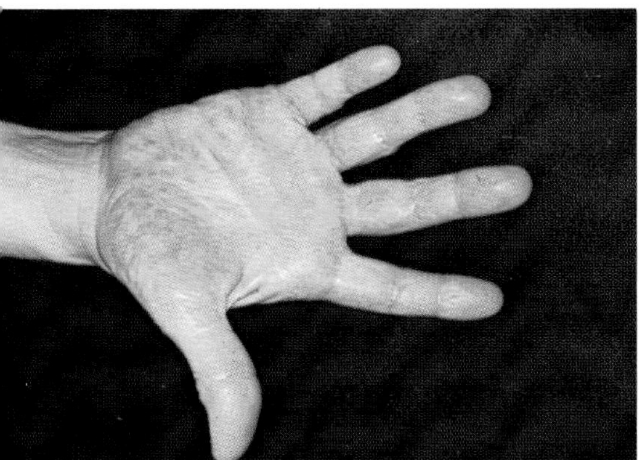

C, Palmar erythema of hyperthyroidism.

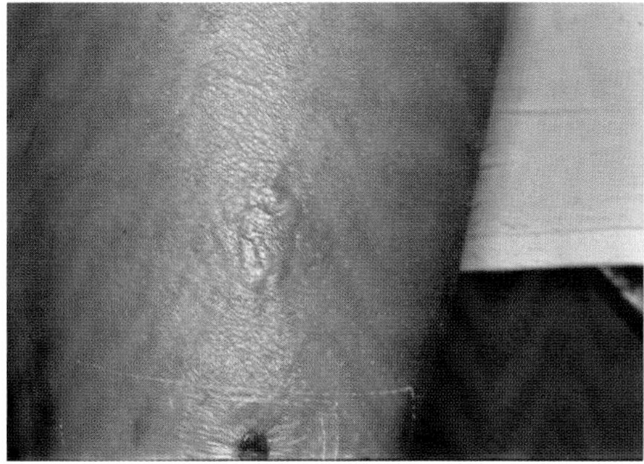

D, Pretibial myxedema. An erythematous waxy-appearing nodule with an irregular surface.

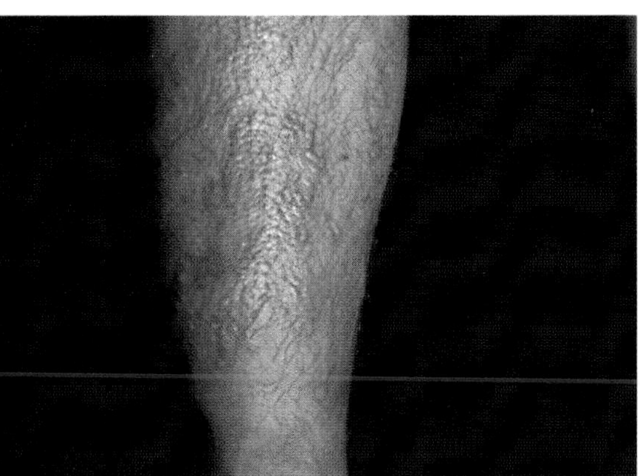

E, Pretibial myxedema. Note the peau d'orange appearance of the skin.

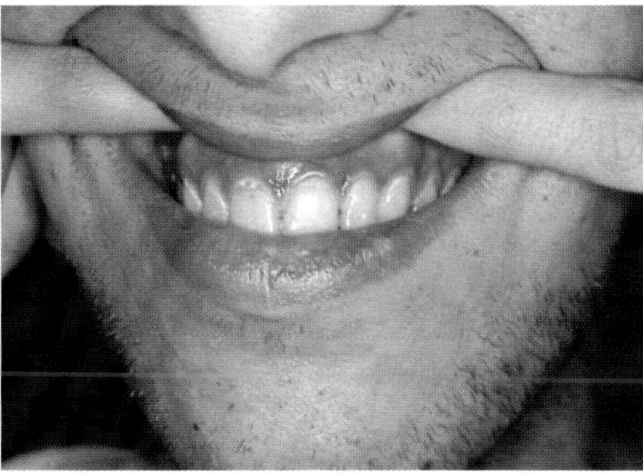

F, Addison's disease. Gingival hyperpigmentation.

cannot close adequately. Edema and vascular congestion of the sclerae develop (chemosis) (Fig. 13–7). Extraocular muscle function becomes impaired with severe proptosis. Infiltration of the retro-orbital tissues and extraocular muscles by lymphocytes, plasma cells, and mucopolysaccharides accounts for the proptosis and derangement of muscle function. The globe is displaced forward and the diameter of the muscles may increase by five to ten times. If the ophthalmopathy is not corrected, the muscle fibers may be destroyed, leading to eventual contractures. Progressive exophthalmos can lead to diplopia, corneal ulceration, and panophthalmitis with loss of visual acuity. Currently the best explanation for the pathogenesis of the ophthalmopathy is cell-mediated immunity to retro-orbital muscle antigen.[10]

The pretibial myxedema component of Graves' disease usually arises after surgical or radio-iodine therapy for thyrotoxicosis. However, pretibial myxedema can develop in the absence of hyperthyroidism[20] as well as during the phase of untreated acute hyperthyroidism. It has also been reported in patients with Hashimoto's thyroiditis, indicating the close relationship between Graves' disease and thyroiditis. Pretibial myxedema may develop within weeks or as long as 28 years after thyroid hyperactivity has been treated.[21] The status of the patients' thyroid function bears no relationship to the development of this component of Graves' disease. The individual may be hyper-, hypo-, or euthyroid at the time pretibial myxedema develops.

The complete syndrome of pretibial myxedema is characterized by plaques on the shins, exophthalmos, and clubbing with or without osteoarthropathy. The preexisting exophthalmos usually becomes worse when the syndrome appears. The clubbing and the bony changes tend to develop late in the course of this syndrome; they are sometimes referred to as thyroid acropachy. Osteoarthropathy is not a common feature of this disorder, and most patients have only clubbing in association with the cutaneous and ocular abnormalities.

The cutaneous manifestation is characterized by flesh-colored, pink, or violaceous plaques and nodules on the shins (Plate 35 *D, E*). Rarely, the plaques and nodules develop on the calves and posterior aspects of the lower legs (Fig. 13–8). These intradermal lesions have a waxy and sometimes translucent quality and are produced by the massive deposition of acid mucopolysaccharides identical to those found in the skin of patients with hypothyroidism and in the retro-orbital tissue of those with exophthalmos and Graves' disease. The main component of the mucopolysaccharides is hyaluronic acid, which is present in amounts 6 to 16 times greater than that found in unaffected skin.[22] As the mucin accumulates, the skin forms nodules or plaques with prominent dilated follicular openings (peau d'orange appearance). In extreme cases, mucin can infiltrate the skin of the entire leg and produce thickened skin with folds overhanging the ankles, which simulates elephantiasis (Fig. 13–9). Siegler and Refetoff reported a patient in whom the deposition of mucin not only produced the typical cutaneous lesions, but also caused entrapment of the branches of the peroneal nerves. This entrapment produced foot drop in one leg and impaired dorsiflexion in the other. The neurological abnormalities disappeared after the cutaneous lesions were successfully treated by topical corticosteroids under occlusive dressings.[23]

Figures 13–10 to 13–12 illustrate the findings in one of our patients. In

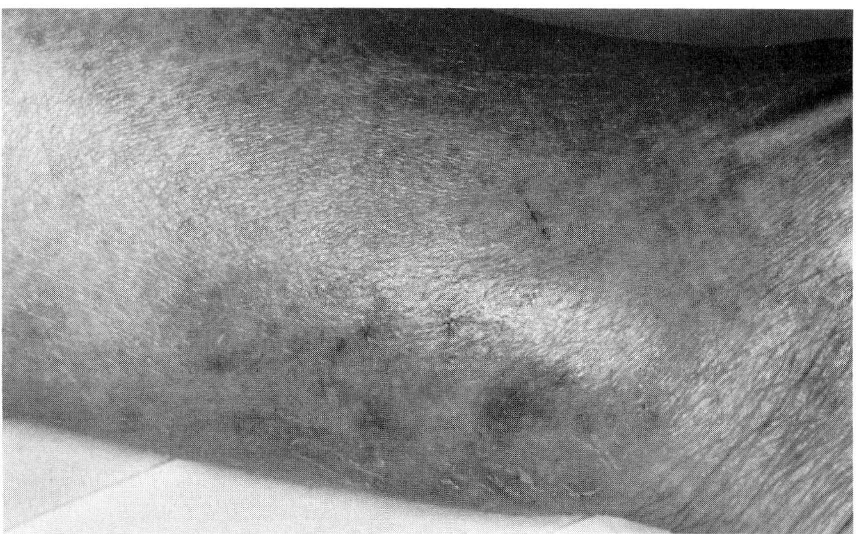

Figure 13–8. Pretibial myxedema. Plaque with foci of purpura involving the posterior lower calf. Atypical location.

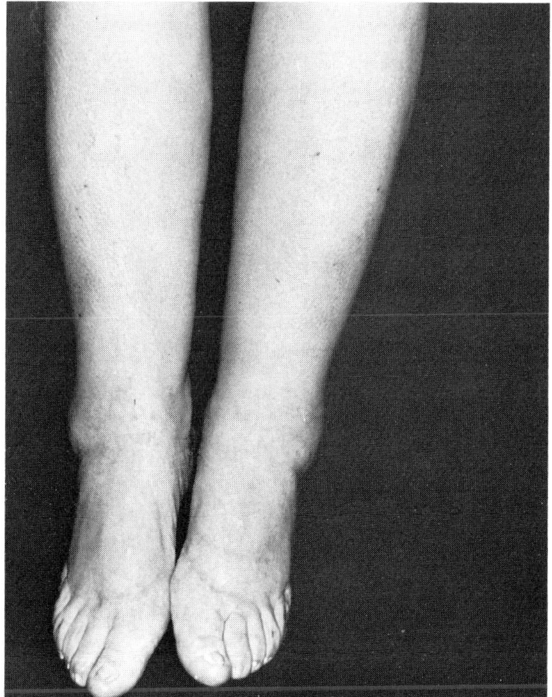

Figure 13–9. Pretibial myxedema. Skin of the entire leg is infiltrated with mucin to produce the cylindrical legs with skin folds overhanging the ankles.

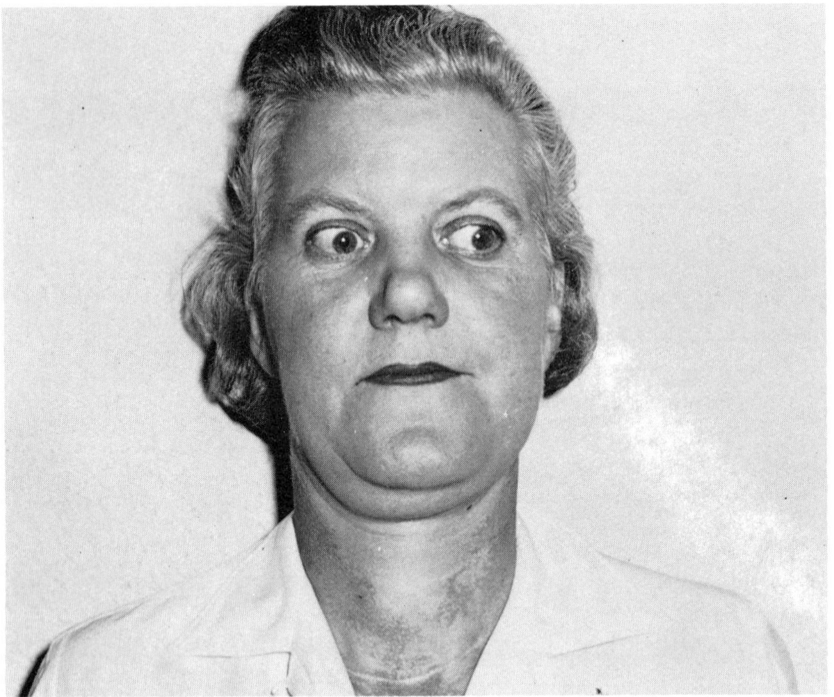

Figure 13–10. Pretibial myxedema. Exophthalmos is present. Facial skin is diffusely infiltrated with mucin and is firm.

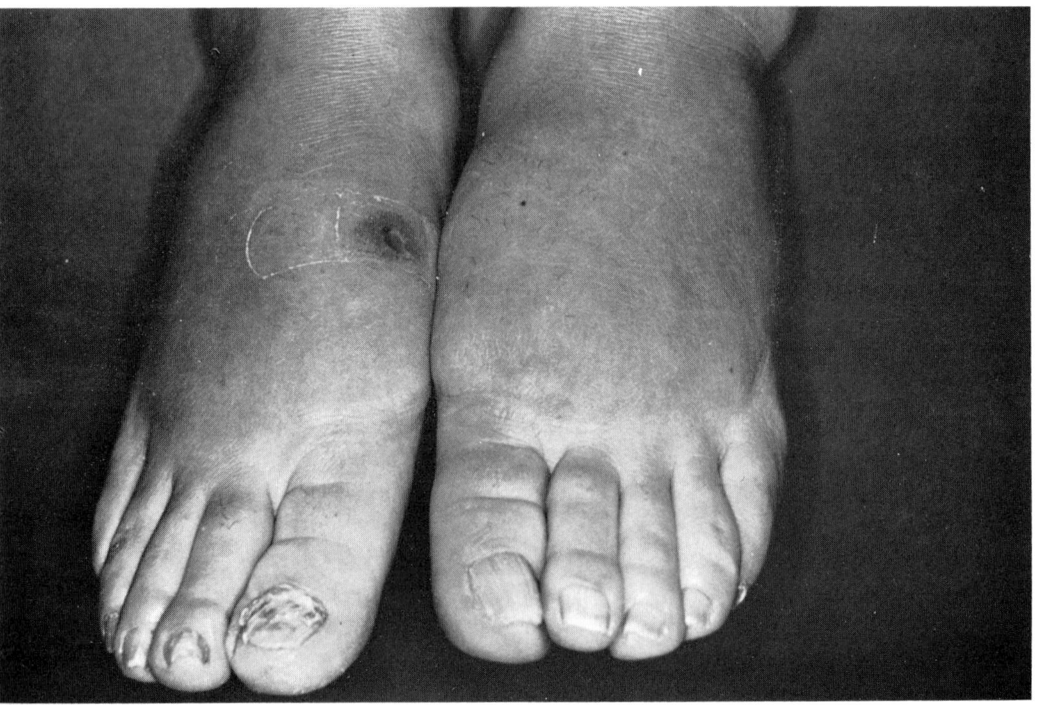

Figure 13–11. Pretibial myxedema. Same patient shown in Figure 13–10. Skin of feet is similarly infiltrated with mucin and is hard to palpation.

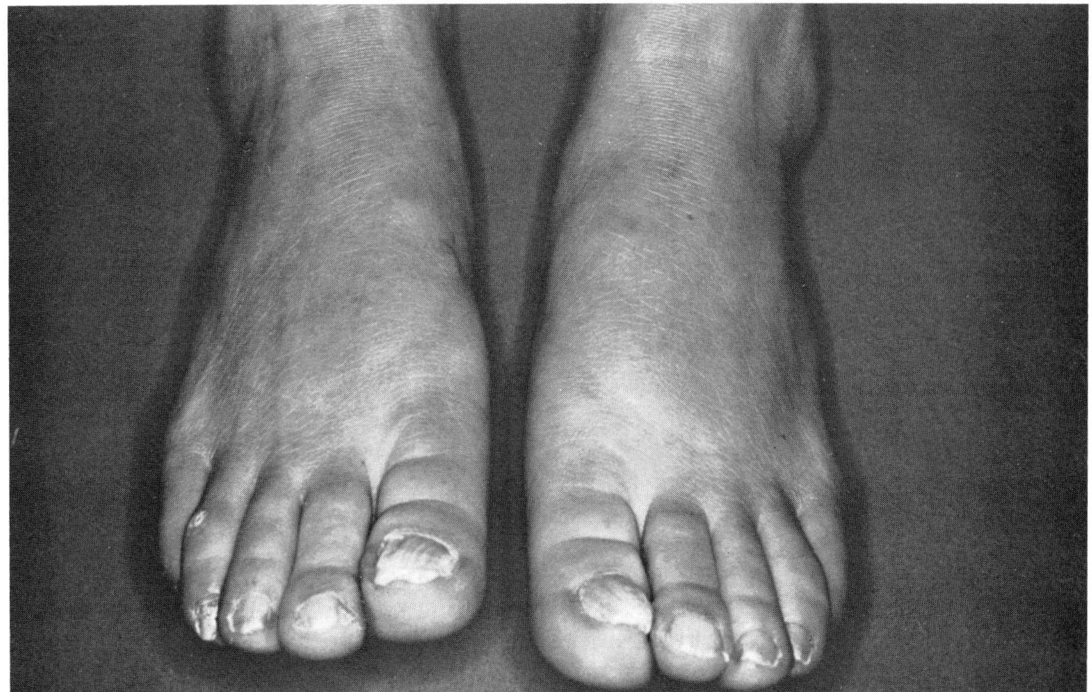

Figure 13–12. Pretibial myxedema. Same patient shown in Figure 13–11. Feet have returned to normal size, and the skin has returned to normal consistency one year after treatment with oral corticosteroids.

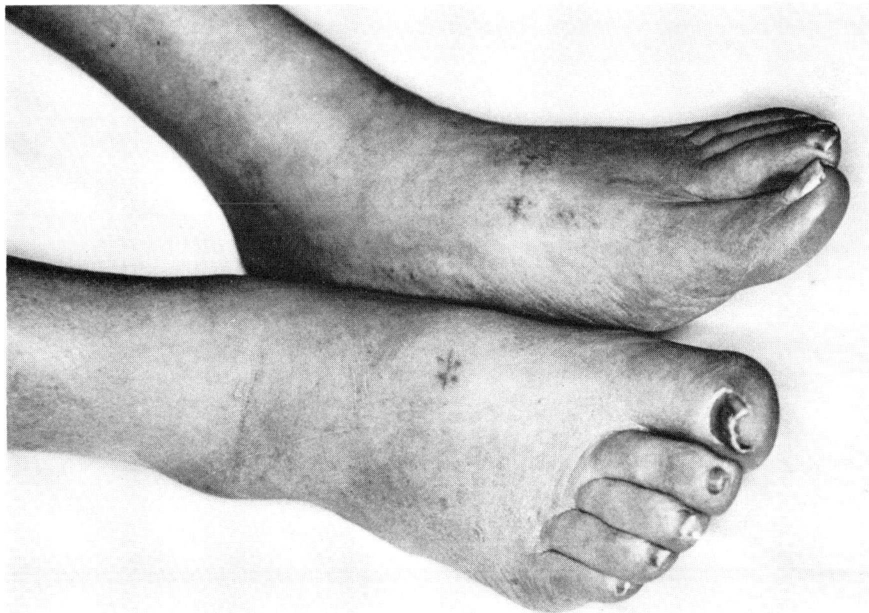

Figure 13–13. Pretibial myxedema. In this patient thyroid function was normal and LATS and thyroid antibodies were absent from the serum. Feet and ankles were diffusely indurated.

addition to the typical lesions on the shins, her face, hands, and feet were massively and diffusely infiltrated by mucin: the facial skin was free of wrinkles; the hands and feet were stony-hard and simulated scleroderma. Desiccated thyroid, which was given to this patient because she was mildly hypothyroid, caused the cutaneous lesions to swell and become painful. Triamcinolone, 4 to 6 mg per day, was administered, and the thyroid medication caused no further difficulties. After one year of combined therapy, the deposition of mucin almost completely disappeared from the hands, feet, and face; and she was subsequently able to wear her rings and shoes comfortably.

Figure 13–13 and Plate 30*C* illustrate an unusual manifestation of pretibial myxedema in a 70-year-old man who had normal thyroid function, no previous history of thyroid disease, and *no* laboratory evidence of LATS or thyroid antibodies. His feet and ankles were diffusely indurated, and the typical pink papules and plaques were present on the shins. On the lateral aspects of both legs extending to the calves there were larger areas of erythema and warmth that simulated cellulitis. In the center of one of these areas there was a small ulceration secondary to a contact dermatitis. Biopsies from the foot, shin, and "cellulitic" area showed the characteristic histologic findings of pretibial myxedema.

Surgical procedures on the nodules or indurated tissues of pretibial myxedema may be followed by deposition of mucin, leading to further enlargement of the involved areas.[24]

It has been proposed that LATS is responsible for the deposition of mucin in the dermis through the mechanism of an antigen-antibody reaction. However, Schermer et al. demonstrated by direct immunofluorescence that immunoglobulins and complement were not present in the cutaneous lesions nor could LATS be isolated from them. They also showed that there was no correlation between the serum level of LATS and the severity of the skin lesions.[9]

A breakthrough in our understanding of the pathogenesis of pretibial myxedema was made by Cheung et al., who showed that the serum of these patients contained a nonimmunoglobulin protein that stimulated skin fibroblasts to produce mucin and proteins.[25] Skin fibroblasts from patients with pretibial myxedema and from normal individuals produced more hyaluronic acid, sulfated mucopolysaccharides, and collagen after exposure to this serum factor than to normal serum. In addition, the pretibial myxedema serum factor stimulated fibroblasts taken from the shins, but not fibroblasts derived from the foreskin or shoulder region of normal individuals or of patients with pretibial myxedema. These studies imply that the fibroblasts in the various regions of the body possess different biologic characteristics and that their growth may be modulated by specific humoral factors. The pathogenesis of the skin lesions in pretibial myxedema appears to be distinct and unrelated to the mechanisms proposed for the other clinical and biochemical features of Graves' disease, Hashimoto's thyroiditis, and hypothyroidism.

HYPOTHYROIDISM

The skin becomes rough and dry in primary myxedema. These changes are most prominent over the extensor surfaces of the limbs; and in the severely affected patients, ichthyosis vulgaris is simulated (Fig.

13–14). In a few patients, hyperkeratosis of the palms and soles has developed. The facial skin is puffy and produces coarse features; the expression is often dull and flat; the tongue is enlarged; and the periorbital skin, especially the infraorbital tissue, is chronically edematous. A spectrum of facial changes can be observed in hypothyroidism (Figs. 13–15 to 13–17).

Because of the deposition of mucin, the feet and hands may become puffy, but never to the extent seen in pretibial myxedema. Although the skin of a patient with myxedema may appear to be thickened because of its coarse and dry quality, objective measurements have shown that the thickness of the skin is normal. The temperature of the skin falls in advanced myxedema. A yellow tint may appear in the skin secondary to carotenemia. Diffuse hair loss is common. The outer third of the eyebrows is shed. The hair is said to become coarse and brittle, and the nails may break easily at the edges. Freinkel and Freinkel showed that deficiency of thyroid hormone was associated with an increased percent-

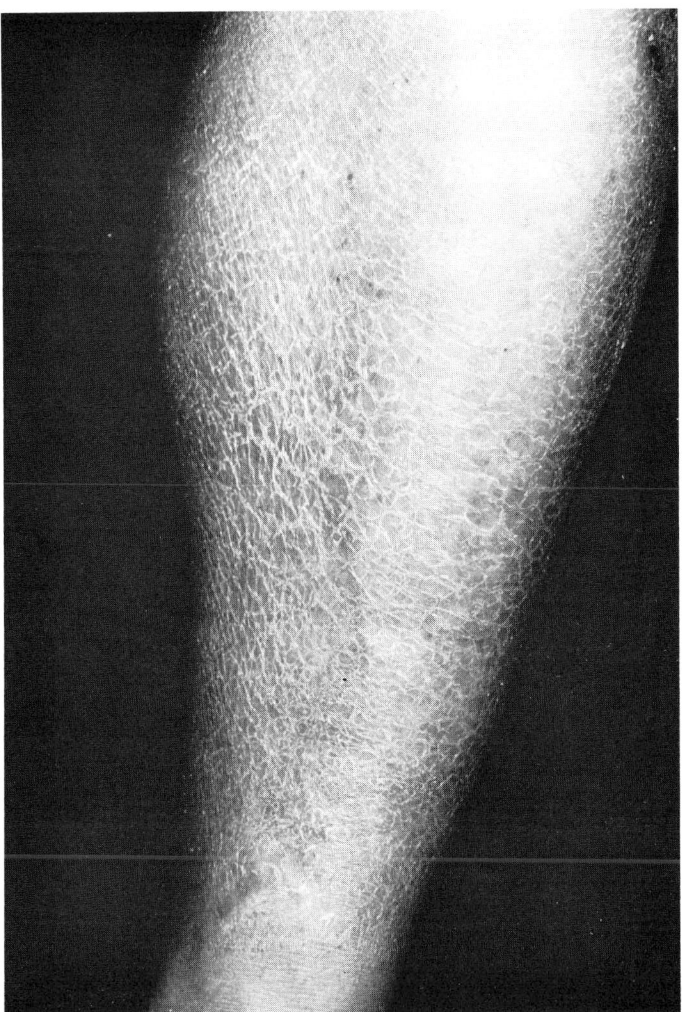

Figure 13–14. Myxedema. Dry skin resembling ichthyosis on extensor surfaces.

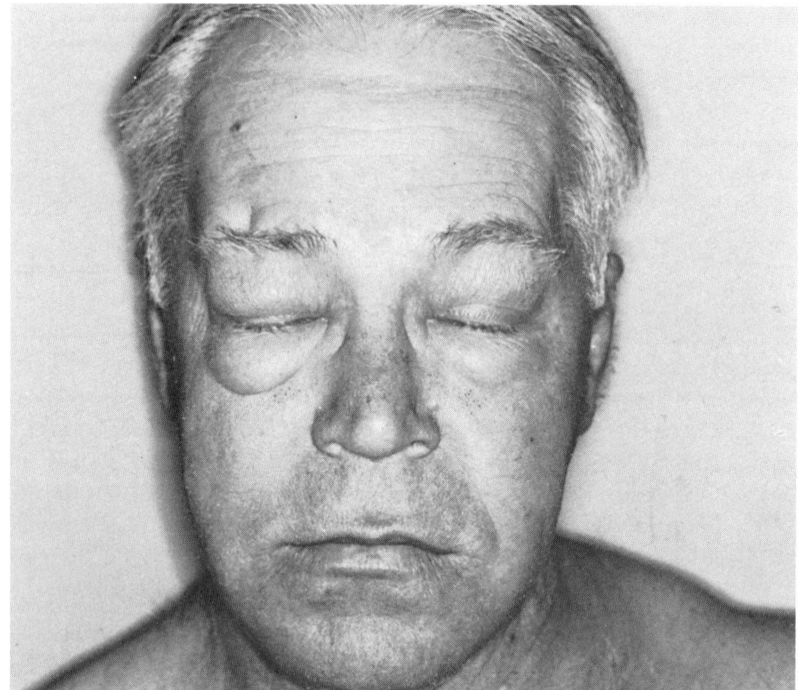

Figure 13–15. Myxedema. Marked periorbital edema.

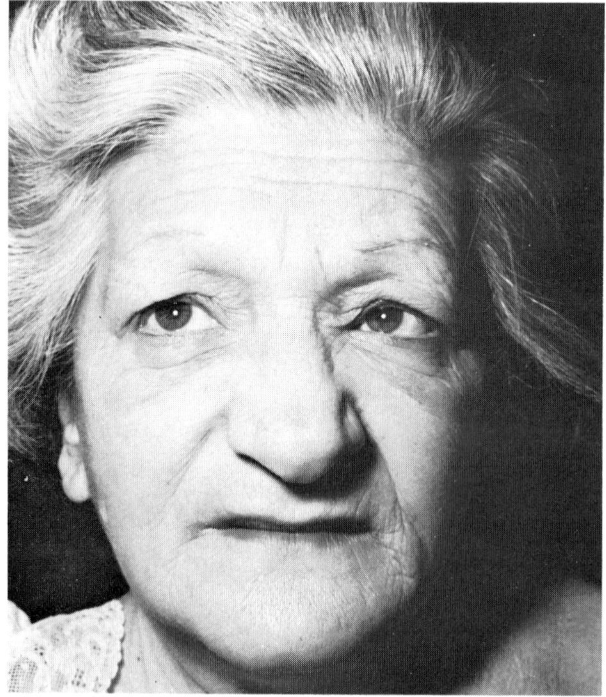

Figure 13–16. Myxedema. Coarse features and mildly puffy lids. (Courtesy of Dr. Ronald Savin.)

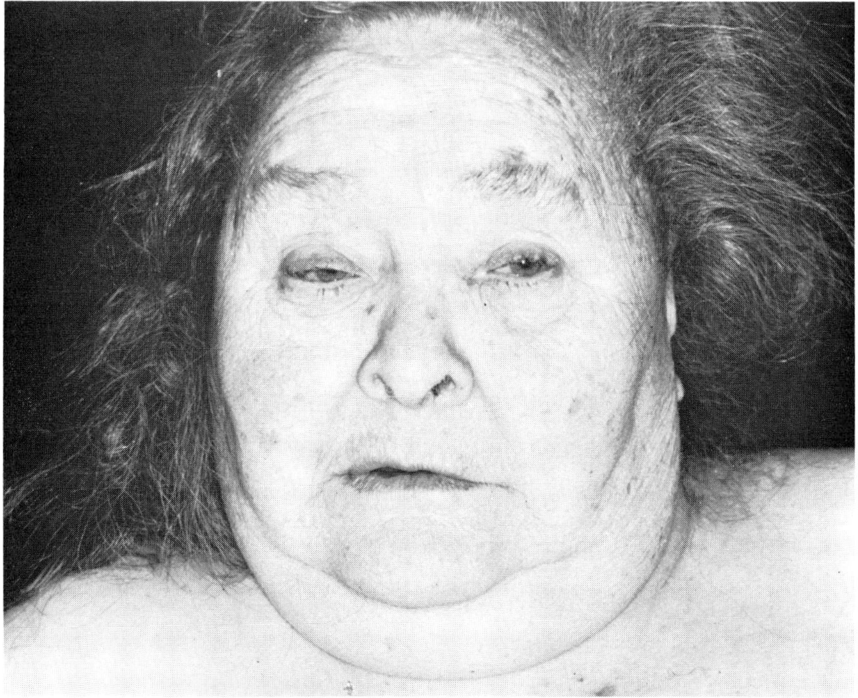

Figure 13–17. Severe myxedema.

age of scalp hair being in the telogen or resting phase of the hair growth cycle. Within eight weeks after treatment with thyroid extract had been started, the telogen/anagen hair ratio began to return to normal. It appears that thyroid deficiency is associated with shortening of the hair growth cycle (premature arrest of the anagen phase) and that hormone replacement is able to initiate new hair growth.[26]

Hypercholesterolemia and hypertriglyceridemia can develop and result in eruptive and tuberous xanthomas, but these are unusual findings.[27]

Purpura and ecchymoses, manifestations of easy bruising on the arms and legs, were observed by Christianson in 9 of 222 patients with myxedema at the Ochsner Clinic over 14 years.[28] The bleeding disappeared following successful thyroid replacement therapy. It is probable that the deposition of mucin in the dermal connective tissue around the capillaries produced weakening of the normal vascular supports.

The presence of chronic periorbital edema is usually a sign of hypothyroidism rather than of an allergic disease.

Congenital hypothyroidism — cretinism — presents a picture that is not easily forgotten; a facies characterized by wide-set eyes, a broad flat nose, large protruding tongue, periorbital puffiness, sparse hair, rough skin, short neck, and a protuberant abdomen with an umbilical hernia.

When hypothyroidism develops secondary to pituitary failure, the cutaneous and hair abnormalities are not as severe as those seen in primary myxedema.

Myxedema may be associated with several types of rheumatic complaints: joint stiffness, arthralgias and myalgias, carpal tunnel syndrome, synovial thickening, noninflammatory joint effusions, and gener-

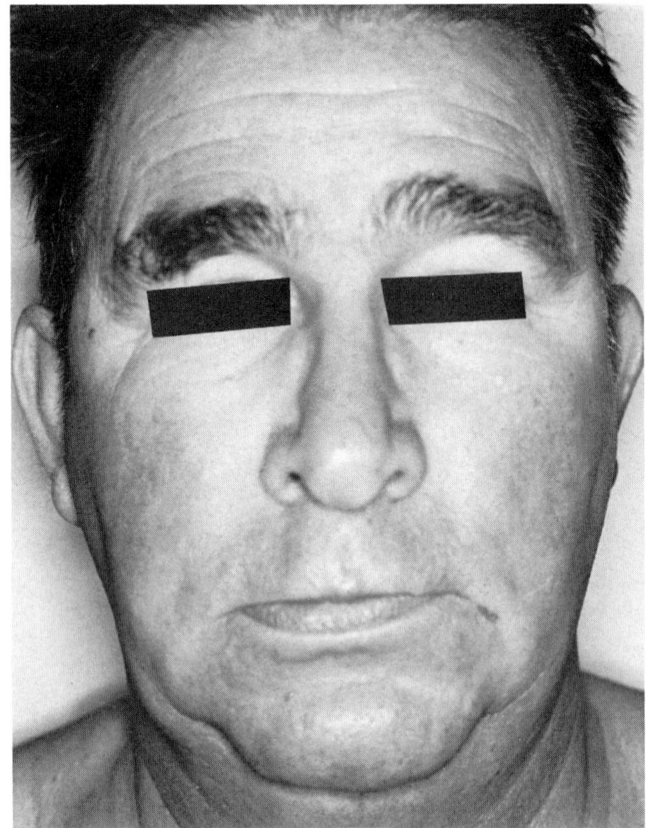

Figure 13–18. Myxedema. Generalized involvement of skin led initially to diagnosis of "stiff-man" syndrome.

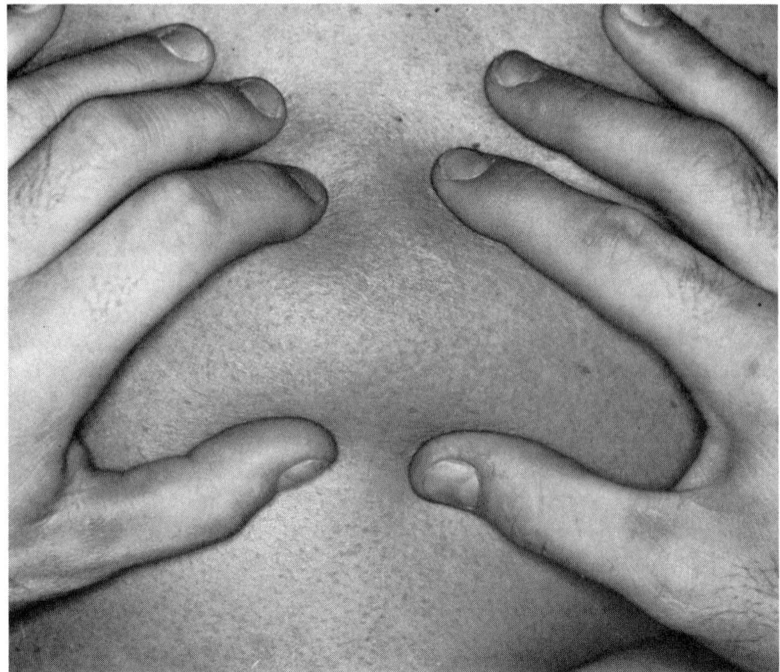

Figure 13–19. Myxedema. Same patient as in Figure 13–18. Skin of back was markedly indurated. Compare with normal individual in Figure 13–20.

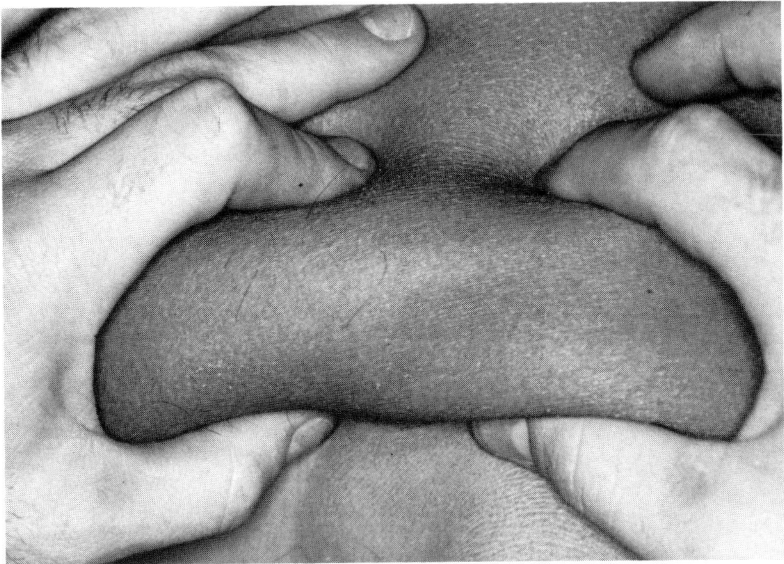

Figure 13–20. Normal individual showing the degree of compression for the skin of the back.

alized stiffness.[29] These signs and symptoms are completely reversible following thyroid hormone replacement. Since many of the complaints are nonspecific, the patient might be thought to be suffering from a rheumatic disease. The following case report illustrates this point.

A 50-year-old man complained of generalized stiffness. He was admitted to the Neurology service for further studies related to the possible diagnosis of "stiff-man" syndrome. On physical examination, he had a slightly puffy face and the skin over his trunk, arms, and legs felt firm (Figs. 13–18 to 13–20). He moved slowly. The clue to the correct diagnosis was the demonstration of an abnormally slow relaxation phase of the Achilles tendon reflex. Skin biopsy showed the characteristic histochemical findings of myxedema. The signs and symptoms promptly disappeared after thyroid hormone replacement was begun.

HYPERPARATHYROIDISM

Functioning parathyroid adenomas produce the signs and symptoms of primary hyperparathyroidism. Cutaneous lesions do not occur in this form of the disease, but there are two external manifestations that will suggest this diagnosis.

Hypercalcemia may produce a white line on the lateral margins of the cornea, so called "band keratopathy" (Fig. 13–21). However, this corneal abnormality is not specific for hyperparathyroidism, since it is also a manifestation of hypercalcemia secondary to vitamin D intoxication and sarcoidosis. The white bands of arcus senilis and juvenilis arise on the superior and inferior margins of the cornea, and in advanced cases they extend and form a complete circle around the edge of the cornea.

Excessive parathormone secretion in hyperparathyroidism can also cause bone cysts, especially in the mandible. These lesions may look like

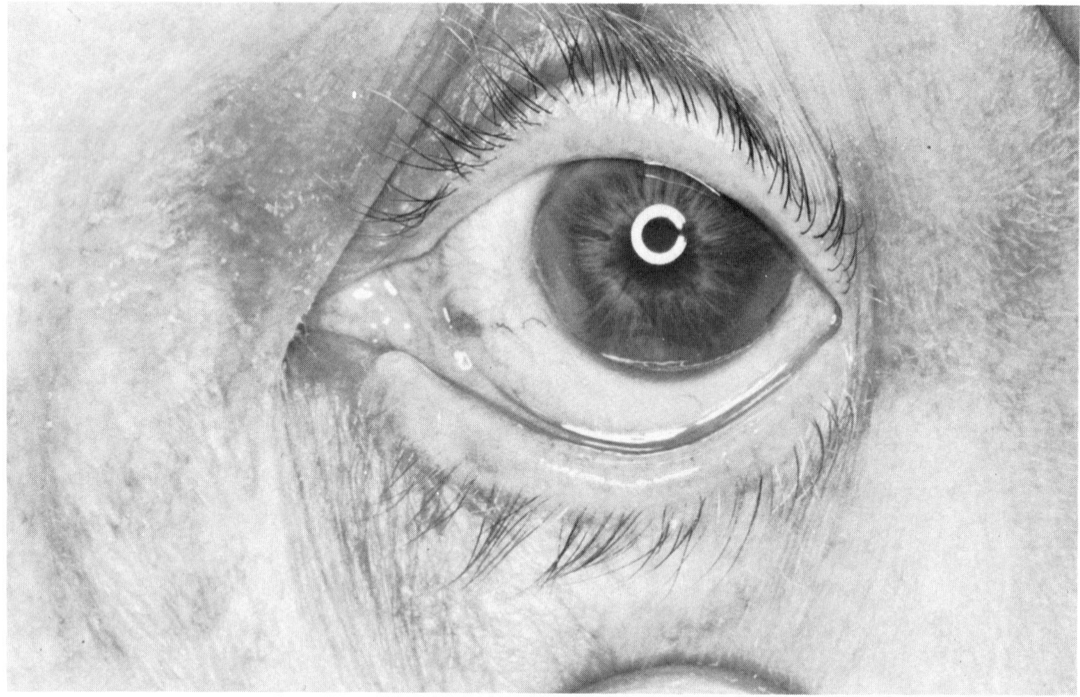

Figure 13–21. Band keratopathy caused by hypervitaminosis D. White bands appear on lateral margins of cornea. Arcus juvenilis and senilis develop on superior and inferior margins in early stages.

an epulis on the gum. Sometimes the cysts may be very large and produce subcutaneous tumors, as illustrated by Deiss.[30] Radiographs of such lesions would suggest the correct diagnosis.

Primary hyperparathyroidism can also be simulated by cancers secreting polypeptides, thereby mimicking the action of parathormone. Hypernephromas and bronchogenic carcinoma account for 60 per cent of all such cancers.[31]

Hyperparathyroidism secondary to chronic renal failure, on the other hand, is associated with cutaneous lesions. As renal glomerular function fails and as the level of serum phosphate rises, the associated fall in serum calcium stimulates the parathyroid glands to become hyperplastic and to hyperfunction. In addition to bone resorption and cyst formation, metastatic calcification can develop in the dermis and subcutaneous tissues and produce grossly visible nodules. In some patients calcification of the vessels has developed, leading to gangrene of the fingers and toes and cutaneous infarction on the lower abdomen and legs.[32, 33] Plate 30*D* illustrates a patient with chronic renal disease who developed persistent cyanosis of the fingers and toes secondary to vascular calcification. Primary hyperparathyroidism may also be associated with vascular calcification that produces similar cutaneous changes.[33]

Several authors have pointed out that severe generalized pruritus in uremia can be abolished by parathyroidectomy.[34, 35] The pruritus seems to be caused primarily by hypercalcemia related to the secondary hyperparathyroidism, and the itching disappears within two to seven days after the glands have been surgically removed. Hypercalcemia in the presence of normal renal function is rarely associated with pruritus.

HYPOPARATHYROIDISM

Parathyroid insufficiency develops either as a complication of thyroid surgery or as a congenital and idiopathic disorder that usually appears in infancy or early childhood but that may appear as late as the thirties and forties. The cutaneous and clinical manifestations of hypoparathyroidism that occur after thyroidectomy are different from those associated with the congenital idiopathic variety of hypoparathyroidism.

Post-thyroidectomy Syndrome

Attacks of hypocalcemia and tetany follow inadvertent removal of parathyroid glands during thyroidectomy. Thinning or complete loss of scalp hair may be associated with tetanic episodes.[36] The nails can also be shed, but it is more common to see horizontal grooves on the nails (Beau's lines) that can be correlated with the acute attacks of hypocalcemia (Fig. 12–29); these grooves appear at the base of the nail about three weeks after the tetanic attack. Although the interval between tetany and hair loss has not been stated in the majority of published reports, it is likely that the hair loss occurred within one to three weeks after the attack in some cases. The likely mechanism is a temporary interruption of keratinization produced by the metabolic stress that leads to narrowing of the hair shaft, which readily breaks. Beau's lines are produced by the same mechanism. Telogen effluvium — the conversion of hairs from the growing (anagen) to the resting (telogen) phase with subsequent shedding three months later — was the probable mechanism in one of Lachmann's patients. Hair loss following pregnancy and high fevers is produced by the same process.

The skin is usually dry and scaly. Occasionally the nails become frayed and brittle at the distal edge. Dent and Garretts observed localized and generalized eczematous eruptions in two patients with post-thyroidectomy hypoparathyroidism.[37] In the same paper they also described generalized eczematous eruptions in two patients with hypocalcemia secondary to celiac sprue. The eczematous eruptions in all four patients disappeared when the serum calcium was raised to normal.

The hair and nail abnormalities in this type of hypoparathyroidism revert to normal when the hypocalcemia is kept under control.

Hyperpigmentation resembling chloasma, pellagra, and that seen in Addison's disease has also been reported with postoperative hypoparathyroidism. However, these ectodermal and pigmentary changes are uncommon. Lachmann, who reviewed 56 cases, found only 4 patients with these complications. He pointed out a more serious problem: 50 per cent of individuals with chronic hypocalcemia developed cataracts.[36]

Impetigo herpetiformis is a rare disorder characterized by crops of sterile pustules associated with fever, toxicity, and high mortality.[38-40] Traditionally, it has been linked with pregnancy and tetany, but cases have occurred in men and in women who were not pregnant. Impetigo herpetiformis has developed in association with postoperative hypoparathyroidism. However, not all cases of impetigo herpetiformis have been associated with hypocalcemia and tetany. Our review of the literature indicates that this disorder cannot be distinguished by clinical or laboratory criteria from pustular psoriasis of von Zumbusch (see p. 740). Pustular psoriasis can be triggered by diverse stimuli, and it is likely that pregnancy and the metabolic stress associated with postoperative hypoparathyroidism are two such triggers.

Idiopathic Hypoparathyroidism

Idiopathic hypoparathyroidism frequently begins in infancy or early childhood, although cases have appeared in adults who were in their third and fourth decades.[41, 42] The parathyroid glands are absent or have been replaced by fat. The presenting systemic features are seizures or tetany. About one quarter to one half of the affected persons have ectodermal defects. The skin is rough, dry, and scaly; frequently the scalp hair is sparse, and the axillary and pubic hair is scant. If hypoparathyroidism develops during the formation of the teeth, various dental abnormalities result: pitting, ridging, or absence of enamel, and hypoplasia or absence of permanent teeth. Dental abnormalities occur in about one third of the patients. Cataracts are found in half of the patients.

The nails are characteristic. The distal half of the nailplate becomes brittle and then crumbles, leaving a proximal nailplate that is covered with irregular longitudinal grooves (Fig. 13–22). In a minority of cases the nail changes are mild: merely brittleness and longitudinal cracking at the distal free edge.

Two other important features of this syndrome include calcification in the region of the basal ganglia and an increase in the width of the lamina dura of the teeth. In hyperparathyroidism, the lamina dura is thinner than normal.

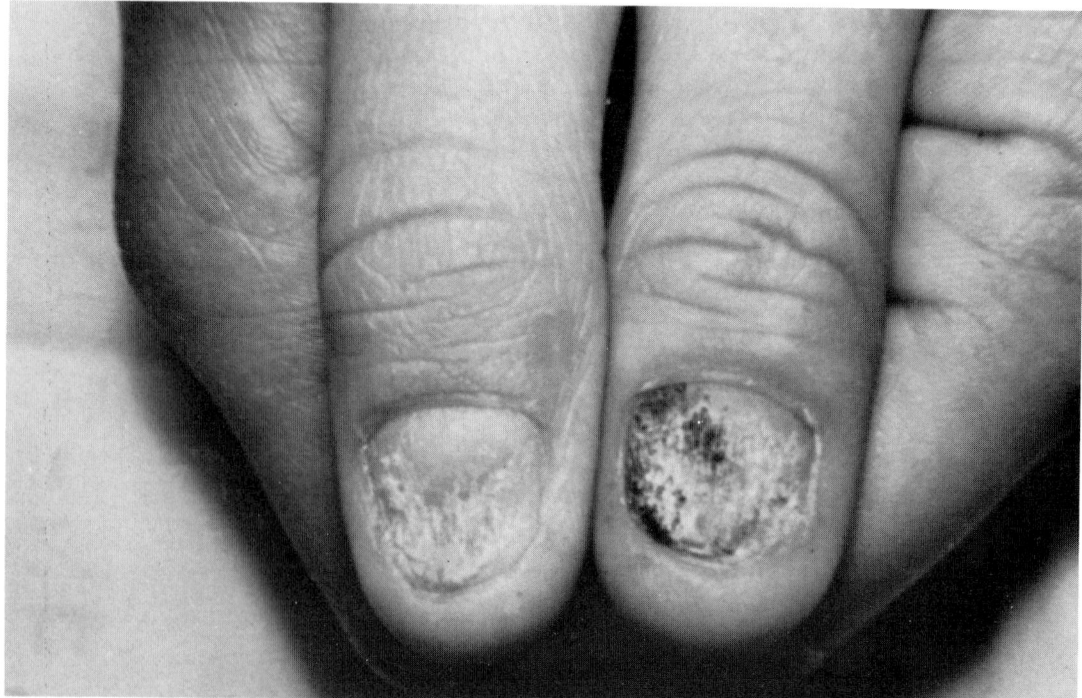

Figure 13–22. Congenital hypoparathyroidism. Distal portion of nails may become ridged, brittle, and crumbly.

Hirano et al. described a 51-year-old man with idiopathic hypoparathyroidism.[43] The patient developed cataracts at age 42; rough and brittle nails and seizures at 44; and a patchy eczematous and erosive dermatitis at 51. The eruption resembled the dermatosis associated with postoperative hypoparathyroidism rather than the skin manifestations of the idiopathic variety. The nails did not become secondarily infected with *Candida albicans*. The patient lost considerable scalp and axillary hair. Within two weeks after beginning treatment with calcium and Vitamin D_2, his eruption disappeared, and his hair and nails began to regrow normally.

Another unusual manifestation of idiopathic hypoparathyroidism was reported by Waisman and O'Regan.[44] Their 11-year-old female patient had the onset of hypoparathyroidism at age three weeks. For several years she had had a generalized erythematous perifollicular eruption on the trunk and proximal portions of the arms. The individual lesions were macules and papules, 2 to 4 mm in size. Following intravenous infusions of calcium salts, the eruption would disappear for about three hours. After the serum calcium level had been restored to normal, the eruption completely disappeared.

Exfoliative dermatitis and psoriasiform dermatitis have also been reported as manifestations of idiopathic hypoparathyroidism.[36, 45]

A curious feature of idiopathic hypoparathyroidism is the development of mucocutaneous candidiasis in 15 per cent of the patients. (Candidiasis does not occur in postoperative hypoparathyroidism.) The candidal infection occurs most frequently in the mouth, on the lips, on the perineum, and in the vagina. The nails are affected less frequently. Systemic infection is unusual; one patient had laryngeal involvement, and another had pulmonary involvement.[41, 46] In at least eight patients the candidiasis preceded the signs and symptoms of hypoparathyroidism; the intervals in three patients were three, six, and ten years.[47]

The reasons for the predisposition to candidiasis in these patients are not known, but they are probably related to two factors. It seems likely that the hair, nail, and skin abnormalities represent an ectodermal defect in association with idiopathic hypoparathyroidism. The abnormal nails and skin may be unable to resist invasion by the ubiquitous yeast, *Candida albicans*. A defect in cell-mediated immunity similar to that found in many cases of chronic mucocutaneous candidiasis appears to be present. Fields et al. and Freinkel and Ashman reported two cases in which cutaneous anergy to Candida was demonstrated.[48, 49] It is of interest that both the thymus and parathyroid glands originate from the same embryonic site: the third and fourth pharyngeal pouches.

Control of the hypoparathyroidism neither clears the ectodermal defect nor permits cure of the yeast infection. Simpson reported that control of hypocalcemia did cause the nail and hair abnormalities to revert to normal in two patients; but judging by the written descriptions, their nail and hair defects were very mild.[50] In another case report, abnormal nails became normal, whereas other nails that had been normal became abnormal without any apparent reason.[51]

The pathogenesis of idiopathic hypoparathyroidism is considered to be related to "auto-immune" mechanisms. This variety of hypoparathyroidism and candidiasis has been associated with Addison's disease, Hashimoto's thyroiditis and Addison's disease, and pernicious anemia and Addison's disease, often on a familial basis. Anti-adrenal antibodies have been found in three siblings with Addison's disease, one of whom also had idiopathic hypoparathyroidism, pernicious anemia, and candidiasis.[52] Vitiligo is also associated with idiopathic hypoparathyroidism.[49, 53] These syndromes have been referred to as a polyglandular auto-immune disease.

PSEUDOHYPOPARATHYROIDISM. Pseudohypoparathyroidism (PH) is a genetic disorder that mimics the clinical and radiographic findings of idiopathic hypoparathyroidism in every way except for the presence of candidiasis.[54, 55] The hypocalcemia and tetany in PH result from renal unresponsiveness to parathormone rather than from parathormone deficiency. The serum level of parathyroid hormone is markedly elevated, and the parathyroid glands are hyperplastic.[56]

Individuals with PH have a characteristic body habitus that readily identifies them. They tend to be short and stocky, have a round face, and exhibit short metacarpals, metatarsals, and, sometimes, short proximal phalanges. The index finger is longer than the middle finger; and when they make a fist, a depression is present where the knuckle should be. Many of the affected individuals are mentally retarded. Subcutaneous calcifications are frequent; in some patients these deposits represent ectopic bone formation and not simply calcinosis. Ectodermal defects are less frequent than in idiopathic hypoparathyroidism.

Pseudopseudohypoparathyroidism (PPH) is probably an incomplete form of PH. Although patients with PPH are physically indistinguishable from persons with PH, the former do not develop hypocalcemia and tetany. Cataracts occur in both PH and PPH.[57, 58]

PH and PPH are thought to be variants, since in the same family some members have PH and others PPH. The transition from PH to PPH in an individual has also been observed.

ADRENAL INSUFFICIENCY

Tuberculosis, histoplasmosis, coccidioidomycosis, and cryptococcosis used to be the etiologic factors in 90 per cent of the cases of Addison's disease. In recent years the infectious bases of adrenal insufficiency have become uncommon; idiopathic cases now predominate. Currently most cases of Addison's disease are assumed to arise on the basis of autoimmune mechanisms.

Diffuse hyperpigmentation, the hallmark of Addison's disease, is most likely produced by the increased secretion of a pigment-promoting peptide(s) from the pituitary. β-MSH had originally been thought to be the responsible peptide, but recent evidence has indicated that the β-MSH peptide is a chemical artifact released from the parent peptide β-lipotropin during extraction procedures (see p. 15). The factors responsible for Addisonian hyperpigmentation are not known at the present time.

The increase in melanotic pigmentation ranges from brown to black and is accentuated on the exposed parts of the body. The face, areolae, genitalia, knees, knuckles, beltline, palmar creases, lips, gums, tongue, buccal mucosa, and areas of friction are the sites of maximum pigmentation (Figs. 13–23 to 13–26; Plate 35*F*). Scars that develop during adrenal insufficiency, as well as pigmented nevi and hair, become darker.

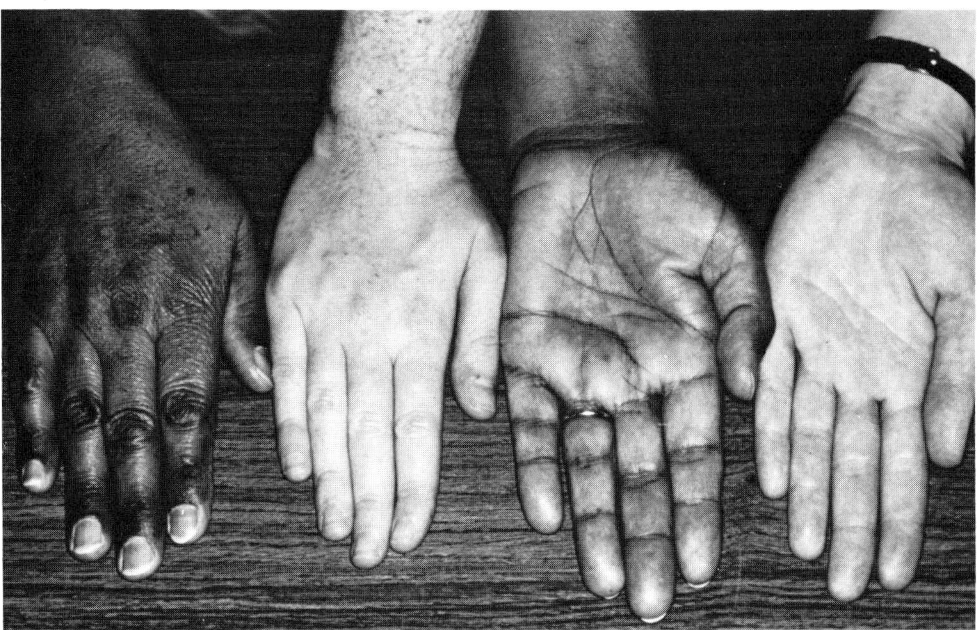

Figure 13–23. Adrenal insufficiency. Hyperpigmentation of skin. Hyperpigmentation is accentuated in palmar creases and over knuckles. Normal person included for comparison.

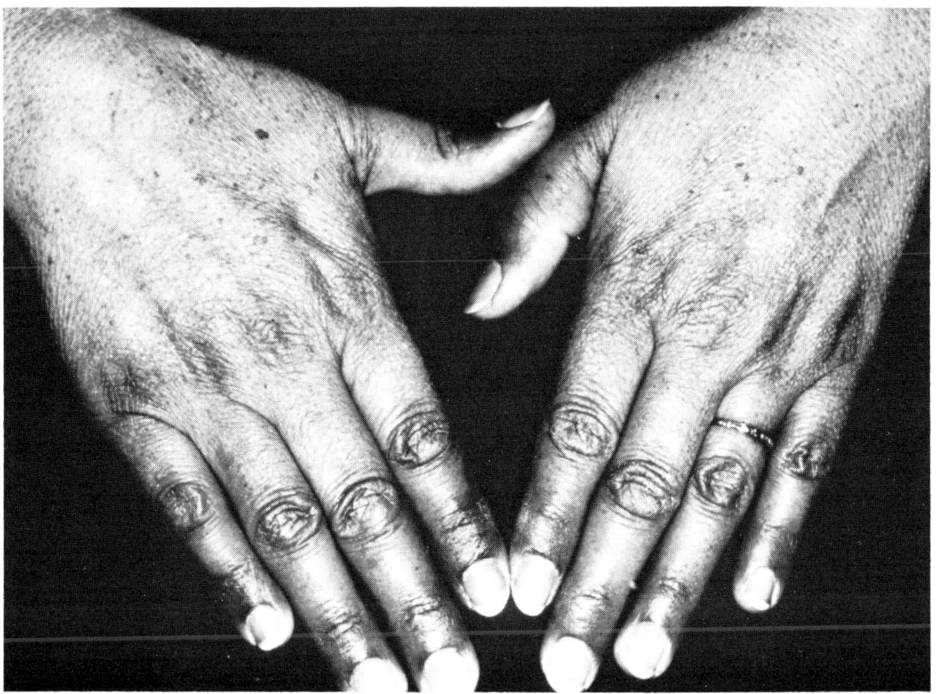

Figure 13–24. Adrenal insufficiency. Hyperpigmentation over knuckles.

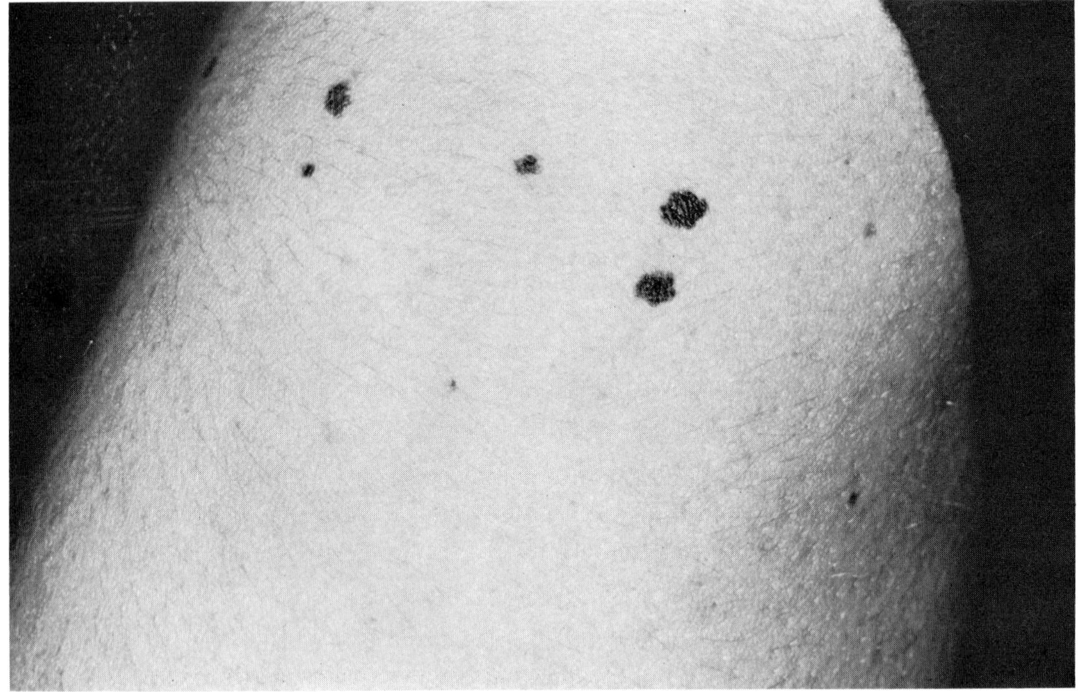

Figure 13–25. Addison's disease. Darkening of preexisting pigmented nevi.

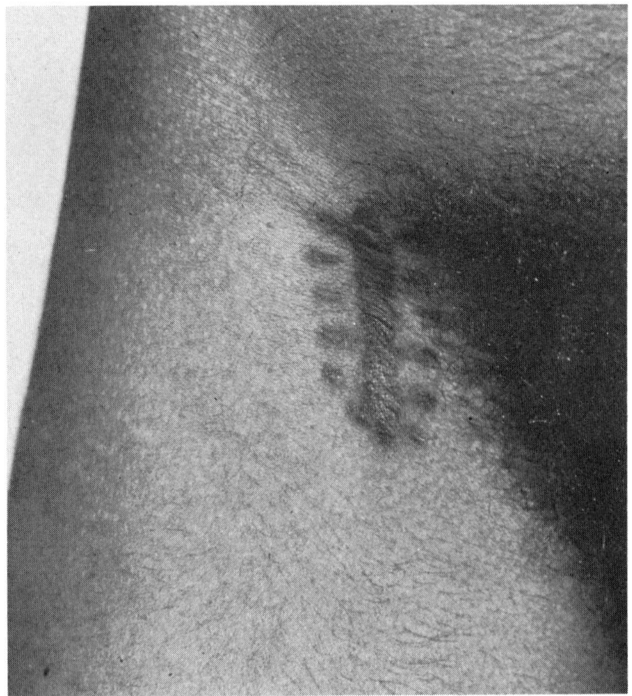

Figure 13–26. Addison's disease. Hyperpigmentation of scar.

Brunettes develop a deeper pigmentation than do blonds. The oral pigmentation develops in spots, rather than diffusely, and is blue or black. There is no strict correlation between the extent and depth of pigmentation and the severity of symptoms in Addison's disease.

Vitiligo develops in 15 per cent of Addisonians; the hyperpigmentation and hypopigmentation can occur together and present a striking picture (Fig. 13–27).[59] Successful treatment of the adrenal insufficiency causes the hyperpigmentation to disappear, and the areas of vitiligo may undergo repigmentation.

Calcification of the ear cartilage has been reported in several cases of Addison's disease, but this sign does not pertain only to adrenal insufficiency, because it has also been observed in acromegaly, hypopituitarism, hyperthyroidism, diabetes mellitus, hypercalcemia secondary to sarcoidosis, and ochronosis. It may also develop following frostbite, trauma, and bacterial chondritis.[2]

Axillary and pubic hair may be lost in some patients.

Buccal hyperpigmentation must be evaluated with the following points in mind. Dark-skinned individuals normally have pigmented spots on the oral mucosa and pigmentation in the palmar creases, both of which are indistinguishable from the pigmentation seen in adrenal insufficiency. The buccal spots in Peutz-Jeghers syndrome are also identical to those of Addison's disease, but the perioral pigmentation differentiates the former from adrenal insufficiency. Cutaneous pigmentation identical to that of Addison's disease occurs in scleroderma and lupus erythematosus, but adrenal function is normal. Hyperpigmentation in association with the electrolyte and urinary steroid findings of Cushing's syndrome usually

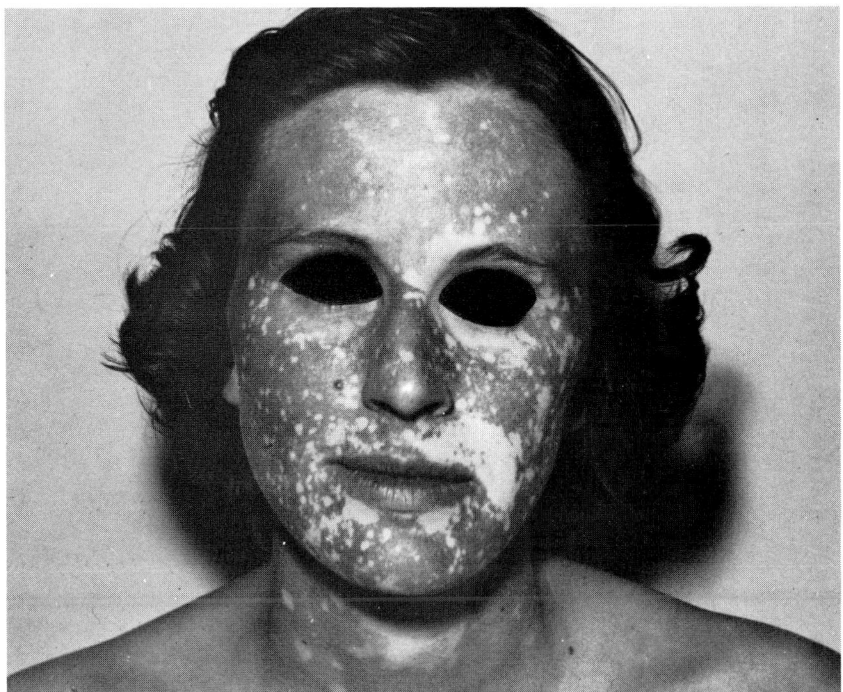

Figure 13–27. Addison's disease. Hyperpigmentation and vitiligo developing together. (Courtesy of Dr. Aaron Lerner.)

indicates the presence of the ectopic ACTH syndrome produced by a nonpituitary tumor. Chronic renal and hepatic diseases can be associated with diffuse hyperpigmentation, and the ingestion of Myleran, actinomycin D, and arsenic can also lead to melanin hyperpigmentation.

ADRENAL HYPERFUNCTION

The adrenal cortex secretes three classes of hormones; glucocorticoids, mineralocorticoids, and compounds with androgenic or estrogenic effects. If only one class of compound is secreted, Cushing's syndrome, aldosteronism, or virilization or feminization syndromes result. Although such pure clinical syndromes exist, it is not unusual to find two or more classes of hormones secreted in any one condition.

Cushing's Syndrome

Fifty to 70 per cent of patients with Cushing's syndrome have bilateral adrenal hyperplasia; 20 to 30 per cent have an adrenal adenoma or carcinoma autonomously secreting cortisol; and about 16 per cent have a nonpituitary tumor secreting ACTH.[60] When an adrenal tumor is present, the remaining adrenal tissue is atrophic. Ten per cent of patients have a pituitary tumor in addition to bilateral adrenal hyperplasia.[61]

Current consensus regarding the pathophysiology of Cushing's syndrome with bilateral adrenal hyperplasia is not too dissimilar from Cushing's original premise that the pituitary gland was at fault. He found basophilic adenomas in many of his patients. Most investigators believe that there is inappropriate control and excessive secretion of corticotropin-releasing factor (CRF) in the hypothalamus. Elevated levels of CRF result in an increased secretion of ACTH by the pituitary gland, which in turn produces bilateral adrenal hyperplasia with increased serum levels of cortisol. This glucocorticoid is responsible for the metabolic and clinical features of Cushing's syndrome. The plasma level of cortisol via a positive feedback mechanism regulates the release of CRF in the normal person; in Cushing's syndrome, this regulating mechanism is probably set at a higher-than-normal level so that CRF production remains chronically excessive and the pituitary gland is continually being driven to secrete increased amounts of ACTH.[61] Recent evidence has suggested that neurotransmitters regulate the release of ACTH.[62] Krieger et al. have proposed that increased levels of serotonin in the hypothalamus may be responsible for the secretion of CRF in some patients with Cushing's syndrome. They were able to treat three patients with cyproheptadine.[63] Sixty per cent of 40 patients with Cushing's syndrome have now been successfully treated with cyproheptadine, an antiserotonin compound.[64]

Chromophobe tumors of the pituitary are more common than the basophilic type in patients affected by Cushing's syndrome with adrenal hyperplasia. These tumors tend to grow rapidly and can even invade suprasellar and parasellar structures. In a few cases these tumors have been malignant, and metastases have developed in the liver, spinal cord, and cervical lymph nodes.[61, 65]

About 16 per cent of patients with Cushing's syndrome develop pituitary tumors or Addisonian hyperpigmentation, or both, following

PLATE 36

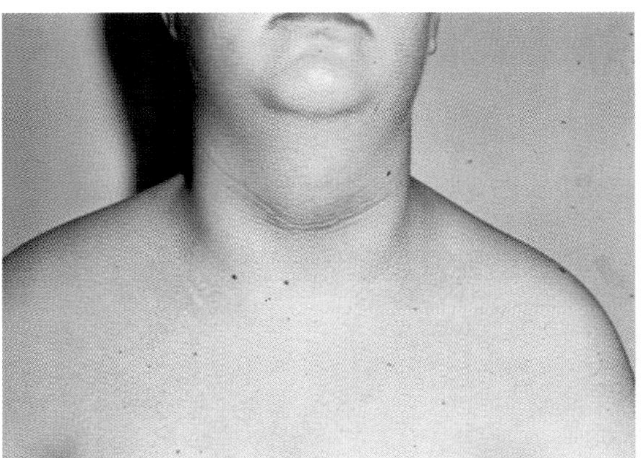

A, Cushing's syndrome. Pigmentation of patient preoperatively. Acanthosis nigricans present on neck.

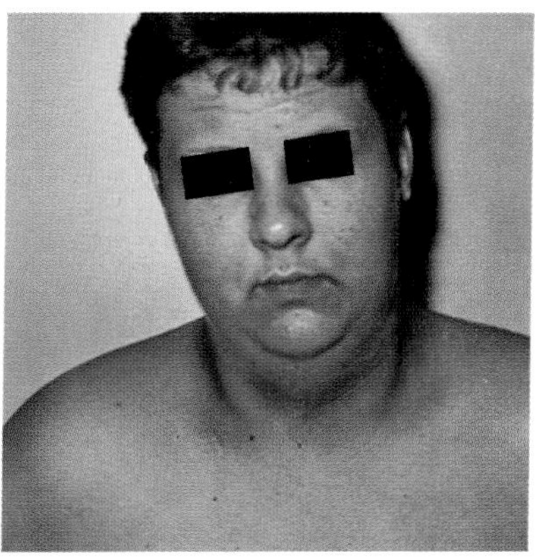

B, Cushing's syndrome. Hyperpigmentation of patient in *A*, six months postoperatively.

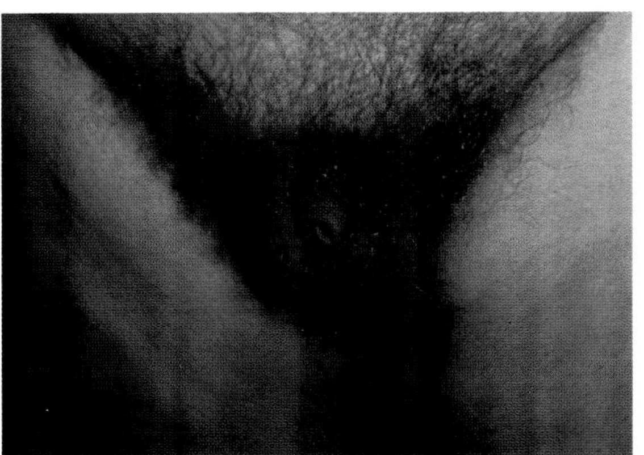

C, Cushing's syndrome. Marked hyperpigmentation of genitalia postoperatively in the patient shown in *B*.

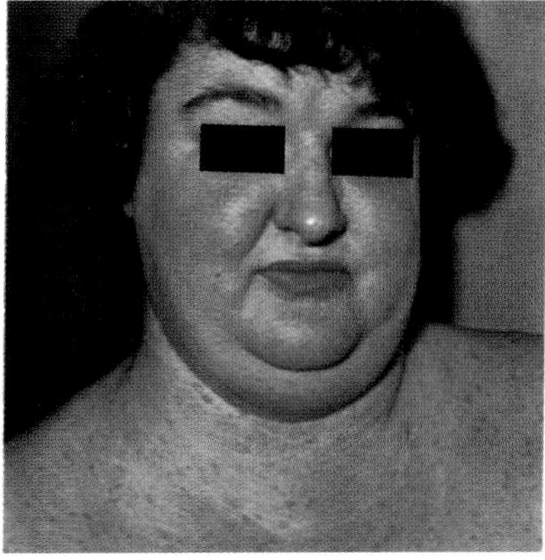

D, Cushing's syndrome. Moon facies, ruddy complexion, and acneiform eruption on chest.

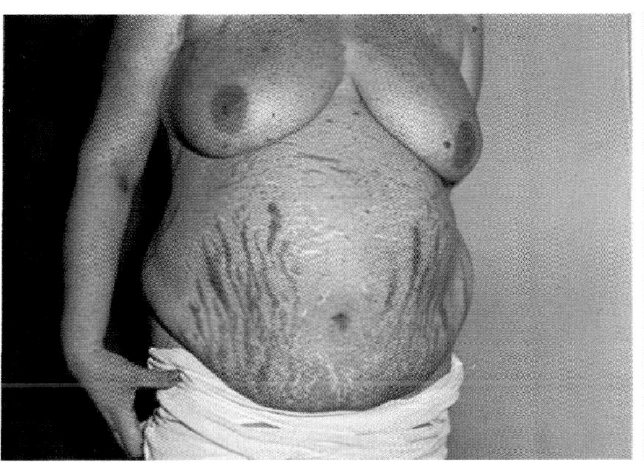

E, Cushing's syndrome. Purple striae.

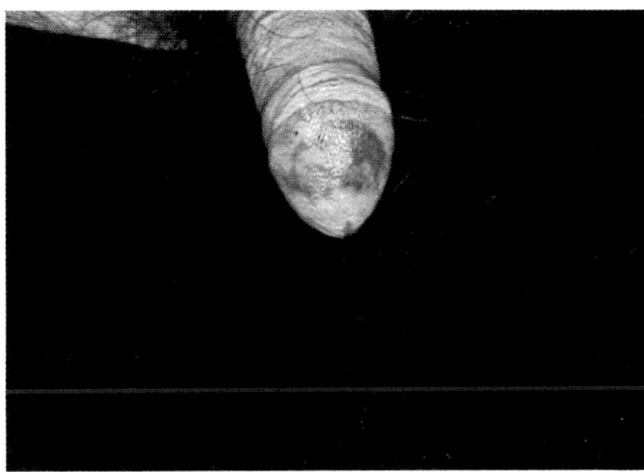

F, Diabetes mellitus. Necrobiosis lipoidica diabeticorum on glans penis. Unusual location.

treatment by bilateral adrenalectomy, in spite of adequate adrenocortical replacement therapy (Plate 36*A–C*). This phenomenon, called Nelson's syndrome, has occurred, on the average, about three years after the surgery, but the range has been from one to eight years.[66] Preoperatively, these tumors may have been too small to visualize; postoperatively, they may have been stimulated to grow by the further increased levels of CRF, which is no longer being influenced by a feedback mechanism. Postoperatively, the tumors could also have arisen *de novo* in a chronically hyperstimulated pituitary gland. The Addisonian pigmentation is most likely produced by increased secretion of a pigment-promoting peptide from the pituitary.

Pituitary tumor formation with hyperpigmentation does not develop after adrenalectomy for other diseases such as disseminated carcinomatosis and adrenal carcinoma.

Patients with Cushing's disease have a round "moon" face with redness and telangiectasia over the cheeks; these features are often accompanied by an increase of fine hair on the face and the extremities (Figs. 13–28 and 13–29; Plate 36*D, E*). The body fat redistributes to produce truncal obesity with contrasting thin arms and legs.[67] Supraclavicular fat pads form. A fatty deposit appears over the back of the neck and is referred to as a "buffalo hump" (Fig. 13–30). Cushing also described the deposition of fat over the anterior cervical area in one of his patients. Lucena et al. have observed this same fatty deposit in three patients treated with oral steroids; they have called this lesion a "dew-

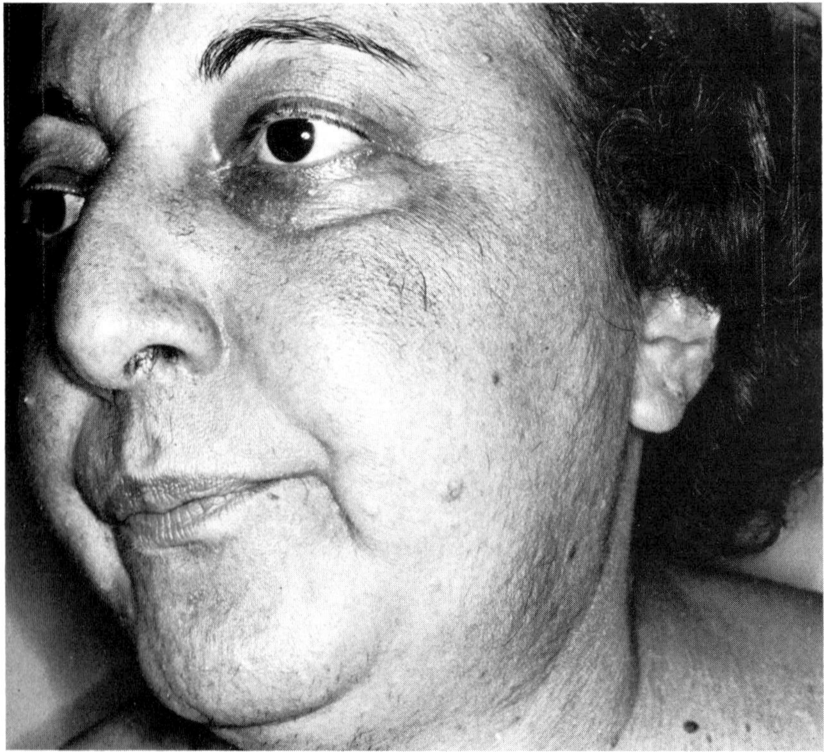

Figure 13–28. Cushing's disease. Moon facies. Telangiectasia on cheeks.

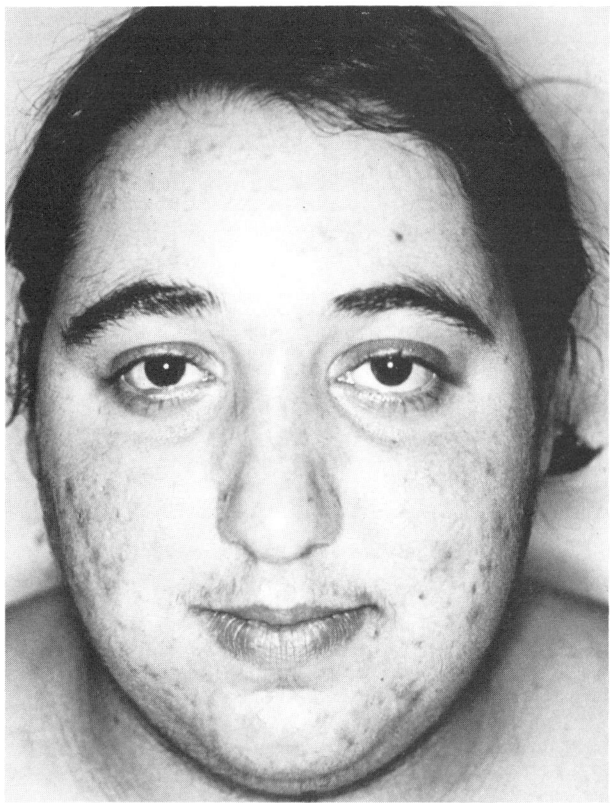

Figure 13–29. Cushing's disease. Moon facies.

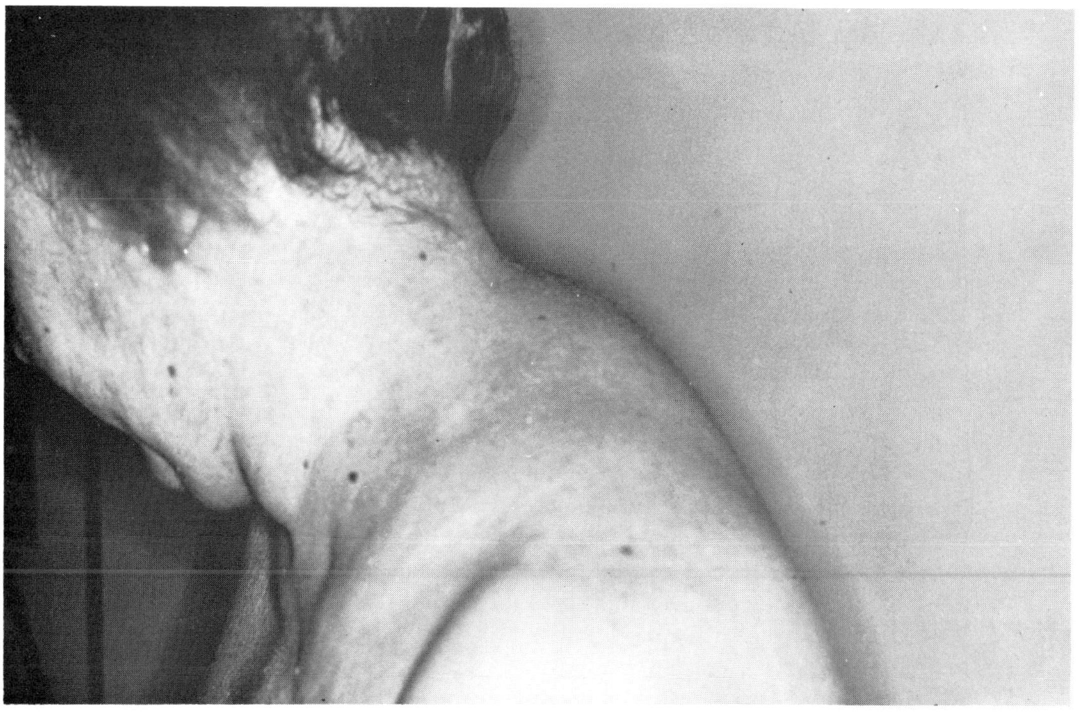

Figure 13–30. Cushing's syndrome. Buffalo hump.

lap.''[68] Santini and Williams described widening of the mediastinum secondary to presumed lipomatosis in two patients. The widening disappeared after bilateral adrenalectomy.[69] The excessive secretion of glucocorticoids produces muscle weakness and wasting, which is partly responsible for the patient's thin limbs; osteoporosis, which leads to vertebral collapse and loss of height; and thinning of the collagen and elastin in the dermis, which causes the purple striae (Plate 36*E*). The clinical impression of atrophic skin in Cushing's syndrome has been verified by direct measurements.[4]

Identical striae can be produced by applying corticosteroids under occlusive material to the skin for several weeks.[70] The dermis becomes atrophic, and the subcutaneous vessels become more easily visible and produce the purple color. In patients with Cushing's syndrome, minor trauma readily produces bruises and ecchymoses because the blood vessels have less support secondary to the decrease in dermal collagen and elastin.[71]

The acne lesions in Cushing's syndrome are perifollicular papules that are produced by hyperkeratosis of the follicular openings (Figs. 13–31 and 13–32). Mild pustule formation can also be seen, but the deep cystic lesions and comedo formation of adolescent acne do not occur. In adults the abrupt onset of true acne vulgaris usually signals the presence of an androgen-secreting tumor.

About 6 per cent of patients with active Cushing's syndrome have Addisonian pigmentation, which further points to the hypothalamus and pituitary gland as the primary sites of pathology in this disease. Mild signs of virilism — frontal balding and clitoral enlargement — appear in some patients, indicating that androgens are also being secreted.

There exists a group of female patients with obesity, red faces, and hirsutism who resemble patients with Cushing's syndrome but who have no demonstrable endocrine disease, as judged by our current laboratory tests.

Individuals with Cushing's disease are predisposed to infection by two common fungi: *Pityrosporon orbiculare*, which produces tinea versicolor, and *Trichophyton rubrum*, which is the usual organism found in chronic mycotic disease of the nails, toe webs, soles and inguinal area.[72] However, in Cushing's syndrome, the *T. rubrum* infection usually disseminates to involve the trunk and buttocks. Following adrenalectomy, tinea versicolor may spontaneously disappear (Figs. 13–33 and 13–34). Burke has demonstrated that some normal persons can be infected with the organism of tinea versicolor only if they have first been given corticosteroids. When the steroids are discontinued, the infection spontaneously remits. The reasons for increased susceptibility to these two common fungal infections are not known.[73]

Brooks and Richards described an unusual type of depigmentation in two West Indian Negroes with Cushing's syndrome.[73] The depigmented patches, which were present on the face, fingers, forearms, and dorsa of the hands, had ill-defined borders and showed varying degrees of pigment loss. Judging by the published photographs, the lesions were not characteristic of vitiligo. A few months after adrenalectomy, complete repigmentation occurred. The authors postulated that the pigment loss was due to selective suppression of ''MSH'' by the high serum cortisol levels.

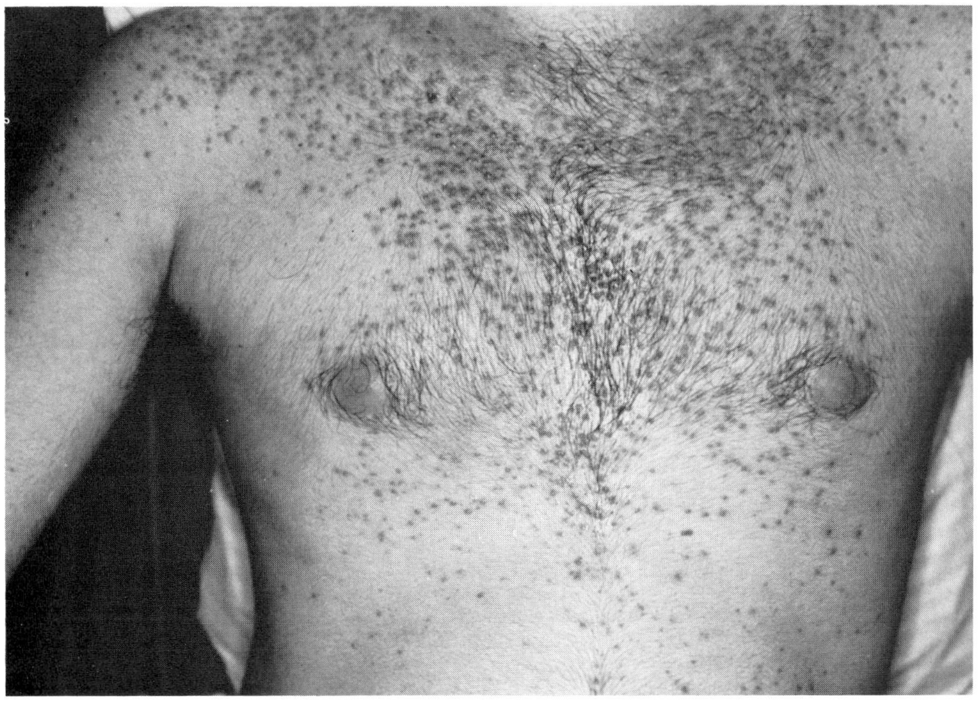

Figure 13–32. Steroid acne. Close-up shows perifollicular papules and pustules.

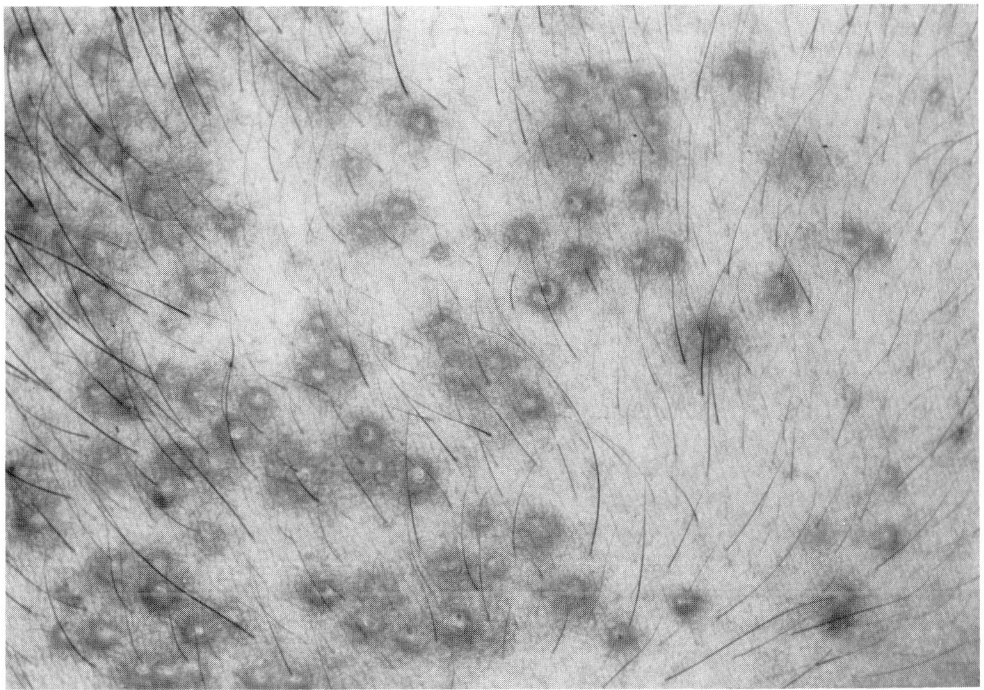

Figure 13–31. Steroid acne.

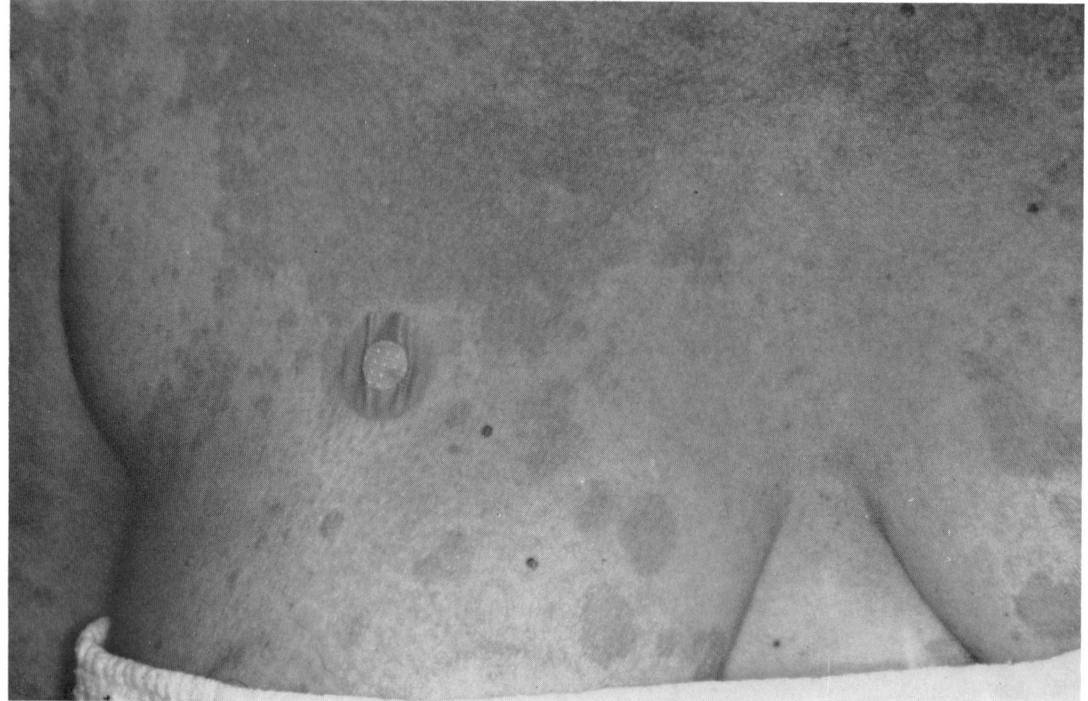

Figure 13–33. Cushing's syndrome. Tinea versicolor is present preoperatively.

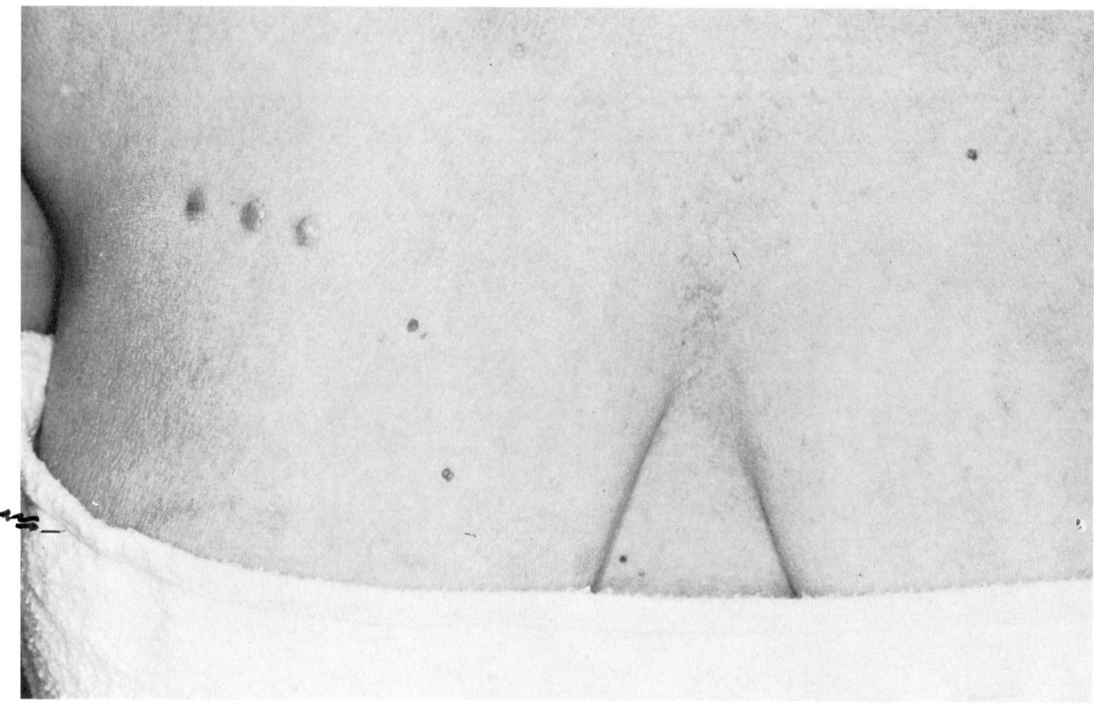

Figure 13–34. Cushing's syndrome. Tinea versicolor has spontaneously disappeared postoperatively. (Figs. 13–33 and 13–34 courtesy of Dr. Ruth Burke.)

Adrenogenital Syndrome

Adrenal virilism results from excessive secretion of adrenal hormones with androgenic activity. It can be produced by adrenal carcinomas, adenomas, and hyperplasias. Features of Cushing's syndrome may be admixed with the virilism. Hirsutism of masculine distribution, clitoral enlargement, amenorrhea, acne vulgaris manifested by comedones, deep cystic and pustular lesions, deep voice, increased muscle mass, and a male habitus are the classic features of virilization in the adult female. Figure 13–35 shows hirsutism and acne in a woman virilized by an androgen-secreting adrenal carcinoma.

The congenital adrenogenital syndrome is a mixture of genetically determined defects involving the hydroxylation of 17-hydroxyprogesterone to hydrocortisone.[75] The most frequently encountered defect is a partial absence of the enzyme required to hydroxylate the C-21 position. Because of low serum levels of cortisol resulting from insufficient synthesis, the pituitary is stimulated via a feedback mechanism to secrete more ACTH that in turn stimulates the adrenal to produce more cortisol. In this process, adequate amounts of cortisol are synthesized, but excessive quantities of adrenal androgens are formed. Girls become virilized, and boys exhibit sexual precocity. If the enzymatic defect at C-21 is complete, then no hydrocortisone or aldosterone can be formed, and a salt-losing syndrome with virilization results.

Masculinization takes the form of pseudohermaphroditism: clitoral hypertrophy or labioscrotal fusion with the formation of a phallic urethra. Pubic and axillary hair appear, and the voice deepens. MSH hyperpigmentation of the skin, areolae, genitalia, palmar creases, and buccal

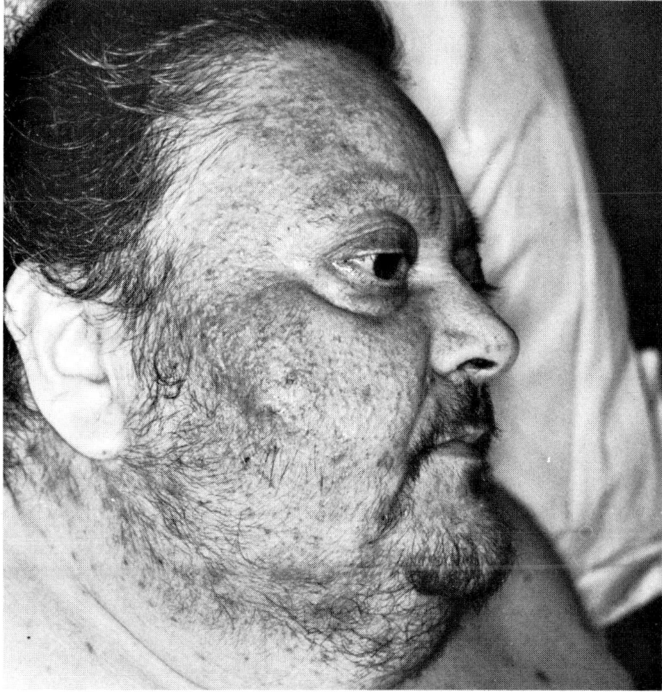

Figure 13–35. Virilization produced by an adrenal carcinoma. Note hirsutism, marked facial comedones, and acne on face.

mucosa develops in some patients. The secondary sex characteristics usually appear by three years of age.

When the enzymatic block is at the C-11 position, one step closer to cortisol, 11-desoxycorticosterone accumulates, and a salt-retention syndrome with hypertension develops in addition to the virilization.

A defect in hydroxylation at the C-3 is present in the variety of adrenogenital syndrome that is least frequently encountered. The affected children die in early infancy, and their genitalia are incompletely differentiated. Males have hypospadias and cryptorchidism.

The differential diagnosis of masculinization includes virilism produced by Leydig's cell tumors in men and arrhenoblastomas in women. True hermaphroditism is excluded by determination of urinary steroid excretion, sex chromatin, and chromosomal patterns. The Stein-Leventhal syndrome also has to be considered. Women with familial hirsutism are the patients most frequently encountered in the differential diagnosis of virilization.

DIABETES MELLITUS

At least 30 per cent of diabetics have some type of cutaneous involvement during the course of their chronic illness.[76] The eruptions arise in a variety of ways: some are caused by infectious agents; some result from vascular, metabolic, or nutritional disturbances; some arise as side effects of medications; and some are idiopathic. In addition, the skin of juvenile diabetics has a different appearance from that of adults with mature-onset disease. The skin of the former is frequently pale with a translucent quality, whereas the skin texture of the latter is usually identical to that of nondiabetics of the same ages.

Patients with diabetes mellitus probably do not have a predisposition to cutaneous bacterial or mycotic infections, but when these infections occur they are usually more severe and more difficult to bring under control than if they developed in a healthy person.[77] The necessity for preventing and vigorously treating bacterial infections stems from the fact that they frequently cause diabetes mellitus to go out of control. It is not unusual for diabetic acidosis to be precipitated by cellulitis and furuncles. Mycotic infections, whether caused by *Candida albicans* or a dermatophyte, are dangerous because they produce breaks in the skin that serve as portals for pathogenic bacteria.

Diabetics in ketoacidosis are especially prone to develop mucormycosis — a saprophyte fungal infection involving the paranasal sinuses and central nervous system. In the early phase of the infection, the nasal turbinates are inflamed and the mucosa necrotic. The eye is painfully inflamed. As the infection progresses, proptosis and ophthalmoplegia develop. Involvement of the cavernous sinus produces headache, lethargy, and cerebral infarction. The fungus spreads through the vascular channels, producing thromboses. Although this infection was originally thought to be caused only by the genus Mucor, other phycomycete species such as Rhizopus can also be pathogenic. Phycomycosis is a more accurate term to describe this dreaded complication of diabetic ketoacidosis. Although almost all cases have occurred in association with ketoacidosis, Sandler et al. described an instance of this infection in a patient

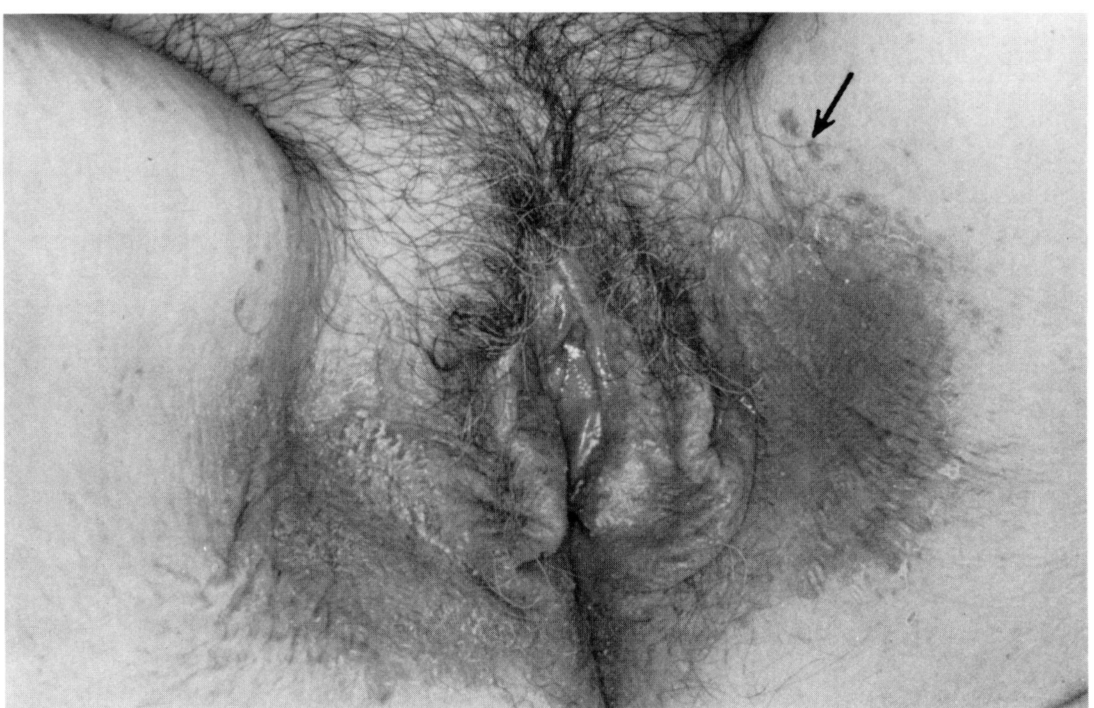

Figure 13-36. Candidiasis. Arrow indicates satellite vesicopustular lesions characteristic of candidiasis.

with well-controlled diabetes.[78] These organisms can also produce hemorrhagic cutaneous infarction secondary to hematogenous dissemination.[79]

Premature peripheral vascular insufficiency secondary to arteriosclerosis is a frequent complication of diabetes mellitus. The earliest signs are loss of hair, shininess, atrophy, and coolness of the skin over the toes. As the condition progresses, gangrene and ulceration secondary to trauma may develop. Bacterial cellulitis and lymphangitis secondary to mycotic infections only aggravate these complications. When peripheral neuropathy is also present, ulcerations may develop because of loss of sensation. The sole is a frequent site for neurotrophic ulcers, which are sometimes called malum perforans.

Generalized pruritus is not a feature of diabetes mellitus. However, it is common for patients to have pruritus vulvae and ani. Usually the perineal pruritus is associated with candidiasis (Fig. 13-36); but glycosuria must also be an important factor because when it is reduced, the itching promptly disappears. Pruritus from any cause, especially in association with dry skin (xerosis), should be vigorously and quickly treated to prevent excoriations that can lead to secondary bacterial infections.

One textbook of endocrinology states that yellow discoloration of the skin secondary to carotenemia is present in 10 per cent of diabetics.[80] However, experience at the Yale-New Haven Medical Center does not support this statement. This statistic must have been obtained many years ago when diabetics were treated with diets low in carbohydrates and high in vegetables and protein. In 1945, Mosenthal and Loughlin reported that only 24 per cent of diabetics in their studies had elevated serum levels of carotene; this is in contrast to investigations carried out in 1930 when 85 per cent of diabetics were so affected.[81] Carotenemia in diabetes mellitus is probably related more often to an increased dietary intake of carotene than to liver dysfunction or uncontrolled hyperlipemia (see p. 612). The hyperlipemia of diabetes usually represents hypertriglyceridemia and not hypercholesterolemia. Carotene is transported in the blood by β-lipoprotein, the carrier of cholesterol.

The therapy of diabetes mellitus can result in cutaneous complications. The sulfonylurea drugs produce a variety of drug reactions: urticaria, erythema multiforme, and photosensitivity eruptions. Lipoatrophy or lipohypertrophy may result from repeated injections of insulin into the same area. These abnormalities of the subcutaneous fat disappear when the sites of injection are rotated. Lipoatrophy produces large hollow depressions in the skin, and lipohypertrophy results in immense lipomas (Figs. 13–37 and 13–38).

The defect in carbohydrate metabolism is not the only abnormality in diabetes. Angiopathy of small vessels is another important pathologic feature. Currently two types of angiopathy are recognized.[82-86] The capillaries in the eye, kidney, and skeletal muscles frequently have thickened walls secondary to increased deposition of basement mem-

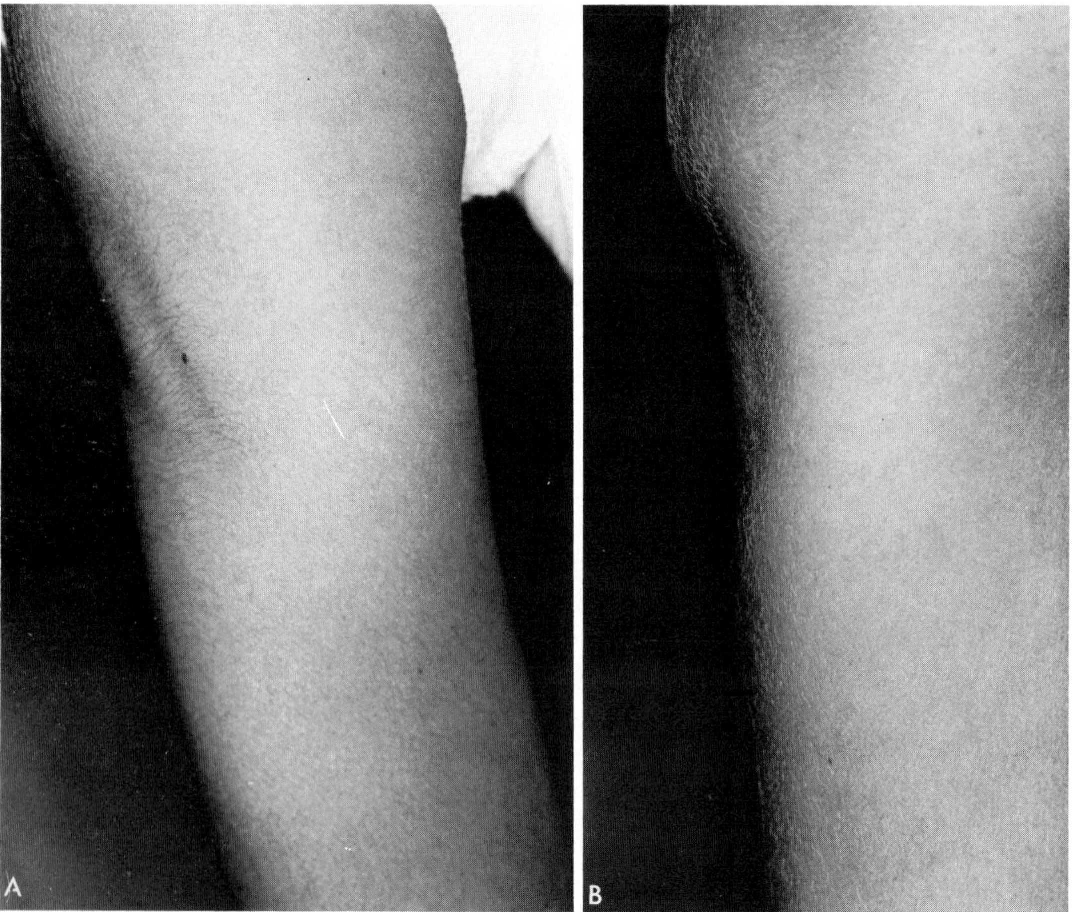

Figure 13–37. *A* and *B*, Diabetes mellitus. Lipoatrophy from insulin injections.

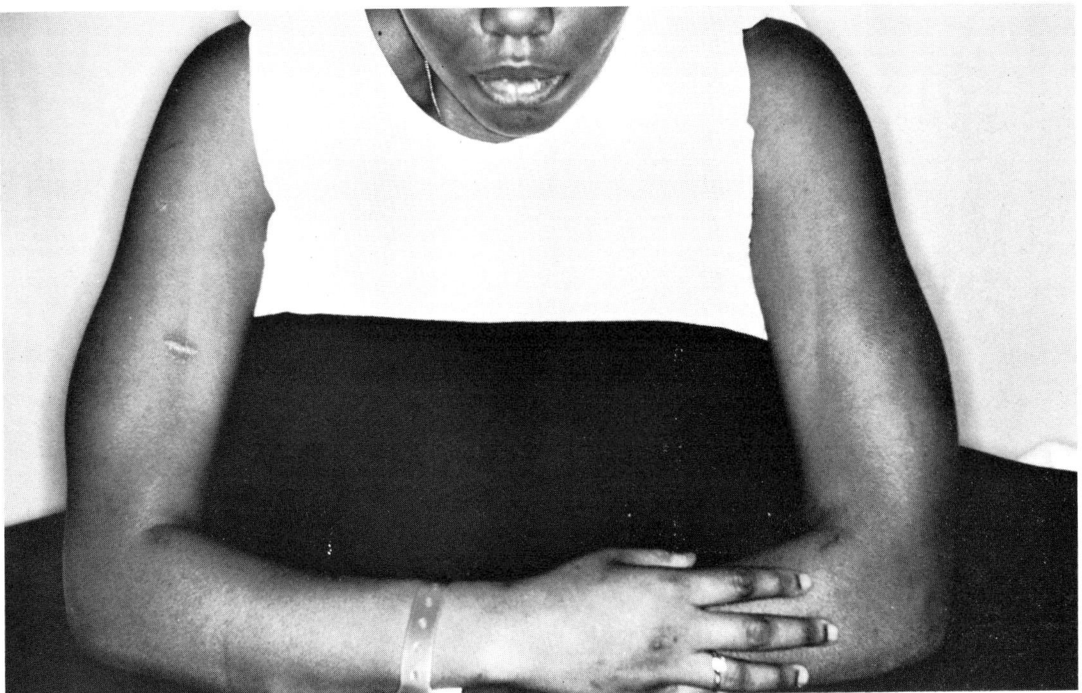

Figure 13–38. Lipohypertrophy in biceps areas from repeated injections of insulin into the same sites.

brane material. These morphologic changes are believed to be the basis for the retinal disease and partly responsible for the renal disease. The arterioles in the nerves and skin may be affected by obliterative endarteritis. Endothelial swelling and intimal proliferation lead to luminal narrowing of the affected arterioles. In addition the vascular walls are thickened because of the deposition of mucopolysaccharides within the basement membrane material. This type of angiopathy is believed to be responsible for the peripheral neuropathy of diabetes and its most characteristic cutaneous lesions, necrobiosis lipoidica diabeticorum (NLD) and shin spots.[87, 88]

NLD occurs three times more often in women than in men; in 90 per cent of patients it is localized to one or both shins. In the remaining individuals, it may be on the trunk, arms, face, or scalp. The glans penis was affected in one of our patients (Plate 36*F*). NLD usually develops in the third or fourth decade, but it may be seen in younger or older individuals; it was observed at birth in one patient. NLD appears in 0.1 to 0.3 per cent of diabetics.[89]

NLD is a sharply demarcated plaque that has a shiny atrophic surface. It begins as a red or red-brown flat lesion that expands slowly. It can be as small as 0.5 cm or as large as 25 cm. The lesions tend to be oval, and several may coalesce to form a large plaque (Plate 37*A–D*; Figs. 13–39 to 13–42).

The active border remains erythematous, but the red-brown center becomes yellow as lipid is deposited. However, the yellow color is almost certainly produced by the accompanying carotene. A vascular pattern develops within the plaque. Dermal vessels become telangiectatic, and the subcutaneous vessels also become visible. The histopathology of

PLATE 37

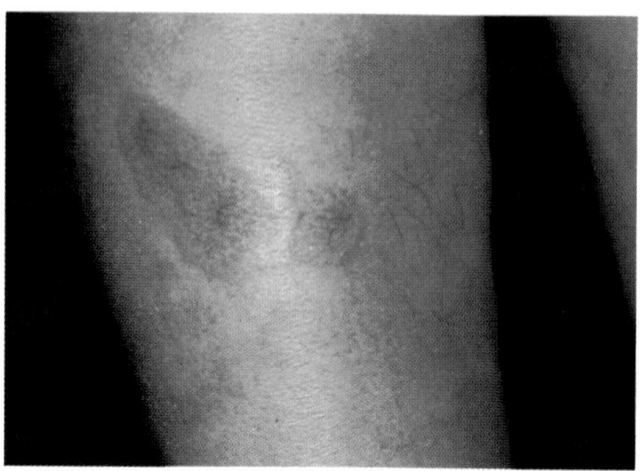

A, Necrobiosis lipoidica diabeticorum (NLD). Telangiectasia in center of lesion, but yellow color has not yet developed.

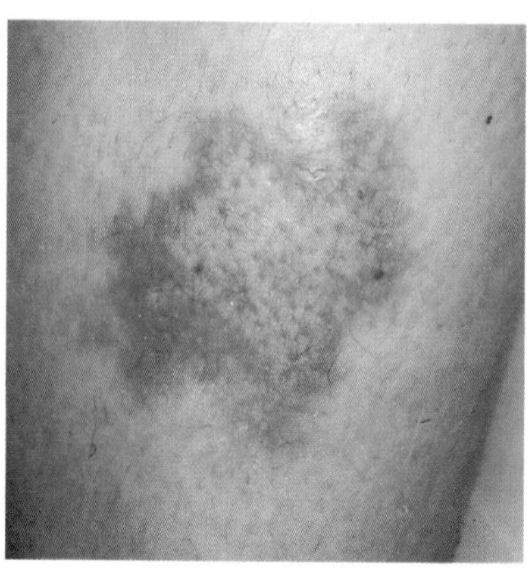

B, NLD Yellow color developing. Border is erythematous.

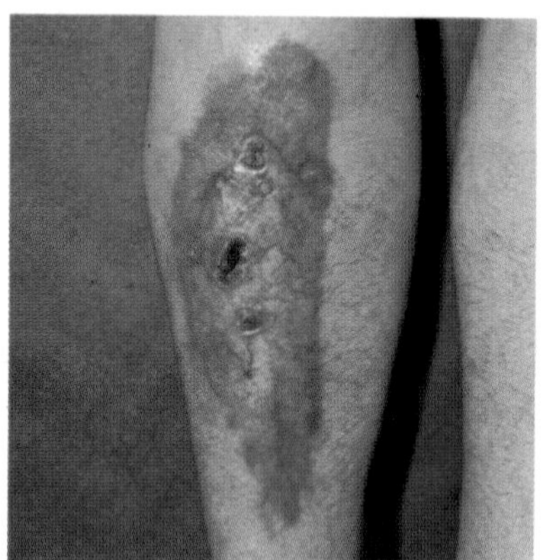

C, NLD. Fully developed lesion. Note prominent dilated blood vessels.

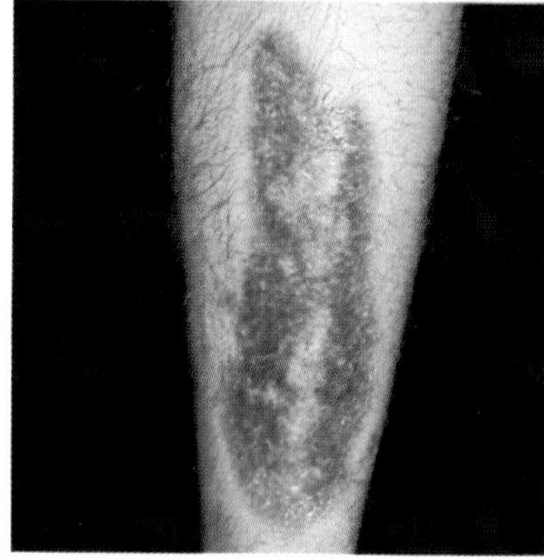

D, NLD. Hyperpigmentation is marked in this lesion of NLD. This is an unusual finding.

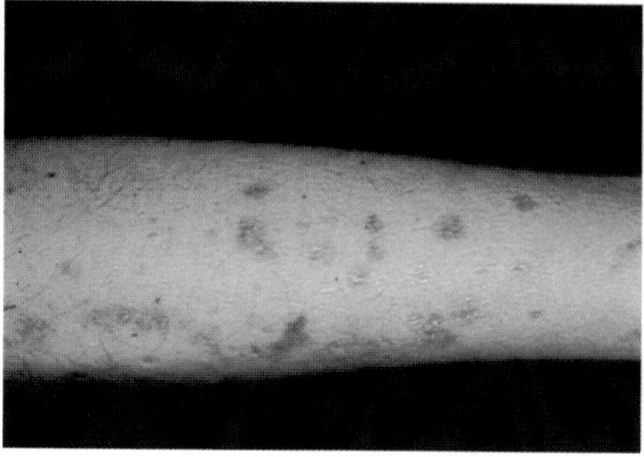

E, Diabetic dermopathy. Hyperpigmented depressed spots on shin.

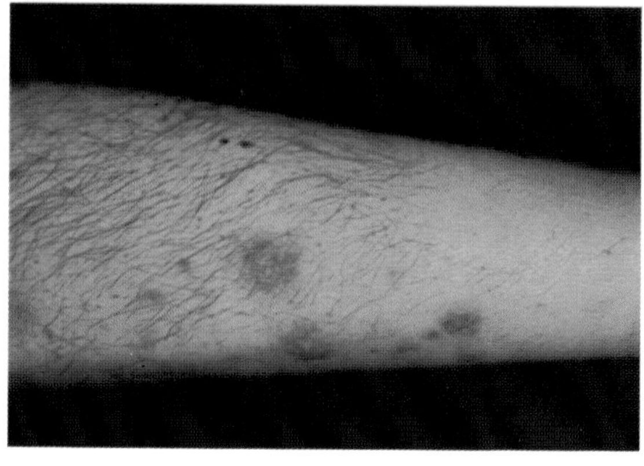

F, Diabetic dermopathy.

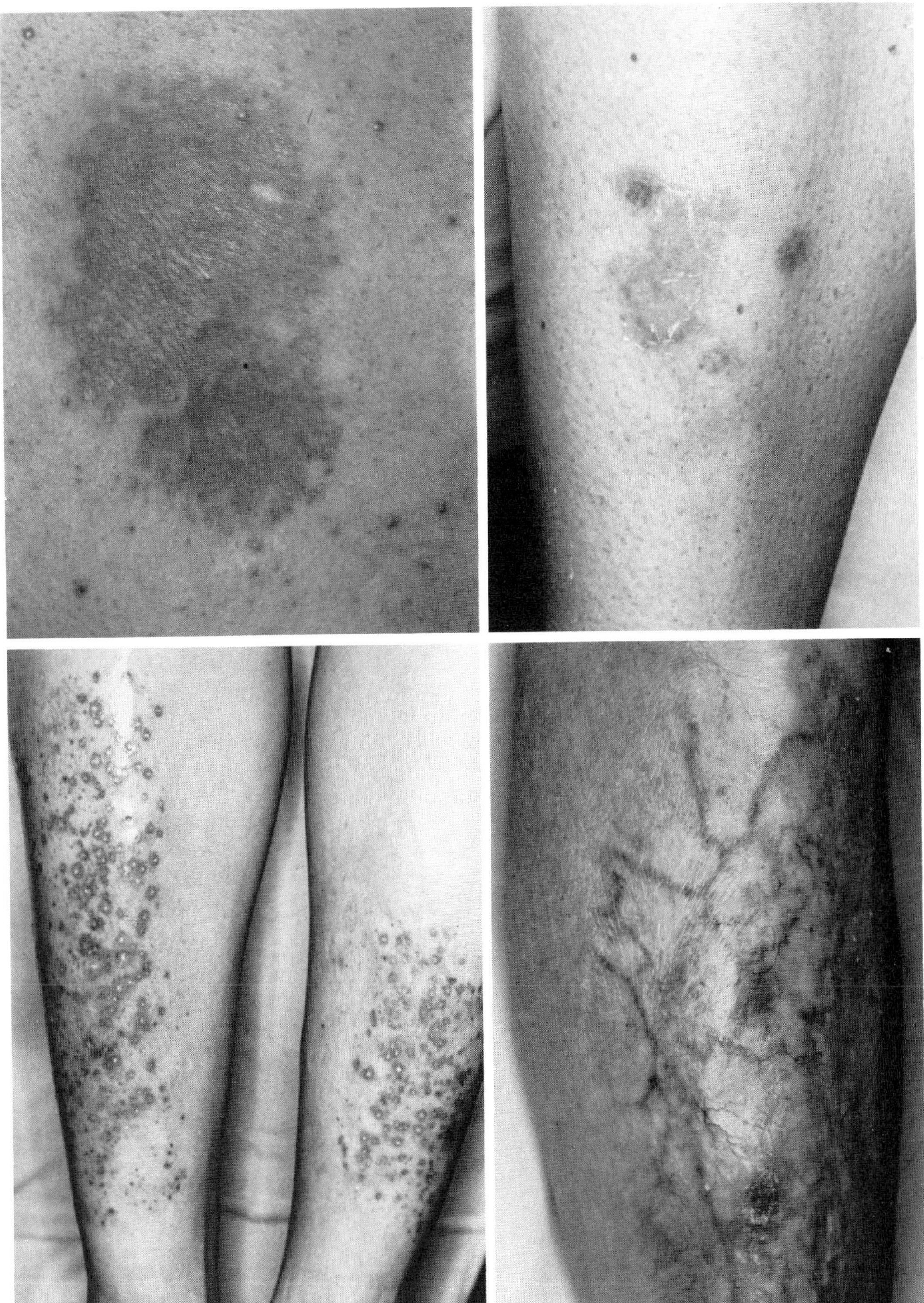

Figure 13–39. Top left. Necrobiosis lipoidica diabeticorum. Coalescence of individual small lesions.

Figure 13–40. Top right. Necrobiosis lipoidica diabeticorum.

Figure 13–41. Bottom left. Necrobiosis lipoidica diabeticorum. Multiple small lesions.

Figure 13–42. Bottom right. Necrobiosis lipoidica diabeticorum. Spontaneous resolution after 10 years. Compare with initial appearance shown in Plate 37*C*.

NLD is that of an obliterative endarteritis, characteristic of diabetic microangiopathy, with secondary necrobiotic changes in the bundles of collagen. A granulomatous reaction with giant cells may occur.[90, 91]

NLD precedes the onset of diabetes in about 15 per cent of patients by about two years (range one half to fourteen years). In 25 per cent of the patients, NLD and diabetes mellitus appear concomitantly; in the rest, NLD appears after diabetes has been diagnosed. In two thirds of the latter group of patients, the interval is less than six years. Spontaneous resolution occurs in 13 to 19 per cent of cases after an average of 6 to 12 years. Resolution or progression of NLD does not appear to be related to the activity of the diabetes. Minor trauma may produce ulcerations in lesions of NLD with healing taking as long as a year.

Muller and Winkelmann studied 171 patients with NLD.[89] Sixty-five per cent of the patients had diabetes mellitus when they were examined initially. Nineteen of the remaining 60 persons were restudied several years later: three had developed diabetes; five had abnormal glucose tolerance tests after pretreatment with prednisone; and six reported that diabetes had developed in a close relative. One of their patients had NLD for 17 years before diabetes mellitus developed. Only 5 of the 19 were untainted by the stigmata of diabetes mellitus. These data suggest that 90 per cent of persons with NLD are either diabetic, will develop diabetes, or have a family history of the disease. Muller and Winkelmann observed that diabetes occurred at an earlier age in those persons with NLD.

The pathogenesis of the endarteritic lesion in NLD has not been established. Two hypotheses have been offered. Some investigators have suggested that an immune complex vasculitis is responsible for the angiopathy because immunoglobulins and complement have been detected in the vascular walls in some cases.[92] However, none of the other histologic features of vasculitis was present: neutrophils, nuclear dust, and fibrin deposition. A more attractive hypothesis involves platelet physiology.[93] Platelets from diabetics show an increased sensitivity to aggregate both spontaneously and when stimulated by ADP, epinephrine, and collagen. In experimental animals, platelet interaction with endothelial lining of large vessels results in the release of a mitogen from platelets that stimulates smooth muscle cell proliferation. This phenomenon is believed to cause intimal proliferation. Clinical observations have suggested that the sensitivity of platelets to aggregation in response to ADP and epinephrine may be correlated with progressive retinopathy and neuropathy. Biopsies of sural nerves in diabetic patients have shown thromboses in the small vessels. Eldor et al. were able to produce resolution in a lesion of NLD by using antiplatelet aggregating agents such as aspirin and dipyridamole.[94] The lesion had been present for four years and was ulcerated. The ulcer healed in three weeks and the entire plaque of NLD disappeared within six weeks, leaving behind a scar. No new lesions appeared during the succeeding eight months while the patient was on therapy. This interesting observation needs to be confirmed.

A second cutaneous sign of diabetes has recently been described under the following terms: shin spot, pigmented pretibial patch, and diabetic dermopathy. This marker begins as red or red-brown papules that evolve into sharply circumscribed atrophic patches that are often hyperpigmented and scaly (Plate 37*E*, *F*). Sometimes only depressed areas with normal skin color are present. Although these lesions are found almost exclusively on the shins, they have also been observed on the forearms. A quick glance at them suggests that trauma is responsible for their development, but this is not the correct explanation. According to Melin and Binkley, and Graham et al., the histologic findings in these lesions were identical to the microangiopathy of diabetes mellitus.[88, 95, 96] Melin and Binkley also believed that these spots were correlated with diabetic retinopathy, nephropathy, and neuropathy. However, Danowski and co-workers were unable to confirm these associations except in men in whom the shin spots seemed to be related to neuropathy.[97] Danowski et al. observed identical cutaneous lesions in 1.5 per cent of normal medical students and in 20 per cent of patients with a variety of endocrinopathies but in whom the glucose tolerance test was normal. About 50 per cent of their juvenile and adult diabetics had shin spots. The possibility that the control subjects might be destined to develop diabetes could not, of course, be unequivocally excluded. Melin and Binkley observed that these spots occurred in 10 to 30 per cent of female diabetics and in 60 to 65 per cent of male diabetics past the age of 30. The age and sex distribution of diabetic dermopathy is very different from that of NLD.

Fisher and Danowski studied the shin spots by light and electron microscopy and histochemical techniques.[98] Although they did not find obliterative endarteritis as others have, they did observe thickening of the arteriolar walls secondary to mucopolysaccharide deposition. All workers agree that the necrobiotic changes of collagen found in NLD are lacking in the shin spots. Fisher and Danowski also observed increased numbers of elastic staining fibers in the dermis, similar to the findings in the skin of patients with chronic renal acidosis.[99] However, the problem of diabetic angiopathy needs to be reevaluated in terms of the most recent ultrastructural criteria dealing with the identification of arterioles, capillaries, and venules.[100, 101]

Granuloma annulare has always been considered to be a dermatologic curiosity. Its morphology is that of rings with clear centers and an elevated border composed of contiguous papules. The etiology is unknown, and the disorder occurs at all ages. Spontaneous resolution is not uncommon and may follow biopsy of a lesion. The histopathology resembles NLD and the rheumatoid nodule in terms of both the angiopathy and the necrobiotic changes of the collagen. Deep subcutaneous lesions of granuloma annulare have been mistaken for rheumatoid nodules.[102] Granuloma annulare may occur as a generalized papular eruption in addition to the classic ringed form (Figs. 13–43 and 13–44).

Reports have suggested that disseminated granuloma annulare may be a sign of diabetes mellitus in adults. However, these observations have not been universally confirmed and the issue needs further study.[103-105] Controversy also exists whether the angiopathy seen in granuloma annulare represents a vasculitis. Although some workers have demonstrated immunoglobulins and complement by direct immunofluorescence in some vessels, the other important histologic features of leukocytoclastic vasculitis have been missing.[106] Other workers have suggested that granuloma annulare may represent a granulomatous disorder produced through the mechanism of delayed hypersensitivity.[107] Since the vascular changes in granuloma annulare resemble those found in NLD and diabetes mellitus, it would be worthwhile to determine whether a disturbance in platelet aggregation could be related to the obliterative endarteritis found in both localized and disseminated granuloma annulare.

The studies of Dawber suggest that there may be an increased

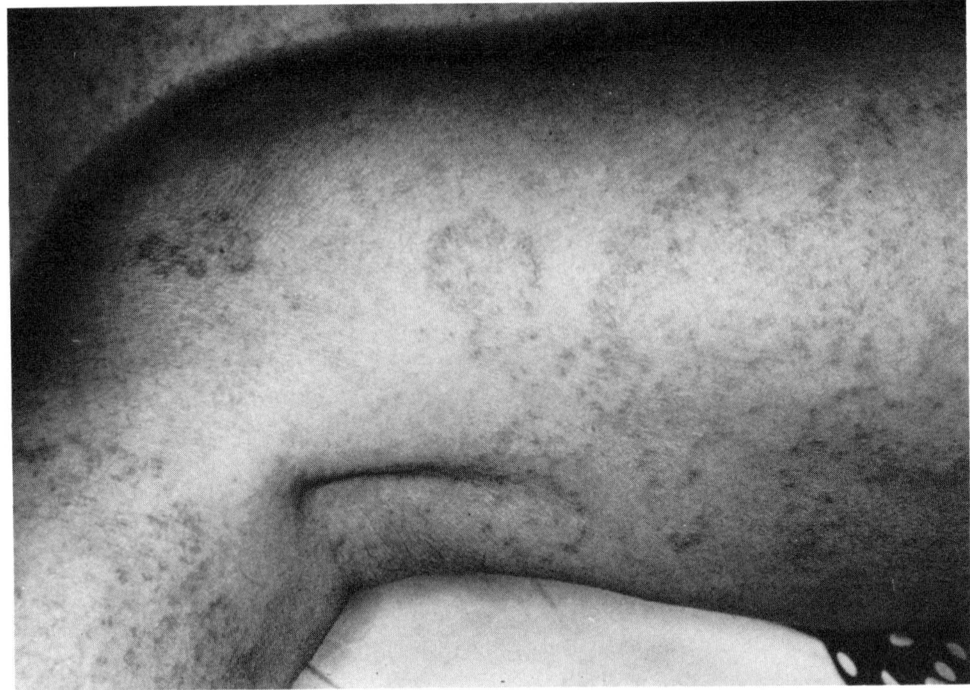

Figure 13–43. Disseminated granuloma annulare in diabetes mellitus. The disseminated papules tend to form rings, but the centers are not completely free of the papules.

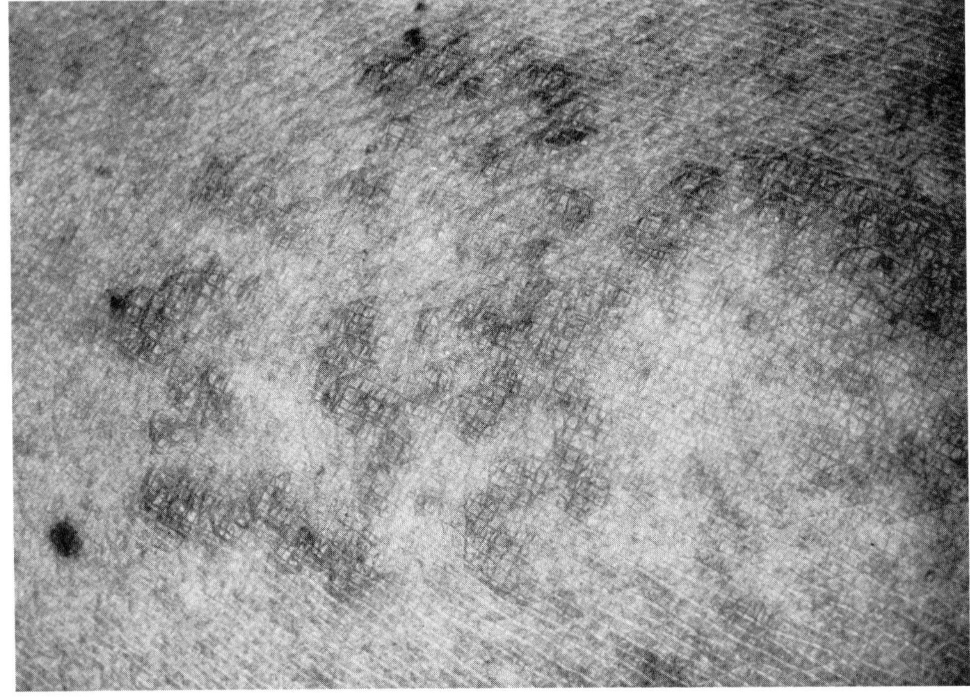

Figure 13–44. Close-up of the granuloma annulare papules in Figure 13–43.

prevalence of vitiligo in diabetes mellitus.[108] He found that 4.8 per cent of 520 patients with diabetes had vitiligo, compared to 0.7 per cent of 443 control subjects. The prevalence of vitiligo in the general population in the United States of America and in Europe is thought to range from 0.14 to 1.0 per cent.[109] Vitiligo was twice more frequent in female than in male diabetics. Also, the vitiligo appeared after age 40 in 76 per cent of the diabetics, and frequently preceded the onset of the diabetes mellitus. Vitiligo usually develops before age 40 in 89 per cent of individuals with this pigmentary disorder. Macaron et al. reported that the prevalence of vitiligo appeared to be increased in juvenile diabetics as well.[110]

Several investigators have described an unusual blistering dermatosis in approximately 30 patients.[111-115] These blisters appear suddenly without accompanying erythema on the fingers, toes, feet, and forearms (Figs. 13–45 and 13–46). They can range in size from several millimeters to several centimeters and may be recurrent. Typically the blister is tense and enlarges to its eventual maximum size within a few days. In my experience, the blister fluid has been viscous and clear. The chemical nature of the fluid has not been determined. The blisters heal without scarring over a six-week period. Although the etiology is unknown, trauma is not believed to play a role. Although many patients have had an accompanying peripheral neuropathy, this complication has not been considered to be important in the genesis of this bullous dermatosis.

The blisters have been shown to be intraepidermal, subcorneal, and subepidermal by routine histologic methods. In a few cases with subepi-

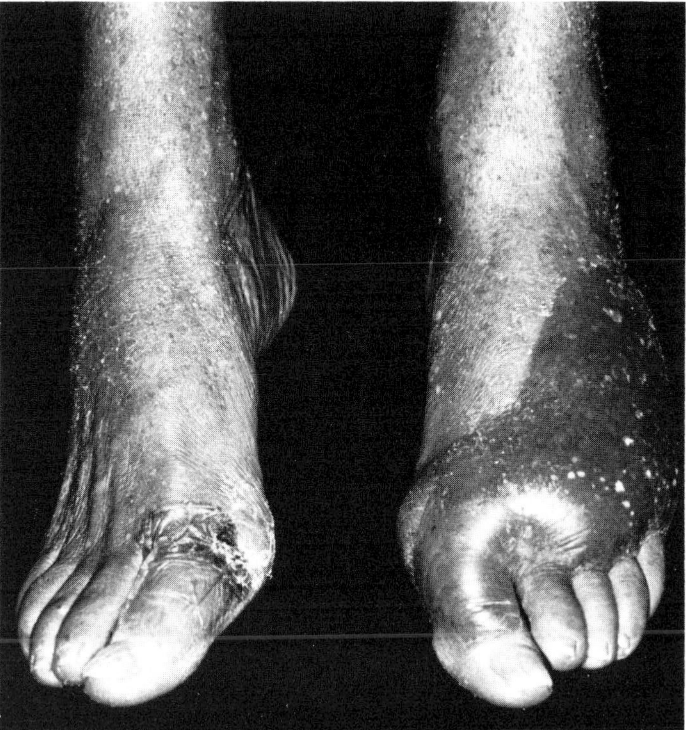

Figure 13–45. Bullous lesions of diabetes mellitus. Blister at base of right great toe has broken and collapsed.

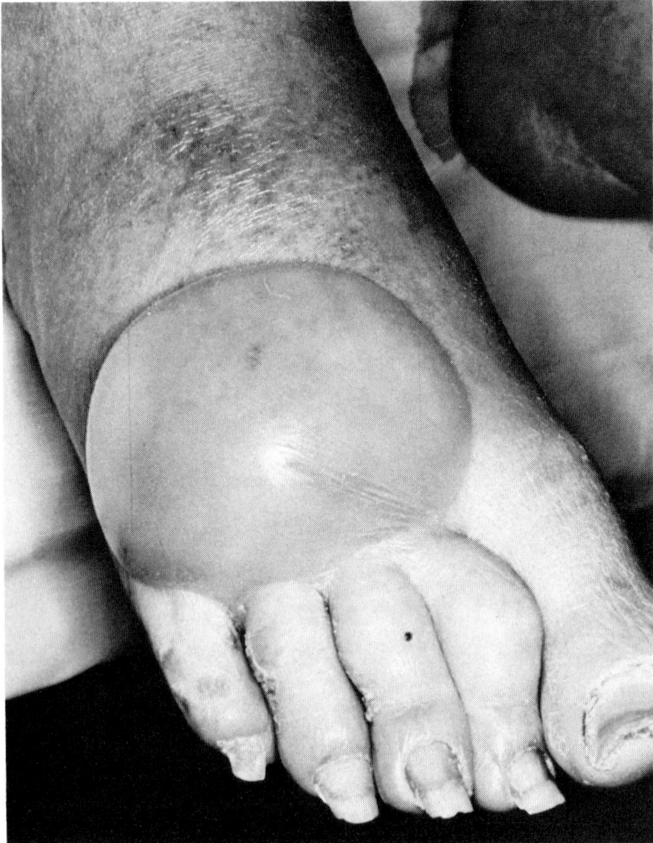

Figure 13–46. Bullous lesion of diabetes mellitus.

dermal blisters, the overlying epidermis was markedly edematous and exhibited foci of epidermal cell degeneration with vesicle formation. An electron microscopic study of one case showed that the blister formation began in the lamina lucida, the zone between the plasma cell membrane of the basal cells and the basal lamina itself.[115] Photosensitivity has been suggested as the initiating factor. In one case, the lesions were provoked by exposure to the sun,[115] and in all cases, the lesions have occurred in sun-exposed areas. Bernstein et al. suggested that an imbalance of Mg^{++} and Ca^{++} created by the underlying diabetes might contribute to a weakening of the dermal-epidermal interface so that sunlight and other stimuli might be able to induce separation with blister formation.[115] Porphyrin abnormalities and bullous pemphigoid have been excluded in this entity.

Eruptive xanthomas arise during the hypertriglyceridemic phase of uncontrolled diabetes mellitus and spontaneously disappear over several weeks after the serum lipid levels have returned to normal (Plate 38*A*). Diabetes mellitus is the most common cause of eruptive xanthomas.

Lipodystrophies

The lipodystrophies comprise a group of uncommon disorders in which there is partial or total absence of subcutaneous fat. (The term

PLATE 38

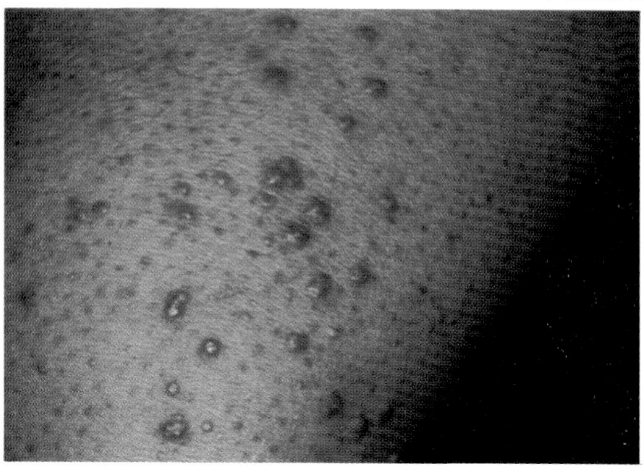

A, Diabetes mellitus. Eruptive xanthomas.

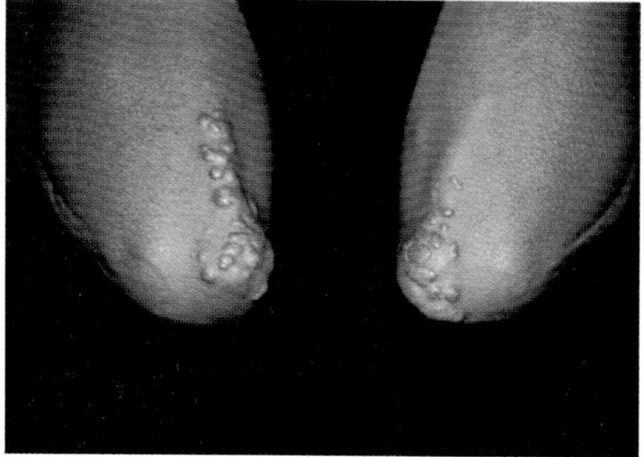

B, Biliary cirrhosis. Tuberous xanthomas.

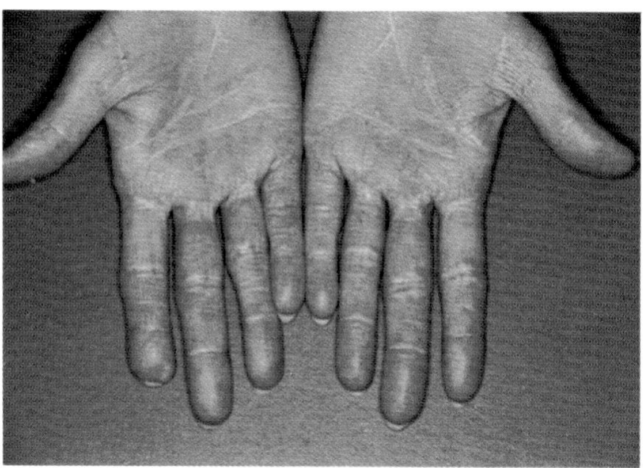

C, Biliary cirrhosis. Flat xanthomas.

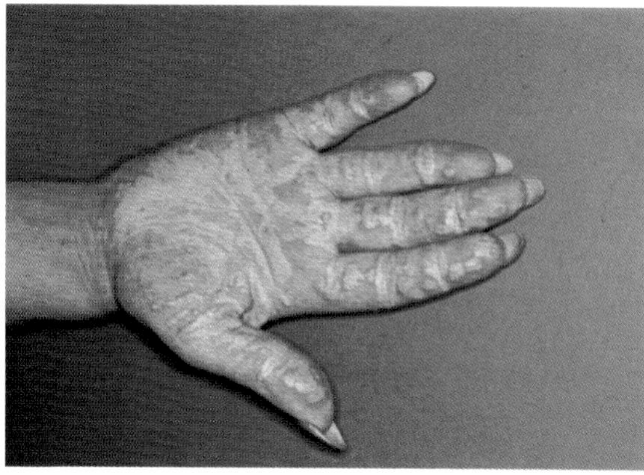

D, Biliary cirrhosis. Flat xanthomas.

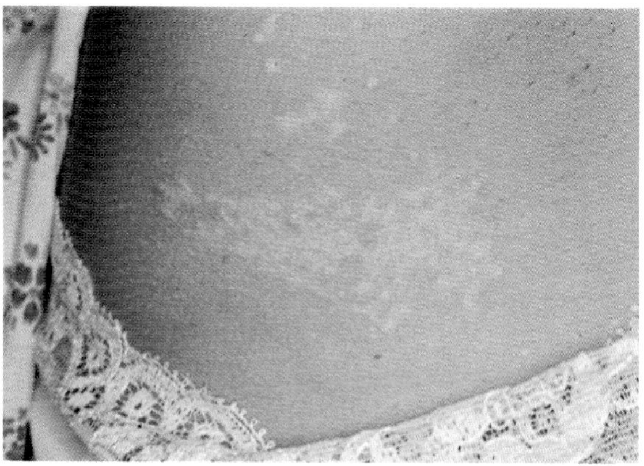

E, Biliary cirrhosis. Flat xanthomas on trunk.

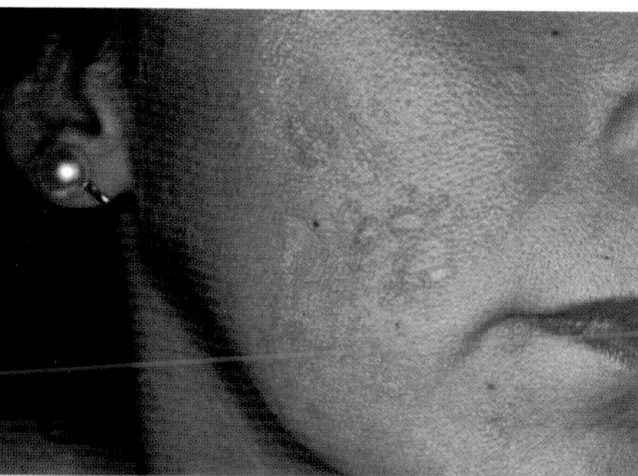

F, Biliary cirrhosis. Flat xanthomas in acne scars.

lipoatrophy is used interchangeably with *lipodystrophy* in the literature.) A significant number of affected individuals develop insulin-resistant diabetes. Acanthosis nigricans is the striking cutaneous marker in some forms of lipodystrophy.

Congenital total lipodystrophy (generalized lipodystrophy) is either present at birth or develops within the first two years of life. In the latter case, the subcutaneous fat disappears over the course of several months. *Acquired generalized lipodystrophy* has appeared in the first to third decades in a few individuals.[116-118] The two forms are considered to be variants of the same entity, even though the *acquired* form lacks some of the clinical features of the *congenital* variety. They are often referred to as the Lawrence-Siep syndrome. The syndrome is thought to be recessively inherited because of its presence in siblings and its association with parental consanguinity in several cases. One case of the *congenital* variety began with abdominal pain and fever of unknown origin in an 18-month-old female infant.[119]

The disorder is characterized by acanthosis nigricans; accelerated somatic growth and bone maturation; increased muscle mass; enlarged penis, clitoris, or labia minora; and generalized hirsutism and hyperpigmentation. In addition, the individuals usually develop hypertriglyceridemia, and hepatomegaly secondary to fatty infiltration that can lead to cirrhosis and fatal hepatic failure. In some, dilatation of cerebral ventricles, cerebral atrophy, seizures, and mental retardation have been present. Insulin-resistant diabetes develops several years after the onset of the syndrome. In addition to complete atrophy of subcutaneous fat, the mesenteric, retroperitoneal, and epicardial fat has also disappeared in some individuals. Only the mammary fat remains. Idiopathic enlargement of the heart and kidney, nephrotic syndrome, and proteinuria with hypertension have been observed in a few patients. The *acquired* form of the disease has lacked the features of hirsutism, hyperpigmentation, genital enlargement, and central nervous system involvement.[116]

Although the etiology and pathogenesis are not known, the best evidence suggests hypothalamic dysfunction. It is well recognized that the hypothalamus exerts important regulatory effects on glucose homeostasis and lipid metabolism.[120] It also contains the feeding centers, which play a vital role in the experimental production of obesity in animals. Lesions produced in the ventromedial nucleus of the rat hypothalamus result in hypertriglyceridemia through as-yet-undetermined mechanisms. The ventromedial and ventrolateral areas of the hypothalamus are the origin of the circuits that directly innervate the liver, pancreas, and adipose tissue through the sympathetic, parasympathetic, and vagus nerves. The fine and immediate regulation of blood glucose is controlled through direct neural innervation of the liver by the autonomic nervous system. Effects of longer duration are mediated through the action of glucagon and epinephrine, which are also under neural control by the autonomic system. Vagal stimulation produces an immediate rise in insulin secretion independent of the blood level of glucose.

Upton and colleagues have implicated the hypothalamus in generalized lipodystrophy more directly by detecting increased concentrations of hypothalamic releasing factors for corticotropin and luteinizing hormone in the blood of these patients.[119, 121] They proposed that the defect in this disorder may be a hypophysial disturbance secondary to an abnormality in dopamine-β-hydroxylase activity, which is the rate-limiting step for the conversion of dopamine to norepinephrine. Dopamine and norepinephrine are believed to modulate the secretion of hypothalamic releasing factors. However, the manner in which the hypersecretion of these releasing factors would produce lipoatrophy or the metabolic disturbances is not understood. These investigators treated one patient with pimozide, a cerebral dopaminergic blocking agent. Within two years after treatment, the blood levels of releasing factors for corticotropin and luteinizing hormone had returned to normal and the subcutaneous fat had begun to reappear in the reverse order in which it had disappeared.[119]

Partial lipodystrophy is much more common and not genetically determined, appearing at any time from childhood to early adult life. It may appear idiopathically, following a febrile childhood illness such as measles or scarlet fever, or following a nonspecific febrile illness.[116, 122-124] As in the other forms of lipodystrophy, women are affected more often than men. The face is *almost* always affected. The neck, arms, chest, and trunk are involved in varying degrees. The fat from the hips or upper thighs to the feet remains. In some individuals, there appears to be an increased deposition of fat around the hips. Variants of partial lipodystrophy exist but are uncommon: subcutaneous atrophy may involve only the buttocks, arms, and legs, with sparing of the face and trunk[125]; hemilipoatrophy affecting half the face or trunk has been described[123]; and Figure 13–47 illustrates a patient in whom only the buttocks and upper thighs were affected. The lipoatrophy is usually permanent, although in one case following scarlet fever in which the face and arms were affected, there was a spontaneous reappearance of the fat eight years later.[122] Generalized hirsutism, hyperpigmentation, and hepatomegaly have been

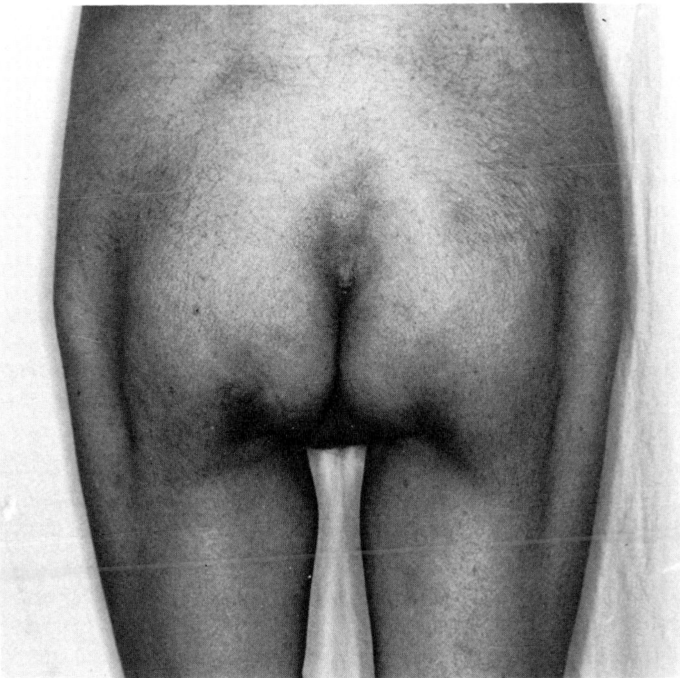

Figure 13–47. Partial lipodystrophy. This woman had lipodystrophy only of buttocks and upper thighs in association with diabetes mellitus.

observed in a few patients with partial lipodystrophy, but acanthosis nigricans was not mentioned.[122] It is not clear whether acanthosis nigricans is truly absent or whether it has simply not been specifically looked for in this variety of lipoatrophy.

Insulin-resistant diabetes may develop several years after the lipodystrophy has appeared.

Membranoproliferative glomerulonephritis secondary to circulating immune complexes can be detected in 40 to 50 per cent of cases.[122, 125] Usually there is an associated decrease in serum levels of C3 with normal levels of C4 and C2 indicating activation of the alternative complement pathway. However, renal disease has developed in the absence of complement abnormalities.[126] In addition, the complement abnormalities are often present without renal disease, suggesting that they precede its development. Since a few patients have had an increased frequency of infections, it has been postulated that the renal disease may be related to immune complexes generated by repeated viral infections.[125] The relationship between the lipodystrophy and the complement abnormalities is obscure.

Although the common form of partial lipodystrophy does not appear to be inherited, Dunnigan et al. described several women in two families with a dominantly transmitted variant of partial lipodystrophy.[127] This variety differed from the common type in that the face was spared while the rest of the body — trunk and limbs — was affected. Also, these patients had one or more of the following: hypertriglyceridemia with tuberous and eruptive xanthomata, hypertrophy of the labia minora, skeletal muscle hypertrophy, and acanthosis nigricans. Insulin-resistant diabetes was present as well. Lillystone and West described another instance of this form of lipoatrophy.[128] If the face were not spared, these cases would be clinically similar to the total lipoatrophy syndrome. Major distinctions, however, are the dominant inheritance pattern found in the Dunnigan variant in contrast to the recessive pattern of the Lawrence-Siep variety, and the absence thus far of hepatomegaly and renal and cardiac abnormalities.

Insulin-resistant diabetes is most commonly caused by high titers of circulating antibodies to insulin. However, insulin-resistant diabetes associated with the lipodystrophy syndromes is produced by a reduced concentration or reduced affinity of the insulin receptor sites in some patients,[129] and by as-yet-unidentified mechanisms in others.[130] Antibodies to insulin receptors have not been detected in any of these patients by the currently available assay.[130]

Insulin-resistant diabetes has also been reported in association with acanthosis nigricans. Kahn et al. described two groups of women with this syndrome which he termed Types A and B.[130, 131] Type A were adolescent girls, some of whom had increased body hair, enlargement of the clitoris, and accelerated somatic growth in addition to acanthosis nigricans. They had features found in congenital lipodystrophy, except for the absence of lipoatrophy. The insulin resistance was associated with decreased numbers of receptors to insulin. Type B were women aged 10 to 60 who had circulating antibodies against insulin receptors in association with features suggesting an underlying autoimmune disease. Pulini et al. described an instance of the type B variant in a 64-year-old black man.[132] Field et al. reported the case of a nonobese black woman with insulin-resistant diabetes and acanthosis nigricans developing at age 15.[133] Over the course of the succeeding 18 months, both the diabetes mellitus and acanthosis nigricans spontaneously disappeared, and her response to insulin also returned to normal.

The cause of the lipoatrophy in both the total and partial varieties has not been determined. However, histologic examination of the atrophic areas in both types shows that the fat cells are present but devoid of cytoplasmic fat.[122, 129] A disturbance in the autonomic nervous innervation of adipose tissue coupled with defective insulin receptors could explain the loss of fat. Defective innervation could determine the observed patterns of total, partial, and hemilipoatrophy. Defective insulin receptors could result in low glucose uptake by the fat cells, with a consequently reduced synthesis of triglycerides as proposed by Oseid et al.[129] Although not all patients with lipoatrophic diabetes have depressed insulin binding,[130] those who do not might have a defect that occurs beyond the receptor site to produce the same result.

ACANTHOSIS NIGRICANS

Acanthosis nigricans is known chiefly for its ominous association with abdominal cancer in adults. However, it occurs much more frequently in a benign setting, especially in children and young adults. Many of these individuals are overweight, so that the term juvenile — or pseudo—acanthosis nigricans is applied to this dermatosis when associated with obesity. In some cases the acanthosis improves moderately with weight reduction. However, since juvenile, or pseudo, acanthosis nigricans is indistinguishable clinically and histologically from acanthosis associated with cancer, it would be best to abandon this terminology and simply diagnose a case as acanthosis nigricans in association with a specific disease. Acanthosis nigricans also occurs as a congenital and familial disorder, and in this instance it probably represents an epidermal nevus and not the acquired disorder, acanthosis nigricans.

Acanthosis nigricans has been considered a possible sign of endocrine disease for many years. The obesity associated with acanthosis in some patients has been postulated to develop on an endocrine basis. Rothman reported the case of a man who had been obese and had had acanthosis nigricans from the age of seven years.[134] When he died in adulthood, he was found to have a basophilic adenoma. No endocrine diseases had been diagnosed during life. The notion that pituitary or hypothalamic derangements might be responsible for both the obesity and acanthosis nigricans was further fostered by two reports of children who developed acanthosis and became obese following trauma that resulted in skull fractures.[135, 136] Brown et al. demonstrated additional links between acanthosis and endocrine disease in a series of 72 patients with acanthosis nigricans.[137, 138] Seventeen of the individuals, mostly children, had one of the following endocrinopathies: acromegaly, gigantism, Cushing's syndrome, Stein-Leventhal disease, adrenal insufficiency, diabetes mellitus, hyperthyroidism, hypothyroidism, and lipodystrophy with hyperlipemia. One patient had a pituitary adenoma. Not all of these patients were obese, and the acanthosis nigricans improved in only a few after the endocrine disease was successfully treated. Brown et al. delineated a syndrome of hirsutism, obesity, amenorrhea, and acanthosis nigricans in five women in whom no endocrine disease could be uncovered.

In an effort to pursue this problem further, Hollingsworth and Amatruda studied 28 massively obese patients.[139] Fourteen had acanthosis nigricans (10 men and 4 women) and 14 did not (12 men and 2 women). In the group with acanthosis there were 2 adolescent girls who weighed 259 and 242 pounds and one man who weighed 283 pounds. The rest were over 300 pounds. The patients without acanthosis nigricans had comparable weights. Both groups of patients had a striking incidence of massive obesity in their families. Eleven of the fourteen patients with acanthosis developed obesity in childhood, and several remembered that their skin lesions had been present before puberty. Only 7 of 14 nonacanthotic patients could date their obesity to childhood. Three of the acanthotic group had suffered significant head trauma that produced unconsciousness. Seven of the nonacanthotic group gave a similar history, and four of them developed obesity in adult life following head injury. Table 13–1 summarizes the data on these patients.

Four women were identified with the syndrome of acanthosis, hirsutism, and amenorrhea. One of them had polycystic ovaries; and in 2 others, similar ovarian disease was believed to be present on the basis of physical examination. None of the nonacanthotic women had these abnormalities.

The only abnormalities of pituitary-adrenal function were found in the four women with acanthosis, hirsutism, and amenorrhea. There was a loss of the diurnal variation in plasma 11-hydroxycorticosteroids. Cushing's syndrome was excluded in these four patients.

Additional support for the link between acanthosis nigricans and endocrine disease includes the cases of generalized lipoatrophy, familial partial lipoatrophy, and insulin-resistant diabetes described previously. The nature of the agent responsible for producing acanthosis nigricans is not known, but it is likely to be a peptide whose origin is in the pituitary or hypothalamus on the basis of the clinical associations that have been described above. Scott et al. reported the case of a 16-year-old black girl who developed acanthosis nigricans in association with a presumed viral encephalopathy that persisted for three months.[140] The acanthosis nigri-

Table 13–1. Acanthosis Nigricans and Obesity

	Obesity With Acanthosis	Obesity Without Acanthosis
Number of patients	14 (10 males, 4 females)	14 (12 males, 2 females)
Onset obesity in childhood	11	7
Family history of obesity	13	11
Head trauma	3	7
Diabetes mellitus	1	1
Abnormal glucose tolerance test	1	0
Cryptorchidism	2	2
Testicular atrophy (postpubertal)	0	1
Thyroid goiter	1	0
Hyperthyroidism	0	1
Hypothyroidism	0	1
Stein-Leventhal syndrome	4	0

cans appeared and disappeared respectively with the onset and remission of the encephalopathy.

In support of the proposal of Rothman[134] and Lerner[141] that the pituitary might be secreting a factor to produce acanthosis nigricans, Nordlund and Lerner produced hyperadrenalism and acanthosis nigricans on the neck, knuckles, and waist line and in the axillae of an obese woman who was being treated with β-MSH and L-dopa for metastatic melanoma.[142] The MSH preparation was a crude extract of bovine pituitaries that contained small amounts of ACTH, unidentified peptides, and a high concentration of β-MSH. After discontinuation of the therapy, the hyperadrenalism and acanthosis nigricans disappeared. The preparation was subsequently purified by passage through a Sephadex column, and when readministered to the same patient, the skin darkened again but the hyperadrenalism and acanthosis nigricans did not recur. The crude MSH had also been administered to other patients who were not obese, and none developed acanthosis nigricans. The obese patient appeared to be particularly responsive to the putative acanthosis nigricans factor present in the crude MSH.

Acanthosis nigricans has also developed following treatment with nicotinic acid, corticosteroids, and diethylstilbesterol.[143] These drugs may be inducing the dermatosis in a predisposed population. Brown et al. noted that their two patients who developed acanthosis nigricans following ingestion of nicotinic acid had major disturbances in lipid metabolism. One patient also had an abnormal glucose tolerance test.[137]

HYPERLIPIDEMIAS

The hyperlipidemic disorders are characterized by persistent elevation of some or all of the plasma lipids: cholesterol, triglycerides, and phospholipids. Xanthomas represent the abnormal accumulations of these substances in skin, tendon, fascia, and periosteum. These same lipids accumulate in the cornea to produce arcus juvenilis and senilis; in the major vessels these accumulations cause atheromatous plaques.

Xanthomas are also associated with disorders in which there are no abnormalities of blood lipids. These so-called "normolipemic xanthomatoses" have been previously discussed under the headings of histiocytosis X, xanthoma disseminatum, nevoxanthoendothelioma, and cerebrotendinous xanthomatosis. They represent disorders that are characterized by histiocytic proliferation with secondary uptake of fat rather than by an error in lipid metabolism. (See Chap. 4.)

Prior to 1967, when the hyperlipidemic diseases were reclassified by Frederickson et al.[144] on the basis of electrophoretic and ultracentrifugal analyses of serum lipoproteins, these disorders had been divided into two major groups: hypercholesterolemia and hyperlipemia, each having familial and acquired subdivisions. In hypercholesterolemia, the fasting serum is clear, but in hyperlipemia it may be lactescent because of increased amounts of triglyceride. In many cases of hyperlipemia, abdominal pain secondary to pancreatitis was present; and in hypercholesterolemia, premature coronary artery disease was characteristic. It soon became apparent that in some families, hypercholesterolemia was accompanied by lactescent serum and that the hyperlipemic variety was a heterogeneous group of familial disorders. The acquired or secondary hyperlipidemias are much more common than the familial types; and they are associated with diabetes mellitus, hypothyroidism, biliary cirrhosis, myeloma, nephrosis, and glycogen storage disease.

The terminology used in this traditional classification has also been confusing. Whereas most clinicians have used the names *hyperlipemia* and *hyperlipidemia* to indicate hypertriglyceridemia, others have used these terms to describe patients with hypercholesterolemia. If one wishes to retain this nomenclature and be unambiguous, then either only *hypercholesterolemia* or only *hypertriglyceridemia* (or both, if applicable) should be used to describe a specific case.

The new classification, based upon an analysis of serum lipoproteins, was thought to divide the familial hyperlipidemic states into five groups, each with its own lipoprotein pattern and clinicopathologic features.[144] These lipoprotein patterns could also be used to describe the serum lipid abnormalities of the acquired hyperlipidemias, except for biliary cirrhosis.

The electrophoretic pattern of serum lipoproteins is shown in Figure 13–48. Four main lipid staining bands are present. At the origin are the chylomicrons (density: <1.006; $S_F >400$) which are made up almost exclusively of dietary triglycerides. The second band is the beta lipoprotein band (low density lipoprotein (LDL); density: 1.006 to 1.063; S_F 0–12), whose lipid fraction contains about 55 per cent cholesterol, 30 per cent phospholipid, and 15 per cent triglyceride. The third band, the prebeta lipoprotein band (very low density lipoprotein (VLDL); density: <1.006; S_F 20–400), moves somewhat faster to the anode and contains 50 per cent triglyceride, 20 per cent cholesterol, and 30 per cent phospholipid. Remnant or intermediate density lipoproteins (IDL) refers to a group of lipoproteins that are not detected in normal electrophoretic patterns. They have the same density as prebetalipoproteins and are composed of equal amounts of cholesterol and triglycerides. When present in abnormally increased amounts they migrate electrophoretically between the beta and prebeta bands. The high density alpha lipoprotein band (HDL) is not involved in the metabolic diseases to be discussed in this section. Elevation of serum cholesterol is primarily associated with an increased amount of beta lipoprotein. Increased plasma triglycerides, which are responsible for the lactescent serum, are correlated with an increase in the prebeta lipoprotein or chylomicron fractions.

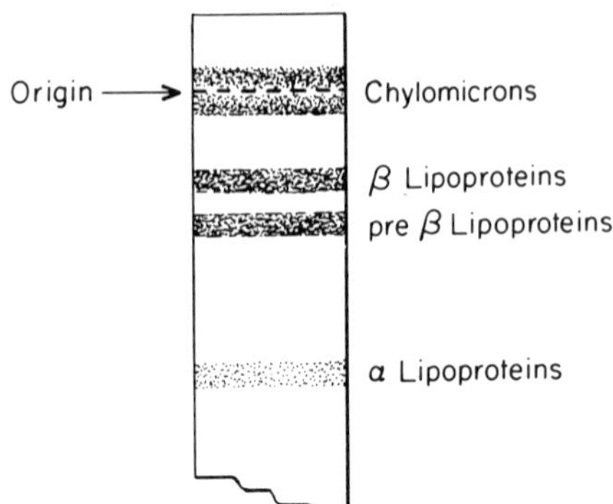

Figure 13–48. Electrophoretic pattern of lipoproteins. (Courtesy of Dr. Robert Scheig.)

The protein component of each class of lipoprotein is composed of several polypeptide chains called apoproteins A, B, C, and E.[145, 146]

The lipoprotein bands detected by electrophoresis are believed to be related to the metabolism of the lipoproteins in the following way.[147] Within the intestinal wall, dietary animal and vegetable fats form triglyceride-rich chylomicrons which become incorporated into lipoprotein complexes that are released into the circulation via the intestinal lymph. The chylomicrons are hydrolyzed by the enzyme lipoprotein lipase (LPL), yielding free fatty acids and glycerol. As hydrolysis continues, the chylomicrons become smaller and form prebetalipoproteins. (Prebetalipoproteins are also derived from synthesis in the gut and liver). Continued hydrolytic action by LPL on the prebetalipoproteins sequentially produces remnant lipoprotein (IDL) and betalipoprotein (LDL), the metabolic end-product of chylomicron hydrolysis.

The metabolic pathways of LDL have recently been unravelled by Brown and Goldstein.[148] Mammalian cells have LDL receptors that allow the betalipoproteins to enter the cells where degradative processes yield cholesterol and phospholipids necessary for membrane synthesis and other metabolic needs. Endogenous cellular cholesterol synthesis is modulated by the enzyme hydroxymethylglutaryl CoA reductase (HMG CoA reductase). Tissue catabolism, hydrolysis of VLDL and IDL, and hepatic synthesis all contribute to the plasma levels of LDL. Betalipoprotein synthesis by the liver is also controlled by HMG CoA reductase. The activity of this enzyme is controlled by the amount of cholesterol absorbed from the diet. High cholesterol diets suppress HMG CoA reductase, resulting in a decreased synthesis of endogenous cholesterol and LDL; low cholesterol intake stimulates HMG CoA reductase activity, leading to increased synthesis of endogenous cholesterol and LDL. The major excretory pathway for cholesterol is through its oxidation to bile salts. Thyroid hormones control this oxidative step. Hyperthyroidism accelerates oxidation and formation of bile salts, resulting in the production of hypocholesterolemia, while hypothyroidism produces the reverse effects — hypercholesterolemia secondary to hyperbetalipoproteinemia.

When the classification of the hyperlipidemias was first proposed it was believed that each of the lipoprotein bands represented molecules under independent metabolic influence.[144] Each lipoprotein pattern was thought to be specific for a monogenic lipid disorder. Five types were recognized at that time and were referred to by Roman numerals I to V. In the past decade, it has become clear that none of the lipoprotein patterns is specific for any one genetic disorder, except perhaps for type 1. The lipoprotein patterns can vary under physiologic and pharmacologic conditions. Lipid levels in the blood are the result of interacting genetic and environmental influences. The lipoprotein patterns are helpful in pointing to a possible genetic disorder in a given patient, but they must be combined with detailed clinical and chemical studies of family members to determine the exact type of genetically determined lipid disorder. Six monogenic lipid disorders are currently recognized.[147, 149, 150] The reader is referred to the excellent review of this topic by Parker.[151]

Cutaneous Manifestations

Cutaneous xanthomas, characteristic of the hyperlipidemias, are categorized as tendinous, tuberous, planar, or eruptive, depending upon their anatomic location and mode of development. The yellow color of xanthomas is almost certainly produced by carotene, although I have not been able to find a published report in which xanthomas were analyzed for this substance. Carotene is responsible for the yellow color of butter and subcutaneous fat.[152] White fat, which is found among some animals, such as the sheep, pig, and goat, does not contain carotene. Krinsky et al. demonstrated that 75 per cent of the blood carotene is transported by low density lipoproteins (S_F 3–9) and the remainder by the high density lipoproteins.[153] Serum carotene concentrations are high when hypercholesterolemia is present.[144]

Tendon xanthomas are firm subcutaneous masses that have a predilection for the extensor tendons of the fingers, patellae, and elbows (Figs. 13–49 and 13–50). The Achilles tendon is one of the most frequently involved sites. The triceps, peroneal, and toe tendons are affected less often. Xanthomas in the extensor tendons of the hands can be detected most easily by examining the clenched fist. This type of xanthoma is produced by a diffuse infiltration of lipid within the tendon; it is not an exophytic tumor on the tendon sheath. The plantar aponeurosis, fascia, and the tibial periosteum can be infiltrated as well. Tendon xanthomas indicate hypercholesterolemia and are found almost exclusively in familial type II and III diseases. We have seen an exception to this rule in two women with biliary cirrhosis and marked xanthomatosis. Both had xanthomas in the Achilles tendon and in the extensor tendons of the hands. Tendon xanthomas may develop in association with normal plasma lipids in two storage diseases: cerebrotendinous xanthomatosis involving cholestanol (see p. 213), and storage disease of plant sterols — beta sitosterol, campesterol, and stigmasterol — absorbed from the diet.[154]

Tuberous xanthomas represent lipid deposits in the dermis and subcutaneous layer. Normally they range from a few millimeters up to about 5 cm; they may be papular, nodular, plaquelike, or pedunculated. Tuberous xanthomas are concentrated over the extensor surfaces of the large joints as well as those of the hand. They can also be found on the buttocks and heels and in the flexures — axillae, antecubital and popliteal fossae, and finger webs[155] (Plate 38*B*). Rarely, the xanthomas may develop about the hair follicles to produce perifollicular papules. Xanthomas can also be scattered over the trunk. Tuberous xanthomas are also formed by the confluence of eruptive xanthomas when hypertriglyceridemia becomes persistent. Tuberous xanthomas are primarily associated with increased serum triglycerides on either a familial or an acquired basis. However, in severe familial type II hypercholesterolemia, tuberous xanthomas may be present in addition to tendon xanthomas in the absence of significant triglyceridemia. Tuberous xanthomas are also common in biliary cirrhosis in which hypertriglyceridemia does not occur. Tuberous lesions may become smaller when serum lipids are lowered; this is in contrast to tendon xanthomas, which remain constant.

Plane xanthomas are flat, yellow or yellow-brown plaques that are distributed chiefly on the palms, face, sides of the neck, and upper trunk (Plate 38*C–F*). When they occur on the eyelids they are called xanthelasma (Plate 39*A*). Plane xanthomas have a marked predilection for palmar creases and surgical and acne scars. The term *xanthoma striatum palmare* has been used when they occur in the palmar creases.

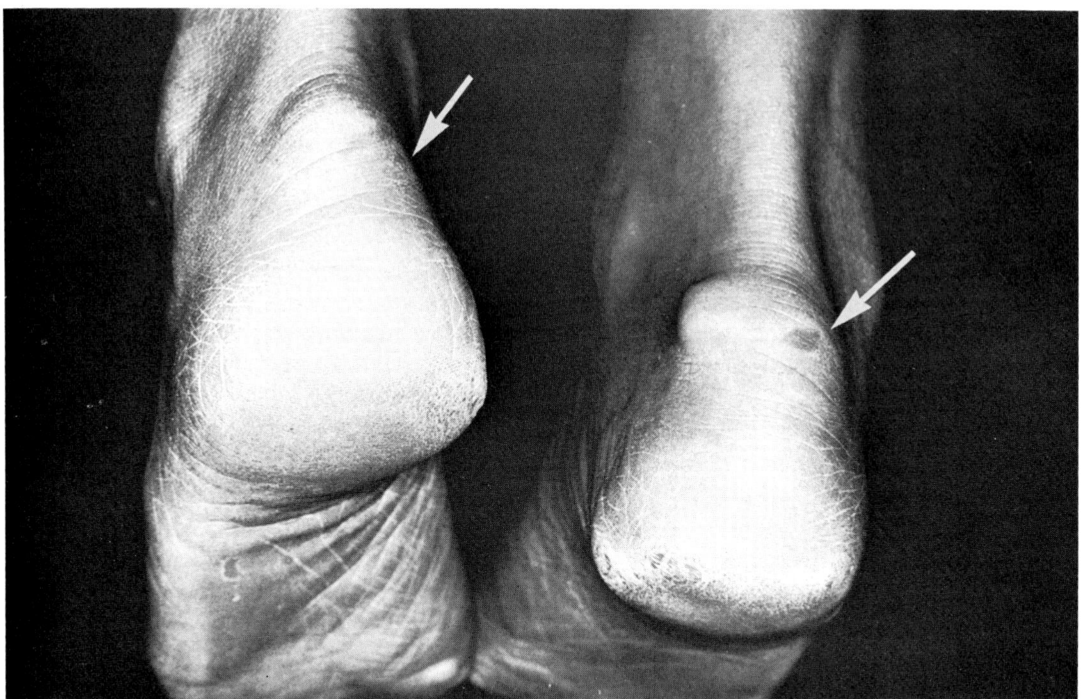

Figure 13–49. Bilateral Achilles tendon xanthomas (arrows) in patient with biliary cirrhosis.

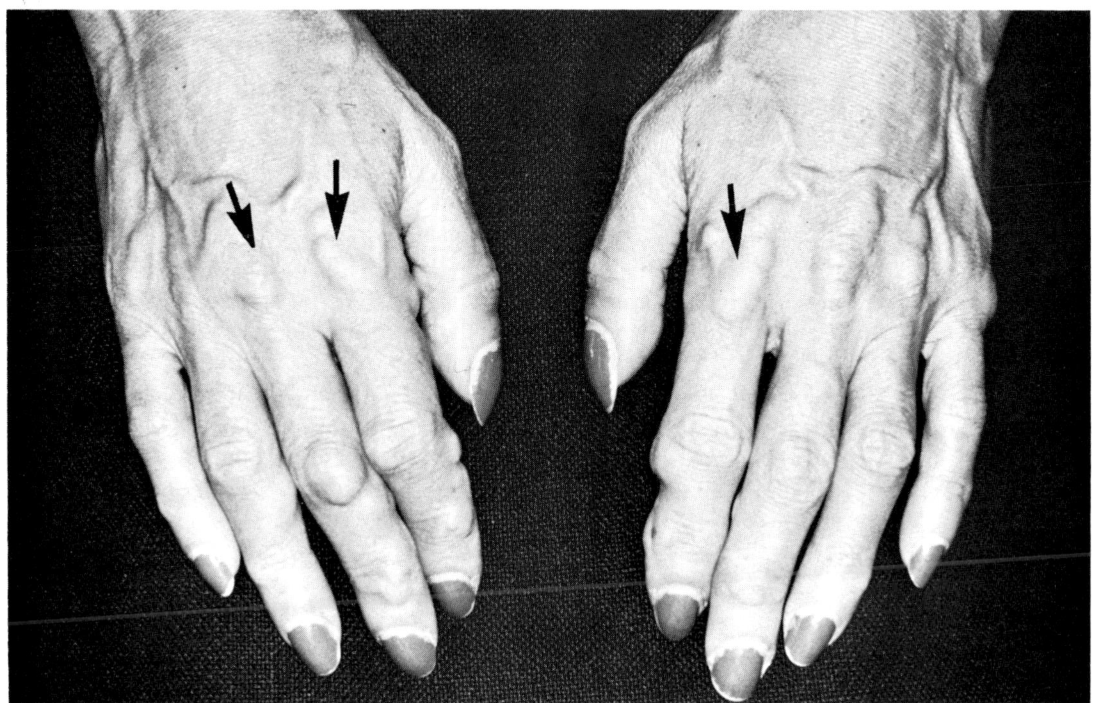

Figure 13–50. Tendon xanthomas (arrows) in extensor tendons of fingers of a patient with biliary cirrhosis. Tuberous xanthomas are also present on fingers.

Frederickson et al. believe that plane xanthomas are restricted to familial type III lipoproteinemias. However, Polano described plane xanthomas in five of eight patients with type IV hyperlipoproteinemia, and Mishkel observed them in five cases of familial type II disease.[156, 157] Plane xanthomas are one of the predominant features of biliary cirrhosis.

Eruptive xanthomas are small red-yellow papules that arise in crops and have an erythematous base (Plate 38*A*). They develop primarily on the buttocks and backs of the thighs and in the body folds. The oral mucosa may also be affected. These xanthomas can arise as a Koebner's phenomenon in areas of trauma. Eruptive xanthomas usually indicate an abrupt increase of serum triglycerides. When the lipids return to a normal level, the xanthomas disappear. If the triglyceridemia persists, the eruptive lesions may enlarge and coalesce to form tuberous lesions. Lipemia retinalis is frequently associated with eruptive xanthomas. When hypertriglyceridemia reaches a certain severity, it may become visible as a pale cast on the retina in association with a marked increase in the light reflex of the retinal vessels. Eruptive xanthomas are found in familial types I, III, IV, and V, but the most frequent cause is the hypertriglyceridemia of uncontrolled diabetes mellitus.

Unfortunately, xanthomas merely indicate the probable presence of hyperlipidemia; the different types of xanthomas cannot be used to make an unequivocal diagnosis of a specific lipoproteinemia. Tendon xanthomas indicate the presence of type II or III disease. Eruptive xanthomas are specific for hypertriglyceridemia, but they do not suggest an etiology. Tuberous xanthomas are found in both hypercholesterolemia and triglyceridemia and are a specific sign *only in association with tendon xanthomas*. This combination indicates severe type II disease with premature ischemic heart disease. Planar xanthomas by themselves are not helpful because they are commonly found in types III and IV, biliary cirrhosis, and rarely in type II. Xanthelasma is the least helpful of all the xanthomas in the clinical diagnosis of the hyperlipidemias (see p. 681).

Clinical Features of the Six Types of Hyperlipoproteinemia[144, 147, 149]

Type I disease is characterized by the presence of a high concentration of chylomicrons in plasma 14 hours or more after the last meal of a normal diet. Other names for this disorder include familial hyperchylomicronemia, fat-induced hyperlipemia, and idiopathic or familial hyperlipemia of the Buerger-Grütz type. This disorder is rare; only about 35 cases have been studied. Both boys and girls are affected, and the diagnosis is often made during the first year of life; however, some patients may not be diagnosed until adulthood.[158] The serum is milky because of an increased chylomicron content when the affected individual is on a normal diet. The defect in this disease is believed to be a faulty removal of chylomicrons from the blood because of deficient lipoprotein lipase activity. This manifests itself as a decrease in plasma postheparin lipolytic activity. About two thirds of the affected children have eruptive xanthomas that disappear when they are fed a low fat diet. Systemic features of this illness include bouts of fever; abdominal pain; and hepatic and/or splenic enlargement. Pancreatitis occurs in about 10 per cent of the patients and may be secondary to the hyperlipemia. Lipemia retinalis is common. These patients do not have abnormal glucose tolerance tests, nor do they show evidence of premature ischemic heart disease or atherosclerosis even after 20 to 30 years of hyperlipemia. Type I appears to be dominantly transmitted.

Type II disease is characterized by an increase in betalipoprotein alone (IIa) or in association with a mild increase in prebetalipoprotein (IIb). In patients with type IIb, the prebetalipoproteins are not increased enough to produce a milky plasma. Synonyms for this disorder include familial hyperbetalipoproteinemia, familial hypercholesterolemia, familial hypercholesterolemic xanthomastosis, and xanthoma tuberosum multiplex. Familial type II disease is dominantly inherited. Serum cholesterol and phospholipids are elevated, although the blood level of triglycerides is usually normal. Whether patients with the "prebeta band" have abnormal glucose tolerance tests or are prediabetic remains to be determined. The over-all incidence of "chemical diabetes" in type II disease is not greater than that believed to be present in the general population.

In the homozygous form of the disease, tendon, fascial and periosteal xanthomas in association with tuberous lesions, xanthelasma, arcus juvenilis, and atherosclerosis of the coronary arteries are characteristic features (Fig. 13–51). The xanthomas usually develop before the third decade, and frequently they are present in the first. These individuals die of ischemic heart disease in their twenties and thirties.[154, 155, 157, 158] The plasma cholesterol level is four to six times normal in homozygous type II disease.

Heterozygotes develop tendon xanthomas in the second and third

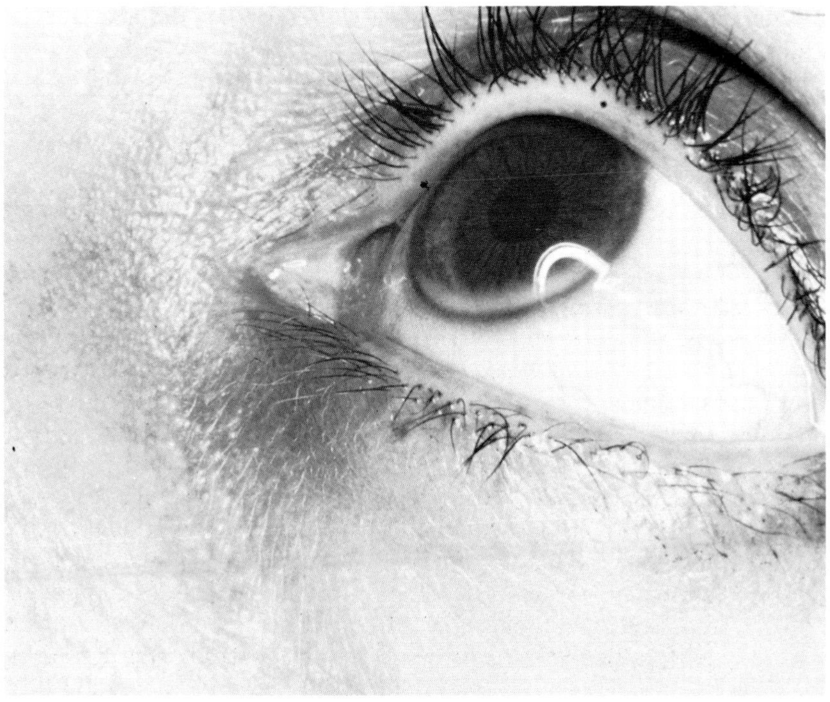

Figure 13–51. Arcus juvenilis in a 30-year-old woman with type II lipoproteinemia.

decades. Tuberous xanthomas are much less common. The levels of plasma cholesterol are two to three times normal. Although studies have indicated that most heterozygotes suffer from coronary artery disease more frequently and earlier than normal individuals,[161-163] Harlan et al. studied a kindred of 1961 individuals who behaved differently.[164] Of 659 carefully evaluated persons, 79 had hypercholesterolemia. None had tuberous xanthomas or heart disease. Tendon xanthomas appeared after age 30. In this family, xanthelasma was found in 27 per cent of the members, arcus in 33 per cent, and tendon xanthomas in 47 per cent.

High density lipoproteins (HDL) appear to be protective against coronary artery disease.[165] This variable may be important in determining the predisposition to heart disease in different kindreds of heterozygous patients.

Goldstein and Brown have demonstrated that the primary metabolic defect resides in the receptor mechanism for betalipoprotein.[166, 167] Using fibroblasts from individuals with homozygous type II disease, they showed that there was either a defect in the binding of LDL to its receptor or an abnormality in one or more of the various steps involved in the internalization of betalipoprotein. These various defects result in LDL not being degraded as rapidly as it should be and endogenous cholesterol synthesis not being subjected to the normal negative feedback control exerted by LDL on the HMG CoA reductase system. Both disturbances result in hyperbetalipoproteinemia. The multiple defects found at the cellular level imply that the type II phenotype is a heterogeneous group of disorders. This has been recognized clinically in one study in which homozygous type II patients were divided into those who responded to diet and drug therapy and those who did not.[168] The responders demonstrated greater binding of LDL to its receptors than did nonresponders; the responders also exhibited suppression of HMG CoA reductase activity in fibroblasts by LDL, while the nonresponders did not.

It has been estimated that probably no more than 5 per cent of individuals with hypercholesterolemia and a type II pattern have *monogenic* familial hypercholesterolemia. Currently, most individuals with a type II pattern are believed to have hypercholesterolemia caused by a combination of environmental and poorly understood polygenic factors.[147, 149] A newly described *monogenic* disorder, familial combined hyperlipidemia, needs to be excluded in such patients (see p. 680). A variety of nongenetic disorders can also produce type IIa patterns: hypothyroidism, nephrosis, Cushing's syndrome, and dysproteinemias.

Type III disease is characterized by an excess of lipoproteins that have beta mobility but *an abnormally low density*. Electrophoresis often shows a broad band that extends from the beta into the prebeta region (broad beta band). When the serum is ultracentrifuged and the supernatant is electrophoresed, it can be demonstrated that most of the lipoprotein band with beta mobility has a density <1.006. The usual beta lipoprotein that is found in type II disease has a density >1.006. This beta band in type III is also called "floating beta" or "β-VLDL" to distinguish it from the normal prebetalipoproteins (α-VLDL) present in blood. In addition to β-VLDL, remnant lipoproteins (IDL) are also increased. β-VLDL has a higher proportion of cholesterol relative to triglyceride than α-VLDL. The apoprotein compositions of both are also different: apoprotein E is relatively or absolutely increased and apoprotein C in relation to B is decreased.[169] Diagnosis depends upon demonstration of the presence of β-VLDL. Unfortunately, electrophoresis demonstrates a broad beta band in only 50 per cent of patients, and it may be present inconsistently in a minority of patients with the other primary hyperlipidemias. A more reliable test requires ultracentrifugation of plasma in order to obtain molecules of density < 1.006 in which VLDL cholesterol can be measured and related to the total plasma triglyceride level. Frederickson et al. have proposed that when plasma levels of triglycerides are between 150 and 1000 mg/dl, a ratio of not less than 0.3 is diagnostic for type III hyperlipoproteinemia.[170]

Synonyms for this entity have included familial hypercholesterolemia with hyperlipemia, carbohydrate-induced hyperlipemia, and essential hyperlipemia. Cholesterol, phospholipids, and triglycerides are all elevated; and the fasting serum is lactescent. A diet rich in carbohydrates will increase the level of triglycerides, and a diet low in carbohydrates can reduce it.

Type III patients have tuberous, eruptive, planar, and tendon xanthomas; xanthelasma; arcus; ischemic heart disease; and peripheral vascular atherosclerosis.[171] Glucose tolerance tests are abnormal in most persons. Affected individuals are frequently obese.

The xanthomas usually develop after age 25.[144, 171] Some of the xanthomas in type III patients have characteristics of both the eruptive and tuberous types and may wax and wane and even disappear in the absence of any obvious change in the plasma lipoprotein pattern. Following effective therapy, the xanthomas disappear.[171]

The biochemical defect in type III has not yet been established, but two hypotheses have been proposed. There may be a defect in the removal of remnant lipoprotein from the circulation or in its conversion to betalipoprotein[147]; or there may be an abnormality involving the synthesis of the apoprotein portion of prebetalipoprotein so that the latter is not metabolized in its normal pathway.[172] Type III disease appears to be a monogenic autosomal dominantly transmitted disorder.[173]

Type IV disease, currently being called familial hypertriglyceridemia, is transmitted as an autosomal dominant trait. The disorder is caused by an increased hepatic synthesis of prebetalipoproteins (VLDL). The nature of the basic defect is not understood.[147] Although most patients exhibit a type IV lipoprotein pattern, a type V pattern may be induced by consumption of a carbohydrate-rich diet, excessive alcohol intake, or oral contraceptives. The development of diabetes mellitus or hypothyroidism will induce a type V pattern also. There appears to be an increased risk of coronary heart disease in these patients.[149] The diagnosis can be made with certainty only in individuals who have affected relatives, since patients with this form of hypertriglyceridemia have no unique clinical or biochemical features that can be used to distinguish them from other persons who suffer from other genetic or nongenetic forms of hypertriglyceridemia. Eruptive xanthomas may occur when the plasma triglyceride levels become markedly elevated. Synonyms for this entity have included familial hyperprebetalipoproteinemia, essential familial hyperlipemia, and carbohydrate-induced hyperlipemia.

Type V is a combination of types I and IV, a fat-induced and carbohydrate-induced hyperlipemia. Other names for this entity have included familial hyperchylomicronemia with hyperprebetalipoproteinemia, mixed hyperlipemia, and combined fat- and carbohydrate-induced hyperlipemia. The clinical features include abdominal pain, eruptive xanthomas, lipemia retinalis, and obesity. Almost every patient has an abnormal glucose tolerance test. Evidence of accelerated atherosclerosis in these patients or their families has not been found. This disorder is not a late manifestation of type I disease. Postheparin lipoprotein lipase and hepatic triglyceride lipase activities in plasma have been shown to be normal.[147] The genetics of this disorder have not been conclusively established, but the data suggest that it could be a monogenic disorder. The evidence does not support the notion that types IV and V are heterozygous and homozygous genotypes, respectively, of the same mutant alleles or that single genes for type I and type IV defects interact to produce type V.

Familial combined hyperlipidemia is a newly discovered monogeneic, dominantly transmitted lipid disorder. It was uncovered in a study of 2520 relatives and spouses of 176 survivors of myocardial infarction.[149] The affected patient has a type IIa, IIb, or IV lipoprotein pattern, but within the family the relatives with hyperlipidemia exhibit a spectrum of lipoprotein patterns — IIa, IIb, IV, or V. This disorder is genetically distinct from familial hypertriglyceridemia because the relatives of the probands exhibit a spectrum of lipoprotein patterns instead of only type IV. It also can be distinguished from familial hypercholesterolemia because the children of individuals with combined hyperlipidemia do not exhibit hypercholesterolemia, as children of familial hypercholesterolemic families do. Individuals with combined hyperlipidemia have an increased incidence of coronary artery disease. The prevalence of tendon and tuberous xanthomas is low. Combined hyperlipidemia was the most common familial lipid disorder found in the survivors of myocardial infarction and their relatives. The next two most common lipid disorders found in this group were *polygenic* hypercholesterolemia and a sporadic form of hypertriglyceridemia.

It must be emphasized that the most common causes of xanthomatosis are the secondary causes rather than the familial disorders that have just been discussed. During the uncontrolled phase of diabetes mellitus, when hypertriglyceridemia develops, eruptive xanthomas appear. The lipoprotein pattern is type IV. Hypothyroidism is not often complicated by xanthomatosis; but when it is, tuberous and eruptive xanthomas are observed. Lipoprotein patterns II and IV develop in untreated hypothyroidism. The hyperlipemia of myxedema responds to treatment with thyroid hormone. The nephrotic syndrome is associated with patterns II and IV, and eruptive xanthomas are the characteristic lesions. Glycogen storage disease is also characterized by eruptive xanthomas and a type IV pattern. Multiple myeloma is sometimes accompanied by patterns II and IV and by tendinous, tuberous, or eruptive xanthomas (see p. 229).

Biliary cirrhosis exhibits a unique pattern of increased plasma levels of cholesterol and phospholipids and normal amounts of triglycerides. The lipoprotein pattern does not fit any of the five types. An unusual lipoprotein is produced in biliary cirrhosis. Its apoprotein consists of albumin and apoprotein C, which allows it to transport large quantities of cholesterol and phospholipids.[174] Tuberous and planar xanthomas and xanthelasma are invariably present. Tendon xanthomas are said not to occur, but we have seen two patients with xanthomas in the Achilles tendons and the extensor tendons of the hands. Infants with atresia of the intrahepatic bile ducts develop xanthomas identical to those observed in biliary cirrhosis.[175] Hyperpigmentation and pruritus, in association with planar and tuberous xanthomas, are pathognomonic for biliary cirrhosis and occur in no other disease. In spite of the striking xanthomatosis and markedly elevated serum levels of cholesterol, ischemic heart disease does not occur with increased frequency in this disorder.

Xanthelasma is the least important sign of hyperlipidemia. Many individuals have prominent xanthelasma without other xanthomas. In at least 50 per cent of such persons, no serum lipid abnormality is found. Pedace and Winkelmann studied 896 patients who had only xanthelasma.[176] Thirty-three per cent of the men and 40 per cent of the women had elevated levels of serum cholesterol. Familial hypertriglyceridemia was present in 12 per cent of the patients, and familial hypercholesterolemia occurred in 4.7 per cent of the patients.

The mechanism of the formation of xanthomas is not completely understood. The most popular view holds that serum lipids infiltrate the tissues, preferentially in areas subject to stress and pressure, and are phagocytized by macrophages that evolve into foam cells.

Polano studied the lipid composition of 27 tuberous, tendinous, and eruptive xanthomas.[156] He found that all the lesions contained proportionally more free fatty acids and more free cholesterol than were present in blood lipids. The eruptive xanthomas showed a lipid pattern different from tendinous or tuberous lesions. The eruptive xanthomas contained more than 10 per cent free fatty acids and reflected in part the blood lipid patterns. However, the lipid profile of the tendinous and tuberous xanthomas could not be correlated with the type of hyperlipoproteinemia in the patient.

Polano also found that although the fatty acid pattern of the triglycerides and the free fatty acids in the blood and xanthomas were approximately the same, the fatty acid profiles of the cholesterol esters in the blood were different from those in the xanthomas. There was proportionally more oleic acid and proportionally less linoleic acid in the cholesterol esters in xanthomas than in the cholesterol esters of plasma. The lipid pattern of early atheromatous plaques in the aorta is similar to that of xanthomas.

Xanthomas seem to reflect in part the degree and the duration of elevation of serum lipids, but not all patients with elevated serum lipids develop xanthomas. It is not possible to completely correlate the presence of xanthomas with lipid levels, even in those patients with eruptive xanthomas.

Parker and Odland have investigated the problem of xanthoma formation by comparing eruptive xanthomas of diabetics with identical lesions produced in rabbits fed high cholesterol diets.[177] The light and electron microscopic findings in these two xanthomas were identical, even though the lipid composition of the lesions was different. Triglyceride was the major lipid fraction in the diabetic xanthoma, whereas cholesterol was the major fraction in the rabbit lesions. Parker and Odland observed that lipoprotein particles permeated vessel walls in the xanthomas; they thus provided evidence to support the popular hypothesis that plasma lipids contribute to the fat accumulating in these lesions. They also showed that the capillary pericyte and dermal macrophage participate in the formation of the foam cell. The lipid droplets were the same size as the chylomicron lipoproteins isolated in humans and rats, and they were identical in the human and rabbit xanthomas. The ability of chylomicron particles to permeate dermal capillaries may be more dependent upon physical form and size than on the nature of their lipid composition.

The Porphyrias

The enzymatic deficiencies responsible for most of the genetically determined porphyric syndromes have been discovered in the past decade. The deficient enzymes are those involved in the biosynthesis of heme. Prior to this time, research emphasis has been directed toward understanding the ALA-synthetase enzyme system, which exhibited increased activity in all forms of porphyria but could not really explain the diversity of specific biochemical abnormalities characteristic of each type of porphyria.[178, 179] Figures 13–52 and 13–53 depict the biosynthetic

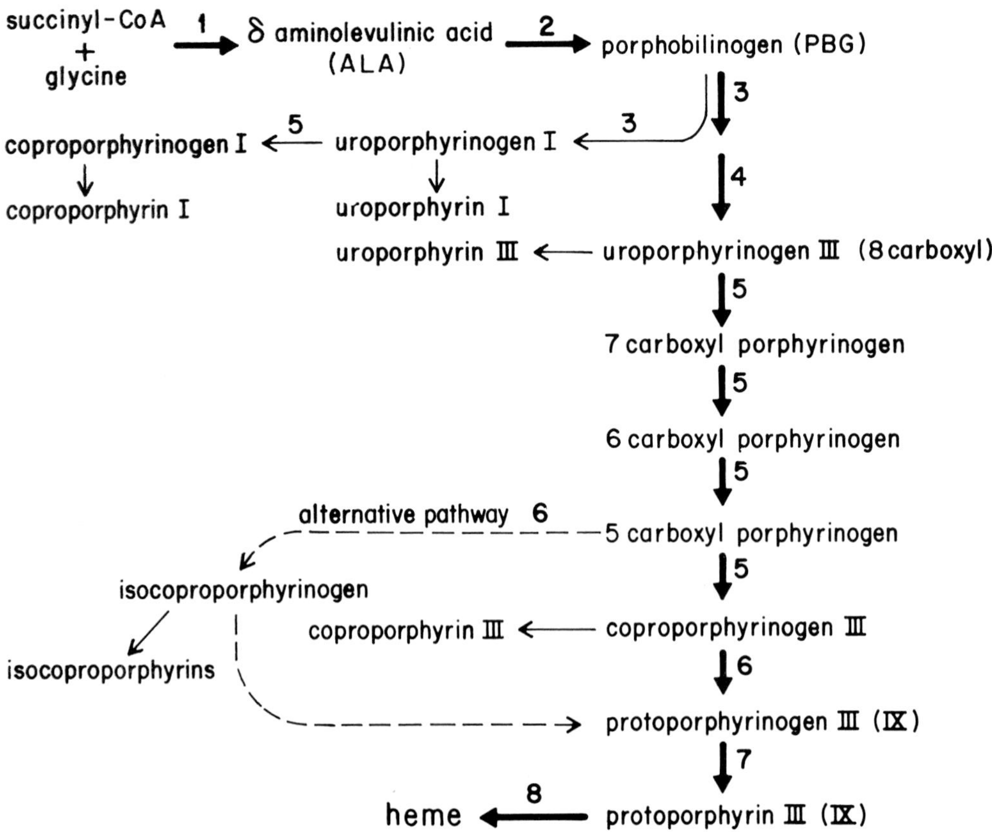

Figure 13–52. Biosynthetic pathway of heme. Bold arrows indicate pathway of heme synthesis. Thin and dashed arrows indicate pathway of porphyrin formation. Enzymes involved in pathways: 1 — ALA synthetase; 2 — ALA dehydrase; 3 — uroporphyrinogen I synthetase; 4 — uroporphyrinogen III cosynthetase; 5 — uroporphyrinogen decarboxylase; 6 — coproporphyrinogen oxidase; 7 — protoporphyrinogen oxidase; 8 — heme synthetase (ferrochetalase).

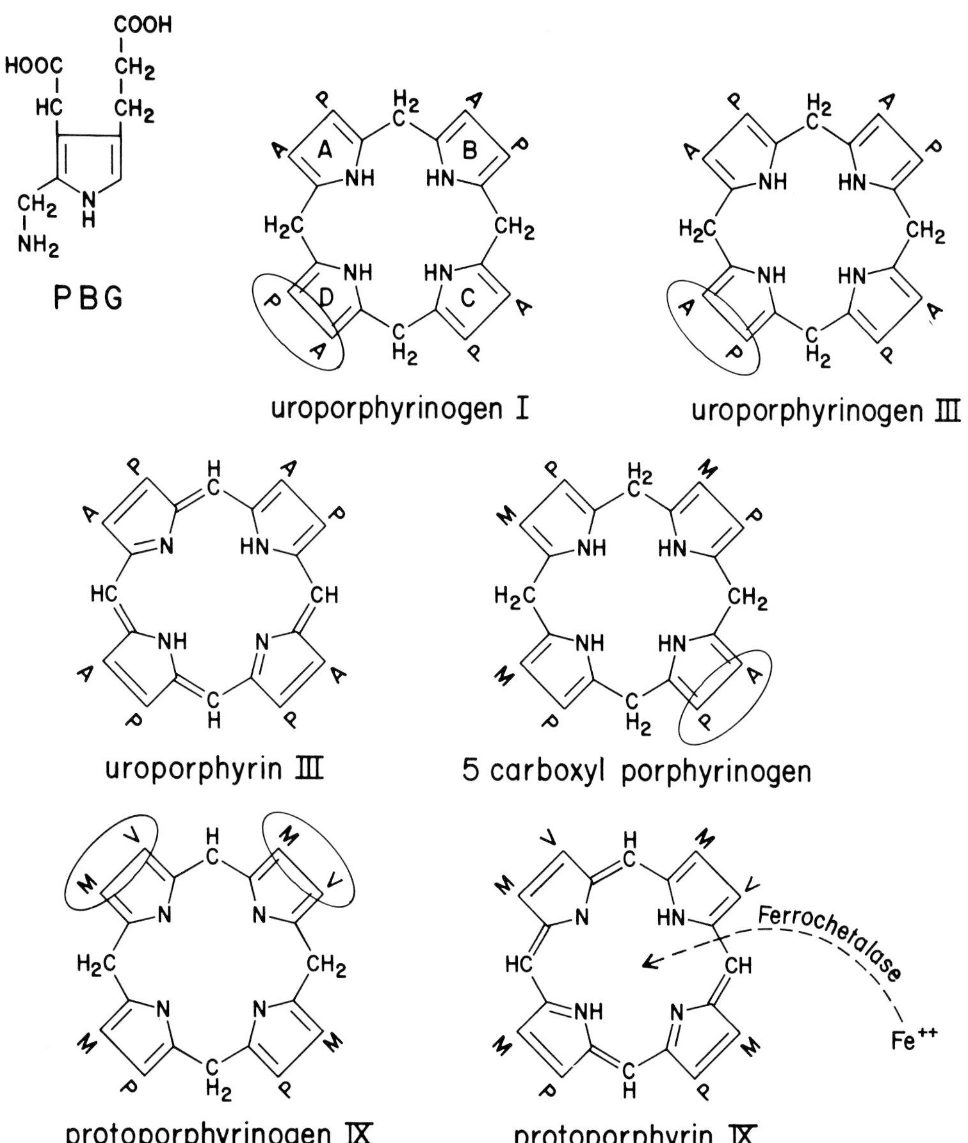

Figure 13–53. Structural formulas of pyrroles involved in heme biosynthesis and porphyria. Prosthetic groups: A—acetic acid; P—propionic acid; M—methyl; V—vinyl. Circled prosthetic groups are discussed in text.

pathway of heme and the structural formulas of the porphyrins and their precursors. Each of the porphyrias represents an inborn metabolic error involving one of the enzymes that participate in the synthesis of heme.

Glycine and succinyl CoA react to form δ-aminolevulinic acid (ALA) under the enzymatic action of ALA-synthetase, the rate-limiting enzyme for heme biosynthesis. Two molecules of ALA are then condensed to form the monopyrrole porphobilinogen (PBG), the source of the tetrapyrroles forming the final product heme. The tetrapyrroles exist in nature as types I or III isomers, the difference being the order of the side chains, acetic acid, and propionic acid in the D ring (Fig. 13–53). Heme is a type III isomer.

Four molecules of PBG are condensed to form uroporphyrinogen III by the interaction of two enzyme systems, uroporphyrinogen I synthetase and uroporphyrinogen III cosynthetase. If uroporphyrinogen I synthetase acts alone, the four molecules of PBG are condensed instead to form uroporphyrinogen I (a type I isomer), which is not an intermediate in the biosynthesis of heme.

Uroporphyrinogen III is converted to coproporphyrinogen III by the enzymatic decarboxylation of all four acetic acid side chains, beginning in the ring D and proceeding sequentially through rings A, B, and C. Uroporphyrinogen decarboxylase is responsible for this conversion. (This same enzyme converts uroporphyrinogen I to coproporphyrinogen I). In addition to the sequential decarboxylation of uroporphyrinogen to coproporphyrinogen, an alternate minor pathway exists which passes from the pentacarboxylic precursor of coproporphyrinogen, the last step in this sequential decarboxylation, to protoporphyrinogen and finally heme. The intermediates in this minor pathway are known as isocoproporphyrinogens and lead to the formation of isocoproporphyrins[179] (Fig. 13–52).

At the next major step, coproporphyrinogen III is converted to protoporphyrinogen III by the decarboxylation and oxidation of two of the four propionic acid side chains to form vinyl groups in rings A and B. The resulting protoporphyrinogen is oxidized to protoporphyrin IX by the removal of six hydrogen atoms. The enzyme coproporphyrinogen oxidase is responsible for the oxidative decarboxylation of the propionyl groups, and the enzyme protoporphyrinogen oxidase is necessary for the final oxidative step. Both protoporphyrinogen and protoporphyrin are type III isomers, but they are usually designated type IX, indicating that they are the ninth isomer of 15 potential protoporphyrinogen and protoporphyrin isomers. Type IX isomer is the only one found in nature. Under the action of ferrochetalase (heme synthetase), ferrous iron is introduced into protoporphyrin to form heme, which is then conjugated to various proteins to form hemoglobin, myoglobin, catalase and cytochromes.

The other *porphyrins* found in the porphyric disorders — uroporphyrins I and III, and coproporphyrins I and III — are by-products formed by irreversible oxidation of their parent porphyrinogen molecules. Porphyrin formation occurs in the tissues where the parent porphyrinogen molecules are synthesized. Under normal physiological conditions, porphyrin formation occurs only to a minimal degree. The true intermediates of heme synthesis are type III porphyrinogens, *not porphyrins*. Also, the catabolism of heme and the hemoproteins leads to bile pigments, but not porphyrins. Although the porphyrias are characterized by enzymatic blocks in heme synthesis, hemoglobin formation remains relatively unimpaired because of compensatory pathways. However, these compensatory paths can obscure the primary genetic enzymatic defect.

Currently, seven types of porphyria are recognized: (1) acute intermittent porphyria, (2) erythropoietic porphyria, (3) porphyria cutanea tarda, (4) hereditary coproporphyria, (5) variegate porphyria, (6) erythropoietic protoporphyria, and (7) congenital erythropoietic coproporphyria. Each type is believed to result from a genetically determined deficiency in one of the enzyme systems involved in the biosynthesis of heme. All of the porphyrias except for acute intermittent porphyria have photo-enhanced or phototoxic cutaneous lesions because of the presence of the photosensitizing tetrapyrrole molecules. Porphyria cutanea tarda, variegate porphyria, and erythropoietic protoporphyria are the porphyric syndromes most commonly encountered in clinical medicine. The porphyrias have also been classified into erythropoietic and hepatic types based upon the major site of porphyrin production. By this criterion, the erythropoietic type includes congenital erythropoietic porphyria, erythropoietic protoporphyria, and congenital erythropoietic coproporphyria. The rest are hepatic porphyrias.

Acute intermittent porphyria is a dominantly transmitted disease in which a deficiency of uroporphyrinogen I synthetase leads to the accumulation of PBG and ALA. Both are excreted in the urine in excessive amounts. Even though PBG and ALA can usually be detected in the urine at all times, acute intermittent porphyria is considered to be a latent benign disease. However, potentially fatal acute attacks can be precipitated by barbiturates, including thiopental anesthesia, griseofulvin, sulfonamides, phenytoin, and meprobamate.[179] Estrogens have produced mixed effects. They have exacerbated the disorder in some women, but have prevented it in others who regularly experienced flares with their menstrual cycle. Experimental studies employing tissue culture and intact animals have shown that barbiturates and other lipid-soluble drugs are relatively weak inducers of ALA synthetase. However, if the biosynthetic pathway of heme is partially blocked, then these drugs become potent inducers of hepatic ALA synthetase. Induction of this enzyme leads to the increased formation and the increased urinary excretion of ALA and PBG present during acute attacks.[180]

The acute attacks, which can last from days to months, are characterized by fever, colicky abdominal pain with vomiting that simulates a variety of surgical conditions, peripheral and cranial neuropathies, and psychoses. Neuropathy can eventuate in paralysis within a few days, but recovery is usual over the course of several months. Paralysis of extremities, dysphonia, dysphagia, and respiratory failure have resulted. Involvement of the autonomic nervous system produces tachycardia out of proportion to the observed fever, labile hypertension, and postural hypotension. The syndrome of inappropriate ADH secretion may develop secondary to hypothalamic damage.

Erythropoietic porphyria (Gunther's disease) is recessively transmitted and characterized by a deficiency of uroporphyrinogen III cosynthetase.[178] Type I uroporphyrinogen and coproporphyrinogen are formed instead of the corresponding type III molecules. The striking clinical feature is marked photosensitivity that begins in infancy. Bullae leading to ulcers and severe scarring appear on the face, ears, nose, scalp, and other exposed areas. Repeated lesions, complicated by secondary infection, produce destruction of terminal phalanges and nails, as well as the nasal and auricular cartilages. The teeth fluoresce red under ultraviolet light and may be colored yellow or brown. Hypertrichosis with fine hairs develops over the face, neck, and extremities. Chronic hemolytic anemia, often with splenomegaly, is a constant feature of the disease.[179] Although the clinical features are associated with the homozygous state, three instances of erythropoietic porphyria with onset in adult life have been reported.[181] It has been suggested that the late onset may be related to the heterozygous state with an acquired or possibly hormonal modification of uroporphyrinogen I synthetase and/or uroporphyrinogen III cosynthetase. The diagnosis of Gunther's disease can be established by measuring the activity of uroporphyrinogen III cosynthetase in red cells and finding

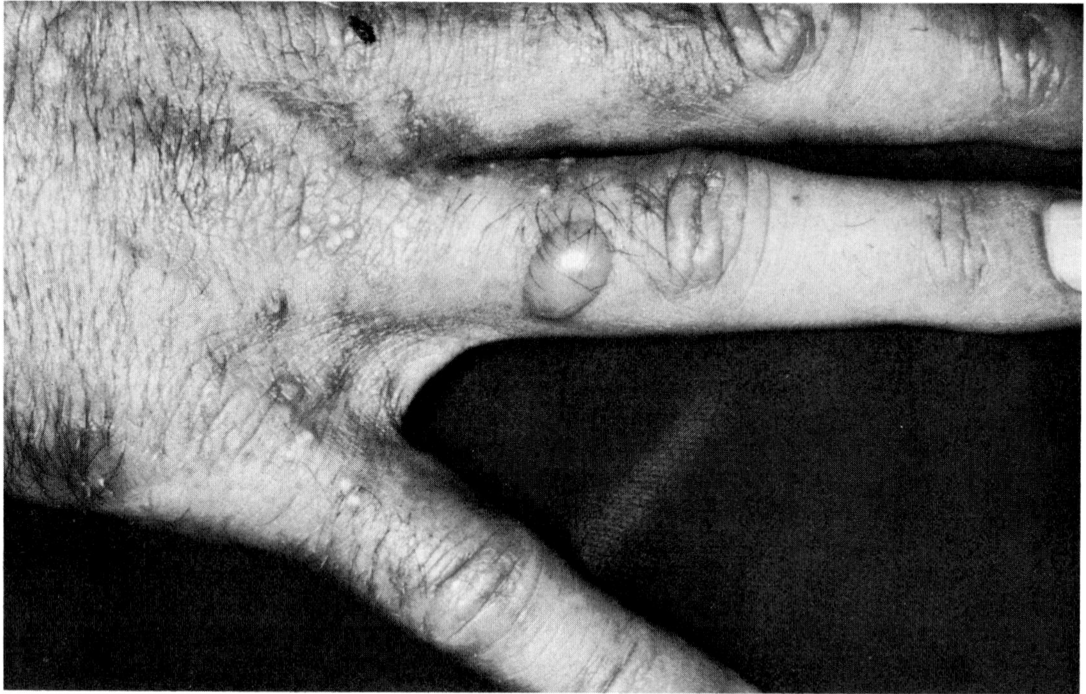

Figure 13–54. Porphyria cutanea tarda. Blisters develop following minor trauma to the skin. Milia are present over the knuckles.

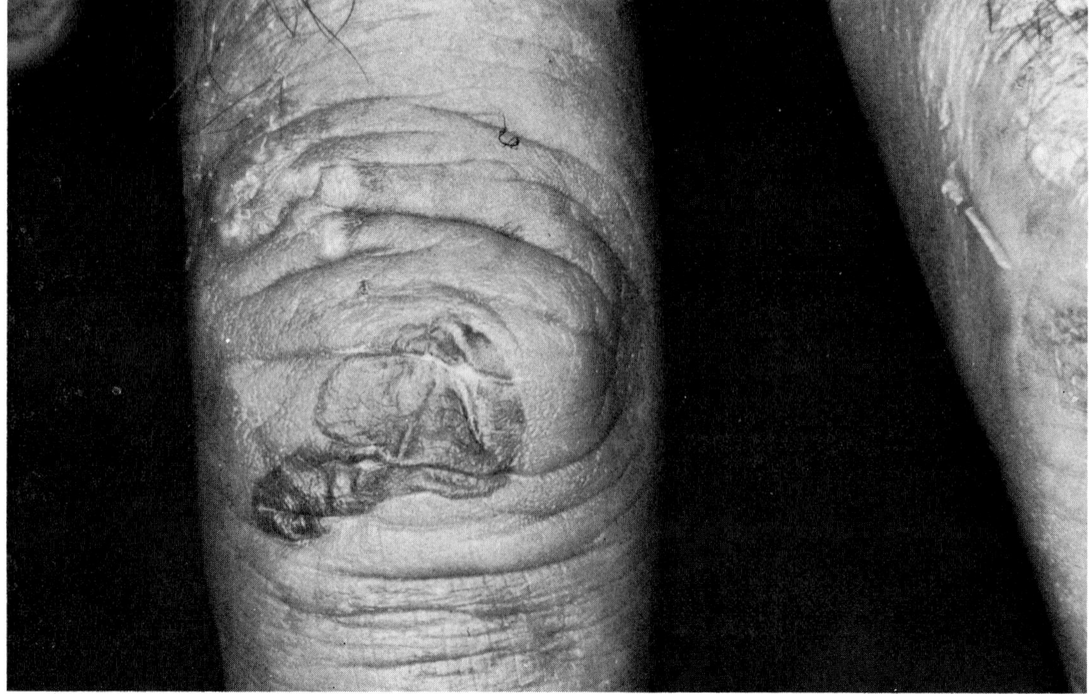

Figure 13–55. Porphyria cutanea tarda. Skin over the knuckle has been sheared off after mild trauma.

increased amounts of uroporphyrin I and coproporphyrin I in red blood cells, plasma, urine, and stool.

Porphyria cutanea tarda is the most commonly encountered variety of porphyria in clinical medicine. Although it most frequently appears in the fifth and sixth decades and in adult men, it has been observed in children and young women in their twenties and thirties.[182, 183] The cutaneous manifestations include extreme skin fragility, resulting in the production of bullae or erosions following minor trauma (Figs. 13–54 and 13–55). Firm traction on the skin can produce shearing similar to the Nikolsky sign. The skin heals with the formation of scars and milia (Figs. 13–56 and 13–57). Milia are epidermal cysts that vary from 1 to 3 mm and appear as white or yellow papules. Skin fragility is most marked on sun-exposed areas such as the face, hands, and bald scalp. The lower extremities and trunk are infrequently affected. Skin fragility in porphyria cutanea tarda is not true photosensitivity — the blisters and erosions are mechanically induced. However, since the predominant sites of involvement are related to exposure to sunlight, porphyrin-induced photosensitivity must play a role in creating the increased fragility of the skin. Some patients with porphyria cutanea tarda do exhibit abnormally increased erythema after ultraviolet light exposure, but a blistering photosensitivity reaction does not develop.

Hypertrichosis around the outer canthi is common in men (Fig. 13–58*A*). In women, increased hair growth tends to develop over the face (Fig. 13–58*B*). In severe cases, increased hair growth may develop on the extremities and trunk. Hyperpigmentation commonly develops on sun-exposed areas. A red-purple suffusion of the head and neck is present in some patients.

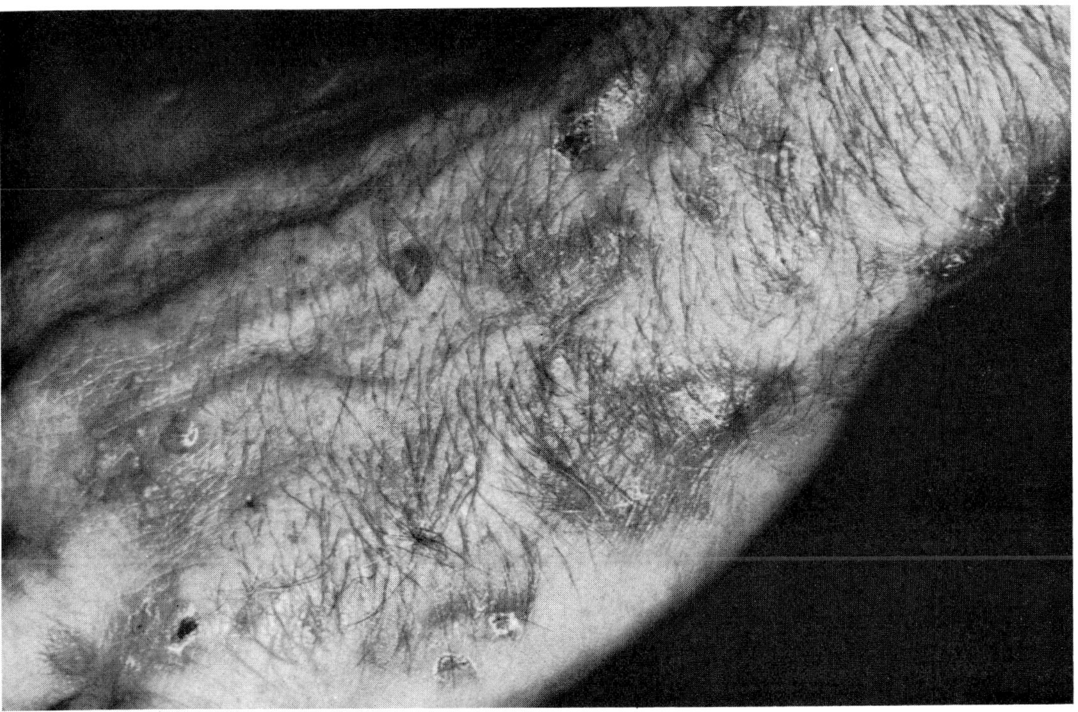

Figure 13–56. Porphyria cutanea tarda. Scars from previous minor injuries.

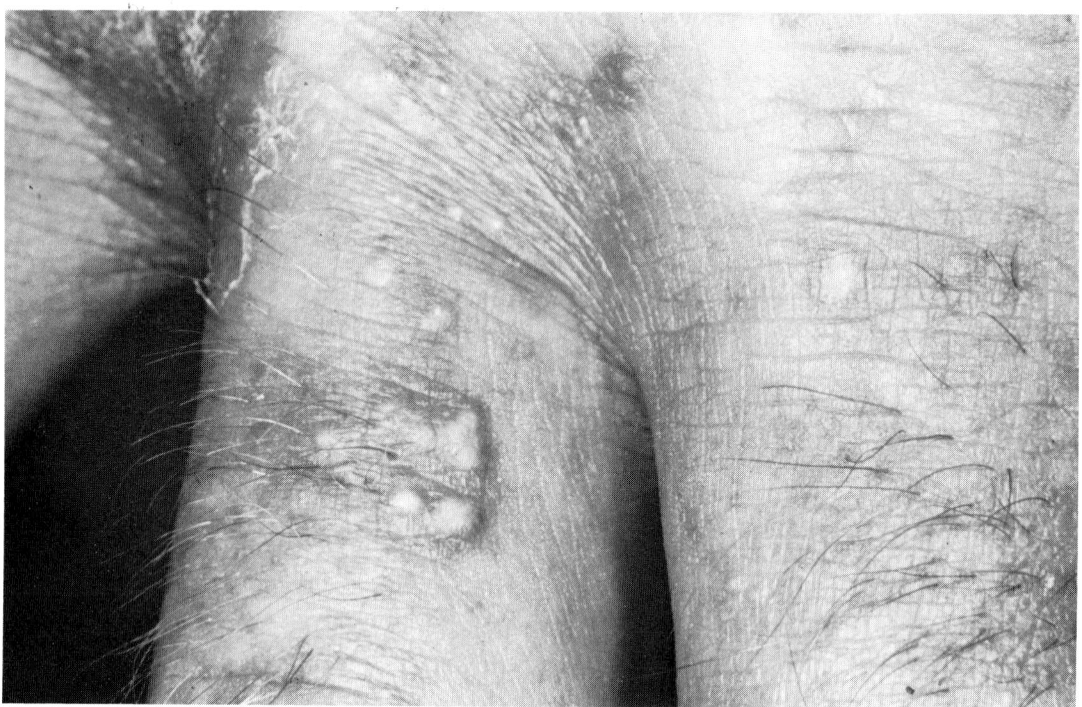

Figure 13–57. Porphyria cutanea tarda. Close-up view of milia that are epidermal cysts.

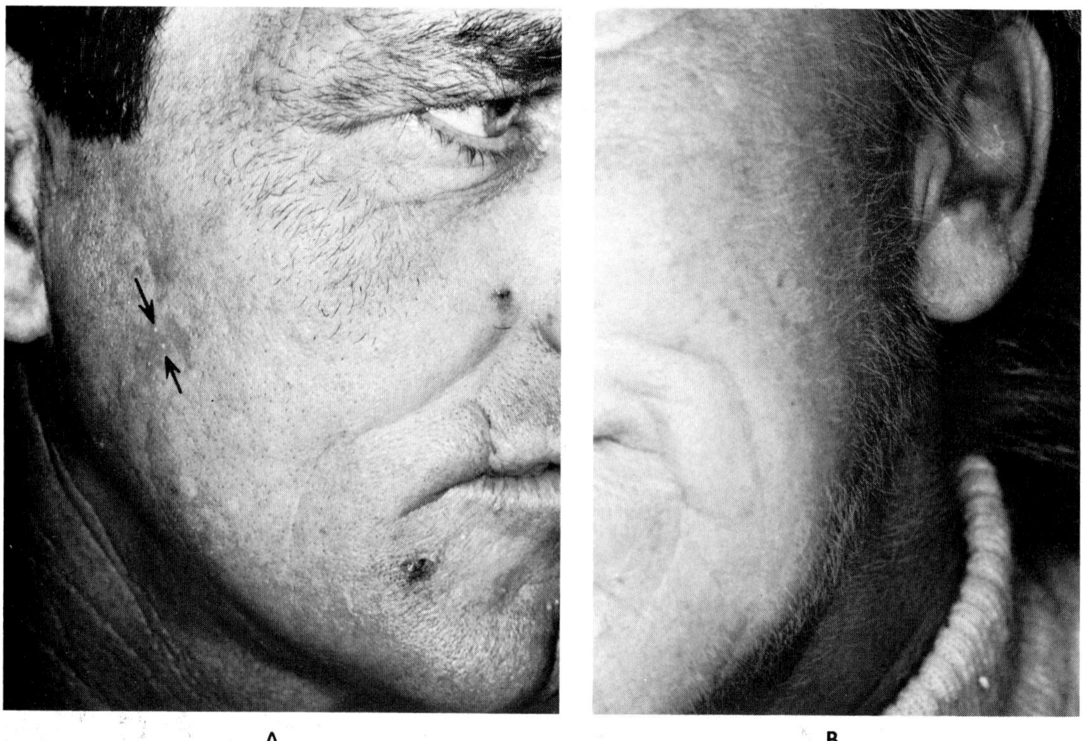

A B

Figure 13–58. *A*, Porphyria cutanea tarda. Hirsutism around the eye. Arrows point to milia in beard area. *B*, Porphyria cutanea tarda. Appearance of increased facial hair growth in affected woman.

In a minority of patients, scleroderma-like changes develop on sun-exposed areas. The skin lesions are clinically and histologically indistinguishable from those of morphea. In some individuals, the process may extend beyond the sun-exposed areas and produce a picture of generalized morphea. Calcinosis cutis with secondary ulceration can develop within these lesions, especially in the preauricular areas. In a series of 40 patients with porphyria cutanea tarda reported by Grossman, seven had morphea-like lesions and three of these had calcinosis cutis.[184] The lesions were present for several years before the clinical onset of porphyria in one person. Figures 13–59 to 13–61 show one of our patients with generalized morphea and calcinosis that had been present for at least 10 years before porphyria cutanea tarda developed. It is not clear whether the morphea-like changes represent an unusual phototoxic response or true morphea induced by the combination of sunlight and the metabolic derangements in porphyria. The sclerodermoid changes improve following successful therapy of the porphyria.[185] However, the development of morphea in some individuals many years before the onset of porphyria cutanea tarda may not be coincidental. The documented association of porphyria cutanea tarda and lupus erythematosus[186] suggests a real association between this form of porphyria and connective tissue diseases.

Current evidence indicates that porphyria cutanea tarda is a sporadic (acquired?) disease in 85 to 90 per cent of cases, and a genetic dominantly transmitted disorder in 10 to 15 per cent. The enzymatic defect has been shown to reside in the uroporphyrinogen decarboxylase system.[187-192] In this form of porphyria, there is hepatic overproduction of four types of

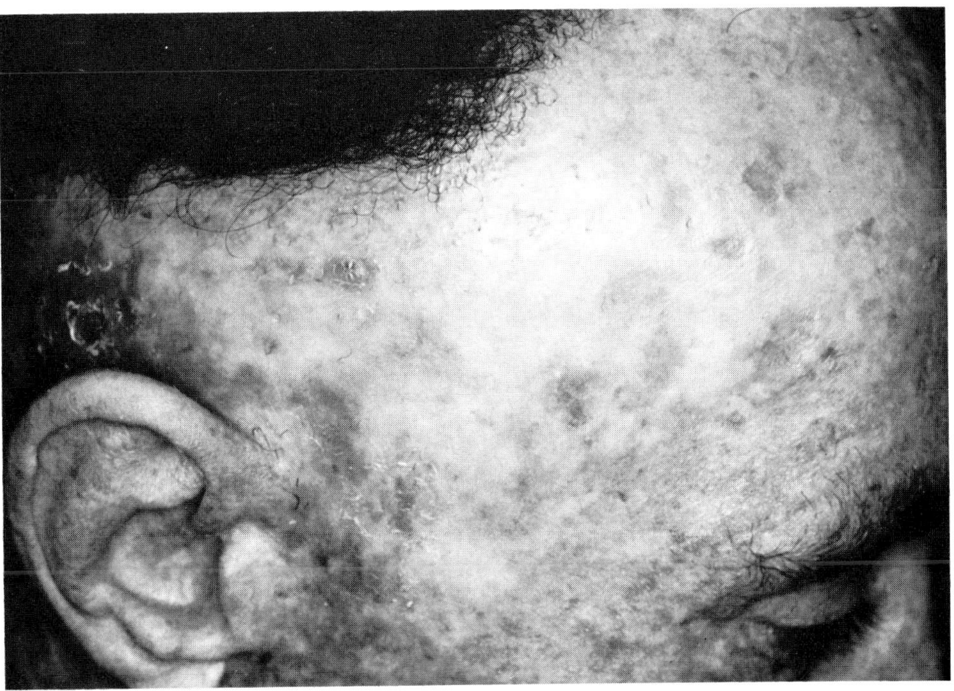

Figure 13–59. Porphyria cutanea tarda. Morphea and calcinosis cutis were present on face and scalp for 10 years before porphyria developed.

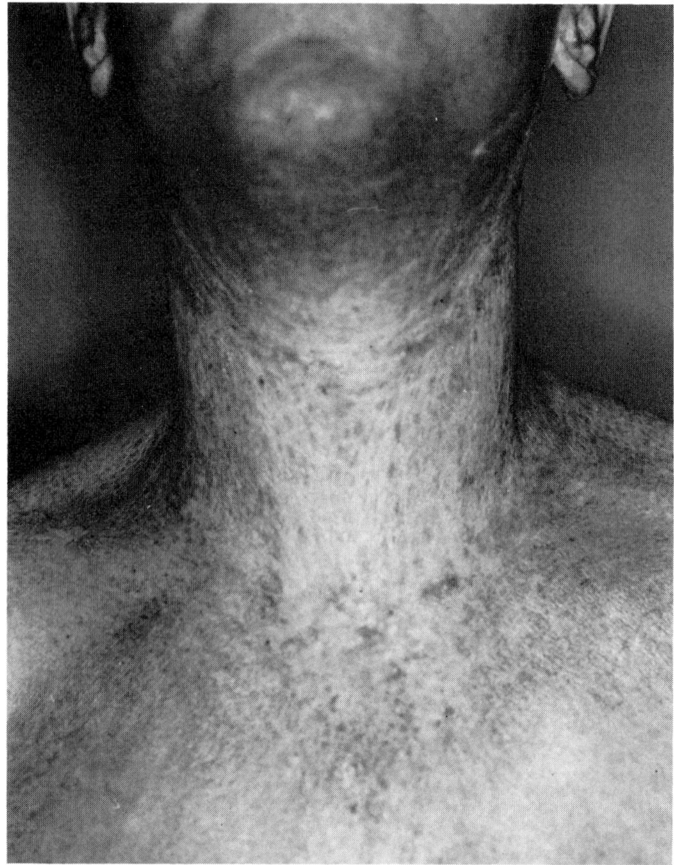

Figure 13–60. Porphyria cutanea tarda. Morphea on neck and chest. Same patient as in Figure 13–59.

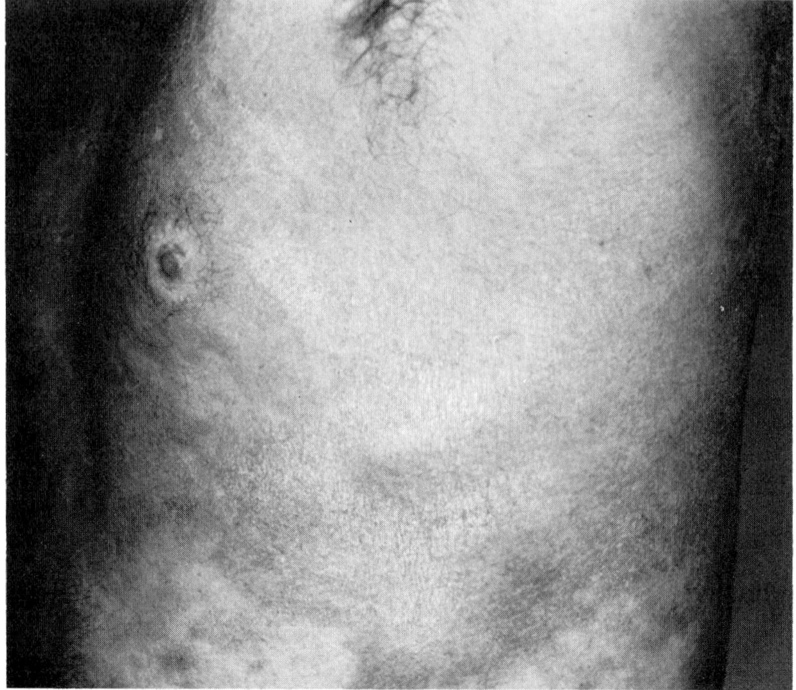

Figure 13–61. Porphyria cutanea tarda. Morphea on trunk. Same patient as in Figure 13–60.

porphyrins which are specifically diagnostic for the disorder: type III uroporphyrin and its 7-carboxyl porphyrin derivative, type I uroporphyrin, type III isocoproporphyrins, and type III coproporphyrin. This complex pattern can be explained by the single enzyme deficiency found in the disease.[187] The urine contains increased amounts of uroporphyrins and their 7-carboxyl derivatives, and lesser amounts of coproporphyrin. Fecal analyses show primarily isocoproporphyrins, coproporphyrins, and 7-carboxyl derivatives of type III uroporphyrin. There is a normal urinary excretion of ALA and PBG.

The genetic form of the disease exhibits a deficiency of uroporphyrinogen decarboxylase in both the liver and erythrocytes, while in the sporadic form, only the liver enzymatic system appears to be affected. The fibroblastic and erythrocytic systems have been shown to be normal.[190] The genetic form of the disease exists in overt, subclinical, and latent forms. The overt phase displays clinical disease accompanied by excessive urinary excretion of uroporphyrins; the subclinical stage, excessive uroporphyrinuria without clinical disease; and the latent form, decreased uroporphyrinogen decarboxylase activity in red cells without clinical or urinary abnormalities.[189] The enzymatic defect alone is not sufficient to produce clinical disease.

Increased body stores of iron and hepatic siderosis are found in most patients with porphyria cutanea tarda.[189] Iron overload is considered to be a major pathogenetic factor in porphyria cutanea tarda because of the clinical benefits of treatment by phlebotomy. Currently, it is believed that both the enzymatic defect and stimuli that produce hepatic siderosis are necessary to produce clinical disease, and if the stimuli are eliminated or controlled the disease will enter remission or be more easily controlled.[189] The cause of the isolated hepatic enzymatic deficiency in the sporadic form of the disease is not known. It remains deficient in postphlebotomy remission.[188, 190] If the sporadic form should also prove to be inherited, then the biochemistry and/or genetics must be more complicated than in the other forms of porphyria in which all the tissues tested have been shown to be affected.[178]

A variety of precipitating conditions are recognized. In adult men, alcoholism with or without hepatic siderosis or cirrhosis is a common association. An enhanced rate of intestinal iron absorption caused by these conditions has been postulated. Estrogen ingestion for treatment of prostatic carcinoma and for birth control measures is becoming a more frequent precipitating event. However, one woman in whom porphyria was induced by estrogens was able to complete a pregnancy without any recurrence of the disease.[183] The onset of porphyria cutanea tarda in a young woman should make one consider the possibility of estrogen-induced porphyria. Prolonged administration of iron will also induce the disease in susceptible individuals. The unintentional ingestion of seed treated with hexachlorobenzene, a fungicide, produced an epidemic of porphyria in Turkey.[193, 194] Although more than 3,000 persons were affected, suggesting that the disease was produced solely by a toxic mechanism, there may have been predisposing factors in some cases. Epidemiologic studies have shown that some of the family members who ingested the fungicide never became ill.[193] Industrial workers in the United States exposed to the manufacture of the fungicides 2,4D and 2,4,5-T, chlorinated hydrocarbons closely related to hexachlorobenzene have developed porphyria.[195] Hexachlorobenzene produces experimental porphyria cutanea tarda in rats. Hepatic uroporphyrinogen decarboxylase activity is decreased, but the enzymatic activity in the erythrocytes remains normal in this experimental model. The pattern of porphyrin excretion and porphyrin accumulation in the rat liver in the experimental disease is similar to that found in the human disease.[196, 197] Primary hepatic tumors such as benign hepatomas and hepatic carcinomas producing a variety of prophyrins have been associated with the syndrome of porphyria cutanea tarda. However, the porphyrin patterns have not been identical to those found in the naturally occurring disorder.[180, 198]

Identical appearing blistering syndromes without any evidence of porphyrin abnormalities have been produced by tetracycline in young women being treated for acne.[199] Nalidixic acid treatment for chronic urinary tract infection has been incriminated in five persons.[200] Patients with chronic renal disease treated by hemodialysis have developed a mechanicobullous eruption indistinguishable from porphyria cutanea tarda.[201, 202] It has been suggested that a photosensitizing agent of as-yet-undetermined type may have been leached out of the tubing to produce this syndrome.[203] Poh-Fitzpatrick et al. reported two patients on hemodialysis who did develop chemically proven porphyria cutanea tarda. They suggested that there may be chemical agents associated with hemodialysis that are capable of inducing hepatic porphyrin synthesis.[204] It is likely that there is a group of persons undergoing dialysis who are at risk of developing this bullous dermatosis of hemodialysis (Fig. 13–62) or true porphyria cutanea tarda. Keczkes and Fan reported four patients with chronic renal failure who developed an identical syndrome without hemodialysis.[205] However, all their patients were taking furosemide, and they concluded that the bullous eruption was a phototoxic reaction secondary to this drug. Therapy of psoriasis with 8-methoxypsoralen and

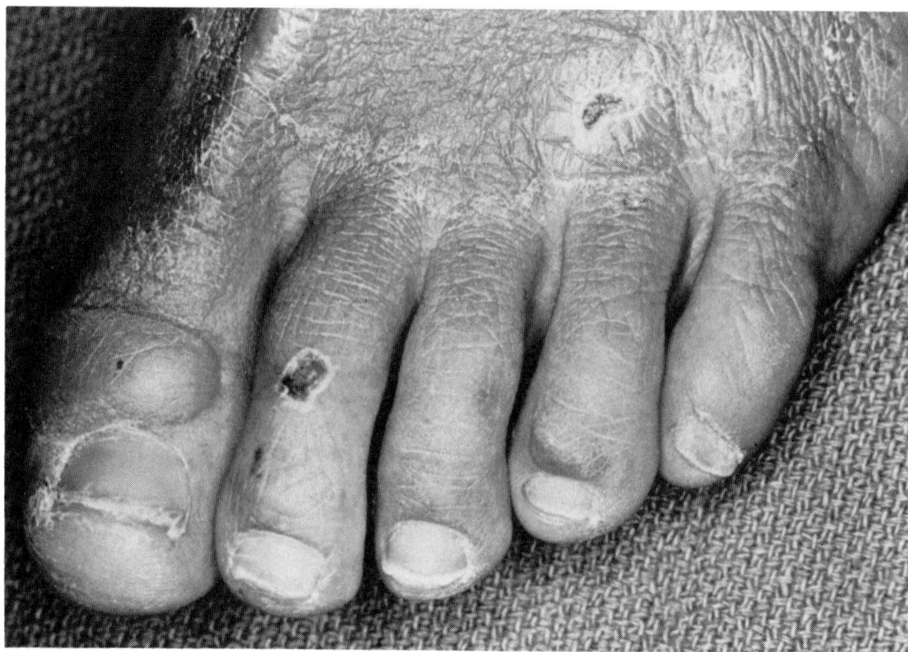

Figure 13–62. Bullous dermatosis associated with hemodialysis.

ultraviolet A (320 to 400 nm) may produce hirsutism and skin fragility identical to that found in porphyria cutanea tarda. Urinary porphyrin excretion has been normal in these individuals.[206]

Treatment of porphyria cutanea tarda by phlebotomy over the course of several weeks is followed by disappearance of the uroporphyrinuria. Several months later, the skin fragility, pigmentation, and hirsutism remits. Total remissions have persisted for at least four to six years.[207] The sclerodermoid changes also improve. Ippen observed that hypertrichosis in some female patients reappeared prior to the detection of renewed uroporphyrinuria heralding relapse. Blister formation and skin fragility reappeared three to six months following biochemical relapse in those patients who could not be appropriately followed.[207]

Phlebotomy is believed to be effective because it partially depletes the body stores of iron, which exerts both inhibitory and stimulatory effects on the enzymes involved in heme synthesis. Iron inhibits uroporphyrinogen decarboxylase but can stimulate ALA synthetase.[208, 209] However, the basic enzymatic deficiency persists in phlebotomy-induced remission.[188, 190]

The antimalarial drugs chloroquine and hydroxychloroquine are also effective in treating this form of porphyria. They cause the liver to release its stores of uroporphyrin.[210, 211] The dose of antimalarial used should be low; otherwise the patient may become violently ill with fever, malaise, leukocytosis, and severe abdominal pain and may suffer severe hepatic damage.[211] Prolonged remissions follow treatment with both high and low doses of antimalarials.[212]

Variegate porphyria and *hereditary coproporphyria* have three features in common: Mendelian dominant trait, cutaneous manifestations indistinguishable from those of porphyria cutanea tarda, and development of acute attacks identical to those of acute intermittent porphyria (Figs. 13–63 and 13–64). Variegate porphyria, however, is more prevalent than hereditary coproporphyria. The two disorders are biochemically distinct. In *variegate porphyria*, the liver produces excessive amounts of protoporphyrin and coproporphyrin, which are excreted in the stool. The amount of stool protoporphyrin is always greater than that of coproporphyrin. The urinary excretion of coproporphyrin is high and that of uroporphyrin only slightly elevated. Isocoproporphyrins are not present. During acute attacks, the levels of PBG and ALA are increased in the urine, but unlike most cases of acute intermittent porphyria, they return to normal or remain only slightly elevated after the acute episode has ended. The abnormal pattern of fecal porphyrin excretion is continuous, permitting the disorder to be diagnosed during periods of relative remission. There are a small number of patients in whom the fecal excretion of porphyrins is borderline or normal, and current methods cannot diagnose variegate porphyria in such patients.[213] An analogous situation has been found in a few patients with acute intermittent porphyria in whom the urinary excretion of porphyrin precursors is normal.[214]

By contrast, in *hereditary coproporphyria* the stool contains more coproporphyrin than protoporphyrin. The pattern of urinary porphyrin excretion in the acute and chronic stages is identical to that of variegate porphyria. The drugs that exacerbate acute intermittent porphyria are also contraindicated in variegate porphyria and hereditary coproporphyria.

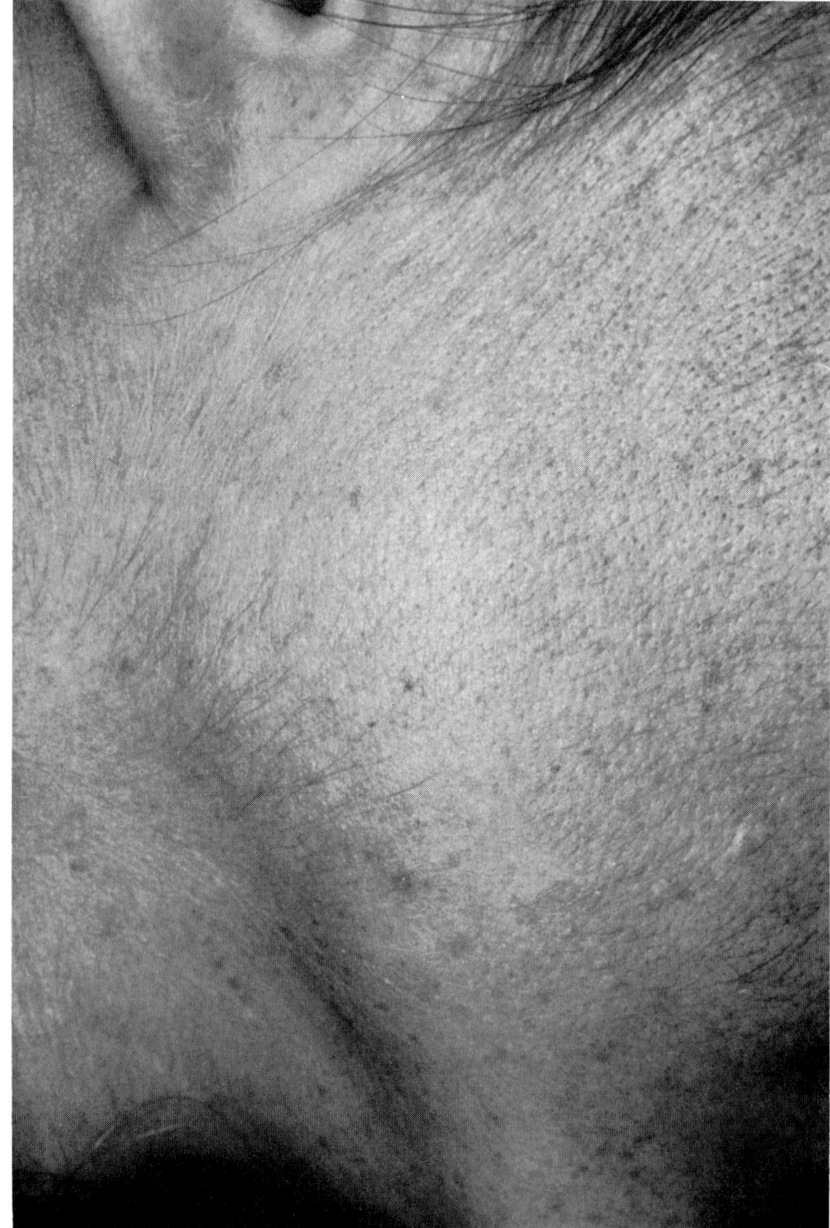

Figure 13–63. Variegate porphyria. Increased facial hair in affected woman is identical to that seen in porphyria cutanea tarda.

Estrogens in the form of birth control pills caused exacerbation of cutaneous lesions in two women with these disorders.[215, 216] However, the blisters arose on sun-exposed areas on the basis of true photosensitivity and not secondary to trauma. The basis for the flares was shown to be cholestatic jaundice caused by the estrogen. Presumably, this hepatic dysfunction produced a diversion from fecal to urinary excretion with resulting high porphyrin levels in the blood and skin predisposing the individuals to a photosensitivity reaction. The occasional worsening of skin manifestations during pregancy in variegate porphyria may have a similar pathogenesis.[217] One of the women with hereditary copropor-

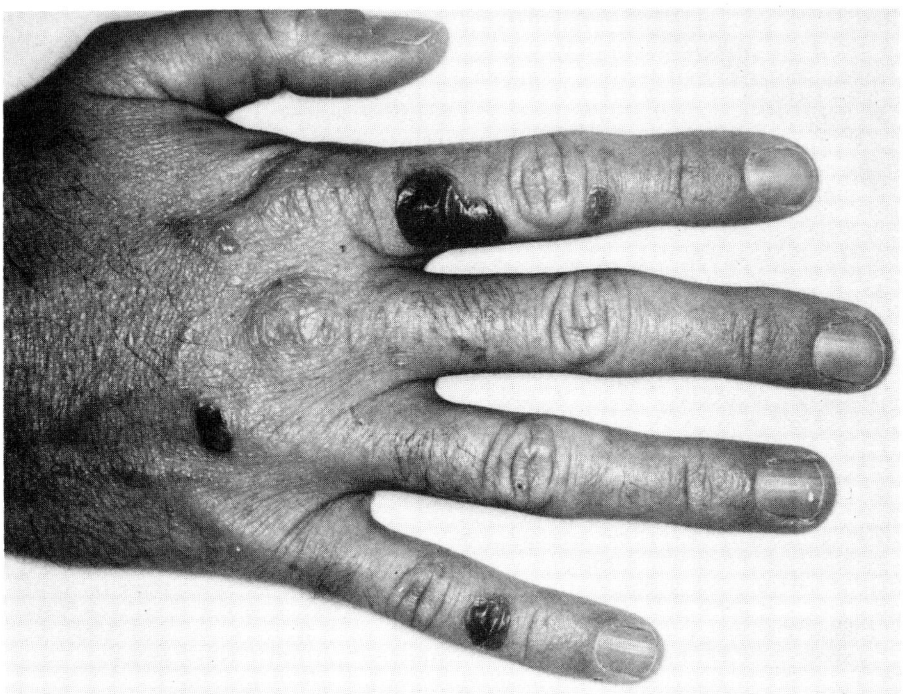

Figure 13–64. Variegate porphyria. Traumatically induced blisters on hands. Same patient as in Figure 13–63.

phyria cited above was later able to complete a pregnancy without any adverse effects on her skin or disease.[216]

The enzymatic defect in *hereditary coproporphyria* is a deficiency in coproporphyrinogen oxidase which allows for the accumulation and subsequent increased urinary and fecal excretion of coproporphyrin III. The enzymatic defect has been demonstrated in cultured skin fibroblasts and in blood lymphocytes. Hereditary coproporphyria remains clinically latent more often than acute intermittent porphyria.[178]

Until recently, studies to elucidate the enzymatic abnormality in *variegate porphyria* have been inconclusive. The accumulation of protoporphyrin suggested a block at the level of heme synthetase (ferrochetalase). Decreased activity of this enzyme was reported in leukocytes and normoblasts but not in muscle cell mitochondria.[213] However, heme synthetase is also deficient in *erythropoietic protoporphyria*. It was not clear how a partial block in the same enzyme could produce two different human porphyrias. Becker et al. suggested that the enzyme mutations in variegate porphyria and erythropoietic protoporphyria might be different: the enzyme in variegate porphyria might be stable but less active, and the molecule in erythropoietic protoporphyria, unstable.[218] However, the enzyme protoporphyrinogen oxidase, which catalyzes the oxidation of protoporphyrinogen to protoporphyrin, had also been proposed as the block, but direct measurements of this enzyme had not been made.[178, 213] In 1980, Brenner and Bloomer demonstrated that heme synthetase activity was normal in cultured fibroblasts from patients with variegate porphyria, and that the activity of protoporphyrinogen oxidase was reduced to 43 per cent of that in normal cells compatible with an autosomal dominant disorder in which there is a structural defect in the gene.[219] As a result of protoporphyrinogen oxidase deficiency, protoporphyrinogen may accumulate in the liver cells of patients with variegate porphyria and be excreted in the bile in excessive amounts. In the feces, it would be oxidized nonenzymatically to protoporphyrin.

Brenner and Bloomer made another important observation. Although the fibroblasts of these patients had decreased activity of protoporphyrinogen oxidase, they did not accumulate excess protoporphyrins under normal culture conditions or after supplementation with δ-aminolevulinic acid and iron. The fibroblasts did not duplicate the abnormality that is believed to be present in the liver cells of patients with this disease. Brenner and Bloomer suggested that the relative activities of the enzymes in the biosynthetic pathway of heme may vary in different tissues and that perhaps it is only in the liver that the deficiency of protoporphyrinogen oxidase activity reduces this step to a level at which protoporphyrinogen accumulates.

It is important to emphasize that the clinical syndrome of acute intermittent porphyria may be a manifestation of acute intermittent porphyria, variegate porphyria, or hereditary coproporphyria. Analysis of stool porphyrins will discriminate among the three. Fecal protoporphyrin and coproporphyrin are not increased in acute intermittent porphyria.

Erythropoietic protoporphyria is dominantly transmitted. Most cases appear before the age of five years, when the individual has his first significant exposure to sunlight. In a few patients, the disease began between 8 to 21 years of age.[220-222] Within a few minutes of exposure to sunlight, the person usually develops mild erythema accompanied by sensations of stinging, burning, or itching. With continued exposure the erythema increases and edema develops, sometimes giving rise to vesicles but more often producing superficial necrosis with crusting. These manifestations have been incorrectly called solar urticaria and solar eczema. Petechiae and purpura may appear in the edematous areas (Figs. 13–65 and 13–66). Repeated attacks produce wrinkled skin around the eyes, radial grooves simulating rhagades around the mouth, and shallow pitted scars on the cheeks, nose, and dorsa of the hands. The skin may become thickened and coarse and develop a lichenoid or cobblestone appearance over the surface (Figs. 13–67 and 13–68). Rarely, some patients have reported increased fragility of the skin in response to minor trauma. Phototoxic reactions involving the nails may also occur. Pain and tenderness under the nailplate are accompanied by separation of the nailplate from the nailbed (onycholysis).

Infants and young children too young to be aware of the nature of their photosensitivity and unable to communicate will cry when they are out in the sun or will rub the affected areas. Because the complaints of stinging and burning at times seem to be out of proportion to the observed erythema, some affected individuals have been erroneously diagnosed as neurotic. Individual tolerance to sunlight exposure varies from a few minutes to several hours. The signs and symptoms of erythropoietic protoporphyria can develop indoors at the window because glass will transmit the 400 to 410 nm wave band to which these patients are sensitive.[223]

Erythropoietic protoporphyria has been considered to be a relatively benign disease. Mild iron deficiency anemia is present in most patients. Hemolytic anemia developed in an exceptional case and improved after

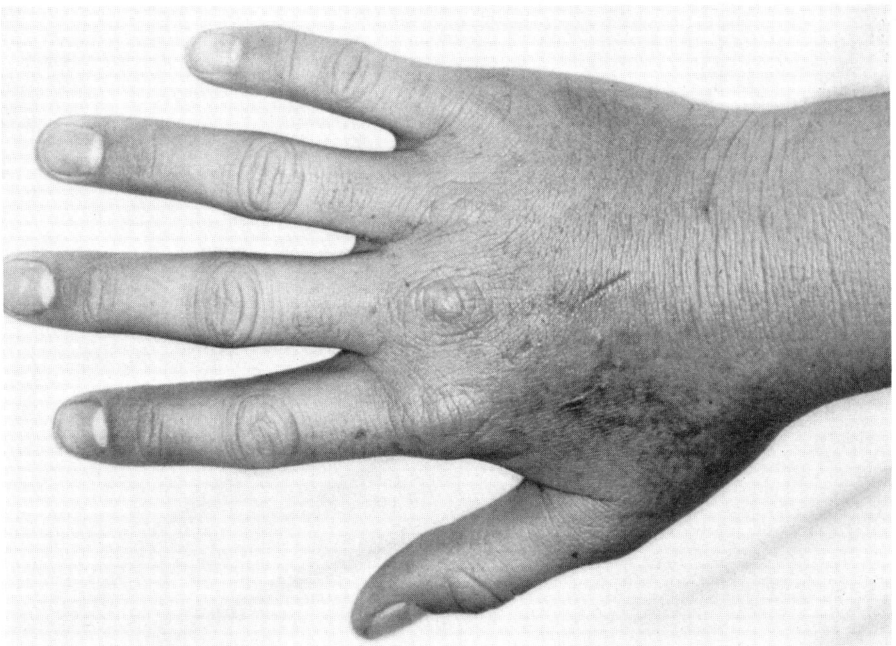

Figure 13–65. Erythropoietic protoporphyria. Purpura developed in areas of erythema and edema provoked by sun exposure in this patient.

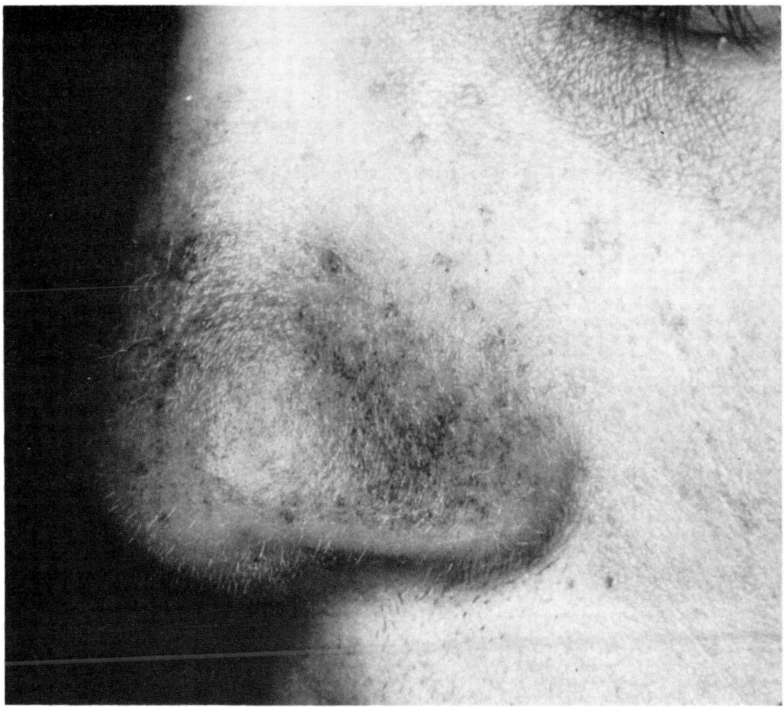

Figure 13–66. Erythropoietic protoporphyria. Same patient as in Figure 13–65. Purpura also developed in nasal lesions.

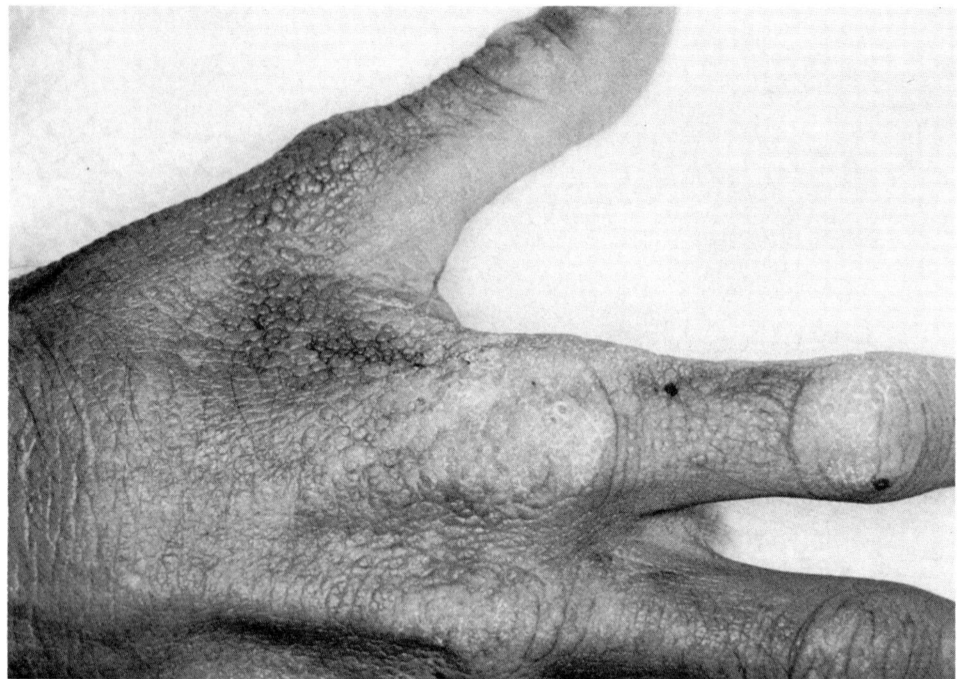

Figure 13–67. Erythropoietic protoporphyria. Skin may be coarse and thick with lichenoid or cobblestone appearance in longstanding cases.

splenectomy.[224] There is an increased prevalence of cholelithiasis because of stones composed primarily of protoporphyrin. However, cirrhosis secondary to marked deposition of protoporphyrin, producing death from hepatic failure within three months after the development of jaundice, has been reported in 15 cases thus far.[225] This complication has occurred in about 5 per cent of reported cases of erythropoietic protoporphyria.[225, 226] However, liver disease without this fatal outcome occurs in a higher but as-yet-undetermined percentage. The protoporphyrin, deposited in crystalline form in the liver, is believed to provoke inflammation and subsequent fibrosis of the hepatic tissues.[225]

The genetic defect has been shown to be decreased activity of ferrochetalase (heme synthetase) which catalyzes the insertion of ferrous iron into protoporphyrin to form heme.[178] The resulting accumulation of protoporphyrin in the reticulocytes leaks into the plasma as these cells mature into erythrocytes. The plasma protoporphyrin is cleared by the liver, with some being excreted into the bile and stool and the rest being deposited in the liver. Although the primary site of protoporphyrin overproduction is in the bone marrow, the liver probably contributes a variable fraction.[227] Although the excessive protoporphyrin accumulation is due principally to deficient heme synthetase activity, it may be modified by the rate of ALA formation in heme-producing tissues and by the availability of iron.[228]

The diagnosis can be made by detecting elevated levels of protoporphyrin in erythrocytes. The red cells also fluoresce orange-red under ultraviolet light but only transiently, in contrast to erythropoietic porphyria, in which the fluorescence is stable. The excretion of urinary porphyrins is normal.

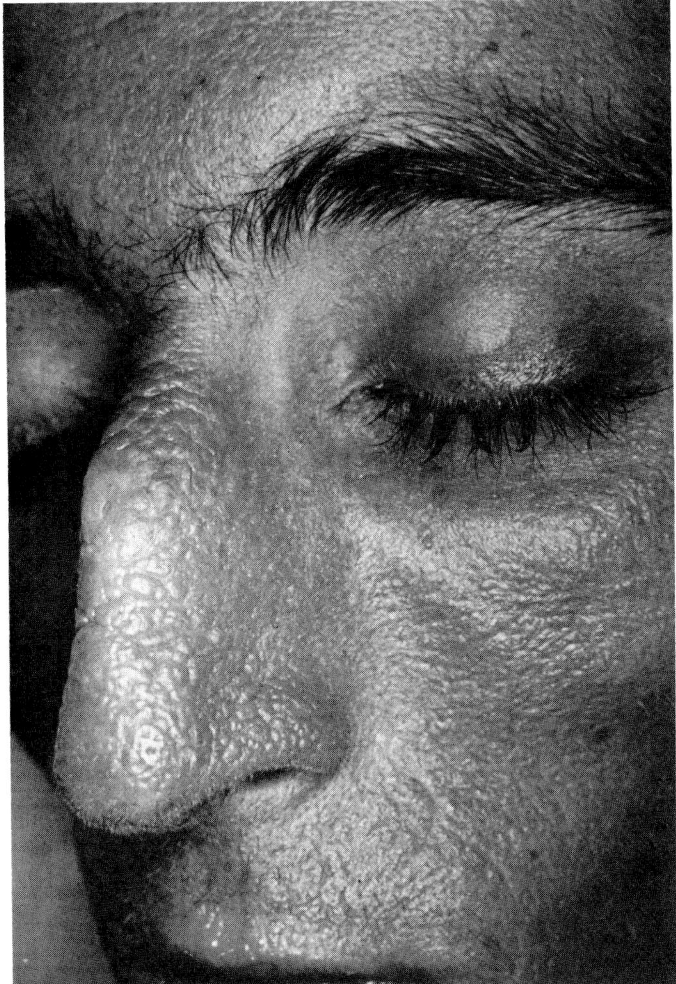

Figure 13–68. Erythropoietic protoporphyria. Same patient as in Figure 13–67. Changes on face identical to those on hands. He also was jaundiced and had severe cirrhosis.

Polymorphous light eruption, solar urticaria, and airborne contact dermatitis can be readily differentiated from erythropoietic protoporphyria on the basis of age of onset, biopsy findings, and laboratory tests. Hydroa aestivale (hydroa vacciniforme) is a rare blistering photodermatosis that forms crusts and eventual varioliform scarring in the same distribution pattern as erythropoietic protoporphyria (Figs. 13–69 and 13–70). Some of these cases were undoubtedly examples of porphyria, but studies have indicated that this photodermatosis does exist as a clinical entity in the absence of detectable porphyrin abnormalities.[229, 230]

Oral beta-carotene has been used successfully to moderate the photosensitivity in erythropoietic protoporphyria. Patients have been able to increase their tolerance to sun exposure by at least threefold. The drug is believed to quench the photoexcited states of protoporphyrin, the singlet oxygen formation, and the free radicals produced by the action of 400 to 410 nm light on the increased levels of protoporphyrin in the skin and red blood cells. The photoexcited molecules, singlet oxygen, and free radicals, which are highly damaging to cells, are believed to be the basis

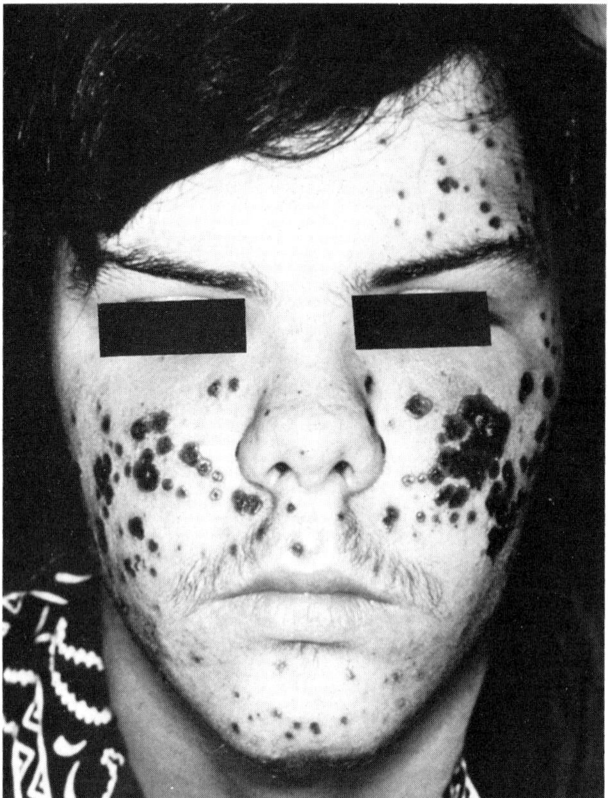

Figure 13–69. Hydroa aestivale. Photosensitivity reaction produces blisters with scarring that resembles smallpox and vaccinia.

for the signs and symptoms of the cutaneous photosensitivity in erythropoietic protoporphyria.[230]

The cirrhosis produced by the deposition of protoporphyrin in the liver was successfully treated by the use of oral cholestyramine, which interrupted the enterohepatic circulation of protoporphyrin and increased its excretion in the stool.[225] In one patient, splenectomy improved the cirrhosis, the severe hemolytic anemia, and the clinical photosensitivity.[224] The administration of iron improves the biochemical abnormality in these patients by allowing the protoporphyrin to be more fully utilized to form heme.[225] Iron is not an injurious agent in this form of porphyria as it is in porphyria cutanea tarda.

Congenital *erythropoietic coproporphyria* is an extremely rare dominantly transmitted disease that is analogous to erythropoietic protoporphyria. The signs and symptoms are similar but less immediate in their appearance after exposure to the sun. Only two patients have been described: a mother with the biochemical abnormality and her 22-year-old daughter with the clinical disorder. The photosensitivity began at age 10 years and was characterized by swelling and redness associated with itching and burning that occurred only after she had been exposed to the sun for a considerable period of time. In addition, the reaction did not occur until several hours after exposure to the sun was over. The face and eyelids were most severely involved and the skin healed without scarring. The red cells fluoresced under ultraviolet light and contained a hundred-

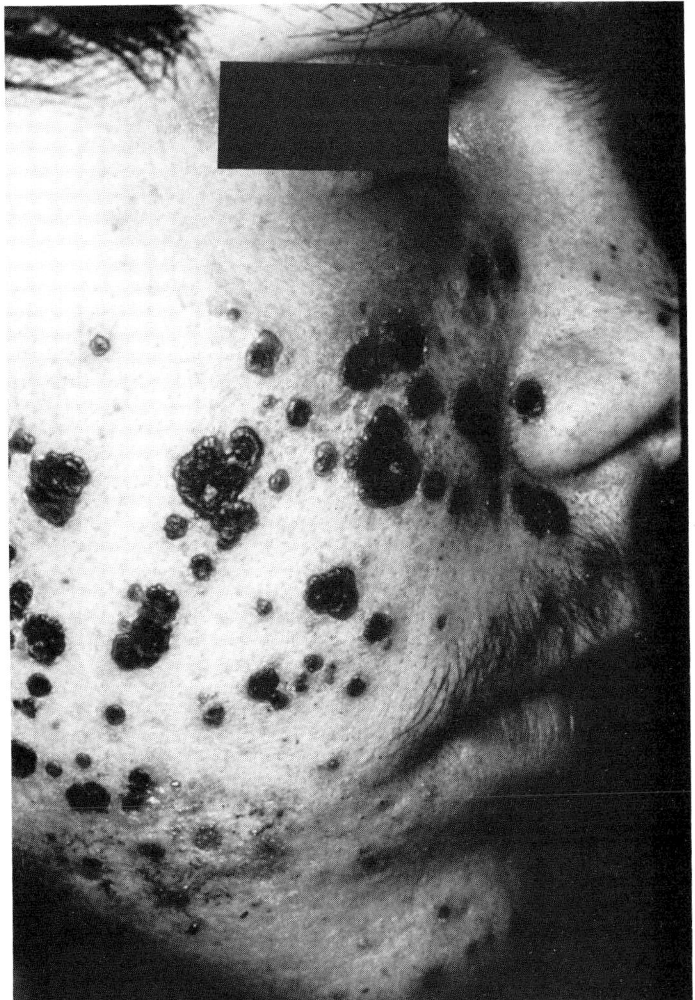

Figure 13–70. Hydroa aestivale. Close-up of lesions in Figure 13–69. Blisters are in healing phase.

Table 13–2. BIOCHEMICAL ABNORMALITIES IN THE PORPHYRIAS

Type*	Enzyme Deficiency	Red Cells†	Urine†	Feces
AIP	Uroporphyrinogen I synthetase	Normal	PBG, ALA	Normal
CEP	Uroporphyrinogen III Cosynthetase	Uro I, Copro I positive, stable fluorescence	Uro I > Copro I	Copro I > Uro I
PCT	Uroporphyrinogen decarboxylase	Normal	Uro III > Copro III	Isocopro III Copro III
HC	Coproporphyrinogen oxidase	Normal	Copro III > Uro III ALA, PBG	Copro III > Proto
VP	Protoporphyrinogen oxidase	Normal	Copro III ALA, PBG	Proto ⩾ Copro III
EPP	Ferrochetalase	Proto > Copro III positive, transient fluorescence	Normal	Proto > Copro III
		Copro III > Proto		
CEC	Unknown	Normal	Normal	

*AIP = acute intermittent porphyria.
CEP = congenital erythropoietic porphyria.
PCT = porphyria cutanea tarda.
HC = hereditary coproporphyria.
VP = variegate porphyria.
EPP = erythropoietic protoporphyria.
CEC = congenital erythropoietic coproporphyria.

†PBG = porphobilinogen.
Uro = uroporphyrin.
Copro = coproporphyrin.
Proto = protoporphyrin
ALA = δ-amino levulinic acid.
Isocopro = isocoproporphyrin.

fold increase in coproporphyrin, but only a two- to threefold increase in protoporphyrin.[231] In erythropoietic protoporphyria, the protoporphyrins are usually increased 10- to 100-fold.[219]

Levine et al. reported a unique observation: the coexistence of two types of porphyria in one family. The father had porphyria cutanea tarda and one of two daughters had erythropoietic protoporphyria. Neither parent nor the other daughter showed biochemical evidence of any porphyria. The paternal grandfather probably had porphyria cutanea tarda.[232]

The biochemical abnormalities of the porphyrias are summarized in Table 13–2

REFERENCES

1. Sarver, M. E., Sabeh, G., Fetterman, G. H., Wald, N., and Danowski, T. S.: Fractional hypopituitarism with giantism and normal sella turcica. N. Engl. J. Med., *271*:1286, 1964.
2. Randall, R. E., Jr., and Spong, F. W.: Calcification of the auricular cartilage in a patient with hypopituitarism. N. Engl. J. Med., *269*:1135, 1963.
3. Daughaday, W. H.: The adenohypophysis. *In* Williams, R. H. (ed.): Textbook of Endocrinology, 4th ed. W. B. Saunders Company, Philadelphia, 1968, p. 73.
4. Sheppard, R. H., and Meema, H. E.: Skin thickness in endocrine disease. A roentgenographic study. Ann. Intern. Med., *66*:531, 1963.
5. Pochi, P.: Personal communication.
6. Lerner, A. B.: Three unusual pigmentary syndromes. Arch. Dermatol., *83*:97, 1961.
7. McKenzie, J. M.: Humoral factors in the pathogenesis of Graves' disease. Physiol. Rev., *48*:252, 1968.
8. Zaidman, G. W., and Shapiro, H.: Ophthalmopathy and thyroid disorders. N. Engl. J. Med., *296*:1003, 1977.
9. Schermer, D. R., Roenigk, H. H., Jr., Schumacher, O. P., and McKenzie, J. M.: Relationship of long-acting thyroid stimulator to pretibial myxedema. Arch. Dermatol., *102*:62, 1970.
10. Volpé, R.: The role of autoimmunity in hypoendocrine and hyperendocrine function. Ann. Intern. Med., *87*:86, 1977.
11. Brown, J., Solomon, D. H., Beall, G. N.,

Terasaki, P. I., Chopra, I. J., Van Herle, A. J., and Wu, S.-Y.: Autoimmune thyroid diseases—Graves' and Hashimoto's. Ann. Intern. Med., *88*:379, 1978.

12. Howel-Evans, A. W., Woodrow, J. C., McDougall, C. D. M., Chew, A. R., and Evans, R. W.: Antibodies in the families of thyrotoxic patients. Lancet, *1*:636, 1967.
13. Hochstein, M. A., Nair, V., and Nevins, M.: Hypothyroidism followed by hyperthyroidism. Occurrence in a patient with elevated antithyroid antibody titer. J.A.M.A., *237*:2222, 1977.
14. Adams, D. D., and Kennedy, T. H.: Evidence to suggest that LATS protector stimulates the human thyroid gland. J. Clin. Endocrinol. Metab., *33*:47, 1971.
15. Onaya, T., Kotani, M., Yamada, T., and Ochi, Y.: New in vitro tests to detect the thyroid stimulator in sera from hyperthyroid patients by measuring colloid droplet formation and cyclic AMP in human thyroid slices. J. Clin. Endocrinol. Metab., *36*:859, 1973.
16. Hall, R., and Stanbury, J. B.: Familial studies of autoimmune thyroiditis. Clin. Exp. Immunol., *2*:719, 1967.
17. Roitt, I. M., and Doniach, D.: A reassessment of studies on the aggregation of thyroid autoimmunity in families of thyroiditis patients. Clin. Exp. Immunol., *2*:727, 1967.
18. Readett, M. D.: Constitutional eczema and thyroid disease. Br. J. Dermatol., *76*:126, 1964.
19. Barrow, M. V., and Bird, E. D.: Pruritus in hyperthyroidism. Arch. Dermatol., *93*:237, 1966.
20. Lynch, P. J., Maize, J. C., and Sisson, J. C.: Pretibial myxedema and nonthyrotoxic thyroid disease. Arch. Dermatol., *107*:107, 1973.
21. Malkinson, F. D.: Hyperthyroidism, pretibial myxedema and clubbing. Arch. Dermatol., *88*:303, 1963.
22. Sisson, J. C.: Hyaluronic acid in localized myxedema. J. Clin. Endocrinol. Metab., *28*:433, 1968.
23. Siegler, M., and Refetoff, S.: Pretibial myxedema — a reversible cause of foot drop due to entrapment of the peroneal nerve. N. Engl. J. Med., *294*:1383, 1976.
24. Rotchford, J. P.: Pretibial myxedema with graft site involvement. Arch. Dermatol., *106*:255, 1972.
25. Cheung, H. S., Nicoloff, J. T., Kamiel, M. B., Spolter, L., and Nimni, M. E.: Stimulation of fibroblast biosynthetic activity by serum of patients with pretibial myxedema. J. Invest. Dermatol., *71*:12, 1978.
26. Freinkel, R. K., and Freinkel, N.: Hair growth and alopecia in hypothyroidism. Arch. Dermatol., *106*:349, 1972.
27. Craig, L. S., Lisser, H., and Soley, M. H.: Report of two cases of myxedema with extreme hypercholesterolemia; one complicated by xanthoma tuberosum. J. Clin. Endocrinol., *4*:12, 1944.
28. Christianson, H. B.: Cutaneous manifestations of hypothyroidism including purpura and ecchymoses. Cutis, *17*:45, 1976.
29. Bland, J. H., and Frymoyer, J. W.: Rheumatic syndromes of myxedema. N. Engl. J. Med., *282*:1171, 1970.
30. Deiss, W. P., Jr.: Diseases of the parathyroid glands. Resident Physician, *13*:55, 1967.
31. Lafferty, F. W.: Pseudohyperparathyroidism. Medicine (Balt.), *45*:247, 1966.
32. Hällgren, R., Wibell, L., Ejerblad, S., Eriksson, I., Johansson, H., Grimelius, L., and Wilander, E.: Arterial calcification and progressive peripheral gangrene after renal transplantation. Acta. Med. Scand., *198*:331, 1975.
33. Winkelmann, R. K., and Keating, F. R., Jr.: Cutaneous vascular calcification, gangrene and hyperparathyroidism. Br. J. Dermatol., *83*:263, 1970.
34. Hampers, C. L., Katz, A. I., Wilson, R. E., and Merrill, J. P.: Disappearance of "uremic" itching after subtotal parathyroidectomy. N. Engl. J. Med., *279*:695, 1968.
35. Massry, S. G., Popovtzer, M. M., Coburn, J. W., Markoff, D. L., Maxwell, M. H., and Kleeman, C. R.: Intractable pruritus as a manifestation of secondary hyperparathyroidism in uremia. N. Engl. J. Med., *279*:697, 1968.
36. Lachmann, A.: Hypoparathyroidism in Denmark. A clinical study. Acta Med. Scand., Suppl. *121*, 1941.
37. Dent, C. E., and Garretts, M.: Skin changes in hypocalcemia. Lancet, *1*:142, 1960.
38. Hvidberg, E.: Impetigo herpetiformis. Dermatologica, *114*:337, 1957.
39. Beek, C. H.: On impetigo herpetiformis. Dermatologica, *102*:145, 1951.
40. Katzenellenbogen, I., and Feuerman, E. J.: Psoriasis pustulosa and impetigo herpetiformis — single or dual entity. Acta Dermat. Venereol., *46*:86, 1966.
41. Forbes, G. B.: Clinical features of idiopathic hypoparathyroidism in children. Ann. N. Y. Acad. Sci., *64*:432, 1956.
42. Steinberg, H., and Waldron, B. R.: Idiopathic hypoparathyroidism: an analysis of 52 cases including the report of a new case. Medicine (Balt.), *31*:133, 1952.
43. Hirano, K., Ishibashi, A., and Yoshino, Y.: Cutaneous manifestations in idiopathic hypoparathyroidism. Arch. Dermatol., *109*:242, 1974.
44. Waisman, M., and O'Regan, S.: Maculopapular eruption in hypoparathyroidism. Arch. Dermatol., *112*:991, 1976.
45. Harrell-Steinberg, A., Ziprkowski, L., Haim, S., Gasni, J., and Levin, M.: Observations on hypoparathyroidism. I. Exfoliative dermatitis as the presenting sign of hypoparathyroidism. J. Clin. Endocrinol. Metab., *17*:1094, 1957.
46. Case Records of the Massachusetts General Hospital (Case 40361). N. Engl. J. Med., *251*:442, 1954.
47. Sutphin, A., Albright F., and McCune, D. J.: Five cases (three in siblings) of idio-

pathic hypoparathyroidism associated with moniliasis. J. Clin. Endocrinol., *3*:625, 1943.

48. Fields, J. P., Fragola, L., and Hadley, T. P.: Hypoparathyroidism, candidiasis, alopecia, and vitiligo. Arch. Dermatol., *103*:687, 1971.
49. Freinkel, R. K., and Ashman, M. S.: Chronic mucocutaneous candidiasis, vitiligo, polyendocrinopathy, pernicious anemia: subacute combined degeneration of the spinal cord. Arch. Dermatol., *113*:693, 1977.
50. Simpson, J. A.: Dermatological changes in hypocalcemia. Br. J. Dermatol., *66*:1, 1954.
51. Kenny, F. M., and Holliday, M. A.: Hypoparathyroidism, moniliasis, Addison's and Hashimoto's diseases. N. Engl. J. Med., *271*:708, 1964.
52. Hung, W., Migeon, C. J., and Parrott, R. H.: A possible autoimmune basis for Addison's disease in three siblings, one with idiopathic hypoparathyroidism, pernicious anemia and superficial moniliasis. N. Engl. J. Med., *269*:658, 1963.
53. McGregor, B. C., Katz, H. I., and Doe, R. P.: Vitiligo and multiple glandular insufficiencies. J.A.M.A., *219*:724, 1972.
54. Albright, F., Burnett, C. H., Smith, P. H., and Parson, W.: Pseudohypoparathyroidism — an example of "Seabright-Bantam syndrome." Endocrinology, *30*:922, 1942.
55. Bronsky, D., Kushner, D. S., Dubin, A., and Snapper, I.: Idiopathic hypoparathyroidism and pseudohypoparathyroidism: case reports and review of the literature. Medicine (Balt.), *37*:317, 1958.
56. Lee, J. B., Tashjian, A. H., Streeto, J. M., and Frantz, A. G.: Familial pseudo-hypoparathyroidism. N. Engl. J. Med., *279*: 1179, 1968.
57. Miles, J., and Elrick, H.: Pseudo- and Frantz, A. G.: Familial pseudohypoparathyroidism. N. Engl. J. Med., *279*: 1179, 1968.
58. Hermans, P. E., Gorman, C. A., Martin, W. J., and Kelly, P. J.: Pseudo-pseudohypoparathyroidism (Albright's hereditary osteodystrophy): a family study. Mayo Clin. Proc., *39*:81, 1964.
59. Forsham, P. H.: The adrenal cortex. *In* Williams, R. H. (ed.): Textbook of Endocrinology, 4th ed. W. B. Saunders Company, Philadelphia, 1968, p. 324.
60. Orth, D. N., and Liddle, G. W.: Results of treatment in 108 patients with Cushing's syndrome. N. Engl. J. Med., *285*:243, 1971.
61. Rovit, R. L., and Duane, T. D.: Cushing's syndrome and pituitary tumors. Pathophysiology and ocular manifestations of ACTH-secreting pituitary adenomas. Am. J. Med., *46*:416, 1969.
62. Krieger, D. T.: Neurotransmitter regulation of ACTH release. Mt. Sinai J. Med. N.Y., *40*:302, 1973.
63. Krieger, D. T., Amorosa, L., and Linick, F.: Cyproheptadine-induced remission of Cushing's disease. N. Engl. J. Med., *293*:893, 1975.
64. Krieger, D. T.: Cyproheptadine for pituitary disorders. N. Engl. J. Med., *295*:394, 1976.
65. Simkin, B., Pamsk, J. F., Palmer, W. S., and Cohen, S.: Cushing's syndrome associated with basophilic carcinoma of the pituitary. Ann. Intern. Med., *56*:495, 1962.
66. Nelson, D. H., Meakin, J. W., and Thorn, G. W.: ACTH-producing pituitary tumors following adrenalectomy for Cushing's syndrome. Arch. Intern. Med., *52*:560, 1960.
67. Ross, E. J., Marshall-Jones, P., and Friedman, M.: Cushing's syndrome: diagnostic criteria. Q. J. Med., *35*:149, 1966.
68. Lucena, G. E., Bennett, W. M., and Pierre, R. V.: "Dewlap." A corticosteroid-induced episternal fatty tumor. N. Engl. J. Med., *275*:834, 1966.
69. Santini, L. C., and Williams, J. L.: Mediastinal widening (presumable lipomatosis) in Cushing's syndrome. N. Engl. J. Med., *284*:1357, 1971.
70. Chernosky, M. E., and Knox, J. M.: Atrophic striae after occlusive corticosteroid therapy. Arch. Dermatol., *90*:15, 1964.
71. Winer, L. H., Kling, D. H., and Levin, G. H.: Ecchymosis in arthritis patients on prolonged corticosteroids. Arch. Dermatol., *86*:654, 1962.
72. Boardman, C. R., and Malkinson, F. D.: Tinea versicolor in steroid-treated patients. Arch. Dermatol., *85*:44, 1962.
73. Burke, R. C.: Tinea versicolor: susceptibility factors and experimental infection in human beings. J. Invest. Dermatol., *36*:389, 1961.
74. Brooks, V. E. H., and Richards, R.: Depigmentation in Cushing's syndrome. Arch. Intern. Med., *117*:677, 1966.
75. Stempfel, R. S., Jr., and Tompkins, G. M.: Congenital virilizing adrenocortical hyperplasia (the adrenogenital syndrome). *In* Stanbury, J. B., Wyngaarden, J. B., and Fredrickson, D. S. (eds.): The Metabolic Basis of Inherited Disease, 2nd ed. McGraw-Hill Book Co., New York, 1966, p. 635.
76. Allen, G. E.: Diabetes mellitus and the skin. Practioner, *203*:189, 1969.
77. Thornton, G. F.: Infections and diabetes. Med. Clin. North Am., *55*:931, 1971.
78. Sandler, R., Tallman, C. B., Kearny, D. G., and Irving, W. R.: Successfully treated rhinocerebral phycomycosis in well controlled diabetes. N. Engl. J. Med., *285*:1180, 1971.
79. Kramer, B. S., Hernandez, A. D., Reddick, R. L., and Levine, A. S.: Cutaneous infarction. Manifestation of disseminated mucormycosis. Arch. Dermatol., *113*:1075, 1977.
80. Williams, R. H.: The pancreas. *In* Williams,

R. H. (ed.): Textbook of Endocrinology, 4th ed. W. B. Saunders Company, Philadelphia, 1968, 781.
81. Mosenthal, H. O., and Loughlin, W. C.: Plasma vitamin A and carotene in diabetes mellitus. J. Mount Sinai Hosp. N. Y., *12*:523, 1945.
82. Bloodworth, J. M. B.: Diabetic microangiopathy. Diabetes, *12*:99, 1963.
83. Dolmam, C. L.: The morbid anatomy of diabetic neuropathy. Neurology, *13*:135, 1963.
84. LeCompte, P. M.: Vascular lesions in diabetes mellitus. J. Chron. Dis., *2*:178, 1955.
85. Bloodworth, J. M. B., Jr., and Molitor, D. L.: Ultrastructural aspects of human and canine diabetic retinopathy. Invest. Ophthalmol., *4*:1037, 1965.
86. Siperstein, M. D., Raskin, P., and Burns, H.: Electron microscopic quantification of diabetic microangiopathy. Diabetes, *22*:514, 1973.
87. Bauer, M. F., Hirsch, P., Bullock, W. K., and Abul-Haj, S. K.: Necrobiosis lipoidica diabeticorum. Arch. Dermatol., *90*:558, 1964.
88. Graham, J. H., Marques, A. S., Johnson, W. C., and Gray, H. R.: Stasis dermatitis. *In* Graham, J. H., Johnson, W. C., and Helwig, E. B.: Dermal Pathology. Harper and Row, Hagerstown, Md., 1972, p. 352.
89. Muller, S. A., and Winkelmann, R. K.: Necrobiosis lipoidica diabeticorum. A clinical and pathologic investigation of 171 cases. Arch. Dermatol., *93*:272, 1966.
90. Rollins, T. G., and Winkelmann, R. K.: Necrobiosis lipoidica granulomatosis. Necrobiosis lipoidica in the non-diabetic. Arch. Dermatol., *82*:537, 1960.
91. Gray, H. R., Graham, J. H., and Johnson, W. C.: Necrobiosis lipoidica, necrobiosis lipoidica diabeticorum, and granuloma annulare. *In* Dermal Pathology, *op. cit.*, p. 417.
92. Ullman, S., and Dahl, M. V.: Necrobiosis lipoidica. An immunofluorescence study. Arch. Dermatol., *113*:161, 1977.
93. Mustard, J. F., and Packham, M. A.: Platelets and diabetes mellitus. N. Engl. J. Med., *297*:1345, 1977.
94. Eldor, A., Diaz, E. G., and Naparstek, E.: Treatment of diabetic necrobiosis with aspirin and dipyridamole. N. Engl. J. Med., *298*:1033, 1978.
95. Melin, H.: An atrophic circumscribed skin lesion in the lower extremities of diabetics. Acta Med. Scand., *176*, Suppl. 423, 1964.
96. Binkley, G. W.: Dermopathy in the diabetic syndrome. Arch. Dermatol., *92*:625, 1965.
97. Danowski, T. S., Sabeh, G., Sarver, M. E., Shelkrot, J., and Fisher, E. R.: Shin spots and diabetes mellitus. Am. J. Med. Sci., *251*:570, 1966.
98. Fisher, E. R., and Danowski, T. S.: Histologic, histochemical and electron microscopic features of the shin spots of diabetes mellitus. Am. J. Clin. Pathol., *50*:547, 1968.
99. Smith, J. G., Jr., Sams, W. M., Jr., and Finlayson, G. R.: Biochemistry and pathology of cutaneous elastic tissue. *In* MacKenna, R. M. B. (ed.): Mod rn Trends in Dermatology, vol. 3. Butterworths, London, 1966, p. 110.
100. Yen, A., and Braverman, I. M.: Ultrastructure of the human dermal microcirculation: the horizontal plexus of the papillary dermis. J. Invest. Dermatol., *66*:131, 1976.
101. Braverman, I. M., and Yen, A.: Ultrastructure of the human dermal microcirculation. II. The capillary loops of the dermal papillae. J. Invest. Dermatol., *68*:44, 1977.
102. Taranta, A.: Occurrence of rheumatic-like subcutaneous nodules without evidence of joint or heart disease. N. Engl. J. Med., *266*:13, 1962.
103. Romaine, R., Rudner, E. J., and Altman, J.: Papular granuloma annulare and diabetes mellitus. Arch. Dermatol., *98*:152, 1968.
104. Dicken, C. H., Carrington, S. G., and Winkelmann, R. K.: Generalized granuloma annulare. Arch. Dermatol., *99*:556, 1969.
105. Haim, S., Friedman-Birnbaum, R., and Shafrir, A.: Generalized granuloma annulare: relationship to diabetes mellitus as revealed in 8 cases. Br. J. Dermatol., *83*:302, 1970.
106. Dahl, M. V., Ullman, S., and Goltz, R. W.: Vasculitis in granuloma annulare. Histopathology and direct immunofluorescence. Arch. Dermatol., *113*:463, 1977.
107. Umbert, P., and Winkelmann, R. K.: Histologic, ultrastructural, and histochemical studies of granuloma annulare. Arch. Dermatol., *113*:168, 1977.
108. Dawber, R. P. R.: Vitiligo in mature-onset diabetes mellitus. Br. J. Dermatol., *80*:275, 1968.
109. Lerner, A. B.: Vitiligo. J. Invest. Dermatol., *32*:285, 1959.
110. Macaron, C., Winter, R. J., Traisman, H. S., Kahan, B. S., Lasser, A. E., and Green, O. C.: Vitiligo and juvenile diabetes mellitus. Arch. Dermatol., *113*:1515, 1977.
111. Rocca, R. P., and Pereyra, E.: Phlyctenar lesions in the feet of diabetic patients. Diabetes, *12*:220, 1963.
112. Cantwell, A. R., and Martz, W.: Idiopathic bullae in diabetics. Bullosis diabeticorum. Arch. Dermatol., *96*:42, 1967.
113. Allen, G. E., and Hadden, D. R.: Bullous lesions of the skin in diabetes. Br. J. Dermatol., *82*:216, 1970.
114. Kurwa, A., Roberts, P., and Whitehead, R.: Concurrence of bullous and atrophic skin lesions in diabetes mellitus. Arch. Dermatol., *103*:670, 1971.
115. Bernstein, J. E., Mendenica, M., Soltani, K., and Griem, S. F.: Bullous eruption of diabetes mellitus. Arch. Dermatol., *115*:324, 1979.

116. Senior, B., and Gellis, S. S.: The syndromes of total lipodystrophy and of partial lipodystrophy. Pediatrics, *33*:593, 1964.
117. Gordon, H., Pimstone, B. L., Keary, P. M., and Gordon, W.: Congenital generalized lipodystrophy with abnormal growth hormone homeostasis. Arch. Dermatol., *104*:551, 1971.
118. Reed, W. B., Ragsdale, W., Jr., Curtis, A. C., and Richards, H. J.: Acanthosis nigricans in association with various genodermatoses. Acta Derm-venereol., *48*:465, 1968.
119. Corbin, A., Upton, G. V., Mabry, C. L., and Hollingsworth, D. R.: Diencephalic involvement in generalized lipodystrophy: Rationale and treatment with the neuroleptic agent pimozide. Acta Endocrinol., *77*:209, 1974.
120. Frohman, L. A.: The hypothalamus and metabolic control. Pathobiol. Annu., *1*:353, 1971.
121. Upton, G. V., and Corbin, A.: Hypothesis: hypothalamic dysfunction and lipoatrophic diabetes. Yale J. Biol. Med., *46*:314, 1973.
122. Eisinger, A. J., Shortland, J. R., and Moorehead, P. J.: Renal disease in partial lipodystrophy. Q. J. Med., *41*:343, 1972.
123. Poley, J. R., and Stickler, G. B.: Progressive lipodystrophy. A clinical study of 50 patients. Am. J. Dis. Child., *106*:356, 1963.
124. West, R. J., Fosbrooke, A. S., and Lloyd, J. K.: Metabolic studies and autonomic function in children with partial lipodystrophy. Arch. Dis. Child., *49*:627, 1974.
125. Sissons, J. G. P., West, R. J., Fallows, J., Williams, D. G., Boucher, B. J., Amos, N., and Peters, D. K.: The complement abnormalities of lipodystrophy. N. Engl. J. Med., *294*:461, 1976.
126. Méry, J. Ph., Kowrilsky, O., Morel-Maroger, L., and Adam, C.: Partial lipodystrophy and glomerulonephritis without complement activation. N. Engl. J. Med., *298*:1034, 1978.
127. Dunnigan, M. G., Cochrane, M. A., Kelly, A., and Scott, J. W.: Familial lipoatrophic diabetes with dominant transmission. Q. J. Med., *43*:33, 1974.
128. Lillystone, D., and West, R. J.: Lipodystrophy of limbs associated with insulin resistance. Arch. Dis. Child., *50*:737, 1975.
129. Oseid, S., Beck-Nielsen, H., Pedersen, O., and Søvik, O.: Decreased binding of insulin to its receptor in patients with congenital generalized lipodystrophy. N. Engl. J. Med., *296*:245, 1977.
130. Flier, J. S., Kahn, R., and Roth, J.: Receptors, antireceptor antibodies and mechanisms of insulin resistance. N. Engl. J. Med., *300*:413, 1979.
131. Kahn, C. R., Flier, J. S., Bar, R. S., Archer, J. A., Gorden, P., Martin, M. M., and Roth, J.: The syndromes of insulin resistance and acanthosis nigricans. N. Engl. J. Med., *294*:739, 1974.
132. Pulini, M., Raff, S. B., Chase, R., and Gordon, E. E.: Insulin resistance and acanthosis nigricans. Report of a case with antibodies to insulin receptors. Ann. Intern. Med., *85*:749, 1976.
133. Field, J. B., Johnson, P., and Herring, B.: Insulin resistant diabetes with increased endogenous plasma insulin followed by complete remission. J. Clin. Invest., *40*:1672, 1961.
134. Rothman, S.: Pituitary basophilism in the juvenile type of acanthosis nigricans. J.A.M.A., *156*:242, 1954.
135. Rothman, S., and Lynfield, Y.: Acanthosis nigricans, juvenile type, combined with necrobiosis lipoidica diabeticorum. Arch. Dermatol., *79*:113, 1959.
136. Bloom, R. E., and Rothman, S.: Juvenile acanthosis nigricans. Arch. Dermatol., *71*:413, 1955.
137. Brown, J., Winkelmann, R. K., and Randall, R. V.: Acanthosis nigricans and pituitary tumors. J.A.M.A., *198*:619, 1966.
138. Brown, J., and Winkelmann, R. K.: Acanthosis nigricans. A study of 90 cases. Medicine (Balt.), *47*:33, 1968.
139. Hollingsworth, D. R., and Amatruda, T. T., Jr.: Acanthosis nigricans and obesity. An endocrine abnormality? Arch. Intern. Med., *124*:481, 1969.
140. Scott, R. W., Klein, A. W., and Layden, J. J.: Acanthosis nigricans associated with a benign encephalopathy. Arch. Dermatol., *109*:78, 1974.
141. Lerner, A. B.: On the cause of acanthosis nigricans. N. Engl. J. Med., *281*:106, 1969.
142. Nordlund, J. J., and Lerner, A. B.: Cause of acanthosis nigricans. N. Engl. J. Med., *293*:200, 1975.
143. Banuchi, S. R., Cohen, L., Lorincz, A. L., and Morgan, J.: Acanthosis nigricans following diethylstilbestrol therapy. Occurrence in patients with childhood muscular dystrophy. Arch. Dermatol., *109*:545, 1974.
144. Fredrickson, D. S., Levy, R. I., and Lees, R. S.: Fat transport in lipoproteins. N. Engl. J. Med., *276*:34, 94, 148, 215, 273, 1967.
145. Alanpovic, P.: Apoproteins and lipoproteins. Atherosclerosis, *13*:141, 1970.
146. Gotto, A. M., Brown, W. V., Levy, R. I., Birnbaumer, M. E., and Fredrickson, D. S.: Evidence for the identity of the major apoprotein in low density and very low density lipoprotein in normal subjects and patients with familial hyperlipoproteinemia. J. Clin. Invest., *51*:1486, 1972.
147. Fredrickson, D. S., Goldstein, J. L., and Brown, M. S.: The familial hyperlipoproteinemias. *In* Stanbury, J. B., Wyngaarden, J. B., and Frederickson, D. S. (eds.): The Metabolic Basis of Inherited Disease, 4th ed. McGraw-Hill Book Co., New York, 1978, p. 604.
148. Brown, M. S., and Goldstein, J. L.:

Receptor-mediated control of cholesterol metabolism. Study of human mutants has disclosed how cells regulate a substance that is both vital and lethal. Science, *191*:150, 1976.
149. Goldstein, J. L., Schrott, H. G., Hazzard, W. R., Bierman, E. L., and Motulsky, A. G.: Hyperlipidemia in coronary heart disease. II. Genetic analysis of lipid levels in 176 families and delineation of a new inherited disorder, combined hyperlipidemia. J. Clin. Invest., *52*:1544, 1973.
150. Hazzard, W. R., Goldstein, J. L., Schrott, H. G., Motulsky, A. G., and Bierman, E. L.: Hyperlipidemia in coronary heart disease. III. Evaluation of lipoprotein phenotypes of 156 genetically defined survivors of myocardial infarction. J. Clin. Invest., *52*:1569, 1973.
151. Parker, F.: Hyperlipidemia and xanthomatosis. *In* Dermatology Update. Reviews for Physicians. Elsevier, New York, 1979, p. 89.
152. Palmer, L. S.: Carotinoids and Related Pigments. The Chromolipoids. Chemical Catalog Company, New York, 1922, p. 125.
153. Krinksy, N. I., Cornwell, D. G., and Oncley, J. L.: The transport of vitamin A and carotenoids in human plasma. Arch. Biochem., *73*:233, 1958.
154. Shulman, R. S., Bhattacharyya, A. K., Connor, W. E., and Frederickson, D. S.: Sitosterolemia and xanthomatosis. N. Engl. J. Med., *294*:482, 1976.
155. Elias, P., and Goldsmith, L. A.: Intertriginous xanthomata in type 2 hyperlipoproteinemia. Arch. Dermatol., *107*:761, 1973.
156. Polano, M. K.: Cutaneous xanthomatosis in relation to the blood lipoprotein pattern. Br. J. Dermatol., *81*: (Suppl. 2) 39, 1969.
157. Mishkel, M. A.: The diagnosis and management of the patient with xanthomatosis. An experience with thirty-five cases. Q. J. Med., *36*:107, 1967.
158. Klatskin, G., and Gordon, M.: Relationship between relapsing pancreatitis and essential hyperlipemia. Am. J. Med., *12*:3, 1952.
159. Crocker, A. C.: Skin xanthomas in childhood. Pediatrics, *8*:573, 1951.
160. Fredrickson, D. S., and Lees, R. S.: Familial hyperlipoproteinemia. *In* Stanbury, J. B. et al. (eds.): The Metabolic Basis of Inherited Disease, 2nd ed. McGraw-Hill Book Co., New York, 1966, p. 458.
161. Slack, J.: Risks of ischaemic heart disease in familial hyperlipoproteinaemic states. Lancet, *2*:1380, 1969.
162. Jensen, J., Blankenhorn, D. H., and Kornerup, V.: Coronary disease in familial hypercholesterolemia. Circulation, *36*:77, 1967.
163. Stone, N. O., Levy, R. I., Fredrickson, D. S., and Verter, J.: Coronary artery disease in 116 kindred with familial type II hyperlipoproteinemia. Circulation, *49*:476, 1974.
164. Harlan, W. R., Jr., Graham, J. B., and Estes, E. H.: Familial hypercholesterolemia, a genetic and metabolic study. Medicine (Balt.), *45*:77, 1966.
165. Streja, D., Steiner, G., and Kwiterovich, P. O., Jr.: Plasma high-density lipoproteins and ischemic heart disease. Ann. Intern. Med., *89*:871, 1978.
166. Goldstein, J. L., and Brown, M. S.: Familial hypercholesterolemia: identification of a defect in the regulation of 3-hydroxy-3 methylglutaryl coenzyme A reductase activity associated with overproduction of cholesterol. Proc. Natl. Acad. Sci., *70*:2804, 1973.
167. Goldstein, J. L., and Brown, M. S.: Familial hypercholesterolemia. A genetic regulatory defect in cholesterol metabolism. Am. J. Med., *58*:147, 1975.
168. Breslow, J. L., Spaulding, D. R., Lux, S. E., Levy, R. I., and Lees, R. S.: Homozygous familial hypercholesterolemia. N. Engl. J. Med., *293*:900, 1975.
169. Kushwana, R. S., Hazzard, W. R., Wahl, P. W., and Hoover, J. J.: Type III hyperlipoproteinemia: diagnosis in whole plasma by apolipoprotein E immunoassay. Ann. Intern. Med., *86*:509, 1977.
170. Fredrickson, D. S., Morganroth, J., and Levy, R. I.: Type III hyperlipoproteinemia: an analysis of two contemporary definitions. Ann. Intern. Med., *82*:150, 1975.
171. Morganroth, J., Levy, R. I., and Fredrickson, D. S.: The biochemical, clinical and genetic features of type III hyperlipoproteinemia. Ann. Intern. Med., *82*:158, 1975.
172. Hall, M. H., Bilheimer, D. W., Phair, R. D., Levy, R. I., and Berman, M.: A mathematical model for apoprotein kinetics in normal and hyperlipemia patients. Circulation, *114*:49, 1974 (Suppl. 3).
173. Hazzard, W. R., O'Donnell, T. F., and Lee, Y. L.: Broad-β disease (Type III hyperlipoproteinemia) in a large kindred. Evidence for a monogenic mechanism. Ann. Intern. Med., *82*:141, 1975.
174. Seidel, D., Alanpovic, P., Furman, R. H., and McConathy, W. J.: A lipoprotein characterizing obstructive jaundice. J. Clin. Invest., *49*:2396, 1970.
175. Ito, J., Sugai, T., and Saito, T.: Atresia of the intrahepatic bile ducts with xanthomatosis. Arch. Dermatol., *96*:53, 1967.
176. Pedace, F. J., and Winkelmann, R. K.: Xanthelasma palpebrum. J.A.M.A., *193*:893, 1965.
177. Parker, F., and Odland, G. F.: Electron microscopic similarities between experimental xanthomas and human eruptive xanthomas. J. Invest. Dermatol., *52*:136, 1969.
178. Gajdos, A., and Gajdos-Torok, M.: The specific enzyme deficiencies in five of the six known varieties of porphyrias. Int. J. Biochem., *9*:917, 1978.
179. Meyer, U. A., and Schmid, R.: The por-

phyrias. *In* Stanbury, J. B., Wyngaarden, J. B., and Fredrickson , D. S. (eds.): The Metabolic Basis of Inherited Disease, 4th ed. McGraw-Hill Book Co., New York, 1978, p. 1166.
180. DeMatteis, F., and Stonard, M.: Experimental porphyrias as models for human hepatic porphyrias. Sem. Hematol., *14*:187, 1977.
181. Weston, M. J., Nicholson, D. C., Lim, C. K., Clark, K. G., Macdonald, A., Henderson, M. A., and Williams, R.: Congenital erythropoietic uroporphyria (Günther's disease) presenting in a middle aged man. Int. J. Biochem., *9*:921, 1978.
182. Welland, F. H., and Carlsen, R. A.: Porphyria cutanea tarda in an 8-year-old boy. Arch. Dermatol., *99*:451, 1969.
183. Gilchrest, B., Pathak, M. A., and Parrish, J. A.: Porphyria cutanea tarda in young women. Arch. Dermatol., *111*:263, 1975.
184. Grossman, M. E.: A ten-year followup of 40 patients with porphyria cutanea tarda. Presented at Resident's Forum, Annual Meeting. American Academy of Dermatology, Dec. 4, 1978.
185. Jablonska, S., and Szczepánski, A.: Scleroderma-like lesions in metabolic disorders. *In* Jablonska, S. (ed.): Scleroderma and Pseudoscleroderma, 2nd ed. Polish Medical Publishers, Warsaw, 1975, p. 478.
186. Cram, D. L., Epstein, J. H., and Tuffanelli, D. L.: Lupus erythematosus and porphyria. Arch. Dermatol., *108*:779, 1973.
187. Elder, G. H.: Porphyrin metabolism in porphyria cutanea tarda. Sem. Hematol., *14*:227, 1977.
188. Kushner, J. P., Barbuto, A. J., and Lee, G. R.: An inherited enzymatic defect in porphyria cutanea tarda. J. Clin. Invest., *58*:1089, 1976.
189. Benedetto, A. V., Kushner, J. P., and Taylor, J. S.: Porphyria cutanea tarda in three generations of a single family. N. Engl. J. Med., *298*:358, 1978.
190. Elder, G. H., Lee, G. B., and Tovey, J. A.: Decreased hepatic uroporphyrinogen decarboxylase in porphyria cutanea tarda. N. Engl. J. Med., *299*:274, 1978.
191. Felsher, B. F., Norris, M. E., and Shih, J. C.: Red-cell uroporphyrinogen decarboxylase in porphyria cutanea tarda. N. Engl. J. Med., *299*:1095, 1978.
192. deVerneuil, H., Aitken, G., and Nordmann, Y.: Familial and sporadic porphyria cutanea. Two different diseases. Hum. Genet., *44*:145, 1978.
193. Peters, H. A.: Hexachlorobenzene poisoning in Turkey. Fed. Proc., *35*:2400, 1976.
194. Schmid, R.: Cutaneous porphyria in Turkey. N. Engl. J. Med., *263*:397, 1960.
195. Bleiberg, J., Wallen, M., Brodkin, R., and Applebaum, I. L.: Industrially acquired porphyria. Arch. Dermatol., *89*:793, 1964.
196. Elder, G. H., Evans, J. O., and Matlin, S. A.: The effect of the porphyrogenic compound hexachlorobenzene on the activity of hepatic uroporphyrinogen decarboxylase in the rat. Clin. Sci. Mol. Med., *51*:71, 1976.
197. San Martin de Viale, L. C., Rios de Molina, M. del C., Wainstock de Calmanovici, R., and Tomio, J. M.: Porphyrins and porphyrinogen carboxylase in hexachlorobenzene induced porphyria. Biochem. J., *168*:393, 1977.
198. Keczkes, K., and Barker, D. J.: Malignant hepatoma associated with acquired hepatic cutaneous porphyria. Arch. Dermatol., *112*:78, 1976.
199. Epstein, J. H., Tuffanelli, D. L., Seibert, J. S., and Epstein, W. L.: Porphyria-like cutaneous changes induced by tetracycline hydrochloride photosensitization. Arch. Dermatol., *112*:661, 1976.
200. Wiskemann, P. L. A., and Schulz, K. H.: Bullöse Photodermatitis durch Nalidixinsäure. Hautarzt, *24*:445, 1973.
201. Gilchrest, B., Rowe, J. W., and Mihm, M. C., Jr.: Bullous dermatosis of hemodialysis. Ann. Intern. Med., *83*:480, 1975.
202. Brivet, F., Drueke, T., Guillemette, J., Zingraff, J., and Crosnier, J.: Porphyria cutanea tarda-like syndrome in hemodialyzed patients. Nephron, *20*:258, 1978.
203. Thivolet, J., Euvrard, S., Perrot, H., Moskovtchenko, J. F., Claudy, A. L., and Ortonne, J. P.: La pseudo-porphyrie cutanée tardive des hemodialyses. Ann. Dermatol. Venereol., *104*:12, 1977.
204. Poh-Fitzpatrick, M. B., Bellet, N., DeLeo, V. A., Grossman, M. E., and Bickers, D. R.: Porphyria cutanea tarda in two patients treated with hemodialysis for chronic renal failure. N. Engl. J. Med., *299*:292, 1978.
205. Keczkes, K., and Farr, M.: Bullous dermatosis of chronic renal failure. Br. J. Dermatol., *95*:541, 1976.
206. Braverman, I. M.: Unpublished observations.
207. Ippen, H.: Treatment of porphyria cutanea tarda by phlebotomy. Sem. Hematol., *14*:253, 1977.
208. Kushner, J. P., Steinmuller, D. P., and Lee, G. R.: The role of iron in the pathogenesis of porphyria cutanea tarda. II. Inhibition of uroporphyrinogen decarboxylase. J. Clin. Invest., *56*:661, 1975.
209. Felsher, B. F., and Kushner, J. P.: Hepatic siderosis and porphyria cutanea tarda: relation of iron excess to the metabolic defect. Sem. Hematol., *14*:243, 1977.
210. Scholnick, P. L., Epstein, J. H., and Marver, H. S.: The molecular basis of the action of chloroquine in porphyria cutanea tarda. J. Invest. Dermatol., *61*:226, 1973.
211. Felsher, B. F., and Redeker, A. G.: Effect of chloroquine on hepatic uroporphyrin metabolism in patients with porphyria cutanea tarda. Medicine, *45*:575, 1966.
212. Taljaard, J. J. F., Shanley, B. C., Stewart-Wynne, E. G., Deppe, W. M., and Joubert, S. M.: Studies on low-dose chloro-

quine therapy and action of chloroquine in symptomatic porphyria. Br. J. Dermatol., *87*:261, 1972.
213. Mustajoki, P.: Variegate porphyria. Ann. Intern. Med., *89*:238, 1978.
214. Meyer, U. A., Strand, J., Doss, M., Rees, A. C., and Marver, H. S.: Intermittent acute porphyria — demonstration of a genetic defect in porphobilinogen metabolism. N. Engl. J. Med., *286*:1277, 1972.
215. Fowler, C. J., and Ward, J. M.: Porphyria variegata provoked by contraceptive pill. Br. Med. J., *1*:663, 1975.
216. Roberts, D. T., Brodie, M. J., Moore, M. R., Thompson, G. G., Goldberg, A., and MacSween, R. N. M.: Hereditary coproporhyria presenting with photosensitivity induced by the contraceptive pill. Br. J. Dermatol., *96*:549, 1977.
217. Freinkel, R. K., and Ashman, M.: Variegate porphyria. Arch. Dermatol., *110*:653, 1974.
218. Becker, D. M., Viljoen, J. D., Katz, J., and Kramer, S.: Reduced ferrochetalase activity: a defect common to porphyria variegata and protoporphyria. Br. J. Haematol., *36*:171, 1977.
219. Brenner, D. A., and Bloomer, J. R.: The enzymatic defect in variegate porphyria. Studies with human cultured skin fibroblasts. N. Engl. J. Med., *302*:765, 1980.
220. Schmidt, H., Snitker, G., Thomsen, K., and Lintrup, J.: Erythropoietic protoporphyria. A clinical study based on 29 cases in 14 families. Arch. Dermatol., *110*:58, 1974.
221. Corbett, M. F., Herzheimer, A., Magnus, I. A., Ramsay, C. A., and Kobza-Black, A.: The long term treatment with β-carotene in erythropoietic protoporphyria: a controlled trial. Br. J. Dermatol., *97*:655, 1977.
222. Zaynoun, S. T., Hunter, J. A. A., Darby, F. J., Zarembski, P., Johnson, B. E., and Frain-Bell, W.: The treatment of erythropoietic protoporphyria. Experience with beta-carotene. Br. J. Dermatol., *97*:663, 1977.
223. Poh-Fitzpatrick, M. B.: Erythropoietic protoporphyria. Int. J. Dermatol., *17*:359, 1978.
224. Porter, F. S., and Lowe, B. A.: Congenital erythropoietic protoporphyria. I. Case reports of clinical studies, and porphyrin analyses in two brothers. Blood, *22*:521, 1963.
225. Bloomer, J. R.: Pathogenesis and therapy of liver disease in protoporphyria. Yale Biol. Med., *52*:39, 1979.
226. Poh-Fitzpatrick, M. B.: Erythropoietic porphyrias: current mechanistic, diagnostic, and therapeutic considerations. Sem. Hematol., *14*:211, 1977.
227. Scholnick, P., Marver, H. S., and Schmid, R.: Erythropoietic protoporphyria: evidence for multiple sites of excess protoporphyrin formation. J. Clin. Invest., *50*:203, 1971.
228. Bloomer, J. R., Brenner, D. A., and Mahoney, M. J.: Study of factors causing excess protoporphyrin accumulation in cultured skin fibroblasts from patients with protoporphyria. J. Clin. Invest., *60*:1354, 1977.
229. Bickers, D. R., Demar, L. K., DeLeo, V., Poh-Fitzpatrick, M., Aronberg, J. M., and Harber, L. C.: Hydroa vacciniforme. Arch. Dermatol., *114*:1193, 1978.
230. Mathews-Roth, M. M., Pathak, M. A., Fitzpatrick, T. B., Harber, L. H., and Kass, E. H.: Beta carotene therapy for erythropoietic protoporphyria and other photosensitivity diseases. Arch. Dermatol., *113*:1229, 1977.
231. Heilmeyer, L., and Clotten, R.: Congenital erythropoietic coproporphyria. German Med. Monthly, *9*:353, 1964.
232. Levine, J., Johnson, W. T., and Tschudy, D. P.: The coexistence of two types of porphyria in one family. Arch. Dermatol., *114*:613, 1978.

14

Connective Tissue

This chapter covers diseases related to the true connective tissues and their components — collagen, elastin, cartilage, and adipose tissue. The arthritides are also included in this section.

DISORDERS OF ELASTIN, COLLAGEN, AND CARTILAGE

Pseudoxanthoma Elasticum

Prior to 1974, pseudoxanthoma elasticum (PXE) was thought to be almost always recessively inherited, with an occasional case showing dominant transmission. In that year, Pope demonstrated the heterogeneity of the syndrome which he divided into two dominant and two recessive types.[1,2] Most of the manifestations of PXE can be attributed to an abnormality in the elastin component of skin, walls of blood vessels, and internal organs. The skin, eyes, and cardiovascular system are affected in this disorder, which occurs twice as often in women as in men. The abnormalities in the skin and eye are not usually recognized before the second decade.[4]

The cutaneous lesions have three manifestations. (1) In the classic or major form, the primary cutaneous lesions are 2- to 4-mm, yellow rhomboidal or oval papules that arise chiefly on the neck and in the axillae, antecubital fossae, and inguinal and periumbilical areas (Fig. 14–1; Plate 39*B*). The palate and the labial, vaginal, and rectal mucosae may also be affected. On the lips, the papules look like the yellow grains of ectopic sebaceous glands observed in Fordyce's condition. The lesions of PXE have even been found by endoscopy on the gastric mucosa. The cutaneous eruption may number only a few papules, or it may be composed of thousands of spots that coalesce to form a yellow reticulated pattern on the neck and in the flexures. The appearance of the eruption is often compared to plucked chicken skin or Moroccan leather. The surface has also been likened to cobblestones. When the skin is severely affected, it may become lax and form redundant folds, especially on the neck and abdominal wall and in the axillary folds. (2) In the minor, more subtle form, the individual papules are much smaller. The eruption occurs in the same locations but is fainter and is described as macular with a golden yellow color. When the skin is stretched, however, the papular component becomes evident. (3) In rare cases, the entire skin may be involved, hanging in folds from the limbs and trunk and appearing too large for the

PLATE 39

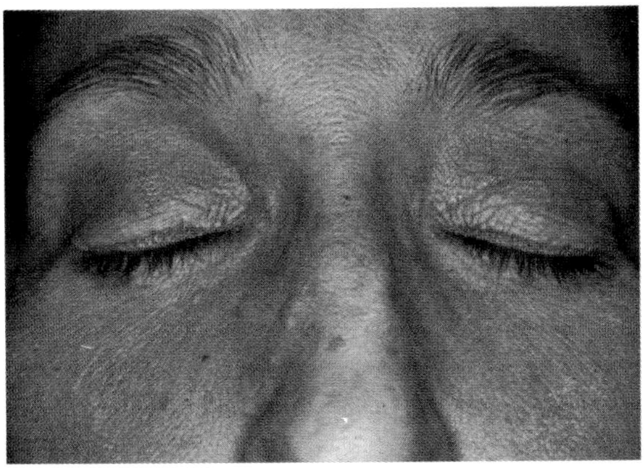

A, Biliary cirrhosis. Xanthelasma.

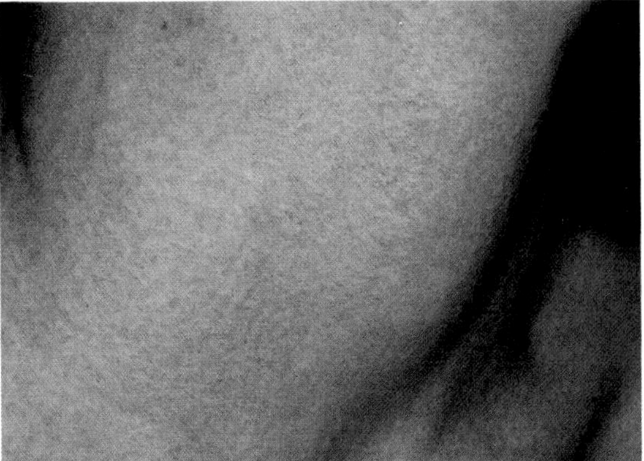

B, Pseudoxanthoma elasticum. Pathognomonic yellowish papules are present over entire neck.

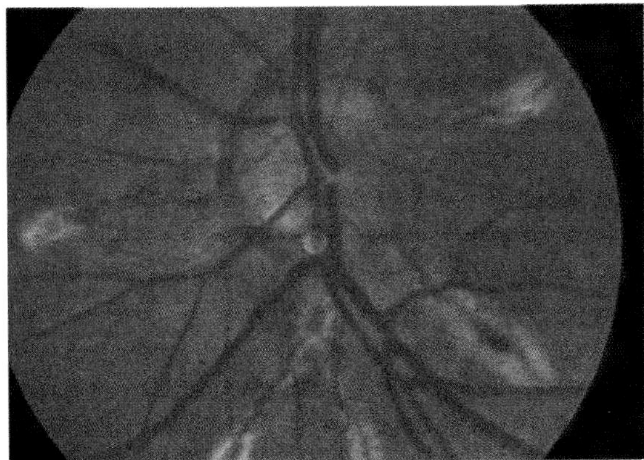

C, Angioid streaks on the retina of a patient with pseudoxanthoma elasticum. They are seen as brown lines that parallel the retinal vessels. (Courtesy of Dr. Thomas Kugelman.)

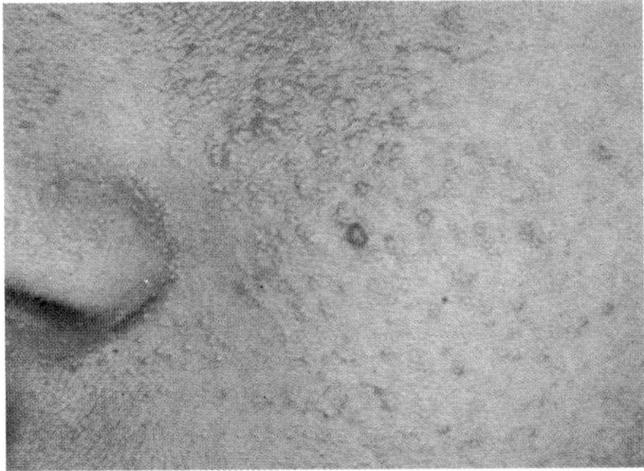

D, Tuberous sclerosis. Early stage in the formation of adenoma sebaceum. Pink papules with fine telangiectasia.

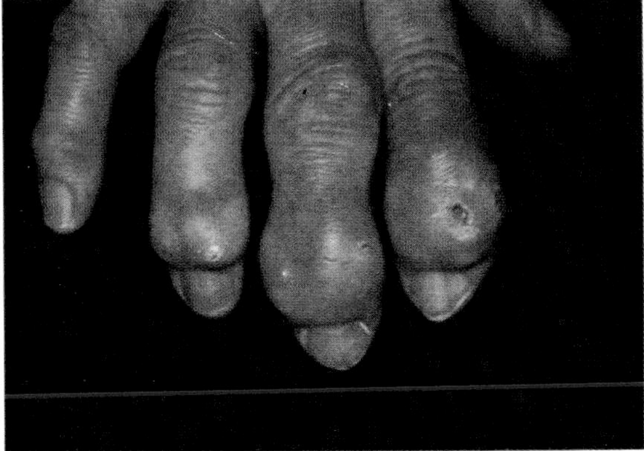

E, Gout.

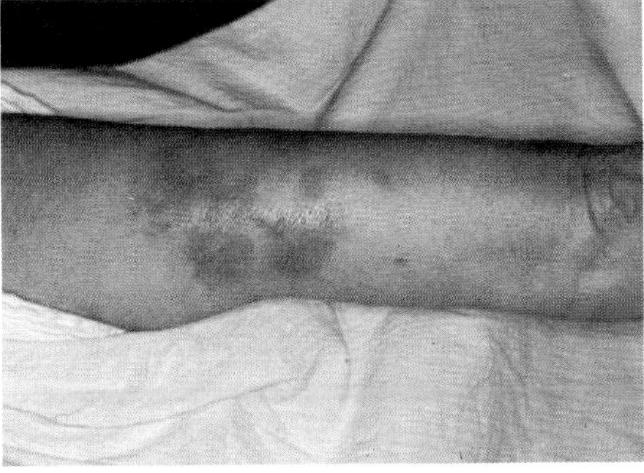

F, Weber-Christian panniculitis affecting the subcutaneous fat of the arm in this patient.

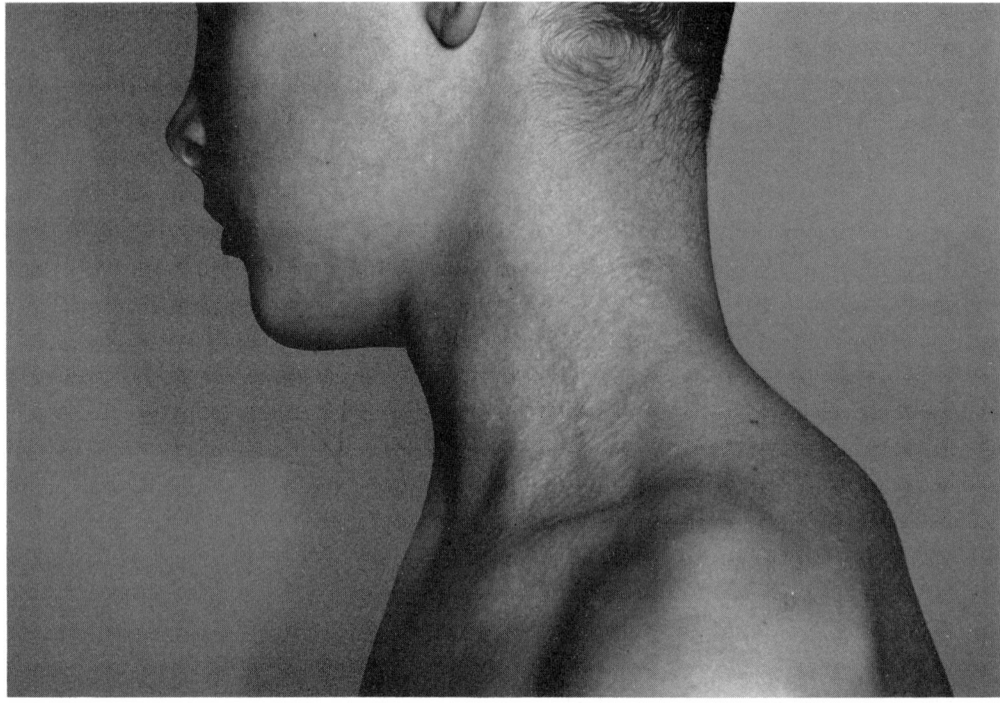

A

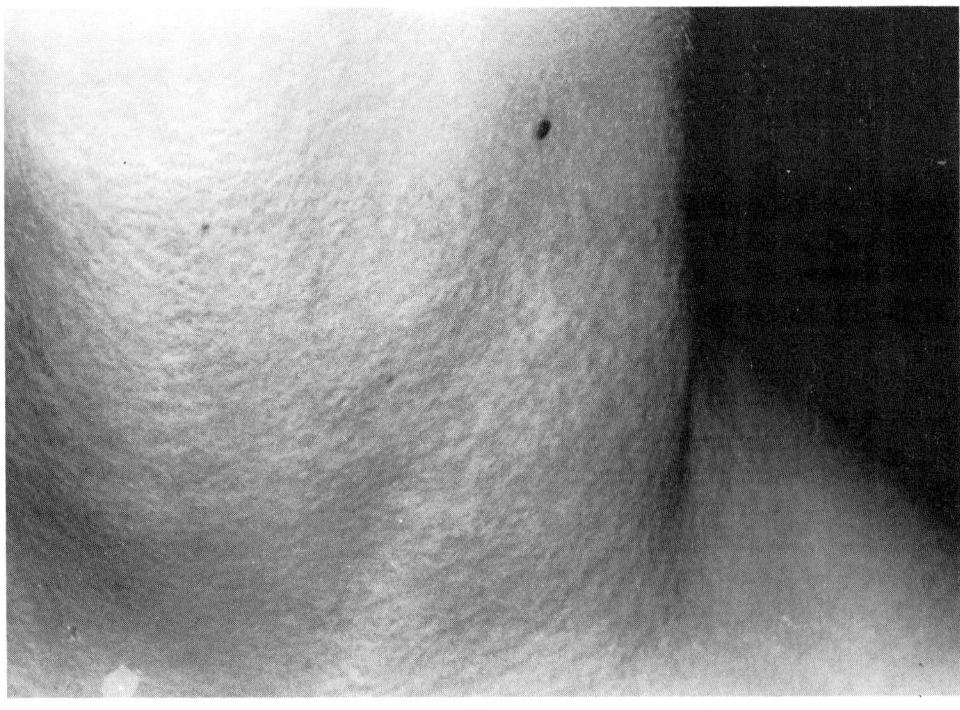

B

Figure 14–1. *A*, Pseudoxanthoma elasticum. Yellow papules on side of neck. *B*, Pseudoxanthoma elasticum. Yellow papules form a reticulated pattern on the neck of this patient.

body. In these instances, the entire skin surface may have an ivory-yellow color.[2]

The histogenesis of these lesions appears to be an increased proliferation of normal elastic fibers that become prematurely and abnormally calcified.[3,5,6] An abnormal deposition of glycosaminoglycans on the elastic fiber has been proposed as the basis for the increased calcification in this disorder.[7] The histopathology of PXE is unique, and the disease is easily diagnosed by biopsy of a cutaneous lesion.

The eye is involved in 75 per cent of patients. The elastic tissue in Bruch's membrane tears, and the subsequent fibrosis during repair produces on the retina broad brown linear bands that simulate vessels. These lines are known as angioid streaks (Plate 39*C*). The retinal vessels are fragile because of the elastic tissue abnormalities in their walls, and hemorrhage often occurs. Partial loss of vision may result from these episodes of hemorrhage and subsequent fibrosis. Less commonly, severe visual impairment, including blindness, may follow progressive retinal scarring, macular degeneration, and chorioretinitis, which are also complications of PXE.

In addition to retinal hemorrhage, there may also be bleeding from gastrointestinal, uterine, urogenital, and subarachnoid sites because of the generalized vascular involvement. Gastrointestinal bleeding is the most common type of hemorrhage observed, and it may be fatal. The media and the intima of the vessels become heavily calcified and are associated with diminished pulses; in the extremities, intermittent claudication results, and angina pectoris develops in the myocardium. However, death from myocardial infarction is unusual. Calcification of vessels in the extremities, myocardium, choroid plexus, and carotid system can be easily demonstrated by radiography.

Hypertension develops in 25 per cent of patients with PXE. In a few patients, the cause has been ascribed to vascular changes in renal arteries.[4]

Hypertension, gastrointestinal bleeding, and peripheral vascular insufficiency can be the presenting signs and symptoms in PXE,[8] and when these occur in children or adults under 30, the diagnosis of PXE should be considered.

The diagnostic skin lesions of PXE develop in childhood, but they are frequently overlooked because of their small size, subtle color, and lack of symptoms.

Although the cutaneous lesions are clinically and histologically pathognomonic for PXE, the angioid streaks are only relatively specific. These retinal lesions are also found in a minority of patients with Paget's disease of bone and sickle-cell anemia, and rarely in Ehlers-Danlos syndrome.[9] The significance of the ocular lesions in these three disorders is unknown.

The features of the four varieties of PXE described by Pope are summarized in Table 14–1. Dominant type I showed the classic "plucked chicken skin" eruption in all cases, and was characterized by severe retinopathy with visual loss, the most severe vascular disease, and hypertension. The more common dominant type II exhibited both the major and minor forms of eruption. Vascular and ocular disease were mild, but there was a high prevalence of blue sclerae, high arched palate, and loose jointedness. In a few patients, the skin was more extensible

Table 14–1. CLINICAL FEATURES OF THE FOUR VARIANTS OF PXE*

	Dominant Type I	Dominant Type II	Recessive Type I	Recessive Type II
Total No. Patients	12	52	54	3
Classic flexural rash	100%	24%	77%	0%
Macular rash	0%	70%	14%	0%
Generalized cutaneous PXE	0%	0%	0%	100%
Angina	56%	0%	0%	0%
Claudication	56%	0%	0%	0%
Hypertension	75%	8%	20%	0%
Hematemesis	8%	4%	16%	0%
Severe choroiditis	75%	8%	35%	0%
Angioid streaks	34%	47%	47%	0%
High arched palate	0%	54%	12%	0%
Blue sclerae	8%	41%	10%	0%
Loose jointedness	0%	35%	6%	0%

*Data from Pope, F. M.: Two types of autosomal recessive pseudoxanthoma elasticum. Arch. Dermatol., *110*:209, 1974.

than normal.[10] Recessive type I was characterized by the classic flexural lesions in most patients, but vascular disease was minimal and retinal disease moderate. Hematemesis was common in the affected women. Recessive type II was very rare, only three patients having been described. They showed universal involvement of their skin, which had a lax, loose-fitting appearance. Systemic complications were not found in these individuals.

Cutis Laxa

Cutis laxa is another disorder of elastic tissue. Cutis laxa may be inherited as a dominant, recessive, or X-linked recessive disorder.[11] It is much less common than PXE. An acquired form of the disease occurs in adults. The abnormalities usually begin at birth or shortly thereafter in most affected persons. The skin sags as if its mass were too large for the frame of the body. With time, large pendulous folds hang down from the face and abdomen, and the children look prematurely aged (Fig. 14–2). The facial cutaneous changes resemble the features of the bloodhound. Repeated plastic surgery is required to correct the lax skin, which worsens with age.

The pathogenesis of this disease is not well understood. Current studies suggest that there is a decrease in the amount of elastic tissue in the skin and rest of the body, as well as an abnormality in the formation of elastin. Electron microscopic studies, in one case each of congenital and acquired cutis laxa, have showed that the microfibrillar component of the elastic fiber was normal, but the protein elastin portion was decreased.[12] Lysyl oxidase activity was shown to be deficient in cultured skin fibroblasts from two males with the presumed X-linked recessive form of cutis laxa. This enzyme deficiency was more apparent when collagen rather than elastin was used as the substrate to assay enzyme activity.[11] The defect in lysyl oxidase would lead to generalized connective tissue weakness because of decreased cross linking in both elastin and collagen.

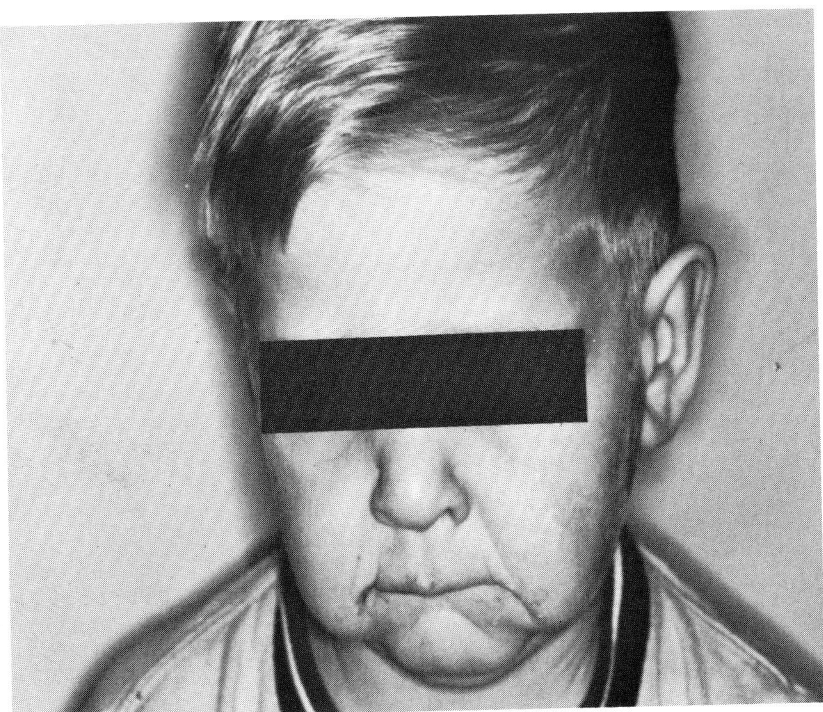

Figure 14–2. Cutis laxa in a four-year-old boy. Note sagging cheeks. (Courtesy of Dr. Sidney Klaus.)

Because of the decrease in the amount of elastic tissue in the skin and body, the term *generalized elastolysis* has been suggested as a name for this disorder.[12a] Most of the reported patients with cutis laxa have had pulmonary emphysema and hernias. Other associated conditions have included pulmonary artery stenosis and diverticula of the gastrointestinal tract.[13]

The lax skin of cutis laxa must be differentiated from the mildly sagging skin of PXE and the pendulous folds sometimes encountered in neurofibromatosis. In PXE, the lax skin is covered with the typical yellow papules; in neurofibromatosis, café au lait spots and cutaneous tumors are usually present elsewhere to indicate that a plexiform neurofibroma is responsible for the sagging folds of skin.

Cutis Hyperelastica (Ehlers-Danlos Syndrome)

Our increasing understanding about the Ehlers-Danlos syndrome is derived directly from the advances in the field of collagen biosynthesis. Collagen is now known to be composed of at least five molecular species, named I, II, III, IV, and V.[14] Each species is composed of three antigenically distinct polypeptide chains (alpha chains). The three chains, which may be identical or different depending upon the collagen species, are coiled around each other like a rope. This coiling continues as the molecules form fibrils and eventually collagen fibers. Antibodies are now available to identify the different types of collagen in various tissues, and the enzymes involved in collagen biosynthesis can be assayed in different disorders to learn about pathogenesis. Table 14–2 lists the collagen species, their tissue distribution, and their molecular composition.

Table 14–2. MOLECULAR SPECIES OF COLLAGEN

Type	Tissue Distribution	Molecular Form
I	bone, tendon, dermis ligament, fascia, uterus, arteries	$[\alpha_1(I)]_2\alpha_2$
II	cartilage	$[\alpha_1(II)]_3$
III	dermis, arteries, uterus	$[\alpha_1(III)]_3$
IV	basement membranes	$[\alpha_1(IV)]_3$
V	dermis, placenta, heart valve	$\alpha A \alpha B$

Type I is composed of three α chains, two identical and one different. The others are composed of three identical chains that are characteristic of their species (designated by the Roman numeral). Type V is a newly discovered species whose molecular composition is not yet defined.

Rarely, the extensibility may be limited to an area of the skin, or one side of the body may be more affected than the other. The extensibility may be limited to the mucous membranes of the mouth and tongue. Individuals affected in this way can touch their noses with the tips of their tongues. The ears of some patients are stretchable and can also be folded into a ball. Laxity of the skin is not present except late in the disease and then only on the palms and soles.

In Ehlers-Danlos syndrome, an abnormality of collagen, rather than elastin, is responsible for the cutaneous and systemic manifestations. The skin feels smooth and rubbery and can be pulled away easily from the underlying structures (Fig. 14–3). When released, the skin snaps back and fits snugly again.

The joints are hyperextensible and easily dislocated. Joint effusions and hemarthroses secondary to trauma from joint instability may occur. Many individuals suffer from habitual dislocation of the hips, patellae, shoulders, radii, clavicles, and temporomandibular joints. Flat feet are common in this syndrome. The combination of hyperextensible skin and joints is responsible for the appellation of "India rubber man," which has been given to these patients (Fig. 14–4).

However, the skin and its blood vessels are extremely fragile. Minor trauma can produce hematomas and gaping "fish-mouth" lacerations. The gums may bleed after brushing the teeth. The dermis has poor tensile strength and cannot hold the sutures needed to repair these wounds. The skin often heals by secondary intention, and cigarette-paper-thin scars with fine wrinkling characteristically form. The resolution of hematomas is accompanied by fibrosis, which produces soft "pseudotumors" (Fig. 14–5). Similar lesions can develop over pressure points on the heels, knees, and elbows. Fragility also affects the major arteries, which may rupture spontaneously or following minor trauma. Intracranial aneurysm, hemothorax, and dissection aneurysm of the aorta are reported examples of such catastrophes. Varicose veins are common in Ehlers-Danlos syndrome.

Abnormalities in collagen biosynthesis and fiber organization form the basis for the different clinical subtypes of the Ehlers-Danlos syndrome delineated by Beighton.[15] One of the defects is believed to be the way in which the bundles of collagen are joined to each other. A loosely, rather

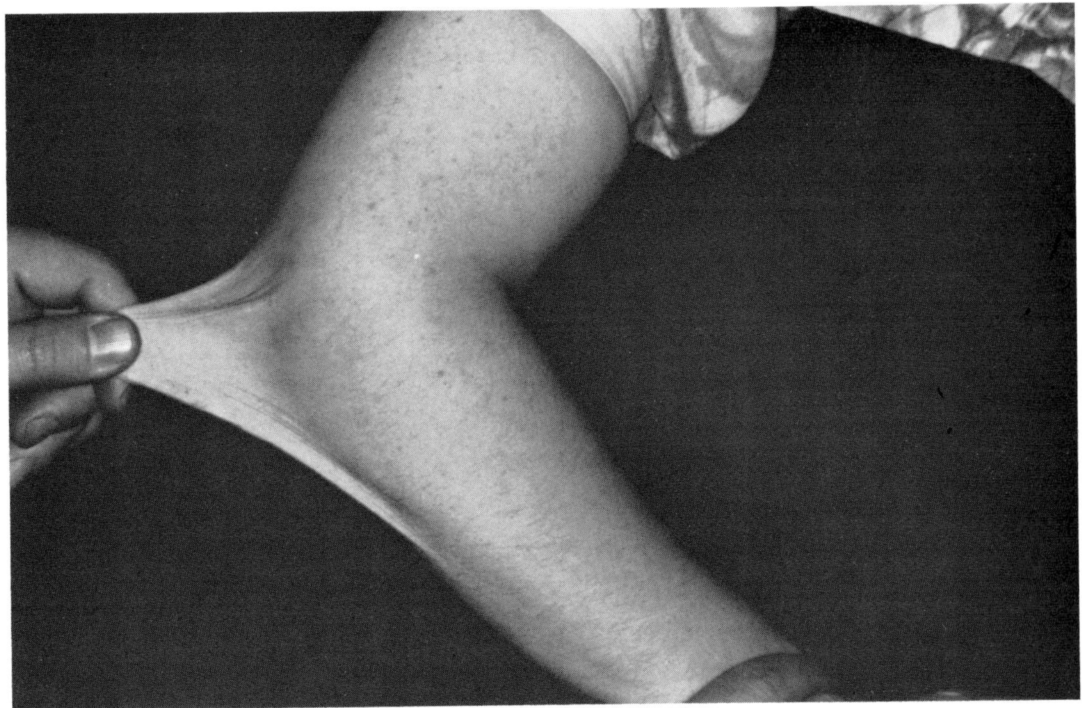

Figure 14–3. Ehlers-Danlos syndrome. Hyperelastic skin.

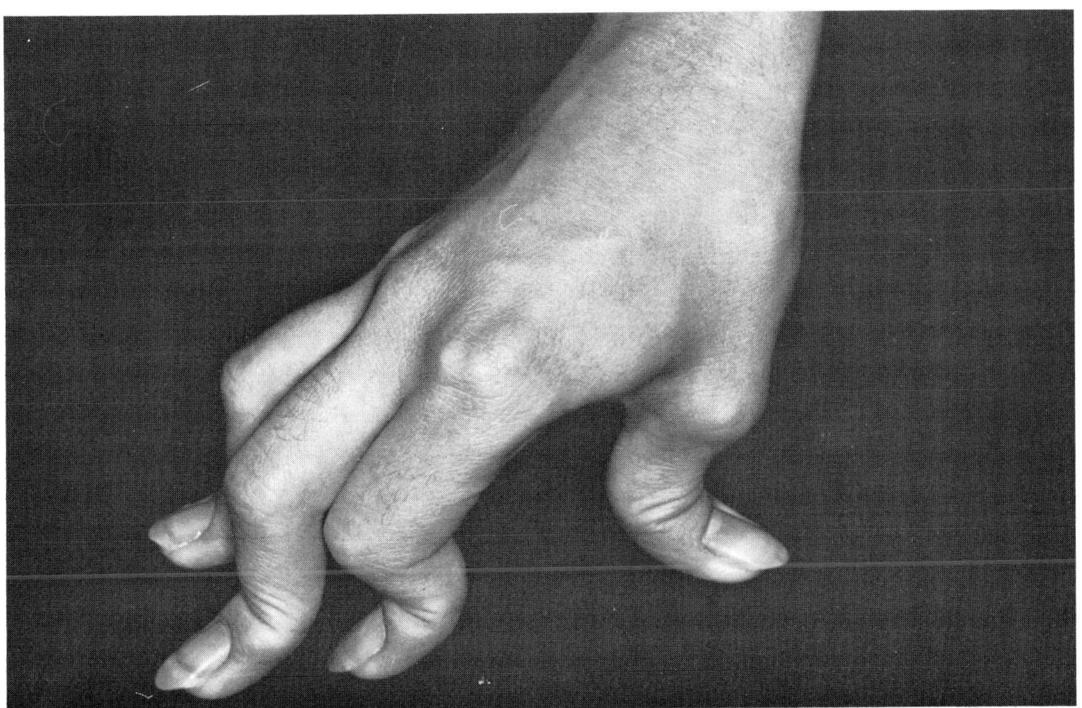

Figure 14–4. Ehlers-Danlos syndrome. Hyperextensible joints.

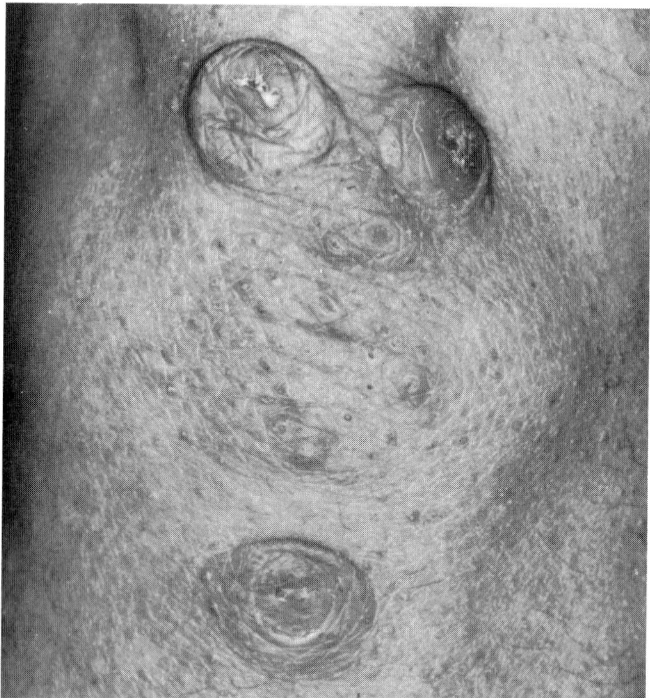

Figure 14–5. Ehlers-Danlos syndrome. Pseudotumor scars on knee.

than tightly knit "wickerwork" organization of collagen bundles has been postulated.[16] This hypothesis is supported by the values for the elastic modulus of the skin in this syndrome measured by Grahame and Beighton.[17] The loose "wickerwork" arrangement allows hyperextensibility of the skin and joints but this does not provide as much tensile strength or support for blood vessels as would be possible with a tighter network. This loose organization of collagen bundles may partly explain some of the other observed features in this syndrome: diaphragmatic and inguinal hernias; diverticula of stomach, duodenum, and colon; rectal prolapse in children under four to five years; spontaneous rupture of the lung; megaesophagus and megacolon; and abnormal fragility of the bowel with gastrointestinal bleeding.[4]

Pregnancy in Ehlers-Danlos syndrome may be complicated by increased bruisability, vulvar and leg varicosities, abdominal hernia, and excessive bleeding from episiotomy. Caesarean section may require a subsequent immediate hysterectomy because of the failure of sutures to hold. Uterine and vaginal ruptures have been reported. Premature births are increased because fragility of fetal tissue leads to early rupture of the membranes.

Like PXE, the Ehlers-Danlos syndrome has also been shown to be heterogeneous. Beighton divided this disorder into five major types,[15] and two additional ones have been added subsequently.

Type I — gravis. Skin hyperextensibility, fragility, and bruising are marked. Joint hypermobility is generalized and severe. At surgery, tissues are found to be friable. Prematurity due to early rupture of fetal membranes is a feature of this variety.

Type II — mitis. Cutaneous and joint manifestations are mild. Hypermobility of joints tends to be limited to the hands and feet. Tissue friability and prematurity are not usually features of this milder type.

Type III — benign hypermobile. Joint hypermobility is generalized and marked. Cutaneous hyperextensibility and other cutaneous features are usually mild. Skeletal deformities are not usually present, but complications of joint hypermobility are frequent. The "floppy mitral valve" syndrome — redundant chordae tendineae and valve cusps — can be associated with this form of Ehlers-Danlos syndrome.

Types I, II, and III are dominantly transmitted. The biochemical defect is unknown.

Type IV — ecchymotic, arterial, or Sack variety. Joint hypermobility is largely limited to the digits, and skin hyperextensibility is minimal or absent. The skin does not feel velvety but is thin and pale with a prominently visible subcutaneous venous pattern. Minor trauma is followed by extensive ecchymoses. Thin, darkly pigmented scars cover bony prominences. The dreaded complications are ruptures of the great vessels and the bowel. Patients with this form have the highest mortality rate and rarely live beyond the second decade. A commonly associated skin lesion in type IV is elastosis perforans serpiginosa. Patients with this form of Ehlers-Danlos syndrome fail to synthesize type III collagen,[11] which is found in high concentrations in the skin, gastrointestinal tract, and aorta. This syndrome exhibits autosomal recessive inheritance.

Type V — X-linked. Joint hypermobility is mild, but skin stretchability is marked. Skin fragility, "cigarette paper" scarring, and bruising occur to a moderate degree. The "floppy mitral valve" syndrome is also associated with this variety. Studies of one family revealed the biochemical defect to be decreased activity of lysyl oxidase. These subjects excreted increased amounts of hydroxylysine glycosides and valylproline in the urine, suggesting an increased turnover of collagen and elastin, respectively, because of a decrease in cross-links. Lysyl oxidase is necessary for cross-linking in both collagen and elastin.[14]

Type VI — ocular form. This variety is an autosomal recessive disorder and is uncommon.[18, 19] The major features are marked cutaneous fragility and hyperextensibility of skin and joints. Recurrent joint dislocation and severe scoliosis result. Because of the marked joint hypermobility, two patients were described as floppy babies and were diagnosed as having amyotonia congenita for several years before the correct diagnosis was made.[18] The pregnancy of one of the patients was complicated by premature rupture of the fetal membranes.[16] The ophthalmologic features include blue sclerae, epicanthal folds, myopia, microcornea with glaucoma, and retinal detachment. Rupture of the globe and intraocular bleeding occur both spontaneously and following minor trauma. In two patients, these latter complications led to blindness and enucleation, respectively.[4, 18, 19] One patient died of a dissecting aneurysm of the aorta.[15] These ocular abnormalities have also developed in individuals who did not have the stigmata of Ehlers-Danlos syndrome, but whose siblings did.[4]

The biochemical defect in this form is a defective lysyl hydroxylase enzyme that is needed to hydroxylate lysine for subsequent cross-linking, after the lysine has been incorporated into the collagen molecule. Ascorbic acid, a cofactor for lysyl hydroxylase, was given in large doses to one of these patients in an effort to correct or improve the enzymatic defect. The initial results have been encouraging.[20] However, there appears to be considerable heterogeneity in the molecular defect in different patients,[14] and some patients diagnosed as having type VI disease appear to have normal lysyl hydroxylase activity.[21]

Type VII. This variety was originally called arthrochalasis multiplex congenita because of the marked loose jointedness. Three patients have been reported, all exhibiting an identical syndrome: multiple joint dislocations, marked joint hypermobility, soft velvety skin which is stretchable and heals with atrophic scars, easy bruisability, short stature, microcornea, and scoliosis. Type VII is transmitted as an autosomal recessive.[22]

Initially, it was believed that type VII was identical to a syndrome found in inbred cattle and sheep called dermatosparaxis, in which the skin is extremely fragile and easily torn. The defect in these animals is a deficiency of procollagen aminoprotease, which is necessary to cleave the nonhelical amino terminal peptide extension of procollagen after it is secreted from the fibroblast. This cleavage is necessary so that the collagen molecules can aggregate properly and become cross-linked to form a strong stable fiber.[23, 24] The early studies in humans suggested that a decrease in procollagen aminoprotease was also present in type VII. However, recent work has indicated that the enzyme is normal and that the abnormality is a structural mutation in one of the three peptide extensions (pro $\alpha 2$) of type I collagen. The mutation prevents the normal enzymatic removal of the aminopeptide from this chain, preventing the collagen molecules from aggregating properly.[25]

Syndromes combining features of Ehlers-Danlos and PXE have been observed in a few patients.[4] The relationship of such syndromes to the seven types is as yet unknown.

Blue sclerae are not pathognomonic of osteogenesis imperfecta but can be seen in cases of Ehlers-Danlos syndrome, PXE, and Marfan's syndrome.

Relapsing Polychondritis

Relapsing polychondritis is a disorder in which there are episodic and recurrent bouts of inflammation involving cartilage throughout the body.[26, 27] The illness is associated with inflammation of the eye and inner ear, as well as with a variety of autoimmune rheumatic disorders. The most frequent presenting clinical features include (1) bilateral auricular chondritis, (2) nasal chondritis, (3) polyarthritis, (4) ocular inflammation, (5) respiratory tract chondritis, and (6) audiovestibular damage. The diagnosis can be made if three or more features are present. Over 160 cases have been reported in the world's literature. The disease occurs equally in men and women and may develop at any age from childhood to the ninth decade, but the average age of onset is in the fifth decade.

The auricular chondritis is characterized by the sudden development of erythema, swelling, heat, and tenderness limited to the cartilaginous portion of the ear (helix, antihelix, tragus, and sometimes the external auditory canal). The surrounding soft tissues may also be inflamed, and regional lymphadenopathy may be present. The inflammation generally persists for five to ten days before spontaneously subsiding. Repeated attacks may lead to induration and nodularity of the ear (Fig. 14–6). If severe, a "cauliflower ear" can be produced. In extreme cases, the

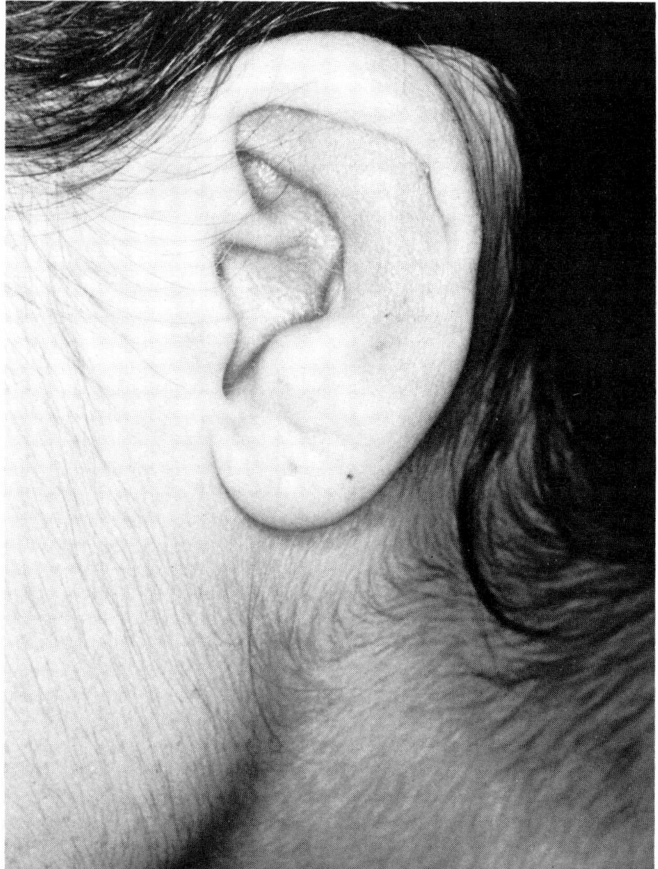

Figure 14–6. Relapsing polychondritis. Induration and nodularity of pinna.

cartilage is completely destroyed, resulting in floppy ears. The ear falls forward because of lack of support, and the external auditory canal may also become soft and collapse on itself. However, in most cases, nodularity and induration are the end result of the recurrent inflammation. Calcification of the ear cartilage develops in up to 40 per cent of cases.

Nasal chondritis develops and behaves like auricular chondritis. The nose and surrounding tissues are red, tender, and swollen during an acute attack. Mild nose bleeds may be an accompanying feature. Recurrent bouts of inflammation lead to collapse of the nasal septal cartilage, producing a "saddle nose" similar to that seen in syphilis (Fig. 14–7).

The arthritis can affect single or multiple joints. The large and small joints of the arms, hips, and knees are most commonly affected. The costochondral junctions and sternomanubrial and sternoclavicular joints can also be involved. Rarely the spine and ankles are affected. The arthritis typically is migratory, nonerosive, and seronegative.

Ocular inflammation involves all segments of the eye, producing conjunctivitis, scleritis and episcleritis, iritis, and chorioretinitis. Chorioretinitis and inflammation of the vitreous may lead to decreased vision. Scleromalacia perforans has been reported.

When the respiratory tract is initially involved, the patient usually complains of hoarseness, sometimes to the point of aphonia, because of inflammation and edema in the glottic, subglottic, and laryngeal areas.

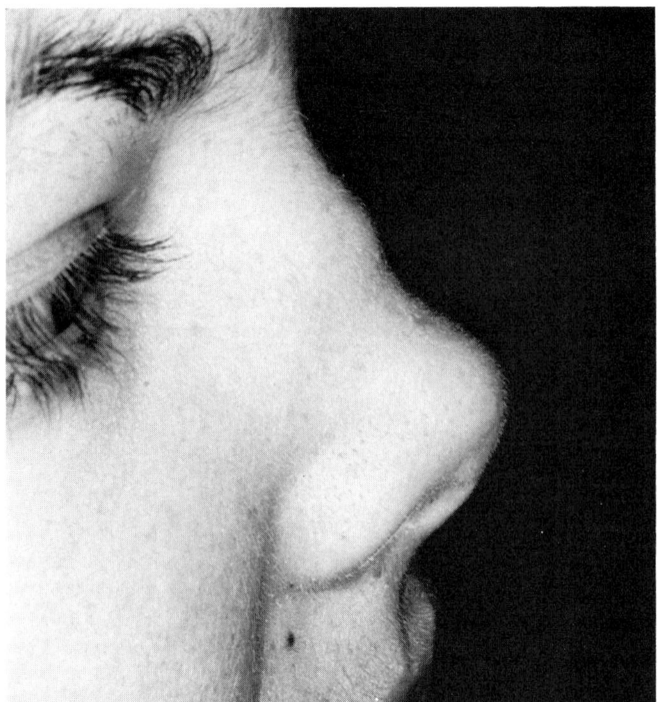

Figure 14–7. Relapsing polychondritis. Collapse of nasal septal cartilage leading to "saddle nose" deformity.

Tracheostomy is sometimes required at this stage because of airway obstruction. Later in the course of the disease, respiratory tract involvement takes the form of inflammation involving the laryngeal and tracheal cartilages. There may be tenderness over the thyroid cartilage or anterior trachea in such circumstances. Inflammation of these cartilages may lead to secondary collapse, requiring tracheostomy.

Audiovestibular involvement begins as an acute event, either unilaterally or bilaterally. The signs and symptoms are those of nausea, vomiting, vertigo, tinnitus, and sensorineural deafness. The auditory damage is usually permanent and resolution, if it occurs, is only partial. The vestibular disturbances usually improve.

In a few patients, the illness begins with fever, weight loss, arthralgias, and myalgias. Such presentations remain diagnostic problems until the more specific signs of relapsing polychondritis appear.

About 30 per cent of patients have an associated rheumatic disease, most commonly adult or juvenile arthritis, Sjögren's syndrome, systemic LE, or autoimmune thyroid disorders. The mortality from relapsing polychondritis ranges from 22 to 30 per cent after an average duration of four years.[26] The most common causes of death have been airway collapse or obstruction, and cardiovascular complications.

The cardiovascular complications consist of aortic insufficiency caused by dilatation of the valvular ring secondary to destruction of the medial elastic layers in the aortic root. The mitral valve may become insufficient for analogous reasons. Valve replacement is often necessary in such circumstances. Aneurysms of the ascending and abdominal aortas can develop and rupture. Necrotizing vasculitis of both large and small vessels is also a feature in some cases of relapsing polychondritis.

Table 14–3. INCIDENCE OF ORGAN INVOLVEMENT IN RELAPSING POLYCHONDRITIS IN 159 PATIENTS*

Type of Involvement	Per Cent
Auricular chondritis	88
Nasal chondritis	72
Thoracic cartilaginous joints	36
Peripheral joints	76
Spondylitis	15
Ocular involvement	65
Respiratory tract involvement	56
Cochlear damage	40
Vestibular damage	26
Aortic insufficiency	6
Mitral insufficiency	3
Pericarditis	2
Myocardial ischemia	1
Aneurysm of large artery	6
Systemic arteritis	6
CNS vasculitis	3
Cutaneous vasculitis	6

*From McAdam, L. P., O'Hanlan, M. A., Bluestone, R., and Pearson, C. M.: Relapsing polychondritis: prospective study of 23 patients and a review of the literature. Medicine, *55*:193, 1976.

Thromboses of the aorta and the carotid and lower extremity arteries can develop as a consequence of a preceding vasculitis or aneurysm formation. Glomerulonephritis is an uncommon manifestation.[26a] Table 14–3 summarizes the prevalence of the main features in this disorder.

The pathology in relapsing polychondritis appears to be an initial loss of matrix and mucopolysaccharides followed by a secondary perichondral inflammatory reaction with neutrophils, lymphocytes, and plasma cells. The cartilage is eventually destroyed and replaced by fibrous tissue.[26, 27] The autopsy of one patient who died from rupture of an abdominal aortic aneurysm showed that the mucopolysaccharides were decreased in the normal-appearing bronchial and tracheal cartilage and the thoracic aortic wall, in addition to the normal-appearing wall of the abdominal aorta close to the aneurysm.[27] The most recent evidence suggests that relapsing polychondritis is an immunologically mediated disorder. Antibodies to type II collagen, but not to the other types, have been detected. The titers correlated with disease activity. The antibodies were directed against *native* type II collagen, rather than denatured collagen, indicating that the antibodies may not be a consequence of inflammation, but rather may be a primary event in pathogenesis.[28] Placental transfer of the disease has been reported.[29] The affected baby had a saddle nose and arthritis of the knees. The arthritis persisted for two years before subsiding. Other workers have demonstrated deposition of immunoglobulins and complement in the inflamed cartilage of a patient with relapsing polychondritis.[30]

Circulating immune complexes have also been detected in patients with relapsing polychondritis.[28] It is possible that the complexes are formed secondary to release of collagen fragments after tissue damage. They may be responsible for the associated arteritis that is believed to be the basis for aneurysms, arterial thromboses, and sensorineural deafness and for the glomerulonephritis.

Dapsone is extremely effective in suppressing the acute chondritis. It is believed to act by inhibiting lysosomal enzymes.[31-33] Proteolysis of cartilage with loss of mucopolysaccharides produced by lysosomal enzymes may be the initial pathologic event. The antibodies to native type II collagen might be the triggering event for this proteolysis. Dapsone has proved to be effective in suppressing the chondritis and episcleritis.[33] It is not yet known whether it will be effective in controlling the major systemic features of the disease.

THE ARTHRITIDES

Rheumatoid Arthritis

The skin of patients with longstanding rheumatoid arthritis is often pale, translucent, shiny, and atrophic. These features are most apparent over the hands and fingers. At first glance, sclerodactyly may be thought to be present, especially if there is arthritic swelling of the proximal interphalangeal joints. However, careful observation will reveal that the skin is thin rather than thick and hidebound as in scleroderma. About 5 per cent of patients with rheumatoid arthritis have cuticular linear telangiectasia identical to that found in LE, scleroderma, and dermatomyositis. Necrotizing angiitis involving the small cutaneous vessels and less often the large muscular vessels may occur and result in hemorrhagic bullae, ulceration, and purpura. The legs are usually affected by the angiitic process. Rheumatoid nodules develop in about 20 per cent of patients. These bumps tend to occur over pressure points; the juxta-articular regions of the elbows are most often affected (Fig. 14–8).

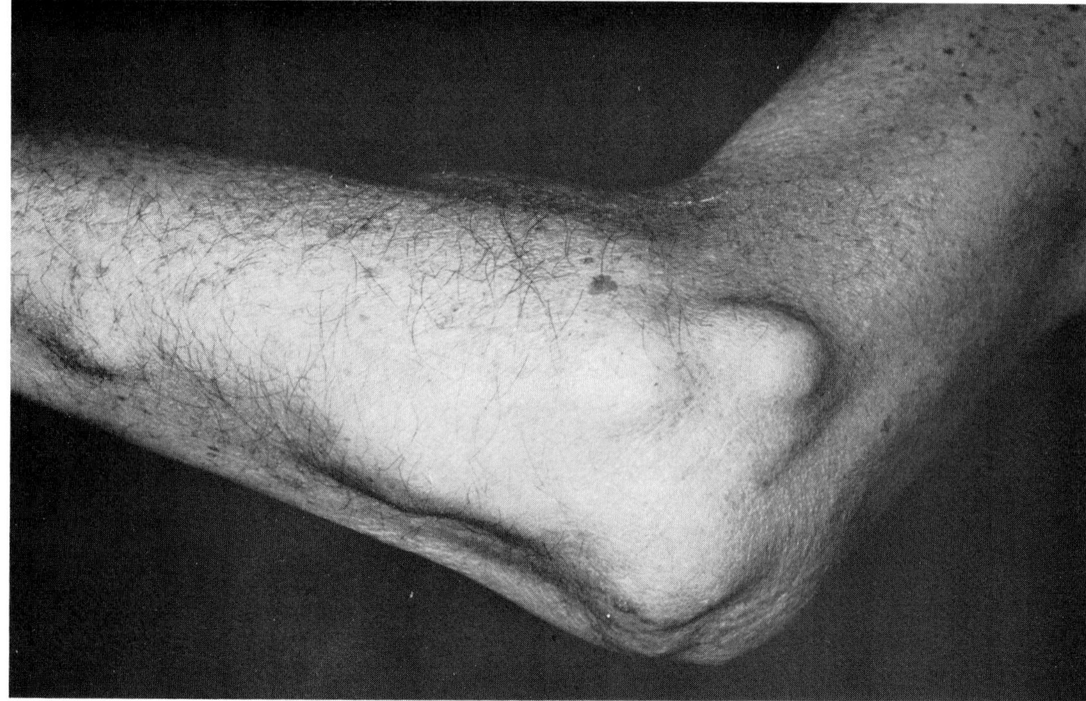

Figure 14–8. Rheumatoid nodules.

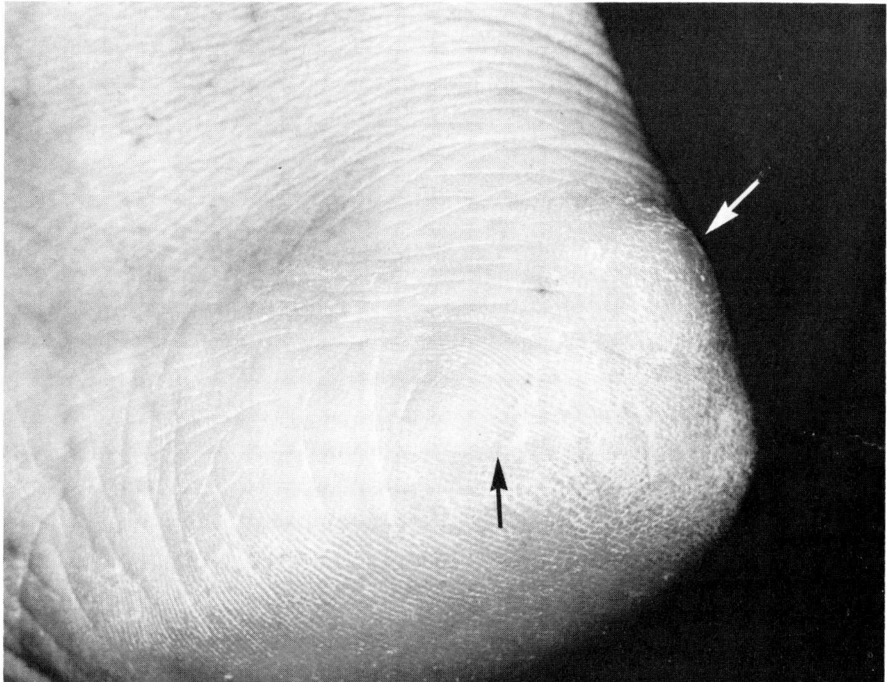

Figure 14–9. Rheumatoid nodules on heel (arrows).

However, any area of skin under chronic pressure can probably develop a rheumatoid nodule (Fig. 14–9). We observed such a lesion in the skin over the thoracic spine of a man who had been confined to bed for several months. Palmar erythema is also a feature of rheumatoid arthritis.

An exanthem that accompanies a daily fever spike is present in 40 per cent of patients with juvenile rheumatoid arthritis (Still's disease). The fever and rash may be present daily for weeks, months, or even years before the arthritis makes its debut (see p. 463). Subcutaneous nodules are less common in Still's disease than in adult rheumatoid arthritis (6 per cent versus 20 per cent).

Reiter's Syndrome

Urethritis, conjunctivitis, iritis, and arthritis are the features of Reiter's syndrome.[34] They may appear together or develop sequentially over the course of several weeks. Cutaneous and mucosal eruptions are present in 50 to 80 per cent of patients. These lesions may develop in association with the other features of the syndrome, or they may arise independently. The attacks of Reiter's syndrome are self-limiting, but relapses are common. During the recurrences, any of the genitourinary, ocular, articular, or cutaneous features may be present together or separately.

The mucocutaneous signs are limited to the palms, soles, and penis and the oral and urethral mucosae in most cases of Reiter's syndrome. However, scattered lesions do appear over the trunk and extremities in some individuals. Rarely, a generalized eruption may develop in association with the palmar, plantar, and penile lesions.

The cutaneous lesions may closely resemble or faithfully mimic those of psoriasis. They can begin as red macules that become scaly (Fig. 14–10), or they may start as broad pustular lakes that can develop scales thick enough to form horns (Figs. 14–11 and 14–12).

The first type of lesion, the red scaly macule, is most frequently found on the glans penis and at the urethral meatus (Figs. 14–13 and 14–14). When several penile lesions are present, they may coalesce into a larger circinate patch (balanitis circinata). Psoriasiform lesions may be found scattered over the scrotum, buttocks, trunk, and extremities. The skin of the fingers and toes may become erythematous, swollen, moist, and scaling (Fig. 14–15). The nails may be yellow and lifted up at their distal margins by subungual hyperkeratosis, as in psoriasis (Fig. 14–16). Even the scalp may display heavy psoriasiform scaling.

The second type of eruption, the heavily cornified lesion, has a predilection for the palms and soles and is usually called keratoderma blenorrhagicum. In the early vesiculopustular stage, the lesions may be indistinguishable from those of pustular psoriasis of Barber, a dermatosis which affects only the palms and soles. (This is a *benign* recurrent pustular eruption that may or may not be related to true psoriasis and must be distinguished from pustular psoriasis of von Zumbusch, an acute generalized toxic form of psoriasis vulgaris — see p. 740). The extreme horn formation that develops in the late phase is unusual in ordinary psoriasis. The uncommon generalized eruption that has occurred in Reiter's syndrome has been characterized by extremely keratotic hornlike lesions rather than by flat psoriasiform patches.

The oral mucosal lesions are superficial asymptomatic erosions that

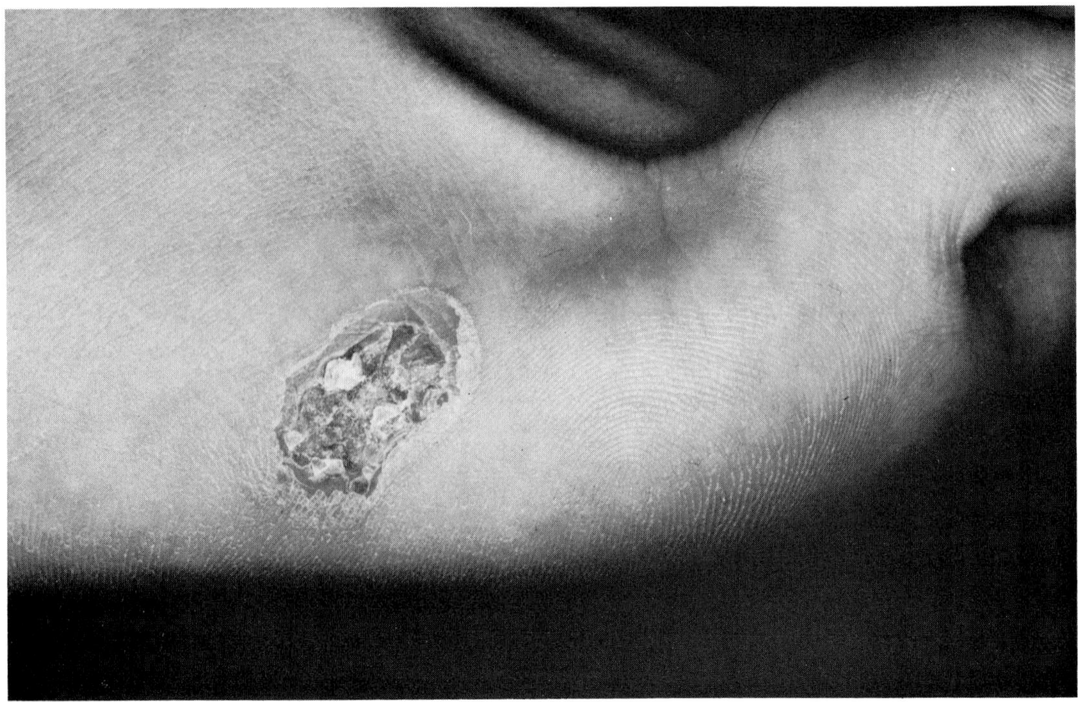

Figure 14–10. Reiter's syndrome. Psoriasiform lesion.

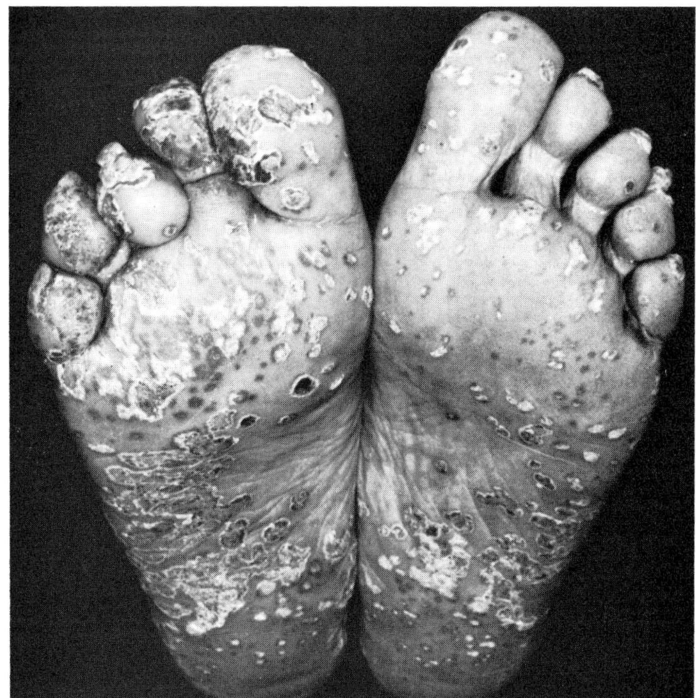

Figure 14–11. Reiter's syndrome. Keratoderma blenorrhagicum.

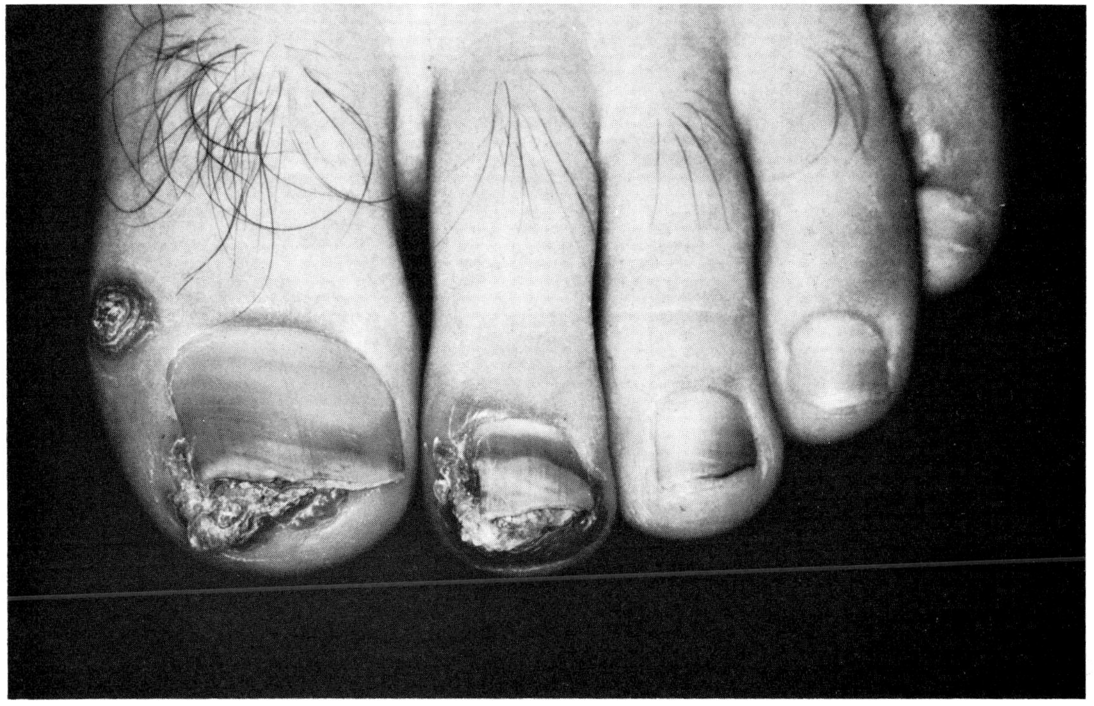

Figure 14–12. Reiter's syndrome. Keratoderma blenorrhagicum.

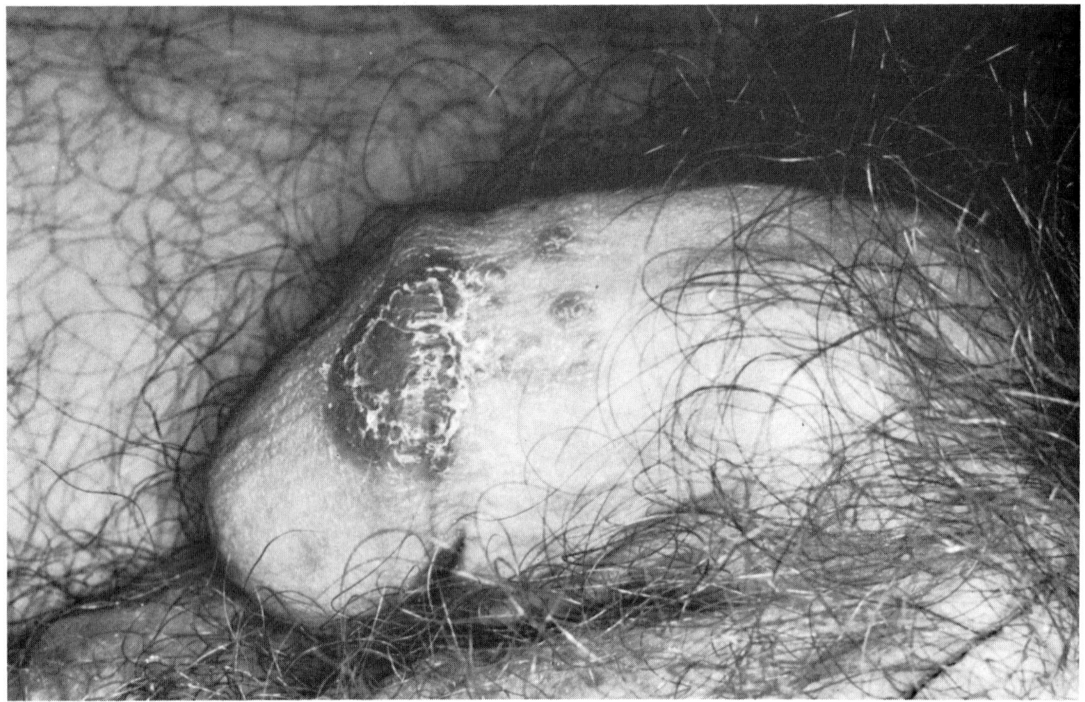

Figure 14–13. Reiter's syndrome. Psoriasiform lesion.

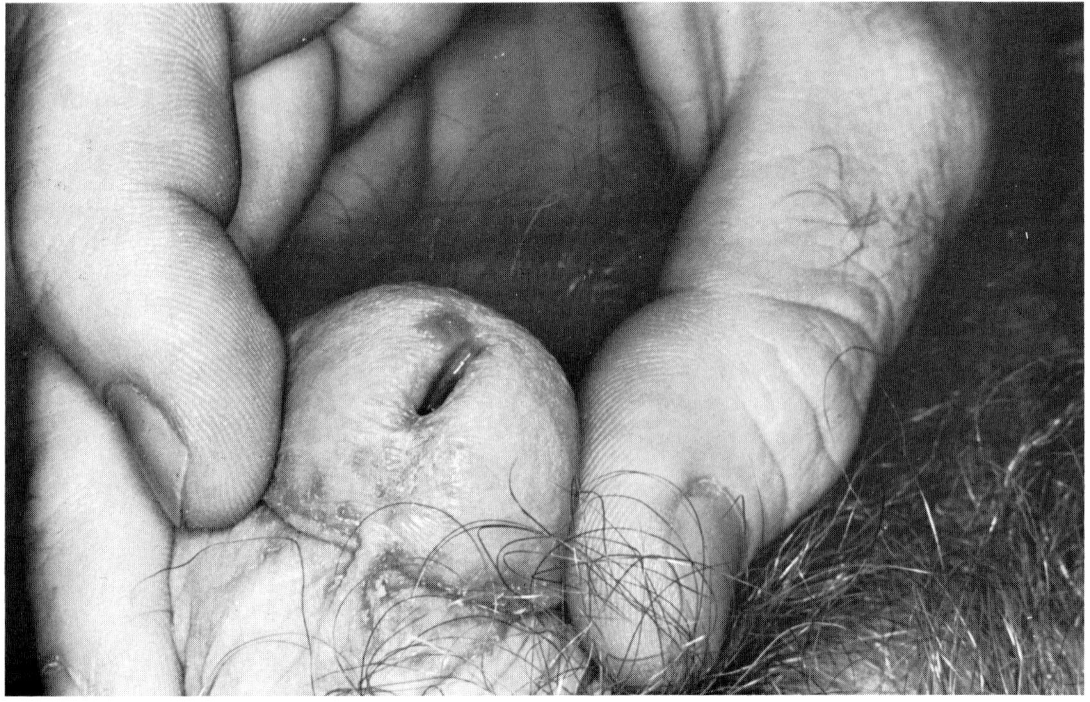

Figure 14–14. Reiter's syndrome. Psoriasiform lesion at urethral meatus.

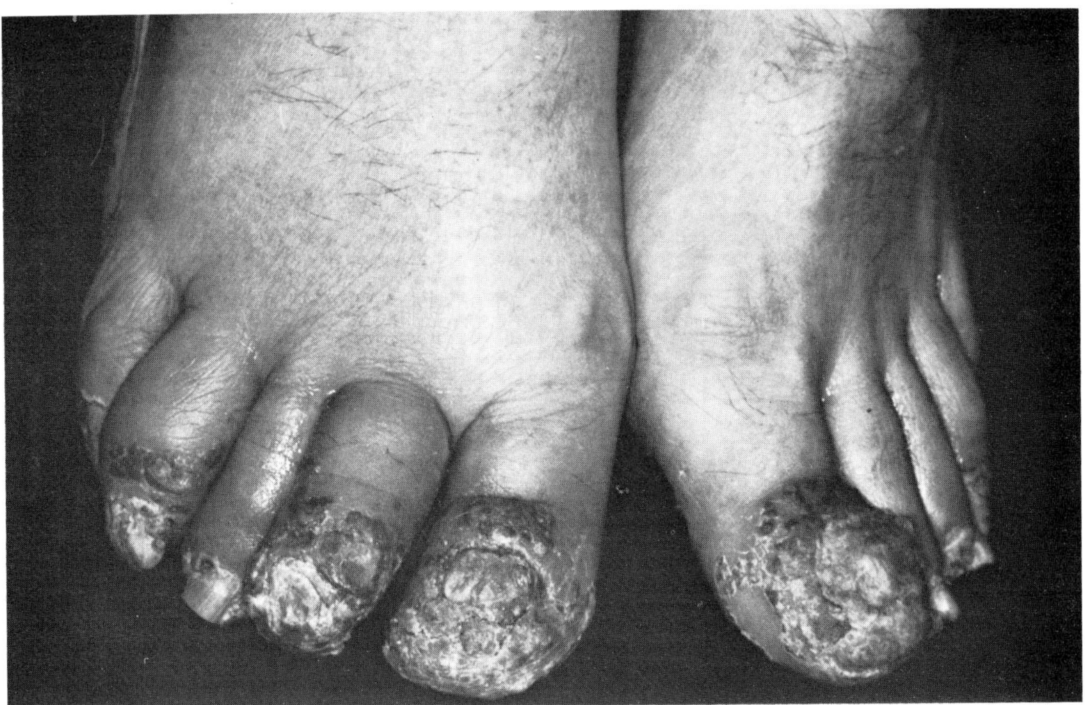

Figure 14–15. Reiter's syndrome. Psoriasiform lesions. Note arthritis in second and fourth toes.

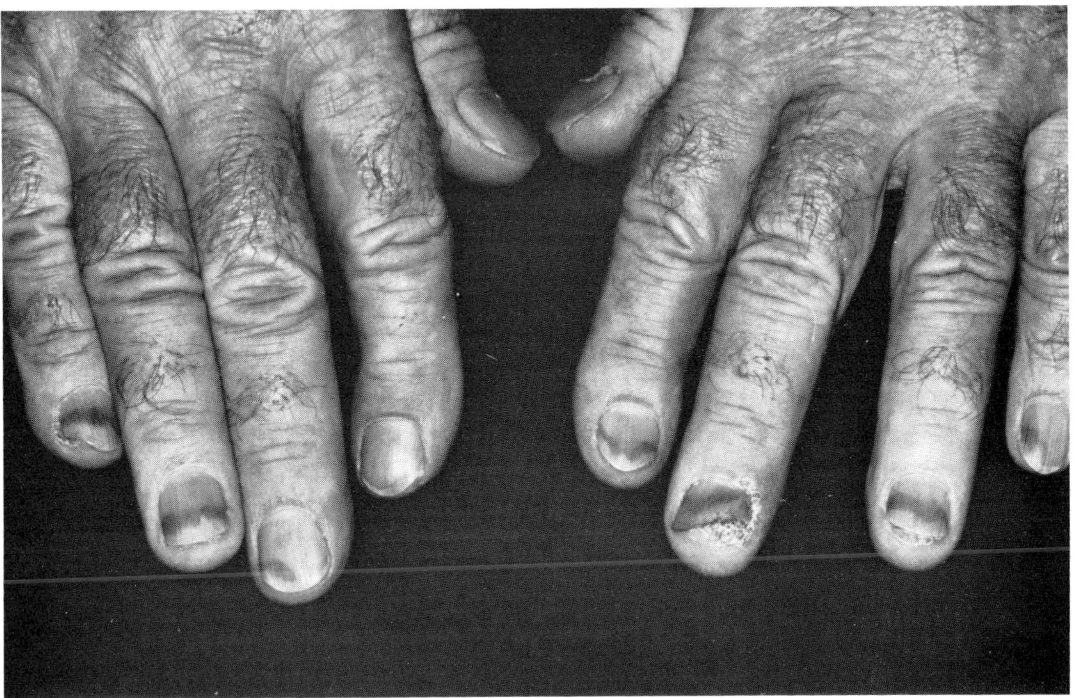

Figure 14–16. Reiter's syndrome. Nail abnormalities are similiar to those of psoriasis.

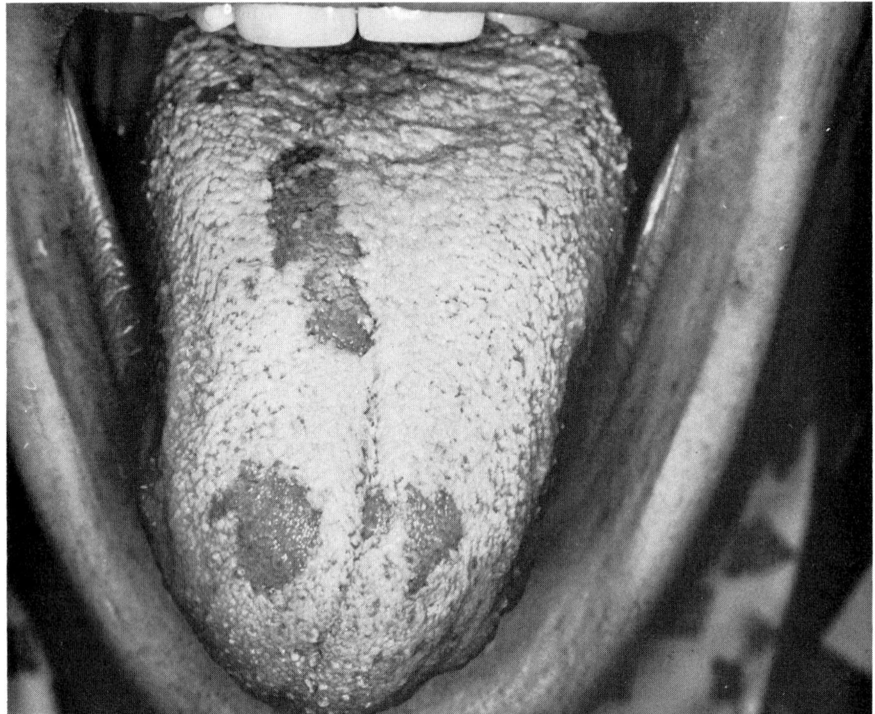

Figure 14–17. Reiter's syndrome. Lingual patches devoid of papillae.

usually persist for only a few days. The tongue may show patches of denuded papillae that superficially resemble geographic tongue (Fig. 14–17).

Reiter's syndrome and psoriasis vulgaris can have identical-appearing cutaneous lesions as described above. The acutely edematous, red, moist, scaling lesions on the fingers and toes of Reiter's syndrome (Fig. 7–92) are indistinguishable from those of pustular psoriasis of von Zumbusch. The histopathologic findings in Reiter's syndrome are identical to those of von Zumbusch disease: massive accumulations of neutrophils within the epidermis forming the spongiform pustule of Kogoj histologically and sterile pustules clinically. At times it is difficult to distinguish clinically between Reiter's syndrome and psoriasis vulgaris or pustular psoriasis of von Zumbusch. However, helpful differentiating points include the following: Reiter's syndrome, in contrast to both forms of psoriasis, occurs almost exclusively in men; psoriasis vulgaris does not have mucosal lesions, conjunctivitis, or urethritis; von Zumbusch disease may exhibit mucosal lesions similar to those of Reiter's syndrome, but it lacks the conjunctivitis, urethritis, and predilection for males. Both Reiter's syndrome and von Zumbusch disease exhibit an increased prevalence of HLA-B27. Psoriasis vulgaris is associated with HLA-B13 and B17. Reiter's syndrome and pustular psoriasis have several features in common and may represent disorders with closely related pathogenetic mechanisms but with different etiologies. There have been several reports of patients who have had seemingly typical attacks of Reiter's syndrome which have later evolved into classic psoriasis vulgaris.[35]

Psoriasis

Arthritis in varying degrees of severity is present in about 30 per cent of psoriatics. It behaves as spondylitis or rheumatoid arthritis in many patients, and some individuals even develop arthritis mutilans. The patterns of arthritis are the same in both psoriasis vulgaris and pustular psoriasis of von Zumbusch and at times may be indistinguishable from those in Reiter's syndrome. However, a significant number of persons have a form of arthritis that appears to be relatively specific for psoriasis. Instead of the proximal finger and toe joints, which are affected in rheumatoid arthritis, the distal interphalangeal joints of the fingers and toes become red, swollen, and painful (Fig. 14–18). Blunt sausage-shaped fingers are produced by active psoriatic arthritis. Rheumatoid factor is absent from the sera of patients with psoriatic arthritis. The activity of any of the varieties of arthritis in psoriasis does not always correlate with the behavior of the cutaneous lesions, nor can distal finger joint involvement be correlated with the presence of psoriatic abnormalities in the nails.

Ochronosis

Ochronosis (alkaptonuria) is an inborn error of tyrosine metabolism. Homogentisic acid accumulates in the tissues and is excreted in the urine because of the absence of homogentisic acid oxidase. Homogentisic acid polymerizes to form a brown-black pigment that is deposited in articular cartilage, intervertebral discs, and many other tissues. Freshly voided

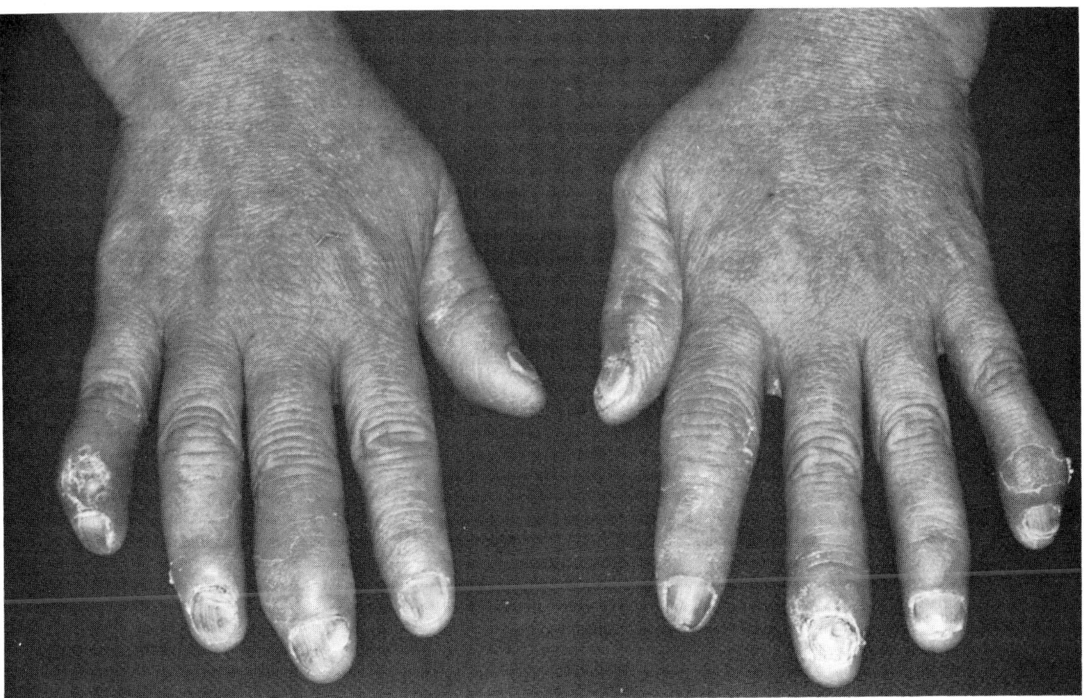

Figure 14–18. Psoriatic arthritis. The distal interphalangeal joints are characteristically involved, and the fingers may become blunt and sausage-shaped.

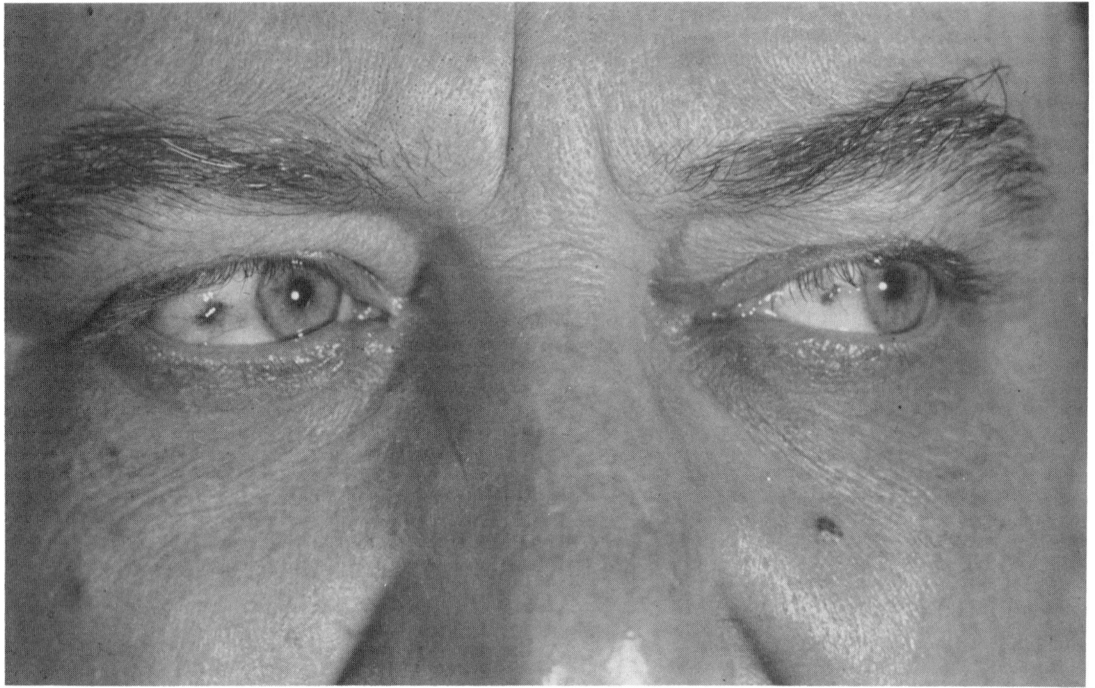

Figure 14–19. Ochronosis. Pigmented spots on sclerae.

urine contains homogentisic acid that polymerizes on standing, turning the urine black.

Spondylitis and osteoarthritis of the major weight-bearing joints are the arthritic complications of ochronosis and are believed to be a direct result of the deposition of the black pigment in the cartilage.[36]

The cutaneous manifestations of ochronosis are produced by the polymerization of homogentisic acid.[37] A 1- to 2-mm brown-black spot of pigment can be found on the sclera midway between the limbus and the outer or inner canthus (Fig. 14–19). The cartilage of the ears becomes irregularly thickened, inflexible, and slate-blue. Sometimes the malar, nasal, axillary, and inguinal skin areas are also hyperpigmented. Even the eardrum and cerumen can be black. The homogentisic acid is secreted in the sweat, where it polymerizes. As a result, the perspiration in the axillary, inguinal, and malar areas may contain pigment that looks like beads of ink on the skin. Clothing may be stained. The fingernails may be blue gray.[38]

Gout

Uric acid accumulates in the skin and in the periarticular tissues to produce the striking cutaneous changes in gout. These accumulations are known as tophi, and they develop chiefly on the helix and antihelix of the ear (Fig. 14–20) and in the olecranon and prepatellar bursae. However, uric acid accumulations can also be found in the tendons of fingers, wrists, toes, and ankles, and even in bone, myocardium, and heart valves. They form the knobby deformities in the skin over joints (Figs. 14–21 and 14–22; Plate 39*E*).

Tophi increase in size and number with the duration of the disease.

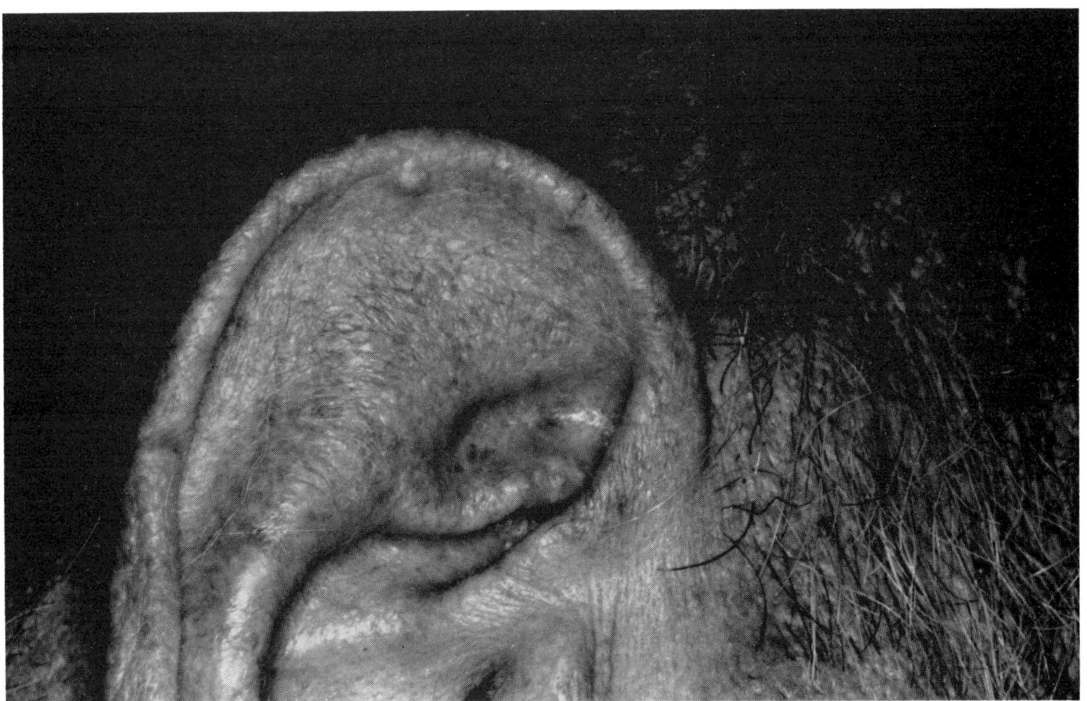

Figure 14–20. Gout. Tophus on ear.

Tophi may be as small as 1 mm or as large as 7 cm. They are white or yellow and may discharge their chalky contents if the overlying skin breaks down. If a lesion is suspected of being a tophus, it should be aspirated, and the contents should be examined by a microscope with polarizing lenses to detect the characteristic birefringence of uric acid crystals (Fig. 14–23).

In acute gouty attacks, the great toe, ankle, or foot is usually involved. The skin over these affected joints is usually hot, dusky red, edematous, and tender to the touch. The appearance simulates an acute bacterial cellulitis, The initial episode of acute gout is often misdiagnosed and treated as a cellulitis.

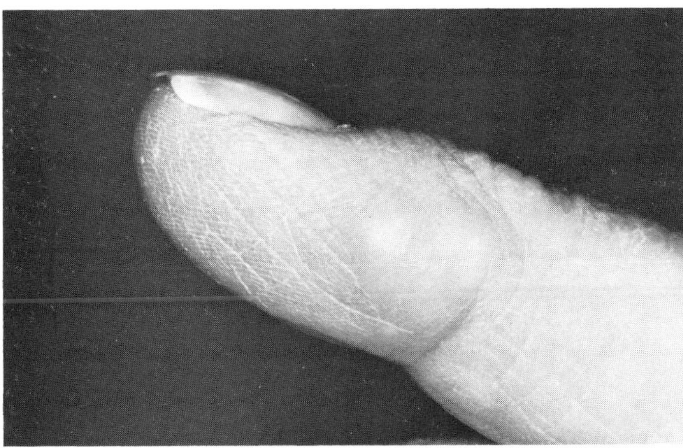

Figure 14–21. Gout. Tophi on finger.

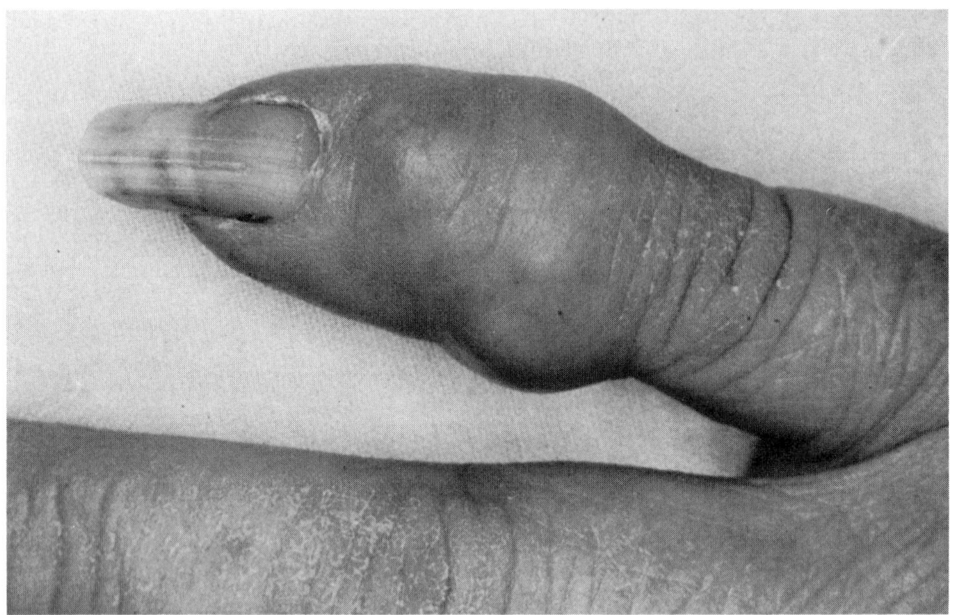

Figure 14–22. Gouty tophi on finger.

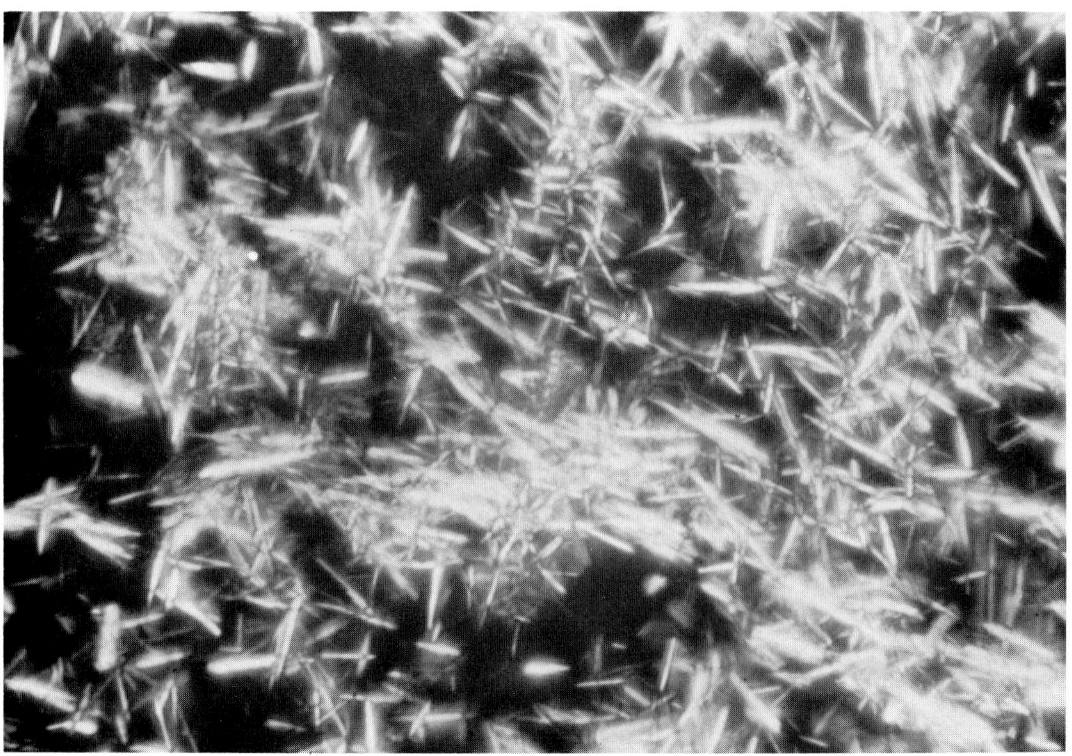

Figure 14–23. Uric acid crystals from tophus photographed with polarizing lenses.

THE PANNICULITIDES

Panniculitis is a term applied to diseases in which the major abnormality is an inflammation of the subcutaneous fat. Fat necrosis is usually present and is often accompanied by severe vascular changes. Arteries and veins of all sizes may show degenerative or proliferative changes and have a dense inflammatory infiltrate in their walls. However, the histologic appearance is not that of leukocytoclastic angiitis, which is discussed in Chapter 8. In some of the panniculitides there is fat necrosis without a significant vascular reaction, and in others there may be edema and a perivascular lymphocytic infiltrate in the fibrous septa between the fat lobules without fat necrosis. A large number of syndromes have been described on the basis of the different histologic patterns and varied clinical manifestations. Unfortunately, few cases have been adequately observed or studied long enough to determine the true nature of these disorders. It is beyond the scope of this section to detail the clinical chaos associated with this group of diseases, and the reader is referred to references that do specify the clinical and histopathologic problems for these disorders.[39-43]

Most patients with panniculitis are women. The clinical lesions are red to violaceous nodules and plaques that have a predilection for the calf of the leg. The bumps may be tender and may ulcerate, or they may remain asymptomatic and intact. They usually arise in groups of two and three, run a course of several weeks, and frequently leave hyperpigmented depressed areas in the skin. The panniculitides tend to be chronic and recurrent. They may, of course, leave no residual marks when they resolve. Pierini et al. have for several years studied and observed a large number of patients with various types of panniculitis. They have come to the conclusion that the various panniculitides represent one disease that has varying clinical expressions and histopathology. They have observed conversion of one type of panniculitis into another.[39] These authors may be correct, and more careful studies such as theirs are needed.

However, from the practical standpoint of diagnosis and management, patients with panniculitis can be placed into the following groups.

1. Erythema nodosum is a form of panniculitis, although fat necrosis does not occur. Perivascular lymphocytic infiltrates with edema in the fibrous septa are the histologic features (see Chapter 9). The lesions resolve without scarring and rarely ever involve the calves of the legs. Subacute nodular migratory panniculitis of Vilanova, Aguade, Perry, and Winkelmann, and erythema nodosum migrans of Bäfverstedt are chronic forms of erythema nodosum.[44]

2. Cold-induced panniculitis is an entity that occurs in children and women. Cold weather produces red nodules and plaques on the calves with a livedo mottling. Systemic diseases are not associated with this group of patients.[40, 45]

3. Circulating lipases from pancreatic carcinoma and acute and chronic pancreatitis can produce fat necrosis that results in red tender subcutaneous nodules that simulate erythema nodosum. Fever, eosinophilia, and joint pain are accompanying features (see p. 39).

4. Panniculitis may be factitial. Patients may have injected foreign material into their skin, or they may have traumatized their limbs or trunk

for a variety of emotional reasons. This possibility should be considered in any case of panniculitis in which the cause is not readily determined.

5. Necrotizing arteritis of small vessels or classic periarteritis nodosa can produce red tender subcutaneous nodules. An adequate excisional biopsy will establish the correct diagnosis. Fever and other systemic signs and symptoms are usually present.

6. Poststeroid panniculitis is a rare entity.[46] Most cases have occurred in children who were on long-term corticosteroid therapy for rheumatic fever. When the steroid dose was discontinued or significantly tapered, subcutaneous nodules appeared one to thirteen days later. The nodules promptly disappeared when the steroid dose was increased again, and in mild cases the nodules disappeared after several months without any therapy. Taranta et al. have suggested that the panniculitis occurred in those areas that showed the greatest accumulation of fat during steroid therapy. The loss of factors leading to the accumulation of fat and the attendant accelerated removal of lipid following the withdrawal of steroids may have injured the fat cells.[47]

7. However, in most patients the panniculitis is of unknown etiology, and it is *not* associated with systemic disease. The histopathology in this group exhibits both fat necrosis and inflammation of arteries and veins. Fibrosis, tuberculoid granulomas, or caseation necrosis is also frequently present in the subcutaneous fat. It is not clear whether the fat necrosis is caused by the observed vascular changes or whether the "vasculitis" is a reaction to the abnormalities in the fat. This varied histopathology has been responsible for the variety of names that have been applied to this chronic recurrent nonspecific panniculitis, e.g., erythema induratum, nodular vasculitis, and Darier-Roussy sarcoid. The majority of patients with this form of panniculitis are women. The lesions are erythematous nodules and plaques that occur chiefly on the calves but that can also develop on the arms and trunk. The eruption is chronic, and the lumps sometimes break down. Pierini et al. suggest the name idiopathic lipogranulomatous hypodermitis for this group of disorders. Rarely, tuberculosis may cause this type of panniculitis. However, culture of the involved tissues and inguinal nodes, if they are enlarged, is necessary to establish the diagnosis of a tuberculous infection. The patient illustrated in Figures 14–24 and 14–25 was initially thought to have idiopathic hypodermatitis, but *Mycobacterium tuberculosis* was eventually isolated from an inguinal node and her panniculitis was cured with antituberculous therapy.

8. Lupus profundus is a variety of panniculitis associated with lupus erythematosus. The lesions are generally well-circumscribed red nodules or plaques that may undergo ulceration (see p. 266).

9. Weber-Christian disease (relapsing febrile nonsuppurative nodular panniculitis) is a rare, but real, entity.[48] The initial histopathologic event seems to be acute fat necrosis that develops in the absence of vascular disease. In the later stages of the disorder, vascular changes develop, but they are never as severe as in idiopathic lipogranulomatous hypodermitis. The cutaneous manifestations are characterized by *crops* of tender or nontender red subcutaneous nodules that are associated with fever, malaise, and sometimes arthralgias (Plate 39*F*). The nodules may break down and leak oil. Usually a depression in the skin, caused by fat necrosis, accompanies the resolution of a lesion. In some patients,

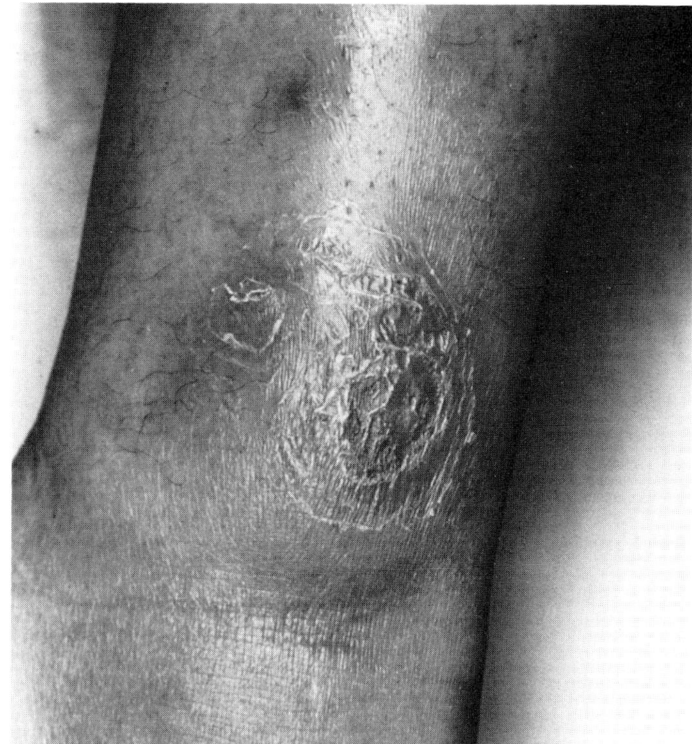

Figure 14–24. Panniculitis over lower ankle caused by infection with *Mycobacterium tuberculosis*.

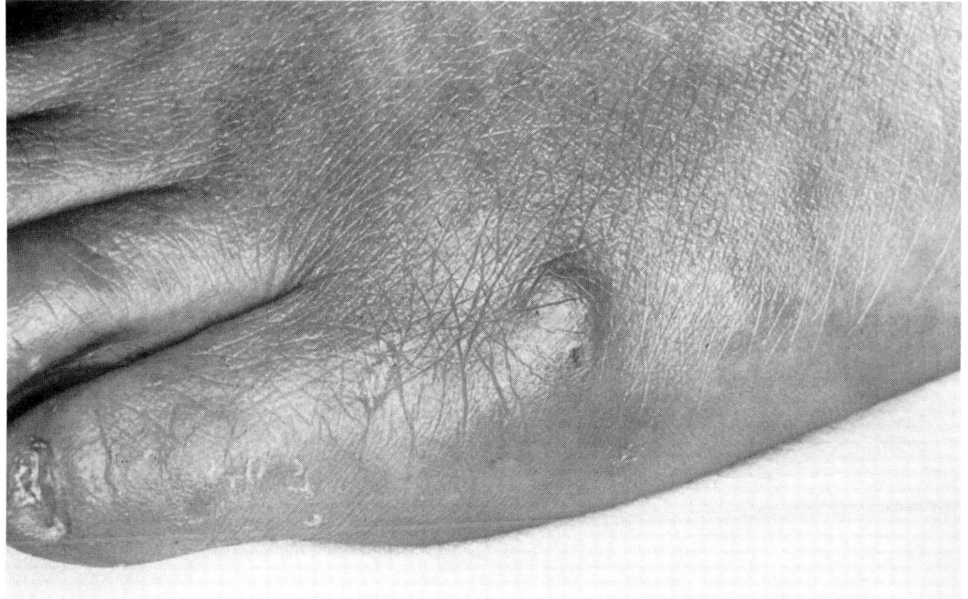

Figure 14–25. Nodule produced by tuberculous panniculitis. Same patient as in Figure 14–24.

visceral fat — mesenteric and pericardial — is also affected. Anemia, leukopenia, generalized lymphadenopathy, and weight loss have occurred in some patients. We cared for one patient who had hypersplenism with leukopenia, anemia, and thrombocytopenia, in association with typical Weber-Christian disease. He died of septicemia after two and one half years of illness. Weber-Christian disease is not as clearly defined in the literature as one would like, since this diagnosis frequently has been applied indiscriminately to the more common nonfebrile nonspecific panniculitis described previously. The diagnosis of Weber-Christian disease should be applied only to cases in which the signs, symptoms, and histopathology are characteristic and in which the specific causes for acute panniculitis summarized above, especially LE, have been excluded. Weber-Christian disease has also been closely mimicked by the immune complex syndrome folowing jejunoileal bypass surgery for morbid obesity.[49]

Similar histopathologic changes in the subcutaneous fat are found in the absence of systemic signs in subcutaneous lipogranulomatosis of Rothmann-Makai. This disorder occurs in children. Its relationship to Weber-Christian disease is unclear. Pierini et al. would group Weber-Christian disease, Rothmann-Makai syndrome, and idiopathic lipogranulomatous hypodermitis into a single entity, but I believe that the evidence for Weber-Christian disease as a separate entity is strong.

REFERENCES

1. Pope, F. M.: Autosomal dominant forms of pseudo-xanthoma elasticum. J. Med. Genet., *11*:152, 1974.
2. Pope, F. M.: Two types of autosomal recessive pseudoxanthoma elasticum. Arch. Dermatol., *110*:209, 1974.
3. Goodman, R. M., Smith, E. W., Paton, D., Bergman, R. A., Siegel, C. L., Otteson, O., Shelley, W. M., Pusch, A. L., and McKusick, V. A.: Pseudoxanthoma elasticum. A clinical and histopathological study. Medicine (Balt.), *42*:297, 1963.
4. McKusick, V. A.: Heritable Disorders of Connective Tissue, 4th ed. C. V. Mosby, St. Louis, 1972.
5. Hashimoto, K., and DiBella, R. J.: Electron microscopic studies of normal and abnormal elastic fibers of the skin, J. Invest. Dermatol., *48*:405, 1967.
6. Hentzer, B., Nielsen, A. O., Johnsen, F., Kobayasi, T., and Danielsen, L.: In vitro calcification of connective tissue from uninvolved skin of patients with pseudoxanthoma elasticum. Arch. Dermatol. Res., *258*:219, 1977.
7. Martinez-Hernandez, A., and Huffer, W. E.: Pseudoxanthoma elasticum: dermal polyanions and the mineralization of elastic fibers. Lab. Invest., *31*:181, 1974.
8. Parker, J. C., Friedman-Kien, A. E., Levin, S., and Bartler, F. C.: Pseudoxanthoma elasticum and hypertension. N. Engl. J. Med., *271*:1204, 1964.
9. Green, W. R., Friedman-Klein, A., and Banfield, W. G.: Angioid streaks in Ehlers-Danlos syndrome. Arch. Ophthalmol., *76*:197, 1966.
10. Harvey, W. P., Pope, F. M., and Grahame, R.: Cutaneous extensibility in pseudoxanthoma elasticum. Br. J. Dermatol., *97*:679, 1975.
11. Uitto, J., and Lichentenstein, J. R.: Defects in the biochemistry of collagen in diseases of connective tissue. J. Invest. Dermatol., *66*:59, 1976.
12. Hashimoto, K., and Kanzaki, T.: Cutis laxa. Ultrastructural and biochemical studies. Arch. Dermatol., *111*:861, 1975.

12a. Goltz, R., Hult, A., Goldfarb, M., and Gorlin, R. J.: Cutis laxa. A manifestation of generalized elastolysis. Arch. Dermatol., *92*:373, 1965.

13. Hayden, J. G., Talner, N. S., and Klaus, S. N.: Cutis laxa associated with pulmonary artery stenosis. J. Pediatr., *72*:506, 1968.
14. Prockop, D. J., Kivirikko, K. I., Tuderman, L., and Guzman, W. A.: The biosynthesis of collagen and its disorders. N. Engl. J. Med., *301*:13, 77, 1979.
15. Beighton, P., Price, A., Lord, J., and Dickson, E.: Variants of the Ehlers-Danlos syndrome: clinical, biochemical, haematological, and chromosomal features in 100 patients. Ann. Rheum. Dis., *28*:228, 1969.
16. Jansen, L. H.: The structure of the connective tissue, an explanation of the symptoms of the Ehlers-Danlos syndrome. Dermatologica, *110*:108, 1955.
17. Grahame, R., and Beighton, P.: Physical properties of the skin in the Ehlers-Danlos

syndrome. Ann. Rheum. Dis., *28*:246, 1969.
18. Pinnell, S. R., Krane, S. M., Kenzora, J. E., and Glimcher, M. J.: A heritable disorder of connective tissue. Hydroxylysine-deficient collagen disease. N. Engl. J. Med., *286*:1013, 1972.
19. Sussman, M. D., Lichtenstein, J. R., Nigra, T., Martin, G. R., and McKusick, V. A.: Hydroxylysine-deficient skin collagen in a patient with a form of Ehlers-Danlos syndrome. J. Bone Joint Surg., *56-A*:1228, 1974.
20. Elsas, L. J., Hollins, B., and Pinnell, S. R.: Hydroxylysine-deficient collagen disease: effect of ascorbic acid. Am. J. Hum. Genet., *26*:28a, 1974.
21. Judisch, G. F., Waziri, M., and Krachmer, J. H.: Ocular Ehlers-Danlos syndrome with normal lysyl hydroxylase activity. Arch. Ophthalmol., *94*:1489, 1976.
22. Lichtenstein, J. R., Martin, G. R., Kohn, L. D., Byers, P. H., and McKusick, V. A.: Defect in conversion of procollagen to collagen in a form of Ehlers-Danlos syndrome. Science, *182*:298, 1973.
23. Lapière, C. M., Lenaers, A., and Kohn, L. D.: Procollagen peptidase; an enzyme excising the coordination peptides of procollagen. Proc. Natl. Acad. Sci. (USA), *68*:3054, 1971.
24. Bailey, A. J., and Lapière, C. M.: Effect of an additional peptide extension of the N-terminus of collagen from dermatosparactic calves on the cross linking of collagen fibers. Eur. J. Biochem., *34*:91, 1973.
25. Steinmann, B., Tuderman, L., Martin, G. R., and Prockop, D. J.: Evidence for a structural mutation of procollagen in a patient with Ehlers-Danlos syndrome Type VII. Eur. J. Pediatr., *130*:203, 1979.
26. McAdam, L. P., O'Hanlan, M. A., Bluestone, R., and Pearson, C. M.: Relapsing polychondritis: prospective study of 23 patients and a review of the literature. Medicine, *55*:193, 1976.
26a. Ruhlen, J. L., Huston, K. A., and Wood, W. G.: Relapsing polychondritis with glomerulonephritis. Improvement with prednisone and cyclophosphamide. J.A.M.A., *245*:847, 1981.
27. Hughes, R. A. C., Berry, C. L., Seifert, M., and Lessof, M. H.: Relapsing polychondritis. Three cases with a clinico-pathological study and literature review. Q. J. Med., *41*:363, 1972.
28. Foidart, J.-M., Abe, S., Martin, G. R., Zizic, T. M., Barnett, E. V., Lawley, T. J., and Katz, S. I.: Antibodies to type II collagen in relapsing polychondritis. N. Engl. J. Med., *299*:1203, 1978.
29. Arundell, R. W., and Haserick, J. R.: Familial chronic atrophic polychondritis. Arch. Dermatol., *82*:439, 1960.
30. Bergfeld, W. F.: Relapsing polychondritis with positive direct immunofluorescence. Arch. Dermatol., *114*:127, 1978.
31. Barranco, V. P.: Inhibition of lysosomal enzymes by dapsone. Arch. Dermatol., *110*:563, 1974.
32. Martin, J. H., Roenigk, H. H., Jr., Lynch, W., and Tingwald, F. R.: Relapsing polychondritis treated with dapsone. Arch. Dermtol., *112*:1272, 1976.
33. Barranco, V. P., Minor, D. B., and Solomon, H.: Treatment of relapsing polychondritis with dapsone. Arch. Dermatol., *112*:1286, 1976.
34. Weinberger, H. S., Ropes, M. W., Kulka, J. P., and Bauer, W.: Reiter's syndrome, clinical and pathologic observations. Medicine (Balt.), *41*:35, 1962.
35. Perry, H. O., and Mayne, J. G.: Psoriasis and Reiter's syndrome. Arch. Dermatol., *92*:129, 1965.
36. O'Brien, W. M., Banfield, W. G., and Sokoloff, L.: Studies on the pathogenesis of ochronotic arthropathy. Arthritis Rheum., *4*:137, 1961.
37. Laymon, C. W.: Ochronosis. Arch. Dermatol. Syph., *67*:553, 1953.
38. Freiberger, H. F., and Pinnell, S. R.: Heritable disorders of connective tissue. *In* Moschella, S. L. (ed.): Dermatology Update, 1979, Reviews for Physicians. Elsevier, New York, 1979, p. 221.
39. Pierini, L. E., Abulafia, J., and Wainfeld, S.: Idiopathic lipogranulomatous hypodermitis. Arch. Dermatol., *98*:290, 1968.
40. Wilkinson, D. S.: The vascular basis of some nodular eruptions of the legs. Br. J. Dermatol., *66*:201, 1954.
41. Montgomery, H., O'Leary, P. A., and Barker, N. W.: Nodular vascular lesions of the legs; erythema induratum and allied conditions. J.A.M.A., *128*:335, 1945.
42. Borrie, P., and Stansfeld, A.: Cutaneous vasculitis. *In* Modern Trends in Dermatology. Vol. 3. Butterworths, London, 1966, p. 182.
43. Förström, L., and Winkelmann, R. K.: Acute panniculitis. A clinical and histopathologic study of 34 cases. Arch. Dermatol., *113*:909, 1977.
44. Perry, H. O., and Winkelmann, R. K.: Subacute nodular migratory panniculitis. Arch. Dermatol., *89*:170, 1964.
45. Solomon, L. M., and Beerman, H.: Cold panniculitis. Arch. Dermatol., *88*:897, 1963.
46. Roenigk, H. H., Jr., Haserick, J. R., and Arundell, F. D.: Poststeroid panniculitis. Arch. Dermatol., *90*:387, 1964.
47. Taranta, A., Mark, H., Haas, R. C., and Cooper, N.: Nodular panniculitis after massive prednisone therapy. Am. J. Med., *25*:52, 1958.
48. Steinberg, B.: Systemic nodular panniculitis. Am. J. Pathol., *29*:1059, 1953.
49. Williams, H. J., Samuelson, C. O., and Zone, J. J.: Nodular nonsuppurative panniculitis associated with jejunoileal bypass surgery. Arch. Dermatol., *115*:1091, 1979.

15

Neutrophilic Dermatoses

There are three striking dermatologic conditions in which the neutrophil is a prominent participant: pustular psoriasis (von Zumbusch), acute febrile neutrophilic dermatosis (Sweet's syndrome), and subcorneal pustular dermatosis (Sneddon-Wilkinson). Each of these entities is characterized by massive neutrophilic migration into the dermis, epidermis, or subcutaneous layer. Collectively, these entities are sometimes referred to as the neutrophilic dermatoses, but they share no similarities with regard to natural history or histopathology. The first two are associated with systemic disease and will be discussed here.

PUSTULAR PSORIASIS (VON ZUMBUSCH)

This disorder arises in two settings: one group of individuals develops pustular psoriasis after many years of psoriasis vulgaris, and the other develops the disease *de novo*. In the extensive series of 104 cases of Baker and Ryan, 60 per cent of individuals had preexisting psoriasis vulgaris.[1] In our series of 11 patients collected since 1970, only three had preexisting psoriasis vulgaris. Females predominate in a ratio of 3:2. Although psoriasis vulgaris tends to appear before the fourth or fifth decades, pustular psoriasis more commonly develops *after* the fourth or fifth and may make its initial presentation in the eighth decade in some individuals. Pustular psoriasis can also develop as early as three to five years of age. In those individuals with preexisting psoriasis vulgaris, one may find a precipitating stress or event to explain the development of the pustular phase. In the *de novo* cases, a causative event is generally not found. Regardless of the setting in which the pustular phase develops, the clinical manifestations are similar. Baker and Ryan have divided them into four major, but not mutually exclusive, groups: the Zumbusch, annular, localized, and exanthematic types.

The *Zumbusch* type is characterized by the sudden development of widespread but discrete areas of warm, painful erythema that become studded with small pustules or large lakes of sterile pus (Figs. 15–1 and 15–2). The pustules are primarily subcorneal collections of neutrophils that characteristically slough off spontaneously after several days or within 24 to 72 hours following topical aqueous compresses (Figs. 15–3 and 15–4). The patches of erythema disappear as well, without leaving any residua. Crops or waves of such lesions affect all portions of the body, including the face and scalp. At times a diffuse erythroderma may develop. Patients may have cycles of such lesions occurring at three- to

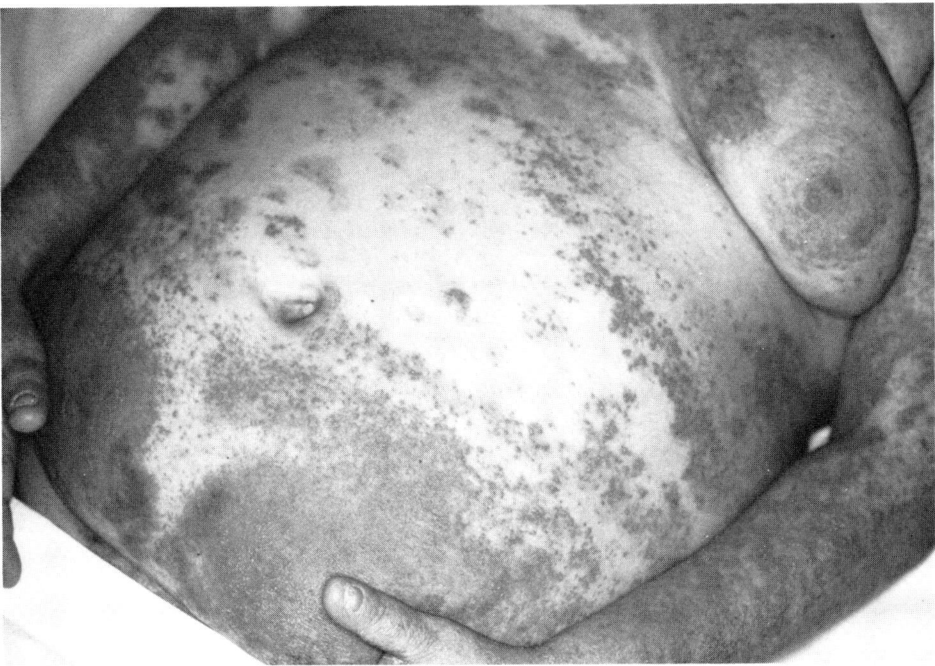

Figure 15–1. Pustular psoriasis (von Zumbusch). Widespread, often painful erythema studded with sterile pustules or large lakes of pus.

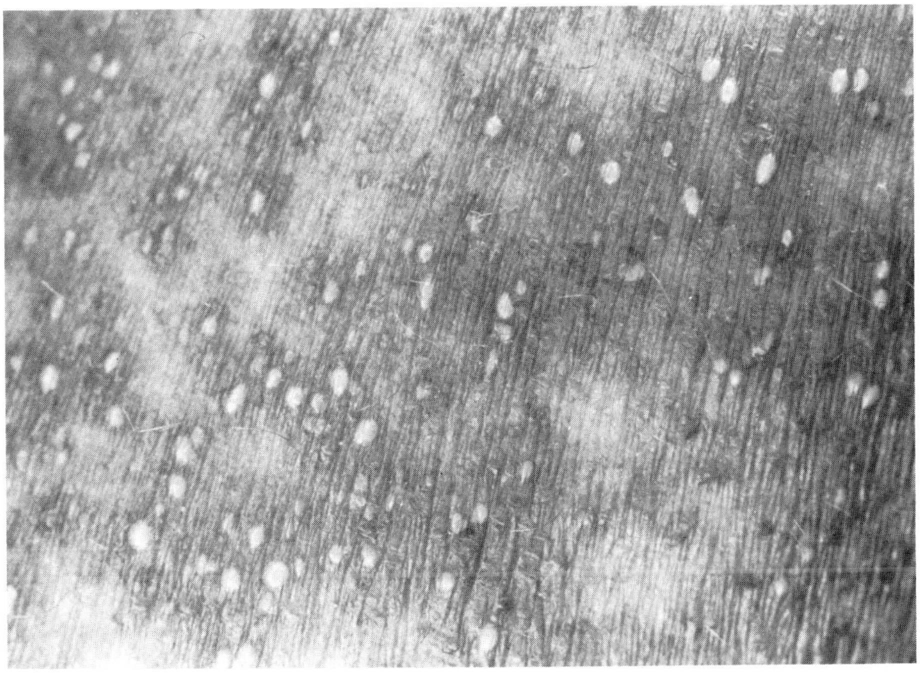

Figure 15–2. Pustular psoriasis (von Zumbusch). Close-up of sterile pustules on base of erythema.

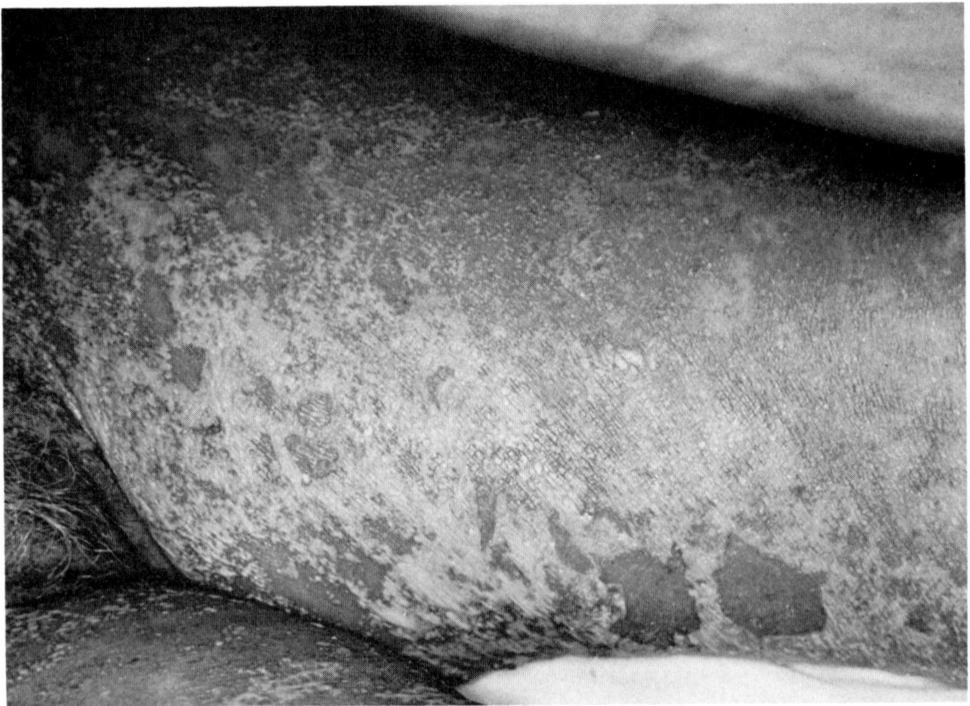

Figure 15–3. Pustular psoriasis (von Zumbusch). Pustules and lakes of pus beginning to slough.

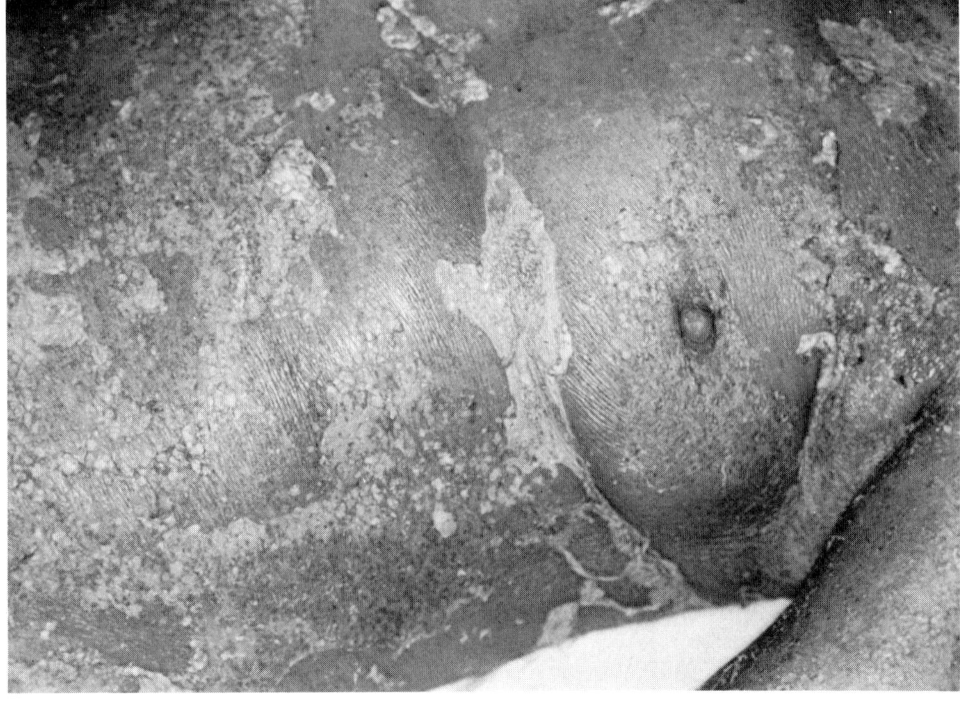

Figure 15–4. Pustular psoriasis (von Zumbusch). Lakes of pus sloughing.

ten-day intervals for several months. Characteristically, as the disease begins to remit over the course of weeks, the crops of lesions become less extensive and less severe. Severe systemic reactions, such as fevers of 100 to 104°F, chills and malaise, accompanied by leukocytosis and neutrophilia, are common in the severe phases of the disease and become milder and eventually disappear as the disorder slowly begins to enter a remission. Remissions usually last for several months but can be as brief as one to two months or as long as 12 to 24 months.

In the *annular* type, arciform and polycyclic rings of erythema studded with pustules appear and advance, leaving behind clear centers (Figs. 15–5 to 15–7). Systemic symptoms are less common with this manifestation of the disease. Patterned lesions can accompany the Zumbusch type, and some patients may have a Zumbusch manifestation with one episode and an annular one with another. The individual patterned lesions may persist for long periods of time — seven to 14 days — and they also arise in crops.

The *exanthematic* type arises *de novo*, is not common, and usually

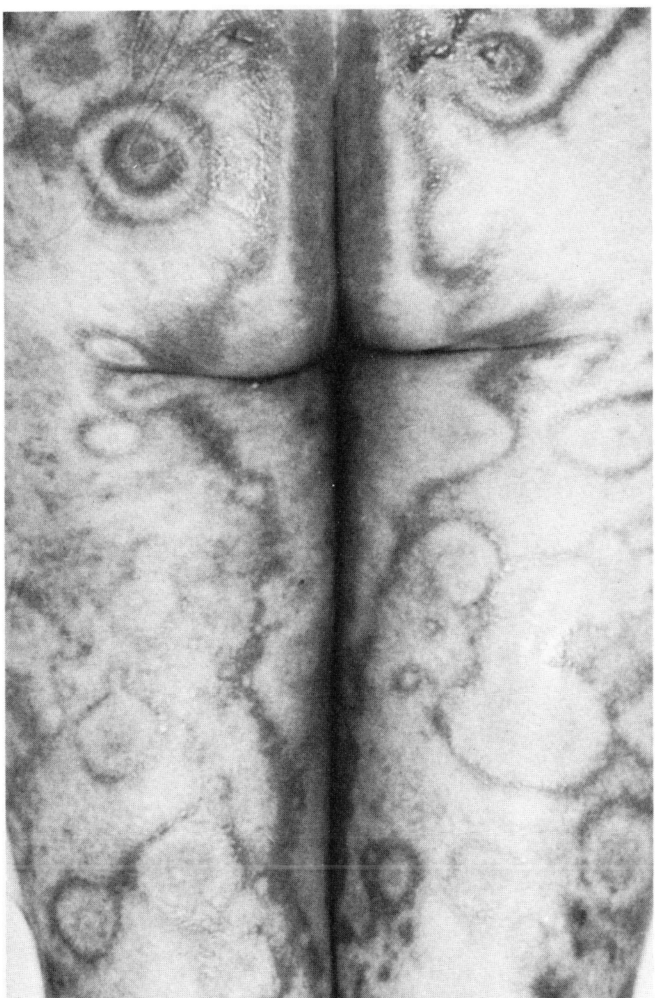

Figure 15–5. Pustular psoriasis (von Zumbusch). Arciform and polycyclic rings.

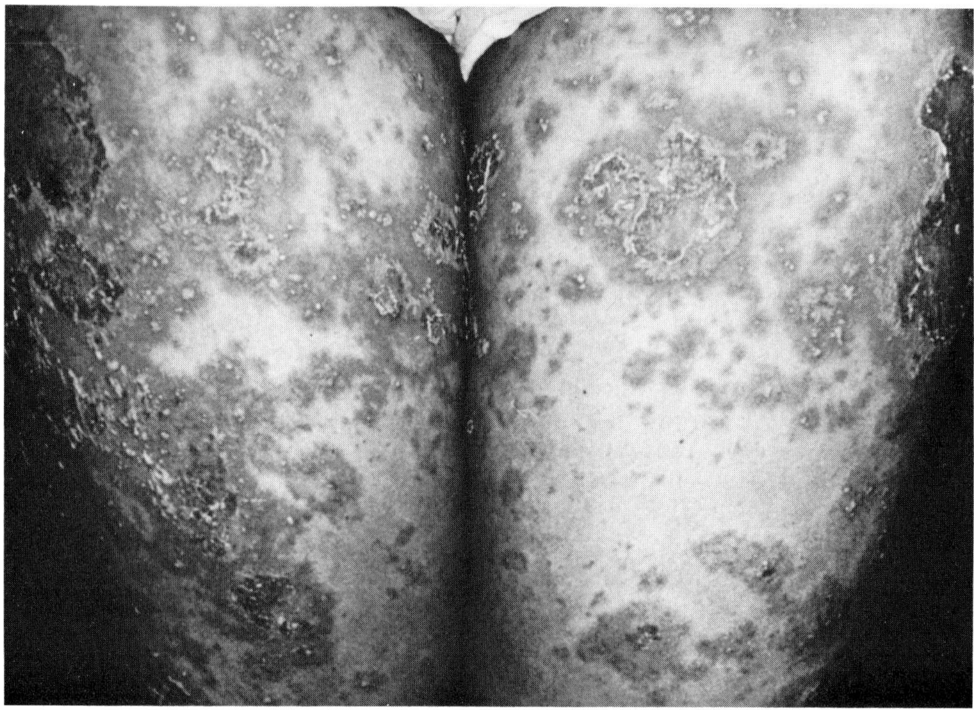

Figure 15–6. Pustular psoriasis (von Zumbusch). Arciform and polycyclic rings studded with pustules.

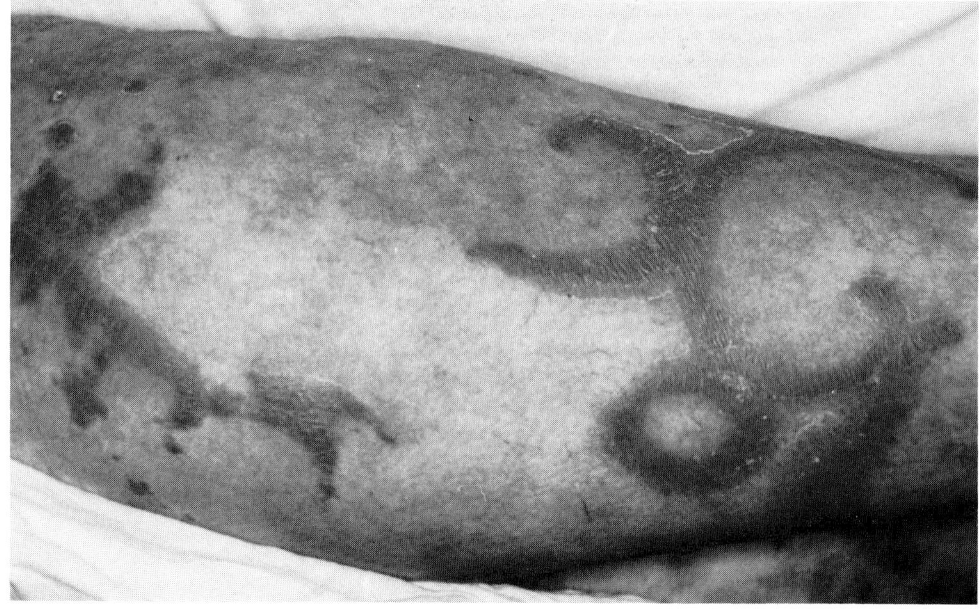

Figure 15–7. Pustular psoriasis (von Zumbusch). Arciform lesions.

follows an upper respiratory infection. It resembles the Zumbusch pattern but usually is a single short-lived episode lasting a few weeks, analogous to the guttate flare of ordinary psoriasis.

The *localized* form represents restricted areas of pustules on or around ordinary psoriatic plaques. In my experience this has been seen most often in patients with psoriasis vulgaris who have overreacted to the Goeckerman regimen or whose skin has been irritated by topical medications. The development of such lesions does not appear to constitute a significant hazard for the development of generalized pustular disease.

In a small number of individuals the pustules are limited to the hands and feet, especially the distal digits and subungual tissues (Figs. 15–8 and 15–9). Such cases have been called acrodermatitis continua of Hallopeau. Foreshortening of the terminal phalanges because of acro-osteolysis secondary to chronic fingertip involvement occurred in one of our patients (Figs. 15–10 and 15–11). In some cases, the disease has been provoked by and limited to pregnancy. In these instances, the disorder has been termed impetigo herpetiformis. Clearly, they are all manifestations of the same disorder: pustular psoriasis (von Zumbusch). In a few patients with pustular psoriasis, the individual lesions have a papulosquamous appearance, but close inspection reveals small pustules beneath the silvery scale (Figs. 15–12 and 15–13). These localized manifestations of the disease are indistinguishable from some of the lesions in Reiter's syndrome.

A frequent accompaniment of the acute eruption is annulus migrans (geographic tongue) (Figs. 15–14 to 15–16).[2] These whitish, arciform, and polycyclic rings may be present on the tongue, buccal mucosa, and

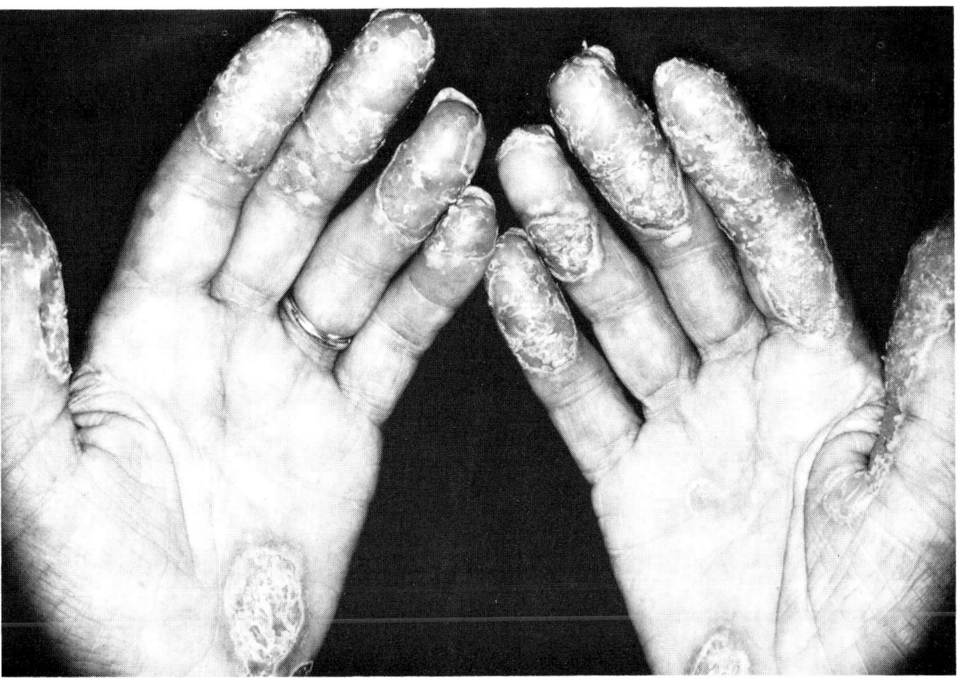

Figure 15–8. Pustular psoriasis (von Zumbusch). Pustules limited to hands, distal digits, and subungual tissues. Also called acrodermatitis continua of Hallopeau. (From O'Keefe, E., Braverman, I. M., and Cohen, I.: Annulus migrans. Identical lesions in pustular psoriasis, Reiter's syndrome, and geographic tongue. Arch. Dermatol., *107*:240, 1973.)

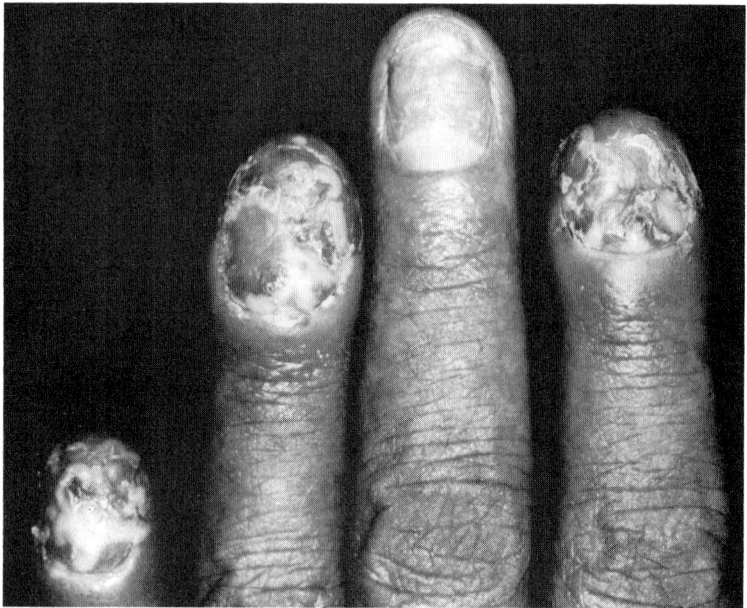

Figure 15–9. Pustular psoriasis (von Zumbusch). Lakes of pus are present under dystrophic fingernails. (From Braverman, I. M., Cohen, I., and O'Keefe, E.: Metabolic and ultrastructural studies in a patient with pustular psoriasis (von Zumbusch). Arch. Dermatol., *105*:189, 1972.)

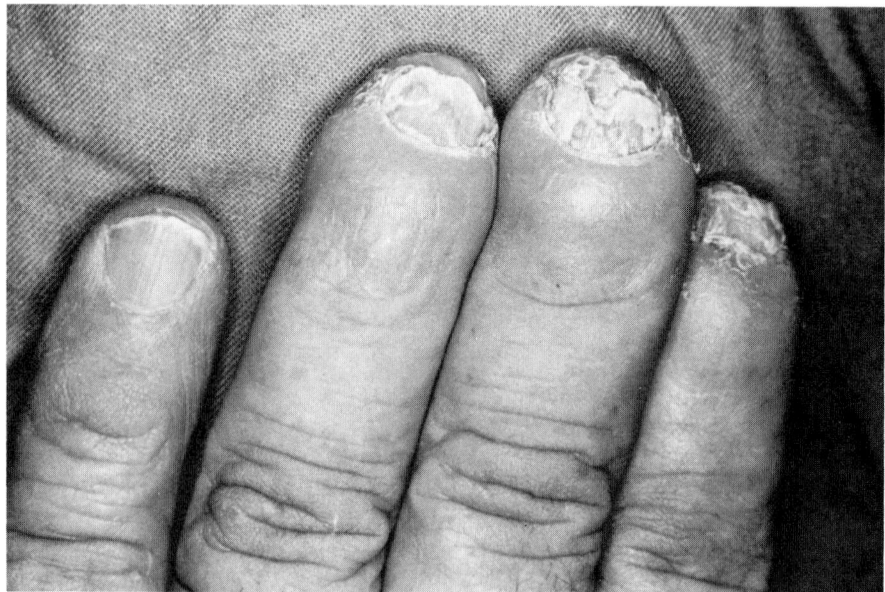

Figure 15–10. Pustular psoriasis (von Zumbusch). Foreshortening of terminal phalanges due to acro-osteolysis.

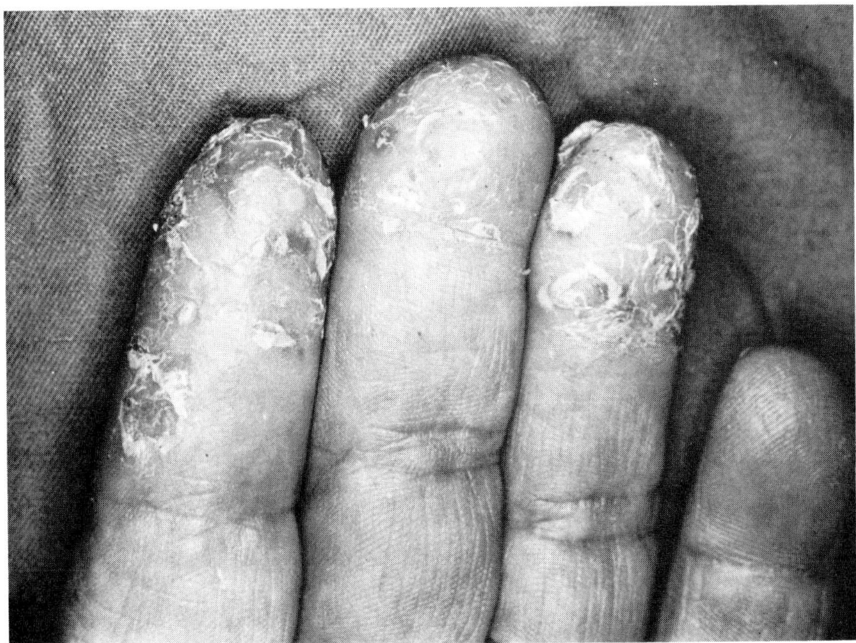

Figure 15–11. Same patient as in Figure 15–10 showing pustule formation on fingertips.

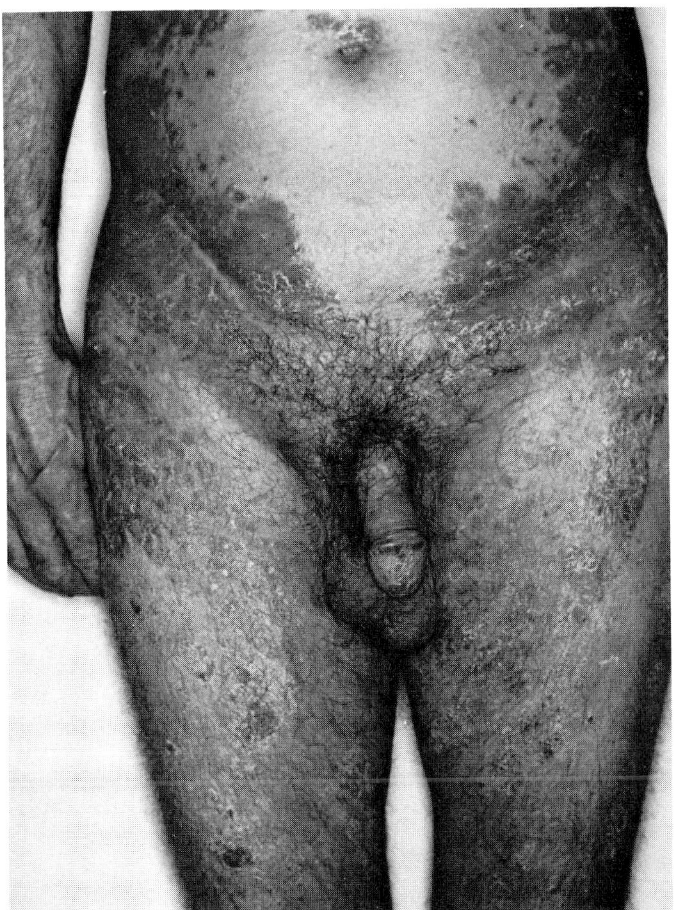

Figure 15–12. Pustular psoriasis (von Zumbusch). Superficially the lesions have a papulosquamous appearance, but inspection reveals small pustules beneath the silvery scale.

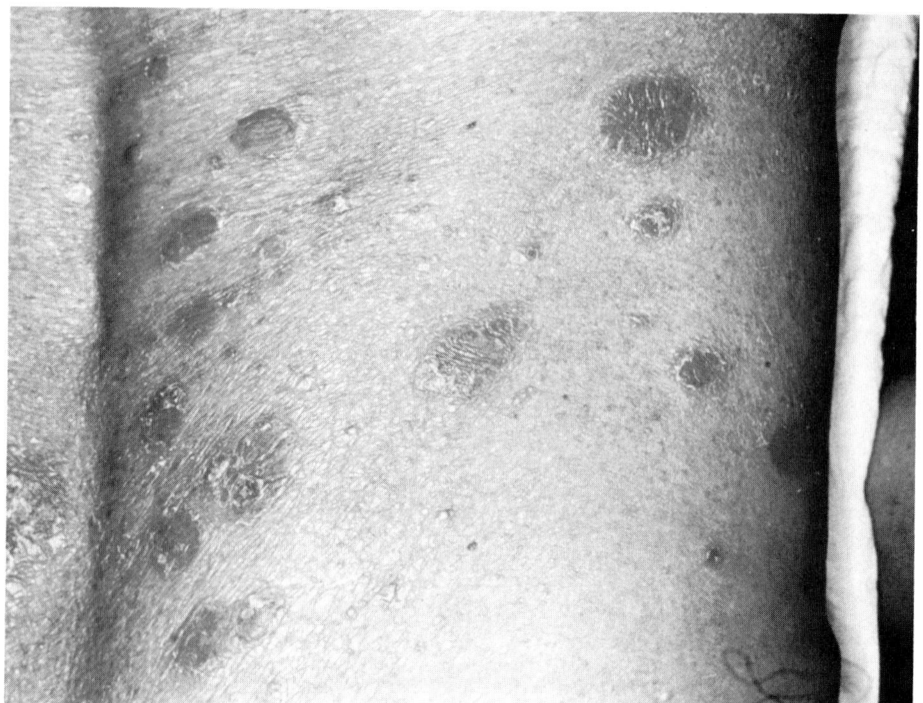

Figure 15–13. Pustular psoriasis (von Zumbusch). Small pustules are present beneath the scales of what appear to be papulosquamous lesions.

gingivae and can be observed to change shape daily. Although they are often present during acute flares, they are not directly related to disease activity because they may be present when the skin is otherwise normal or only minimally affected. Baker and Ryan described erosions, blisters, and pustules in the oral cavity and on the lips of patients with pustular psoriasis.[1]

Considerable cutaneous edema may develop during the acute phase of pustular psoriasis. Misdiagnoses of congestive heart failure, cellulitis, and thrombophlebitis may be made at these times. The edema that develops suddenly usually disappears just as rapidly when the acute episode begins to remit. These wide swings in cutaneous vascular permeability may be associated with profound and at times irreversible changes in the systemic circulation (see below).

There are clearly provocative factors in those cases of pustular psoriasis arising in patients with long-standing psoriasis vulgaris. Baker and Ryan found that withdrawal or reduction in dose of corticosteroids prescribed previously for various reasons was associated with the development of pustular psoriasis in one third of their patients. Identical observations have been made in Japan.[3] The immediate inciting events of the *de novo* disease were generally never detected, but in a few cases an upper respiratory infection or pregnancy was implicated. Emotional tension may be a precipitating factor.[4,5] Lithium carbonate taken for manic-depressive psychosis provoked generalized pustular psoriasis in a patient with previously stable psoriasis vulgaris.[6]

Arthritis was a feature in 30 per cent of patients — a prevalence similar to that observed in psoriasis vulgaris. The clinical features of the arthritis were identical in both forms of psoriasis.

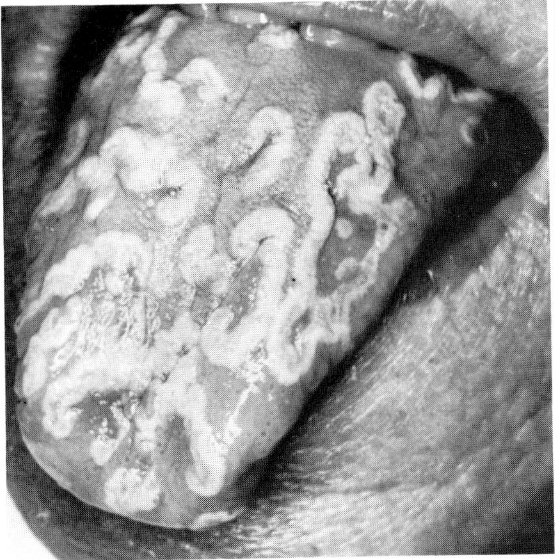

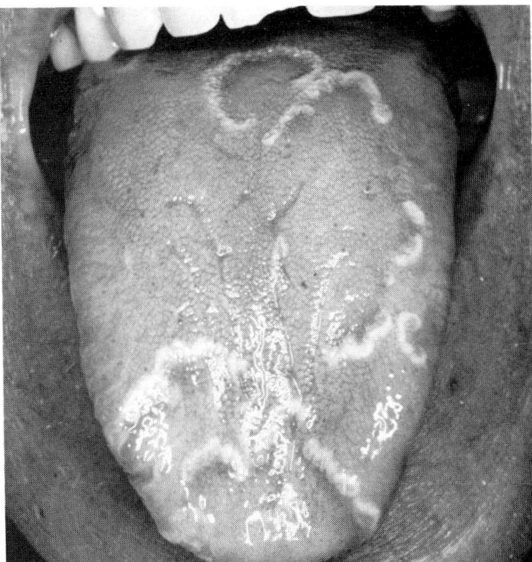

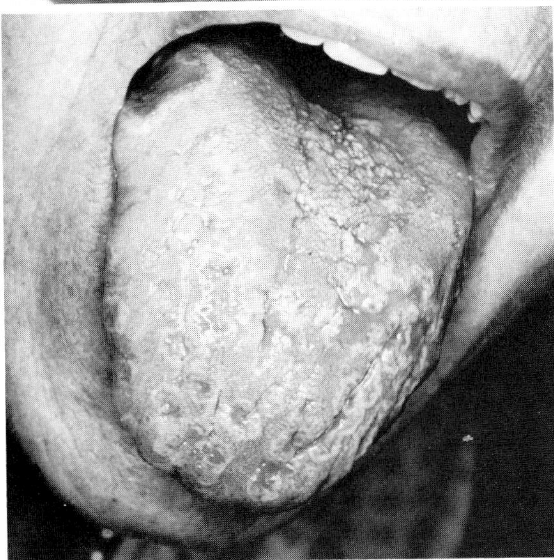

Figure 15–14. Top left. Pustular psoriasis (von Zumbusch). Annulus migrans (geographic tongue). (From O'Keefe, E., Braverman, I. M., and Cohen, I.: Annulus migrans. Identical lesions in pustular psoriasis, Reiter's syndrome, and geographic tongue. Arch. Dermatol., *107*:240, 1973.)

Figure 15–15. Top right. Pustular psoriasis (von Zumbusch). Annulus migrans. (From O'Keefe, E., Braverman, I. M., and Cohen, I.: Annulus migrans. Identical lesions in pustular psoriasis, Reiter's syndrome, and geographic tongue. Arch. Dermatol., *107*:240, 1973.)

Figure 15–16. Bottom left. Pustular psoriasis (von Zumbusch). Annulus migrans.

Most clinicians dealing with this disease have the clinical impression that pustular psoriasis has become more common since the 1960's. The reasons are not known, but the increasing and widespread use of topical and parenteral corticosteroids is believed to be an important factor.

The hallmark of pustular psoriasis is the spongiform pustule of Kogoj found in the upper layers of the epidermis. The earliest lesion — a patch of erythema without pustules — shows dilated capillaries filled with neutrophils and accompanied by a perivascular infiltrate made up chiefly of lymphocytes with only a few neutrophils. As the lesion evolves within the next 24 hours, a massive emigration of neutrophils develops from the vessels into the dermis and epidermis.[4] The epidermal cells become edematous and necrotic, leaving only cellular walls visible. The neutrophils accumulate within the interstices of the cellular walls which form a spongelike network. As the pustule increases in size, the cellular walls disintegrate, resulting in the formation of a large cavity, but the spongiform appearance persists at the periphery. Electron microscopic studies of the early and late lesions have not revealed any obvious abnormalities of neutrophils or epidermal cells.[7]

Psoriasis vulgaris and pustular psoriasis appear to differ only in a quantitative way; e.g., psoriasis vulgaris has small collections of neutrophils in the stratum corneum called Munro's microabscesses, in contrast to von Zumbusch disease, in which massive collections of neutrophils produce the characteristic histologic and clinical pustules. The underlying pathogenetic mechanisms are probably identical. Buetner and colleagues found complement and immunoglobulins in the stratum corneum of psoriatic plaques in ordinary psoriasis, which they related to the presence of anti–stratum corneum autoantibodies present in both psoriatic and normal persons.[8, 9] Tagami and Ofuji demonstrated that the scales of psoriasis vulgaris and pustular psoriasis contained a potent leukotactic substance that might be a cleavage product of C5.[10] They proposed that this factor developed as a result of an antigen-antibody reaction in the stratum corneum. Lazarus et al. demonstrated that psoriatic plaques contained increased amounts of a serine proteinase that can cleave complement to produce C5 cleavage products that are chemotactic for neutrophils.[11] They further showed that noninvolved psoriatic skin, normal skin, and skin from a patient with pityriasis rubra pilaris all had significantly smaller amounts of this chemotactic factor. Although the skin lesions in pustular psoriasis have not been examined in an identical fashion, it seems likely that these proteinases would be found there as well. Another source of chemotactic factor in the psoriatic epidermis is the metabolites of arachidonic acid.[12]

Electron microscopic studies have demonstrated that there are gaps between the endothelial cells of the capillaries within the dermal papillae and between the endothelial cells of the postcapillary venules in the horizontal subpapillary vascular plexus in both the involved and uninvolved skin of persons with psoriasis vulgaris and pustular psoriasis.[7, 13-15] Such gaps would permit the passage of plasma proteins, including complement and immunoglobulins, from the vascular space into the dermis and epidermis in the absence of inflammation.

Neumann and Hard have shown that the microabscesses in psoriasis vulgaris and the spongiform pustules of von Zumbusch disease are intimately related to the ostium of the intraepidermal sweat ducts.[16] On the basis of their studies employing serial sectioning of microabscesses and spongiform pustules, they have proposed that the epidermal cells of the sweat duct are damaged and become detached from each other, thereby permitting the epidermal sweat duct to collapse. The fully developed pustule is a wedge-shaped structure with its base in the stratum corneum and its vertex protruding into the epidermis. Shelley et al. were able to induce pustules with the identical histopathologic findings by the intradermal injection of killed Group A streptococci in a patient with pustular psoriasis.[17] Munro's microabscesses in psoriasis vulgaris are found over the ostia of the sweat ducts. Other investigators have shown that the ostia of the sweat ducts in psoriatic plaques are plugged by keratinous material that is believed to result in decreased sweating from the plaques.[18] The role of the eccrine sweat duct in the accumulation of neutrophils within the psoriatic lesion merits further study.

Although several hypotheses can be constructed to explain the pathogenesis of the spongiform pustule, the following is proposed as a possible explanation for the observed phenomenon. The patches of erythema reflecting vasodilatation are accompanied by increased vascular permeability that allows additional plasma to percolate into the epidermis. The accumulation of plasma may stress the epidermal sweat duct unit in a manner analogous to miliaria, in which the intraepidermal sweat duct ruptures with leakage of sweat because of poral occlusion. If epidermal cell damage around the ostia were to develop and be accompanied by increased proteinase activity, then neutrophils would be attracted into the epidermis to produce the spongiform pustule. If the maximal proteinase activity were found in epidermal cells adjacent to the ostia, the wedge-shaped spongiform pustule and Munro's microabscesses found in psoriasis vulgaris could be logically explained.

The initial stimulus producing the patches of erythema is unknown. The erythema is characterized by vasodilatation, a perivascular accumulation of lymphocytes, and intravascular accumulation of neutrophils.[4] Fever is usually, but not always, present at this time. The neutrophilia often found at this time both in the peripheral blood and in the cutaneous lesion may represent a response not to an epidermal chemotactic factor but rather to the stimulus that is responsible for producing the flare of the disease. The subsequent emigration of neutrophils to produce the spongiform pustule would be a secondary response to events generated by the initial erythema and fever. Granulocytosis produced by steroid therapy or intercurrent infections has been proposed as the initial stimulus in some patients.[4]

The phenomenon of cutaneous erythema simulating erysipelas, in association with fever and leukocytosis, is a characteristic of both familial Mediterranean fever[9] and Sweet's syndrome (see below). In both of these entities there are neutrophilia and marked emigration of neutrophils from the vessels into the dermis without significant epidermal invasion. Consideration should be given to the possibility that pustular psoriasis is a disorder in which the initial events of fever, neutrophilia, and erythema produce a secondary reactive process affecting the epidermis.

Hyperkeratosis does not develop in pustular psoriasis as it does in psoriasis vulgaris, perhaps because the rapid and extensive pustule formation causes the stratum corneum to desquamate prematurely. In support of this proposal, one can cite the patients with pustular psoriasis who have slowly developing papulosquamous lesions without accompanying erythema. Reiter's syndrome may be a manifestation of this phenomenon also because the lesion of keratoderma blenorrhagicum is characterized by a spongiform pustule with marked hyperkeratosis that develops slowly without accompanying erythema, and is also self limited, disappearing spontaneously after several months. Tongue lesions similar to those of pustular psoriasis also occur in Reiter's syndrome. Both pustular psoriasis and Reiter's syndrome are associated with haplotype HLA–B27, whereas psoriasis vulgaris is not.

Hypocalcemia is often present in pustular psoriasis. It is related to the associated hypoalbuminemia and does not generally result in tetany. The hypoalbuminemia and associated hypocalcemia tend to become more pronounced during acute flares of the disorder. The hypoalbuminemia appears to be on the basis of increased catabolism and persists during remissions.[7, 20, 21]

The hemodynamic aspects of pustular psoriasis can be acute, severe, and fatal. Massive shifts of fluid into the skin frequently develop with the onset of erythema, producing marked edema. This phenomenon is responsible for the frequent misdiagnoses of cellulitis and thrombophlebitis at the onset of a flare of pustular psoriasis. However, more profound changes may develop. Warren et al. reported a patient whose acute flare of pustular psoriasis was accompanied by a sudden decrease in plasma volume, oliguria, hypotension, and hepatic and renal failure.[22] The patient recovered following hemodialysis. No precipitating events were found. Warren et al. postulated that the massive leak of plasma proteins from the capillaries into the skin produced the observed edema and that the proteins were subsequently lost from the skin via the pustular exudate. This resulted in the decreased plasma volume that was responsible for the hypotension, and the associated acute renal tubular necrosis. One of our patients developed an identical clinical syndrome but did not recover. She developed an *Escherichia coli* septicemia and died in shock before hemodialysis could be instituted. These sudden and unpredictable shifts in fluid from intra- to extravascular compartments plus the unknown effects from increased catabolism of albumin make pustular psoriasis a potentially serious medical disease.

The endothelial cell gaps do not disappear following therapy. The cause and mechanism of their formation is not known, but the ultrastructural appearance of the gaps is identical to that produced by the intradermal injection of histamine, serotonin, or bradykinin. However, there is no evidence as yet that these mediators play a significant role in the pathogenesis of psoriasis. Our own ultrastructural studies have shown that the mast cells remain intact and are not degranulated in their perivascular locations within the lesions of pustular psoriasis and psoriasis vulgaris. Platelet aggregation was not seen within the psoriatic vessels in acute lesions, but occasionally fibrin deposition was found at the apices of the capillary loops in the dermal papillae.[13, 14]

Elevated serum alkaline phosphatase levels have been reported in pustular psoriasis.[7] In one of our patients this enzyme elevation was associated with a concomitant elevation of 5′–nucleotidase, indicating that the liver was the major source of the elevated serum alkaline phosphatase. This excluded the possibility that the major portion of the elevated alkaline phosphatase represented increased osteoclastic activity resulting from hypocalcemia. Liver biopsies in other patients with pustular psoriasis have shown a periportal leukocytic infiltrate. Such a pericholangitis may account for the increased serum level of the enzyme.[23]

Treatment of pustular psoriasis is difficult and unpredictable. There are no agents that will consistently induce a remission. Methotrexate is helpful in controlling the illness when it is mildly active, but never in the severe acute flares. Parenteral steroids are indicated in the acute episodes when the patient is critically ill.[20]

Pustular psoriasis is a serious and potentially fatal disease. Toxic epidermal necrolysis can be a complication of pustular psoriasis (see p. 503). The extent and severity of the accompanying metabolic and cardiovascular derangements have not yet been completely determined. Ryan and Baker have also emphasized the potential seriousness of this disease by pointing out that 26 of 155 patients in their series died either from the disease or from the consequences of its treatment. Eight of the 26 died from uncontrollable pustular psoriasis.[24]

SWEET'S SYNDROME (ACUTE FEBRILE NEUTROPHILIC DERMATOSIS)

Sweet's syndrome is characterized by multiple warm, painful, discrete red plaques or papules that characteristically arise on the face, neck, upper chest, arms, and legs (Figs. 15–17 and 15–18; Plate 30*E*). They may appear in crops. The skin from the upper chest to the thighs tends to be spared. High fever, leukocytosis, and neutrophilia frequently accompany the development of these cutaneous lesions and the affected individuals feel ill. The plaques and papules frequently have a mammillated surface simulating vesicles. True vesicles or pustules sometimes do develop on the surface. There is a tendency for the plaques to develop partial clearing as the border slowly advances. The border sometimes develops vesicles or pustules as well. Rarely the plaques undergo superficial ulcerations with formation of crusts (Figs. 15–19 to 15–22). Although the lesions are usually multiple, solitary lesions have developed on the face. The multiple lesions have been diagnosed as cellulitis, erythema nodosum, vasculitis, erythema elevatum diutinum, erythema multiforme, and panniculitis at the time of presentation before their true nature was established. The plaques may be as large as 8 cm in diameter, and occasionally, the lesions have involved the entire extensor surface of the forearm or the dorsum of the foot. The lesions heal without scarring, although they may leave behind a reddish-brown color produced by deposition of hemosiderin.

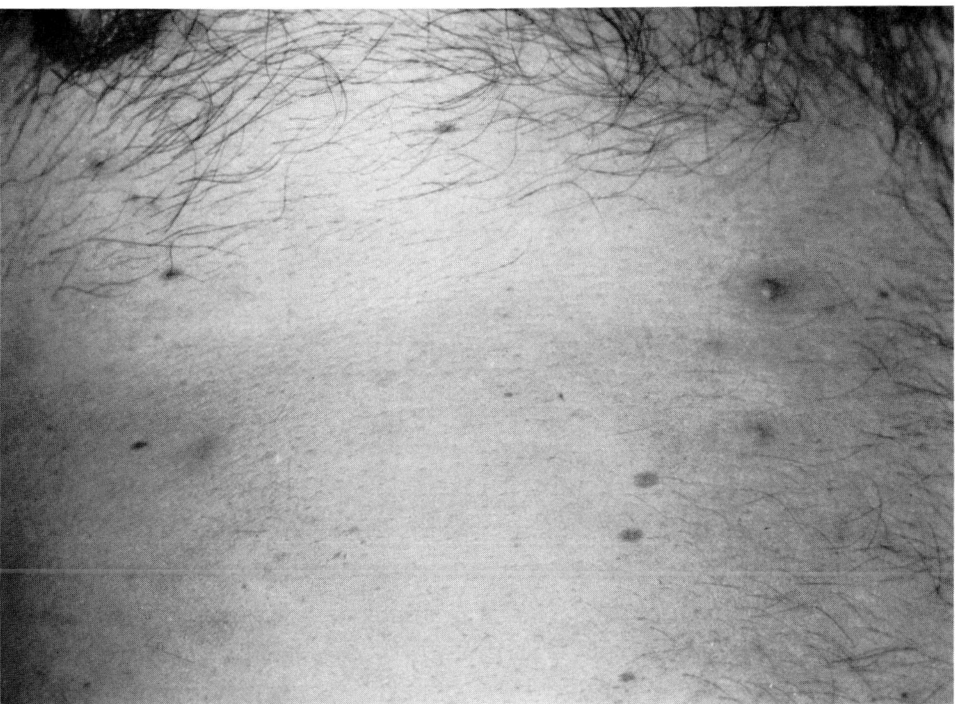

Figure 15–17. Sweet's syndrome. Papulopustules on chest.

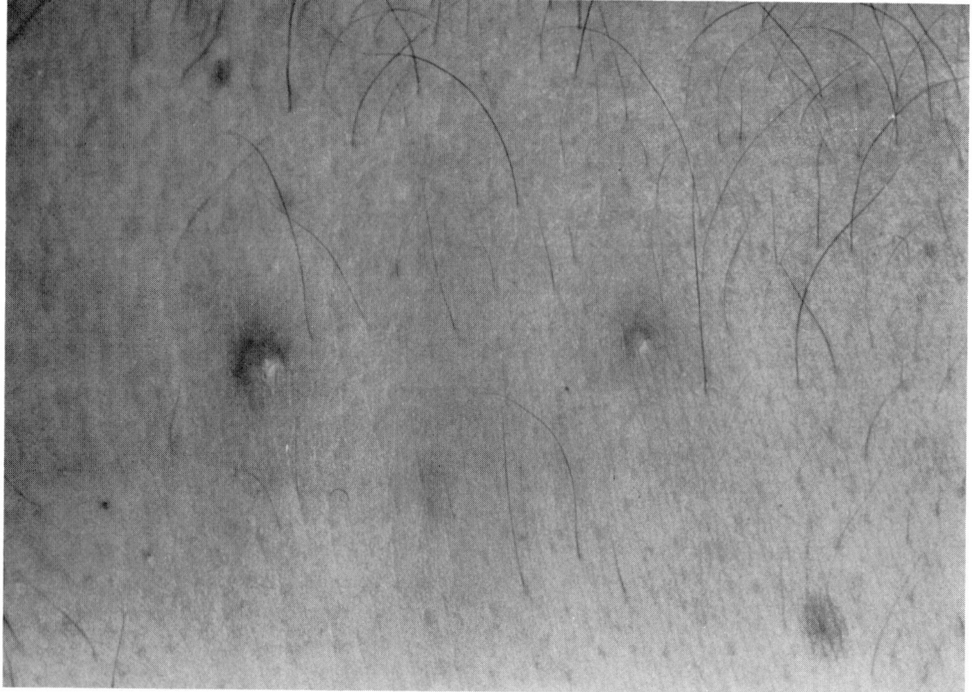

Figure 15–18. Sweet's syndrome. Close-up of papulopustules.

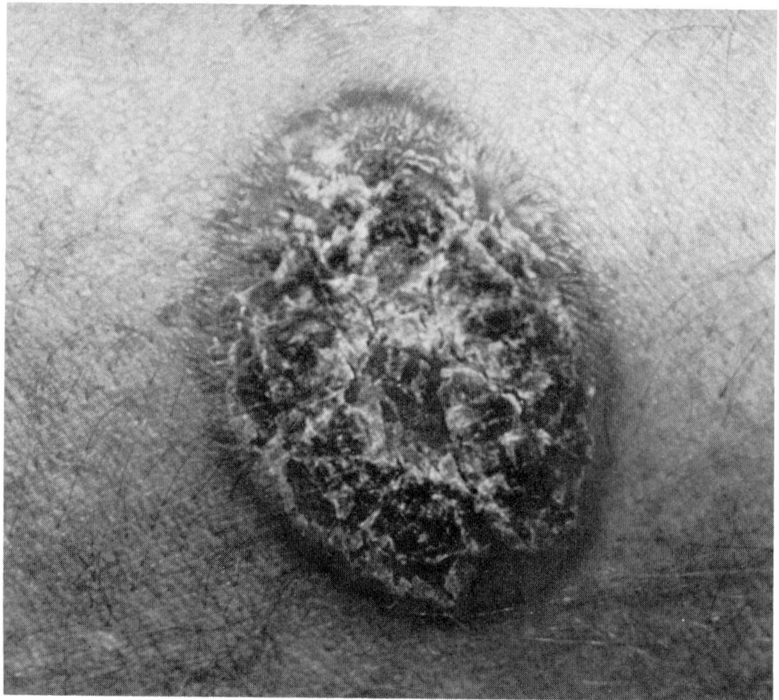

Figure 15–19. Sweet's syndrome. Plaque undergoing superficial ulceration with crust formation. (Courtesy of Dr. Bencel Schiff.)

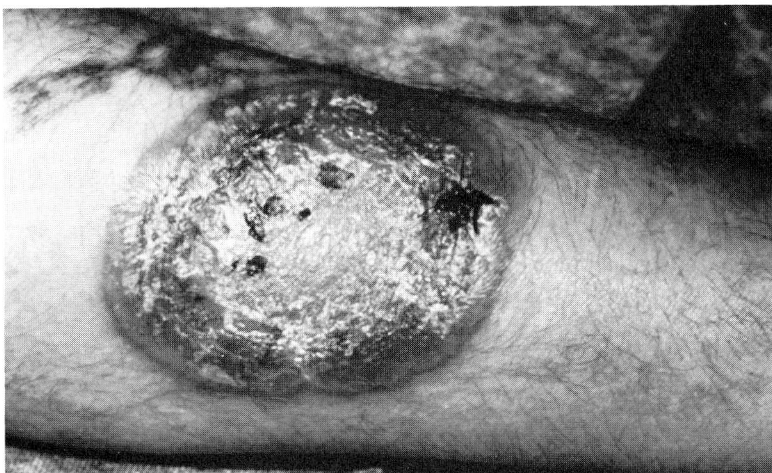

Figure 15–20. Sweet's syndrome. Ulcerated crusting plaque developing partial clearing in center as it expands. Evolution of lesion shown in Figure 15–21. (Courtesy of Dr. Bencel Schiff.)

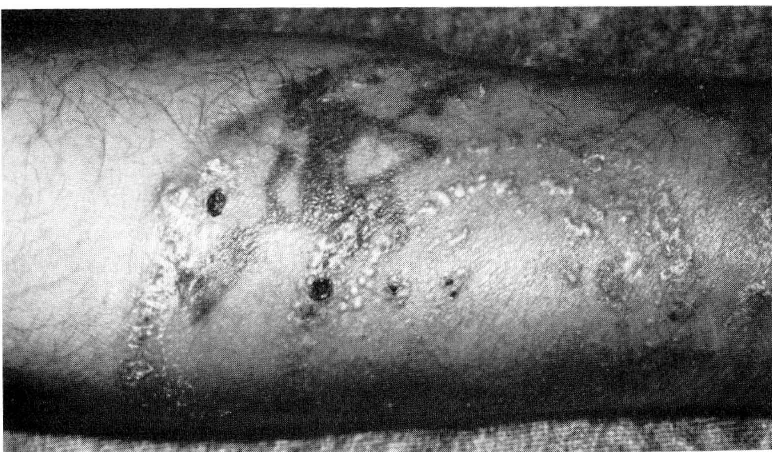

Figure 15–21. Sweet's syndrome. Plaque developed three concentric rings containing pustules with normal skin in between as it continued to expand. (Courtesy of Dr. Bencel Schiff.)

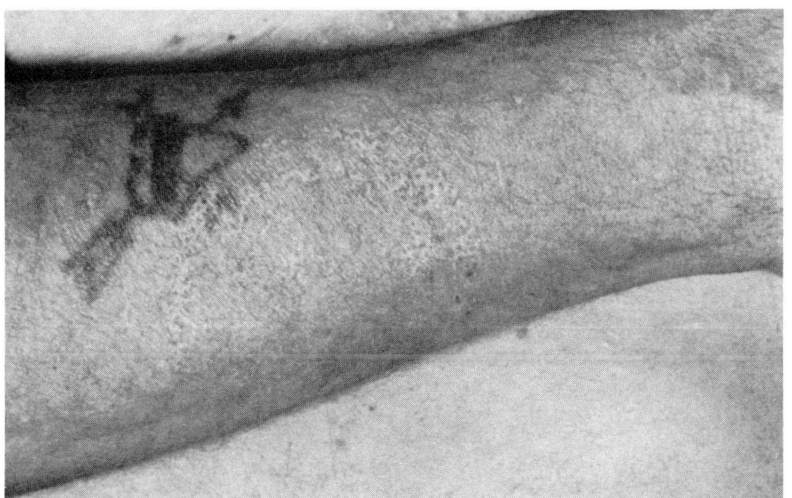

Figure 15–22. Sweet's syndrome. Same patient as in Figure 15–21. Lesions disappeared after prednisone therapy. (Courtesy of Dr. Bencel Schiff.)

In at least half of the reported cases, now totalling about 66, there has been a preceding febrile illness, usually an upper respiratory infection or pharyngitis. Infection by beta-hemolytic streptococci has been incriminated in only a few of these instances. Acute histoplasmosis was the associated event in one case and postvaccination reactions in two others. Seven individuals had an associated leukemia (five with acute myelogenous leukemia) and two with acute blastic leukemia. Metastatic adenocarcinoma from an unknown site and testicular cancer were present in two other individuals.[25-42]

Myalgia, polyarthralgia, and polyarthritis of large joints, both in symmetrical and asymmetrical distributions, have been associated with the cutaneous lesions in several patients.[31, 32, 43, 44] Episcleritis has been an accompaniment of these musculoskeletal complaints. In the largest series, comprising 18 patients, rheumatic complaints were present in 50 per cent of the patients.[31] Two patients had an acute nephritis that parallelled the course of their Sweet's syndrome.[28, 36]

The clinical features of the disease occur in the following frequencies based upon the analysis by Gunawardena et al.[31]: fever occurred in 83 per cent; elevated erythrocyte sedimentation rate in 87 to 94 per cent; ocular involvement in 4 to 72 per cent; leukocytosis in 59 to 79 per cent; musculoskeletal complaints in 12 to 56 per cent; and albuminuria in 11 to 16 per cent of the reported cases. Females are affected seven times more frequently than men.

Sweet's syndrome appears to be composed of four clinical subsets.[25-45] Most of the reported cases belong to the first subset. In this group the syndrome developed one to three weeks following an infectious disease or following vaccination. In two patients the syndrome developed less than one week after the precipitating event. In a few patients the disease subsided spontaneously without therapy within one to four weeks. In the others, prednisone produced a rapid clearing of lesions, which did not recur if the prednisone was tapered over the course of several weeks or months. Too rapid a taper was associated with recurrence. A second subset was composed of a minority of patients in whom recurrent episodes appeared over months to years without any obvious initiating event. In these cases, steroids were used to treat repeated attacks. A third subset has been associated with malignancies, and the patients in this group have experienced the same striking permanent remissions as the individuals who developed Sweet's syndrome after an infectious illness. The fourth group is represented by three individuals who have had a long history of chronic recurrent arthritis in association with Sweet's syndrome.

If untreated, the lesions of Sweet's syndrome may increase in size slowly or rapidly and can persist for one to 12 months. Although the plaques of Sweet's syndrome can be present for many months, they eventually do resolve spontaneously without any scarring.

In three patients, the lesions were initiated by trauma.[30, 34, 46]

The histopathology of the skin lesions shows dense perivascular collections of neutrophils, many of which have undergone leukocytoclasis. Neutrophils are also scattered diffusely throughout the dermis among the collagen bundles. The papillary dermis may be markedly edematous and the epidermis may be spongiotic, thereby giving rise to the pseudovesicular and mammillated appearance of the cutaneous lesions.[43, 46] Massive collections of neutrophils may extend from the dermis into the epidermis to produce clinical pustules, but spongiform pustules are not formed. The neutrophilic emigration may involve the subcutaneous vessels as well. Although the vessels are very dilated, there is no evidence of vascular wall necrosis or deposition of fibrinoid material. There are no histologic features to implicate a vasculitic origin for these lesions. Immunofluorescent examination of the skin lesions in two cases failed to detect immunoglobulins or complement around the vessels or at the dermal-epidermal junction.[35, 44] Serum complement has been normal in those individuals who have been tested.

The association of this syndrome with preceding infections of viral, streptococcal, and fungal etiology and with leukemias and vaccinations implicates an underlying immunologic mechanism. The clinical association of arthralgia and arthritis and the two instances of concomitant renal disease also support the concept of an underlying immune complex mechanism in Sweet's syndrome. Although the histologic findings in Sweet's syndrome are not those of a leukocytoclastic vasculitis, the underlying mechanism could still be related to immune complexes. We should not assume that circulating immune complexes can produce only leukocytoclastic vasculitis. The vascular lesions in erythema multiforme and Mucha-Habermann disease, which are not vasculitic, appear to be produced by circulating immune complexes.[48, 49] Unless vascular lesions are examined for immunoglobulins and complement by immunofluorescent techniques within the first 24 hours of their development, the immunoreactants will have been removed from the tissue and will have become undetectable. Examination of an early lesion by electron microscopy and the use of the histamine technique to trap circulating immune complexes in the cutaneous vessels are two techniques that can be used to pursue this possibility.[47]

Although the lesions in Sweet's syndrome develop almost exclusively in sun-exposed areas, there is no experimental or other clinical evidence to implicate a role for photosensitivity.

The lesions of Sweet's disease respond dramatically to oral prednisone. Relapses are rare if the patient is treated for several weeks or months before the dose is slowly reduced to zero. Indomethacin was strikingly effective in a patient with acute histoplasmosis and Sweet's syndrome in whom steroids were contraindicated.[32]

Although the diagnosis of Sweet's syndrome is properly applied to disorders with the typical features described above, I have seen three individuals with the characteristic cutaneous and histologic lesions of this entity in whom some of the clinical features have been atypical. Whether these cases represent atypical examples of Sweet's syndrome or a closely related neutrophilic dermatosis will be determined by their subsequent courses and by future published reports of similar cases.

The patient illustrated in Figures 15–17 and 15–18 and Plate 30*E* is a 54-year-old man who suffered from bouts of fever, polyarthritis of the small joints of the hands, and cutaneous lesions appearing as papules, sterile pustules, and subcutaneous nodules resembling erythema nodosum. Each episode lasted from two to ten days and occurred at intervals of one to several months over the course of six years. Histologic examination of papules and pustules showed a marked perivascular and diffuse dermal infiltrate of neutrophils without evidence of vasculitis or spongiform pustule formation in the epidermis. The erythema nodosum–like lesions showed an identical infiltrate in the septa of the fat without evidence of fat necrosis or lobular involvement. Leukocytosis was never present, and his illness was unreponsive to corticosteroid therapy. After a course of six years, he was diagnosed as having a leukemia of the Di Guglielmo variety. Since the time of that diagnosis, his attacks have been less severe and less frequent. The other diagnosis considered for this man was Weber-Christian disease. However, there was never any histologic or clinical evidence of fat necrosis, the erythema nodosum–like lesions never produced scarring when they resolved, and most of his cutaneous lesions were erythematous papules and sterile pustules.

The person shown in Figures 15–19 to 15–22 was presented by Dr. Bencel Schiff at a meeting of the New England Dermatological Society on April 4, 1980. The patient is a 49-year-old man with a 17-year history of episodic arthritis, conjunctivitis, and dysuria consistent with Reiter's syndrome. One year before presentation at this meeting, he developed a discrete round plaque with a dusky red elevated border and a central area of crusting after an upper respiratory infection. The lesion slowly expanded, producing three concentric rings with active borders and normal skin in between. This occurred while he was on oral prednisone therapy for two months. The prednisone was discontinued and therapy with dapsone was initiated. The lesion resolved completely one month later. Two months before presentation, he developed two new lesions on his extremities following an upper respiratory infection. In one of the plaques the center flattened and became hypopigmented with fine wrinkling indicative of atrophy. This developed over the course of two months in the absence of treatment. Fever and leukocytosis were not features of his illness. The histologic features of the lesions were characteristic of Sweet's syndrome.

The third case was presented by Dr. Louis Fragola at the same meeting. The patient is a 64-year-old man whose illness began 18 months earlier, within a few weeks after his inferior vena cava was ligated because of pulmonary emboli caused by thrombophlebitis of the legs. He developed crops of dusky red macules and papules on his lower legs and irregularly outlined red plaques on his upper back and neck. Papulopustules were present in some of the plaques. The crops occurred at intervals of one to two months and individual lesions persisted for two to four weeks before spontaneously resolving. Biopsies showed the typical changes of Sweet's syndrome. He never had fever or leukocytosis, and his eruption was only moderately well controlled by oral corticosteroids. Work-up at this time revealed pancytopenia (hematocrit 30, white blood cells 3800–4900, and platelets 60,000–80,000) secondary to myelofibrosis. His physicians speculated that he may have had polycythemia vera preceding the development of myelofibrosis. The phlebitis with pulmonary emboli may have represented a manifestation of polycythemia vera that was not diagnosed at the time.

REFERENCES

1. Baker, H., and Ryan, T. J.: Generalized pustular psoriasis. A clinical and epidemiological study of 104 cases. Br. J. Dermatol., *80*:771, 1968.
2. O'Keefe, E., Braverman, I. M., and Cohen, I.: Annulus migrans. Identical lesions in pustular psoriasis, Reiter's syndrome, and geographic tongue. Arch. Dermatol., *107*:240, 1973.
3. Yasuda, T., Ito, M. Mizuno, A., Kitamura, N., and Ohtaki, N.: Internal factors and pustular psoriasis. *In* Farber, E. M., and Cox, A. J. (eds.): Psoriasis, Proceedings of Second International Symposium. Yorke Medical Books, New York, 1977, p. 140.
4. Kingery, F. A. J., Chinn, H. D., and Saunders, T. S.: Generalized pustular psoriasis. Arch. Dermatol., *84*:912, 1961.
5. Tolman, M. M., and Moschella, S. L.: Pustular psoriasis (Zumbusch). Arch. Dermatol., *81*:400, 1960.
6. Lowe, N. J., and Ridgway, H. B.: Generalized pustular psoriasis precipitated by lithium carbonate. Arch. Dermatol., *114*:1788, 1978.
7. Braverman, I. M., Cohen, I., and O'Keefe, E.: Metabolic and ultrastructural studies in a patient with pustular psoriasis (von Zumbusch). Arch. Dermatol., *105*:189, 1972.
8. Beutner, E. H., Jablonska, S., Jarzabek-Chorzelska, M., Marciejowska, E., Rzesa, G., and Chorzelski, T. P.: Studies in immunodermatology. VI. IF studies of autoantibodies to the stratum corneum and of *in vivo* fixed IgG in stratum corneum of psoriatic lesions. Int. Arch. Allergy Appl. Immunol., *48*:301, 1975.
9. Jablonska, S., Chorzelski, T. P., Jarzabek-Chorzelska, M., and Beutner, E. H.: Studies in immunodermatology. VII. Four compartment system studies of IgG in stratum corneum and of stratum corneum antigen in biopsies of psoriasis and control dermatoses. Int. Arch. Allergy Appl. Immunol., *48*:324, 1975.
10. Tagami, H., and Ofuji, S.: Leukotactic properties of soluble substances in psoriatic scale. Br. J. Dermatol., *95*:1, 1976.
11. Lazarus, G. S., Yost, F. J., Jr., and Thomas, C. A.: Polymorphonuclear leukocytes: possible mechanism of accumulation of psoriasis. Science, *198*:1162, 1977.
12. Hammarstrom, S., Hamberg, M., Samuelsson, B., Duell, E. A., Stawiski, M., and Voorhees, J. J.: Increased concentrations of nonesterified arachidonic acid 12L-hydroxy-5,8,10,14-eicosatetraenoic acid, prostaglandin E_2, and prostaglandin F_2 in epidermis of psoriasis. Proc. Nat. Acad. Sci. (USA), *72*:5130, 1975.
13. Braverman, I. M.: Electron microscopic studies of the microcirculation in psoriasis. J. Invest. Dermatol., *59*:91–98, 1972.
14. Braverman, I. M.: Microcirculation in psoriatic skin. J. Invest. Dermatol., *62*:493, 1974.
15. Mottaz, J., Zelickson, A. S., Thorne, E. G., and Wachs, G.: Blood vessel changes in psoriatic skin. Acta. Dermatol. Venereol., *53*:195, 1973.
16. Neumann, E., and Hard, S.: The significance of the epidermal sweat duct unit in the genesis of pustular psoriasis (Zumbusch) and the microabscesses of Munro-Sabouraud. Acta. Dermatovenereol., *54*:141, 1974.
17. Shelley, W. B., Wood, M. G., and Beerman, H.: Pustular psoriasis elicited by streptococcal antigen and localized to the sweat pore. J. Invest. Dermatol., *65*:466, 1975.
18. Johnson, C., and Shuster, S.: Eccrine sweating in psoriasis. Br. J. Dermatol., *81*:119, 1969.
19. Azizi, E., and Fisher, B. K.: Cutaneous manifestations of familial Mediterranean fever. Arch. Dermatol., *112*:364, 1976.
20. Worm, A.-M., and Rossing, N.: Transcapillary escape rate of albumin and plasma volume in patients with varying degree of psoriasis. Br. J. Dermatol., *97*:423, 1977.
21. Braverman, I. M.: The neutrophilic dermatoses. *In* Moschella, S. L. (ed.): 1979. Review for Physicians. Elsevier, New York, 1979, p. 255.
22. Warren, D. J., Winney, R. J., and Beveridge, G. W.: Oligaemia, renal failure, and jaundice associated with pustular psoriasis. Br. Med. J., *2*:406, 1974.
23. Shelley, W. B.: Generalized pustular psoriasis induced by potassium iodide. J.A.M.A., *201*:133, 1967.
24. Ryan, T. J., and Baker, H.: The prognosis of generalized pustular psoriasis. Br. J. Dermatol., *85*:407, 1971.
25. Bard, J. W.: Acute neutrophilic dermatosis. Cutis, *17*:93, 1976.
26. Brenan, J. A.: Acute febrile neutrophilic dermatosis (Sweet). Aust. J. Dermatol., *10*:186, 1969.
27. Crow, K. D., Kerdel–Vegas, F., and Rook, A.: Acute febrile neutrophilic dermatosis. Sweet's syndrome. Dermatologia, *139*:123, 1969.
28. Evans, S., and Evans, C. C.: Acute febrile neutrophilic dermatosis — two cases. Dermatologica, *143*:153, 1971.
29. Goldman, G. C., and Moschella, S. L.: Acute febrile neutrophilic dermatosis (Sweet's syndrome). Arch Dermatol., *103*:654, 1971.
30. Greer, K. E., Pruitt, J. L., and Bishop, G. F.: Acute febrile neutrophilic dermatosis (Sweet syndrome). Arch. Dermatol., *111*:1461, 1975.
31. Gunawardena, D. A., Gunawardena, K. A., Ratnayaka, R.M.R.S., and Vasanthanathan, N. S.: The clinical spectrum of Sweet's syndrome (acute febrile neutrophilic dermatosis) — a report of eighteen cases. Br. J. Dermatol., *92*:363, 1975.
32. Hoffman, G. S.: Treatment of Sweet's syndrome (active febrile neutrophilic dermatosis) with indomethacin. J. Rheumatol., *4*:201, 1977.

33. Holst, R., and Mobacken, H.: Acute febrile neutrophilic dermatosis (Sweet's syndrome). Report of two cases and review of the literature. Acta Dermatovenereol., *51*:63, 1971.

34. Klock, J. C., and Oken, R. L.: Febrile neutrophilic dermatosis in acute myelogenous leukemia. Cancer, *37*:922, 1976.

35. MacKie, R. M.: Sweet's syndrome. A further case of acute febrile neutrophilic dermatosis. Dermatologica, *149*:69, 1974.

36. Matta, M., Malak, J., Tabet, E., and Kurban, A. K.: Sweet's syndrome: systemic associations. Cutis, *12*:561, 1973.

37. Meiers, H. G.: Akute febrile neutrophile Dermatose. Hautarzt, *23*:111, 1972.

38. Pipard, C., and Delannoy, A.: Syndrome de Sweet et leucémie myéloide aigue. Ann. Dermatol. Venereol., *104*:160, 1977.

39. Purdy, M. J., and Fairbrother, G. E.: Case reports: acute febrile neutrophilic dermatosis of Sweet. Aust. J. Dermatol., *12*:172, 1971.

40. Raff, M., and Santler, R.: Akute febrile neutrophile Dermatose (Sweet syndrome). Hautarzt, *23*:415, 1972.

41. Raimer, S. S., and Duncan, W. C.: Febrile neutrophilic dermatosis in acute myelogenous leukemia. Arch. Dermatol., *114*:413, 1978.

42. Shapiro, L., Baraf, C. S., and Richheimer, L. L.: Sweet's syndrome (acute febrile neutrophilic dermatosis). Arch. Dermatol., *103*:81, 1971.

43. Sweet, R. D.: An acute febrile neutrophilic dermatosis. Br. J. Dermatol., *76*:349, 1964.

44. Trentham, D. E., Masi, A. T., and Bale, G. F.: Arthritis with an inflammatory dermatosis resembling Sweet's syndrome. Am. J. Med., *61*:424, 1976.

45. Whittle, C. H., Beck, G. A., and Champion, R. H.: Recurrent neutrophilic dermatosis of the face — a variant of Sweet's syndrome. Br. J. Dermatol., *80*:806, 1968.

46. Sweet, R. D.: Further observations on acute febrile neutrophilic dermatosis. Br. J. Dermatol., *80*:800, 1968.

47. Braverman, I. M., and Yen, A.: Demonstration of immune complexes in spontaneous and histamine-induced lesions and in normal skin of patients with leukocytoclastic angiitis. J. Invest. Dermatol., *64*:105, 1975.

48. Kazmierowski, J. A., and Wuepper, K. D.: Erythema multiforme: immune complex vasculitis of the superficial cutaneous microvasculature. J. Invest. Dermatol., *71*:366, 1978.

49. Clayton, R., and Haffendin, G.: An immunofluorescence study of pityriasis lichenoides. Br. J. Dermatol., *99*:491, 1978.

16

Pregnancy and the Menstrual Cycle

The skin and its appendages are affected in a variety of ways during pregnancy. It is convenient to divide the cutaneous changes into three groups: those changes in the skin that most pregnant women exhibit and that are considered to be *normal*; those dermatoses that are unique to the gravid state; and those preexisting dermatoses that are either positively or negatively influenced by pregnancy. Dermatoses associated with the menstrual cycle are also discussed in this chapter.

NORMAL CUTANEOUS CHANGES OF PREGNANCY

Pigmentation

Hyperpigmentation is a commonly recognized sign of pregnancy. Although it occurs to some degree in virtually all women, it is more common in brunettes than in blonds. Generalized hyperpigmentation may develop, but it is far more common to see localized areas of melanin hyperpigmentation: the nipples and areolae; the umbilicus; the linea alba, which becomes the linea nigra; the axillae; and vulvar and perianal areas. Estrogen and progesterone seem to be hormones mainly responsible for the pigmentary changes in pregnancy.[1, 2] In individuals of fair complexion these pigmentary changes fade after pregnancy, but in individuals with darker skins some degree of hyperpigmentation remains permanently.

The mask of pregnancy, originally referred to as *chloasma* but now more appropriately termed *melasma,* also develops more often in brunettes than in blonds. Melasma is a splotchy and irregular melanin hyperpigmentation that characteristically develops on the forehead, cheeks, temples, and upper lip (Fig. 16–1). This pigmentary disorder is most likely related to estrogen and progesterone, since identical changes are seen with the use of the contraceptive pill containing these hormones, especially in brunettes. Although melasma usually lightens considerably or may even disappear completely in some women after pregnancy, it usually persists to some degree. With successive pregnancies, melasma may recur or increase in extent. Although melasma is usually associated with pregnancy, it or an identical-appearing pigmentary disorder can also be found in nonpregnant women who have not taken birth control pills and in some men.

Preexisting pigmented moles (nevi) and freckles often darken during pregnancy. Some nevi may increase in size and new nevi may form. The

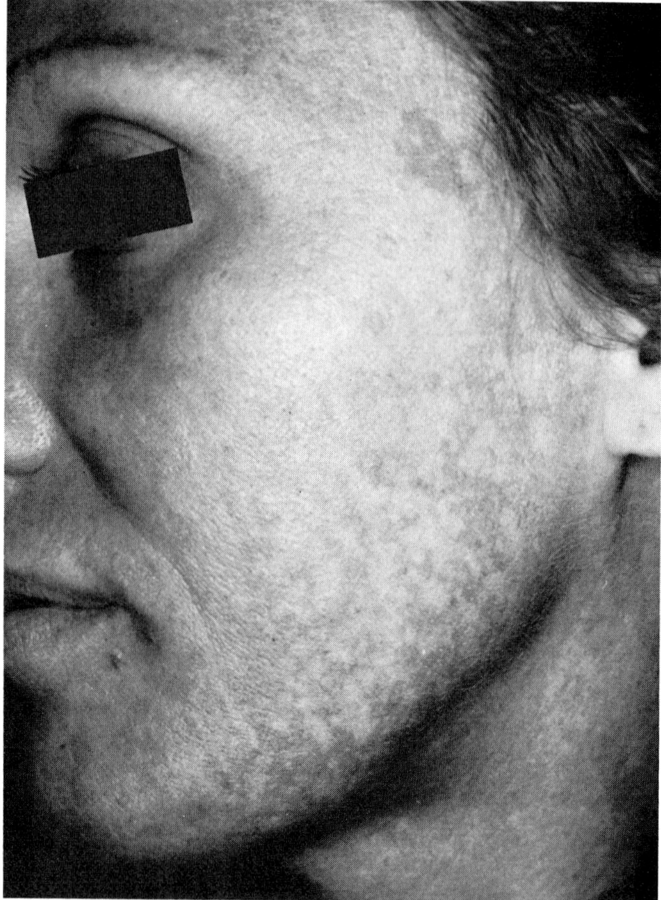

Figure 16–1. Melasma.

increase in pigmentation and size sometimes prompts surgical excision. The increased clinical activity of the lesion is often accompanied histologically by markedly increased junctional activity of the nevus cells and at times the pathologist may consider the possibility of an early melanoma in the differential diagnosis. However, after pregnancy the nevi usually regress to some extent, and the junctional activity reverts to a banal appearance.

Hair

Postpartum hair loss is commonplace and is considered a minor nuisance by those who have previously passed through it and a major catastrophe by those who are experiencing it for the first time. The growing phase (anagen) of an individual hair is two to six years. The hair bulb eventually involutes and is retracted up into the middle of the hair follicle when it enters the resting phase (telogen). After about three months a new hair bulb forms in the depth of the same follicle and as the new hair shaft grows, it ejects the old one. Each shed hair is replaced by a new one. Normally 15 to 20 per cent of scalp hair are in telogen.[3]

Lynfield showed that in the second and third trimesters only 10 per cent of hairs were in telogen.[4] During the first weeks post partum more hairs entered telogen than usual (30 per cent after nine weeks), thus explaining the clinical observation that postpartum hair loss is seen two to four months after childbirth. It usually continues for 6 to 24 weeks, but rarely it may persist for 15 months.[5]

Hair is lost diffusely from the scalp, but there is accentuation of loss along the anterior hair line. Virtually all the hair is replaced after several weeks unless some other process intervenes. The occasional woman who subsequently develops patterned hair loss (analogous to male-patterned alopecia) may incorrectly connect the onset of irreversible hair loss with an episode of postpartum hair loss.

Kligman coined the term *telogen effluvium* to describe this type of hair shedding.[3] The same mechanism operates in hair loss following febrile illnesses such as typhoid fever, scarlet fever, and pneumonia, and severe emotional stress.

Increased hair growth during pregnancy is a rare event, and when observed it has been associated with signs of virilization such as acne, deep voice, and clitoral enlargement. In some of these cases an arrhenoblastoma was present and in others bilateral ovarian enlargement was discovered. In one case, virilization disappeared post partum in association with a spontaneous decrease in the size of the ovaries, and in another, the ovarian enlargement was shown to be produced by hyperplasia of lutein cells.[6]

Turunen et al. reported three women (out of 33,000 successful pregnancies) who developed increased facial hair over the zygomas, jaws, arms, legs, shoulders, areolae, midline of the abdomen, and pubic area.[7] There was deepening of the voice, but no other signs of virilization were described. The hair spontaneously fell out a few days post partum. These workers found increased urinary 17-ketosteroids and androgens in association with decreased 17-β-dehydrogenase activity in the placentas.

Connective Tissue

Striae gravidarum develops in most pregnant women. The striae appear chiefly on the lower abdomen and on the breasts. Initially they are pink or purple but soon become white. They never disappear, and they leave white depressed irregular bands in the skin. For many years, it was believed that they were produced *solely* by the stretching of the skin during pregnancy. Observations that striae also developed in Cushing's syndrome, in growing nonobese adolescents of both sexes, and with the use of topical steroids under occlusive dressings have cast doubts on this theory. Poidevin showed that the *degree* of skin distention was not directly related to the formation of striae, and that striae could develop in the absence of significant stretching.[8] Nevertheless, it is currently believed that a combination of stretch and a "striae factor" is required for the production of striae. Although it has not been proven, adrenocortical hyperactivity is frequently proposed as the "striae factor."

"Skin tags" or fibroma molle are small pedunculated fibromas that develop on the neck and in the axillae during pregnancy. They are benign overgrowths of skin that tend to involute somewhat after delivery.

Blood Vessels

Pregnancy produces its most impressive effects on the vascular system, especially of the skin. There is an increase in vascular permeability as well as in vascular proliferation. Local venous congestion of the vestibule and vaginal mucosa are early signs of pregnancy. Edema of nondependent areas unrelated to toxemia is common. Arteriolar proliferation with extensive branching of the associated capillary bed results in the formation of spiders, which are commonly found as early as two months and continue to appear into the ninth month. Typically, they disappear within a few weeks after childbirth. Erythema on the midpalmar, hypothenar, and thenar areas is also common. The erythema may be splotchy or uniform. It is indistinguishable from the palmar erythema seen in hyperthyroidism and hepatic cirrhosis. Systemic LE may appear for the first time during pregnancy and can also be associated with palmar erythema. However, in systemic LE the erythema is frequently composed of discrete macules or papules and extends onto the finger tips, whereas in pregnancy the palmar erythema is diffuse and usually spares the digits. The palmar erythema of pregnancy also vanishes post partum.

Venous varicosities occur in a significant number of women in both the vulvar and the rectal areas. Although the gravid uterus with pressure on large vessels is important, hereditary valvular incompetence has also been suggested as playing an important role. Saphenous vein varicosities and superficial venous telangiectasias in the shape of "starbursts" or linear patterns become more prominent during pregnancy and regress only slightly post partum.

Vascular proliferation in pregnancy reaches its greatest development with the formation of capillary hemangiomas. They occur chiefly on the head and neck and are considered to be unusual below these areas.[9, 10] The most common sites of involvement are the gingivae, where the developing angiomas are referred to as "pregnancy tumors." Small hemangiomas have been observed on the tongue, upper lip, eyelid, and other areas of the head and neck. Preexisting hemangiomas have been seen to increase in size during pregnancy. The hemangiomas become smaller post partum but do not recede completely.

DERMATOSES UNIQUE TO PREGNANCY

Traditionally, a number of dermatoses have been related to pregnancy in a cause-effect relationship. The natural history of some of these entities is fairly well understood, but the underlying mechanisms and etiologies are unknown.

Herpes Gestationis

Herpes gestationis is an intensely pruritic, blistering eruption of variable morphology that usually appears during the second or third trimester and spontaneously remits within a few weeks postpartum in most instances.

The disorder is uncommon and is estimated to occur once in 3000 to 5000 pregnancies.[11, 12] Pruritus may precede the development of skin lesions by as much as a week, but usually they appear together. More often than not, the eruption begins periumbilically and spreads to involve the trunk and extremities, including the palms and soles. Lesions on the mucous membranes are uncommon.

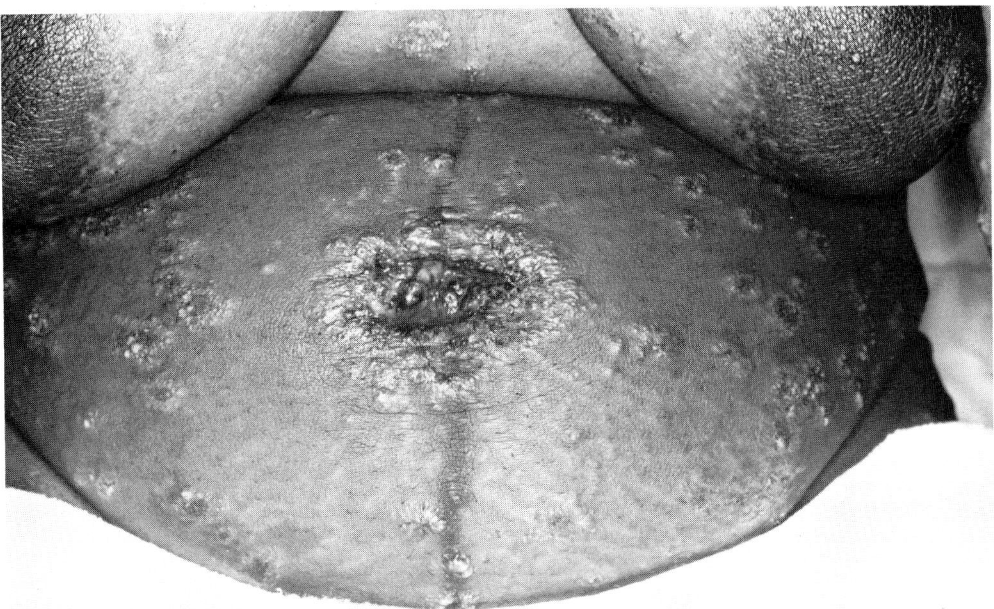

Figure 16–2. Herpes gestationis. Urticarial plaques from which clusters of vesicles and bullae are arising. In this patient they were most fully developed periumbilically.

The lesions are basically erythematous, urticarial plaques from which single or multiple vesicles and bullae often arise. The blisters may develop in the center or around the periphery of the plaques (Figs. 16–2 and 16–3).

The erythematous plaques can be clinically indistinguishable from the iris or target lesions of erythema multiforme (Fig. 16–4).[12, 13] The plaques also can resemble ordinary urticaria. Sometimes the papules and plaques expand with formation of vesicles and bullae along the circumfer-

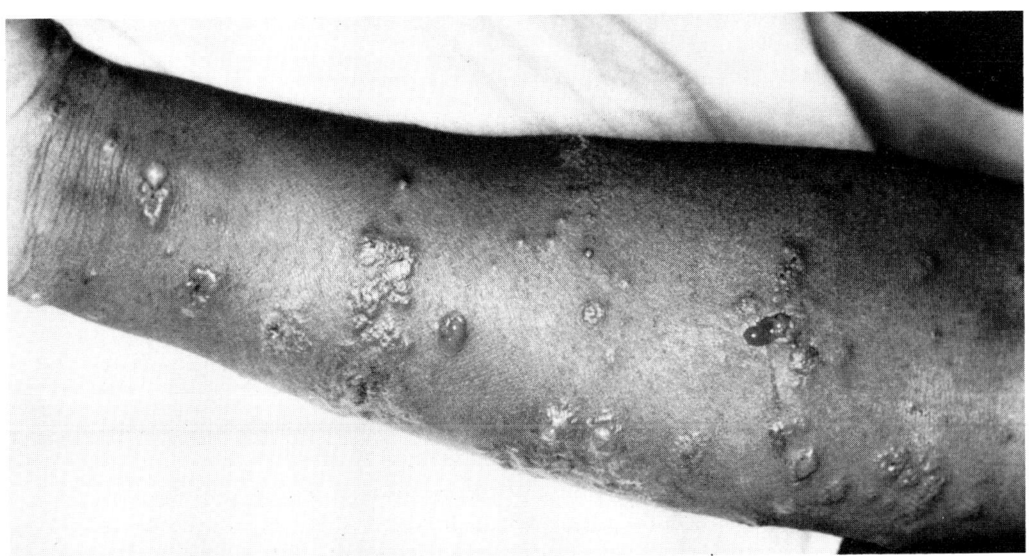

Figure 16–3. Herpes gestationis. Same patient as in Figure 16–2.

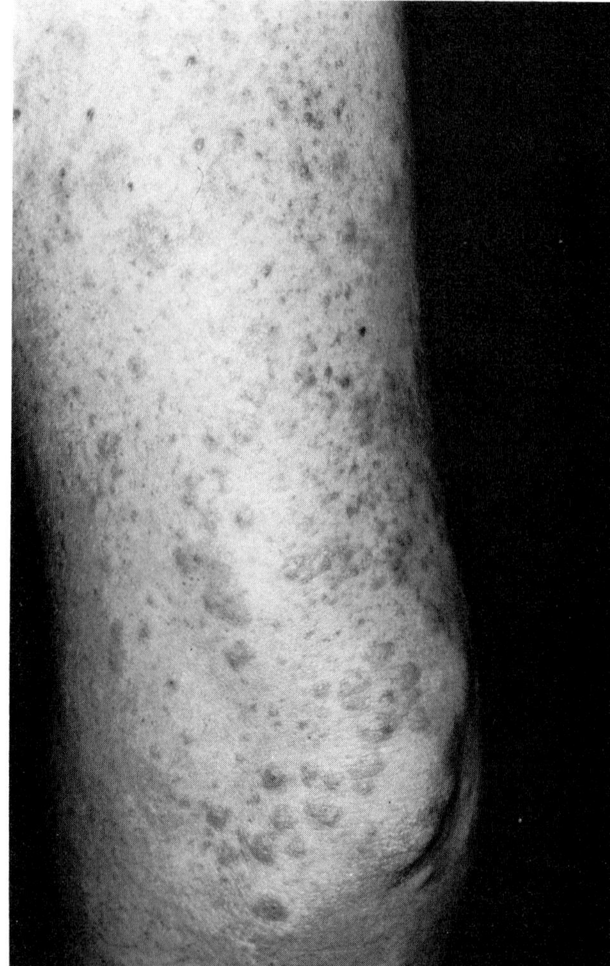

Figure 16–4. Herpes gestationis. Lesions resemble those of erythema multiforme.

ence and at other times they enlarge, leaving behind relatively clear centers simulating the lesions of erythema annulare centrifugum (Fig. 16–5). Individual plaques may fuse to produce polycyclic or gyrate lesions.

Herpes gestationis tends to erupt in crops, and individual lesions tend to subside spontaneously after one to two weeks. The disease may be mild with few lesions and tolerable pruritus, or it may spread rapidly with unrelenting itch. Although the itching can be severe, secondary infection with impetigo and pustule formation is very uncommon.

The disease usually begins in the fourth or fifth month but has been reported as early as two weeks[14] and as late as three to five days post partum.[12, 15] A fluctuating course with exacerbations and relative remissions can be seen during pregnancy. Significant flares can develop post partum.[15] In the average case, the disorder subsides spontaneously within a few days to four weeks post partum, but it can persist for up to 16 weeks. Post partum, the disease may flare repeatedly with the menstrual cycle before spontaneously entering remission. In one case, the disease

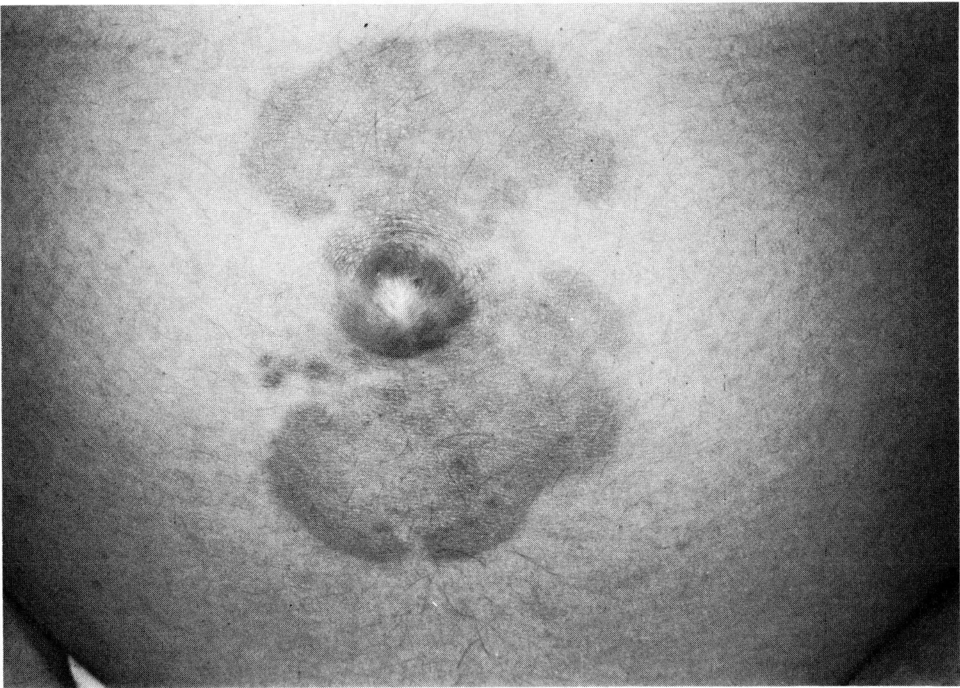

Figure 16–5. Herpes gestationis. In this patient, the lesions resembled those of erythema annulare centrifugum. The histologic features were those of subepidermal bulla formation.

continued for 18 months in this fashion before resolving.[16] One of our patients had persistently active disease for one year post partum, requiring oral steroids for control, before she entered remission. Black reported at the 1977 annual meeting of the Pacific Dermatological Association that in three of his ten patients, the disease was still persistent three to seven years post partum.[17] Birth control pills can produce exacerbations of the disease during states of remission or mild activity.[15, 18, 19]

Although the probability of recurrence with each pregnancy is high, this does not invariably happen, nor does the severity of the disease necessarily become worse with each subsequent pregnancy. One of our patients whose first episode persisted for one year post partum had two subsequent pregnancies, each of which was accompanied by milder and milder courses of herpes gestationis. In the second and third pregnancies corticosteroid therapy was not required, and the disease terminated promptly within a few days post partum.

Histologically, the cutaneous lesions in herpes gestationis show a subepidermal blister with a perivascular collection of lymphohistiocytic cells and eosinophils around the upper and, sometimes, deep dermal vessels.[20] These findings had been confused with those of erythema multiforme and dermatitis herpetiformis in the past. Herpes gestationis was believed to be a manifestation of one of these entities in pregnancy. However, since 1973, it has become clear on the basis of immunofluorescent findings that herpes gestationis is a distinct entity unrelated to those disorders. Direct immunofluorescent examination of lesional and normal skin reveals a linear band of C3, sometimes accompanied by IgG, at the dermal-epidermal junction. In addition, virtually all patients have a circulating IgG which fixes C3 to the basement membrane zone of normal skin by an *in vitro* complement binding technique. This IgG is referred to as the herpes gestationis (HG) factor. In a minority of patients, a circulating antibody directed against the basement membrane zone is also found. These immunofluorescent findings clearly separate herpes gestationis from classic erythema multiforme.[15, 21, 23] The pattern of immunofluorescence by light and electron microscopy strongly suggests that herpes gestationis is most closely related to bullous pemphigoid.[18, 24] Some differences exist. In herpes gestationis, HG factor exists in higher titer than the circulating antibasement membrane zone antibody when the latter is present, whereas in bullous pemphigoid the converse is true.[23]

Before 1973, herpes gestationis was diagnosed on the basis of cutaneous lesions that resembled erythema multiforme, dermatitis herpetiformis, or bullous pemphigoid in association with pregnancy. Oral lesions were reported in occasional patients, suggesting that erythema multiforme might also be a manifestation of the gravid state. By applying these immunofluorescent findings to all bullous eruptions developing in pregnancy, it will be possible to establish whether erythema multiforme or some other as-yet-undefined blistering diseases can also appear during this period. Since immunologically defined herpes gestationis can exhibit iris lesions indistinguishable from those of erythema multiforme,[13] it is difficult to dismiss the possibility that such cases may represent a variant of erythema multiforme.

In 1969, on the basis of a literature review, Kolodny had suggested that maternal and fetal morbidity and mortality were not increased in herpes gestationis.[16] Lawley et al. reviewed their own cases and those published since 1973 in which immunofluorescent findings were used as one of the diagnostic criteria.[15] They found that women who had circulating antibasement membrane zone antibody had a more severe clinical course and needed higher doses of steroids for effective suppression of their bullous disease. They also noted that substantial blood eosinophilia was correlated to some extent with the severity of disease activity. These two prognostic factors need to be reevaluated in future series. Lawley et al. found that fetal morbidity and fetal mortality were increased. Stillbirths occurred in 3 of 39 (7.7 per cent) — six times higher than the rate in the general population. However, there was not an abnormally high rate of spontaneous abortions (1 of 39). Premature births occurred in 8 of 35 live births (23 per cent). The normal rate in the population is 5 to 10 per cent. Four infants were born with skin lesions compatible with herpes gestationis. In two, direct immunofluorescence showed C3 along the basement membrane zone. Indirect immunofluorescent studies of the sera in three infants showed HG factor in two and antibasement membrane zone antibody of the IgG class in one. No comment was made about the immunofluorescent markers in the mothers of the respective babies.

We have made the diagnosis of herpes gestationis in four patients in the past 10 years before the immunologic markers were discovered. A fifth patient was diagnosed with immunologic confirmation. These five patients have had seven healthy babies in as many pregnancies.

In the past pyridoxine deficiency has been proposed as an etiology for this disorder because some patients had been successfully treated with this vitamin.[14, 25] Rh factor isosensitization has also been proposed but not confirmed.[26] At present, it appears that herpes gestationis is either bullous pemphigoid or a closely related disease that can be initiated by pregnancy or birth control pills. It can continue chronically or cyclically with the menstrual cycle post partum for months to years. The behavior of this disease is strikingly similar to cases of autoimmune progesterone dermatitis (see p. 774).

Impetigo Herpetiformis

Impetigo herpetiformis is another rare disease that traditionally has been classified among the unique dermatoses of pregnancy. It is a superficial sterile pustular eruption on an erythematous base that is accompanied by fever, signs of toxicity, hypocalcemia, and sometimes tetany. Remissions occur post partum and recurrences in succeeding pregnancies are likely. The disease may be fatal. Only 100 cases have been reported. In reality, impetigo herpetiformis represents pustular psoriasis of von Zumbusch precipitated by pregnancy.

Although the first description of impetigo herpetiformis were in pregnant women[27] or in women following thyroidectomy,[28, 29] later papers described men and older women and even children with this condition.[30, 31] A significant number of patients said to have impetigo herpetiformis had previously had classic psoriasis with plaques.[31, 32] Patients who developed a generalized pustular eruption and were also pregnant or hypocalcemic often were placed in the category of impetigo herpetiformis because of these associated findings, while males or females not of childbearing age were said to have pustular psoriasis of von Zumbusch. Sometimes conditions were diagnosed as impetigo herpetiformis rather than pustular psoriasis because eosinophils were present in the intraepidermal spongiform pustules characteristic of the disease.[32, 33] However, this distinction may not be valid because neutrophils as well as mast cells contain a low molecular weight eosinophilic chemotactic factor.[34] Eosinophils could be attracted to the spongiform pustules that are composed entirely of neutrophils. Careful surveys indicate that pustular psoriasis of von Zumbusch and impetigo herpetiformis cannot be separated on the basis of sex, age, pregnancy, histopathology, clinical course, therapeutic response, or laboratory findings[33, 35-39] (see p. 740).

Papular Dermatoses of Pregnancy

Several dermatoses characterized by pruritic papules have been described in association with pregnancy. The relationships among them are still unclear.

Papular dermatitis of pregnancy, first described by Spangler et al.,[40] is a generalized severely pruritic papular eruption which occurred in 0.026 per cent of births. As of 1971, about 15 patients had been reported.[41]

The eruption consists of individual erythematous papules 3 to 5 mm in diameter with a smaller papule at the apex. New lesions appear in small numbers, never in crops and never grouped. At the time of examination, most of the papules will have been excoriated. Individual lesions heal spontaneously after seven to ten days, leaving spots of hyperpigmentation.

The disorder is limited to pregnancy and can appear as early as the first month or as late as the last. The disease disappears promptly post partum but usually recurs with successive pregnancies. No manifestations of systemic disease have been described with this disorder. In three patients reported by Spangler and Emerson[41] itching persisted for a few weeks after parturition. Dilatation and curettage were performed with successful removal of retained placental tissue, and the pruritus promptly subsided after this procedure.

A number of placental and endocrinologic clues have been uncovered in this entity.[40, 41] Patients with this disorder develop inflammatory responses to intradermal injections of extracts of placentas from others with this disease but not from placentas of normal individuals. In the last trimester of pregnancy, urinary chorionic gonadotropin levels are markedly elevated; plasma cortisol levels are reduced; plasma cortisol half-life is shortened; and urinary levels of estriol are reduced — a reversal of findings in normal pregnancy, suggesting an estrogen deficiency in this syndrome. Five of the 12 patients in the original report were Rh-negative.

In the original report of Spangler et al.[40] the overall fetal loss was reported as 27 per cent based upon a review of 37 previous pregnancies in the 12 patients. However, 8 of the 11 fetal deaths — abortions and still births — occurred in the absence of any skin disease in the mother. In only three fetal deaths did the mother have papular dermatitis. It remains to be determined whether this disorder is truly associated with a high fetal mortality.[42, 43]

The diagnosis of papular dermatitis of pregnancy is suggested by the presence of severe *intractable* pruritus, accompanied by individual papules that continually appear in a scattered distribution. High levels of urinary chorionic gonadotropin levels in the last trimester, low urinary estriol, and low plasma cortisol levels confirm the clinical diagnosis.

Prurigo of pregnancy was described by Nurse in 1968.[44] He reported 40 women who developed pruritic papules either early (25 to 39 weeks) or late (39th week) in their pregnancies. The excoriated papules occurred chiefly on the proximal parts of the limbs and upper trunk (Figs. 16–6 and 16–7). The syndrome disappeared within three to four weeks after delivery. Recurrences in subsequent pregnancies were unusual and there was no significant fetal loss (2.5 per cent). The prurigo of Besnier[45] and prurigo annularis of Davies[46] seem to be identical to the prurigo of pregnancy described by Nurse. Nurse performed no laboratory tests on his patients, so that it is not known whether his patients' condition could have been a mild variant of the entity described by Spangler et al.[40]

Lawley et al. have delineated a syndrome that they have entitled *pruritic urticarial papules and plaques of pregnancy* (PUPPP).[47] Seven women exhibited an identical clinical syndrome of red urticarial papules and plaques that began on the abdomen and spread to involve the thighs (Figs. 16–8 and 16–9). The buttocks, legs, and arms were less frequently affected. Truncal lesions were rarely seen above the midthorax, and the face was never affected. In spite of marked pruritus, excoriations were rare. A narrow pale halo often surrounded the papules. PUPPP developed in the last trimester (27th to 40th week) and promptly disappeared within two weeks after delivery. There were no abnormal hematologic or urinary findings, including serum chorionic gonadotropin levels. Direct immunofluorescent examination of lesional and normal skin was negative for

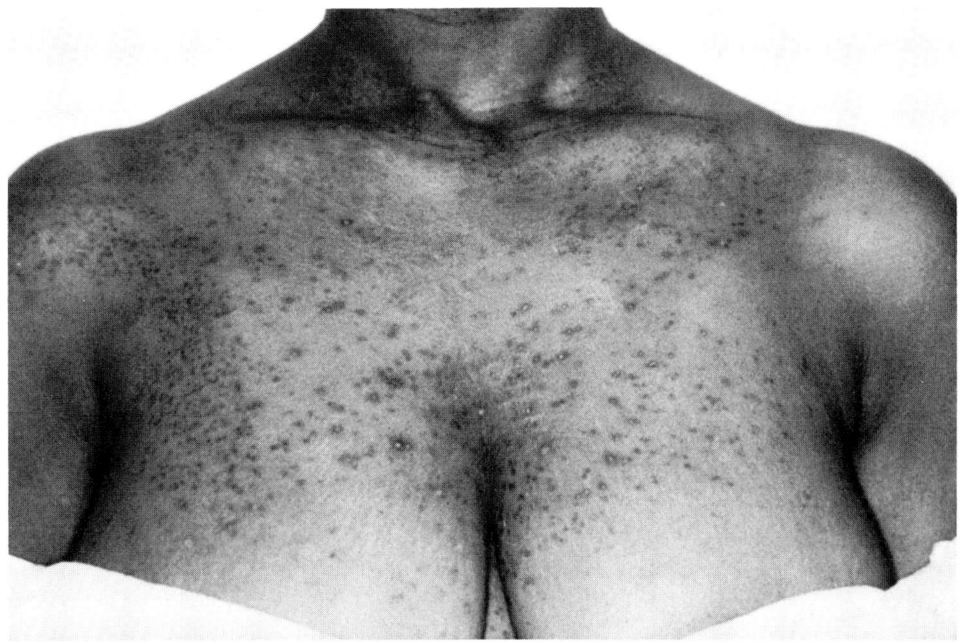

Figure 16–6. Prurigo of pregnancy.

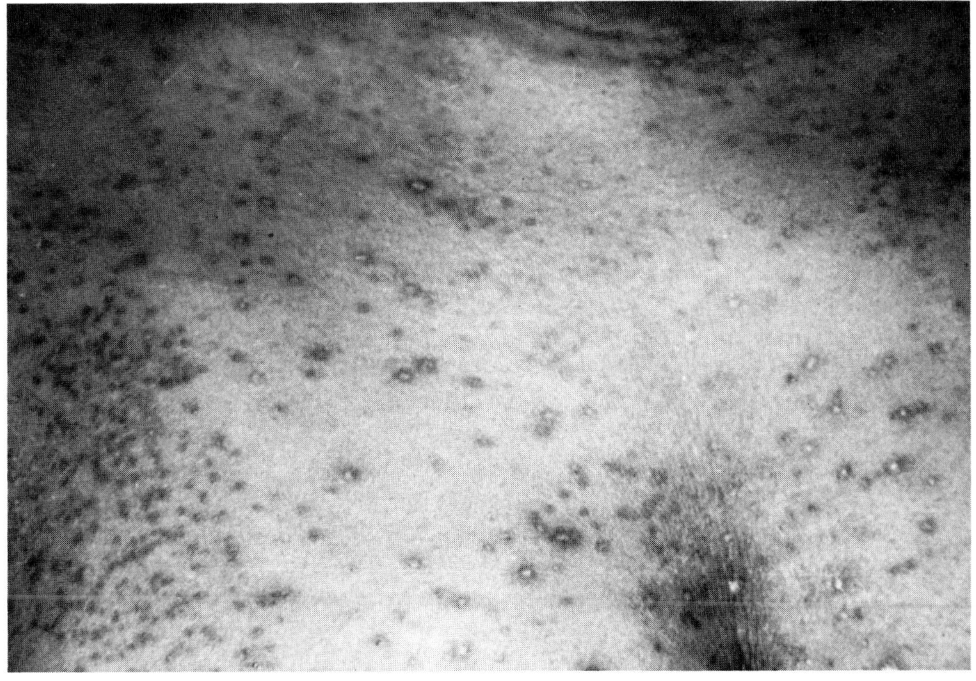

Figure 16–7. Prurigo of pregnancy. Close-up of lesions in Figure 16–6 shows them to be excoriated papules.

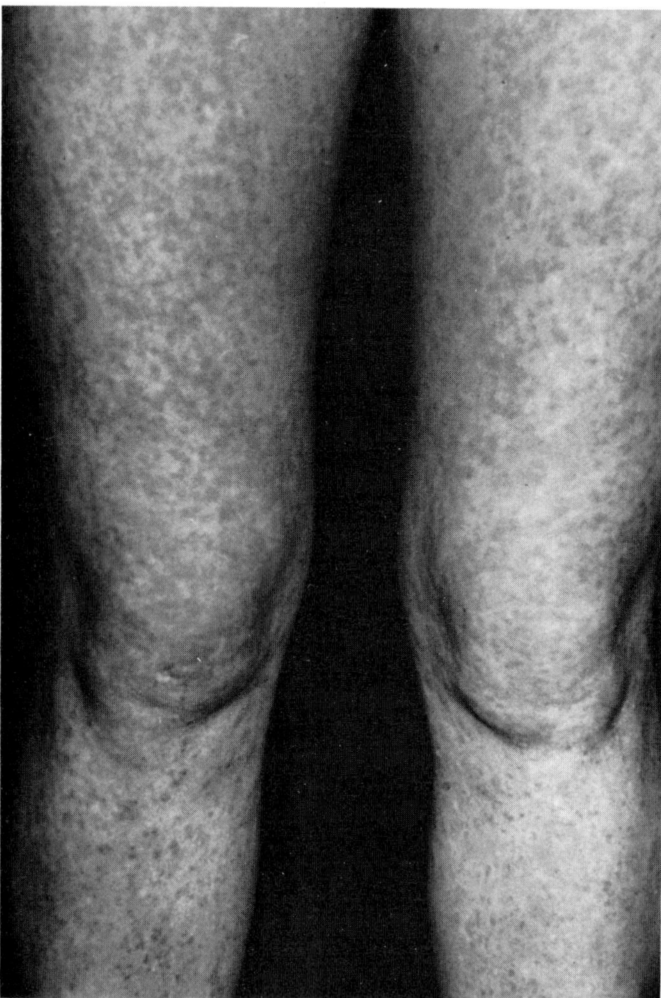

Figure 16–8. PUPPP syndrome. Urticarial papules and plaques on legs and thighs. (From Lawley, T. J., Hertz, K. C., Wade, T. R., Ackerman, A. B., and Katz, S. I.: Pruritic urticarial papules and plaques of pregnancy. J.A.M.A., *241*: 1696, 1979.)

immunoglobulins and complement. Histologically, the skin lesions showed perivascular collections of lymphohistiocytic cells, including a few eosinophils around the superficial and sometimes deep vascular plexuses. Mild spongiosis may be present. PUPPP appears to be distinct from the other pruritic papular dermatoses of pregnancy, and should be able to be distinguished from them on the basis of clinical and morphologic features. The urticarial papules of PUPPP can resemble some of the early lesions of herpes gestationis, but differentiation can be made easily by direct immunofluorescent examination for immunoreactants and by routine histology. PUPPP may be identical to Bourne's toxemic rash of pregnancy based upon the description of the clinical lesions and their distribution. However, the details of individual cases, histopathology, and laboratory data are lacking in Bourne's report.[48] The small number of patients in the series of Lawley et al. preclude any evaluation of possible maternal and fetal complications. Lawley et al. believe that PUPPP may be the most common variety of the pruritic dermatoses of pregnancy, which has not been previously recognized because of its generally late appearance, brief duration, and excellent response to topical steroid therapy.

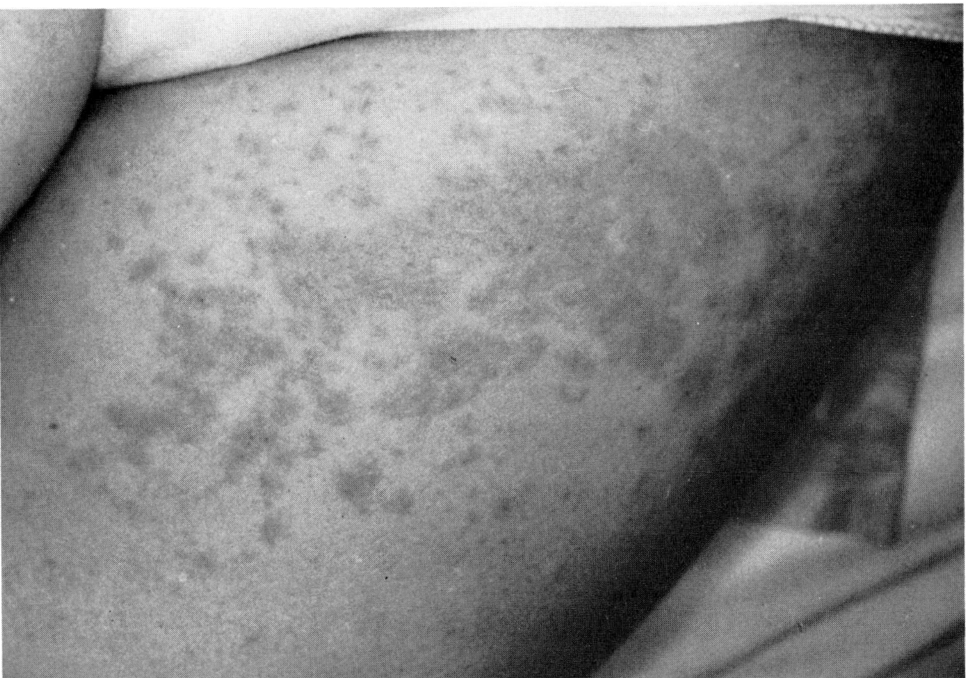

Figure 16–9. PUPPP syndrome. In this patient, the lesions were limited to lower abdomen and upper thighs. They began three weeks before delivery and resolved spontaneously two weeks post partum. Same patient as in Plate 30*F*.

Intrahepatic Cholestasis of Pregnancy

Intrahepatic cholestasis of pregnancy (pruritus gravidarum) produces generalized pruritus that may or may not be eventually accompanied by jaundice. The disorder usually begins in the third trimester, but it may appear as early as the twentieth week of pregnancy. The pruritus and jaundice, if present, promptly disappear after delivery. The pruritus usually precedes the development of jaundice by two to three weeks. The prevalence of this disorder varies from 0.06 to 0.43 per cent of all completed pregnancies.[49] The probability of recurrence in succeeding pregnancies is high. In the series of Rencoret and Aste it was 47 per cent.[49]

This diagnosis should be considered when one evaluates generalized pruritus in the absence of a specific eruption. Liver function tests reveal elevated alkaline phosphatase and bilirubin in the presence of normal flocculation tests and transaminase levels. Other forms of liver disease need to be excluded before this diagnosis can be made.

Estrogens play a role in the impairment of the excretory function of the liver because the syndrome can be reproduced in these affected women by administering the contraceptive pill after pregnancy.

No maternal deaths due to cholestatic jaundice have been recorded. Several series have reported premature labor in as many as 30 per cent of cases. Opinions on fetal loss vary, however. In some series, there were no deaths, and in others the percentage was as high as 37. The main causes of death were intrapartum asphyxia and respiratory distress syndrome. No obvious fetal abnormalities have been found. Because of the high incidence of fetal distress in some series, Rencoret and Aste urge that fetal monitoring in labor should be available to patients with recurrent cholestasis, particularly for those with a history of fetal loss.[49] The reasons for the variability of fetal loss in different series need to be studied further in order to determine if they are directly related to cholestatic jaundice.

The differential diagnosis of pruritus in pregnancy includes not only the entities mentioned above but also all those factors capable of producing pruritus in the nonpregnant state. These include drug reactions, scabies, irritation from woolen and synthetic fibers, ichthyosis, xerosis (winter itch), emotional disturbances, moniliasis of the anogenital region, and underlying lymphoma. In many instances, hard scratching produces excoriations that are erythematous and papular and causes the accompanying traumatically induced edema. The scratch-papule, as a secondary lesion, must be kept in mind in the evaluation of pruritus.

PREEXISTING DERMATOSES AND PREGNANCY

Pregnancy has an adverse effect on neurofibromatosis. Swapp and Main[50] studied 10 women who had 24 pregnancies. In 5 of the 10 cases, the lesions of neurofibromatosis were seen for the first time during pregnancy. In the other patients, café-au-lait spots and neurofibromas were found to increase in size and number. After delivery, considerable regression of the tumors occurred.

In pregnancy, about one half of patients with psoriasis vulgaris enter a remission. Only a small percentage become worse.[51] The behavior of acne vulgaris in pregnancy is unpredictable. Condylomata acuminata frequently become larger and more numerous.[52, 53] In exceptional cases, the condylomata have become so large that vaginal delivery was not possible and caesarean section had to be performed.

The Menstrual Cycle

At least 15 women have been reported with dermatoses that cyclically flare seven to ten days before the menstrual cycle begins, and tend to disappear following menstrual flow. These dermatoses, classified under the category of autoimmune progesterone dermatitis, have taken the form of urticaria, papules, pustules, and dishidrotic eczema-like eruptions. Some patients have had erythema multiforme with oral involvement.[54] Russell and Thorne reported the case of a woman with premenstrual flares of erythema multiforme since age 14, which became worse during pregnancy and finally disappeared with the artificial induction of the menopause by irradiation at age 49.[12]

These dermatoses can be provoked or exacerbated by the injection of progesterone and suppressed by estrogen. These patients develop a delayed hypersensitivity reaction by intradermal injections of progesterone, suggesting that an autoimmune reaction to this hormone is the cause of these dermatoses. It may be significant that six of seven patients reported by Hart had taken progestins (synthetic progesterone-like compounds) in the form of birth control pills prior to the onset of their eruptions.[54]

The premenstrual flares seen in patients with herpes gestationis fall into the general category of autoimmune progesterone dermatitis. It would be worthwhile to inquire about the prior use of progestins in patients with herpes gestationis, as well as to perform skin tests to determine whether delayed hypersensitivity to progesterone is present.

In patients with any type of cyclic eruption related to the menses, the entity of autoimmune progesterone dermatitis should be strongly considered.

REFERENCES

1. Snell, R. S., and Bischitz, P. G.: The effect of large doses of estrogen and estrogen and progesterone on melanin pigmentation. J. Invest. Dermatol., *35*:73, 1960.
2. Snell, R. S.: The pigmentary changes occurring in the breast skin during pregnancy and following estrogen treatment. J. Invest. Dermatol., *43*:181, 1964.
3. Kligman, A. M.: Pathological dynamics of human hair loss. Arch. Dermatol., *83*:175, 1961.
4. Lynfield, Y. L.: Effect of pregnancy on the human hair cycle. J. Invest. Dermatol., *35*:323, 1960.
5. Schiff, B. L., and Kern, A. B.: A study of postpartum alopecia. Arch. Dermatol., *87*:609, 1963.
6. Friedman, I. S., Mackles, A., and Daichman, I.: Development of virilization during pregnancy. J. Clin. Endocrinol. Metab., *15*:1281, 1955.
7. Turunen, A., Pesonen, S., and Ziliacus, H.: Hormone assays during recurrent excessive hair growth in pregnancy. Acta Endocrinol., *45*:447, 1964.
8. Poidevin, L. O. S.: Striae gravidarum. Their relation to adrenal cortical hyperfunction. Lancet, *2*:436, 1959.
9. Rose, T. R.: The hemangiomata of pregnancy. J. Obst. Gynecol. Br. Empire, *56*:364, 1949.
10. Letterman, G., and Schwiter, M.: Cutaneous hemangiomas of the face in pregnancy. Plastic Reconstruct. Surg., *29*:293, 1962.
11. Crawford, G. M., and Leeper, R .W.: Diseases of the skin in pregnancy. Arch. Dermatol., *61*:753, 1950.
12. Russell, B., and Thorne, N.: Herpes gestationis. Br. J. Dermatol., *69*:753, 1957.
13. Bushkell, L. L., Jordon, R. E., and Goltz, R. W.: Herpes gestationis. New immunologic findings. Arch. Dermatol., *110*:65, 1974.
14. Coupe, R. S.: Herpes gestationis. Arch. Dermatol., *91*:633, 1965.
15. Lawley, T. J., Stingl, G., and Katz, S. I.: Fetal and maternal risk factors in herpes gestationis. Arch. Dermatol., *114*:552, 1978.
16. Kolodny, R. C.: Herpes gestationis. Am. J. Obstet. Gynecol., *104*:39, 1969.
17. Black, M. M.: The enigma of herpes gestationis. Trans. Pacific Dermatologic Association, 1977, p. 15.
18. Honigsmann, H., Stingl, G., Holubar, K., and Wolff, K.: Herpes gestationis: fine structural pattern of immunoglobulin deposits in the skin in vivo. J. Invest. Dermatol., *66*:389, 1976.
19. Lynch, F. W., and Albrecht, E. J.: Hormonal factors in herpes gestationis. Arch. Dermatol., *93*:446, 1966.
20. Hertz, K. C., Katz, S. I., Maize, J., and Ackerman, A. B.: Herpes gestationis. A clinicopathologic study. Arch. Dermatol., *112*:1543, 1976.
21. Provost, T. T., and Tomasi, T. B., Jr.: Evidence for complement activation via the alternate pathway in skin diseases. I. Herpes gestationis, systemic lupus erythematosus, and bullous pemphigoid. J. Clin. Invest., *52*:1779, 1973.
22. Jordon, R. E., Yeine, K. C., Tappeiner, G., Bushkell, L. L., and Provost, T. T.: The immunopathology of herpes gestationis. Immunofluorescence studies and characterization of "HG factor." J. Clin. Invest., *57*:1426, 1976.
23. Katz, S. I., Hertz, K. C., and Yaoita, H.: Herpes gestationis. Immunopathology and characterization of the HG factor. J. Clin. Invest., *57*:1434, 1976.
24. Yaoita, H., Gullino, M., and Katz, S. I.: Herpes gestationis. Ultrastructure and ultrastructural localization of in vivo-bound complement. Modified tissue preparation and processing for horseradish peroxidase staining of skin. J. Invest. Dermatol., *66*:383, 1976.
25. Fosnaugh, R. P., Bryan, H. G., and Orders, R. L.: Pyridoxine in the treatment of herpes gestationis. Arch. Dermatol., *84*:90, 1961.
26. Cawley, E. P., Wheeler, C. E., and Wilhite, P. A.: Herpes gestationis and the Rh factor. Southern Med. J., *45*:827, 1952.
27. Hebra, F.: Schwangerschaft dem Wochenbette und bei Uterinalkrankheiten der Frauen zu beobachtende Hautkrankheiten. Wien. Med. Wochenschr., *22*:1197, 1872.
28. Hvidberg, E.: Impetigo herpetiformis. Dermatologica, *114*:337, 1957.
29. Feiwel, M., and Ferriman, D.: Impetigo her-

petiformis. Proc. R. Soc. Med., *50*:393, 1957.

30. Beek, C. H.: On impetigo herpetiformis. Dermatologica, *102*:145, 1951.
31. Katzenellenbogen, I., and Feuerman, E. J.: Psoriasis pustulosa and impetigo herpetiformis — single or dual entity? Acta Dermatovenereol., *46*:85, 1966.
32. Tolman, M. M., and Moschella, S. L.: Pustular psoriasis (Zumbusch). Arch. Dermatol., *81*:400, 1960.
33. Moslein, P.: Impetigo herpetiformis — Psoriasis pustulosa — Acrodermatitis continua Hallopeau. Arch. Klin. Exp. Dermatol., *208*:410, 1959.
34. Czarnetski, B. M., König, W., and Lichtenstein, L. M.: Eosinophil chemotactic factor (ECF) I. Release from polymorphonuclear leukocytes by the calcium ionophore A23187. J. Immunol., *117*:229, 1976.
35. Champion, R. H.: Generalized pustular psoriasis. Br J. Dermatol., *71*:384, 1959.
36. Koch, F.: Zur Frage der Identität von Impetigo herpetiformis, Psoriasis pustulosa, und Psoriasis vulgaris. Hautarzt, *3*:165, 1952.
37. Danboldt, N.: Kasuistischer Beitrag zur Frage Psoriasis pustulosa — Impetigo herpetiformis. Acta Dermatovenereol., *18*:150, 1937.
38. Soltermann, W.: Familiare Psoriasis pustulosa unter dem Bilde der Impetigo herpetiformis. Dermatologica, *116*:313, 1958.
39. Ingram, J. T.: Pustular psoriasis. Arch. Dermatol., *77*:314, 1958.
40. Spangler, A. S., Reddy, W., Bardawil, W. A., Roby, C. C., and Emerson, K.: Papular dermatitis of pregnancy: A new clinical entity? J.A.M.A., *181*:577, 1962.
41. Spangler, A. S., and Emerson, K.: Estrogen levels and estrogen therapy in papular dermatitis of pregnancy. Am. J. Obstet. Gynecol., *110*:534, 1971.
42. Otterson, W. N.: Diethylstilbestrol in management of papular dermatitis of pregnancy. Am. J. Obstet. Gynecol., *113*:570, 1972.
43. Spangler, A. S., and Emerson, K.: Diethylstilbestrol in management of papular dermatitis of pregnancy. Reply to Colonel Otterson. Am. J. Obstet. Gynecol., *113*:571, 1972.
44. Nurse, D. S.: Prurigo of pregnancy. Aust. J. Dermatol., *9*:258, 1968.
45. Costello, M. J.: Eruptions of pregnancy. N.Y. J. Med., *41*:849, 1941.
46. Davies, J. H. T.: Prurigo annularis. Br. J. Dermatol., *53*:143, 1941.
47. Lawley, T. J., Hertz, K. C., Wade, T. R., Ackerman, A. B., and Katz, S. I.: Pruritic urticarial papules and plaques of pregnancy. J.A.M.A., *241*:1696, 1979.
48. Bourne, G.: Toxemic rash of pregnancy. Proc. R. Soc. Med., *55*:462, 1962.
49. Rencoret, R., and Aste, H.: Jaundice during pregnancy. Med. J. Australia, *1*:167, 1973.
50. Swapp, G. H., and Main, R. A.: Neurofibromatosis in pregnancy. Br. J. Dermatol., *88*:431, 1973.
51. Gruneberg, T. H.: Psoriasis und Schwangérschaft, Hautarzt, *3*:155, 1952.
52. Young, R. L., Acosta, A. A., and Kaufman, R. H.: The treatment of large condylomata acuminata complicating pregnancy. Obstet. Gynecol., *41*:65, 1973.
53. Powell, L. C., Jr.: Condyloma acuminatum. Clin. Obstet. Gynecol., *15*:948, 1972.
54. Hart, R.: Autoimmune progesterone dermatitis. Arch. Dermatol., *113*:426, 1977.

17

Nervous System

This chapter deals with both neurocutaneous syndromes and the psychologic aspects of human behavior related to dermatologic diseases. Many of the neurocutaneous syndromes have abnormalities of cutaneous pigmentation as their identifying markers, reflecting the common origin of the nervous system and the melanocytes from the neural crest. Emotional factors not only influence the natural history and behavior of some skin diseases, but significant disturbances in mental health can produce tell-tale signs in the skin.

NEUROCUTANEOUS DISORDERS

Tuberous Sclerosis

The complete syndrome of tuberous sclerosis (epiloia) exhibits epilepsy, mental retardation, a facial lesion called adenoma sebaceum, periungual and subungual fibromas, shagreen patches, white macules, tumors on the retina (phakomas), and calcification in the area of the basal ganglia. Formes frustes of this entity are common. Tuberous sclerosis is inherited in a dominant fashion.

The characteristic lesion is adenoma sebaceum — pink or flesh-colored papules that arise in the nasolabial folds and on the cheeks and that may be accompanied by fine telangiectasia (Fig. 17–1; Plate 39*D*). These lesions grow in size and multiply with age. The term *adenoma sebaceum* is a misnomer because the lesions represent hamartomas composed of fibrous and vascular tissues. The accurate term is *angiofibroma*. The sebaceous glands that are present merely represent the normal constituents of the skin that have been trapped in the lesions.

Angiofibromas also develop under and around the nails (ungual fibromas) and on the gums (Figs. 17–2 to 17–4). On the forehead and scalp these lesions may be as large as several centimeters. In these locations the tumors are mostly fibrous, and the vascular component is minimal (Fig. 17–5).

Shagreen patches are flesh-colored soft plaques or clusters of nodules that are usually found in the lumbosacral area but that can occur anywhere on the trunk (Fig. 17–6). The surface may be pebbly or look like pigskin with prominent follicular openings. These lesions represent foci of increased amounts of collagen.

The phakomas in the retina represent tumors of glial tissue. Similar tumors that develop at the base of the brain and become calcified are referred to as "tubers." Hamartomas also appear in the lung and kidney,

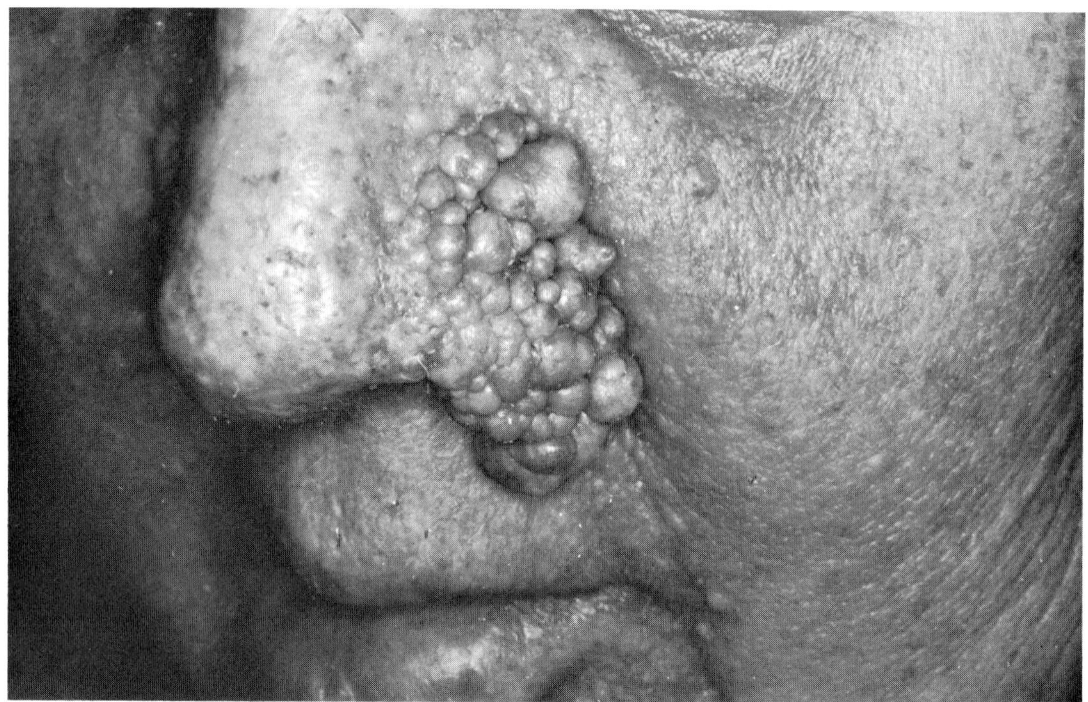

Figure 17–1. Tuberous sclerosis. Florid adenoma sebaceum.

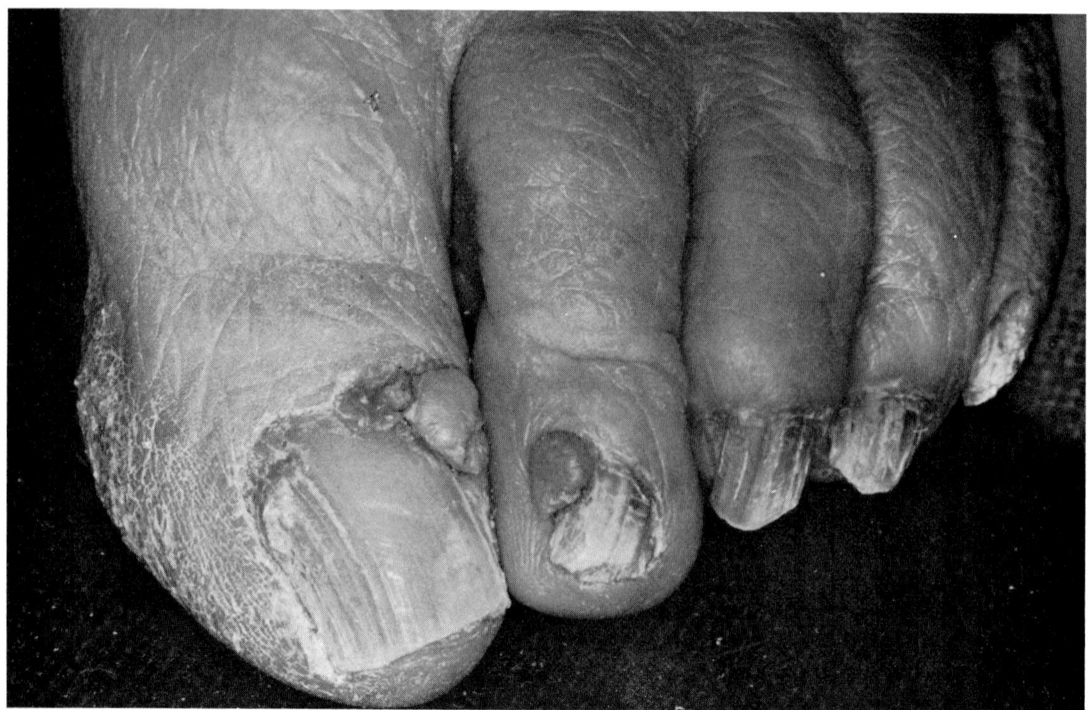

Figure 17–2. Tuberous sclerosis. Ungual fibromas.

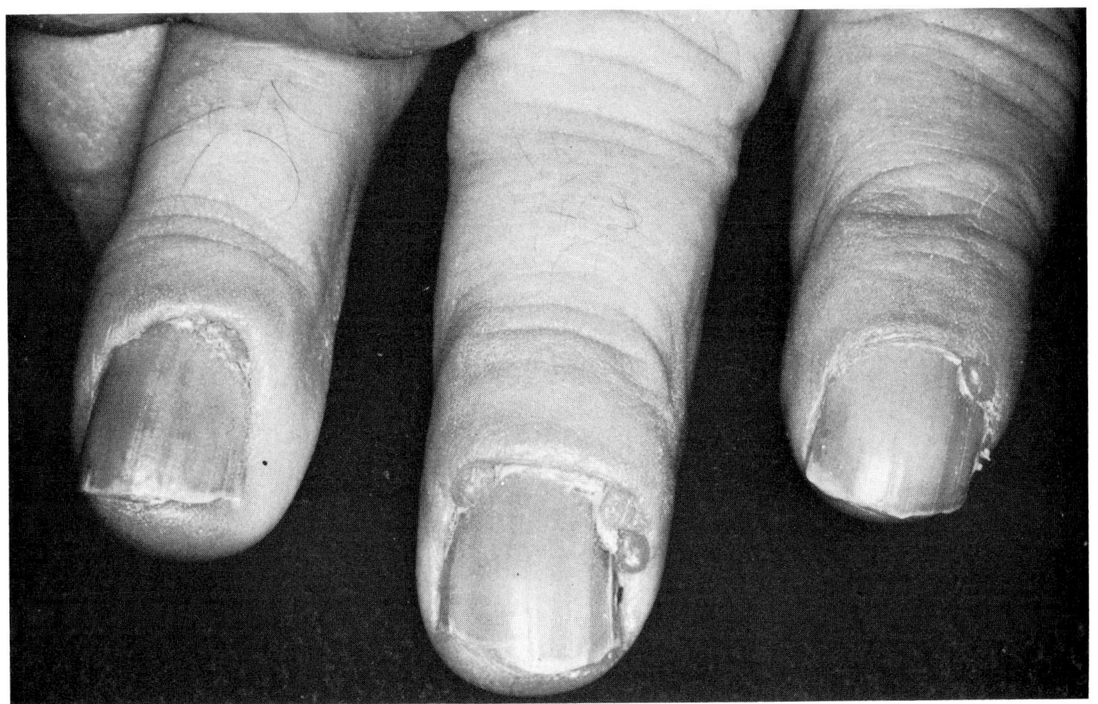

Figure 17–3. Tuberous sclerosis. Ungual fibromas.

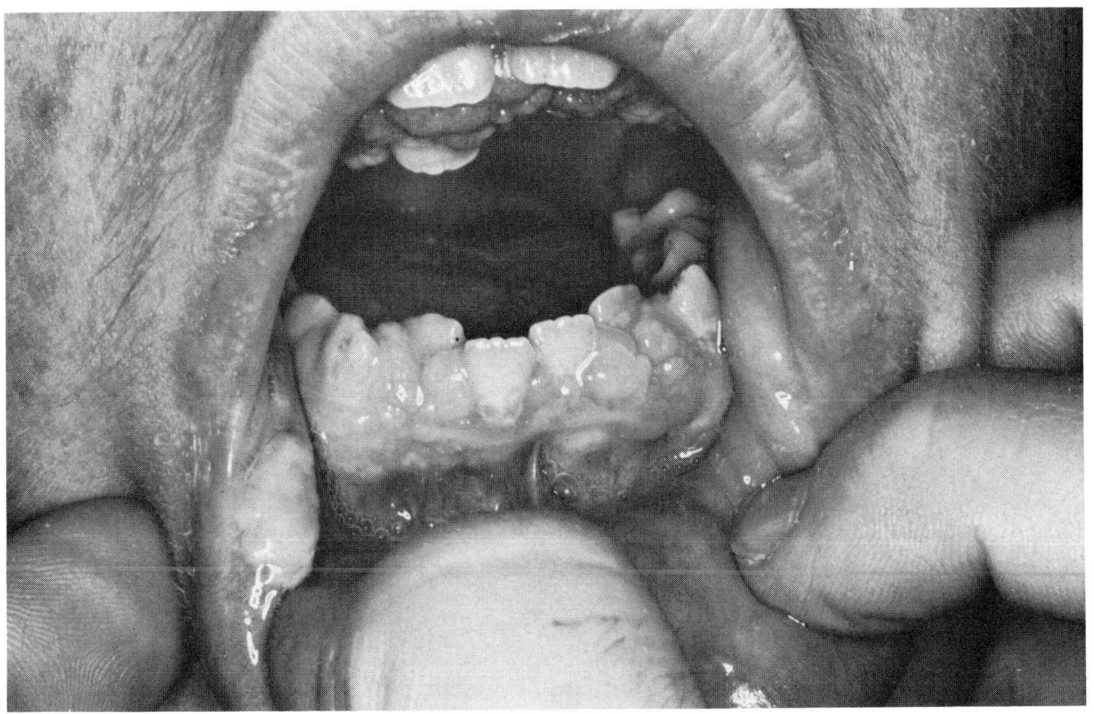

Figure 17–4. Tuberous sclerosis. Gingival fibromas.

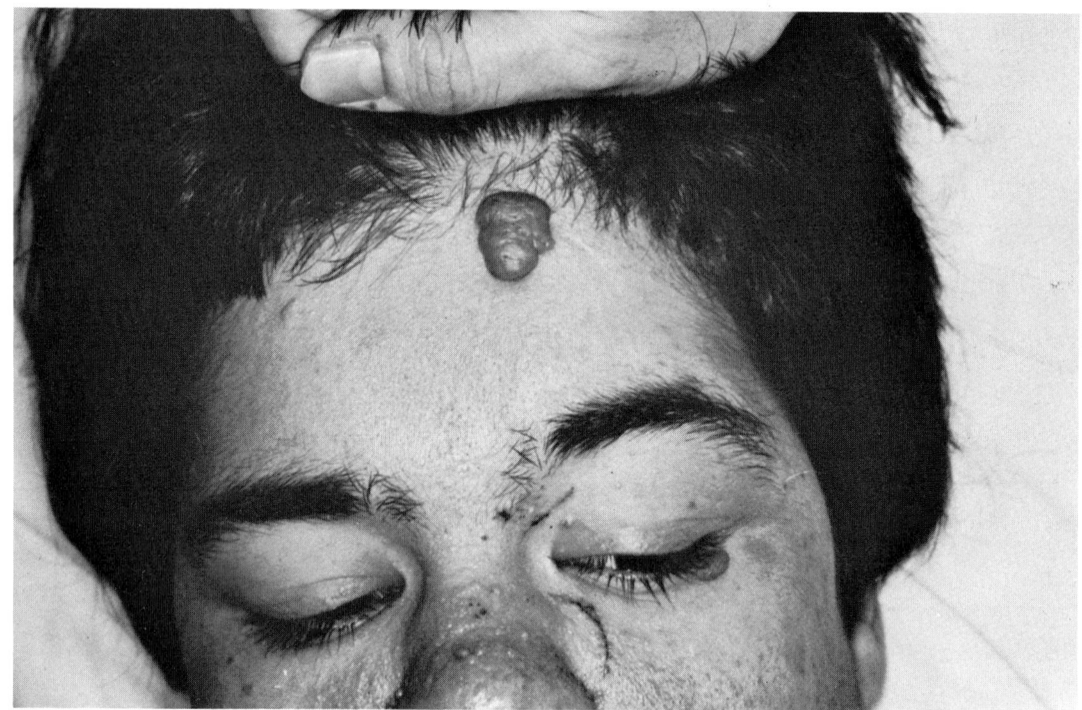

Figure 17–5. Tuberous sclerosis. Fibroma.

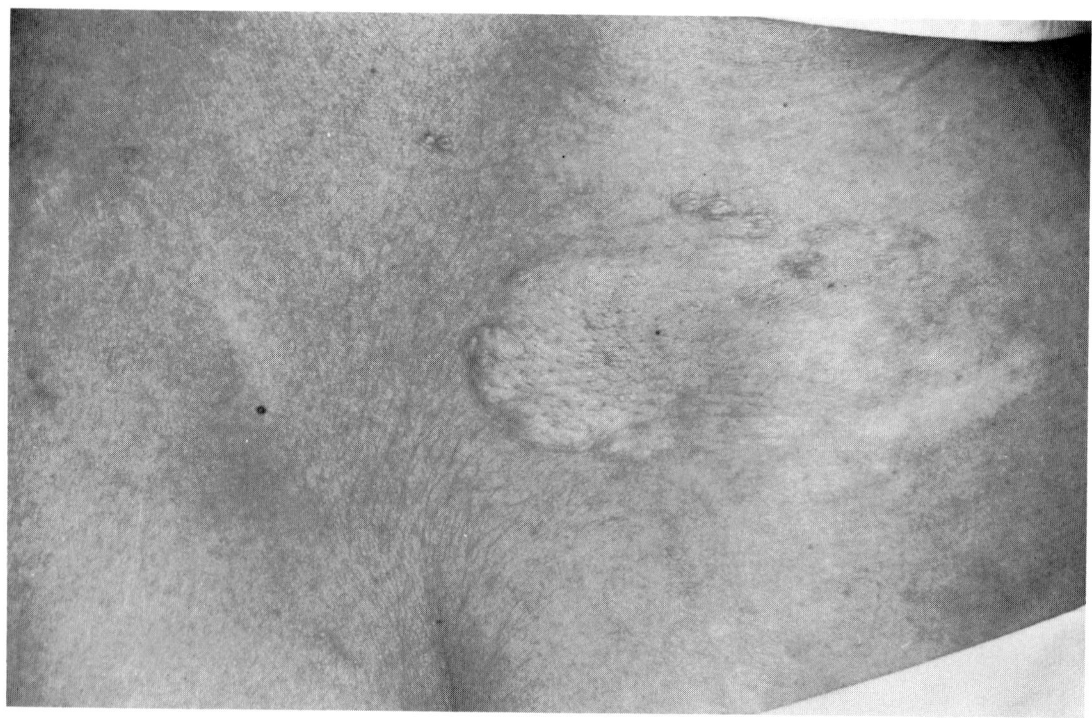

Figure 17–6. Tuberous sclerosis. Large shagreen patch with adjacent smaller plaques above right buttock.

and rhabdomyomas develop in the heart. None of these tumors is, or becomes, malignant.

Lagos et al. published a representative series of 71 patients with tuberous sclerosis. The incidence of these various findings was as follows: seizures, 93 per cent; adenoma sebaceum, 83 per cent; mental retardation, 62 per cent; phakomas, 53 per cent; calcification in the brain, 51 per cent; shagreen patches, 21 per cent; and ungual fibromas, 16 per cent.[1]

The diagnosis of tuberous sclerosis is easily made when these characteristic features are present, but one usually has to wait until the child is at least two years old. Adenoma sebaceum usually appears from two to five years of age; only 13 per cent of children have these lesions in the first year of life. The ungual fibromas and shagreen patches develop in late childhood or early adult life. Calcification in the brain is generally not present in the first year of life. Therefore, it would be helpful if a marker of this disease appeared at birth or shortly thereafter to enable a physician to make the diagnosis of tuberous sclerosis in infants who had myoclonic seizures, epilepsy, or retardation of development.

The white macule seems to be such a cutaneous clue. It is usually present at birth and probably persists throughout life. Chao and the team of Gold and Freeman were the first to point out the significance of this white spot. Since then many other clinicians have confirmed their observations.[2-4] White macules are found on the trunk and extremities and are present in about two thirds of patients with tuberous sclerosis.

Hurwitz and Braverman examined 23 children and adults with tuberous sclerosis and found white spots in 18; in many patients, the spots had been noted at birth.[5] The white spots were oval, leaf-shaped (lance-ovate), or had an over-all oval shape with highly irregular margins. This last configuration was the one most frequently encountered (Figs. 17–7 and 17–8). Only 20 per cent of the lesions were shaped like the leaf of the mountain ash. The spots varied in size from 4 mm to 7 cm, but the majority ranged from 1 to 3 cm in the longest dimension. The macules were concentrated over the abdomen, back, and anterior and lateral surfaces of the legs. The number of white spots ranged from one in a single patient to 32 in another. All of our patients, except one, had at least three or more white lesions. The individual with the single spot had a 7-cm hypopigmented macule with irregular margins on the medial surface of the left knee.

Since the completion of this study, a 16-year-old boy with tuberous sclerosis was seen, whose mother was certain that the white spots appeared at age 13 years.

Although white, the macules are not completely depigmented; they do not have the milk-white color of vitiligo. In one of our patients, the white spots showed evidence of tanning during the summer. Perifollicular pigment was present in the center and on the periphery of some lesions (Fig. 17–9). In addition to the characteristic leukoderma, three patients had hundreds of 2- to 3-mm hypopigmented guttate macules (white freckles) on the legs (Fig. 17–10). Another interesting formation was seen in two individuals: café au lait–like spots and depigmented macules of the same size and configuration were present side by side (Fig. 17–11).

In lightly pigmented skin, especially over the buttocks and lower back, the hypopigmented macules may be missed unless one looks carefully. Some clinicians have found that the use of a Wood's light aids in the discovery of these white spots.[4]

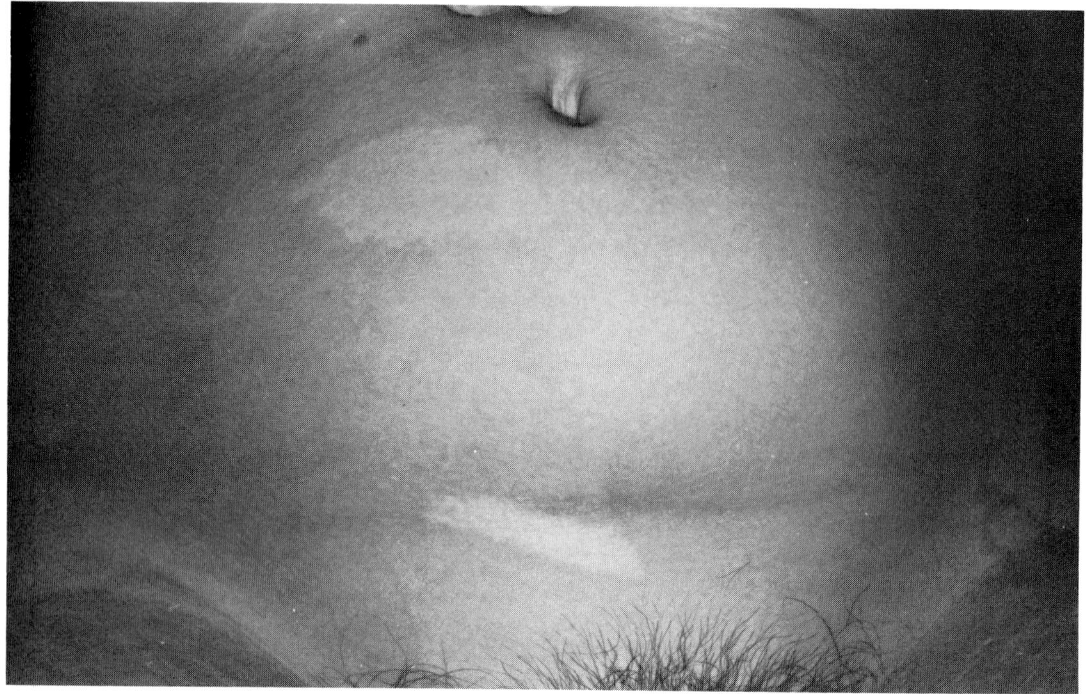

Figure 17–7. Tuberous sclerosis. White macules.

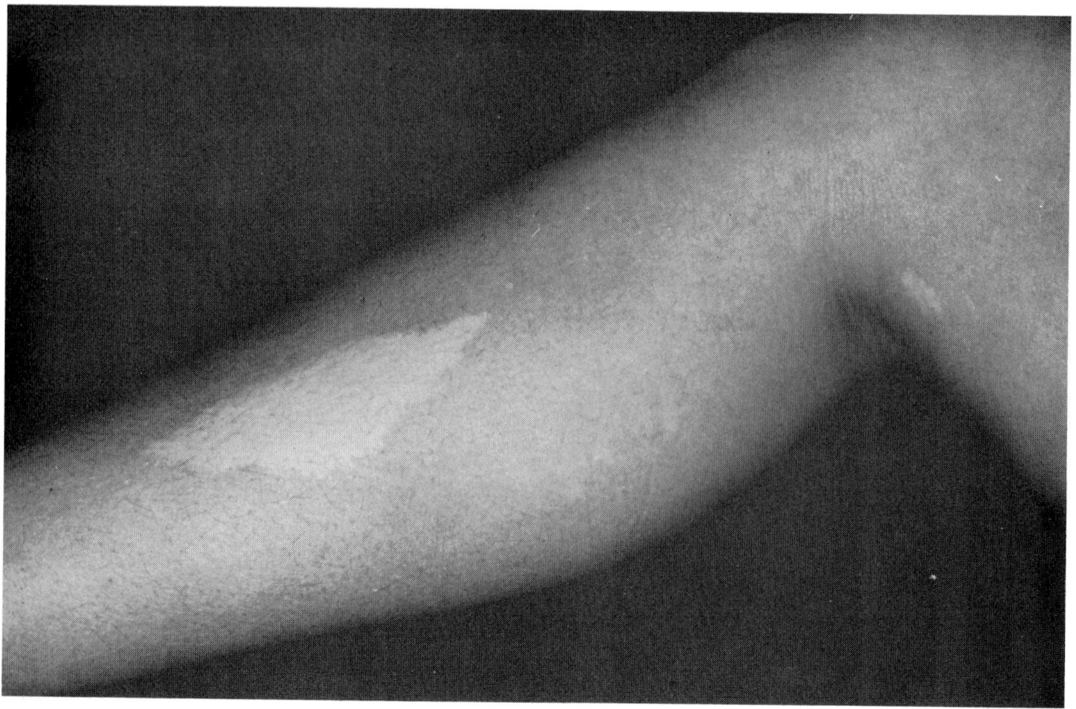

Figure 17–8. Tuberous sclerosis. White macules.

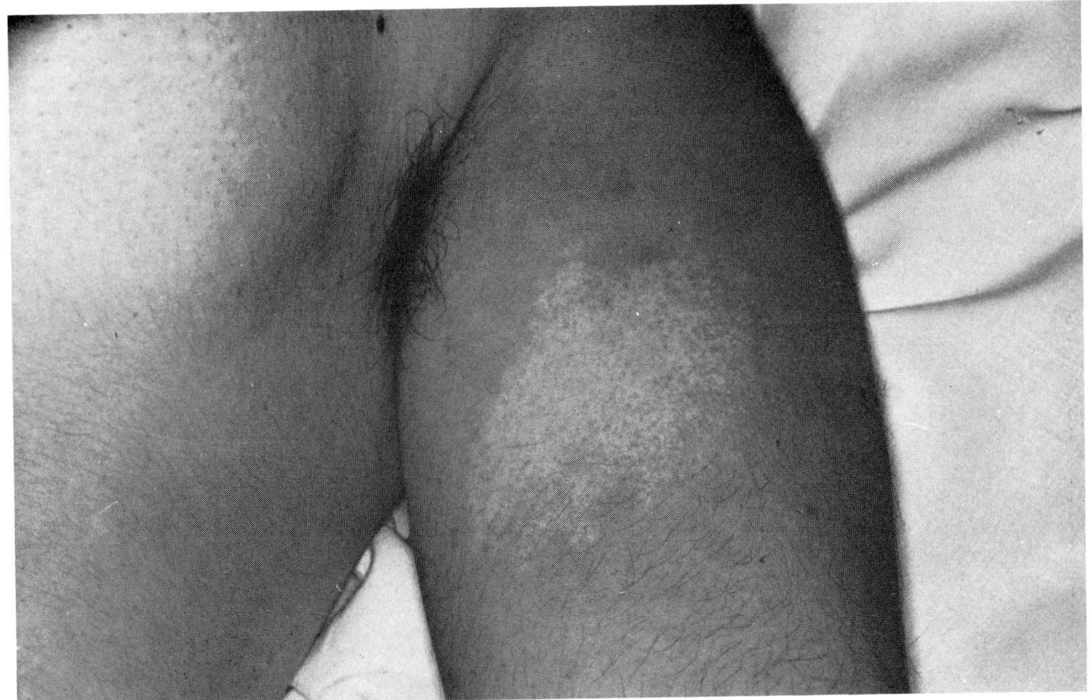

Figure 17–9. Tuberous sclerosis. White macule with perifollicular pigmentation.

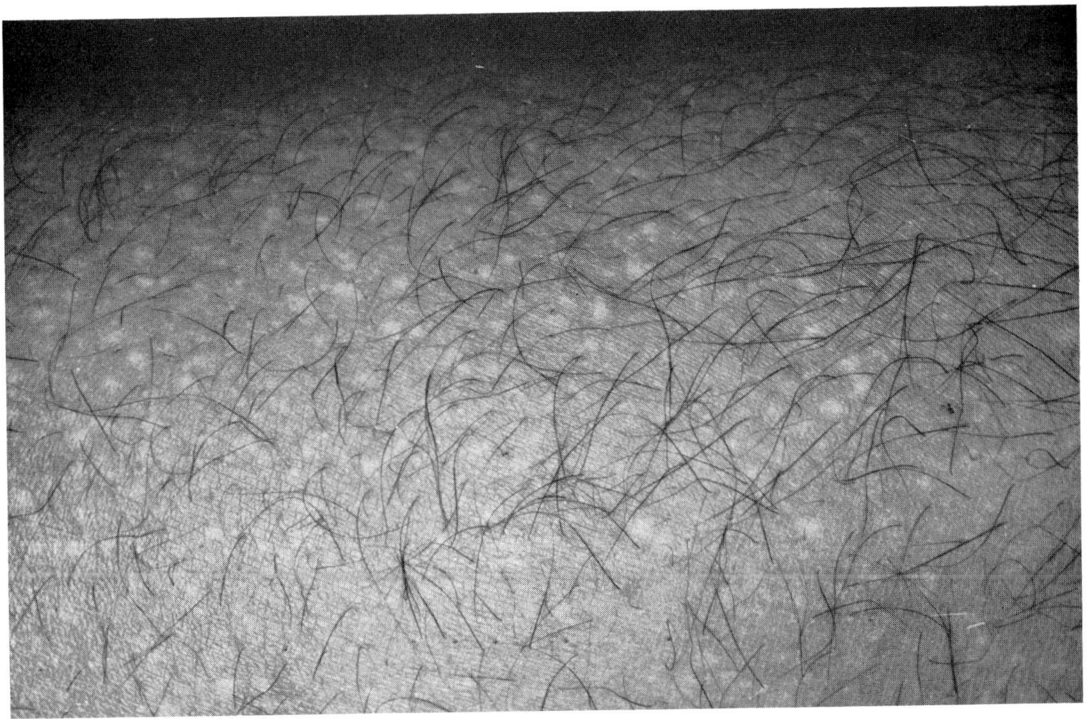

Figure 17–10. Tuberous sclerosis. Speckled hypopigmentation (white freckles).

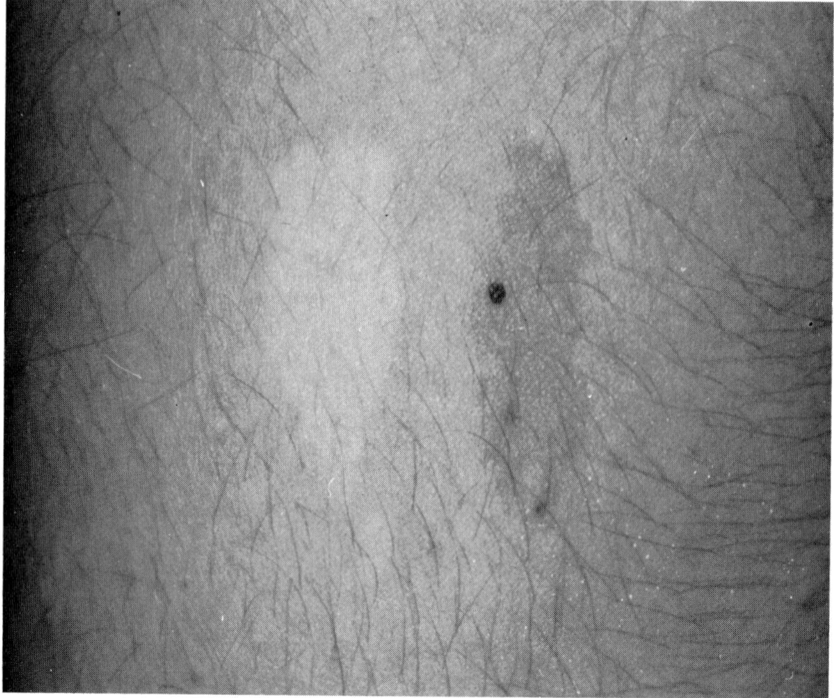

Figure 17–11. Tuberous sclerosis. Café au lait–like spot and white macule of similar configuration side by side.

For controls in this study, 155 children were examined. Fifty-five youngsters had neurologic disorders exclusive of tuberous sclerosis — disorders such as seizures, cerebral palsy, and mental retardation — and attended the neurology clinic at the Yale-New Haven Medical Center. Their ages ranged from 6 months to 16 years. One hundred randomly selected neurologically normal children of comparable ages who were attending the pediatric clinic were similarly studied. Of the 55 neurologically handicapped children, none had the hypopigmented macules of tuberous sclerosis. Of the 100 randomly selected normal children, one child had an ash leaf–shaped white spot that measured 2.5 by 0.75 cm. This patient was 16 months old and had neither a history of seizures nor a family history of tuberous sclerosis. Long-term observation will determine the significance of the hypopigmented macule in this child. None of the 155 children had speckled hypopigmentation.

Although speckled hypopigmentation (white freckles) can be found occasionally in normal persons, its presence in 3 of 23 patients with tuberous sclerosis and its absence in 155 control children suggest that it too may be a sign of the disease. Butterworth had also described white freckles in a case of tuberous sclerosis.[6]

Fitzpatrick et al. were able to discriminate between the white macules of tuberous sclerosis and vitiligo by light and electron microscopic studies.[14] In vitiliginous spots, the melanocytes are absent or reduced in number, whereas in the leukoderma of tuberous sclerosis the melanocytes are present in normal numbers, but the size of the melanosomes and their melanin content appear smaller.

The prevalence of café au lait spots in our patients with tuberous

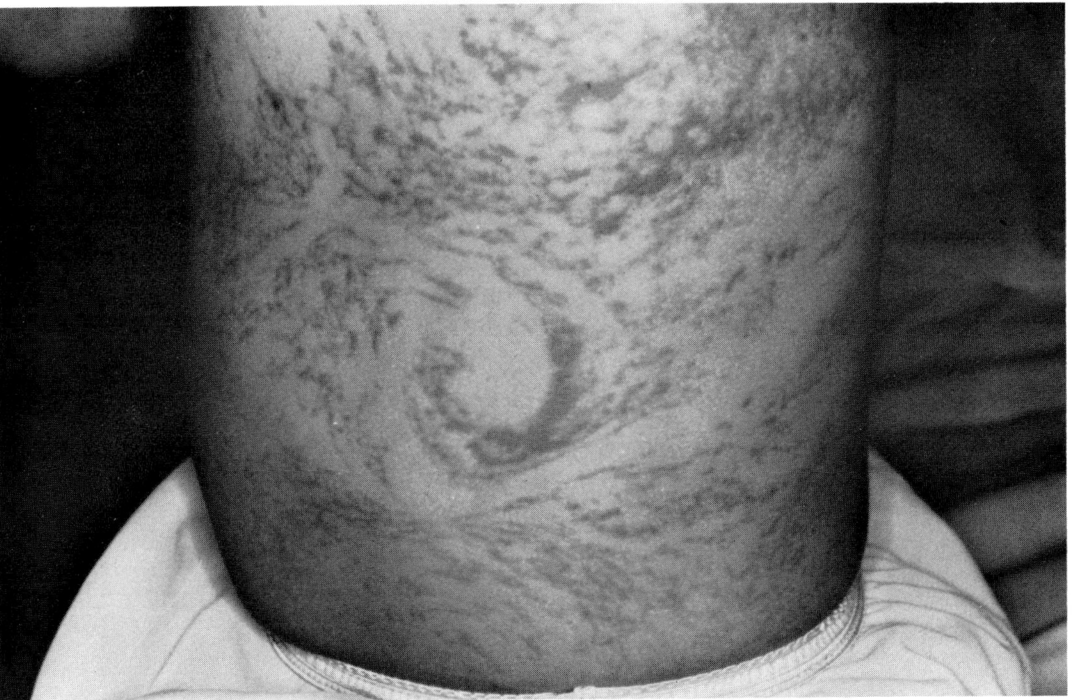

Figure 17–12. Incontinentia pigmenti. Characteristic whorled pattern of hyperpigmentation.

sclerosis was also studied. Twenty-six per cent of these persons had café au lait spots, in contrast to 15 per cent of the neurologically handicapped children and 5 per cent of the normal youngsters. However, no child in any of the groups had more than one or two spots, except for one child who had three spots. Café au lait spots are diagnostic of neurofibromatosis, but only when six or more lesions are present. The significance of café au lait spots in tuberous sclerosis is unknown. Indeed, it is not even known whether the lesions called café au lait spots in tuberous sclerosis or in normal persons are identical to the similar appearing pigmented macules in neurofibromatosis.

Incontinentia Pigmenti

Incontinentia pigmenti (Bloch-Sulzberger type) is a much less common disease and occurs almost exclusively in females. The disease begins within the first two weeks of life in 90 per cent of cases, and within six weeks, in 96 per cent. It is often present at birth. Rarely, the disease may begin as late as two years.[7, 8] Macular hyperpigmentation in a whorled, spidery, splattered, or flecked pattern is present on the trunk (Fig. 17–12). The pigmentation is sometimes preceded by a bullous or linear verrucose dermatitis that spontaneously disappears after several weeks. The pigmentation, which is the hallmark of the disease, may fade in adult life. The bullous and linear verrucose dermatitis may leave atrophic and depigmented patches and streaks after they fade. Eosinophilia greater than 5 per cent, ranging up to more than 45 per cent, was present in 75 per cent of 165 cases in which it was measured.[8] Eosinophils are also prominent in the dermis and epidermis of the skin lesions. The significance of the eosinophilia is not understood.

Approximately 80 per cent of affected children have one or more of the following congenital defects: alopecia, delayed or impaired dentition, cataracts, microcephaly, spastic paralysis, strabismus, epilepsy, or mental retardation. Ocular abnormalities resulting in significant visual loss or frank blindness have occurred in 19 per cent of cases.[8]

Carney's survey of the world's literature on incontinentia pigmenti revealed a positive family history in 55 per cent of the cases.[8] Because almost all of the affected individuals are female, a theory of X-linked dominant trait, lethal for males, has been proposed for this neurocutaneous syndrome.

Two children with incontinentia pigmenti and recurrent bacterial infections have been shown to have defective neutrophil chemotaxis.[9, 10]

Hypomelanosis of Ito

Hypomelanosis of Ito (incontinentia pigmenti achromians) looks like a negative image of incontinentia pigmenti.[11] Because of this appearance, it was considered to be a variant of incontinentia pigmenti by some workers, although Ito, who originally coined the name, believed it represented a bilateral systematized depigmented nevus (nevus depigmentosus).[12] Now that more than 30 cases have been reported, enough differences have been detected for hypomelanosis of Ito to qualify as an entity distinct from incontinentia pigmenti. However, at least 50 per cent of the cases have at least one abnormality involving the ocular, musculoskeletal, or central nervous systems.[11, 13]

The distinguishing features of hypomelanosis of Ito include (1) depigmented areas that are not preceded by inflammatory lesions, although they tend to repigment with age analogous to the hyperpigmented patches of incontinentia pigmenti which lighten and disappear with age; (2) males who are affected; (3) absence of histologic findings of pigment incontinence, in contrast to incontinentia pigmenti; and (4) based upon three reports, autosomal dominant transmission.[14-16]

Some workers define nevus depigmentosus as a congenital, permanent, discrete hypopigmented patch that lacks a swirling pattern,[11] while others are less restrictive in their definition and consider hypomelanosis of Ito to be a manifestation of nevus depigmentosus[17, 18] (Figs. 17–13 and 17–14). Electron microscopic studies have demonstrated differences in melanin pigmentation between the white spots of tuberous sclerosis, nevus depigmentosus (which includes cases of hypomelanosis of Ito), and piebaldism.[18] Regardless of the nosologic niche of hypomelanosis of Ito, it must be recognized that it is an important neurocutaneous syndrome.

Although in most cases of hypomelanosis, the hypopigmented whorled pattern may represent areas of depigmentation, this did not appear to be the case in our patient illustrated in Figure 17–15. We compared the "depigmented" whorls on the trunk with the facial pigmentation by reflectance meter measurements and found them to be identical. In our patient, irregularly but widely distributed patches of hyperpigmentation developed over the trunk in such a fashion that whorled patterns of normally pigmented skin resulted. Figure 17–16 shows an identical whorled pattern of normal pigmentation produced by hyperpigmentation in a patient with dyskeratosis congenita. Griffiths and Payne described an

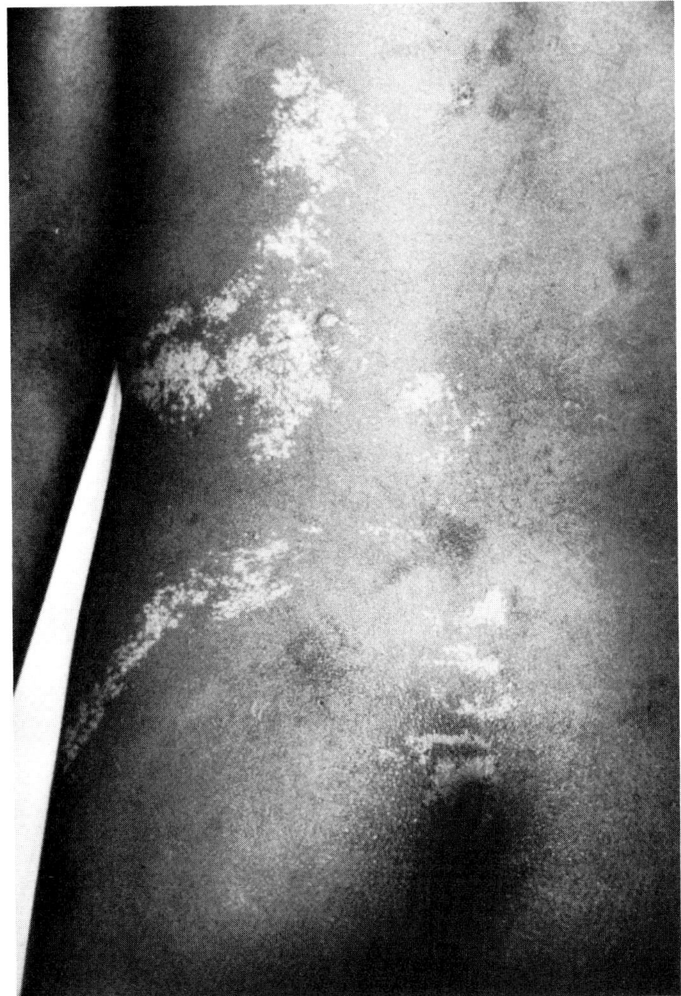

Figure 17–13. Nevus depigmentosus. Discrete hypopigmented patches lacking swirling pattern.

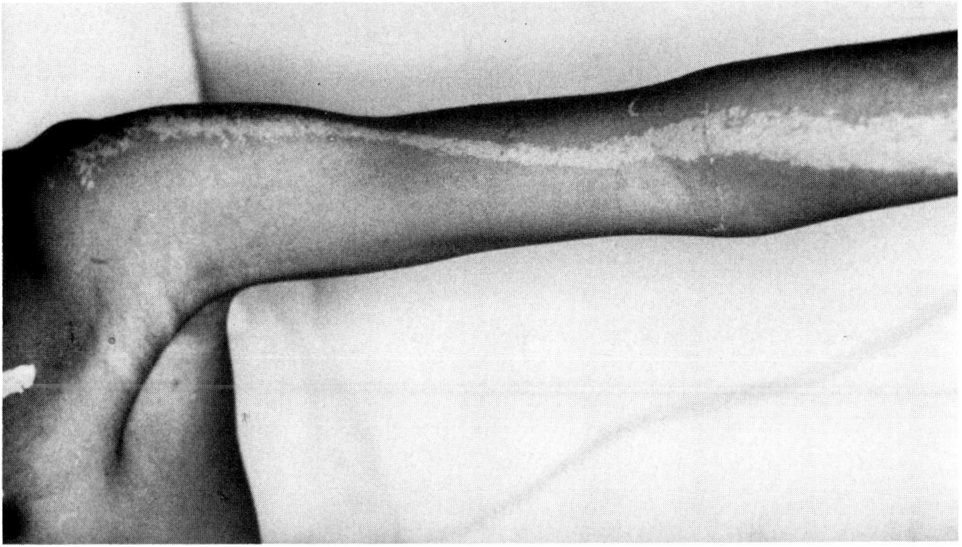

Figure 17–14. Nevus depigmentosus. Linear hypopigmented band.

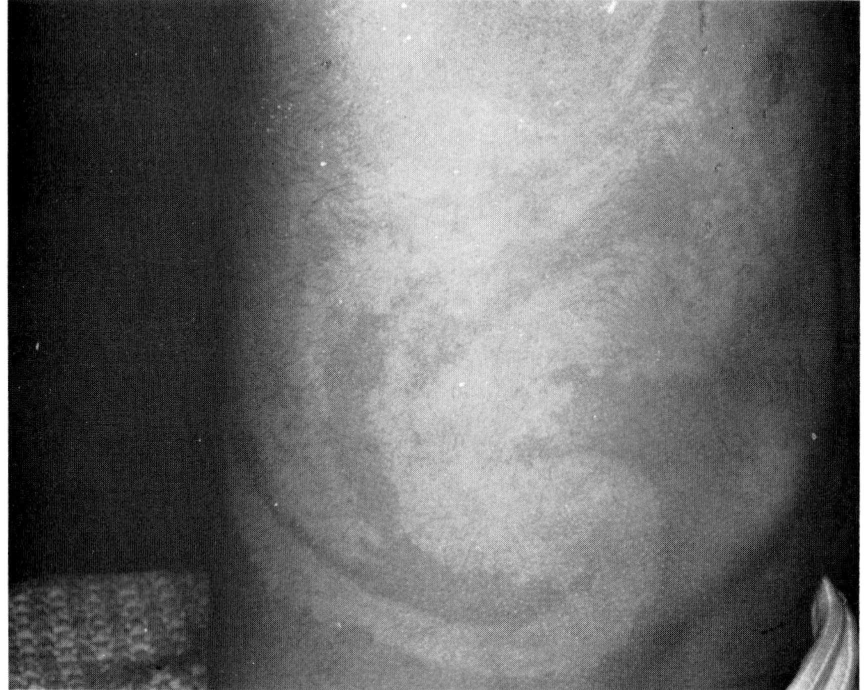

Figure 17–15. Incontinentia pigmenti achromians (Ito). Negative image of whorled pigmentary pattern.

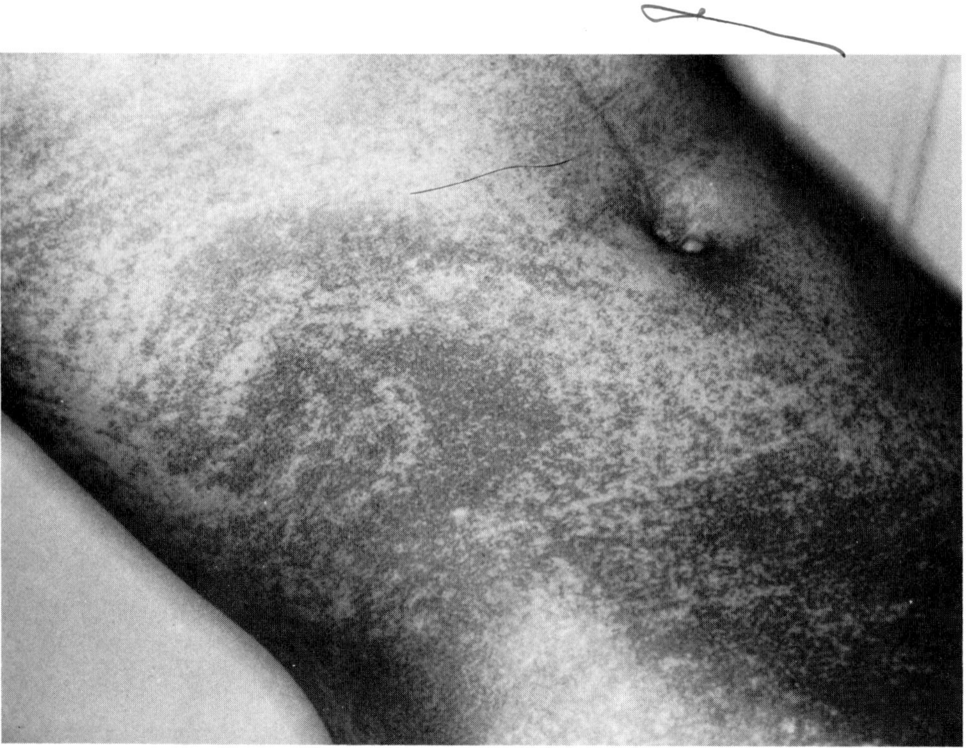

Figure 17–16. Whorled pattern of normal pigmentation, produced by hyperpigmentation in a patient with dyskeratosis congenita, simulating hypopigmentation in hypomelanosis of Ito.

individual with hypomelanosis of Ito in which there were both hypopigmented areas and hyperpigmented patches that produced swirls of normal pigmented skin.[19] It is likely that both hypopigmentation and hyperpigmentation are present in some patients with hypomelanosis of Ito. Measurements of pigmentation by reflectance meters can settle these points in future cases.

Neurofibromatosis (von Recklinghausen's Disease)

Neurofibromatosis, with its features of café au lait spots and cutaneous neurofibromas, is well known to all medical students and physicians (Figs. 17–17 to 17–19). The disease is inherited in a dominant fashion. Crowe et al. have shown that the existence of six or more café au lait spots that are greater than 1.5 cm. indicates the presence of neurofibromatosis.[20] Seventy-eight per cent of patients with this disease have six or more café au lait spots (Fig. 17–20). Axillary "freckling" is another diagnostic sign of neurofibromatosis. The freckles are 1- to 4-mm café au lait spots (Fig. 17–21). Some patients have generalized "freckling" and less than the required six large spots, but this finding is nevertheless just as significant. Café au lait spots can be present at birth, but they increase in number and size with age. The cutaneous neurofibromas often do not appear until late childhood or puberty, and they also increase in size and number with age. The neurofibromas are Schwann's cell tumors derived from the nerve sheath. When small, the neurofibromas may have a violaceous hue, but as they enlarge they become flesh-colored and may be covered with "freckles" or café au lait spots. Before they become large they can be invaginated into the skin with moderate digital pressure. This maneuver is sometimes called "buttonholing" and is almost specific for neurofibromas. Large neurofibromas can be pedunculated or broad based. Some patients have thousands of tumors, whereas others have only a few.

Neurofibromas may also grow in a diffuse (plexiform) fashion and cause localized enlargement of underlying bone and soft tissues; they may cause marked drooping or laxity of the skin in that area.

Neurofibromas and café au lait spots can also be localized to a small area or be unilateral.[21] Neurofibromas frequently develop on the iris, where they form yellow-brown spots (Fig. 17–22 and 17–23; Plate 40*A*).[21a]

In pregnancy, neurofibromas may increase in size and number, or may appear for the first time. Regression is common after the pregnancy has been completed. Swapp and Main noted that 10 of 11 consecutive pregnant women with neurofibromatosis became hypertensive during their pregnancy. There was no evidence of pheochromocytoma, nor was any other cause uncovered. The hypertension disappeared after delivery.[22]

Malignant degeneration of neurofibromas occurred in 2 per cent of the patients in Crowe's series. When malignancy develops, the histology is that of a fibrosarcoma.

Neurofibromas also arise in bone, in the gastrointestinal tract, and in the retroperitoneal sites. They may cause chronic blood loss from the gastrointestinal tract. In the central nervous system, the optic (II) and auditory (VIII) cranial nerves are the sites of predilection. Crowe's data indicate that the fewer café au lait spots a person has, the more likely he is

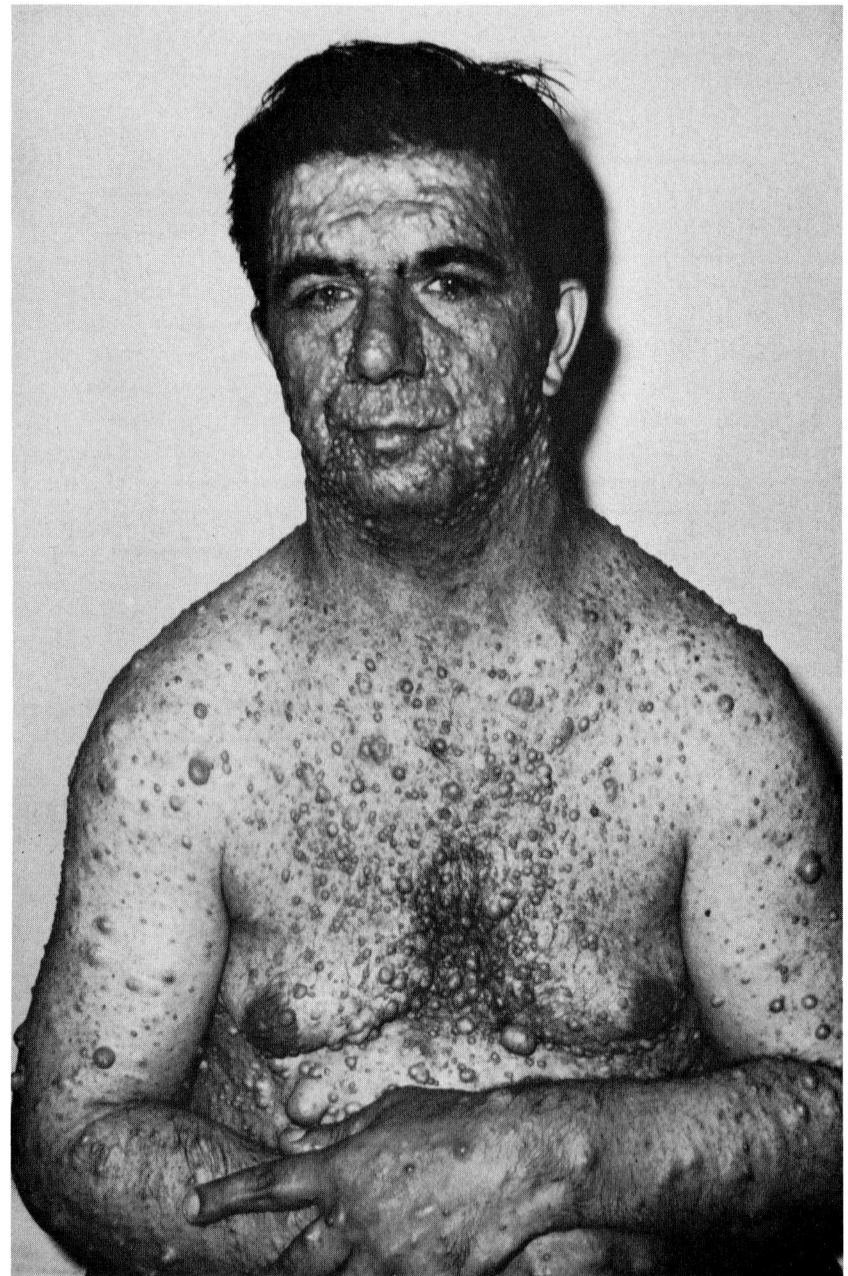

Figure 17–17. Neurofibromatosis. Severe form of the disease.

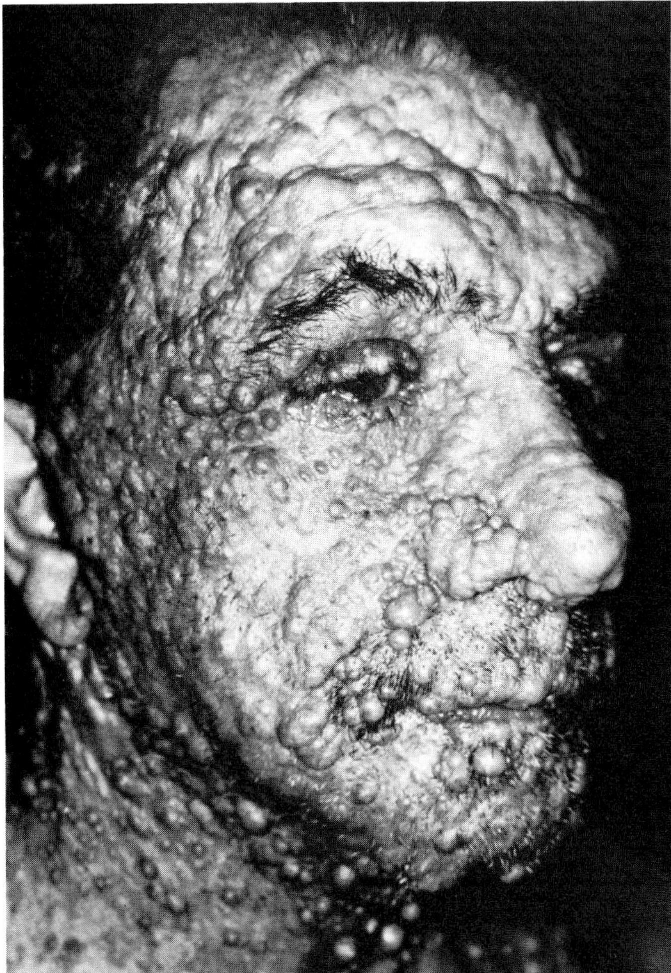

Figure 17–18. Neurofibromatosis. Same patient shown in Figure 17–17 20 years later.

to have neurofibromas in the central nervous system, intrathoracic area, or retroperitoneal area. Also, the individual's pattern of café au lait spots is similar to that of his affected siblings.

Mental retardation and epilepsy are additional features of von Recklinghausen's disease. Five to 20 per cent of patients with pheochromocytoma have neurofibromatosis, but only one out of 223 patients with neurofibromatosis in Crowe's studies had a pheochromocytoma.

The data of both Crowe et al. and Young et al. indicate that neurofibromatosis is a heterogeneous disorder.[20, 23] Three forms presently exist: (1) Central variety. Bilateral acoustic neuromas develop in the absence of significant numbers of café au lait spots and neurofibromas. In the large kindred of Young et al. upon which the concept of a central variety is based, four cases had one to three neurofibromas and only one to two café au lait spots. Ninety-five per cent of the acoustic neuromas encountered in medical practice are unilateral and occur sporadically. However, the acoustic neuromas that occur in 5 per cent of patients with

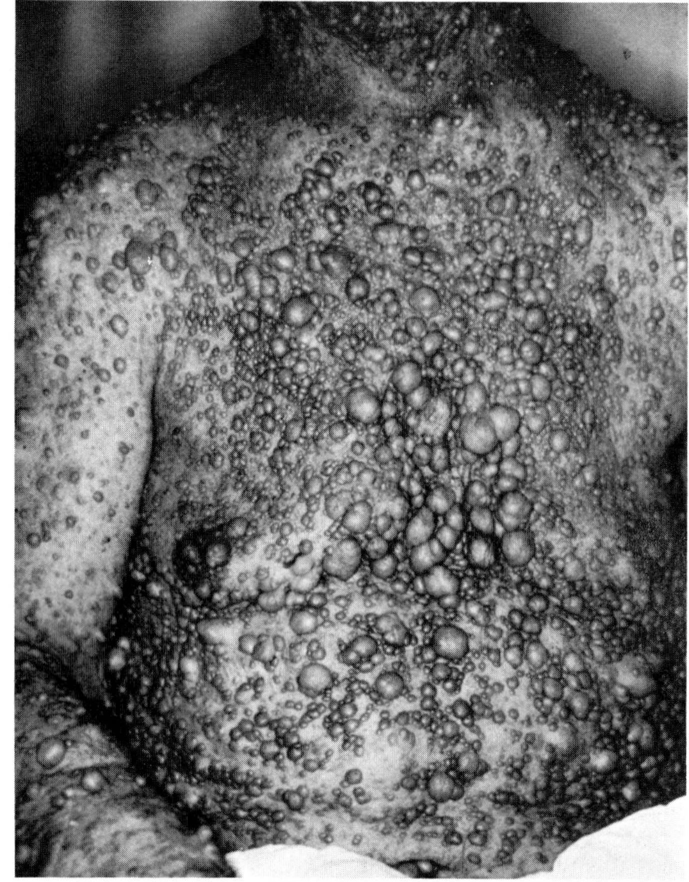

Figure 17–19. Neurofibromatosis. Same patient shown in Figure 17–17 20 years later.

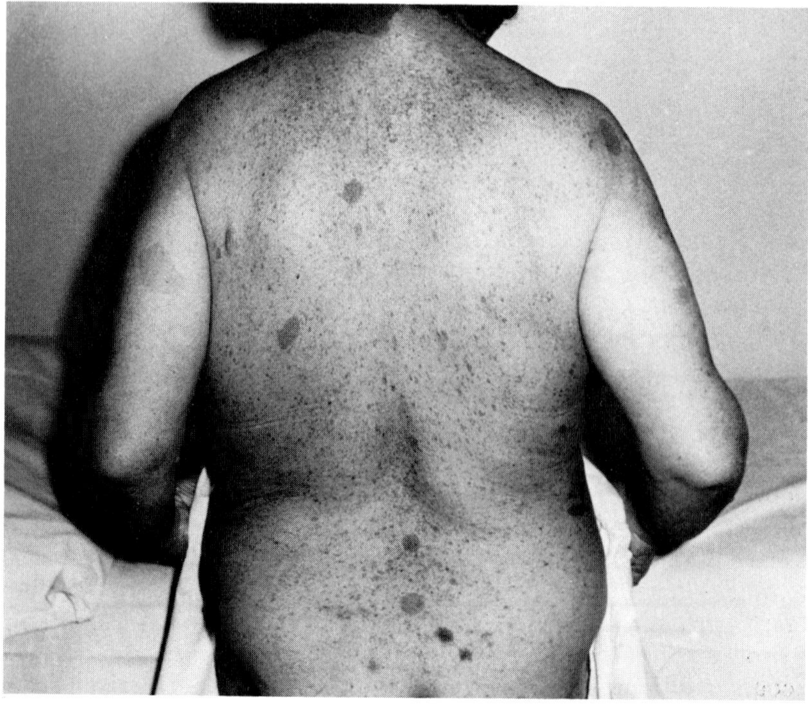

Figure 17–20. Neurofibromatosis. Café au lait spots on trunk.

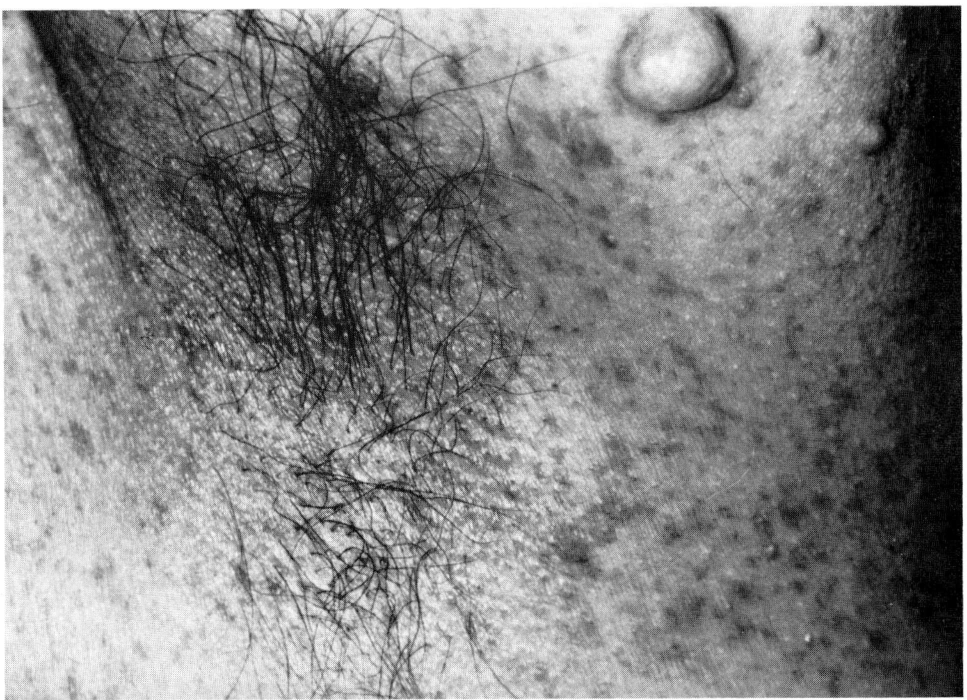

Figure 17–21. Neurofibromatosis. Axillary freckling.

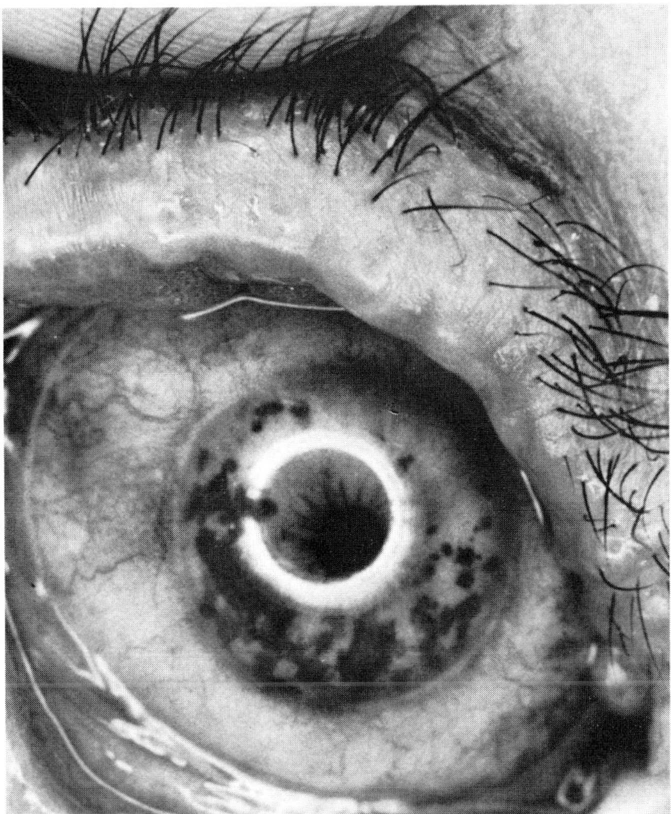

Figure 17–22. Neurofibromatosis. Neurofibromas on iris produce yellow-brown spots.

PLATE 40

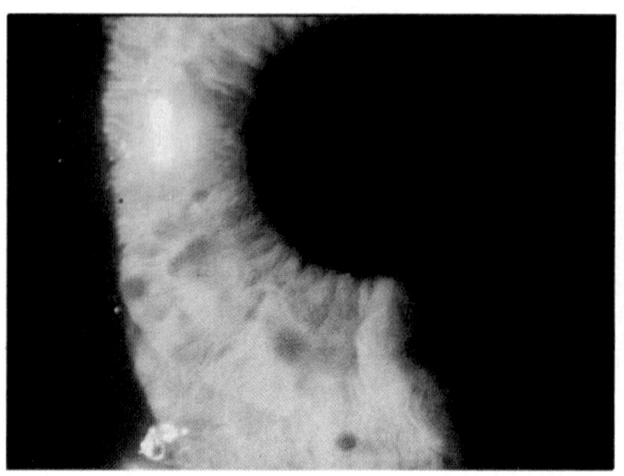

A, Neurofibromatosis. Neurofibromas in the iris produce yellow-brown spots.

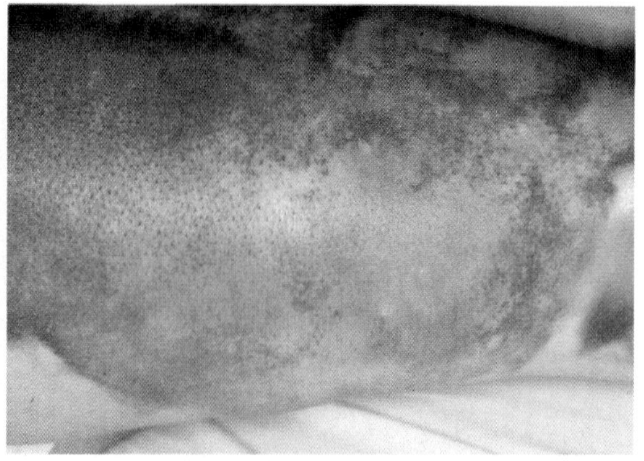

B, Autoerythrocyte sensitivity. Erythema and tenderness surrounded by extensive purpura which is beginning to resolve. Tender erythema precedes the appearance of purpura in this syndrome.

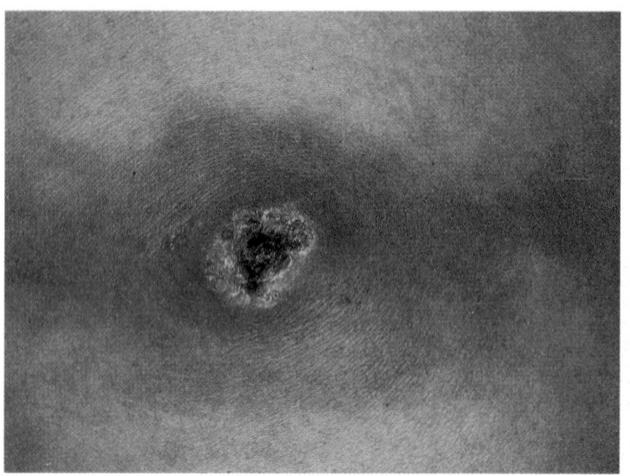

C, Staphylococcal abscess (furuncle). Marked erythema around center which has become necrotic and extruded its core of pus.

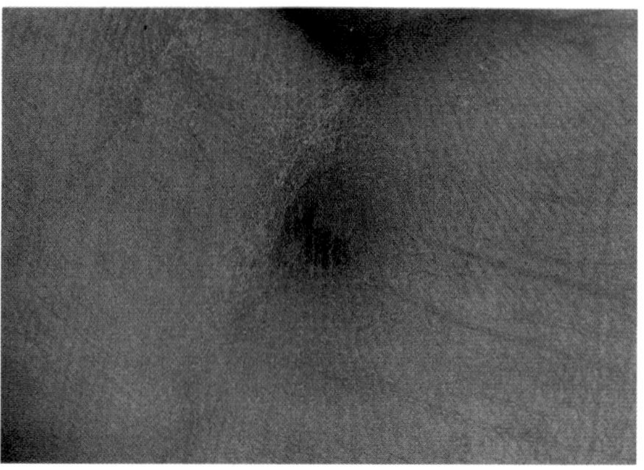

D, Disseminated gonococcemia. Papulovesicle on palm with irregular area of purpura in center.

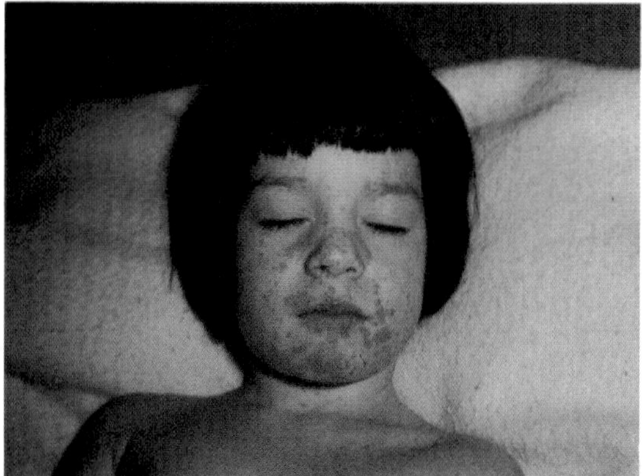

E, Measles (rubeola). Duration eight hours. Discrete red urticarial macules and papules are present at this stage.

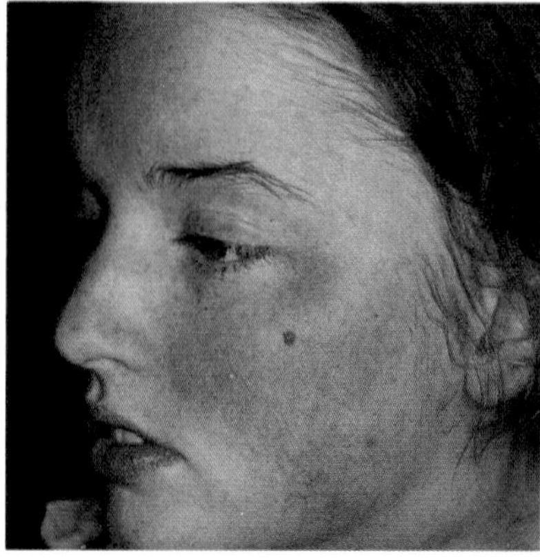

F, Fifth disease (erythema infectiosum). Cheeks are bright red, giving the appearance of having been slapped.

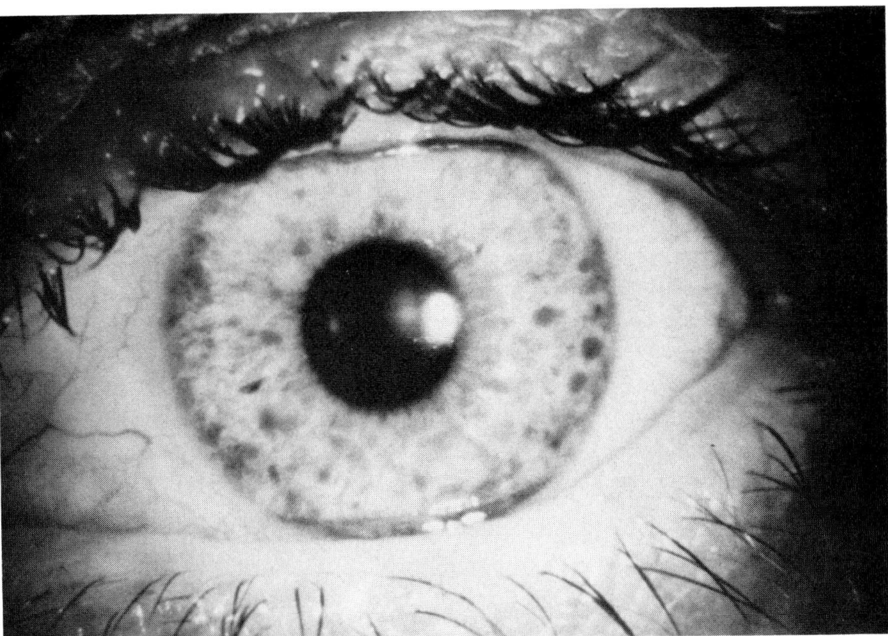

Figure 17–23. Neurofibromatosis. Neurofibromas on iris.

neurofibromatosis are bilateral.[23] (2) Peripheral variety. Many neurofibromas and café au lait spots are present, but there is minimal central nervous system involvement. (3) Mixed variety. Combination of central and peripheral involvement does occur, but it is less common than the central and peripheral varieties. Its prevalence is not yet known.

Recent studies have shown that the sera of patients with the central variety contain nerve growth factor activity that is immunologically identical to nerve growth factor (NGF) isolated from mouse salivary gland.[24] "Nerve growth stimulating activity," unrelated to NGF, was found in patients with the peripheral variety of the disease.[25] In this latter study, some individuals at risk for the central variety had elevated serum levels of NGF. These assays hold promise for furthering our understanding of the pathogenesis of this neurocutaneous syndrome.

Café au lait–like spots also occur in Albright's syndrome (polyostotic fibrous dysplasia with sexual precocity in girls). However, these pigmented macules tend to have a markedly irregular border and are dark brown in contrast to the smooth outline and light brown color of the spots in neurofibromatosis. In Albright's syndrome, axillary freckling does not occur; and the café au lait spots tend to develop over the neck and buttocks, are less than six in number, and often develop over the affected bones. Sexual precocity is not a feature of neurofibromatosis. Confusion between Albright's syndrome and neurofibromatosis may occur rarely. If it does, histologic examination of the café au lait spots for the presence of giant pigment granules in the melanocytes and epidermal cells may prove helpful. They are present in the pigmented spots of von Recklinghausen's disease but they are rare in Albright's syndrome.[26]

Multiple Lentigines Syndrome

The multiple lentigines syndrome is a dominantly transmitted disorder that is probably related to an abnormality involving cells of the neural crest.[27, 28] Affected individuals are covered with hundreds of light tan, dark brown, or black lentigines ranging from pinpoint size to several centimeters (Figs. 17–24 to 17–26). The lentigines are present everywhere, including the palms and soles, with only the oral mucosa apparently being spared. Lentigines are present at birth, but they become obvious at about two to five years of age. They increase in number with age, and there is a marked increase at puberty. The lentigines can also be found on the irides.

A variety of abnormalities are found in affected individuals, leading Moyanhan and Polani to coin the term *leopard syndrome* as a mnemonic device: L, lentigines; E, electrocardiographic conduction defects; O, ocular telorism; P, pulmonary stenosis; A, abnormalities of genitalia; R, retardation of growth; D, deafness. The syndrome has a variable expression.

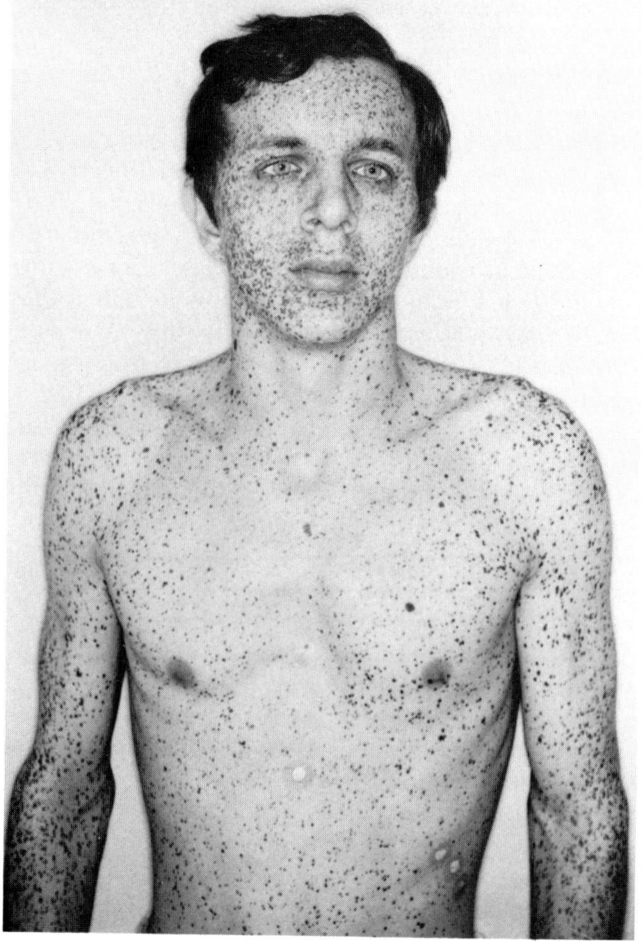

Figure 17–24. Multiple lentigines syndrome. Lentigines on face and upper chest. Hypertelorism.

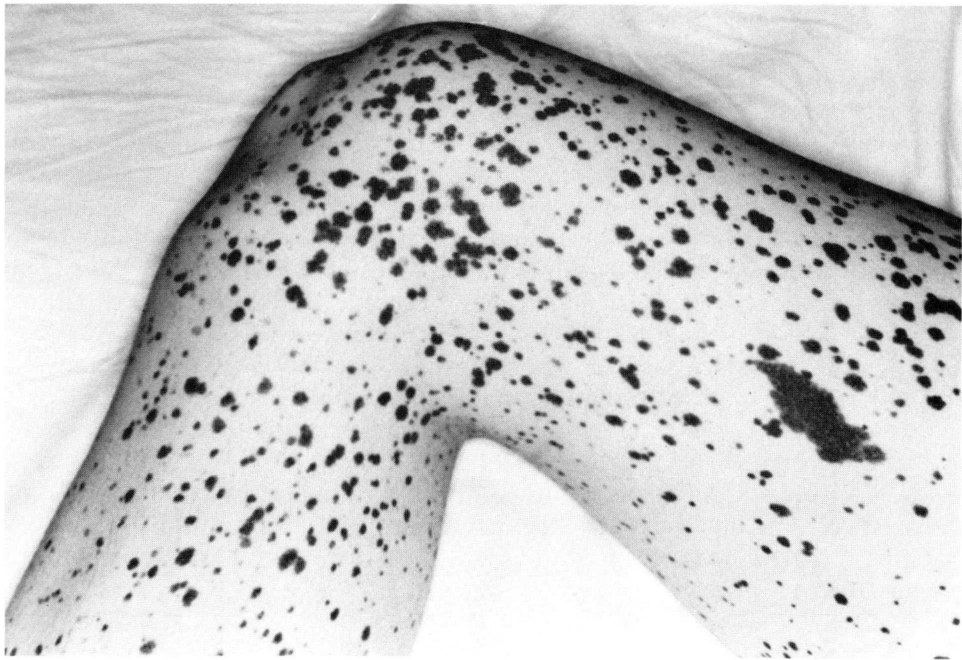

Figure 17–25. Multiple lentigines syndrome. Close-up of lentigines on leg.

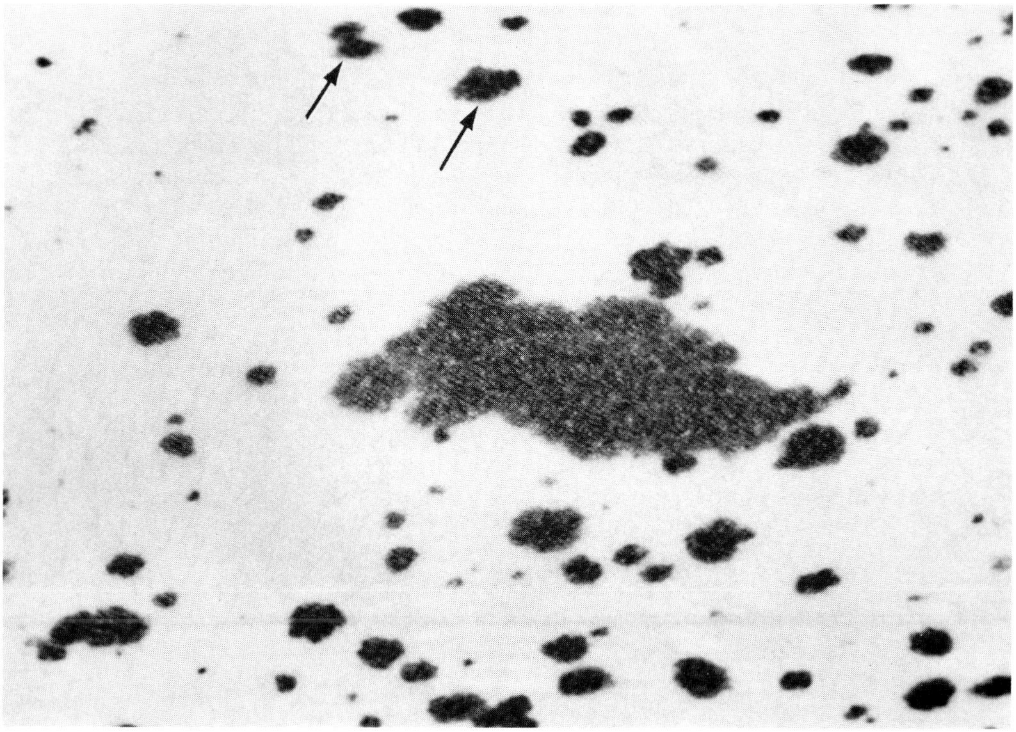

Figure 17–26. Multiple lentigines syndrome. Close-up of individual lentigines. Some have a speckled pattern of pigmentation (arrows).

As our understanding of this syndrome has increased, it has become apparent that the main abnormalities include an obstructive cardiomyopathy, usually caused by subaortic valvular stenosis, and occasionally accompanied by obstruction to the right outflow tract[27]; myocardial conduction defects that may be partial or complete hemiblocks; electrocardiographic patterns simulating myocardial infarction[29, 30]; mental retardation, deafness, and small stature. Other abnormalities noted in patients have included asymmetrical skull, broad nares, high arched palate, pectus excavatum, retarded bone age, strabismus, hypospadias, hypoplasia of ovaries, scanty sex hair, undescended testes, slow peripheral nerve conduction, and abnormal slowing of the electroencephalogram.[27, 28, 31]

An abnormality involving the neural crest elements could explain the major features of this syndrome because these cells play a role in the development of the inner ear and the sympathetic nervous system that richly innervates the heart.

Most cases of obstructive cardiomyopathy are inherited as a dominant trait.[32] Is this one pole of the multiple lentigines syndrome or is it a closely related genetic disorder, analogous to the relationship between the Sipple syndrome (MEN type 2) and MEN type 3? The multiple lentigines syndrome is not an entirely benign disorder, because several patients have died from the progressive cardiomyopathy.[27]

The Waardenberg syndrome is an analogous disorder in which neural deafness is associated with a white forelock and depigmented spots elsewhere on the body. Piebaldism and partial albinism can also be associated with deafness.

Epidermal Nevus Syndrome

The epidermal nevus is a congenital malformation. Histologically one sees only epidermal hyperplasia. However there is probably a dermal influence in the lesion because it always recurs following superficial destructive procedures. Nevus cells are not present and the lesion is not related to the pigmentary system. The usual epidermal nevus can display a verrucous or finely papillated surface, or it may be composed of closely set papillary elevations. The epidermal nevus may be a solitary plaque or it may be arranged in a linear streak or band that is continuous or interrupted when it is extensive (Figs. 17–27 to 17–29). It is often unilateral and may course over the entire side of the body. Less commonly, it is bilateral. Other terms for the extensive form are nevus unius lateris and linear nevus. Solomon et al. have pointed out that the *extensive* epidermal nevi, larger than 10 cm, appear to be associated with osseous and central nervous system abnormalities. Of 23 patients, 18 had skeletal abnormalities; 10, central nervous system abnormalities; and 9, both types. The skeletal abnormalities included scoliosis, spina bifida, enlarged limbs, and localized gigantism. The central nervous system defects included arteriovenous malformations, mental retardation, cranial nerve palsies, and motor paralyses.[33] Although there have been 13 instances of benign and malignant tumors reported in association with the epidermal nevus syndrome, it is not established whether the association is fortuitous or real.[34] The tumors have been present at birth or have developed from 15 months to 43 years later.

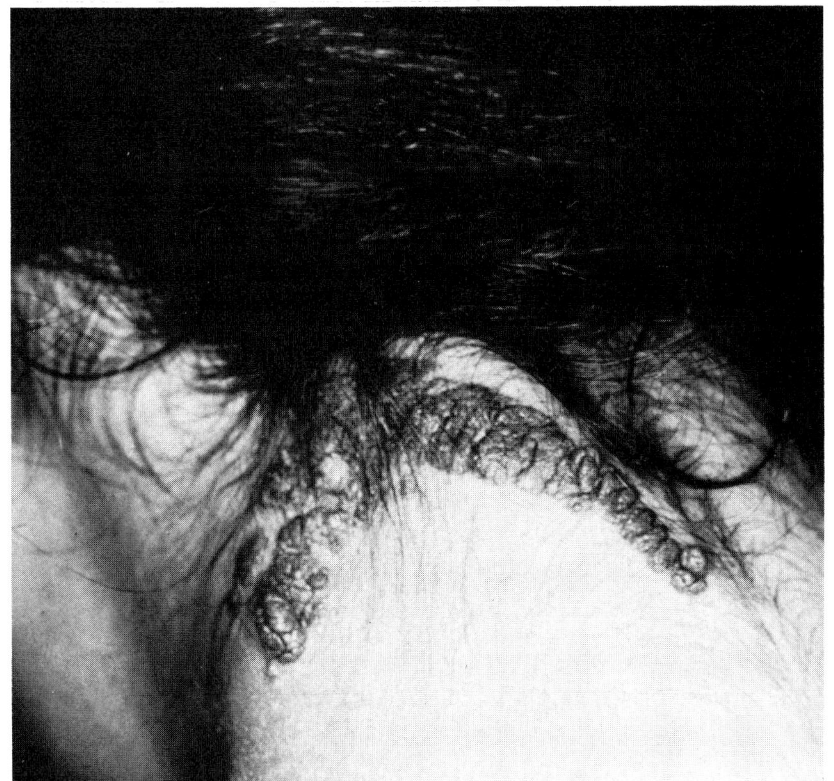

Figure 17–27. Epidermal nevus. Papillated surface.

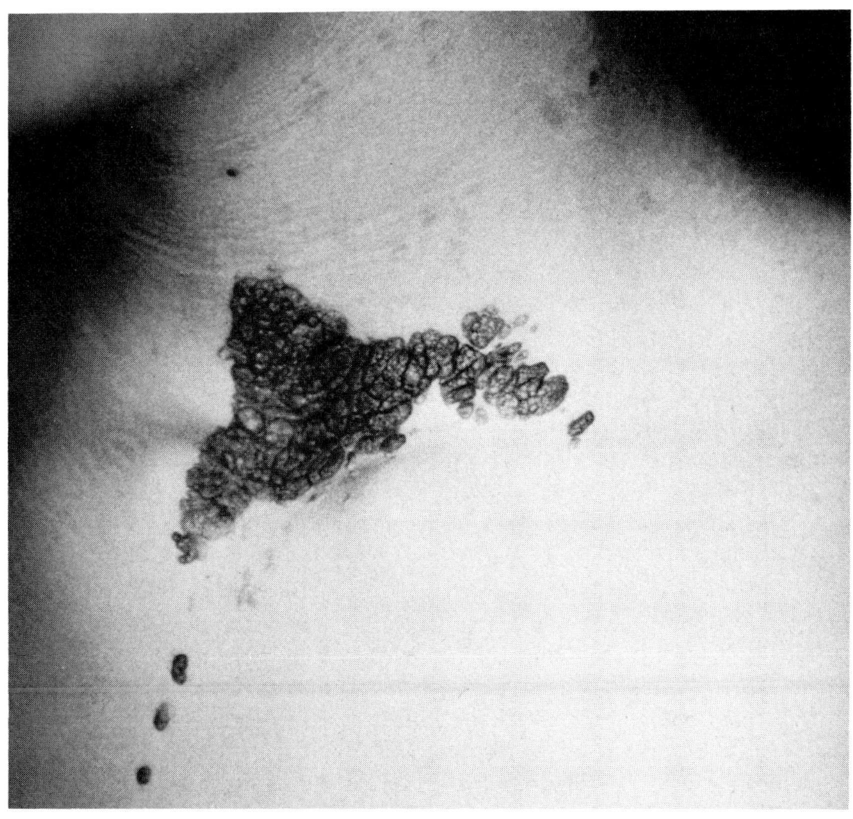

Figure 17–28. Epidermal nevus. Same patient shown in Figure 17–27.

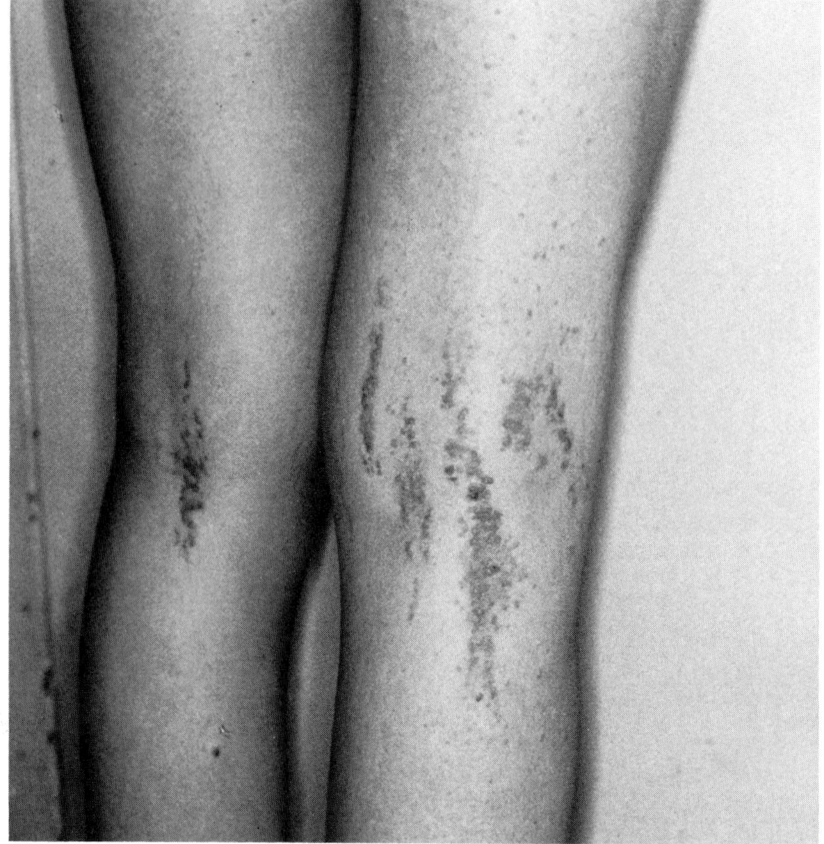

Figure 17–29. Epidermal nevus. Linear verrucous bands.

THE PSYCHE AND THE SKIN

Emotional factors play an important role in dermatologic diseases. Individuals under psychological stress may have exacerbations of their psoriasis, atopic dermatitis, dishidrotic eczema, and sometimes urticaria. Successful coping with emotional stresses may lead to improvement and relative remissions of these dermatoses. Pruritus from any cause becomes worse when the individual is under stress. In some individuals, pruritus vulvi and ani and localized lichen simplex chronicus are a manifestation of underlying psychological tension. The way in which the psyche can modulate inflammatory skin diseases is not understood.

Psychological stresses, much greater than those usually encountered in daily life and more aptly referred to as psychiatric disturbances, can lead to tell-tale signs in the skin. Such lesions fall into the category of factitial dermatitis.[35] The affected individuals, however, deny that they are responsible for the cutaneous lesions. Often the lesions represent a cry for help from individuals who are unable to directly deal with or seek medical help for their severe emotional problems. Persons exhibiting Münchausen's syndrome or who are malingerers, however, *consciously* act to deceive others with fraudulent disease or by deliberately worsening preexisting disease.

Factitial disease in its mildest form includes neurotic excoriations, prurigo nodularis produced by constant rubbing and scratching, and trichotillomania (Figs. 17–30 and 17–31). It is usually possible for the physician and the patient to control and reverse these problems through simple counselling.

A more serious problem usually exists when the factitial dermatoses take the form of large ulcerations and extensive purpura, which the patient states arise spontaneously with minimal or no preceding symptoms or are present in the morning upon awakening. Ulcerations that have bizarre and unnatural configurations and distribution patterns or that persist and recur in sites of excellent blood supply should make one consider the possibility of factitial disease (Figs. 17–32 to 17–34). Individuals who inject foreign material into the skin to produce red tender nodules usually are malingerers or cases of Münchausen's syndrome because this is done at the conscious level.

The most serious psychiatric disturbances are found in the patients who have delusions of parasitosis. These individuals are psychotic. They tear, dig, and rip at their skin to remove the crawling bugs and snakes that they believe are living and reproducing there. As evidence, they bring in the supposed living creatures and their eggs and excreta wrapped in paper tissues and in bottles. Examination reveals lint, crusts, and bits of skin. These patients are almost impossible to treat psychiatrically. However, medical support and treatment for the factitial lesions without trying to dissuade the patients from their beliefs about the origin of the cutaneous lesions proves to be successful in helping them cope with their lives.

Factitial disease is usually self-evident or should be suspected when the lesions do not correspond to known dermatologic disorders, do not heal under appropriate therapy, or regularly recur at times of severe emotional stress. Suggesting a face-saving explanation to the patient for the origin of the factitial lesions is the first step toward communication and acceptance by the patient of the need for psychiatric consultation and therapy. Confronting the individual with his or her responsibility for the production of the lesions will cause an irreversible break in the physician-patient relationship.

The Gardner-Diamond syndrome (autoerythrocyte sensitivity, psychogenic purpura, painful bruising syndrome) is an organic illness with prominent psychiatric manifestations.[36, 37] This disease has probably engendered more debate over whether it is an organic disease or a psychiatric syndrome than any other comparable disorder in medicine. The illness has occurred exclusively in women from adolescence to the sixth decade. It is characterized by crops of painful, warm, red, sometimes slightly edematous patches that become ecchymotic over the course of several hours to one day (Figs. 17–35 to 17–37; Plate 40*B*). The purpura may begin on the periphery of the *red* patch and spread to involve the rest of the area, or it may involve the entire lesion at once. These ecchymotic areas tend to increase in size and may become as large as 15 cm in diameter. They typically form on the extremities, but no part of the skin surface is immune. The ecchymoses are very painful and the patient may require analgesics and narcotics. When the lesions develop around the ankles and knees, it is not unusual for the patient to use crutches because of pain and limitation of movement. The individual lesions last for one to two weeks before fading, and crops develop at irregular intervals of days to months.

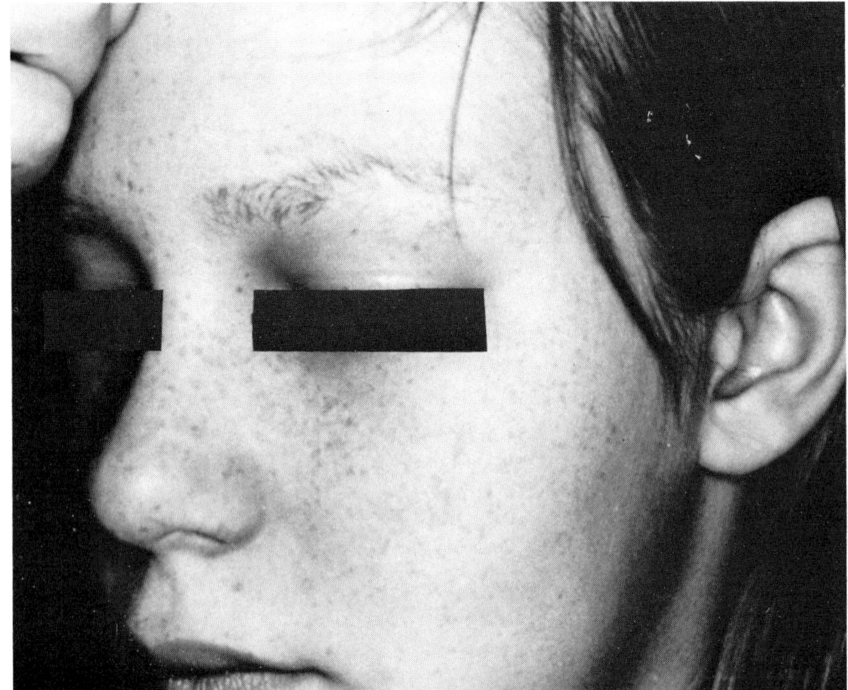

Figure 17–30. Trichotillomania involving eyebrows.

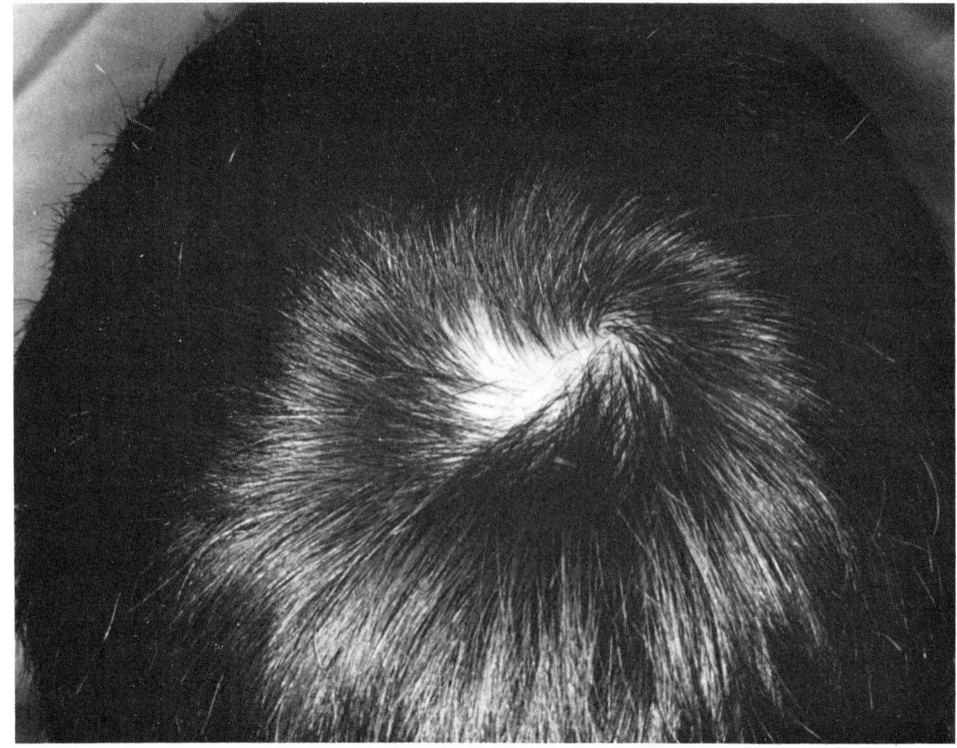

Figure 17–31. Trichotillomania involving vertex of scalp.

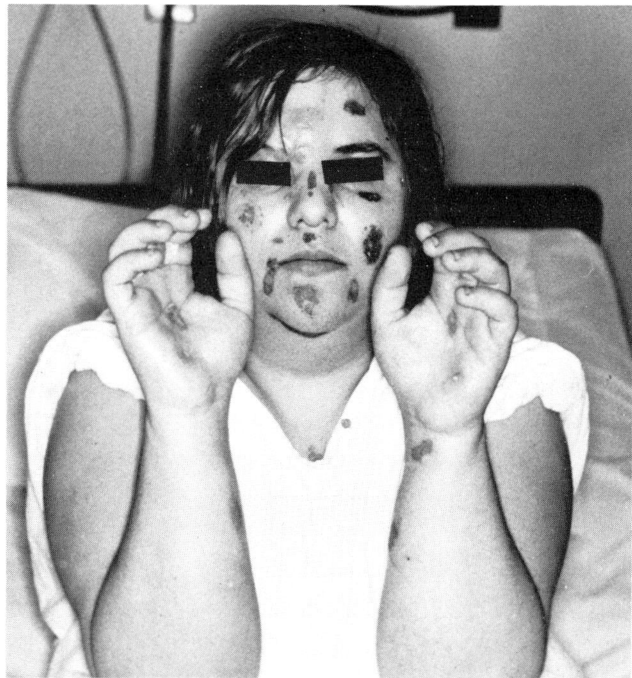

Figure 17–32. Facititial disease. Bizarre pattern of facial ulcerations.

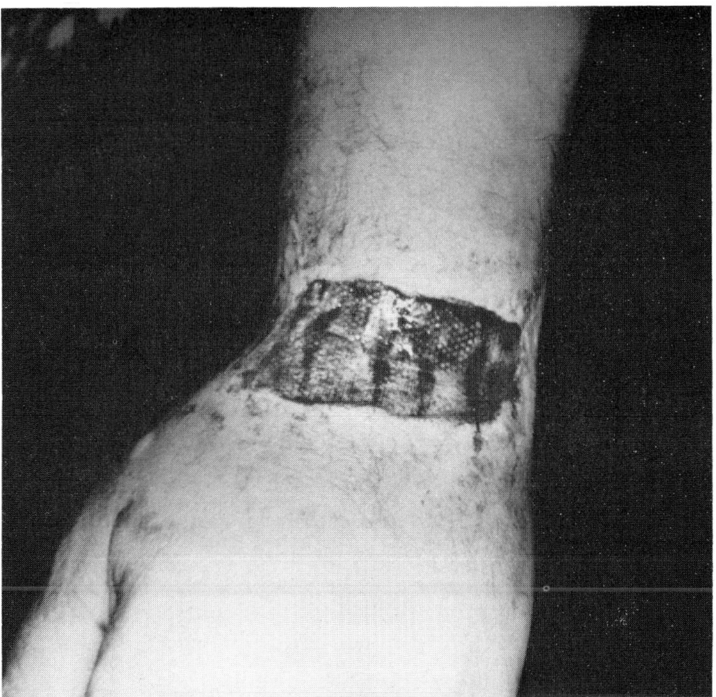

Figure 17–33. Factitial disease. Rectangular ulceration on wrist. Ulcers do not develop naturally with 90 degree corners.

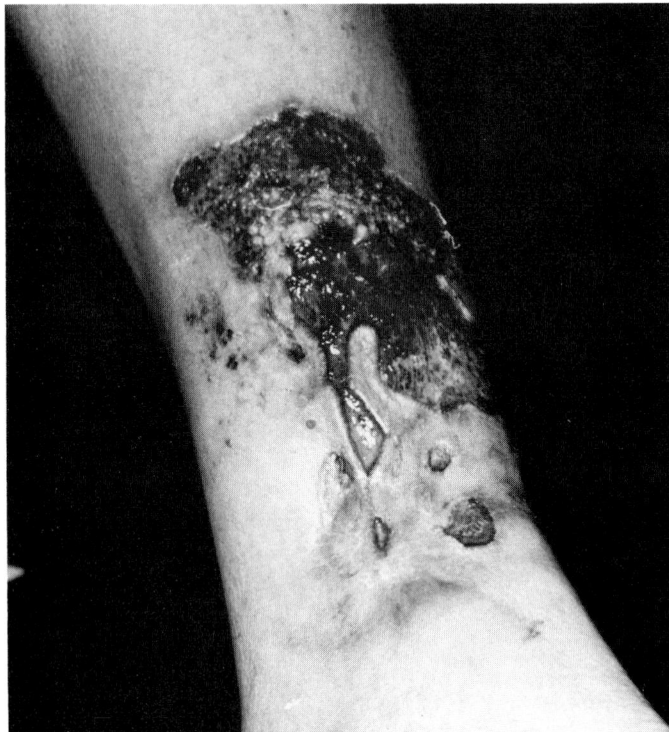

Figure 17–34. Factitial disease. Self-inflicted ulceration. Note unnatural angulation of right lower edge.

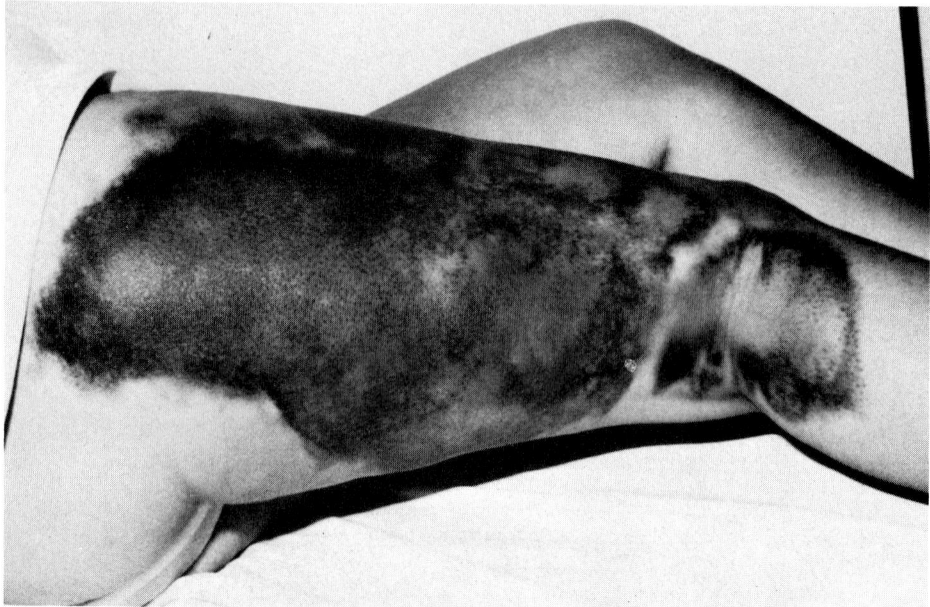

Figure 17–35. Autoerythrocyte sensitivity. Bright red erythema precedes appearance of purpura. See Plate 40*B*.

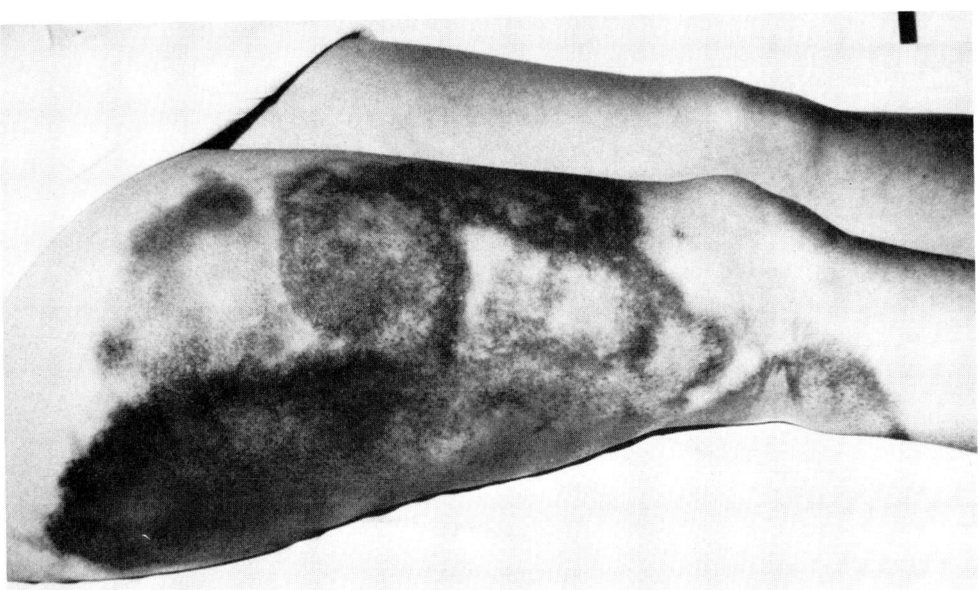

Figure 17–36. Autoerythrocyte sensitivity. Same patient as in Figure 17–35 showing extent of purpura.

The disorder needs to be differentiated from factitial purpura, which is often confused with the Gardner-Diamond syndrome. The distinguishing feature is the painful *bright erythema* which precedes the appearance of the ecchymosis. Extensive purpura, whether produced accidentally or factitiously by trauma, is *not* preceded by painful warm erythema. It was this observation that led Gardner and Diamond to propose this syndrome as a distinct entity.

Most cases have developed following significant trauma, either as

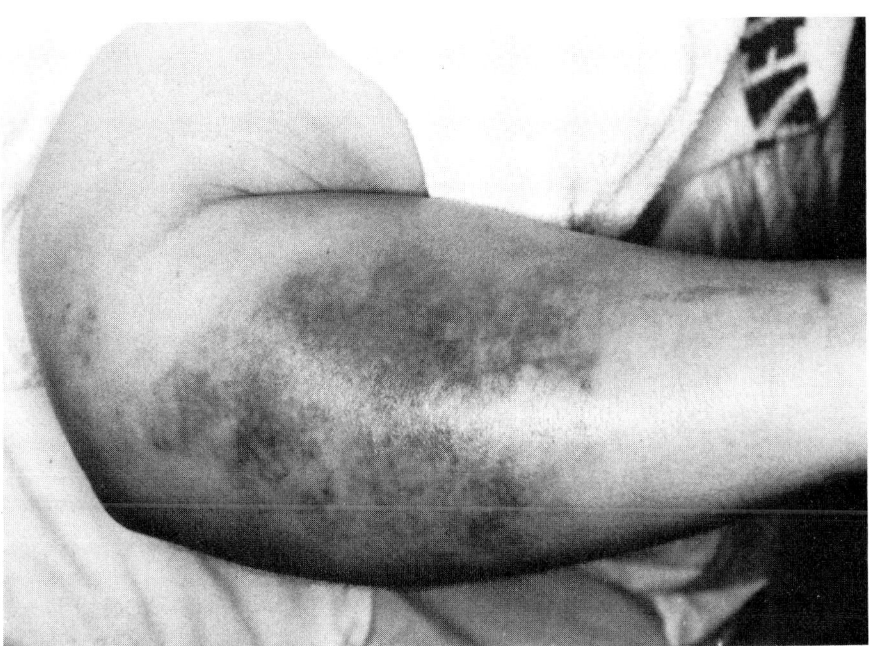

Figure 17–37. Autoerythrocyte sensitivity.

injuries, surgical procedures, or spontaneous abortions.[37] The lesions then develop after minor trauma or spontaneously.

Most of the patients have exhibited masochistic or hysterical signs and symptoms: paresis, paresthesias, headache, diplopia, abdominal pain, chest pain, myalgias.[38] Hypnosis can inhibit or influence the development of the ecchymoses in some patients.[39] These factors have led some clinicians to view this disorder as a cutaneous manifestation of severe emotional stress, but the mechanism by which this is accomplished is unknown.

In addition to the psychiatric manifestations, some patients have exhibited hemoptysis, melena, vaginal bleeding, and hematuria, none of which was adequately explained in the specific cases.[36, 37]

Gardner and Diamond and others since have demonstrated that the intradermal injection of autologous red cells will reproduce lesions in most but not all cases.[36, 37] In some instances the skin of the forearm reacted, but the skin of the back did not. Groch et al. and Boxley have shown that phosphatidyl serine derived from the red cell membrane could reproduce the lesion when injected intradermally. Histological examination of the induced lesion showed a leukocytoclastic angiitis.[40, 41] Some patients with this syndrome have reacted to DNA injections but not to red blood cells,[42] and others have shown positive responses to platelets, PPD, histamine, and sex hormones.[37] The mechanism underlying this disorder is not understood, and the vagaries of the skin tests suggest that the underlying mechanisms may be heterogeneous or may be the final common pathway to a variety of etiologic agents. These vagaries have also suggested to some physicians that these cases actually represent factitial purpura.[43] However, there are enough instances of positive skin tests in individuals who have been carefully observed to exclude the factitial production of a positive skin test to overcome these objections.[39]

At least one aspect of the syndrome, the orificial bleeding, appears to have an explanation. In one case of this illness, an associated chronic glomerulonephritis was shown to be caused by circulating immune complexes that behaved as a cryoprotein. It contained red cell antigen. The renal glomeruli were shown to contain deposits of red cell antigen, C3, and host immunoglobulins by direct immunofluorescence.[44] It is likely that immune complex vasculitis is responsible for the other bleeding phenomena in this disorder. Evidence for delayed hypersensitivity to red cell antigen was demonstrated in another case.[45] Of uncertain significance are morphologic changes found in the red cells of three patients by electron microscopy: club-shaped red cells with retained cellular organelles and elevations in the plasma membrane.[46]

The prognosis and natural history of this disorder have not been well delineated, but it is clear that in some patients the disease becomes less active and probably disappears. Spontaneous remissions may last for months to years, during which affected individuals may develop occasional small areas of painless ecchymoses.[37]

The evolution of the spontaneous lesion from a red spot to purpura that extends over a considerable distance strongly supports the concept that these patients have developed a hypersensitivity response to red cells or some other factor(s) released by trauma. The evolution of the lesions suggests a cascade of inflammation initiated by a small initial stimulus. Histologic examination of the lesion produced by the intradermal injection of phosphatidyl serine shows a leukocytoclastic vasculitis, but biopsy of a spontaneous lesion shows only a massive hemorrhage into the dermis and subcutaneous tissue. These changes would obscure any initial vasculitic process that might be present. The reasons for the psychiatric manifestations are not known, but not all patients with this syndrome are so disturbed. Two of these patients seen at the Yale-New Haven Medical Center recently were judged by psychiatric consultants to be normal. These two patients developed their disease after trauma. One had torn her knee cartilage in an accident and the other was kicked in the knee, which led to an organized hematoma in the bursa that had to be surgically removed six months later.

It is likely that most individuals with this syndrome have discovered that they develop an unusually violent inflammatory response to trauma, especially to minor injury. This reaction is then used for secondary gain by many of them. The psychiatrically disturbed person with the Gardner-Diamond syndrome probably uses this phenomenon to derive secondary gain more often than the normally adjusted individual who is affected by this disorder. However, it needs to be reemphasized that not every patient with this disorder is hysterical or masochistic. At times lesions do arise spontaneously, producing pain and disability to which affected individuals react with a normal emotional response.

REFERENCES

1. Lagos, J. C., and Gomez, M. R.: Tuberous sclerosis: reappraisal of a clinical entity. Mayo Clin. Proc., *42*:26, 1967.
2. Chao, D. H.-C.: Congenital neurocutaneous syndromes in childhood. J. Pediatr., *55*:447, 1959.
3. Gold, A. P., and Freeman, J. M.: Depigmented nevi: the earliest sign of tuberous sclerosis. Pediatrics, *35*:1003, 1965.
4. Fitzpatrick, T. B., Szabo, G., Hori, Y., Simone, A. A., Reed, W. B., and Greenberg, M. H.: White leaf-shaped macules. Earliest visible sign of tuberous sclerosis. Arch. Dermatol. *98*:1, 1968.
5. Hurwitz, S., and Braverman, I. M.: White spots in tuberous sclerosis. J. Pediatr., *77*: 589, 1970.
6. Butterworth, T.: In discussion of case: Tuberous sclerosis with adenoma sebaceum of skin, mucous membrane lesions, and epithelial nevus. Presented by Hambrick, G. W., Jr., and Brown, A. C.: Arch. Dermatol. *97*:206, 1968.
7. Kitamura, K., Fukushiro, R., and Miyabayashi, T.: Incontinentia pigmenti in Japan. Introduction of twenty-one observed cases. Arch. Dermatol. Syph., *69*:667, 1954.
8. Carney, R. G., Jr.: Incontinentia pigmenti. A world statistical analysis. Arch. Dermatol., *112*:535, 1976.
9. Dahl, M. V., Matula, G., Leonards, R., and Tuffanelli, D. L.: Incontinentia pigmenti and defective neutrophil chemotaxis. Arch. Dermatol., *111*:1603, 1975.
10. Jessen, R. T., Van Epps, D. E., Goodwin, J. S., and Bowerman, J.: Incontinentia pigmenti. Evidence for both neutrophil and lymphocyte dysfunction. Arch. Dermatol., *114*:1182, 1978.
11. Jelinek, J. E., Bart, R. S., and Schiff, G. M.: Hypomelanosis of Ito ("Incontinentia pigmenti achromians"). Arch. Dermatol., *107*:596, 1973.
12. Ito, M.: Studies on melanin XI. Incontinentia pigmenti achromians, a singular case of nevus depigmentosus systematicus bilateralis. Tohoku J. Exp. Med., *55*(Suppl):57, 1952.
13. Schwartz, M. F., Jr., Esterly, N. B., Fretzin, D. F., Pergament, E., and Rozenfeld, I. H.: Hypomelanosis of Ito (incontinentia pigmenti achromians): A neurocutaneous syndrome. J. Pediatr., *90*:236, 1977.
14. Rubin, M. B.: Incontinentia pigmenti achromians. Multiple cases within a family. Arch. Dermatol., *105*:424, 1972.
15. Grosshans, E. M., Stoebner, P., Bergoend, H., and Stoll, C.: Incontinentia pigmenti achromians (Ito). Dermatologica, *142*:65, 1971.
16. Cram, D. L., and Fukuyama, K.: Unilateral systematized hypochromic nevus. Arch. Dermatol., *109*:416, 1974.
17. Maize, J. C., Headington, J. T., and Lynch, P. J.: Systematized hypochromic nevus. Incontinentia pigmenti achromians of Ito. Arch. Dermatol., *106*:885, 1972.
18. Jimbow, K., Fitzpatrick, T. B., Szabo, G., and Hori, Y.: Congenital circumscribed

hypomelanosis: a characterization based on electron microscopic study of tuberous sclerosis, nevus depigmentosus and piebaldism. J. Invest. Dermatol., *64*:50, 1975.

19. Griffiths, A., and Payne, C.: Incontinentia pigmenti achromians. Arch. Dermatol., *111*:751, 1975.
20. Crowe, F. W., Schull, W. J., and Neel, J. V.: A Clinical, Pathologic and Genetic Study of Multiple Neurofibromatosis. Charles C Thomas, Springfield, Ill., 1956.
21. Miller, R. M., and Sparkes, R. S.: Segmental neurofibromatosis. Arch. Dermatol., *113*:837, 1977.

21a. Riccardi, V. M.: Pathophysiology of neurofibromatosis. IV. Dermatologic insights into heterogeneity and pathogenesis. J. Am. Acad. Dermatol., *3*:157, 1980.

22. Swapp, G. H., and Main, R. A.: Neurofibromatosis in pregnancy. Br. J. Dermatol., *80*:431, 1973.
23. Young, D. F., Eldridge, R., and Gardner, W. J.: Bilateral acoustic neuroma in a large kindred. J.A.M.A., *214*:347, 1970.
24. Siggers, D. C., Boyer, S. H., and Eldridge, R.: Nerve-growth factor in disseminated neurofibromatosis. N. Engl. J. Med., *292*:1134, 1975.
25. Shenkein, I., Bueker, E. D., Helson, L., Axelrod, F., and Dancis, J.: Increased nerve-growth-stimulating activity in disseminated neurofibromatosis. N. Engl. J. Med., *290*:613, 1974.
26. Benedict, P. H., Szabo, G., Fitzpatrick, T. B., and Sinesi, S. J.: Melanotic macules in Albright's syndrome and in neurofibromatosis. J.A.M.A., *205*:618, 1968.
27. Polani, P. E., and Moynahan, E. J.: Progressive cardiomyopathic lentiginosis. Q. J. Med., *41*:205, 1972.
28. Selmanowitz, V. J., Orentreich, N., and Felsenstein, J. M.: Lentiginosis profusa syndrome (multiple lentigines syndrome). Arch. Dermatol., *104*:393, 1971.
29. Walther, R. J., Polansky, B. J., and Grots, I. A.: Electrocardiographic abnormalities in a family with generalized lentigo. N. Engl. J. Med., *275*:1220, 1936.
30. Matthews, N. L.: Lentigo and electrocardiographic changes. N. Engl. J. Med., *278*:780, 1968.
31. Nordlund, J. J., Lerner, A. B., Braverman, I. M., and McGuire, J. S.: The multiple lentigines syndrome. Arch. Dermatol., *107*:259, 1973.
32. Clark, C. E., Henry, W. L., and Epstein, S. E.: Familial prevalence and genetic transmission of idiopathic hypertrophic subaortic stenosis. N. Engl. J. Med., *289*:709, 1973.
33. Solomon, L. M., Fretzin, D. F., and Dewald, R. L.: The epidermal nevus syndrome. Arch. Dermatol., *97*:273, 1968.
34. Dimond, R. L., and Amon, R. B.: Epidermal nevus and rhabdomyosarcoma. Arch. Dermatol., *112*:1424, 1976.
35. Lyell, A.: Cutaneous artifactual disease. J. Am. Acad. Dermatol., *1*:391, 1979.
36. Gardner, F. H., and Diamond, L. K.: Autoerythrocyte sensitization. A form of purpura producing painful bruising following autosensitization to red blood cells in certain women. Blood, *10*:675, 1955.
37. Ratnoff, O. D., and Agle, D. P.: Psychogenic purpura: a re-evaluation of the syndrome of autoerythrocyte sensitization. Medicine, *47*:475, 1968.
38. McDuffie, F. C., and McGuire, F. L.: Clinical and psychological patterns in autoerythrocyte sensitivity. Ann. Intern. Med., *63*:255, 1965.
39. Agle, D. P., Ratnoff, O. D., and Wasman, M.: Studies in autoerythrocyte sensitization. The induction of purpuric lesions by hypnotic suggestion. Psychosomatic Med., *29*:491, 1967.
40. Groch, G. S., Finch, S. C., Rogoway, W., and Fisher, D. S.: Studies in the pathogenesis of autoerythrocyte sensitization syndrome. Blood, *28*:19, 1966.
41. Boxley, J. D.: Autoerythrocyte sensitization (painful bruising) syndrome. Proc. R. Soc. Med., *64*:1196, 1971.
42. Schwartz, R. S., Lewis, F. B., and Dameshek, W.: Hemorrhagic cutaneous anaphylaxis due to autosensitization to deoxyribonucleic acid. N. Engl. J. Med., *267*:1105, 1962.
43. Stocker, W. W., McIntyre, O. R., and Clendenning, W. E.: Psychogenic purpura. Arch. Dermatol., *113*:606, 1977.
44. McIntosh, R. M., Ozawa, T., Persoff, M., Altshuler, J. H., Guggenheim, S., and Boedecker, E.: Immune-complex nephritis with autoerythrocyte sensitization. N. Engl. J. Med., *296*:1265, 1977.
45. Kalden, J. R., Hoffken, B., and Stangel, W.: Immune mechanism in Gardner-Diamond syndrome. N. Engl. J. Med., *297*:1350, 1977.
46. Oei, S. J., deVries, E., Cats, A., Hamminga, L., and van Vloten, W. A.: Abnormal circulating red blood cells in the painful bruising syndrome. Arch. Dermatol. Res., *263*:227, 1978.

18

Infections

This chapter reviews the skin manifestations of the major infectious diseases encountered in clinical medicine. For more detailed information about the diseases themselves, the reader is referred to comprehensive texts dealing with this subject.[1-5]

THE FEBRILE PATIENT

One is often confronted by an acutely ill febrile patient who has nonspecific complaints of malaise, headache, arthralgias, and myalgias. The history and initial laboratory findings may not be helpful, but a careful examination of the skin may reveal a diagnostic sign or a clue to the correct diagnosis. Most of the infectious diseases encountered in medical practice present with one of the following cutaneous manifestations.

Pustular Lesions

Staphylococcal infections of the skin often produce superficial pustules (pyoderma) or deep abscesses (furuncles, carbuncles) (Plate 40*C*). A more diffuse involvement of the dermis and subcutaneous fat manifests itself as cellulitis. The staphylococci gain a foothold when the surface of the epidermis is disrupted, either as microscopic breaks in normal skin or as major defects caused by inflammatory exudative dermatoses, vesicular viral disorders, and surgical or traumatic wounds. When the staphylococcal infections are restricted in extent and depth, fever and systemic signs are absent, but when they are more extensive, fever, leukocytosis, and even septicemia with rigors may develop.

Staphylococcal septicemia may exist in the absence of any obvious cutaneous or internal focus. Its presence can often be inferred by finding lesions characteristic of septic emboli to the skin. Staphylococcal septic emboli are usually 1- to 2-mm pustules surrounded by a wide red flare (Fig. 18–1). Only rarely do these emboli enlarge to form abscesses and furuncles (Fig. 18–2). If thrombocytopenia is present, the pustules may be surrounded by purpura. Staphylococcal sepsis can be accompanied by conjunctival petechiae and can also be the trigger for DIC (Figs. 18–9 to 18–16).

Erythematous Lesions

Streptococci, chiefly beta-hemolytic group A, also invade the skin and underlying tissues through microscopic breaks and exudative derma-

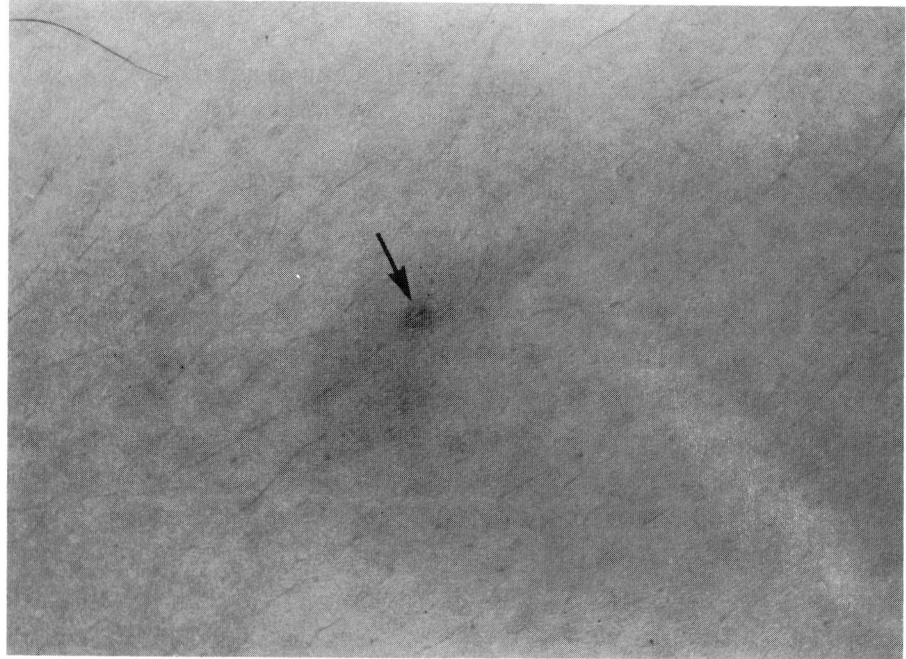

Figure 18–1. Septic embolus produced by staphylococci. Small pustule (arrow) surrounded by wide ring of erythema.

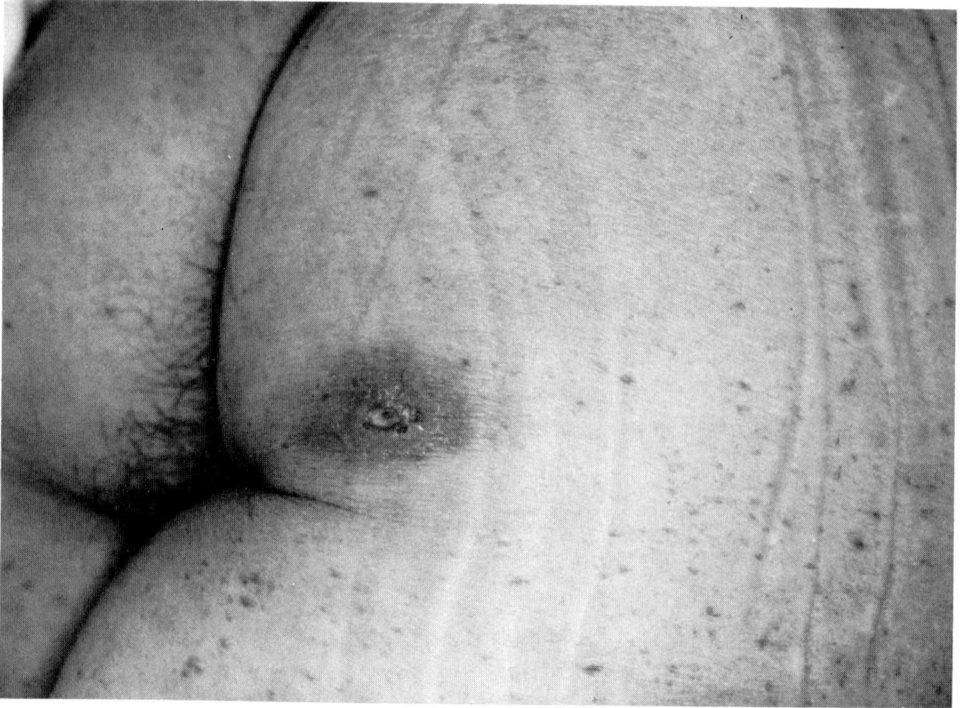

Figure 18–2. Septic embolus produced by staphylococci enlarged to form abscess. Rare occurrence.

toses, surgical and traumatic wounds, and burns, and at parturition. They may accompany staphylococci present in pyoderma and impetigo. The streptococcal infections most frequently responsible for producing a febrile systemic illness are cellulitis, erysipelas, and scarlet fever. In cellulitis, the involved skin is red, hot, and edematous, often with poorly defined borders (Fig. 18–3). Both the dermis and subcutaneous layer are affected. In contrast, the lesion of erysipelas has sharply defined edematous borders and extends more rapidly (Fig. 18–4). Vesicles and bullae may develop on the surface. The streptococci spread through the dermal lymphatics in both cellulitis and erysipelas, but in the latter the infection is confined to the dermis. Although erysipelas frequently develops as a solitary lesion on the face, often spreading to produce a "butterfly" pattern over the cheeks (Plates 12*D* and 17*F*), it can develop as multiple areas and occur anywhere on the body. Multiple attacks of cellulitis and erysipelas can lead to impairment of lymphatic drainage, which in turn predisposes the area to subsequent infections. A vicious circle is established. Recurrent episodes of streptococcal cellulitis and erysipelas are relatively common. On the lower extremities, these repeated infections produce dermal fibrosis and lymphedema in combination with epidermal hyperplasia to create elephantiasis nostras (Figs. 18–5 and 18–6). Such individuals require daily prophylactic doses of penicillin or erythromycin to prevent or minimize these repeated infections. Figure 18–3 shows early elephantiasis in a large pendulous fold of abdominal skin that has been subjected to repeated episodes of cellulitis.

In rare cases, the streptococci may invade the subcutaneous fat and the deeper fascial layer, resulting in thromboses of deep vessels that produce gangrene of the overlying tissues. The initial cutaneous lesion

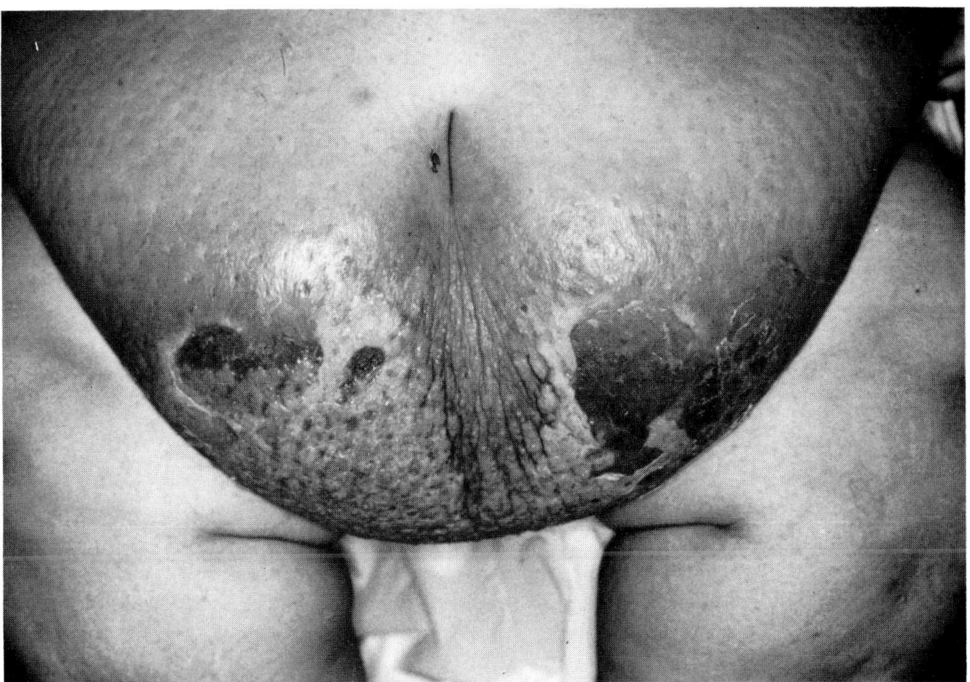

Figure 18–3. Cellulitis in large pendulous fold of abdominal skin produced by beta-hemolytic streptococci.

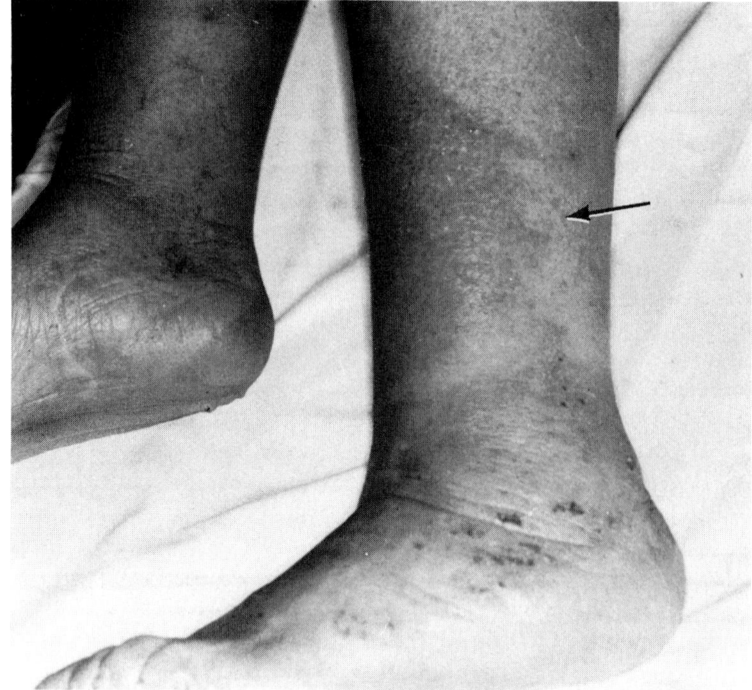

Figure 18–4. Erysipelas on leg produced by beta-hemolytic streptococci. Sharply defined edematous borders (arrow).

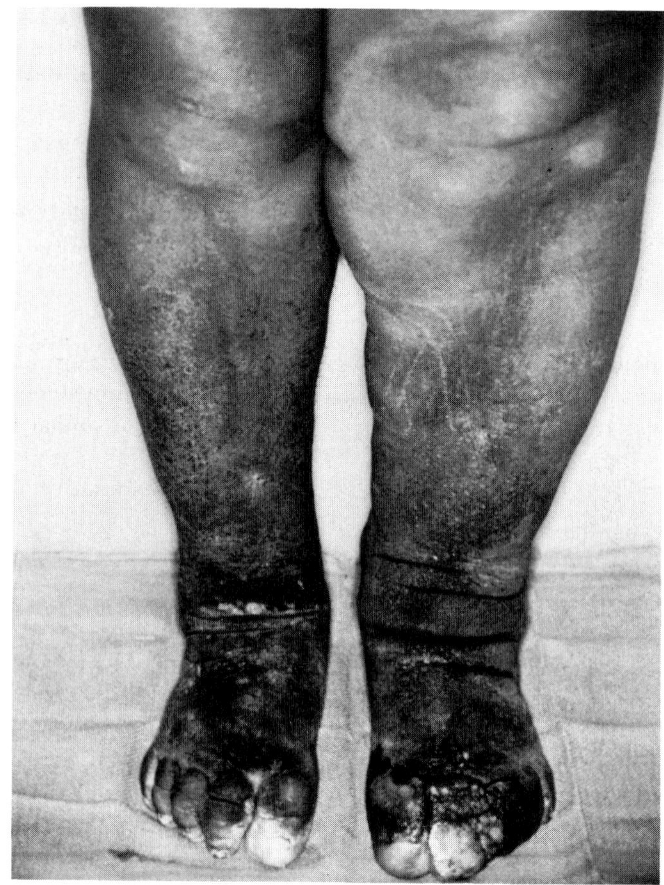

Figure 18–5. Elephantiasis nostras produced by recurrent streptococcal infections.

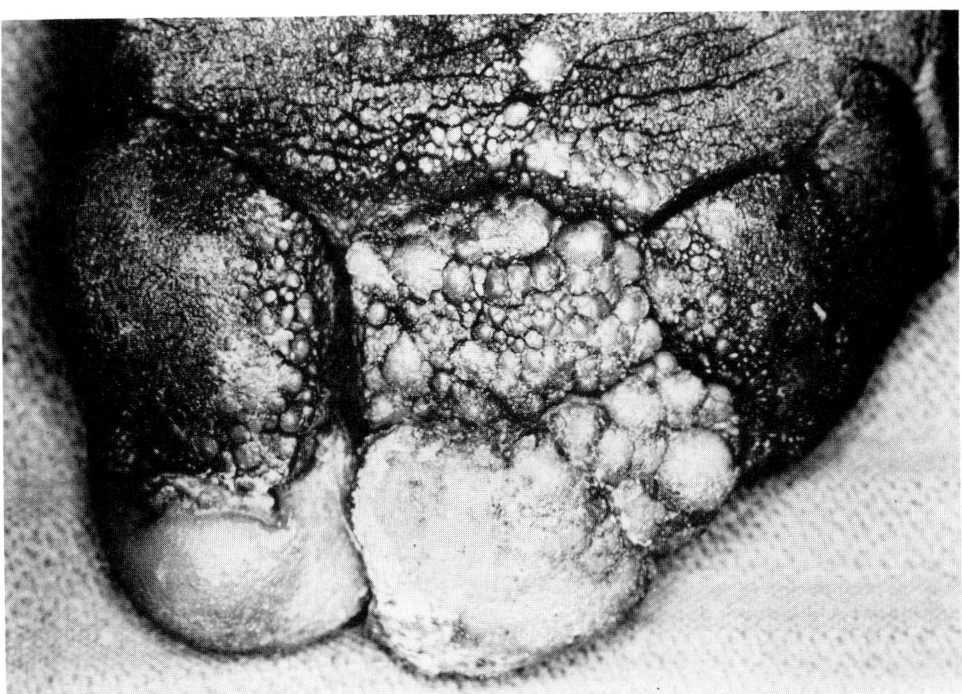

Figure 18–6. Elephantiasis nostras. Close-up of Figure 18–5 to show verrucous and papillomatous appearance of skin surface.

resembles erysipelas, but between the second and fourth day the skin becomes dusky and evolves into frank gangrene with eventual sloughing. Streptococcal gangrene (necrotizing fasciitis) is rapidly progressive and often fatal.[6, 7] The involved areas need to be incised and opened widely, and massive antibiotic therapy should be initiated. Streptococcal septicemia and metastatic abscesses are associated with this variety of streptococcal infection. Other bacteria (anaerobes, pseudomonas, staphylococci), usually as a mixed infection, can also produce necrotizing fasciitis.[7]

In the differential diagnosis of cellulitis, other infectious agents need to be considered in addition to streptococci and staphylococci. Septicemia with *Hemophilus influenzae* type B can produce similar lesions in children under two years of age.[8] The bacterial focus is usually in the pharynx, middle ear, or elsewhere in the upper respiratory tract. The cellulitis is usually a solitary plaque with an erythematous or bluish-purplish hue and an irregular edematous border. It can be indistinguishable from streptococcal erysipelas. Rarely, adults with epiglottitis and other forms of upper respiratory infection caused by *H. influenzae* have developed identical illnesses.[9] The patches of cellulitis usually develop on the neck, chest, and face. Pneumococci can also produce cellulitis in infants. Cellulitis can also be a manifestation of disseminated cryptococcal infection.[10, 11] Plate 14*B* shows an example of this phenomenon in a patient with underlying multiple myeloma. All instances of disseminated cryptococcal infection involving the skin have occurred in immunocompromised hosts. Metastatic carcinoma to the skin produced by lymphatic spread resembles erysipelas (Plates 1*C*,*D*) but lacks the systemic features of fever and malaise. Erysipeloid is caused by a gram-positive bacterium,

Erysipelothrix insidiosa (rhusiopathiae), which is traumatically introduced into the skin of the hands or wrists of individuals who handle infected organic matter. These persons include kitchen workers, meat dressers, and others who handle salt water fish, shellfish and poultry.[12, 13] Erysipeloid typically occurs during the summer and is characterized by a painful violaceous patch that develops at the site of injury within one week. The violaceous patch spreads centrifugally with a distinct elevated border from which the organisms can be isolated. As the area of cellulitis increases, central clearing often develops. Erysipeloid is usually a self-limited infection of two to four weeks, but in uncommon cases it has continued to spread for several months, involving most of the cutaneous surface before ending. Fever and arthritis are uncommon. Rarely, a syndrome of endocarditis, arthritis, and purpura has developed. Erysipeloid is distinguished from erysipelas by the lack of fever and other constitutional symptoms and the tendency toward central clearing.

Unlike staphylococcal sepsis, the hematogenous spread of streptococci does not appear to be associated with septic emboli to the skin. However, suppurative lesions can develop in the joints, pericardium, endocardium, meninges, brain, and bone. Streptococci can invade tissues locally to produce peritonsillar and retropharyngeal abscesses; paranasal sinusitis that can lead to meningitis and brain abscesses; and suppurative cervical lymphadenitis, mastoiditis, and otitis media. Streptococcal invasion is more likely to occur in children than in young adults, and more likely in scarlet fever than in ordinary streptococcal pharyngitis.[14]

Scarlet fever is produced by an erythrogenic toxin elaborated by certain strains of beta-hemolytic streptococci. Although the streptococcal infection is usually in the pharynx or tonsils, it also can arise in surgical and traumatic wounds, in burns, and in the reproductive tissues at childbirth. The rash appears first on the neck, upper chest, and back and later spreads to the lower back, upper extremities, abdomen, and lower extremities. The rash is characterized by diffuse erythema interspersed with many red puncta that represent more intense inflammation around the openings of the hair follicles, producing an appearance of red "goose bumps" (Fig. 18–7). The face is flushed and there is a circumoral pallor. Commonly, a stippled petechial eruption is present on the soft palate and anterior tonsillar pillars one day before and for one to two days after the rash has appeared. The tongue has a white coating with swollen red papillae protruding through (white strawberry tongue). This white coating represents damaged lingual epithelium because it rapidly desquamates, leaving behind a red tongue with prominent swollen red papillae (red strawberry tongue). Petechiae may be present on the legs and in a linear array in the antecubital fossae (Pastia's sign), reflecting increased capillary fragility associated with the rash. The petechiae can be reproduced at this stage by the application of a tourniquet (Rumpel-Leede's sign). The skin begins to desquamate any time from five days to two to three weeks after the onset of the rash. The peeling begins on the neck, upper chest and back, or on the tips of the fingers and toes at the free margins of the nails.[15] Large sheets of skin may come off as casts from the palms and soles.

This desquamation is not specific for scarlet fever because it can follow any severe febrile illness (Fig. 18–8). This pattern of desquamation is also a feature of the mucocutaneous lymph node syndrome. The

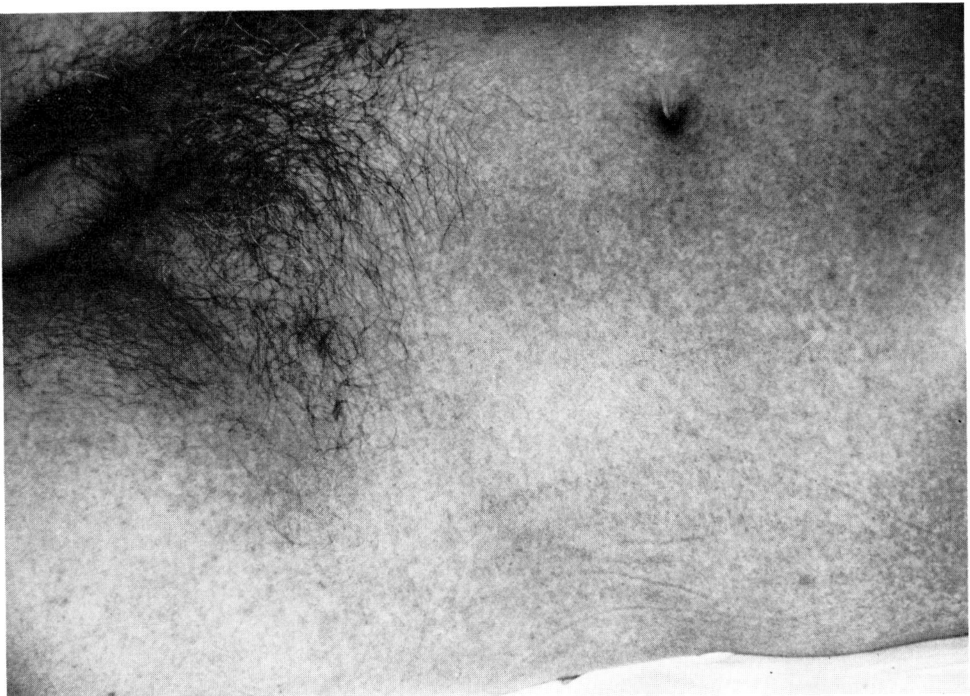

Figure 18–7. Scarlet fever.

petechial enanthem can also be seen in infectious mononucleosis and rubella.

Certain strains of staphylococci produce an erythrogenic toxin that is responsible for the clinical picture of scarlet fever, including the enanthem. In some cases, the erythrogenic toxin appeared to be identical to that of streptococcal scarlet fever, while in others it was not.[16-18]

The enteric fevers, typhoid and paratyphoid, are characterized by rose spots: discrete, *round*, red macules, 1 to 4 mm, that appear in crops

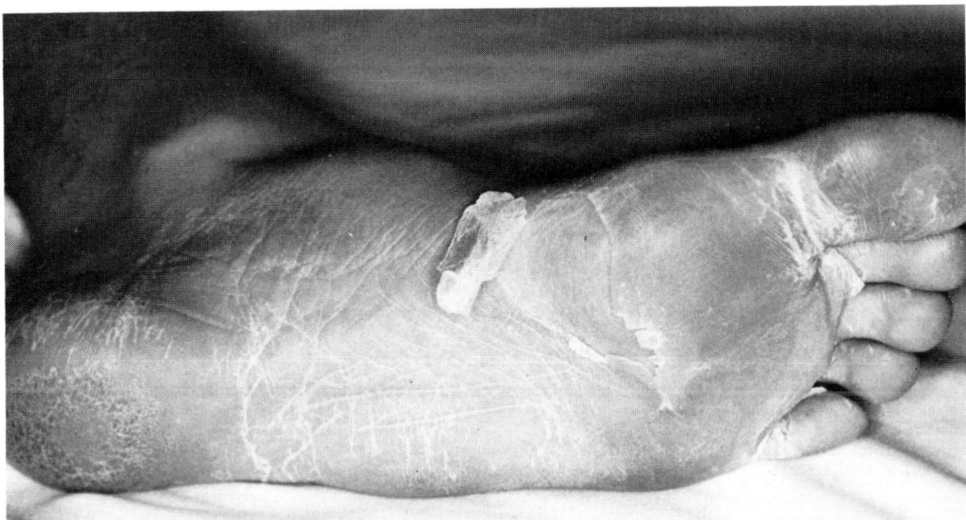

Figure 18–8. Desquamation of skin following severe febrile illness caused by staphylococcal infection.

over the abdomen and chest and may extend to the back and proximal parts of the limbs during the second to third week of the illness. They last for three to four days and disappear. The rose spots are larger in paratyphoid fever, and tend to be maculopapular, so that the rash may be mistaken for measles or infectious mononucleosis. The rose spots are believed to be bacterial emboli to the superficial cutaneous capillaries.[19]

Purpuric Lesions

Purpura and petechiae are the major manifestations of infections caused by the meningococcus, gonococcus, *Escherichia coli*, Klebsiella, Pseudomonas, and Rickettsia. These hemorrhagic phenomena are usually produced by septic emboli, but they can also be clinical signs of disseminated intravascular coagulation (DIC). DIC can be triggered by gram-positive, gram-negative, viral, and rickettsial organisms as well as by tissue injury and neoplasms.[20] The two major signs of DIC, a potentially devastating disorder, are widespread purpura (Fig. 8–43) and extensive areas of hemorrhagic infarcts involving any area of the body but showing a predilection for the extremities (Figs. 18–9 to 18–16). DIC often begins with persistent cyanosis of various portions of the extremities. There may be involvement of digits alone, hands and feet alone, or the distal extremities from the fingers and toes to the lower forearms and legs, respectively. The cyanotic areas often become edematous with formation of hemorrhagic bullae. The most distal portions may develop gangrene (Figs. 18–12 and 18–15). Although petechiae and small patches of purpura are also commonly seen in DIC, they are minor features of the clinical picture. As coagulation factors are consumed in DIC, the initial thrombotic events may be followed by large, painful, subcutaneous hematomas and bleeding from wound and venipuncture sites. The histopathology of the purpuric lesions in DIC is characterized by dermal vessels filled with fibrin thrombi in the absence of inflammation. These biopsy findings can be diagnostically useful in cases in which the coagulation tests for DIC are equivocal or in which differentiation from vasculitic syndromes is necessary. (See page 427 for further discussion.)

Acute meningococcemia is characterized by the development of indurated, gun metal gray patches of purpura that have an irregular (infarctive) pattern. They may develop bullae and ulcerate, and can occur anywhere on the skin (Figs. 18–44, 18–17, and 18–18). Although individual lesions have the same morphology as those of DIC, they are usually less edematous, smaller, and develop bullae less often than those of DIC. Petechiae also appear in acute meningococcemia and are present in addition to the infarctive purpuric areas. Occasionally, a transient erythematous maculopapular eruption resembling measles may appear before the main purpuric eruption develops.

The initial purpuric rash is caused by meningococcal invasion of endothelial cells in large dermal and subcutaneous vessels with subsequent injury leading to increased capillary permeability and localized thrombosis (localized DIC) that results in cutaneous infarction. In many cases, the massive gram-negative bacteremia triggers a generalized DIC with massive bleeding into the skin, adrenals, and other organs, producing the Waterhouse-Friderichsen syndrome (Figs. 18–19 and 18–20). This syndrome, which is usually rapidly fatal, is not a manifestation of adrenal

Text continued on page 821

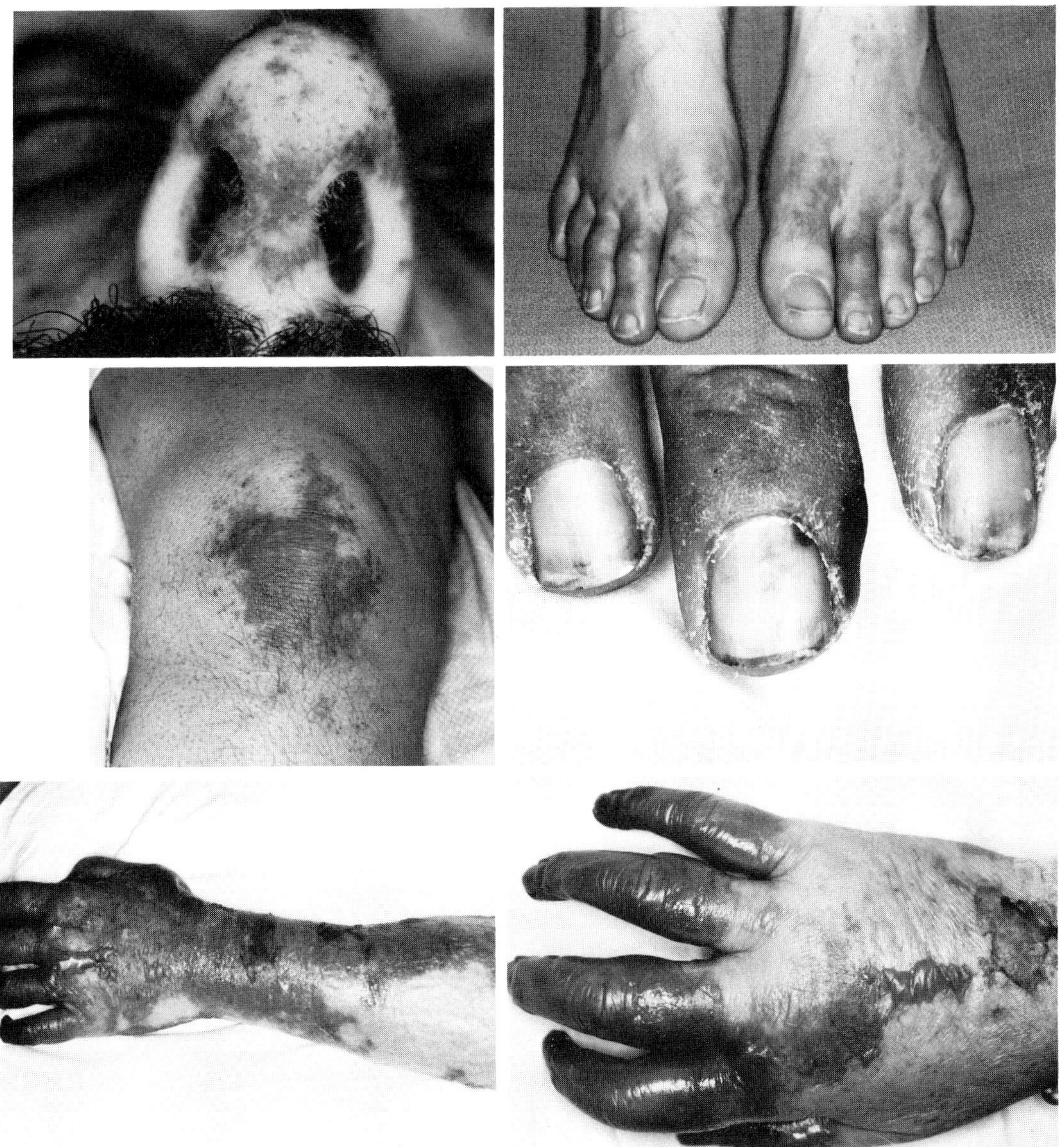

Figure 18–9. Top left. Disseminated intravascular coagulation (DIC) producing purpura on nose. Patient had pneumococcal septicemia in association with pneumococcal meningitis.

Figure 18–10. Top right. DIC. Same patient as in Figure 18–9. Purpuric lesions on feet.

Figure 18–11. Center left. DIC. Irregular purpuric area on knee in patient with a gram-negative bacteremia.

Figure 18–12. Center right. DIC. Digital gangrene in patient with staphylococcal septicemia.

Figure 18–13. Bottom left. DIC. Hemorrhagic bullous infarction of hand and forearm in patient with bacteremia.

Figure 18–14. Bottom right. DIC. Same patient as in Figure 18–13 to show close-up of hemorrhagic bullae and gangrene on fingers and hand.

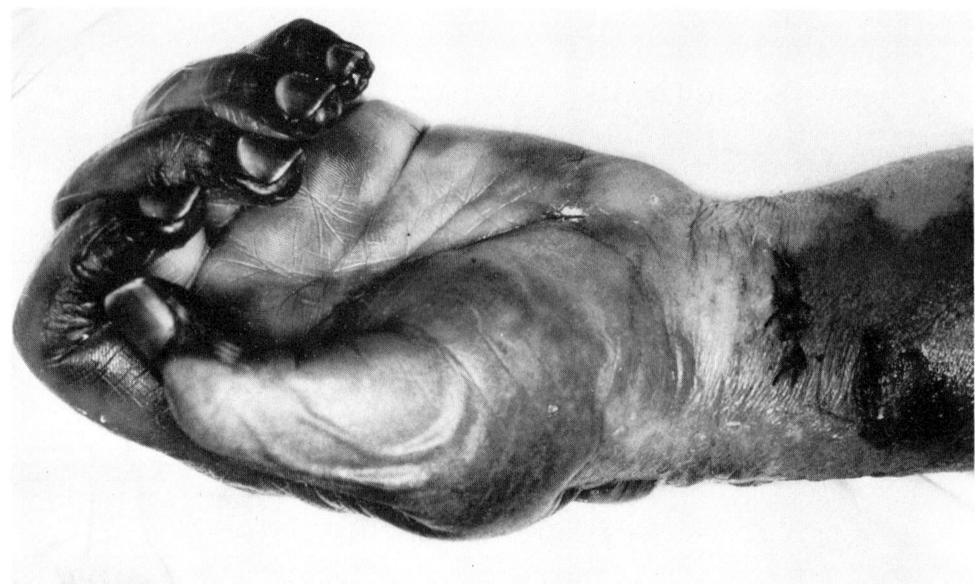

Figure 18–15. DIC.

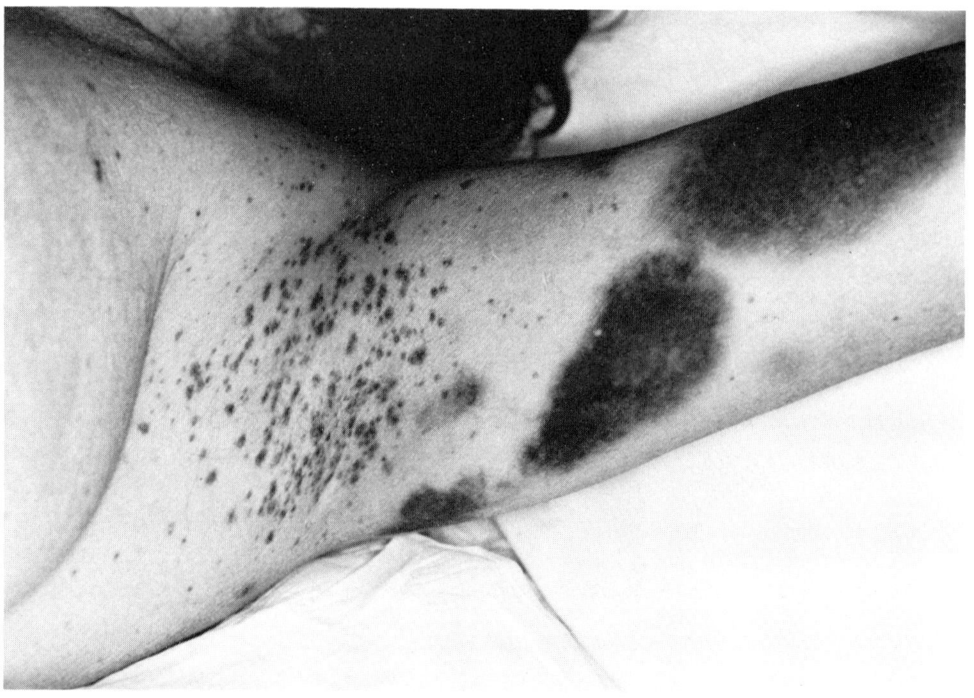

Figure 18–16. DIC in patient with acute leukemia.

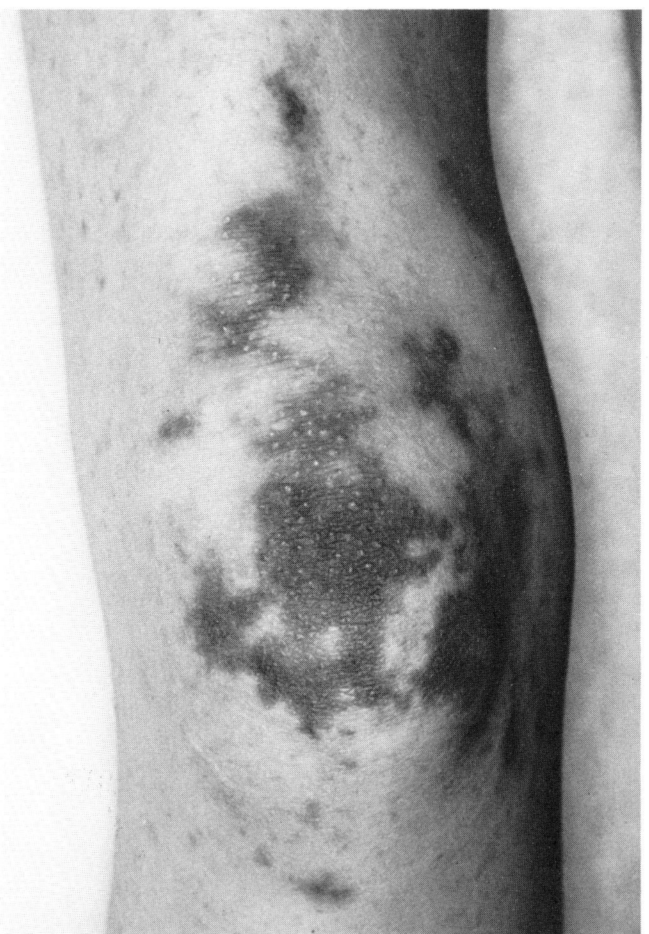

Figure 18–17. Acute meningococcemia. Indurated "gun metal" gray patches of purpura with an irregular (infarctive) pattern.

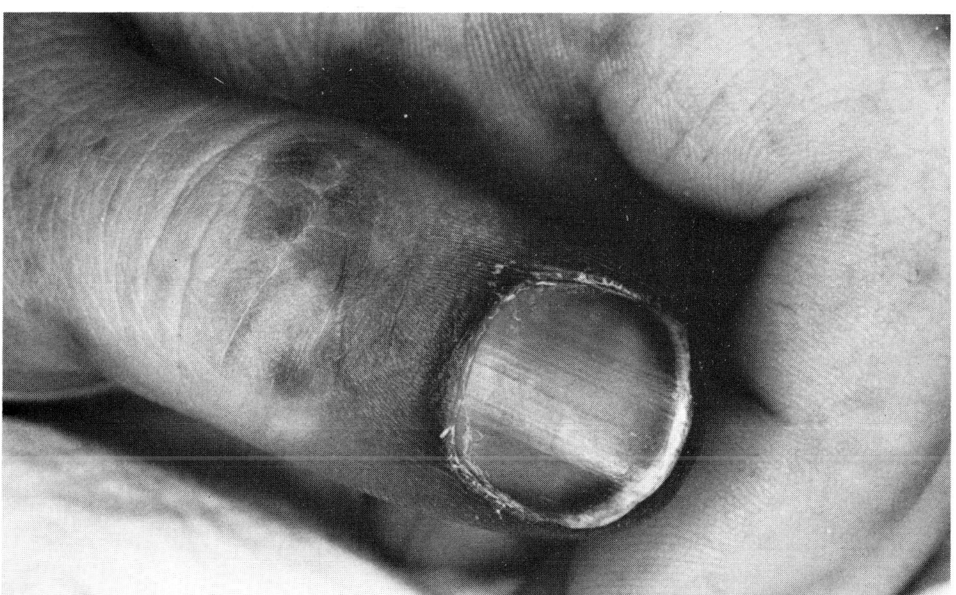

Figure 18–18. Acute meningococcemia. Digital involvement.

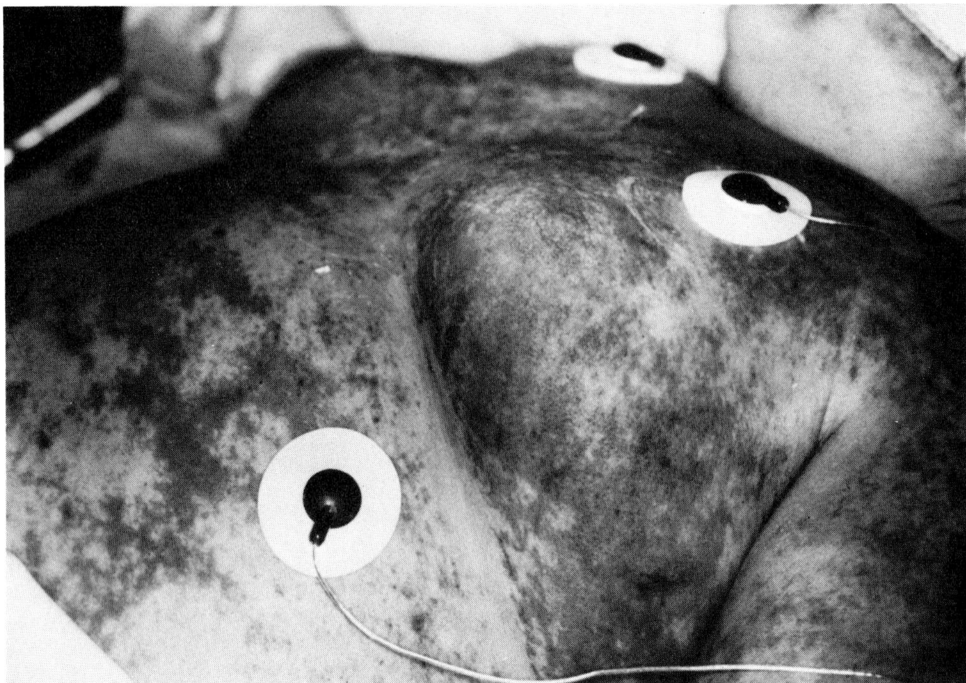

Figure 18–19. Acute meningococcemia with DIC (Waterhouse-Friderichsen syndrome).

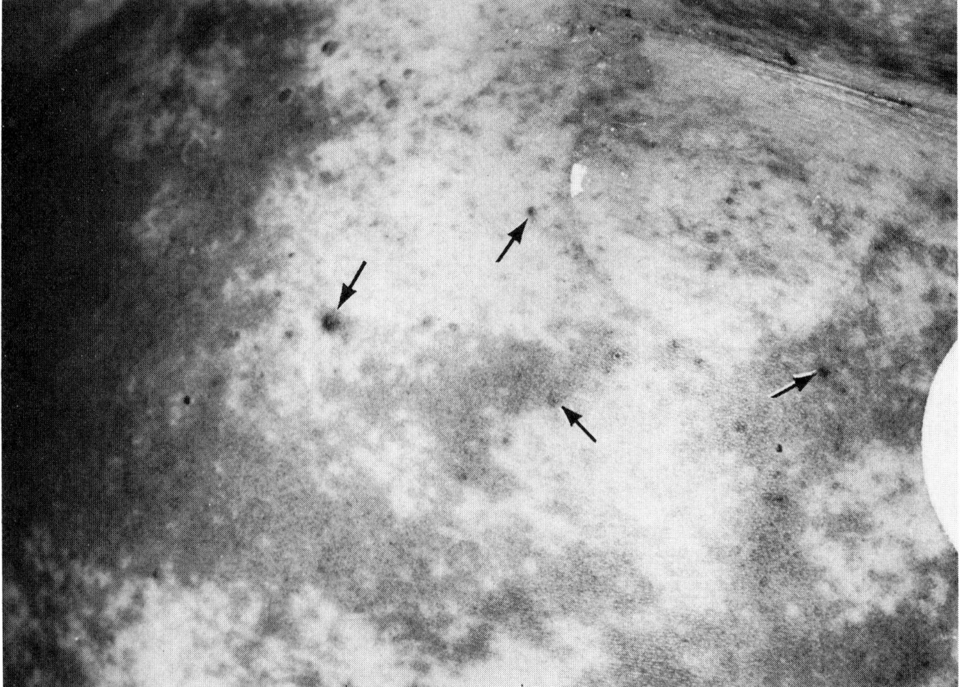

Figure 18–20. Acute meningococcemia. Close-up of Figure 18–19. Small purpuric spots (arrows) were caused by meningococci and broad purpuric areas were produced by DIC.

insufficiency, but rather a result of the gram-negative endotoxemia. Acute meningococcemia may begin with either gun metal gray lesions or DIC. At times, both types of lesions are present at the onset.

The combination of meningitis and purpura is almost always a sign of acute meningococcemia, but important exceptions occur. ECHO and Coxsackie viruses, which are etiologic agents for aseptic meningitis, are usually accompanied by an erythematous maculopapular eruption. However, a petechial rash (without the infarctive pattern) sometimes develops.[21] There is a single report of a 3½-year-old girl with acute bacterial meningitis and the Waterhouse-Friderichsen syndrome caused by the gonococcus.[22]

Chronic meningococcemia is not a virulent disease. It is an uncommon relapsing febrile illness persisting for two to three months and characterized by acute bouts of fever. joint pains, and skin lesions. The eruption has a predilection for the trunk and extensor surfaces of the extremities, but it can also appear on the hands and feet.[23, 24] The most common initial skin lesion is an erythematous macule or papule. The macules evolve into papules and nodules that develop a purpuric area at the summit of the elevated lesions. The initially formed papules develop a similar central hemorrhage. Less frequently the cutaneous lesions have been petechiae, purpuric spots, pustules, and erythematous nodules resembling erythema nodosum. Biopsy of lesions has demonstrated leukocytoclastic angiitis. Since the lesions always coincide with attacks of fever and septicemia, the lesions may represent an immune complex vasculitis secondary to the hematogenous release of bacterial antigen. However, the lesions are clinically indistinguishable from those of disseminated gonococcemia in which the skin lesions are thought to represent septic emboli or possibly localized DIC.

Disseminated gonococcemia occurs in 1 to 3 per cent of patients with gonorrhea. Typically, it is a subacute febrile illness characterized by arthralgias, arthritis, tenosynovitis, and skin lesions that have a predilection for the extremities, palms, fingers, and soles (Figs. 18–21 to 18–23 and Plate 40*D*). The eruption varies from erythematous papules with irregularly shaped purpura in their centers to vesiculopustules with an erythematous halo. The organisms can be identified in the skin lesions by direct immunofluorescent techniques but cannot be cultured.[25] The histologic changes in the vessels are those of a leukocytoclastic vasculitis with thrombosis.[26] The histology is compatible with septic emboli or a localized DIC secondary to endothelial cell damage by bacteria. Circulating immune complexes can be detected in disseminated gonococcemia.[27] They are believed to be responsible for the initial arthritis in the syndrome and perhaps for the associated acute glomerulonephritis noted in the prepenicillin era. A small number of patients with disseminated gonococcemia have hematuria, suggesting that an immune complex nephritis may be another complication of this syndrome.[26] It should be emphasized that bacterial cultures are necessary to distinguish the syndrome of chronic meningococcemia from chronic gonococcemia.

Septicemia with gram-negative organisms — *E. coli,* Klebsiella, and Pseudomonas — is usually a life-threatening condition that can be recognized on the basis of the associated cutaneous lesions. These three organisms produce septic emboli of a characteristic appearance: erythematous wheals and papules that develop irregular areas of purpura (Plate

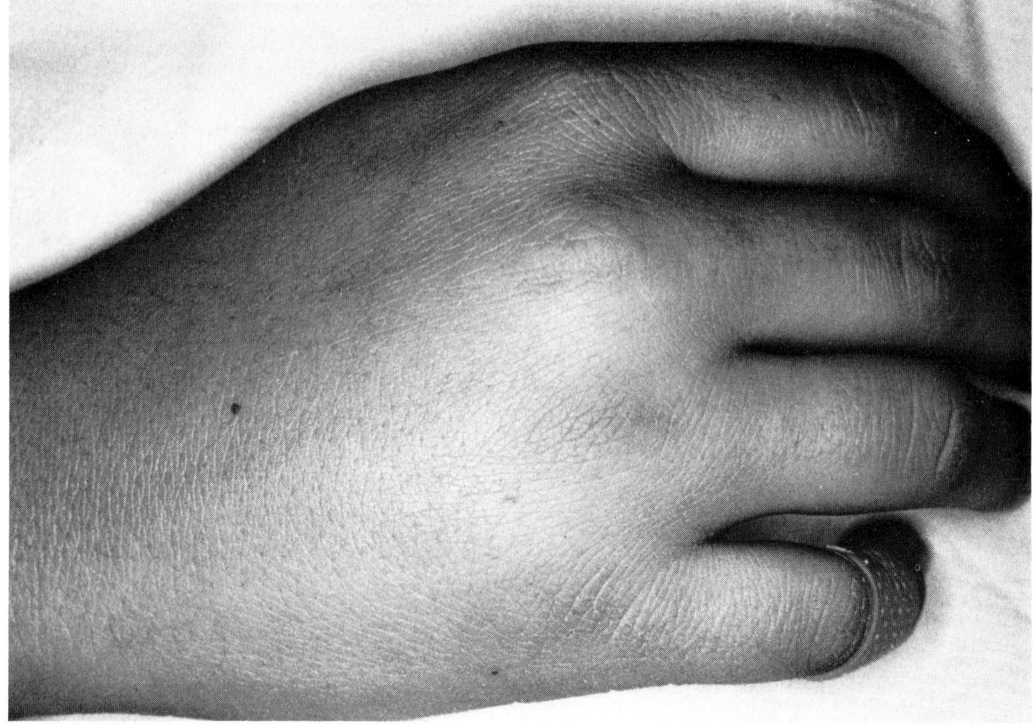

Figure 18–21. Acute disseminated gonococcemia. Swelling of hand with tenosynovitis.

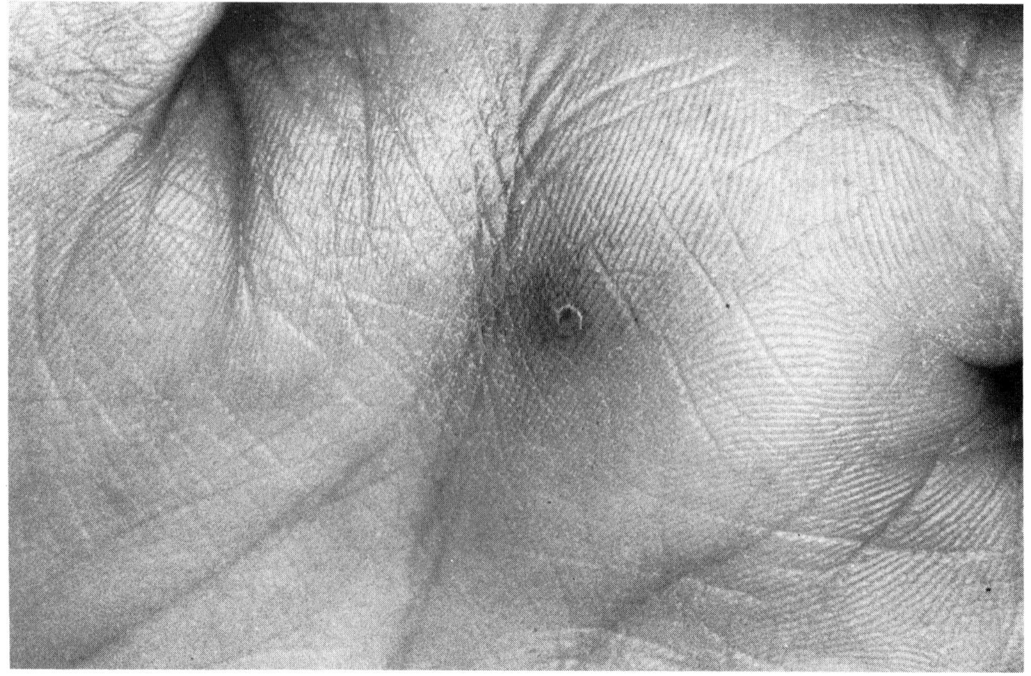

Figure 18–22. Acute disseminated gonococcemia. Vesicopustule with erythematous halo on palm.

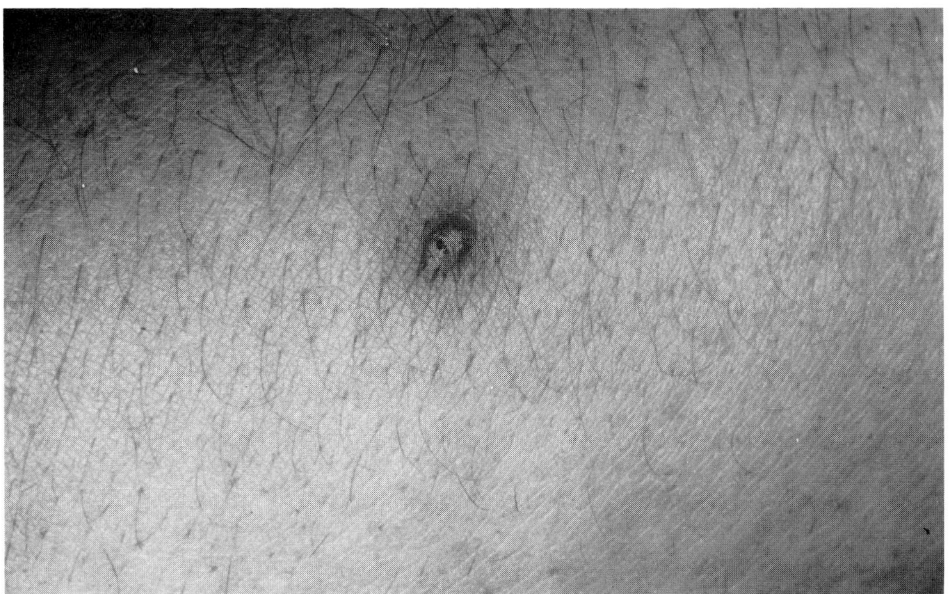

Figure 18–23. Acute disseminated gonococcemia. Vesicopustule on forearm.

41*A*,*B*). The lesions may become necrotic and form ulcers with undermined purpuric edges — echthyma gangrenosum — a condition observed most frequently in debilitated patients with lymphoma and leukemia (Plate 41*C*). The morphology of a wheal or papule with an irregular purpuric area in its center or periphery appears to be a specific sign of septicemia with gram-negative organisms: gonococcus, meningococcus, *E. coli,* Klebsiella, and Pseudomonas. Rarely, identical lesions can be produced by septic emboli of *Candida albicans*. I have not observed such lesions in sepsis with gram-positive organisms. Gram-negative sepsis is frequently accompanied by DIC.

Rocky Mountain spotted fever caused by *Rickettsia rickettsii* and spread by tick bite is characterized by a pink macular rash, 1 to 4 mm in diameter, that initially develops on the palms, soles, hands, feet, wrist, and ankles and then spreads to involve the rest of the body. The rash appears from the second to fourth day of the illness and becomes petechial and purpuric over the course of 24 to 48 hours (Fig. 18–24). In severe cases, the eruption can become confluent, superficially simulating the rash of acute meningococcemia. The mucous membranes can be affected as well. Severe cases can be complicated by the development of DIC.

The rash of epidemic typhus, which is caused by *Rickettsia prowazekii* and transmitted by the body louse, begins on the fourth to seventh day of the illness as a pink macular eruption on the trunk and in the axillae and spreads to the rest of the body, sparing the palms, soles, and face. Over the course of a few days, the rash becomes petechial and purpuric. Although the eruptions of these two most important rickettsial diseases can be extensive and purpuric, they lack the morphology of the hemorrhagic lesions seen in gram-negative sepsis. They also do not exhibit the infarctive patterns found in acute meningococcemia, unless DIC supervenes in a severe case. The rash in these two rickettsial disorders is

PLATE 41

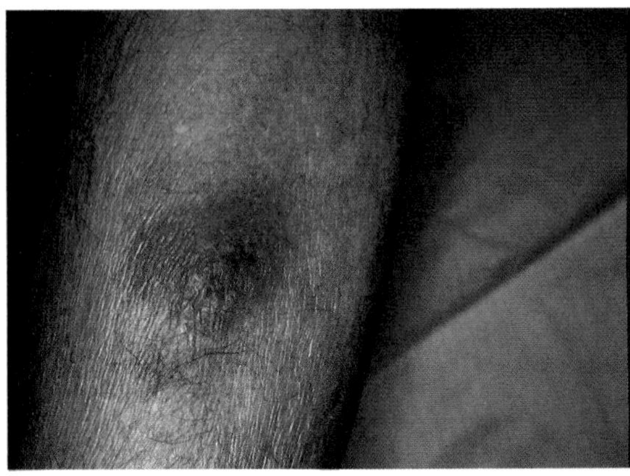

A, Ecthyma gangrenosum caused by Klebsiella. Purpura in center of red urticarial plaque. Early lesion.

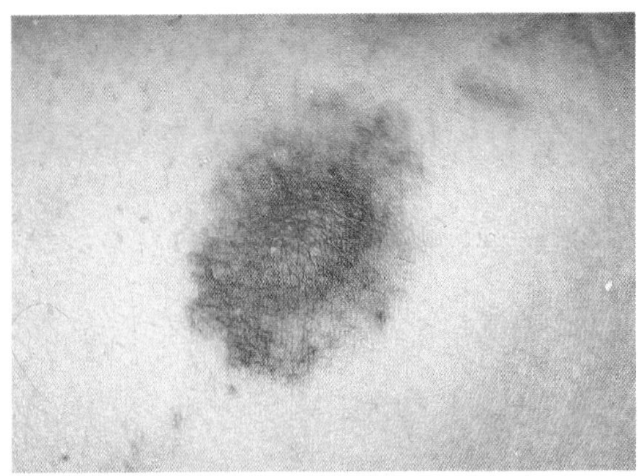

B, Ecthyma gangrenosum caused by Klebsiella. Dusky center. Purpura on border.

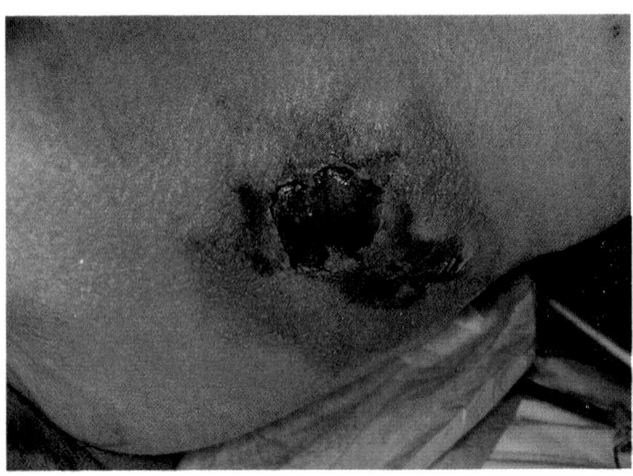

C, Ecthyma gangrenosum caused by *Pseudomonas aeruginosa* on thigh of patient with leukemia. Center of purpuric area has ulcerated. Surrounding area is red, edematous, and forming bullae.

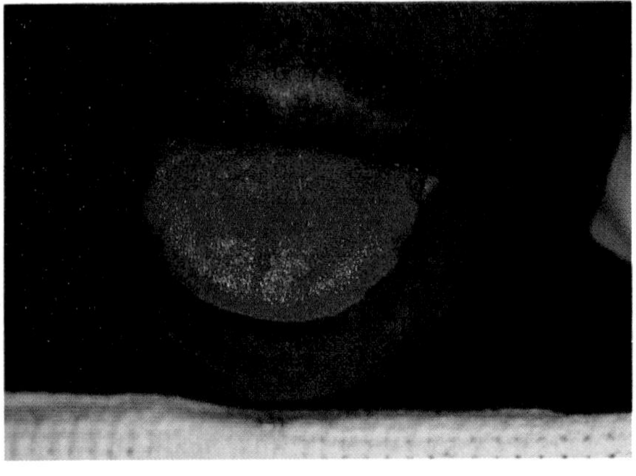

D, Mucocutaneous lymph node syndrome. Tongue is red and resembles the strawberry tongue of scarlet fever. Same patient as in Figures 18–84 to 18–87.

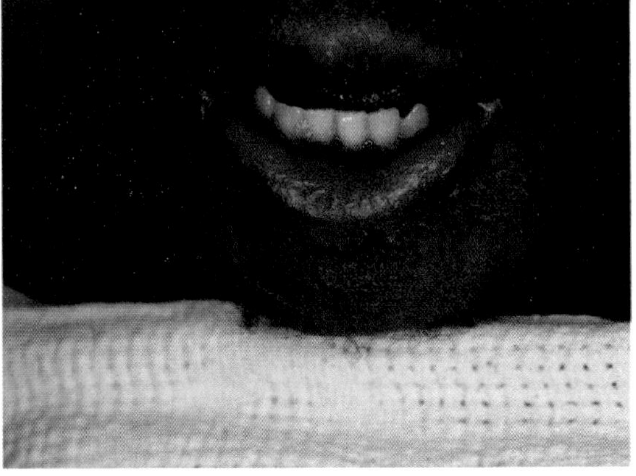

E, Mucocutaneous lymph node syndrome. Lips are red.

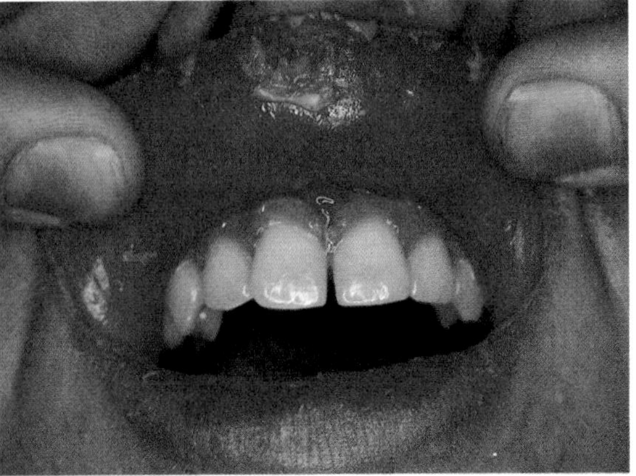

F, Chronic mucocutaneous candidiasis. Candidal infection was confined to lips, which were chronically bright red with desquamation.

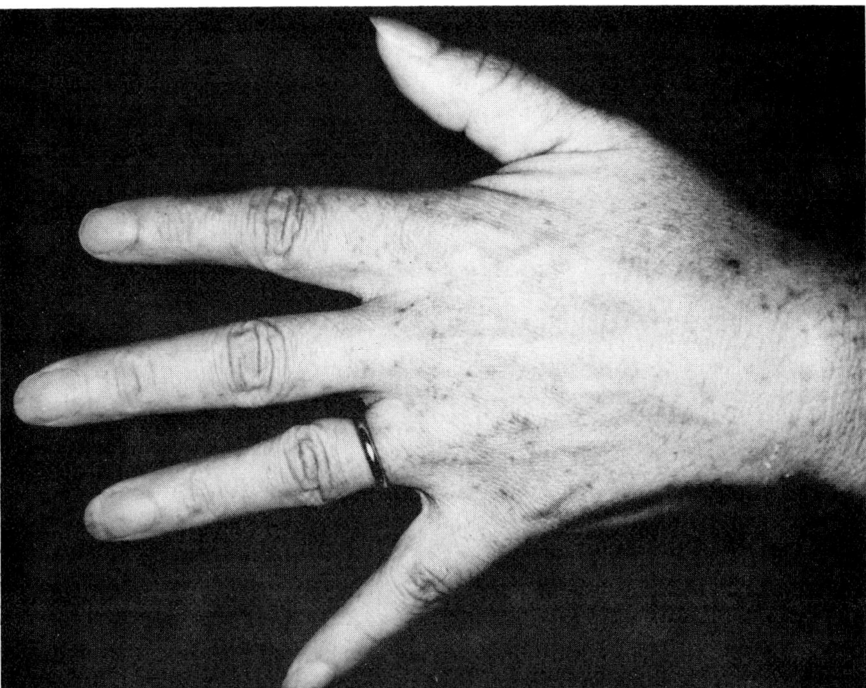

Figure 18–24. Rocky Mountain spotted fever. Small purpuric spots on hand.

produced by the direct invasion of the vascular endothelial cells by the organisms, with subsequent thrombosis and necrosis of the microcirculatory vessels.

Maculopapular Lesions

Erythematous maculopapular eruptions as a manifestation of infectious disease usually are indicative of an underlying viral infection. Drug reactions can mimic these eruptions, but it is usually possible to make the correct diagnosis on the basis of the evolution of the eruption and the associated clinical features. A drug rash usually develops almost simultaneously over the entire body surface, although its intensity may increase with time and its initial appearance may be in the flexures before becoming generalized. Viral exanthems usually start in a characteristic location and spread in a predictable way to involve other areas of skin. If one sees a maculopapular eruption only in its fully developed form without the benefit of an accurate history describing its development, then it may be impossible to distinguish between a drug eruption and a viral exanthem. Only the subsequent course of the illness will determine the correct diagnosis.

The rash of measles (rubeola) follows a three- to four-day prodrome of fever, conjunctivitis, coryza, and cough. The posterior auricular, cervical, and occipital lymph nodes are enlarged. The rash begins as a discrete erythematous maculopapular eruption behind the ears and along the hairline that quickly spreads onto the face and then to the trunk. At first the eruption consists of discrete lesions (Figs. 18–25 and 18–26; Plate 40*E*), but by the second day the rash has become more extensive and the

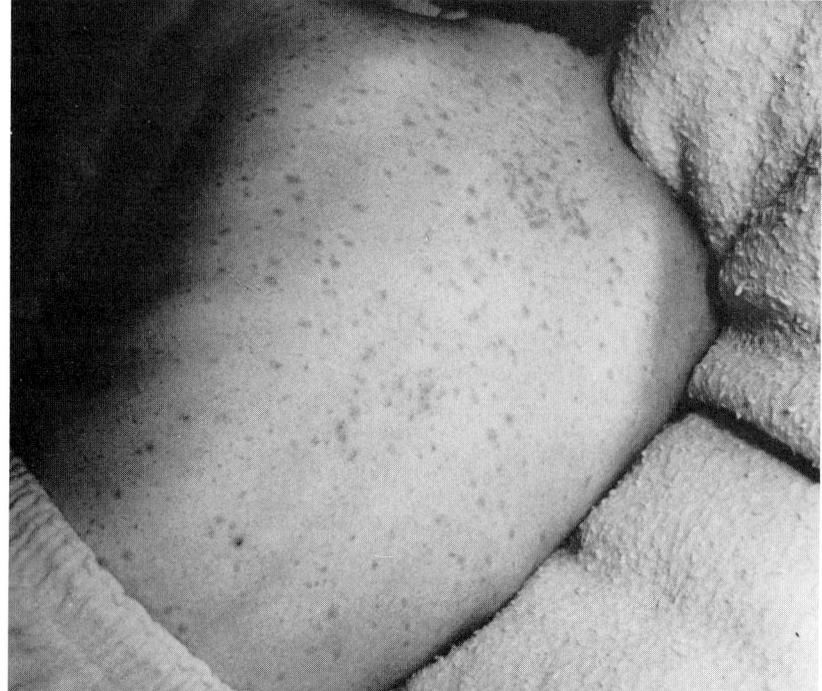

Figure 18–25. Measles (rubeola). Appearance of rash eight hours after onset.

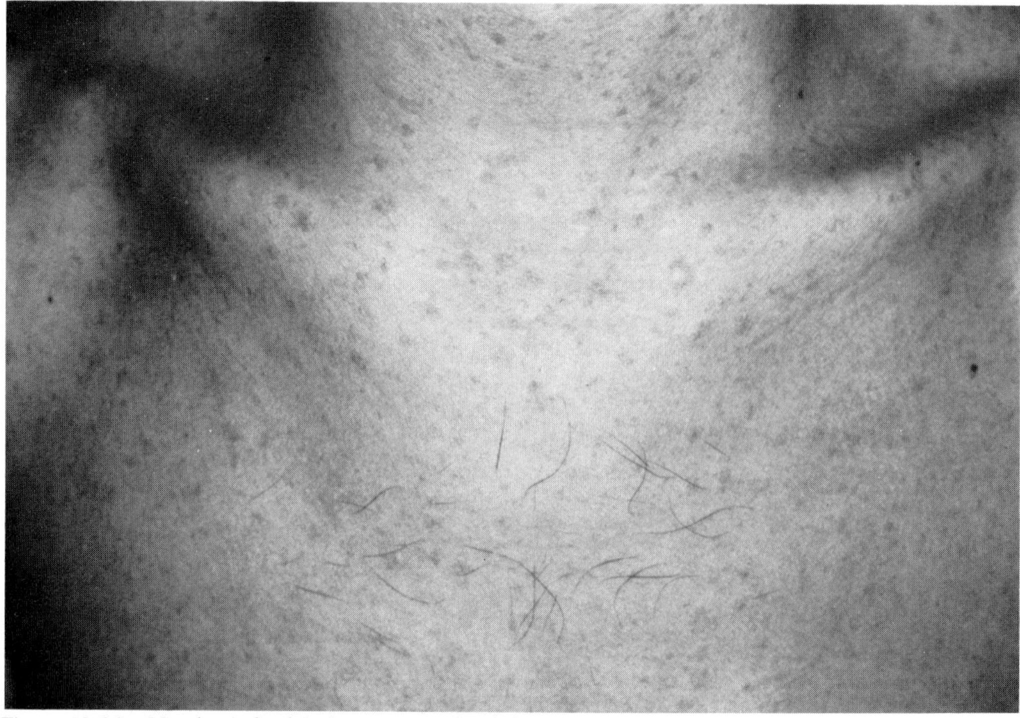

Figure 18–26. Measles (rubeola). Appearance of rash less than 24 hours old. Discrete maculopapular lesions.

individual lesions have become confluent (Fig. 18–27). Koplik's spots, 1- to 2-mm white to bluish white puncta on an erythematous base, are characteristically present on the buccal mucosa opposite the premolars before and during the initial development of the exanthem (Figs. 18–28 and 18–29). Koplik's spots can also develop over the entire buccal mucosa, as well as the palate, inner surfaces of the lips, palpebral conjunctivae, and even on the vaginal mucosa.[28] Koplik's spots are pathognomonic for measles and disappear as the exanthem develops. Occasionally during the three- to four-day prodrome, there may be a transient rash resembling that of scarlet fever, rubella, or measles. Measles varies from a mild to severe disease, and the rash reflects disease activity. In severe cases, the rash may be complicated by petechiae or purpura. Severe measles may trigger DIC to produce black measles — hemorrhagic cutaneous infarcts and bleeding from mucosal surfaces.[4] In the usual case, the rash fades from above downwards and leaves behind a mild brownish staining produced by the deposition of hemosiderin. Even in the mildest cases of measles, there is enough extravasation of red cells secondary to increased vascular permeability to produce this characteristic staining, which disappears after a few weeks. The Koplik's spots and the rash of measles may be either a delayed hypersensitivity reaction to the second viremia that occurs in the disease,[29] or a manifestation of nonimmunologic tissue injury to the circulating virus. Both the Koplik's spots and the rash show collections of perivascular lymphocytes in the dermis and multinucleated giant cells in the mucosal epithelium and

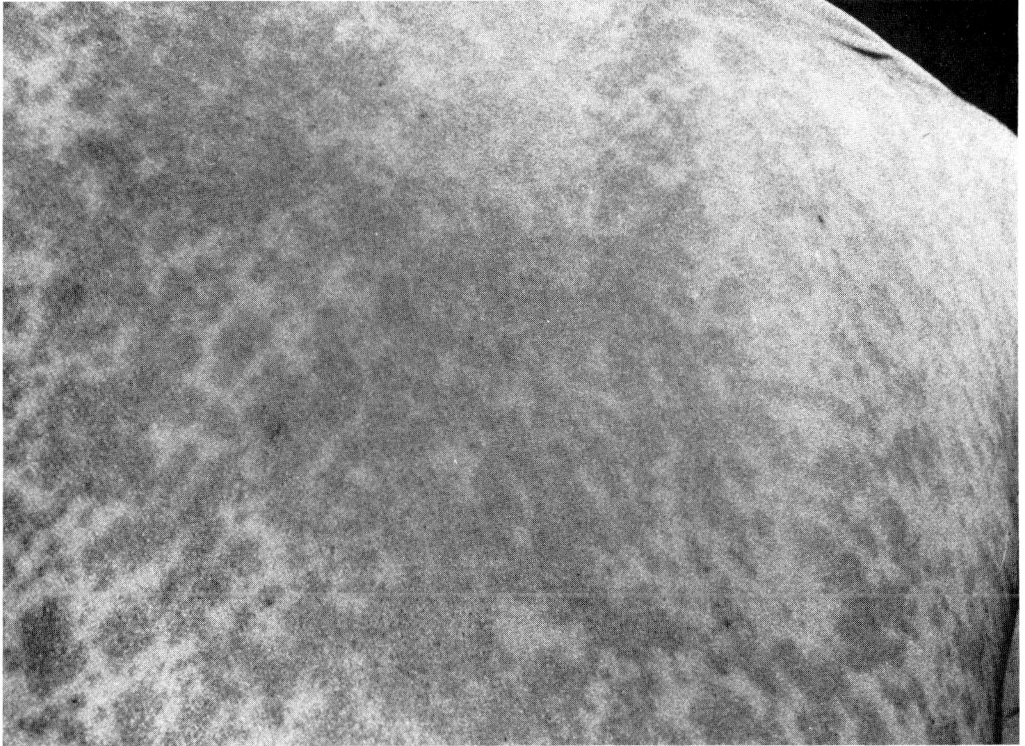

Figure 18–27. Measles (rubeola). Coalescence of measles rash over the back on third and fourth days.

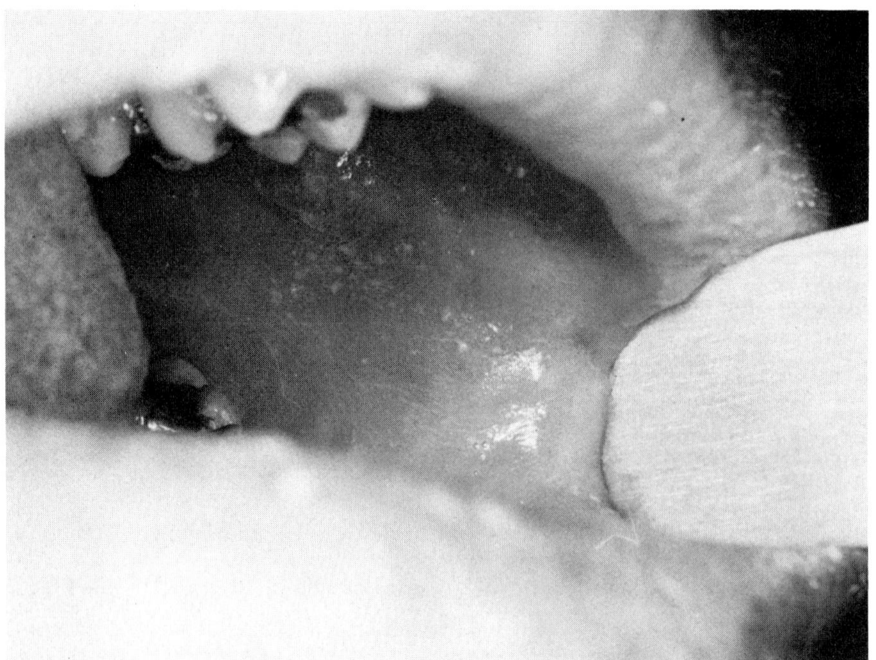

Figure 18–28. Measles (rubeola). Koplik's spots on buccal mucosa. One- to two-mm white or bluish-white elevated puncta, resembling grains of sand, on an erythematous base.

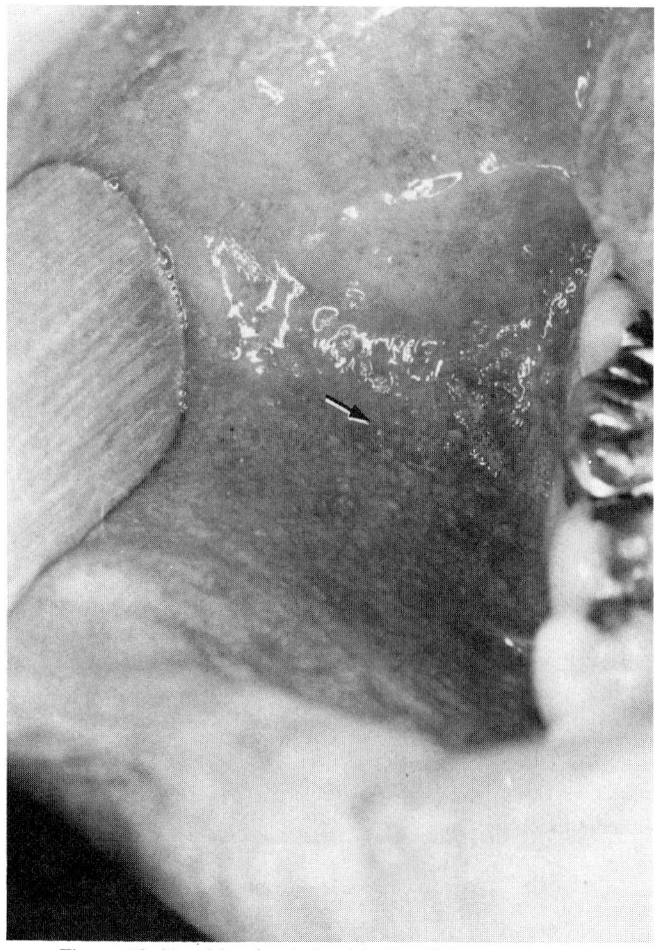

Figure 18–29. Measles (rubeola). Koplik's spots (arrow).

epidermis. The giant cells have been shown by electron microscopy to contain tubular structures characteristic of measles virus.[28]

An atypical form of measles arises in individuals who either have been immunized with killed measles vaccine or have received killed measles vaccine followed at a later date by live virus vaccine, and who several years later are exposed to wild measles virus. These individuals develop a prodrome of fever and malaise for one to two days, followed by a rash that begins *peripherally*. The eruption has been described as urticarial, maculopapular, hemorrhagic, and vesicular. The illness is characterized by high fever, edema of the extremities, interstitial pulmonary infiltrates, and, rarely, pleural effusion. The course of atypical measles is more prolonged and more severe than that of ordinary measles.[30] The pathogenesis is believed to be a hypersensitivity response to measles virus in a partially immune host. Both immune complex[31] and delayed hypersensitivity mechanisms[30] have been implicated.

German measles (rubella) may have a mild prodrome of coryza and cervical adenopathy. Posterior auricular and occipital lymphadenopathy is sometimes present. The rash of rubella is also maculopapular, but it is pink rather than red and lasts for only about three days, in contrast to five to six days in rubeola (Fig. 18–30). Although it spreads in the same manner as in measles, it usually disappears from the face by the second day. The trunk lesions become confluent by the second day and have disappeared by the third. Although Koplik's spots do not develop, one

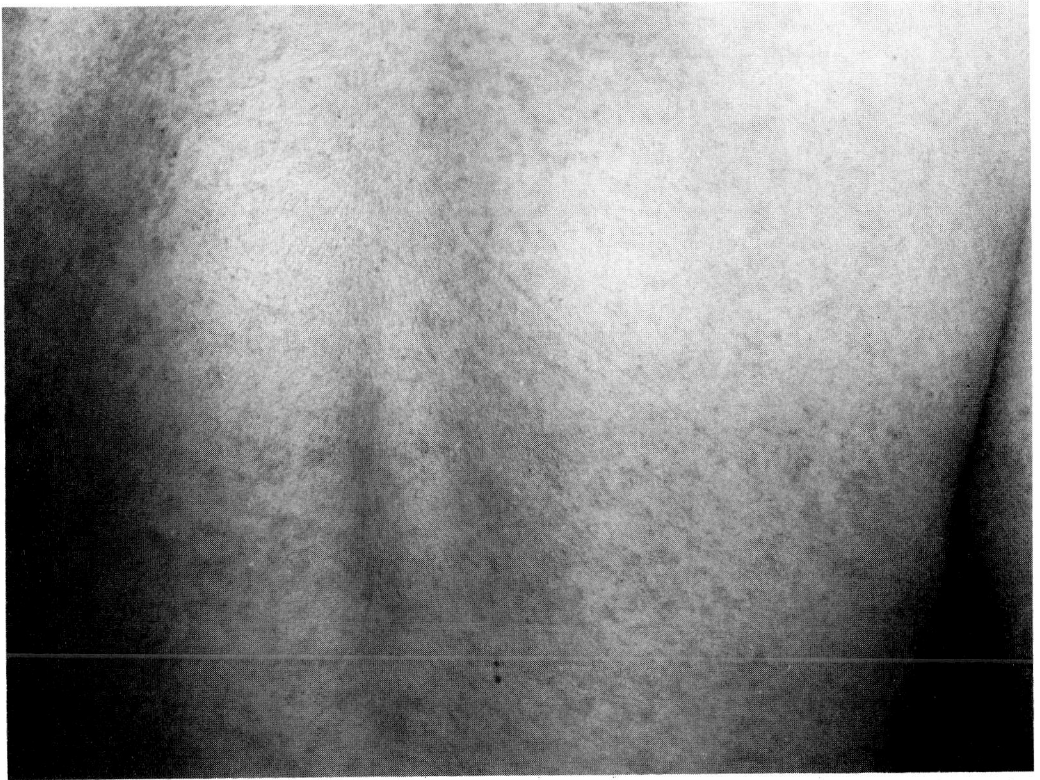

Figure 18–30. German measles (rubella). Maculopapular eruption that is less erythematous and less intense than in rubeola.

may see petechiae on the soft palate. Brown staining by hemosiderin does not occur as the rash fades. Thrombocytopenic purpura may develop as a complication of rubella and can persist for weeks to months. It is thought to be immunologically mediated.[32]

Roseola (exanthem subitum), a presumed viral infection, is characterized by a three- to four-day course of high fever and cervical, occipital, and posterior auricular adenopathy. Symptoms are few, but febrile convulsions may develop. The fever subsides by crisis and is followed by a maculopapular rash resembling rubella that persists for one to two days. However, the rash begins on the trunk and may either remain limited to this area or extend to the neck, upper extremities, face, and lower limbs (Figs. 18–31 and 18–32).

Fifth disease (erythema infectiosum) is also believed to be of viral etiology, although it is not always accompanied by fever.[33] When fever is present it is mild and the patient may have slight malaise. The rash begins on the cheeks as an intensely warm, red, nontender flush that can have raised borders simulating erysipelas. The facial appearance is often referred to as "slapped cheeks" (Plate 40*F*). On the second day, a maculopapular eruption, often in a reticulated pattern appears on the extensor surfaces of the upper and lower extremities and spreads to the flexor surfaces of the distal extremities, the buttocks, and the trunk (Figs. 18–33 to 18–35). The eruption may also appear on the palms and soles. The chest tends to be spared. The average duration of the rash is about six days, but it may persist for up to four weeks. In a minority of cases, the rash appears on the extremities before it develops on the face. As the eruption fades, it forms a more prominent reticulated or lacy pattern over the limbs and trunk before disappearing completely (Fig. 18–35). Arthritis and arthralgias may accompany this disorder. The illness tends to be more severe in adults than in children. It is common for adults to have fever, adenopathy, and arthritis, especially of the knees and wrists.[34, 35] For several weeks after the eruption has disappeared, the rash may recur briefly following trauma, exposure to the extremes of temperature, and excessive exposure to sunlight.

The exanthems caused by the enteroviruses, ECHO and Coxsackie, can be confused with drug eruptions if seen at the height of their development. However, if their evolution is determined, then the correct diagnosis ought to be made most of the time. Three types of exanthems are produced: (1) Rubelliform (morbilliform). The rash characteristically begins on the face and spreads to the neck, chest, and extremities. The exanthem is associated with fever. The rash is composed of 1- to 3-mm pink macules that are transient in most areas, except for the face (cheeks and chin), where they can persist for up to five days and sometimes longer. There is no adenopathy of the posterior cervical and auricular nodes in ECHO 9 infection, a finding that can be helpful in differentiating this illness from rubella. However, in ECHO 9 and Coxsackie A9 infections, petechiae may be a manifestation of the illness. If meningeal signs are also present, a diagnosis of acute meningococcemia may be made incorrectly. A maculopapular eruption affecting primarily the distal extremities and palms and soles can be seen in infections with ECHO viruses 2, 4, 11, 19, and 25 and Coxsackie A9. In approximately 50 per cent of infections with Coxsackie A9, adenopathy of the posterior cervical and occipital nodes develops, simulating rubella.[20] (2) Roseoliform eruptions. ECHO virus, 11, 16, and 25 and Coxsackie B1 and B5 have been associated with a roseola-like syndrome. The eruption, composed of

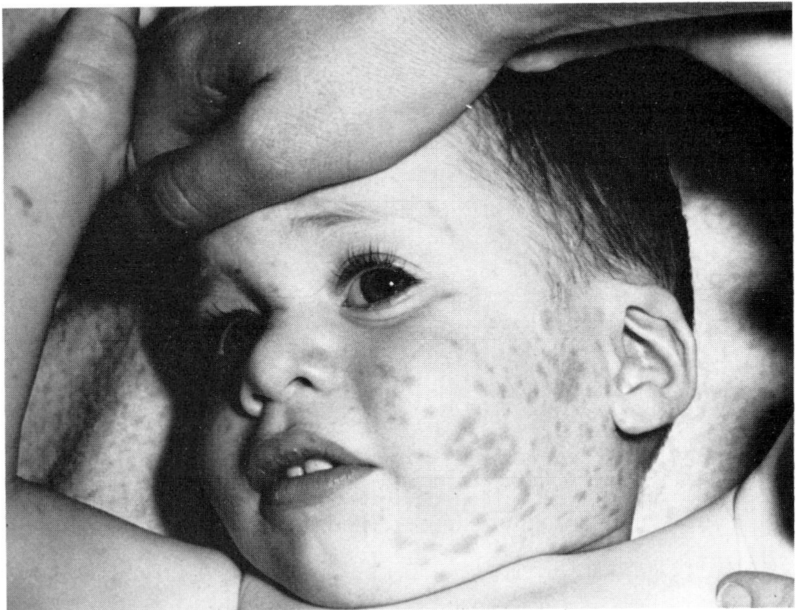

Figure 18–31. Roseola (exanthem subitum). Facial rash resembles early stage of measles.

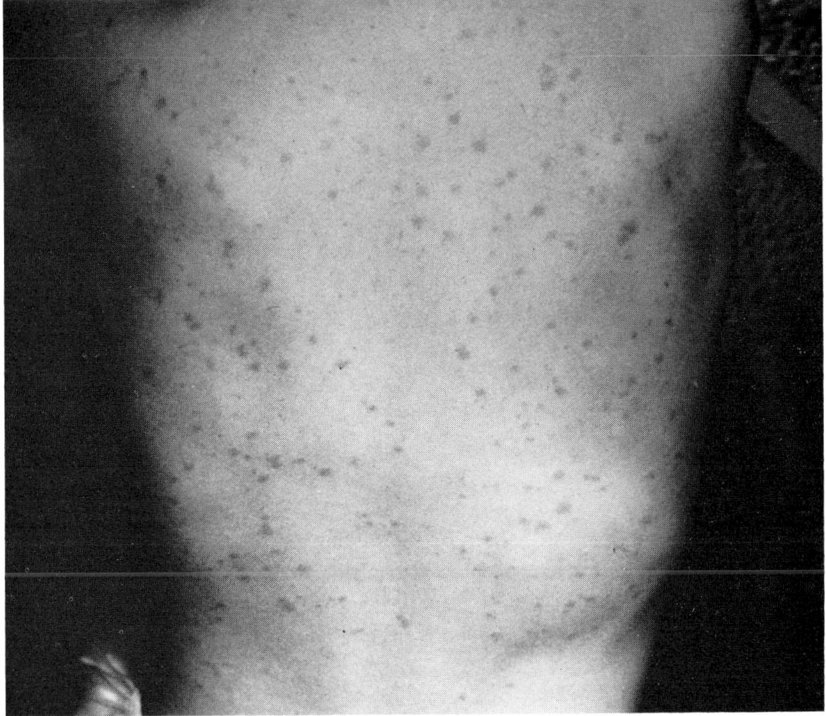

Figure 18–32. Roseola (exanthem subitum). Rash resembles early stage of measles.

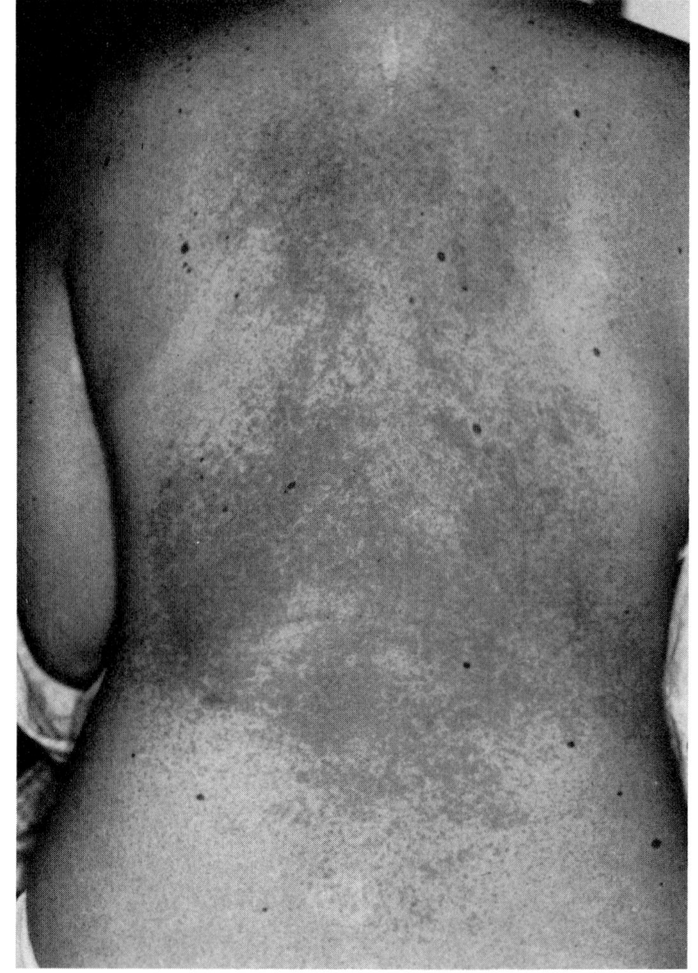

Figure 18–33. Fifth disease (erythema infectiosum). Appearance of rash on back.

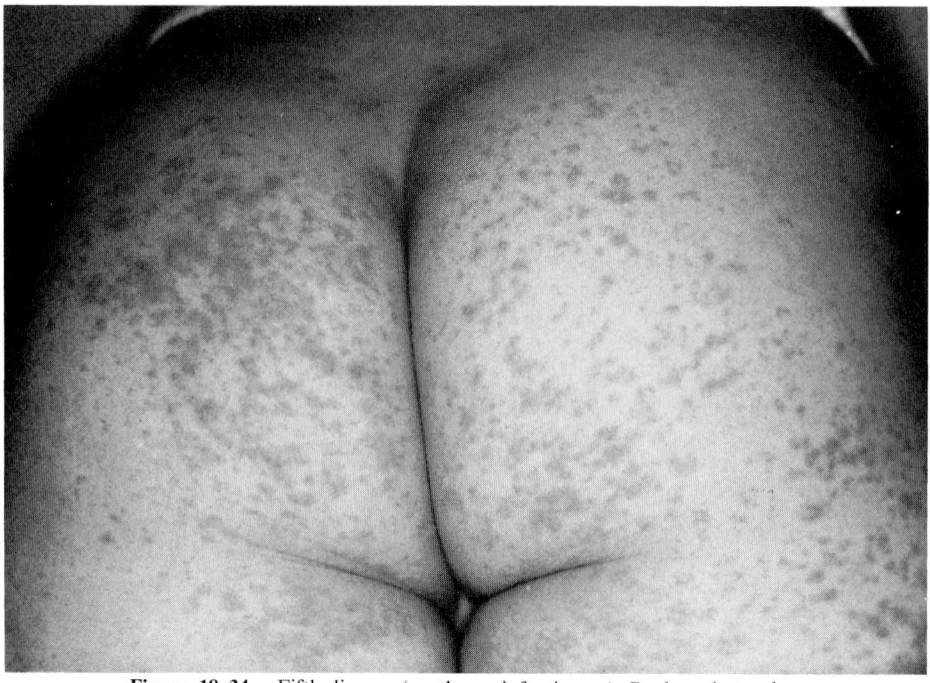

Figure 18–34. Fifth disease (erythema infectiosum). Rash on buttocks.

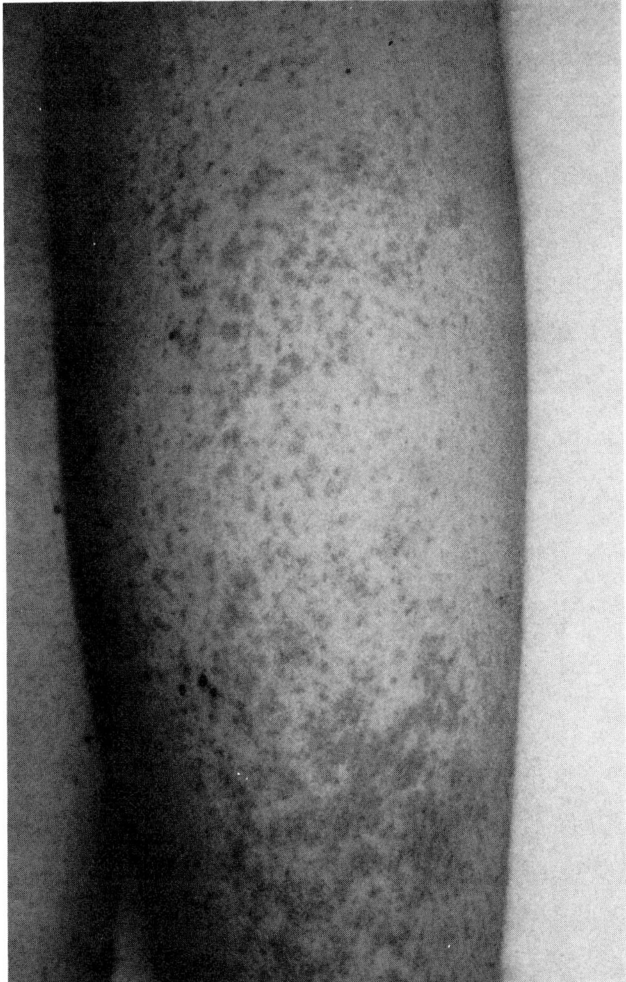

Figure 18–35. Fifth disease (erythema infectiosum). Reticulated pattern developing on upper calf.

0.5- to 1.5-cm pink macules, appears after defervescence, as in roseola, but it differs by starting on the face and upper chest and sometimes spreading to the extremities. It also persists longer — sometimes up to five days. ECHO 16 disease is also known as *Boston exanthem.* (3) Vesicular exanthems. Coxsackie A16, and less commonly types A5, A10, B2, and B5, cause *hand, foot, and mouth disease*. This febrile illness is distinctive because of the development of vesicles on the buccal mucosa, palate, and tongue, and in the majority of cases by vesicle formation on the hands, feet, palms, and soles (Figs. 18–36 and 18–37). Occasionally vesicles may develop on the genitalia, buttocks, and proximal portions of the extremities. The vesicles are often tender and surrounded by a prominent red halo. The lesions last for about one week and the illness is mild.

Herpangina, a closely related disorder, is caused by Coxsackie types A1–6, 8, 10, 16, and 22, and less commonly by several type B Coxsackie strains and ECHO viruses. Fever, headache, vomiting, and sore throat develop suddenly. The pharynx and tonsils are mildly red with minimal exudate. The diagnostic *enanthem* begins as vesicles with red halos on the

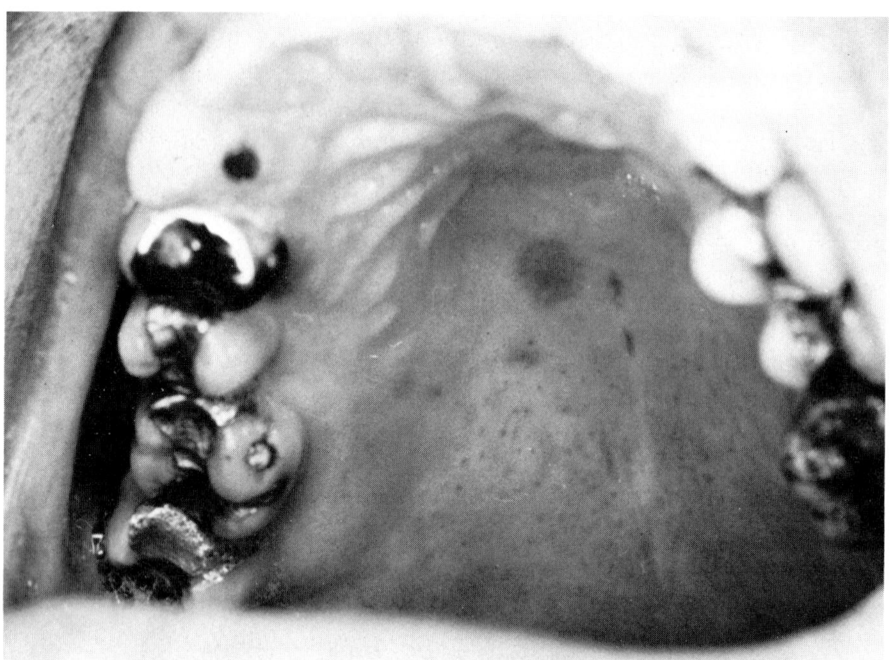

Figure 18–36. Hand, foot, and mouth disease. Coxsackie infection. Vesicles with erythematous halos on palate in 25-year-old woman.

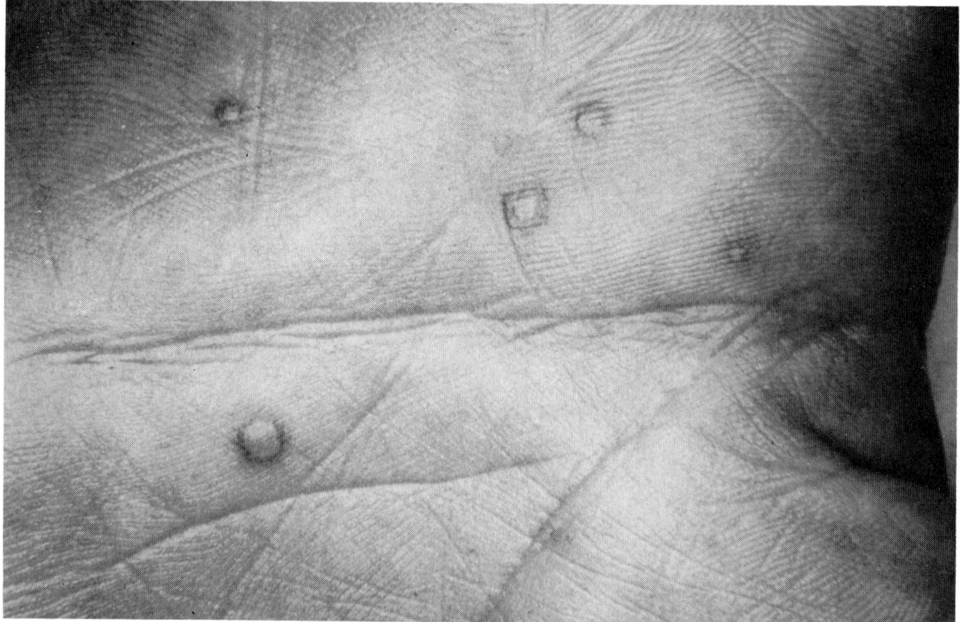

Figure 18–37. Hand, foot, and mouth disease. Same patient as in Figure 18–36. Vesicles on palm.

soft palate between the uvula and the tonsils. They can also develop on the tonsils, posterior pharyngeal wall, and buccal mucosa. Over the course of 24 hours, the vesicles evolve into superficial ulcers measuring 2 to 4 mm. The fever subsides in two to four days, but the ulcers may persist for up to one week. Acute lymphonodular pharyngitis is a variant of herpangina. White or yellow papules occur in the same distribution but do not undergo ulceration.

The prodromal phase of hepatitis B infections may be characterized by urticarial, maculopapular, or petechial eruptions that are produced by an underlying immune complex mechanism (see p. 416). Hepatitis B infection is also believed to be the major cause of *papular acrodermatitis of childhood* (Gianotti-Crosti syndrome).[36, 37] In this syndrome, nonpruritic erythematous papules 1 to 5 mm in diameter erupt symmetrically on the face, buttocks, and limbs (Figs. 18–38 and 18–39). They rarely appear on the trunk. The lesions appear over the course of a few days and do not become confluent. The mucous membranes are unaffected. Occasionally, the papules may be purpuric. The skin lesions persist for two to three weeks, and lymphadenopathy of axillary and inguinal nodes can persist for two to three months. Children two to six years old are primarily

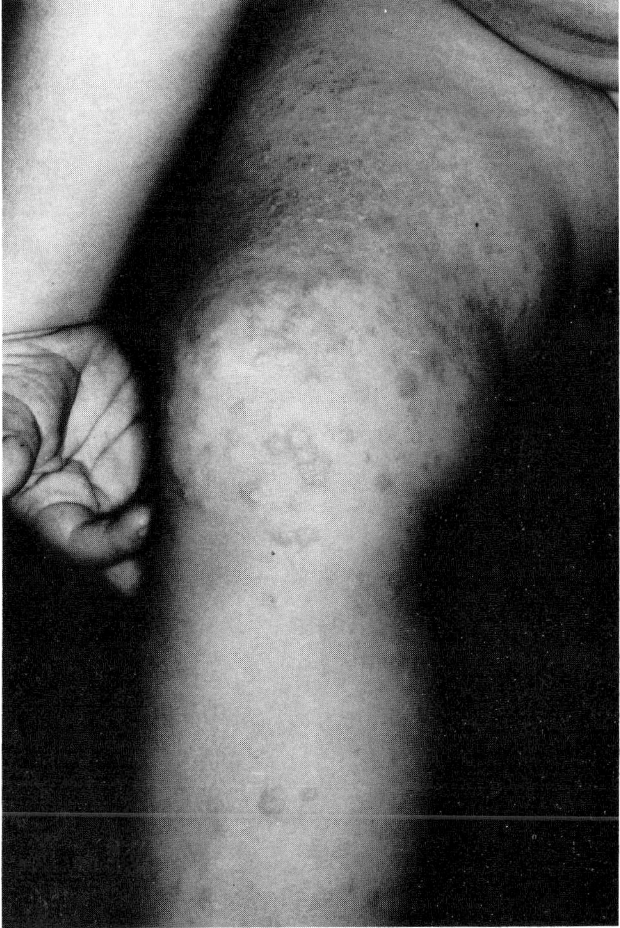

Figure 18–38. Papular acrodermatitis of childhood (Gianotti-Crosti syndrome). Non-pruritic erythematous papules.

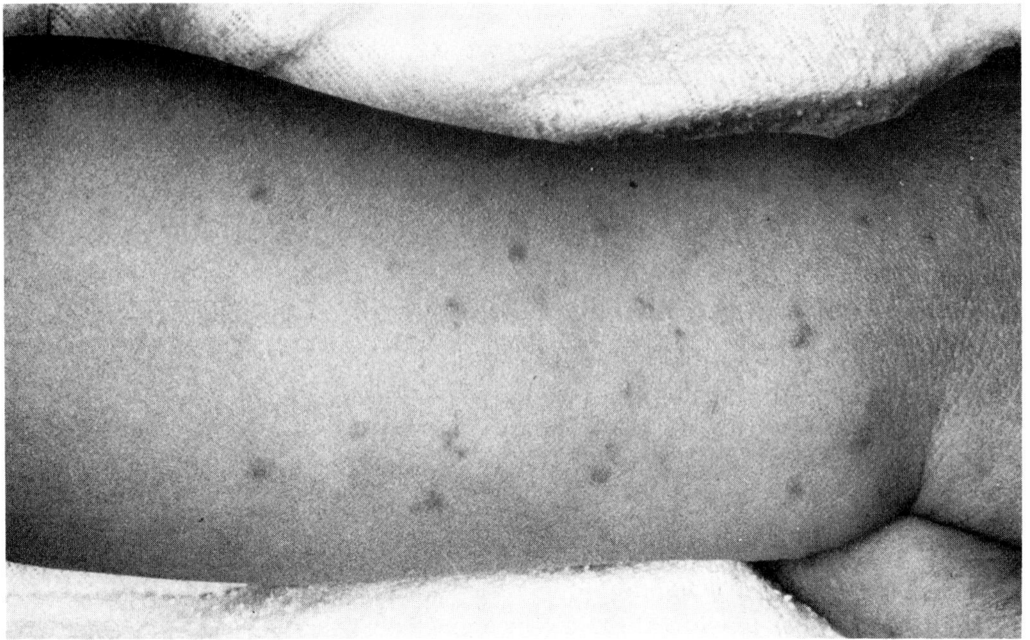

Figure 18–39. Papular acrodermatitis of childhood (Gianotti-Crosti syndrome). Nonpruritic erythematous papules. Same patient as in Figure 18–38.

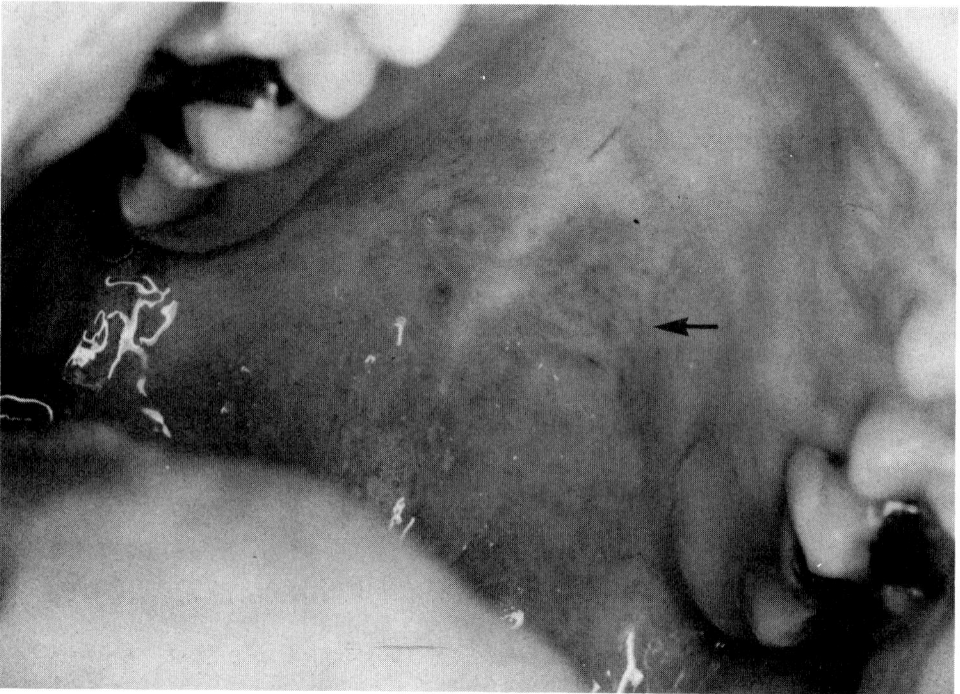

Figure 18–40. Infectious mononucleosis. Petechiae at junction of hard and soft palates (arrow).

affected. Hepatitis, usually anicteric, develops coincident with the rash or one to two weeks later. Gianotti-Crosti syndrome is a naturally occurring disease found in children who have never received injections or blood transfusions. The disorder is associated with hepatitis B surface antigenemia, subtype ayw. The histopathology of the cutaneous lesions is characterized by a perivascular infiltrate of monocytes and lymphocytes. There is no evidence of an underlying vasculitis.

Infectious mononucleosis is associated with an exanthem in about 5 per cent of cases. It usually resembles rubella but may simulate scarlet fever in severe cases. Urticarial lesions and petechiae are present in some patients.[38] The rash of infectious mononucleosis develops in the second to third week of the illness. During this time, petechiae can be found at the junction of the hard and soft palates in 25 to 60 per cent of patients (Fig. 18–40). However, this is not pathognomonic of infectious mononucleosis because similar-appearing petechial enanthems develop in rubella, streptococcal pharyngitis, and other viral diseases. Virtually all patients with infectious mononucleosis who are treated with ampicillin develop a *pruritic* maculopapular eruption five to eight days later.[39] The rash begins on the trunk and spreads to the face and extremities. It becomes generalized on the third and fourth days and involves the palms and soles. The eruption may also appear after the ampicillin has been discontinued.

Vesicular Lesions

Chickenpox (varicella) should pose no difficulties in diagnosis. The development of fever and vesicles coincides in children, but in adults there may be a one- to two-day prodrome of fever, headache, sore throat, and malaise. A scarlatiniform rash may be present during the prodrome. The vesicles of chickenpox appear in crops over the course of seven to ten days. They can range in size from 2 to 5 mm and appear on the skin like a drop of water or a glass bead. At least one or two vesicles develop on the hard palate, uvula, or tonsillar pillars in most cases. The vesicles typically arise as macules, pass through a clear and cloudy vesicular phase, and eventually develop crusts and disappear (Figs. 18–41 and 18–42). The main complications of varicella are staphylococcal and streptococcal impetigo and cellulitis and streptococcal scarlet fever. Severe cases of varicella can trigger DIC. In adults, chickenpox is often complicated by varicella pneumonitis.

Hand, foot, and mouth diseases should not be confused with chickenpox because of the unique distribution of the vesicles and their morphology. Rickettsialpox is an acute febrile illness characterized by an initial cutaneous lesion and a papulovesicular rash. The disease is transmitted by a mite infested with *Rickettsia akari*, whose reservoir is the common house mouse. The initial lesion, a red papule which develops central vesiculation, arises at the site of the bite a few days before the onset of fever, headache, photophobia, chills, anorexia, and a generalized but sparse eruption. The rash is characterized by erythematous macules and papules, some of which develop a central vesicle. The rash may involve any part of the body, including the palms, soles, and oral mucosa. The illness lasts about one week and so does the rash.

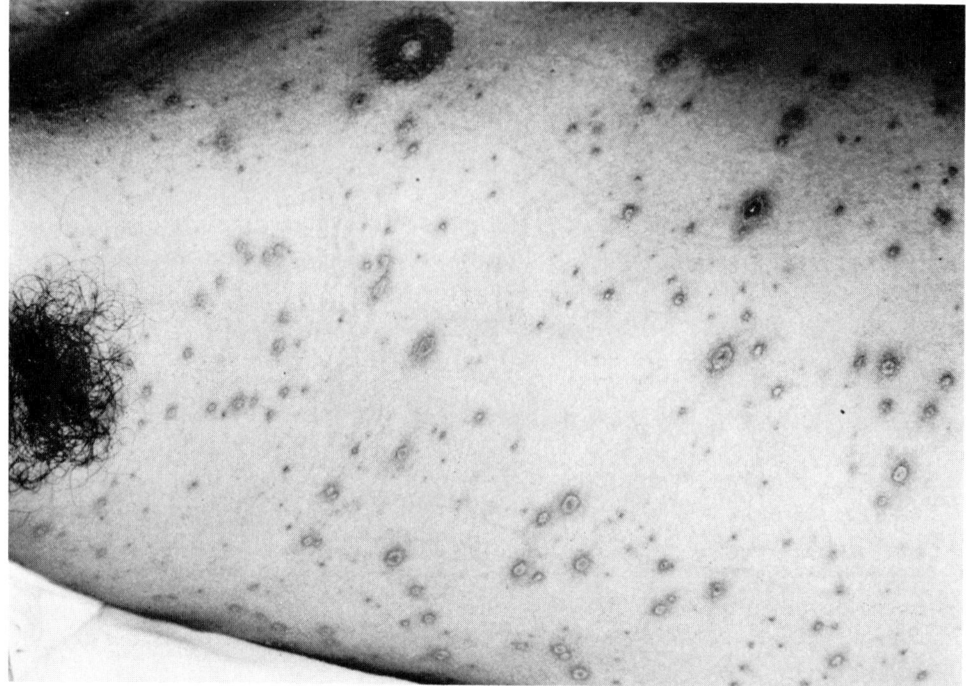

Figure 18–41. Chickenpox (varicella). Vesicles in various stages of development. Many umbilicated vesicles are present. A few crusted vesicles are present near midline of abdomen.

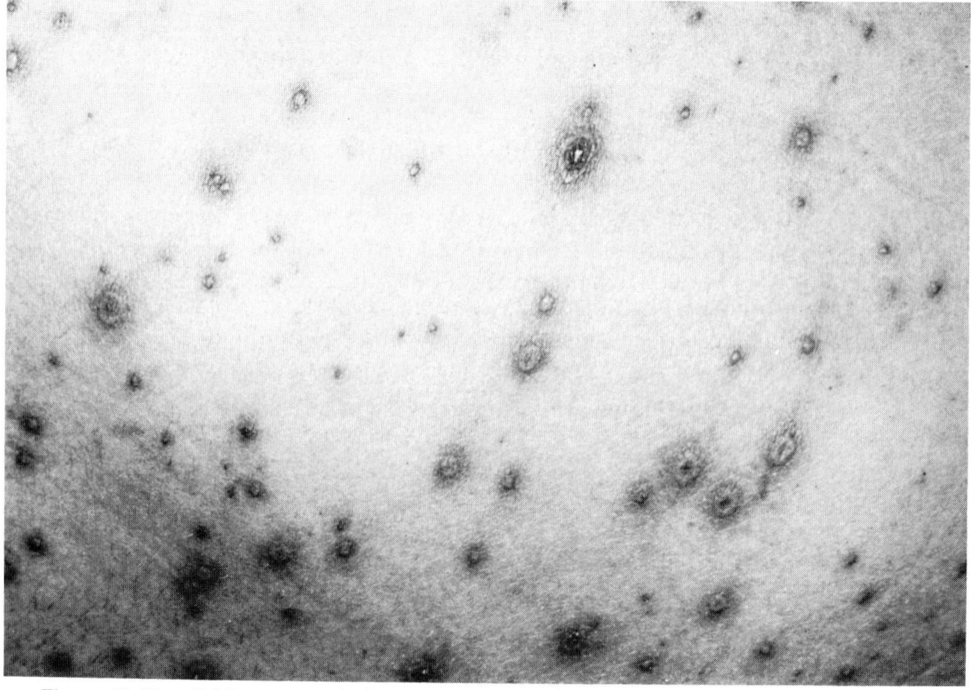

Figure 18–42. Chickenpox (varicella). Closeup of umbilicated vesicles shown in Figure 18–41.

Facial Swelling

Mumps presents a distinctive picture of unilateral or bilateral parotid gland swelling. The other salivary glands may be affected as well. The differential diagnosis includes staphylococcal parotitis. Differentiation can be made by compressing the parotid gland: in staphylococcal parotitis, pus can be expressed from Stensen's duct, while in mumps no secretions are present. If the sublingual salivary glands are affected, the tongue may be swollen, and if the submandibular glands are involved, presternal edema may be present. Both the lingual swelling and presternal edema are thought to be secondary to lymphedema caused by lymphatic obstruction from the enlarged salivary glands.

Most instances of acute infectious disease with cutaneous manifestations will fall into one of the above categories. However, one encounters disorders characterized by persistent fever of more than three weeks duration in which no obvious infectious cause is present. Such cases, which are labelled as FUO (fever of unknown origin), usually require extensive investigations to discover the cause of the fever. Several series of FUO cases have shown that an infectious cause is present in 21 to 43 per cent; collagen–vascular disease in 13 to 19 per cent; neoplasms (lymphoma and leukemia) in 6 to 31 per cent; and undiagnosed disorders in 7 to 40 per cent.[40-45] The most commonly associated infections were hepatic and subphrenic abscesses, osteomyelitis, subacute bacterial endocarditis, cholangitis, cholecystitis, empyema of the gallbladder, perinephric abscess, tuberculosis, histoplasmosis, cryptococcosis, and brucellosis. Noninfectious causes included drug reactions with cutaneous signs, factitial fever, active cirrhosis, regional enteritis, sarcoidosis, temporal arteritis, hypernephroma, atrial myxoma, and hepatoma. Fever also followed the use of bypass pumps in major surgical procedures. Several of the above entities can be associated with cutaneous lesions that are diagnostic by their recognition or can lead to the correct diagnosis by biopsy. Punch biopsies of the skin are useful not only for establishing a diagnosis through histopathologic findings but also for determining etiologic infectious agents by culturing the biopsy specimen.

SPECIFIC DISORDERS

Staphylococcal Scalded Skin Syndrome

Staphylococcal scalded skin syndrome (SSSS, Lyell's syndrome) is usually an acute febrile illness that develops in children under five years of age.[46-48] The etiologic agent is a phage group 2 staphylococcus which elaborates an exotoxin that cleaves the epidermis at the granular cell layer without producing epidermal cell necrosis. Several clinical forms of the syndrome are recognized. (1) Bullous impetigo is a localized form of the disease in which staphylococci are limited to the areas of involved skin where their exotoxin produces large purulent bullae. The neutrophils settle out from the blister fluid to produce definite fluid cell layers (Fig. 18–43). (2) The generalized form of the disease is preceded by purulent conjunctivitis and rhinorrhea, otitis media, or simply rhinorrhea and a reddened pharynx without purulent tonsillitis. Staphylococci can be isolated from these foci. Within a few hours to one to four days after these

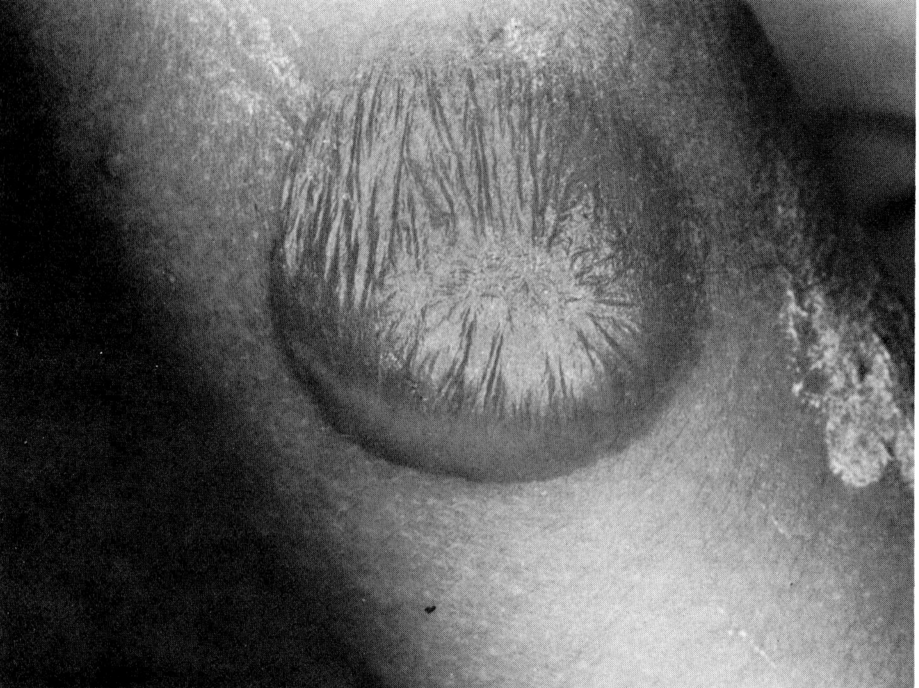

Figure 18–43. Bullous impetigo. Neutrophils have settled out as a layer at bottom of blister.

prodromes, erythema, which is often tender, develops over the central portion of the face, in the flexures, and over the trunk. In neonates there may be total erythroderma. Flaccid bullae develop within 24 to 48 hours and large sheets of skin begin to desquamate, revealing a moist red base that quickly dries (Figs. 9–52 and 9–53). Recovery usually takes place within a week. The bullae are not always apparent so that the erythema may appear to be followed by desquamation. On the face, the bullae break quickly, producing crusted patches resembling impetigo around the eyes, nose, and mouth. The flaccid bullae are more easily seen on the trunk. The mucosa is never involved, although the lips are sometimes mildly red with minor peeling. (3) In some patients the erythema is confined to the face and flexures and the typical large sheets of desquamation are not seen. Instead, minor fissures with desquamation develop in the skin creases. Sometimes in others with extensive erythema, bullae and desquamation also do not occur. Instead a fine fissuring with mild desquamation develops. Although this variety of SSSS has been called "scarlatiniform," the other characteristic features of scarlet fever are lacking: strawberry tongue, facial flushing, and circumoral pallor.[46] True scarlet fever produced by staphylococci does exist and it should not be confused with this abortive form of SSSS.[16-18] Pustules rarely develop in SSSS, except in the diaper and periumbilical areas of neonates.[47] Figures 18–44 and 18–45 illustrate pustules and minimal desquamation in a three-year-old girl with SSSS.

Although SSSS occurs chiefly in children, a number of adults have developed the syndrome. With the exception of one adult who seemed to be a healthy and normal individual,[49] the rest of the affected persons appeared to be immunosuppressed, immunodeficient, or ill with severe

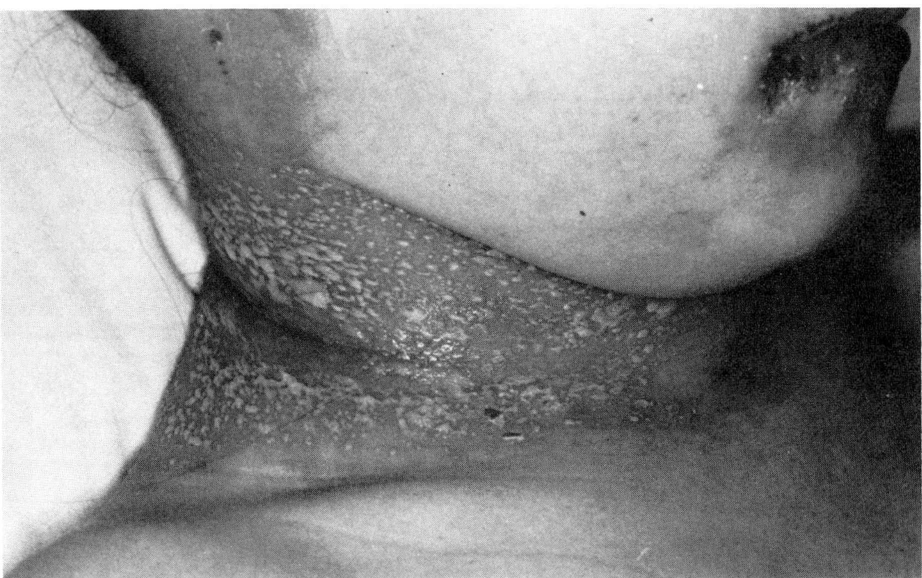

Figure 18–44. Staphylococcal scalded skin syndrome. Pustules and minimal desquamation in a three-year-old girl.

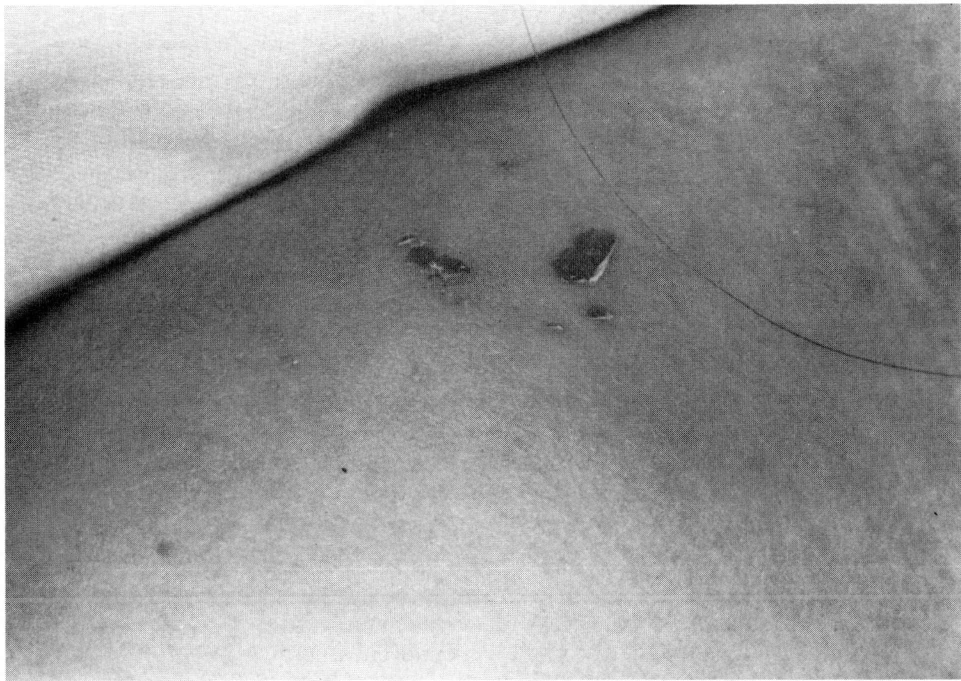

Figure 18–45. Staphylococcal scalded skin syndrome. Minimal desquamation. Same patient as in Figure 18–44.

staphylococcal septicemia. Some of the patients had renal insufficiency.[48-51] SSSS can be reproduced in newborn mice by injection of exotoxin, but adult mice have to be nephrectomized in order for the exotoxin to produce its results. Intradermal injection of exotoxin into adult humans will produce local blisters.[48, 52]

Toxic epidermal necrolysis (TEN) needs to be distinguished from SSSS. TEN is primarily a disease of adults that also begins acutely with tender erythema leading to flaccid bullae and severe desquamation (Figs. 9–49 to 9–51). The oral mucosa is often involved. Some patients with TEN also exhibit features of erythema multiforme. The pathogenesis of TEN involves basal cell necrosis with the production of subepidermal bullae rather than a superficial epidermal split as in SSSS. TEN occurs as a reaction to drugs or as a manifestation of a graft-vs-host reaction.[53] Experimentally, the disease has been reproduced in animals by inducing the graft-vs-host phenomenon.[54] The mortality from TEN is at least 50 per cent, whereas in SSSS it has been less than 2 per cent in recent years. The epidermal split in TEN is equivalent to a second degree burn. Just as SSSS can develop in adults, TEN can occur in children.[48]

Impetigo and Pyoderma

Impetigo is a superficial infection located beneath the stratum corneum of the skin produced by streptococci or staphylococci alone or in combination. When the infection penetrates the entire epidermis, an ulcerated crusted lesion, termed ecthyma, is produced. If the infection develops in the hair follicles, recognized by hairs emerging through pustules, the term folliculitis is applied. Collectively these processes are referred to as pyodermas.

Although staphylococcal and streptococcal impetigo are said to be easily distinguished by their clinical appearance, it is usually difficult to do so. Classically, staphylococcal impetigo produces large flaccid bullae which contain purulent material that forms fluid-cell layers on standing (Fig. 18–43). Milder lesions begin as bullae that quickly collapse to form a thin varnish-like crust (Figs. 18–46 and 18–47). Streptococcal impetigo starts as a red macule that becomes vesicular because of its subcorneal location. However, this phase is transient and rarely recognizable clinically. The vesicles become pustules, slowly enlarge, and break down to form thick honey-colored crusts that appear to be stuck to the surface of the skin (Fig. 18–48). These lesions slowly expand if untreated. However, staphylococci can be found in such lesions as well. There is still controversy concerning whether staphylococci initiate this type of lesion, with streptococci being secondary invaders, or vice versa.

The pyodermas are important because when they are produced by certain nephritogenic strains of streptococci they are followed by acute glomerulonephritis in 10 to 15 per cent of cases about two to three weeks later.[55] This complication of streptococcal infections occurs primarily in children under six years of age during the summer and early fall. Nephritogenic strains of streptococci responsible for pharyngitis produce acute glomerulonephritis in young school-age children during the winter months. Subsequent episodes of streptococcal infections in individuals who have developed nephritis rarely produce another episode of acute glomerulonephritis. Rather, they exacerbate the course of the existing

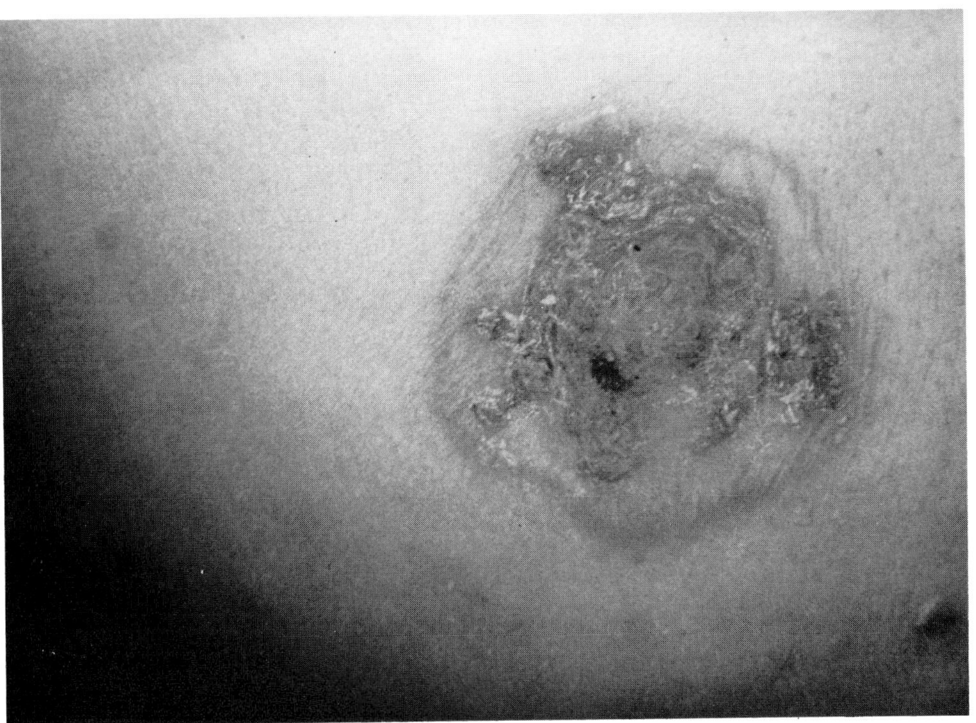

Figure 18–46. Impetigo. Early lesion. Bullous edge with crust formation.

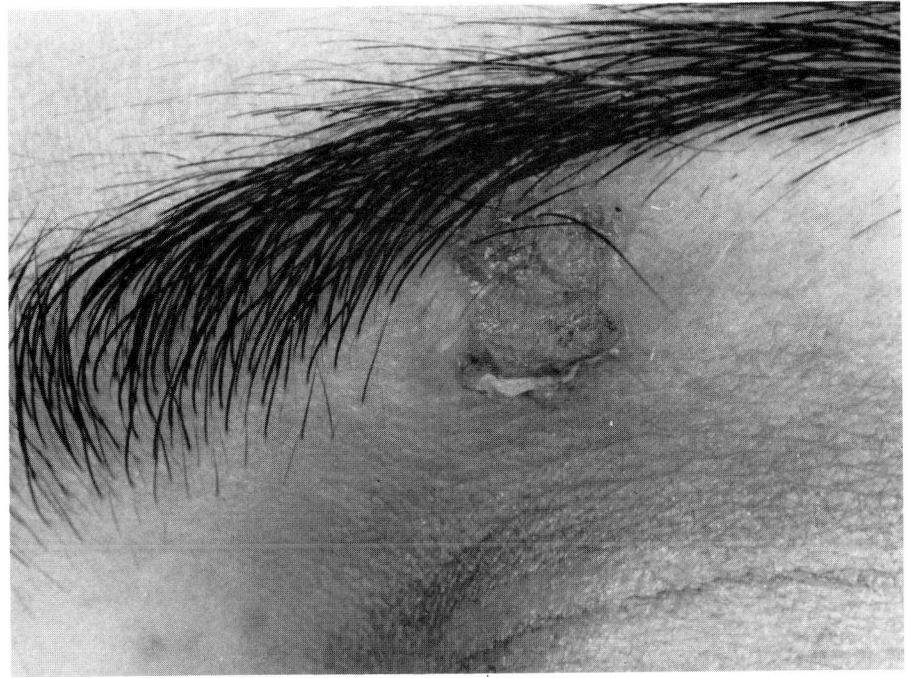

Figure 18–47. Impetigo. Early lesion. Crust forming over collapsed bulla.

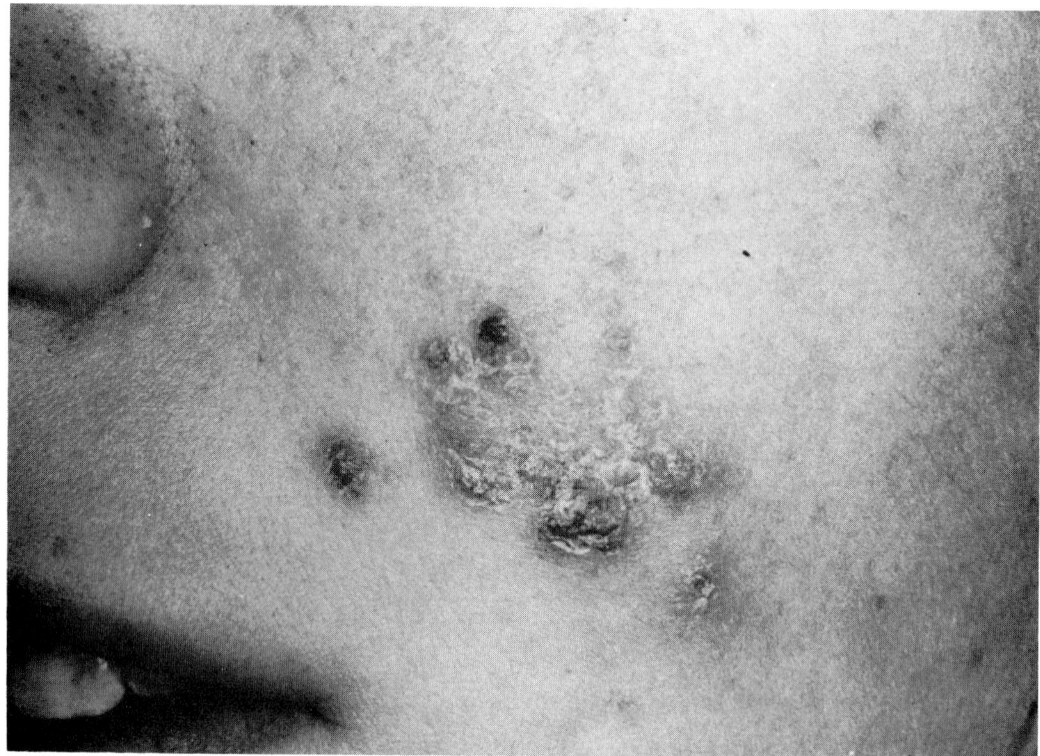

Figure 18–48. Impetigo. Thick, honey-colored crusts appear to be stuck on surface of skin.

chronic glomerulonephritis. Although rheumatic fever follows streptococcal pharyngitis, it does not develop after streptococcal pyodermas. There is no evidence that adequate therapy of an individual with streptococcal pyoderma will prevent glomerulonephritis, which is a hypersensitivity response to the streptococcus. The failure to prevent nephritis is probably related to the fact that patients rarely seek medical help for pyodermas that are less than seven to ten days old.

Streptococci usually colonize normal skin about 10 days before impetigo starts, usually after minor trauma or an abrasion. In about 30 per cent of children with impetigo, streptococci colonize the upper respiratory tract two to three weeks later. Streptococci can also produce a primary cellulitis with lymphangitis — a red tender streak that ascends to regionally enlarged tender nodes. The lymphangitic syndrome is often associated with fissures in the toe webs produced by tinea pedis, as well as with minor trauma to the skin. A variety of dermatoses provide portals of entry for streptococci and staphylococci: atopic dermatitis and other varieties of eczema, recurrent herpes simplex, and scabies.

Although pustules, abscesses, and folliculitis usually indicate a *Staphylococcus aureus* infection, not all instances of such lesions represent a primary bacterial infection. One syndrome, which I will call itching folliculitis for want of a better term, is characterized by crops of folliculitis on the trunk, extremities, and sometimes the scalp (Figs. 18–49 and 18–50). The disorder is very pruritic and can continue for months to years. Culture of the folliculitis reveals either normal flora or *Staphylococcus epidermidis*. This syndrome responds dramatically to oral tetracycline or erythromycin and can be completely suppressed by daily

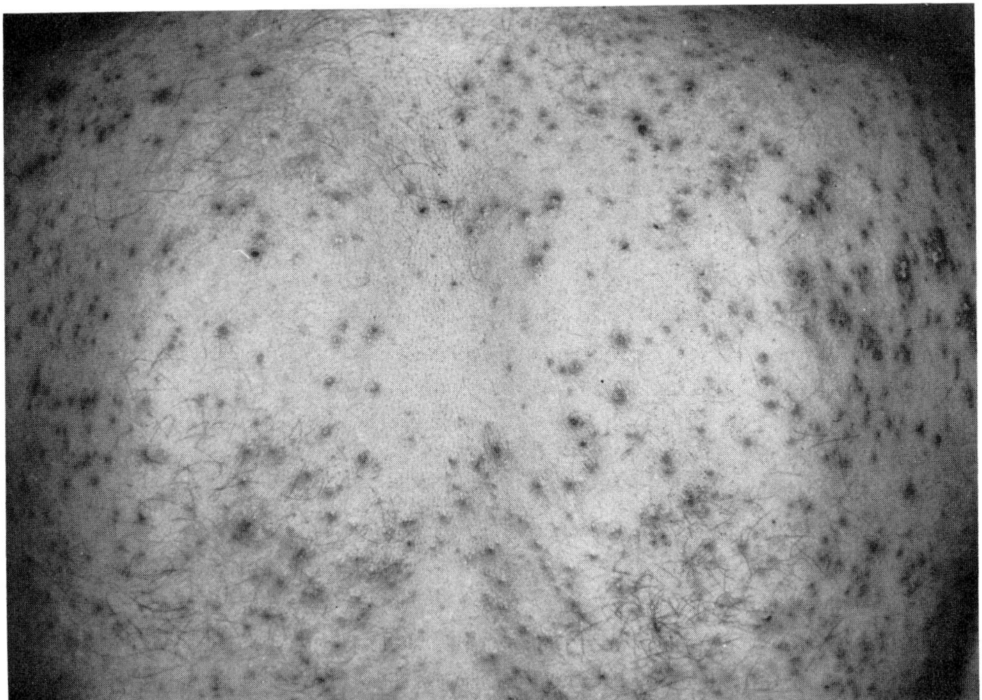

Figure 18–49. Itching folliculitis.

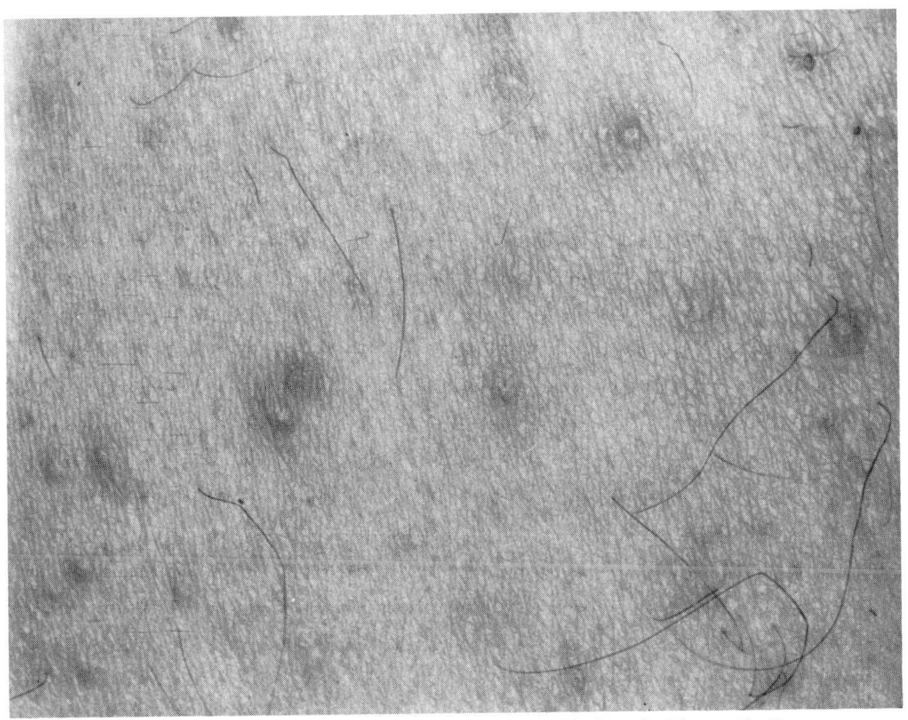

Figure 18–50. Itching folliculitis. Close-up of lesions in Figure 18–49.

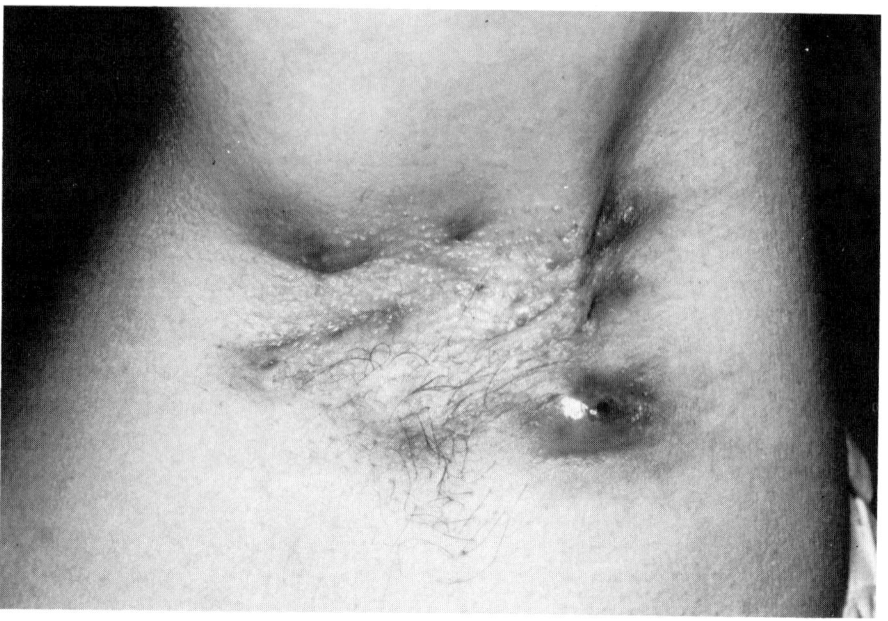

Figure 18–51. Hidradenitis suppurativa. Abscesses, purulent nodules, and scars from previous lesions.

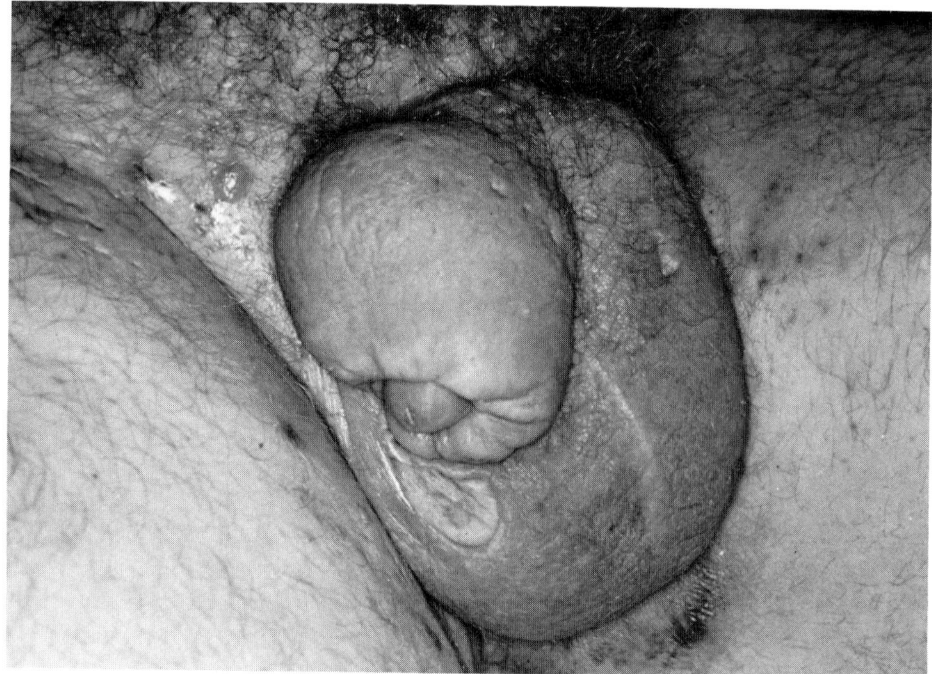

Figure 18–52. Hidradenitis suppurativa. Lymphedema of genitals from lymphatic fibrosis.

low-dose therapy, as in acne vulgaris. Hidradenitis suppurativa is a chronic inflammatory disease with acute exacerbations involving the apocrine sweat glands in the axillae and groins. Abscesses, purulent nodules, and draining sinuses with pseudoepitheliomatous hyperplasia develop in these areas (Fig. 18–51). The disorder is thought to represent a dysfunction of apocrine glands that are secondarily infected, because of the many different bacteria that can be isolated from the pus. The disease can be reasonably well controlled with long-term tetracycline or erythromycin therapy in most cases, as in acne vulgaris. In severe cases, surgical excision of the involved areas is necessary to cure the disorder. Some patients with hidradenitis also have severe acne conglobata on the face, scalp, and trunk. Hidradenitis of the groins can lead to lymphatic fibrosis with lymphedema producing marked swelling of the genitalia, as shown in Figure 18–52.

Chronic tooth abscesses form fistulous tracts to the skin that can open anywhere along the course of the underlying mandible. The fistula may have pursued a circuitous route and its opening on the skin can be far away from the underlying dental abscess. The cutaneous opening may be mistaken for a chronic pustule or even an ulcerated epidermal tumor. Removal of the abscessed tooth will result in prompt closure and disappearance of the tract.

Bacterial Endocarditis

Bacterial endocarditis is associated with several cutaneous signs: conjunctival and palatal petechiae; subungual (splinter) hemorrhages; Roth's spots — oval pale areas surrounded by hemorrhage near the optic disc; Osler's nodes; and Janeway's lesions (Figs. 18–53 to 18–55). Osler's

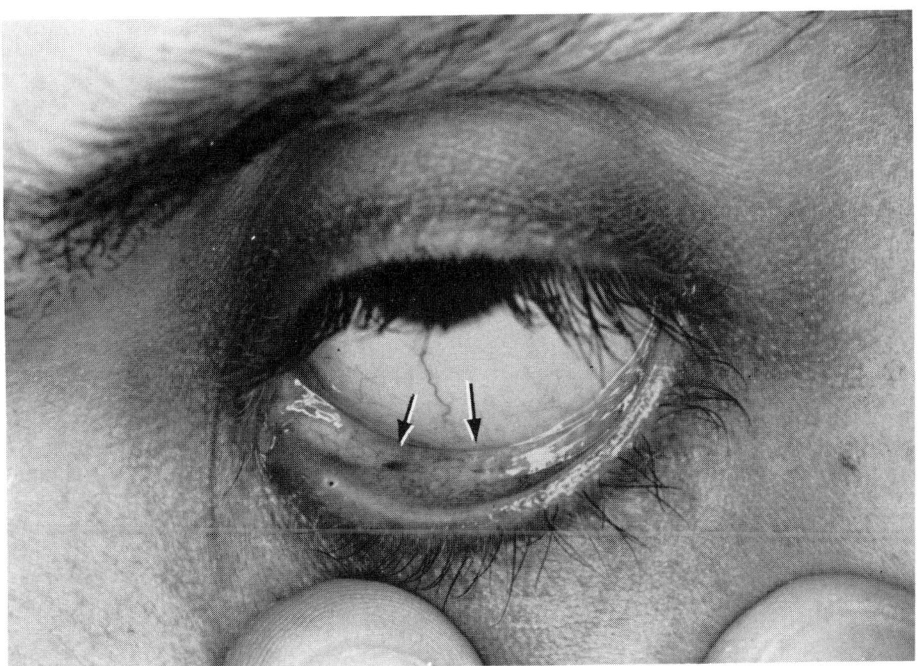

Figure 18–53. Conjunctival petechiae (arrows).

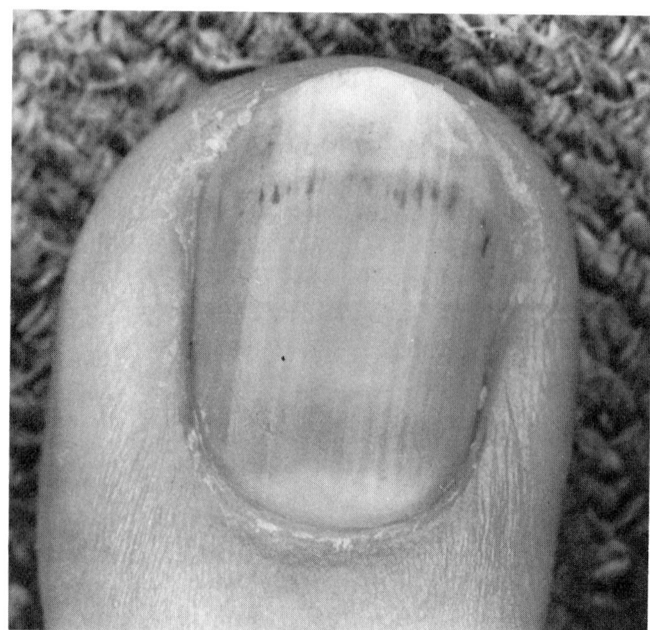

Figure 18–54. Splinter hemorrhages.

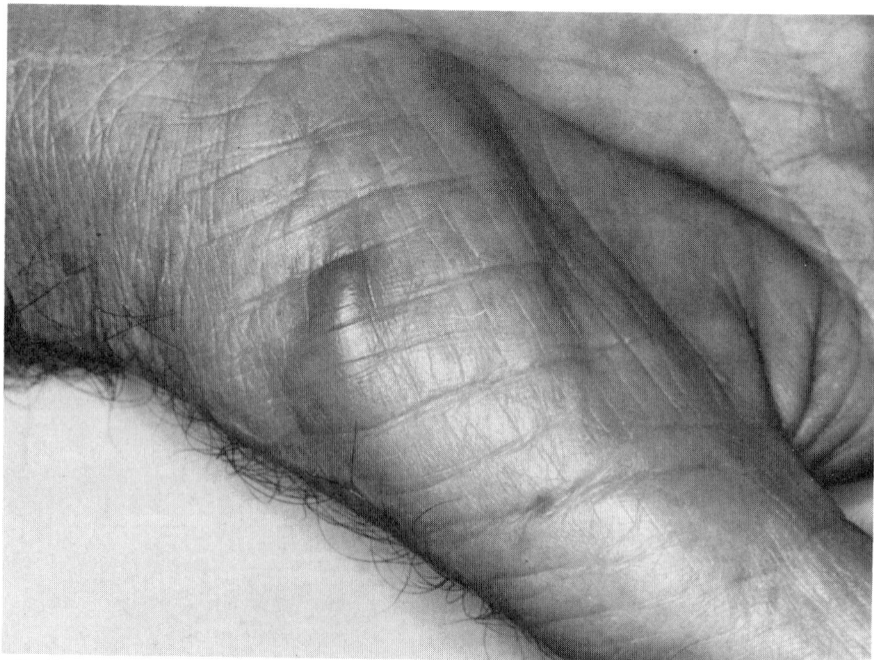

Figure 18–55. Janeway lesion on palm of patient with staphylococcal infection around base of prosthetic aortic valve. This red nodule showed leukocytoclastic vasculitis on biopsy.

nodes have been defined as *tender* erythematous spots with opaque centers that appear on the pulps of the finger tips and toes. Janeway's lesions are *nontender* red or hemorrhagic macules or nodules that develop on the palms and soles.[56] It was originally thought that all these signs were produced by septic or sterile emboli from the valvular vegetations. Current evidence indicates that the Osler and Janeway lesions occurring in acute bacterial endocarditis caused by *S. aureus* are most likely caused by septic (bacterial) emboli. The organisms can be isolated from the cutaneous lesions and histologically thrombi can be demonstrated.[57] In subacute bacterial endocarditis, the Osler and Janeway lesions have the histologic appearance of leukocytoclastic vasculitis. Thrombi are not present and organisms cannot be isolated from the lesions.[58] The evidence is strong that Osler's nodes, Janeway's lesions, and probably even the petechiae, splinter hemorrhages, and Roth's spots are manifestations of an immune complex mechanism generated by chronic bacterial infection.[59-61] Histologically the Roth spot represents a large focal collection of neutrophils surrounded by red blood cells in the nerve fiber and outer plexiform layers of the retina. This formation is thought to be produced by necrotizing inflammation of small vessels. Histologic evidence for septic or aseptic emboli as etiologic factors has not been

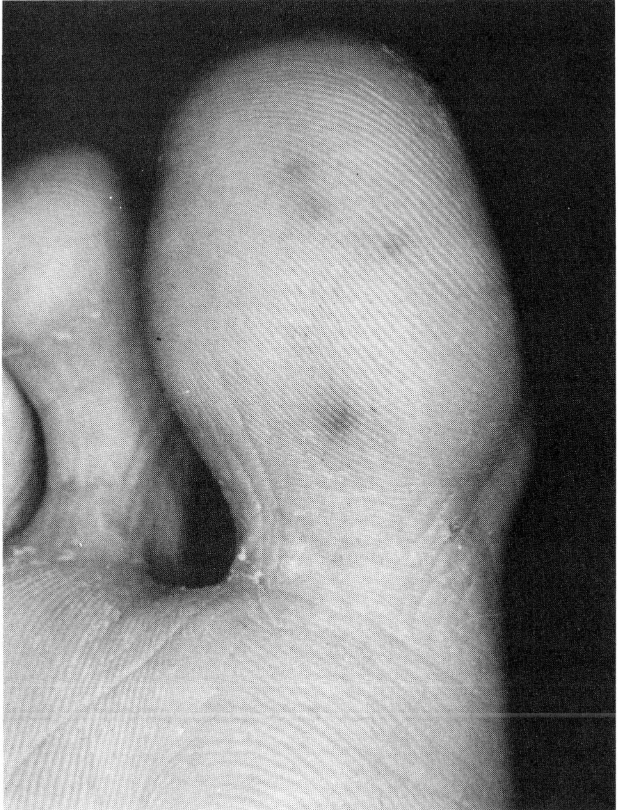

Figure 18–56. Purpuric spots caused by particulate emboli from candidal vegetation on cardiac valve in drug abuser with candidal endocarditis. Biopsy showed PAS-positive material in small dermal vessels without findings of leukocytoclastic vasculitis.

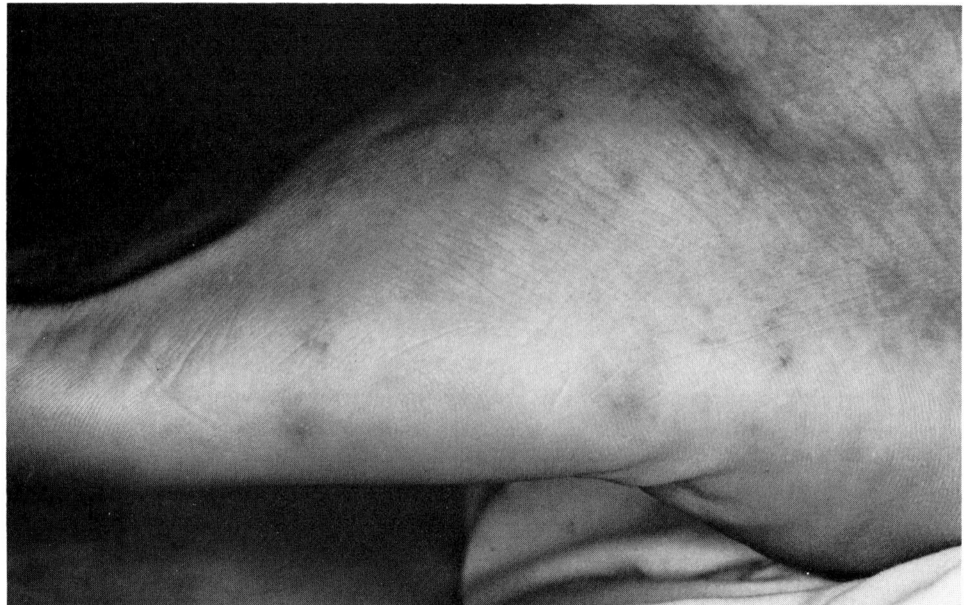

Figure 18–57. Purpuric lesions on foot of patient shown in Figure 18–56. Conjunctival petechiae in Figure 18–53 are from same patient.

found.[60] The glomerulonephritis associated with subacute bacterial endocarditis has also been shown to be an immune complex disorder and not the result of embolization from valvular vegetations.[61, 62]

Although splinter hemorrhages are one of the manifestations of bacterial endocarditis, they are also found in trichinosis, following trauma to the nails and fingers, and as incidental idiopathic abnormalities in normal persons. Splinter hemorrhages by themselves are a weak indicator of any underlying disorder.[62a]

We studied two patients with bacteremia related to the cardiovascular system. Both had Janeway's lesions that were sterile (Fig. 18–55). Light microscopy showed leukocytoclastic vasculitis, and electron microscopy demonstrated immune complexes in the vessel walls.[63] Circulating complexes were trapped in the vessels of normal skin made permeable by histamine (see p. 417). One patient had an *S. epidermidis* infection around the base of a prosthetic aortic valve, and the other had a similar infection in an aortic graft that was required following an abdominal knife wound. The role of immune complexes in chronic infection has been discussed earlier (see p. 421). The main distinction between Osler's node and Janeway's lesion is tenderness, which may be explained by vasculitic involvement of the glomus body in thefinger tip.[58]

However, septic emboli and sterile particulate emboli producing conjunctival petechiae and peripheral purpuric spots do occur in "endocarditis syndromes" (Figs. 18–53, 18–56, and 18–57). These disorders include acute bacterial endocarditis secondary to *S. aureus,* atrial myxomas, and Candida endocarditis that develops in drug abusers and following open heart surgery.[57]

Herpes Simplex

Herpes simplex virus exists as two serologic types, HSV-1 and HSV-2, with the former producing most of the cutaneous lesions above the waist, and the latter responsible for the majority below the waist.[64] The increase in herpes simplex infections in recent years can be explained in large part by the increase in genital herpes (HSV-2). Primary herpes simplex infection in most individuals is subclinical. However, months to years later, recurrent attacks may ensue. In a minority, the primary attack produces a severe illness chiefly affecting the mucous membranes. In between the acute infectious episodes of herpes simplex, the virus is believed to be dormant in a noninfectious state in sensory ganglia. The virus has been isolated from trigeminal, sacral, thoracic, superior cervical, and vagus ganglia.[65-68] However, the virus has also been isolated from the saliva, tears, urethra, and secretions from the prostate and seminal vesicles of healthy individuals during disease-free intervals. Labial herpes is often precipitated by intense exposure to ultraviolet light, menstruation, and emotional stress. Current evidence suggests that the herpes virus infects the skin or mucous membranes, travels to the regional sensory ganglion where it resides until reactivated, and then travels back down the nerve to reinfect the appropriate tissue, causing clinical disease. The inability to isolate the virus from the skin or mucous membranes during disease-free intervals makes it less likely that these tissues are a reservoir. The mechanism by which ultraviolet light triggers labial herpes is not understood, but a neural reflex initiated by intense light exposure might explain this phenomenon.

Herpes simplex produces several clinical syndromes. *Neonatal infection* often develops in prematurely delivered infants of mothers who have active herpes infection of the cervix, vulva, or perineum. The illness is characterized by a disseminated infection of the brain, eye, liver, adrenal, and other organs, leading to death in 50 per cent of affected infants.[64, 69, 70] Cesarean section is usually indicated in situations in which the mother has active herpes and rupture of the membranes has not yet occurred or has been present for less than six hours. However, each case needs to be individually evaluated.[71] In more than 50 per cent of affected infants herpetic skin lesions are present. They may be localized to the scalp or buttocks or may be generalized. In some infants an erythematous macular rash may precede the appearance of vesicles. In a minority of cases, neonatal infection has been localized to the skin, eyes, mouth, or central nervous system.[64]

Primary hepetic infection occurs chiefly in children between the ages of one and four years, but it may appear for the first time in early adult life. The primary infection is usually a febrile illness with involvement of the oral and genital mucosae. The illness varies greatly in severity and it may be accompanied by cervical adenopathy. Involvement of the mouth, tongue, gums, and vulva produces clusters of discrete, punched-out ulcerations or a polycyclic ulcerated appearance when the vesicles become confluent (Figs. 18–58 to 18–61). Regional adenopathy is often present. The duration of the illness is two to three weeks. The mucosal lesions are sometimes difficult to distinguish from erythema multiforme by clinical findings alone. The skin may become involved by inoculation of virus from mucosal sites, but visceral dissemination is rare. However, in the newborn and in immunocompromised hosts, oral herpetic infection may extend to involve the esophagus, lungs, liver, other visceral organs, and brain. Primary infection occurs only once. Subsequent attacks of recurrent herpes simplex are not usually accompanied by fever or constitutional symptoms.

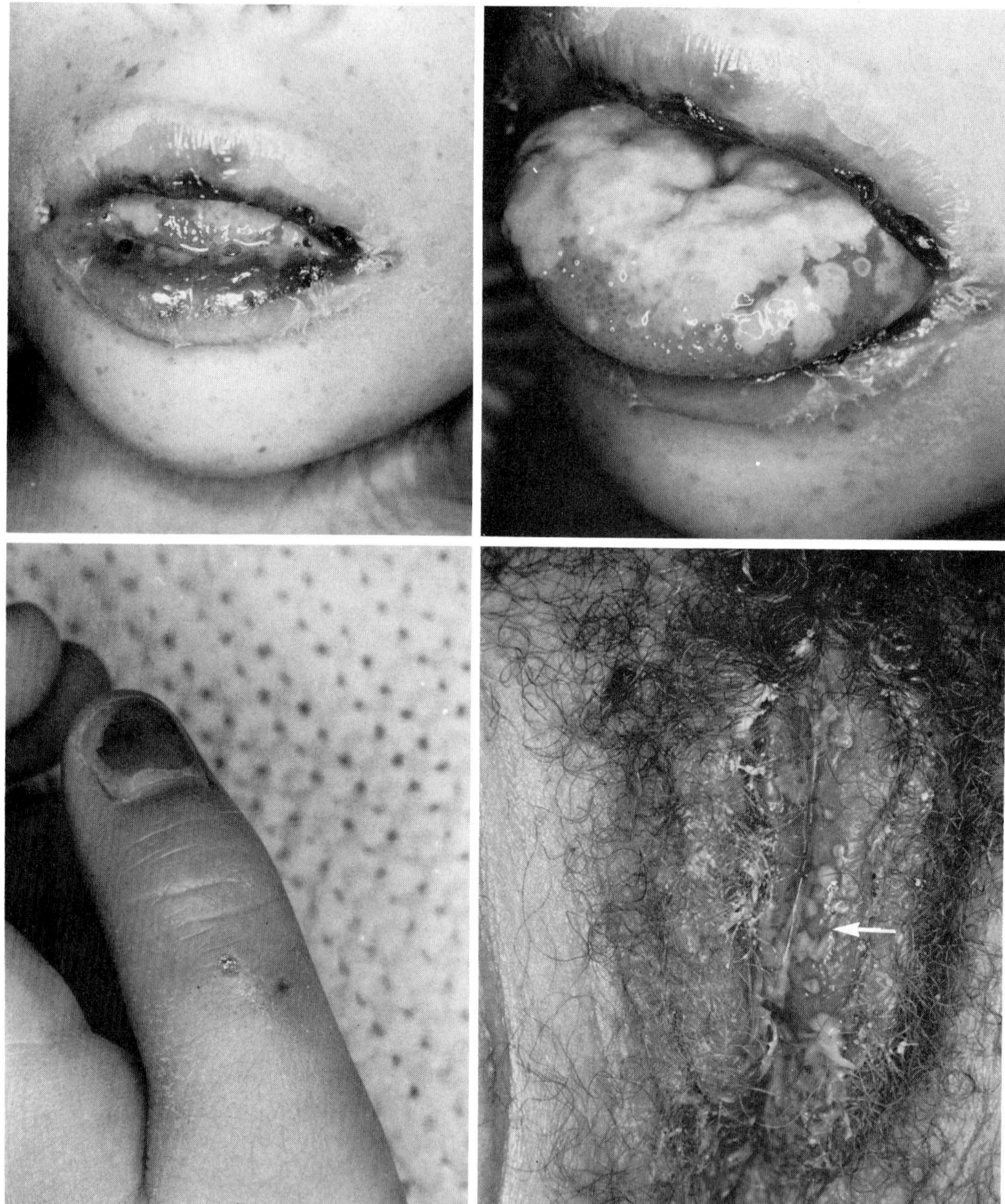

Figure 18–58. Top left. Primary herpes simplex infection.

Figure 18–59. Top right. Primary herpes simplex infection. Same patient as in Figure 18–58.

Figure 18–60. Bottom left. Primary herpes simplex infection on thumb in same patient as in Figure 18–58. Most likely it arose by inoculation from sucking on thumb.

Figure 18–61. Bottom right. Primary herpes simplex infection. Vulvovaginitis in 23-year-old woman. Herpetiform lesions (arrow) are secondarily infected.

Recurrent herpes simplex manifests itself as clusters of vesicles on the lips, around the mouth, and on the buttocks and genitalia (Fig. 18–62). Numbness or tingling often precedes the appearance of the blisters. The vesicles break quickly and often become impetiginized. Herpes runs a course of seven to ten days before resolving. Scarring is rare. Recurrent herpes simplex occasionally produces oral ulcers. However, most instances of mucosal ulceration represent aphthous stomatitis (Figs. 18–63 and 18–64). Recurrent oral herpetic lesions are typically clustered and tend to locate in areas where the mucosa is tightly applied to the underlying periosteum: hard palate, attached gingivae, and the alveolar ridge of the maxilla and mandible (Fig. 18–64). Aphthae or canker sores are characteristically located in areas where the mucosa is freely movable: lips, buccal mucosa, tongue, tonsillar pillars, and soft palate.[72] However, there is considerable overlap in distribution between the two. Although uncommon, recurrent herpes simplex can appear in a dermatome, leading to a misdiagnosis of recurrent zoster.[73-75] Recurrent herpes simplex may be associated with encephalitis and meningitis.[76, 77] Herpes simplex is frequently precipitated by fever, intense exposure to ultraviolet light, emotional stress, menstruation, and section of trigeminal nerve for trigeminal neuralgia. The individual with active herpes simplex and perhaps even the healthy person who is shedding virus from the mouth or genitals are sources for a variety of special herpetic inoculation syndromes.

Herpetic Inoculation Syndromes. Herpes simplex can be introduced into the skin through minor breaks to produce a local infection that is likely to become recurrent later. Herpetic whitlow is an infection of the fingers, especially the paronychial area, occurring chiefly in young persons exposed to oral secretions. It occurs most commonly in physicians and nurses who handle catheters used for aspirating respiratory secretions and in others providing mouth and dental care. Wearing rubber gloves should

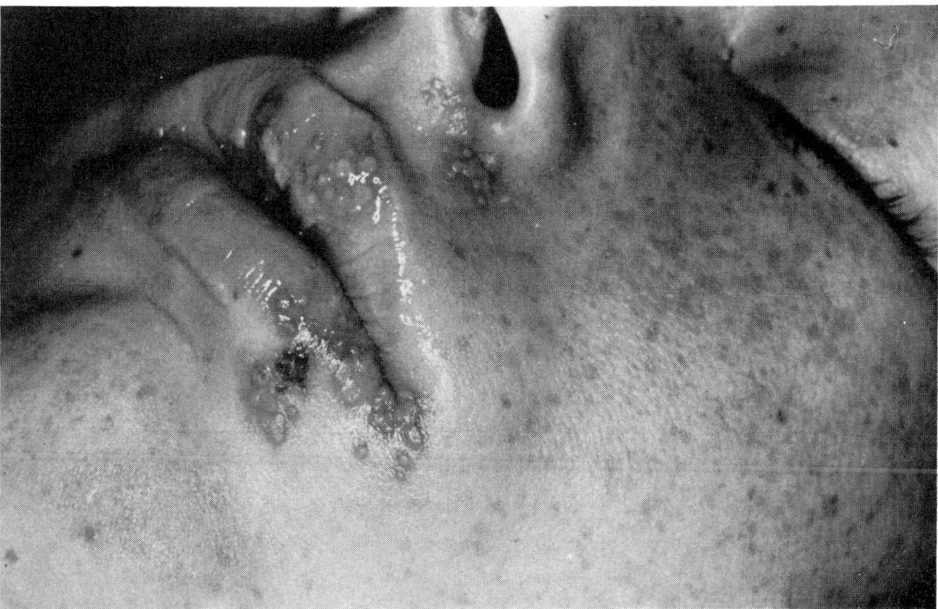

Figure 18–62. Recurrent herpes simplex.

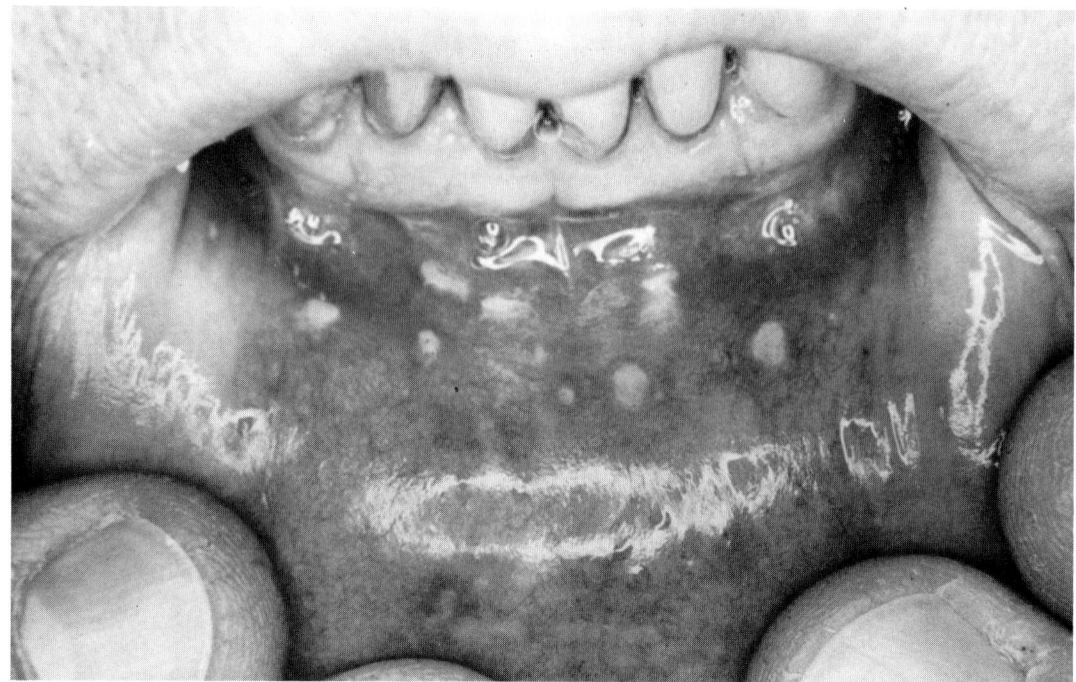

Figure 18–63. Aphthous stomatitis in an otherwise healthy man.

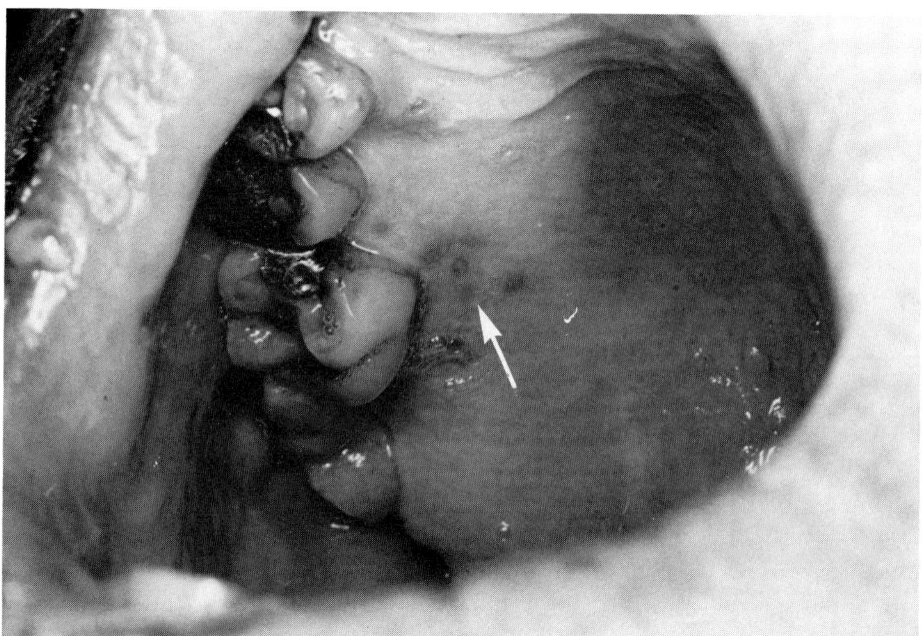

Figure 18–64. Recurrent herpes simplex on oral mucosa. Uncommon event. Cluster of eroded vesicles on alveolar ridge (arrow).

virtually eliminate this type of infection. The whitlow is characterized by erythema, swelling, and vesicles, usually on the finger tip or around the base of the nail. The vesicles become turbid, simulating a bacterial infection (Fig. 18–65). Lymphangitis and tender axillary lymphadenopathy may be present as well. The duration of the infection may be 10 to 20 days.[78] Recurrent herpes simplex on the fingers and hand can also be associated with lymphangitis and lymphadenopathy in the absence of bacterial infection.[79] Wrestlers can develop a widespread cutaneous herpetic infection in areas of abraded skin during a match if they are exposed to a source of herpes virus (herpes gladiatorum).[80] Genital herpes following sexual contact is another inoculation syndrome. Individuals with atopic dermatitis are prone to develop herpetic infections in areas of active eczema and, rarely, in their normal-appearing skin as well. In such patients, it may appear simply that the eczema has flared for unknown reasons, but close inspection will reveal punched-out ulcerations produced by transient vesicles (Figs. 18–66 and 18–67). This syndrome (Kaposi's varicelliform eruption, eczema herpeticum) may be mild or severe. It can be characterized by high fever, adenopathy, and severe toxicity. Usually the disease is self-limiting after a course of one to two weeks. Rarely, it proves fatal because of generalized viral dissemination or secondary bacterial infection.[81]

Vaccinia virus can produce the same syndrome in individuals with atopic dermatitis, but this type of infection should not be seen again now that vaccinations are no longer indicated in medicine. Zoster virus does not infect atopic dermatitis. In addition to atopic patients, individuals with seborrheic dermatitis, Darier's disease, Wiskott-Aldrich syndrome, pem-

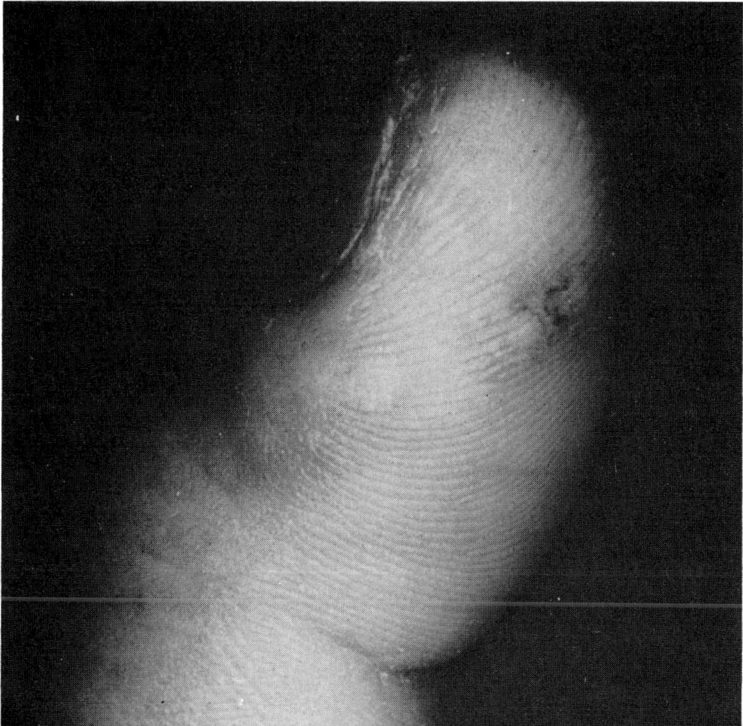

Figure 18–65. Herpes simplex infection. Herpetic whitlow.

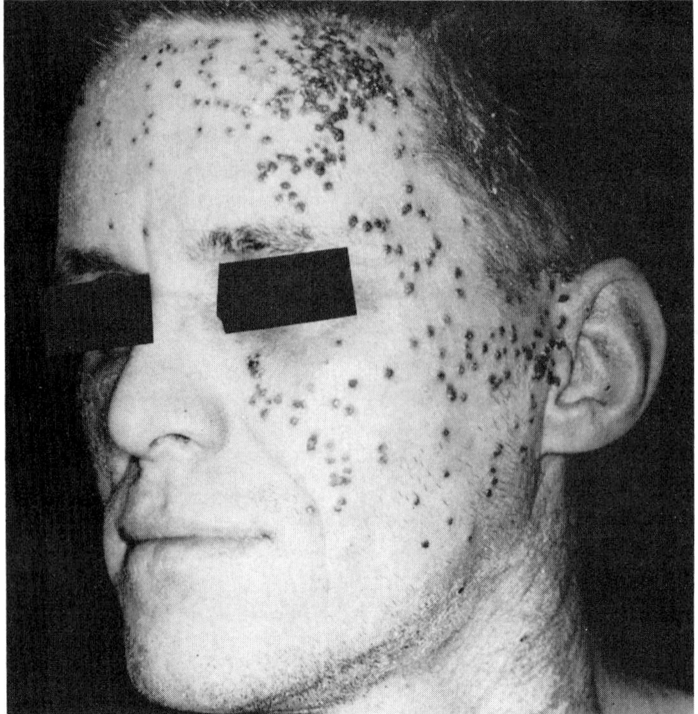

Figure 18–66. Eczema herpeticum. Atopic dermatitis secondarily infected by herpes simplex.

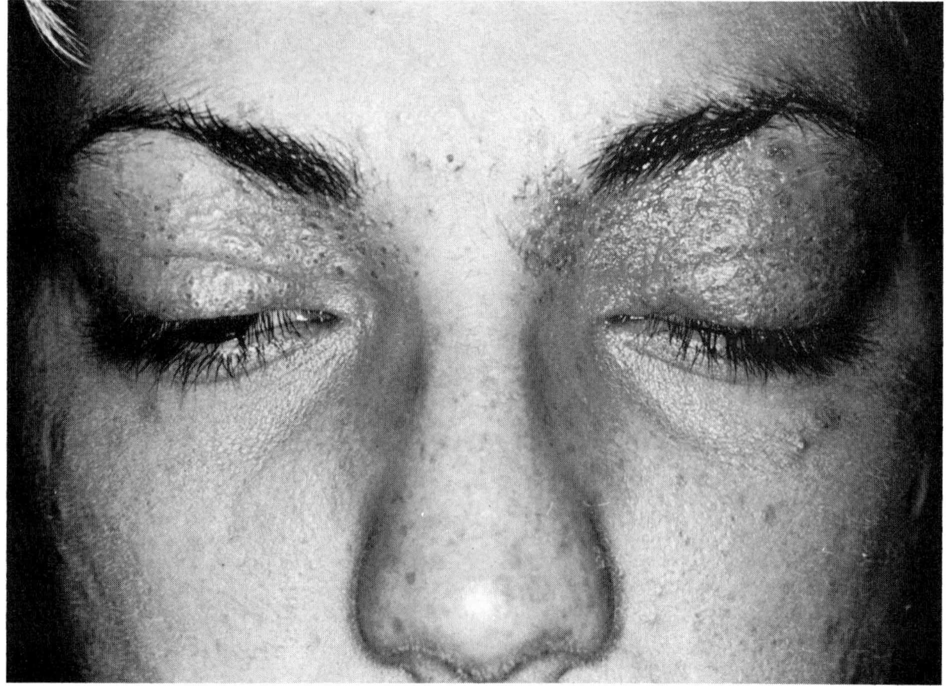

Figure 18–67. Eczema herpeticum on eyelids. Umbilicated and eroded vesicles are present.

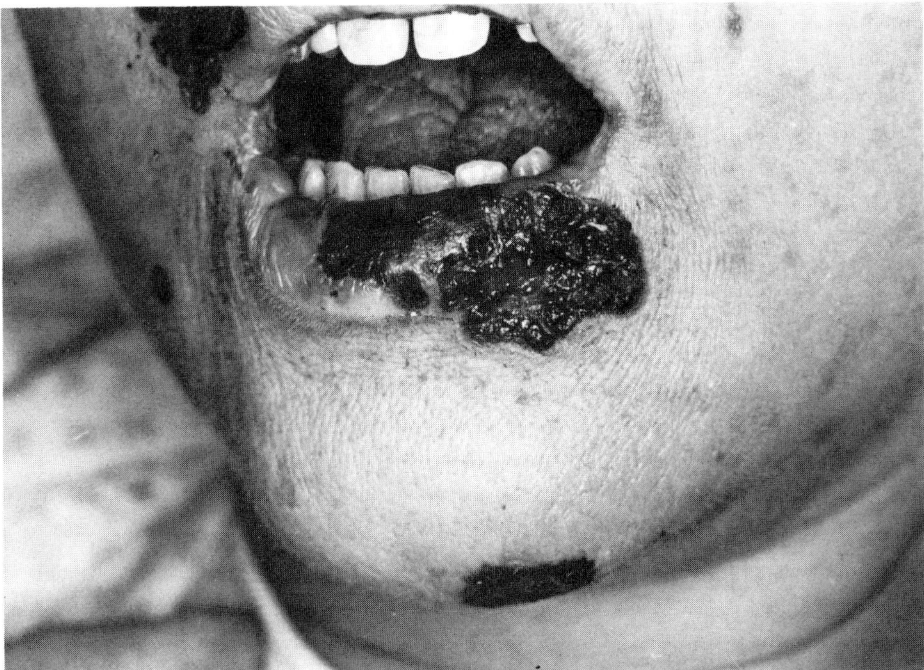

Figure 18–68. Chronic herpes simplex infection producing slowly expanding ulcers in patient with malignant lymphoma.

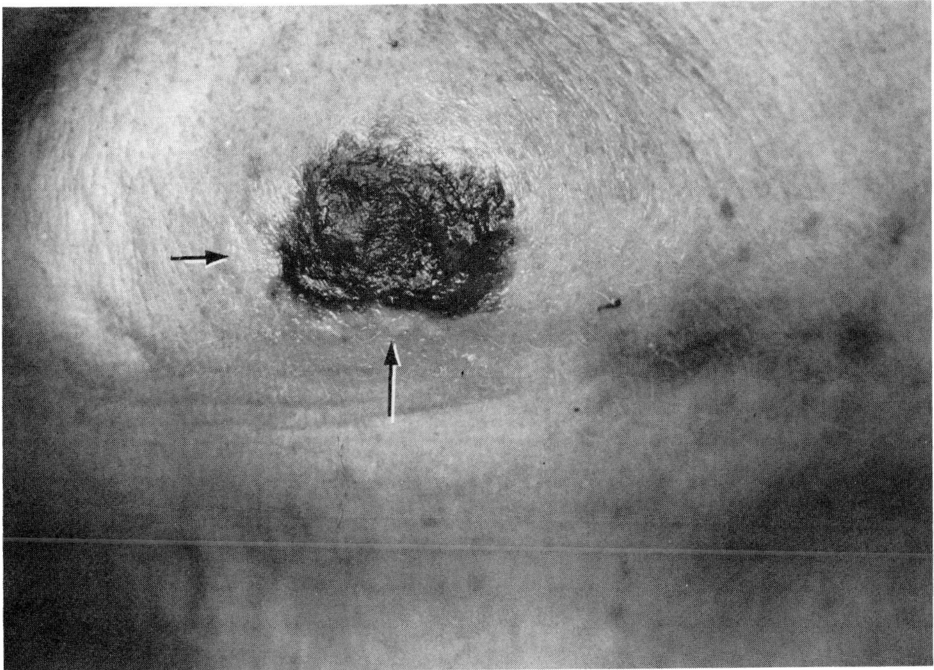

Figure 18–69. Chronic herpes simplex infection. Close-up of lesion on chin in patient shown in Figure 18–68. Vesicles on border producing a "bubbly" surface rather than frank blisters (arrows).

phigus, and congenital ichthyosiform erythroderma may develop the syndrome of eczema herpeticum. Burned patients are also predisposed to herpes simplex infections, especially in areas of healing second degree burns and in the donor sites. The herpetic infection may become disseminated.[82] Patients immunocompromised either by drugs or by associated lymphomatous-leukemic disorders are vulnerable to infections with herpes simplex. There may be continuous recurrences of the usual herpetic lesions about the mouth and nose and in the perineum; persistence of typical lesions for weeks to months; or development of ulcerations of these sites. Often the clustered vesicles break down to form slowly expanding ulcers with vesicular border that may not heal spontaneously for several months (Figs. 18–68 and 18–69). Generalized herpetic ulcers and Kaposi's varicelliform eruption appear to be less common manifestations.[83-85]

Herpes simplex infections may produce unusual manifestations in immunocompromised patients. Figure 3–7 shows a young woman with Hodgkin's disease who developed a hemorrhagic zoster with dissemination. Herpes simplex was isolated from the disseminated vesicles but not from the dermatomal lesions. Another unusual example of disseminated simplex in an immunocompromised patient is illustrated in Figures 18–70 to 18–72. This patient had a 10-year history of mycosis fungoides characterized by plaques and eczematous patches. She developed sudden onset of fever, malaise, and ulcerations in the groins, lower abdomen, and back. The ulcers developed without any clinically obvious blister formation. At first the ulcerations were thought to represent breakdown of skin diffusely infiltrated by mycosis fungoides. Biopsies and cultures of the ulcerations

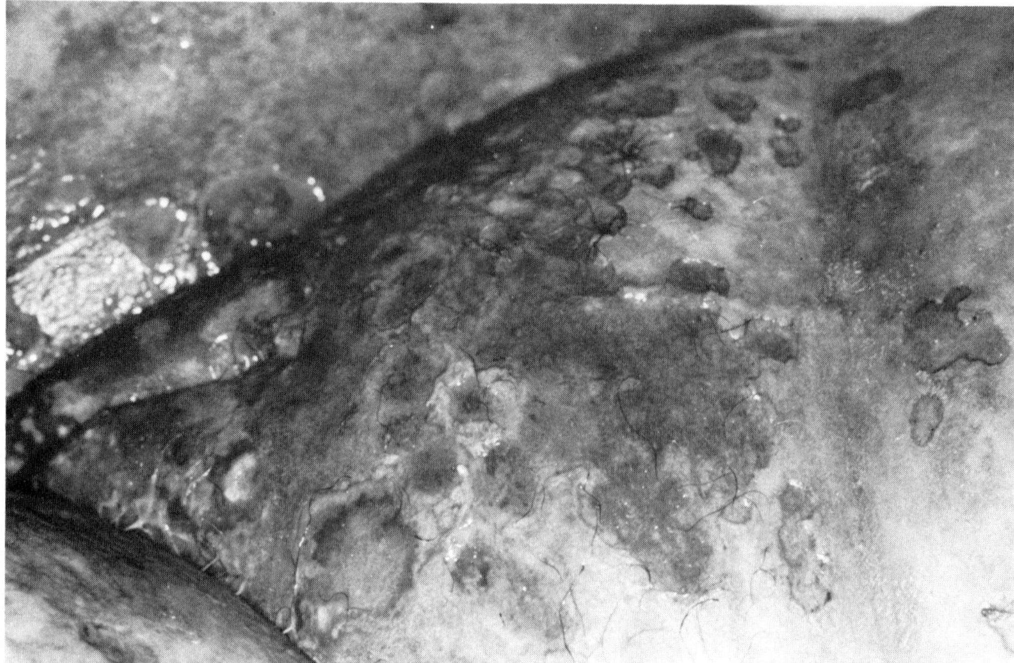

Figure 18–70. Disseminated herpes simplex infection producing ulcerations on lower abdominal wall and pubic area in patient with mycosis fungoides. Ulcerations are polycyclic. A vesicular border was not present.

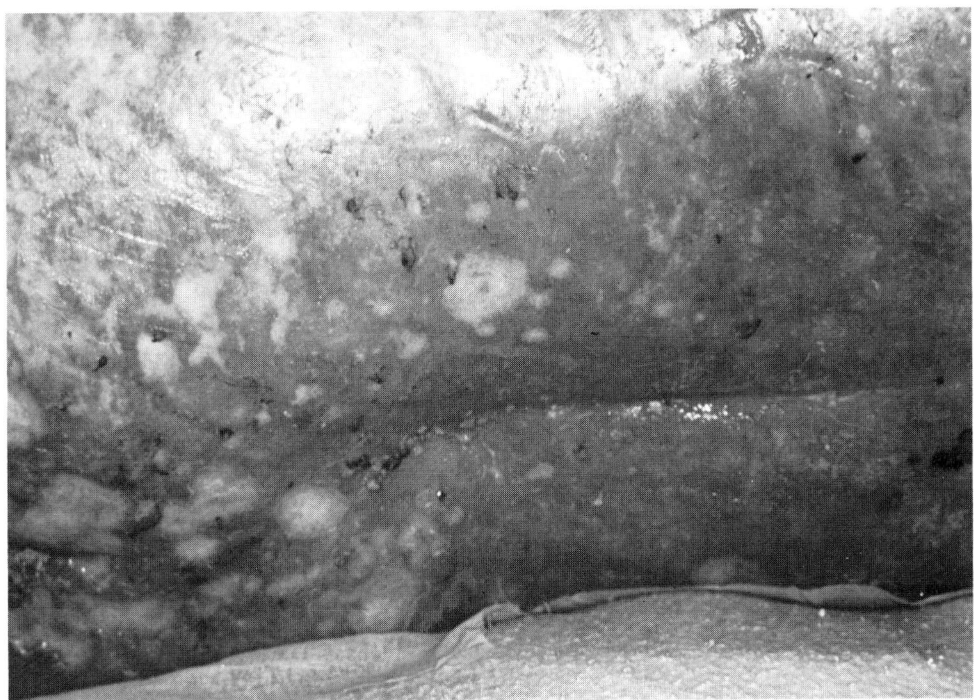

Figure 18–71. Disseminated herpes simplex infection on mid- and lower back of patient shown in Figure 18–70.

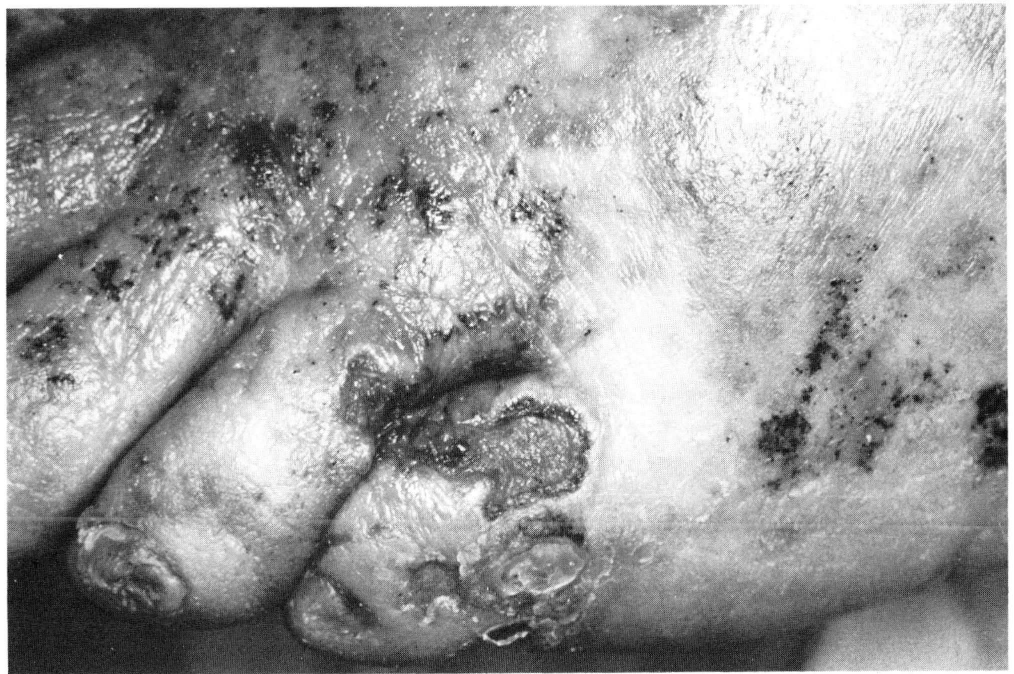

Figure 18–72. Disseminated herpes simplex infection. Same patient as in Figure 18–70.

showed that they were caused by herpes simplex. There was no sign of a mycosis fungoides infiltrate in the ulcers. Closer inspection of the ulcers disclosed their polycyclic configuration, indicating their herpetiform etiology. The earliest lesions were edematous patches without vesicles that quickly ulcerated. In this particular case, the herpes virus was producing herpetiform ulcerations without passing through a clinically obvious vesicular phase. Rapidly appearing ulcerations, especially of polycyclic configuration, should alert one to the possibility of herpes simplex infection in an immunocompromised host.

One of our patients had a patch of herpes simplex, verified by culture on the cheek, for five months during her pregnancy. It disappeared post partum.

Herpes Zoster

Herpes zoster represents a reactivation of varicella virus which had entered cutaneous sensory nerves during chickenpox, traveled to the dorsal root ganglia, and remained there for a variable period in a noninfectious state. Upon reactivation the virus traveled back down the sensory nerves to involve the skin with its characteristic pattern of clustered vesicles. The vesicles in zoster vary in size within a herpetiform cluster, in contrast to herpes simplex, in which the vesicles are relatively

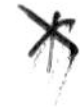

uniform in diameter and shape (Fig. 3–6). This is a useful clinical sign for distinguishing herpes zoster from herpes simplex that occurs in a dermatomal pattern. Zoster can also develop as edematous plaques resembling hives (Fig. 18–73). Close inspection of these plaques reveals a bubbly or fine cobblestone surface produced by small vesicles embedded in an edematous plaque. These lesions often do not evolve any further; they simply resolve from this point over the course of one to two weeks.

At least 50 per cent of patients with ordinary zoster will have a viremia producing a mild cutaneous dissemination of no consequence (Figs. 18–74 and 18–75). As many as 20 to 30 vesicles may be present outside the primary dermatomal lesion without this presentation being considered abnormal. More extensive dissemination, however, is characteristic in lymphoma, leukemia, and mycosis fungoides and may be fatal. Figures 3–8 to 3–11 show a patient with mycosis fungoides who developed a small area of zoster on the neck and shoulder that ulcerated within three days and was followed by a dissemination that covered his entire skin surface. The development of hemorrhagic zoster or immediate ulceration often portends a more severe course than normal, including dissemination. Such necrotic zoster lesions often occur in persons with underlying diseases ranging from severe diabetes mellitus and atherosclerosis to lymphomatous disorders.

Although the zoster virus resides in the sensory ganglia, upon reactivation it may infect the anterior horn cells and produce motor paralysis. The autonomic nervous system may also be affected in this manner. The most common motor paralyses are those affecting the seventh and eighth cranial nerves; involvement of the ninth and tenth is rare. The Hunt syndrome is one of the most common: unilateral facial paralysis, loss of taste on the anterior two thirds of the tongue on the same side, and a herpetic eruption over the concha and external auditory meatus (Figs. 18–76 to 18–79). Zoster vesicles may appear on the pinna or

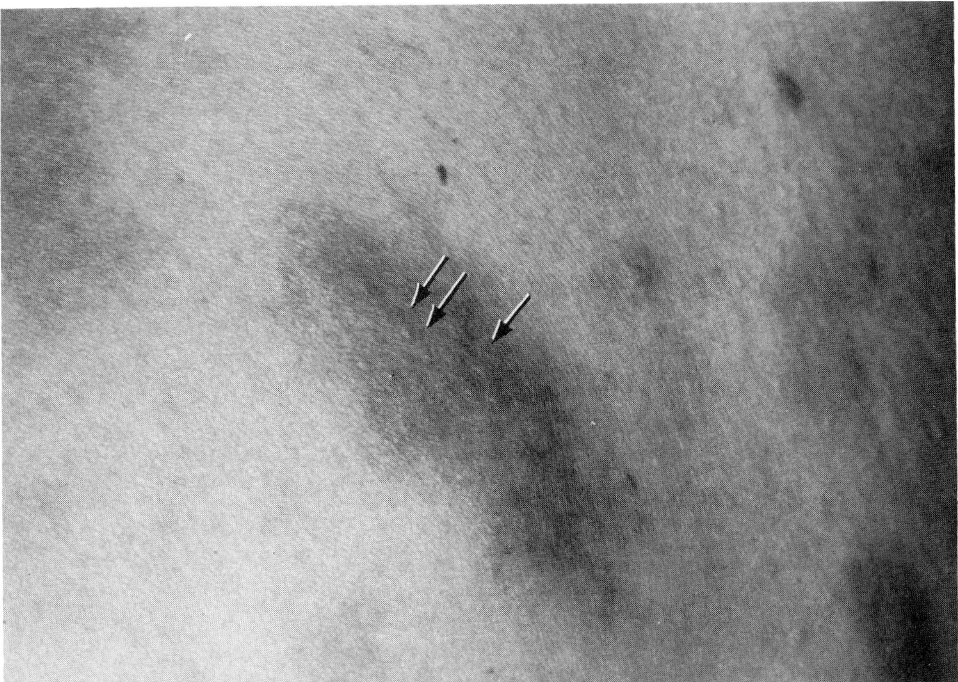

Figure 18–73. Herpes zoster. Vesicles (arrows) may produce a "bubbly" surface on an edematous plaque instead of frank blisters.

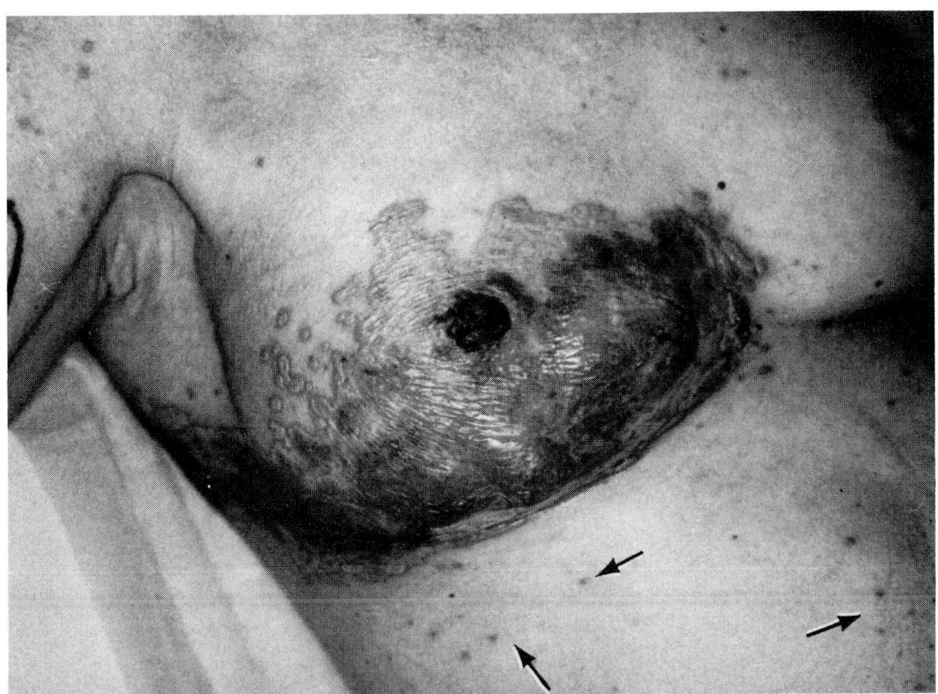

Figure 18–74. Herpes zoster. Mild dissemination (arrows).

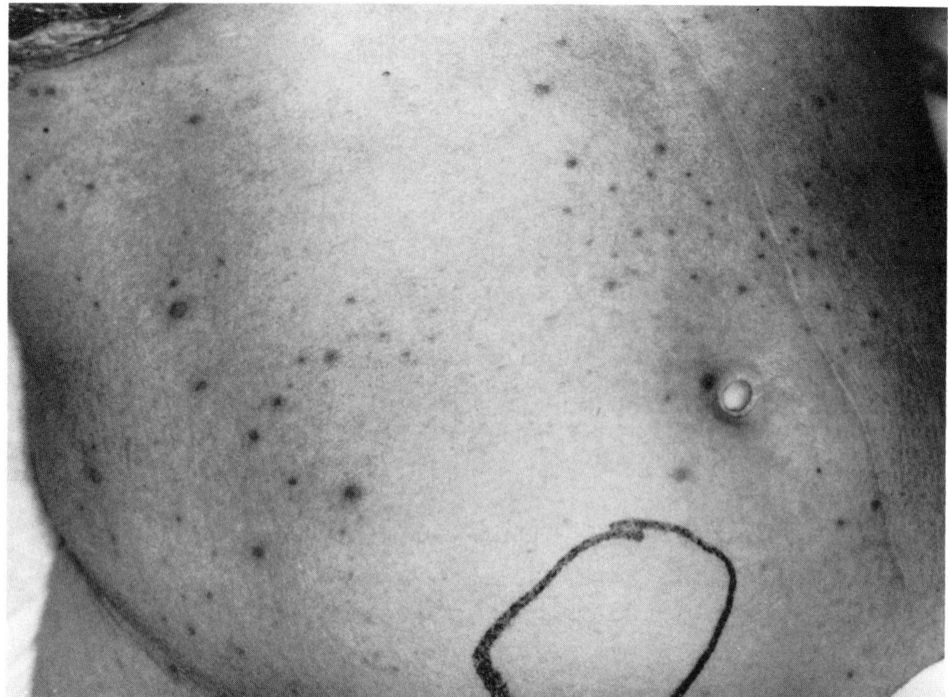

Figure 18–75. Herpes zoster. Same patient as in Figure 18–74. Disseminated lesions resemble chickenpox.

tympanic membrane. In some patients with this syndrome, the eighth nerve is also involved, resulting in vertigo and hearing loss. Auditory nerve involvement and seventh nerve (Bell's) palsy can occur alone as well as in combination. Recovery from motor paralyses is usually complete. Autonomic nerve involvement often manifests itself as bladder dysfunction: dysuria, acute retention, or both. Hematuria secondary to bladder mucosal ulceration is often present. Gastrointestinal tract involvement presents as spasm, hypotonia, or ileus. In about 5 per cent of patients, fever, malaise, and headache are present, indicating mild aseptic meningitis. Regional adenitis may develop with an attack of zoster.

Herpes zoster is frequently preceded by pain and paresthesias. The pain can mimic that of cholecystitis, renal colic, myocardial infarction, and pleurisy, and the correct diagnosis sometimes may not be made for as long as four to five days because of the interval between pain and the telltale lesions. Segmental pain without the eventual development of zoster is rare. Postherpetic neuralgia is uncommon in patients under age 40, but occurs in approximately 50 per cent of patients older than 60. Although postherpetic neuralgia usually resolves spontaneously within one to three months, it may persist for years in occasional individuals, resulting in depression, narcotic addiction, and even suicide.

Zoster involving the first division of the trigeminal nerve is potentially a serious disease. If the tip of the nose is also involved, there is high probability that there will also be ocular involvement (Figs. 18–80 and 18–81). The tip of the nose and the eye are innervated by the nasociliary branch of the trigeminal nerve. Conjunctivitis, keratitis, and iridocyclitis may occur. When the keratitis is severe, extensive scarring with impairment of vision results. Secondary bacterial infection of the eye may

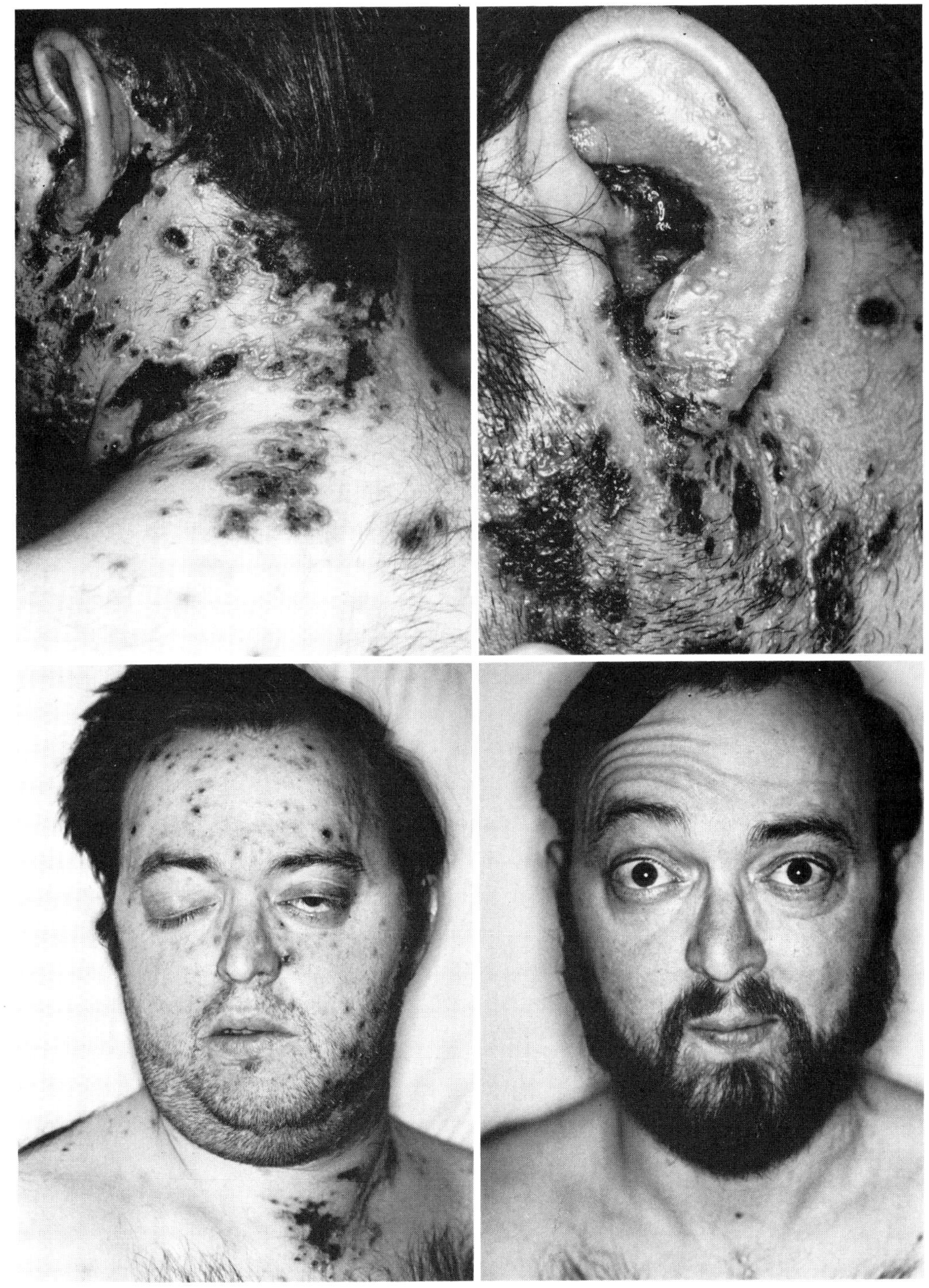

Figure 18–76. Top left. Hunt syndrome.

Figure 18–77. Top right. Hunt syndrome. Involvement of pinna and external auditory meatus.

Figure 18–78. Bottom left. Hunt syndrome. Facial paralysis. Patient cannot close eyelid.

Figure 18–79. Bottom right. Hunt syndrome. Eyelid control was regained upon recovery, but patient is still unable to wrinkle forehead.

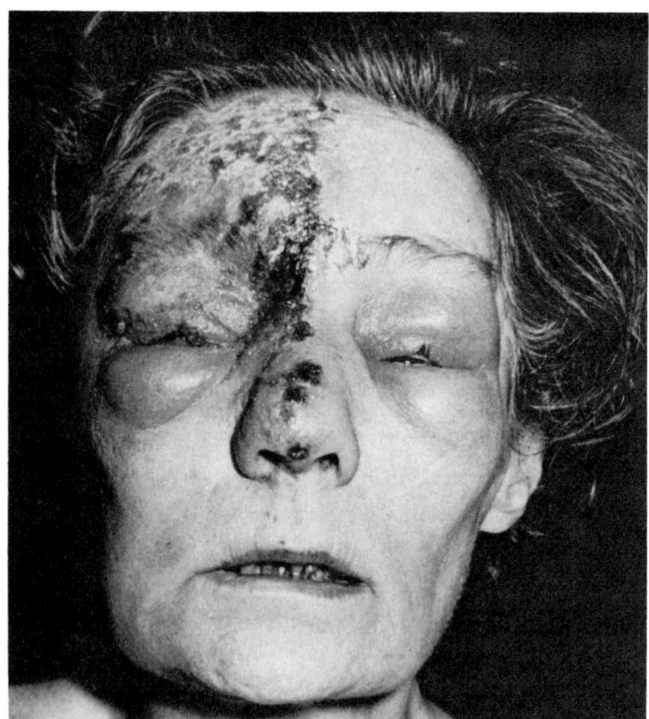

Figure 18–80. Herpes zoster ophthalmicus. Vesicle on tip of nose is usually associated with ocular involvement.

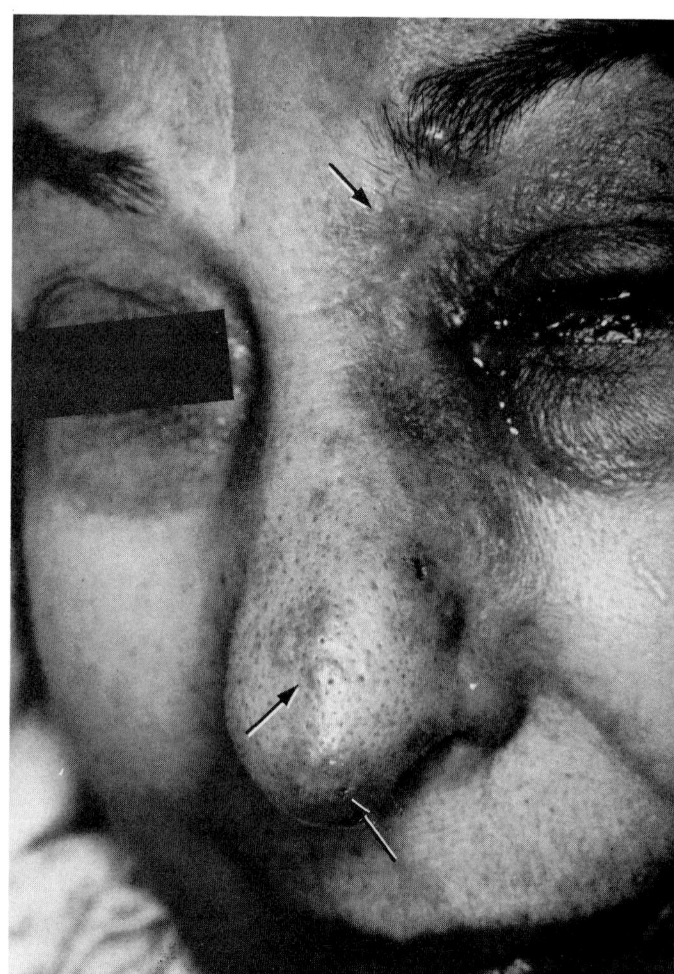

Figure 18–81. Herpes zoster ophthalmicus. Mild involvement. Arrows indicate herpetiform lesions.

produce even greater ocular destruction. Involvement of the trigeminal nerve can also be associated with palsies of the third, fourth, and sixth cranial nerves, producing ophthalmoplegia, iridoplegia, or ptosis.

Second and third attacks of zoster occur, but they usually arise in dermatomes different from those involved in the original episode. If more than one dermatome is involved during an individual attack, they are contiguous. The vesicles of zoster are infectious and will cause chickenpox in susceptible individuals, but they do not transmit zoster.

Mucocutaneous Lymph Node Syndrome

Mucocutaneous lymph node syndrome (MLNS), also known as Kawasaki's disease, is a disorder of uncertain etiology and nosology. Since 1970, over 18,000 cases of MLNS have been recorded in Japan, and since 1974, the disease has been reported all over the world.[86-88] The principal features of the disorder include fever of 38 to 40°C for one to two weeks unresponsive to antibiotics; bilateral conjunctival congestion; reddening of the lips with subsequent fissuring and erosions; diffuse erythema of the oral and pharyngeal mucosa; lingual erythema with prominence of the papillae simulating a strawberry tongue; erythema of the palms and soles with firm edema of the hands and feet appearing on the third to fifth day; a generalized eruption described as scarlatiniform, morbilliform, or, rarely, urticarial resembling erythema multiforme; and desquamation of the skin during the second or third week of illness when the rash begins to fade (Figs. 18–82 and 18–83). Although the peeling and shedding of the skin characteristically begin under the free edges of the

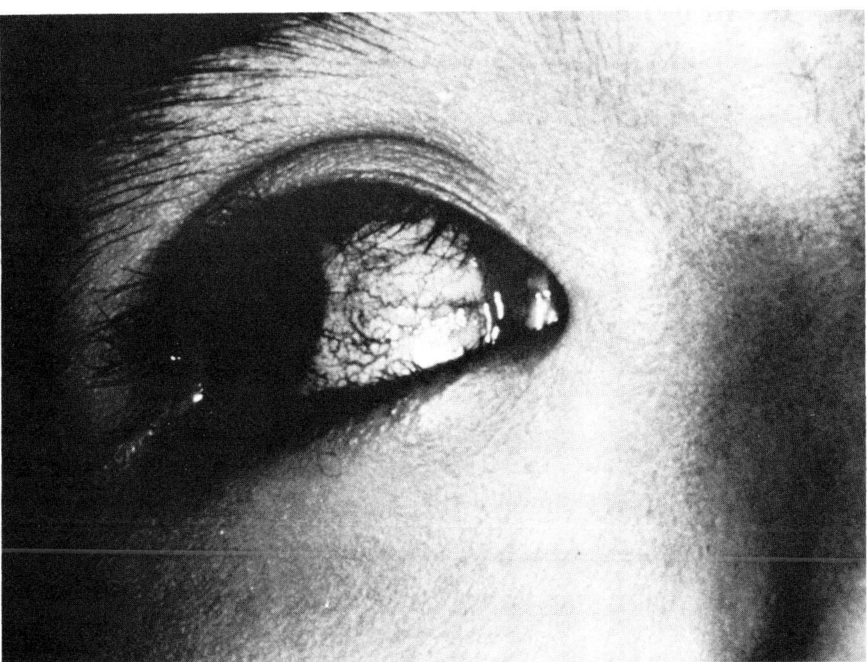

Figure 18–82. Mucocutaneous lymph node syndrome. Conjunctival vascular congestion. (From Hurwitz, S.: Clinical Pediatric Dermatology. Philadelphia, W. B. Saunders Company, 1981, p. 397.)

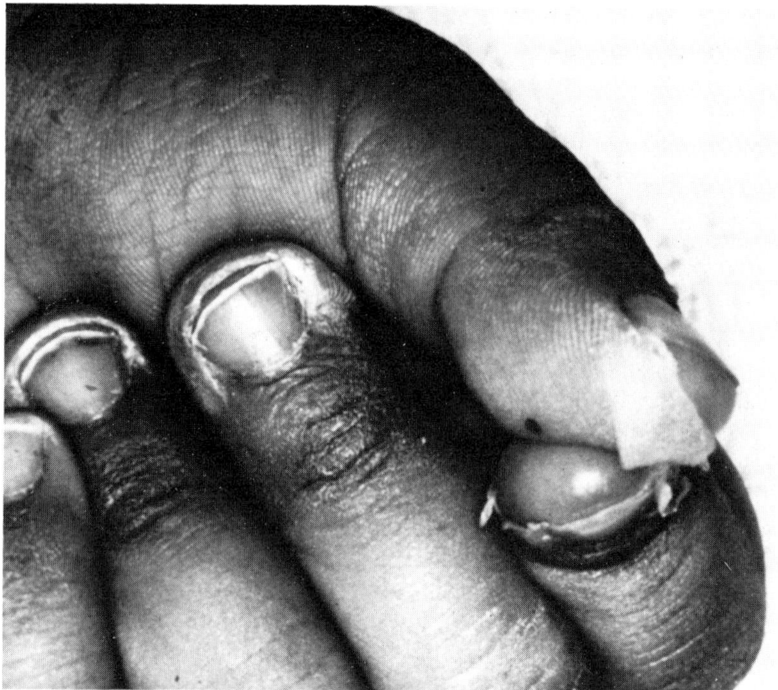

Figure 18–83. Mucocutaneous lymph node syndrome. Peeling and shedding of skin of finger tips. (From Hurwitz, S.: Clinical Pediatric Dermatology. Philadelphia, W. B. Saunders Company, 1981, p. 399.)

fingernails and toenails, they also occur elsewhere over the body. Acute enlargement of the cervical lymph nodes without suppuration also is a feature of MLNS. This illness has a predilection for children under two years of age, but it can be seen in those as old as 10 to 13 and is now being reported in young adults up to age 30. These principal signs and symptoms occur in over 90 per cent of cases, with the exception of lymphadenopathy, which has been reported in about 50 to 75 per cent. Other associated features include arthralgias, arthritis, urethritis, aseptic meningitis, diarrhea, and mild jaundice in 4 to 40 per cent. Nonspecific electrocardiographic changes are found in 20 to 70 per cent of cases.[86, 87]

Approximately 1 to 2 per cent of children have died suddenly during the third or fourth week of the illness while they were convalescing and appeared to be healthy. The most recent survey in Japan indicates that such deaths have decreased to 0.4 per cent.[88] The fatalities are caused by arteritis of the major coronary arteries. Aneurysms and thromboses develop, leading to arrhythmias, infarction, and myocarditis. The aneurysms of the coronary arteries have been reversible in children who have not succumbed at this stage of the illness. Identical vascular changes are found in other major arteries: bronchial, brachial, iliac, splenic, pancreatic, hepatic, mesenteric, and paratracheal. Kawasaki's disease is now generally agreed to be identical to infantile polyarteritis nodosa.[89]

A constellation of laboratory findings characterizes this illness. In most patients there is leukocytosis, increased sedimentation rate, and, in the third week, thrombocytosis, In many, the serum level of IgE is elevated, reaching a peak on days 7 to 14 and returning to normal after one to two months.[90] Sterile pyuria or proteinuria or both are often found.

Histologic examination of lymph nodes and skin lesions in the early case reports were described as showing nonspecific follicular hyperplasia and nonspecific inflammation without evidence of vasculitis, respectively.[91-93] However, later studies have reported lymphoid depletion, vascular proliferation, and immunoblasts along with foci of necrosis and thrombi in the lymph nodes.[93a] Cases have now been reported in young adults as old as 30 years.[94-99] The etiology remains unclear, but in one patient the disease appeared to be associated with a primary Epstein-Barr virus infection[98] and in another, with a possible drug reaction to phenytoin.[99] In this latter patient, a lymph node exhibited changes interpreted as a severe immunoblastic or hyperimmune reaction. Pertinent to this observation is a recent case of ours.

A 24-year-old black man developed fever, cervical lymphadenopathy, a scarlatiniform rash, and all the other mucocutaneous features of this syndrome (Plate 41*D*, *E*; Figs. 18–84 to 18–87). He came to the emergency room after the illness had been present for two weeks. In addition to the fever and rash he was noted to be markedly jaundiced. Over the next four days, desquamation began to develop on the chest and on the hands and feet, but his jaundice became worse and he developed acute respiratory distress and died in coma. At autopsy, he was found to have subacute hepatic necrosis and the changes of angioimmunoblastic lymphadenopathy (AIL) in the lymph nodes, which were enlarged throughout his body. The skin eruption showed the histologic findings of AIL as well.[100] At the time of admission four days earlier, skin biopsies had been obtained to exclude the possibility of a necrotizing vasculitis. These first biopsies showed a nonspecific perivascular mononuclear cell infiltrate without evidence of vasculitis. Immunofluorescent examination of these initial lesions was negative for immunoglobulins and complement. Within four days the histologic changes in the skin had progressed to those found in AIL. Our patient had taken no medications prior to his illness, and there was no evidence for an underlying connective tissue disease or an infectious etiologic agent.

The etiology of Kawasaki's disease is unknown.[101] In spite of the fact that no consistent infectious agents, environmental toxins, or drug reactions have been incriminated, MLNS must be an infectious disease because more than 18,000 cases have been reported since 1970 and it is worldwide in distribution. Its status is identical to the pneumonia known as Legionnaire's disease when it was first reported in large numbers. It took at least a year of intensive investigation by teams of different specialists before the etiologic agent *Legionella pneumophilia*, a new gram-negative bacterium, was discovered. MLNS presents two striking features: (1) The rash is uncannily similar in many of its features to that of scarlet fever, both in its appearance and mode of resolution. Scarlet fever also shows desquamation beginning at the tips of the fingers and toes.[15] (2) The development of both necrotizing arteritis resembling polyarteritis nodosa and AIL appears to be responsible for the fatalities in this

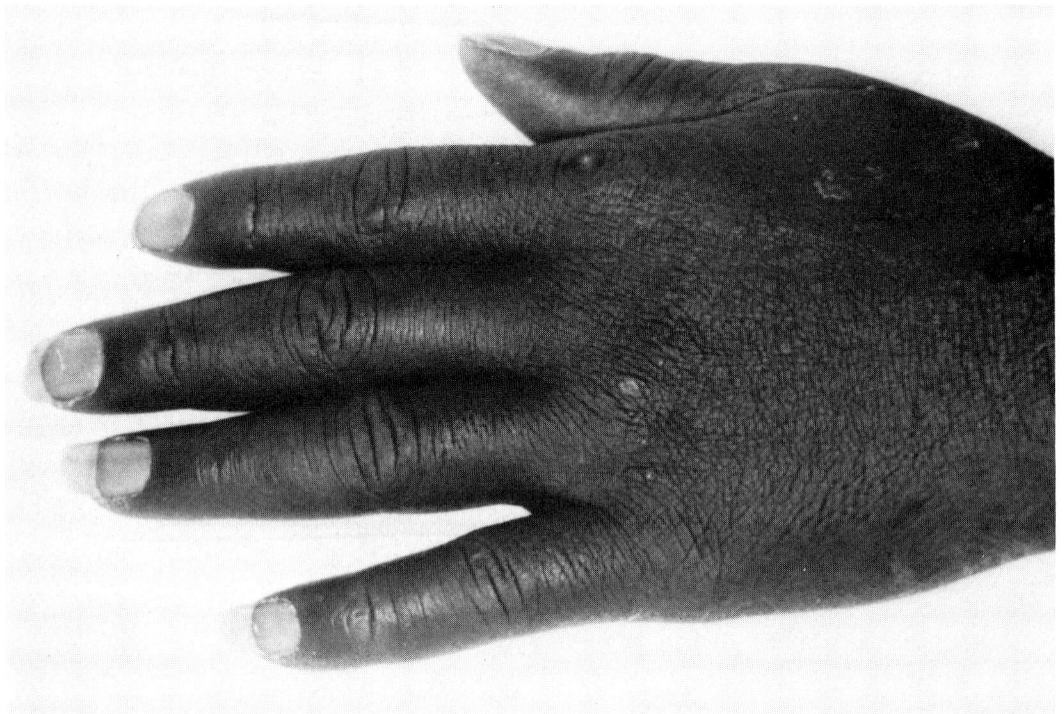

Figure 18–84. Mucocutaneous lymph node syndrome. Edema of hands in 24-year-old black man. Figures 18–84 to 18–87; Plate 41*D* and *E* are of same patient.

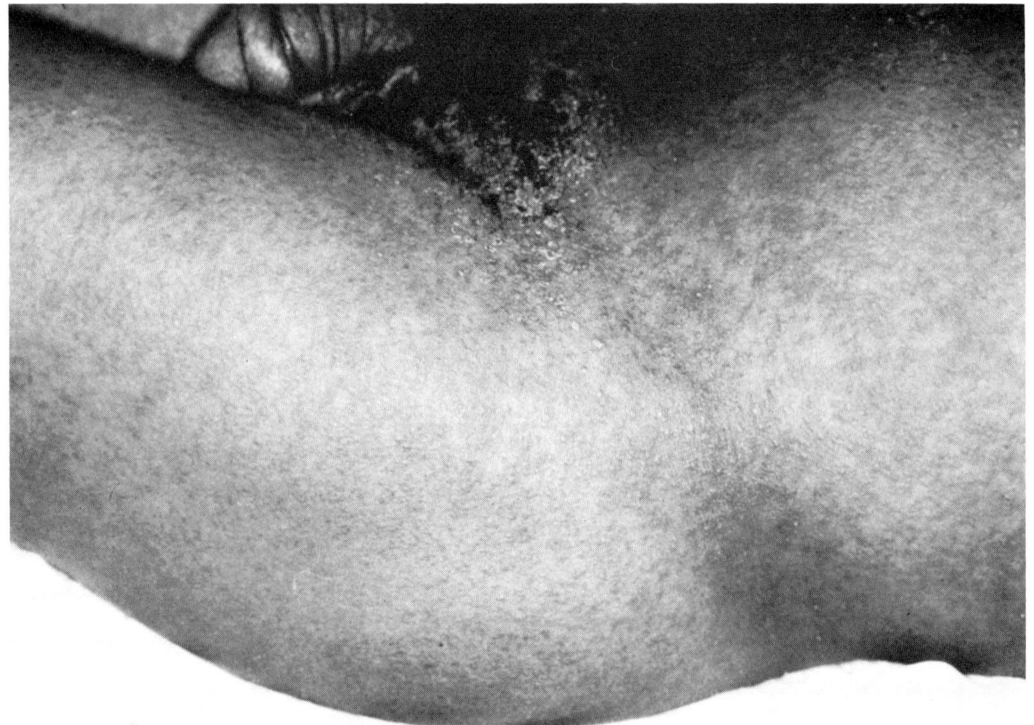

Figure 18–85. Mucocutaneous lymph node syndrome. Scarlatiniform eruption.

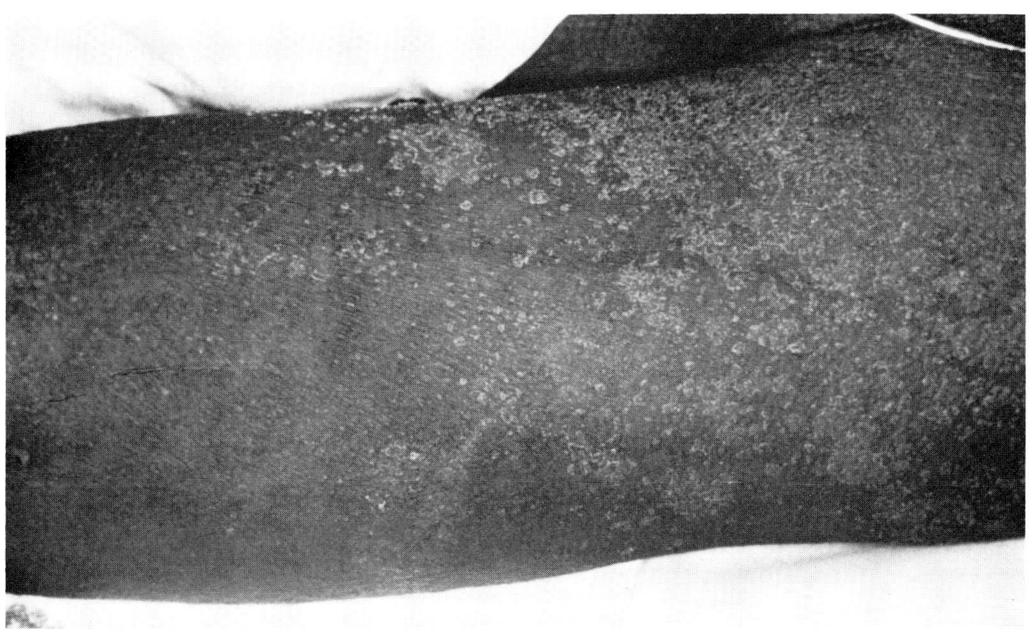

Figure 18–86. Top. Mucocutaneous lymph node syndrome. Desquamation of skin.

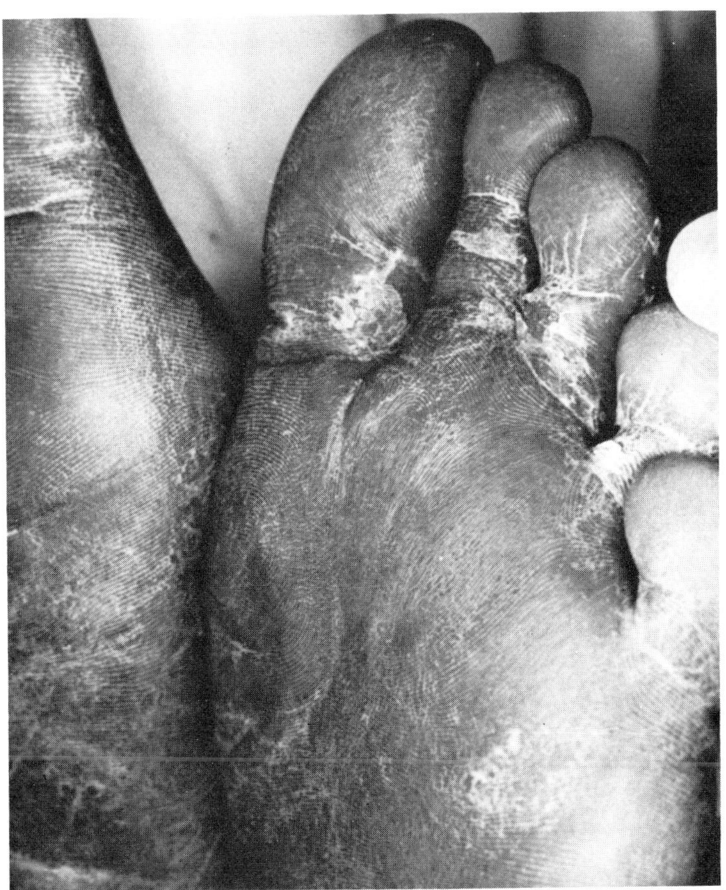

Figure 18–87. Mucocutaneous lymph node syndrome. Peeling of skin over toes.

syndrome. It seems likely to me that there is an infectious agent that produces an erythrogenic toxin responsible for the cutaneous features and that in a few predisposed individuals hypersensitivity reactions develop that may prove fatal. Because of the close resemblance of the cutaneous lesions and some of the clinical features of AIL to MLNS,[100] it is possible that MLNS and some cases of AIL are manifestations of hypersensitivity to the same infectious agent. The histopathology of the lymph nodes in MLNS needs to be reevaluated because the first cases were studied before AIL was described. The description of the lymph nodes in recent case reports is compatible with AIL except for the presence of necrotic foci and thrombi.[93a] The relationship of MLNS and AIL to infection may be analogous to that of periarteritis nodosa following infection with hepatitis B virus.

Chancriform (Inoculation) Syndromes

In several bacterial, viral, and fungal infections the etiologic agent is inoculated into the skin, producing a primary lesion in association with varying degrees of lymphangitic spread and regional adenopathy. Although the fingers, hands, and distal extremities are often the sites of inoculation, the point of entry may occur anywhere so that the overall clinical appearance may not readily point to a chancriform syndrome.

Sporotrichosis develops chiefly in farmers, foresters, gardeners, florists, and miners who handle soil, timber, and vegetation. Straw, marsh hay, rose thorns, and sphagnum moss can all be contaminated by the fungus *Sporothrix schenckii*.[102] In one case the infection developed on the auricle of a brick mason who was probably inoculated there by fragments of contaminated bricks projected into the air while he was splitting them.[103] A painless papule develops at the site of inoculation and slowly enlarges to form an ulcer or crusted lesion. New nodules spring up along the lymphatic channels draining the initial site (Fig. 18–88). Rarely, the regional nodes become enlarged, but usually the diagnosis is made before this stage is reached. Occasionally the inoculation site slowly enlarges to form a plaque and lymphangitic spread does not occur (Fig. 18–89). The diagnosis is made by culture of the lesions.

Mycobacterium marinum (balnei) is an atypical mycobacterium that produces an identical (sporotrichoid) pattern of spread (Figs. 18–90 and

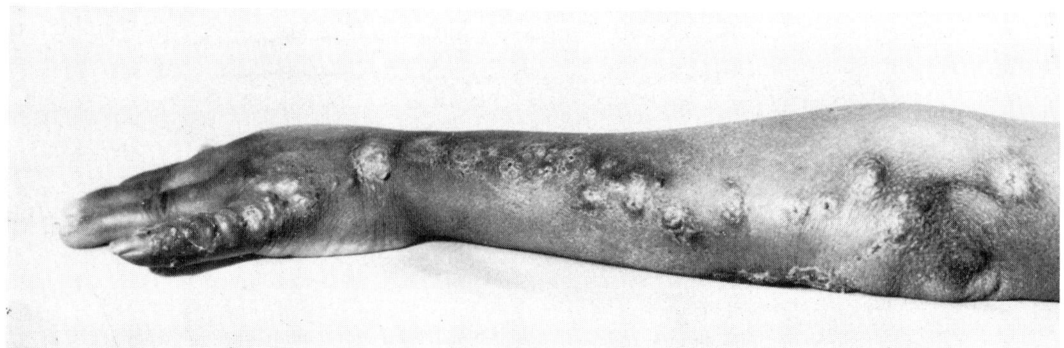

Figure 18–88. Sporotrichosis. Linearly arranged inflammatory nodules on arm. (From Moschella, S. L., Pillsburgy, D. M., and Hurley, H. J., Jr.: Dermatology. Philadelphia, W. B. Saunders Company, 1975, p. 693).

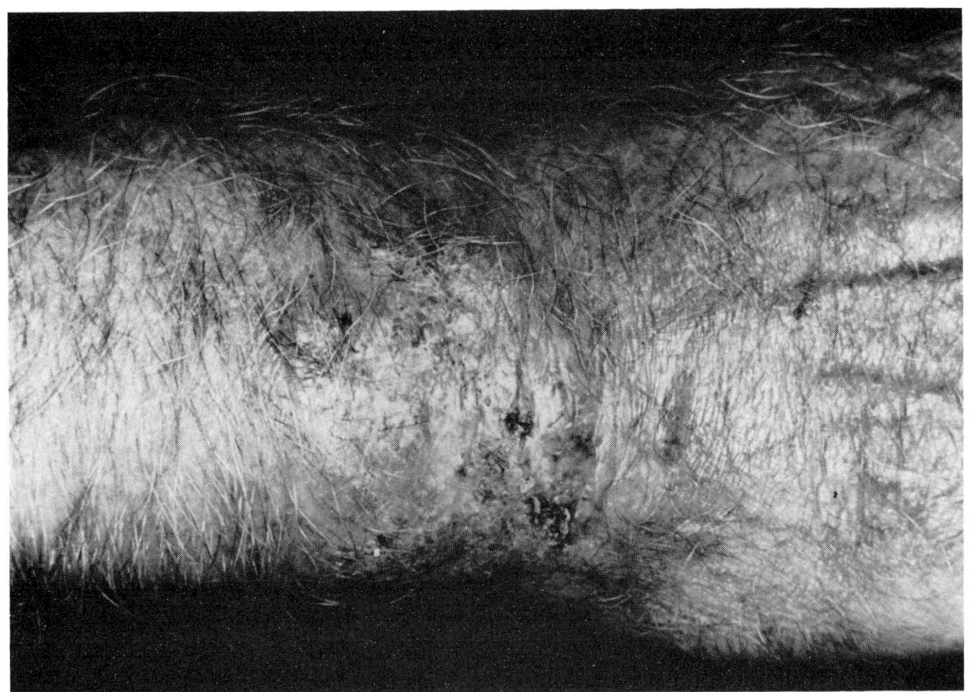

Figure 18–89. Sporotrichosis. Plaque form on wrist.

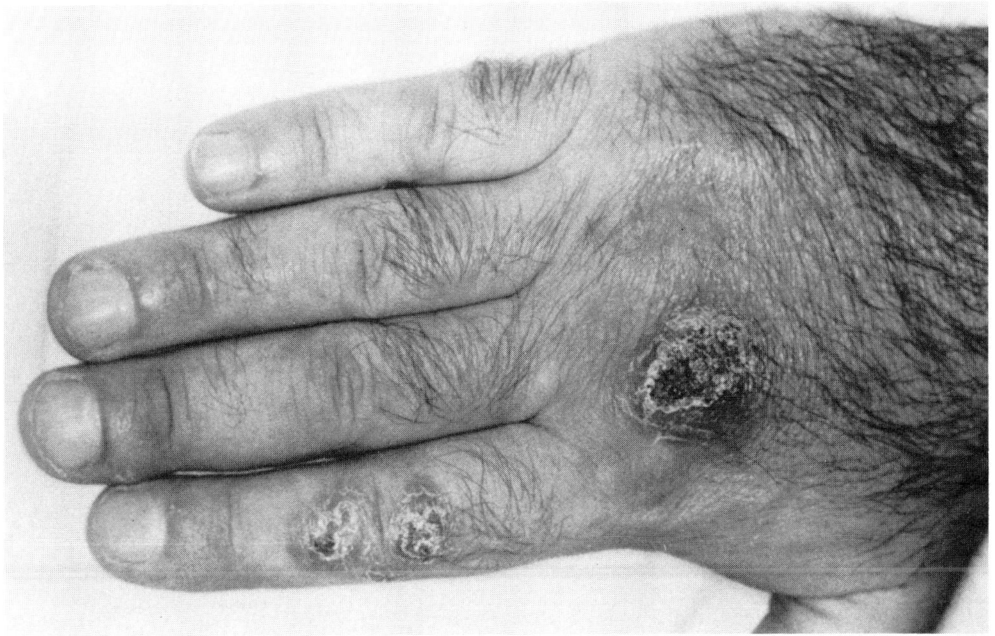

Figure 18–90. Mycobacterium marinum (balnei). Sporotrichoid pattern. Infection acquired from fish tank.

18–91). However, the regional lymph nodes have never been reported to be involved. The atypical mycobacteria are found in fish tanks and in salt and fresh water. In one epidemic of this infection, the organisms were present in a community swimming pool made of rough stone walls.[104] Two hundred and ninety individuals were infected with the organism following abrasions by the stone walls, giving rise to the term *swimming pool granuloma* for this entity. Solitary lesions may occur, but the sporotrichoid pattern is more common. The disease is self-limiting, with healing occurring from several months to as long as three years later. The organism can be cultured from the skin lesion which exhibits a granulomatous reaction.

Herpetic whitlow can be associated with lymphangitis and lymphadenopathy, mimicking a bacterial infection (Fig. 18–65). Recurrent attacks, especially when they occur in nurses, physicians, and dentists, should alert one to this entity.

Tuberculous chancres can arise in the skin or mucous membranes of those individuals with no prior exposure to *M. tuberculosis*. The organism is usually introduced into the skin of exposed areas, especially the extremities, through a break in the skin. Although the syndrome is found chiefly in children, adult cases are becoming relatively more common. Children usually acquire the syndrome by being in close contact with persons having active pulmonary tuberculosis, whereas adults often are infected through accidental inoculations. Laboratory technicians may accidentally inoculate themselves and physicians may acquire the infection while performing postmortem examinations or giving mouth-to-mouth resuscitation. The inoculation site may give rise to a papule or nodule that evolves into a nontender indolent ulcer (chancre); a papule that develops a superficial ulceration with crusting; or a deeper crusted

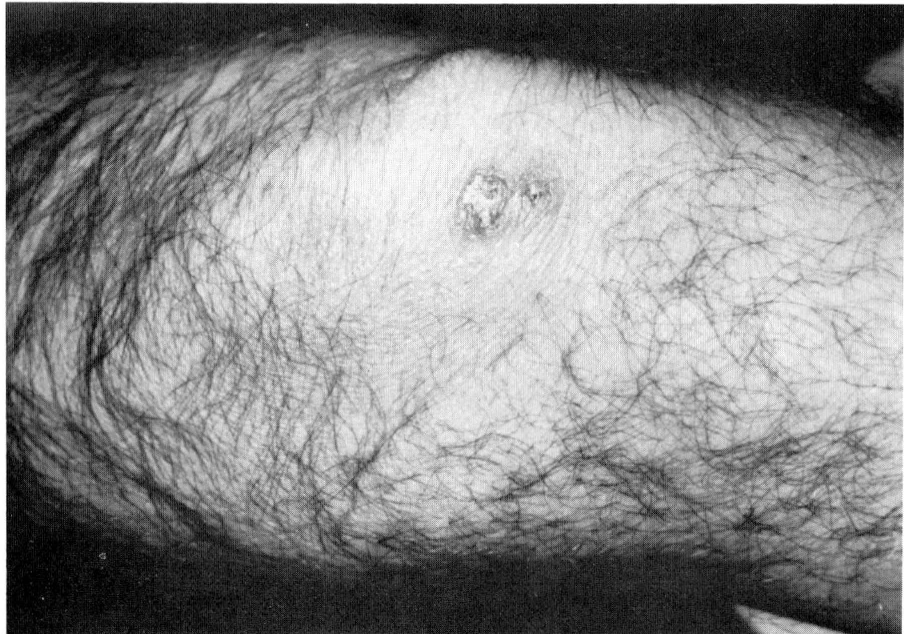

Figure 18–91. Mycobacterium marinum (balnei). Nodules on elbows part of sporotrichoid pattern. Same patient as in Figure 18–90.

erosion resembling ecthyma. Usually the syndrome is recognized by the combination of the primary lesion with regionally enlarged tender nodes (Figs. 18–92 and 18–93). However, sometimes the primary lesion heals and only the regional adenopathy is present. Conjunctival and oral mucosal lesions may not be considered to be tuberculous until regional adenopathy appears.

Individuals who have had a prior exposure and have developed a high degree of cell-mediated immunity to the mycobacterium can develop a different type of inoculation syndrome: tuberculosis verrucosa cutis. The lesions may begin and remain as small verrucous papules resembling ordinary warts, or they may gradually increase in number and coalesce to form round or oval, red-brown, hyperkeratotic warty plaques (Figs. 18–94 and 18–95). Small pustules can develop in the plaques so that they become exudative and resemble blastomycosis, iododerma, bromoderma, and pyoderma vegetans. Spontaneous healing can occur in the centers of the lesions, but a protracted benign course is usual unless the lesions are treated by excision or antibiotic therapy. Regional adenopathy and lymphangitis do not develop. The small verrucous lesions are often referred to as "prosector's warts" when they occur in medical personnel such as students and pathologists. If the inoculation should occur in an individual who has or develops poor cell-mediated immunity to the organism, the regional nodes may break down and drain to the overlying skin, producing scrofuloderma.

Cat scratch disease, which is probably viral in origin, is also characterized by the development of a small edematous papule with central necrosis in association with regional adenopathy. It is a self-limiting disorder.

Syphilis can produce a true chancre, identical to genital chancres, on the finger, lip, tongue, or any area of the body. However, syphilis can also produce a painful paronychia with regional adenopathy as the primary lesion. This variety of syphilitic infection is frequently confused with ordinary bacterial paronychia (Fig. 18–96).

Anthrax typically produces a painless, solitary ulcer that is found chiefly in persons who handle raw imported wool and other products contaminated with the highly resistant spores of *Bacillus anthracis*. The face, neck, and arms are the usual sites of involvement. A painless papule develops at the site of inoculation, enlarges, and becomes vesicular. A wide zone of brawny red edema surrounds the lesion. The vesicular center becomes hemorrhagic and necrotic and forms a black eschar. Low-grade fever and malaise accompany the infection.

In tularemia, the fingers and hands, which are primarily affected, develop an ulcerated papule or nodule at the site of inoculation in association with painful regional adenopathy. The disease occurs chiefly in hunters who have contact with the tissues and body fluids of animals infected with *Francisella tularensis*. The disease can also be transmitted by the bite of an infected tick, in which case the site of entry is usually on the leg, genitalia, buttocks, or trunk. If contaminated water or inadequately cooked meat is the source of the infection, then tularemia may manifest itself as a systemic infection.

Histoplasmosis, coccidioidomycosis, cryptococcosis, and North American blastomycosis can also produce inoculation syndromes, but they are more common following laboratory accidents than natural

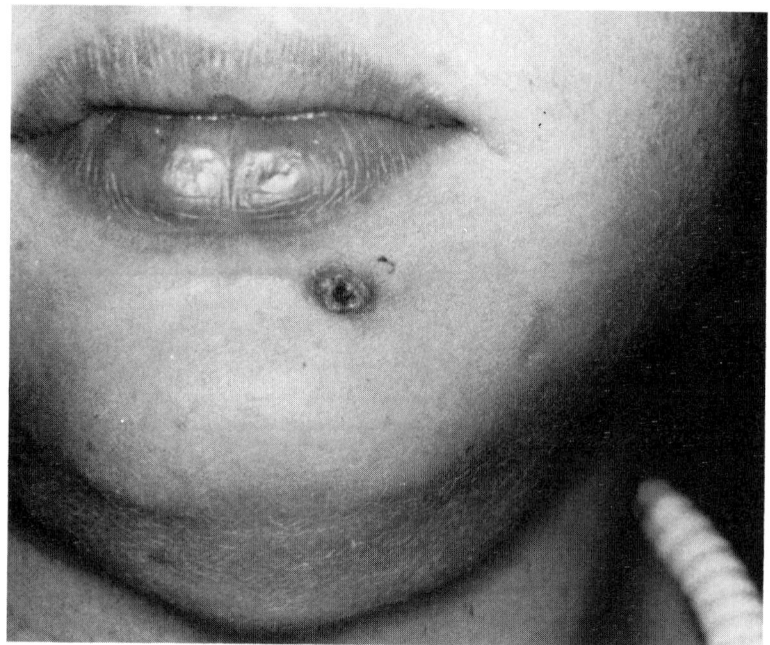

Figure 18–92. Tuberculosis. Tuberculous papule with central necrosis and crusting (chancre). Acquired from a relative.

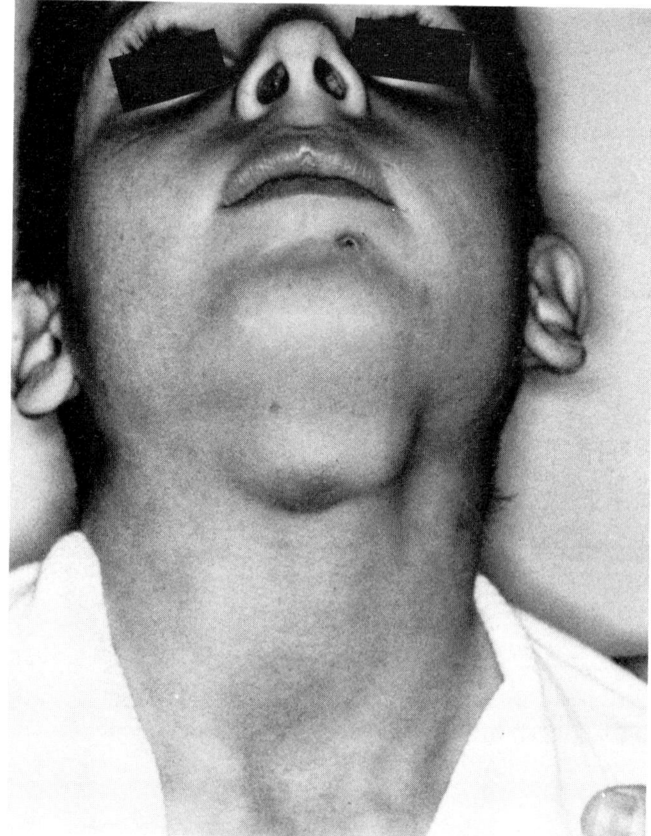

Figure 18–93. Tuberculosis. Same patient as in Figure 18–92. Enlarged submandibular node in association with tuberculous chancre on chin.

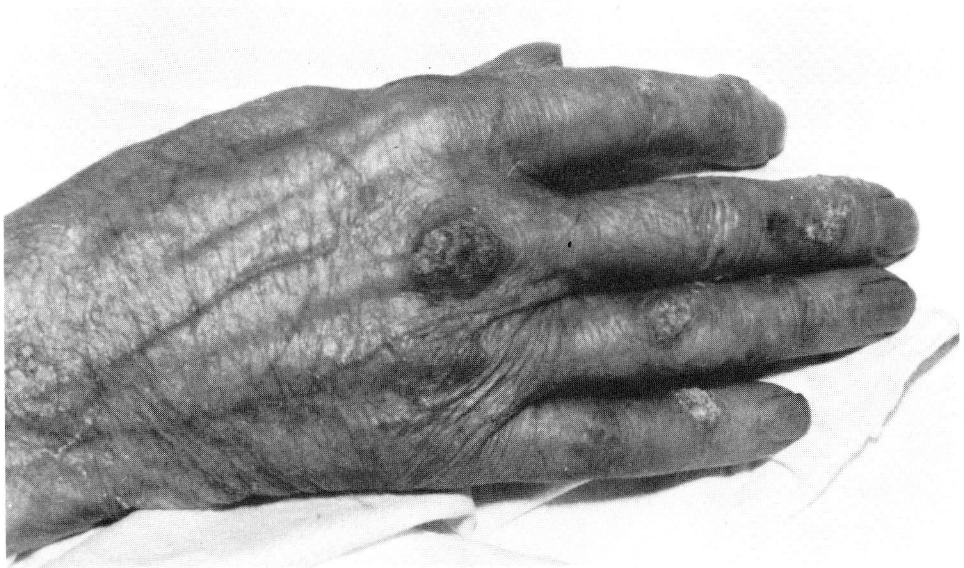

Figure 18–94. Tuberculosis verrucosa cutis. Hyperkeratotic warty plaques. (Courtesy of Dr. Paul Lucky.)

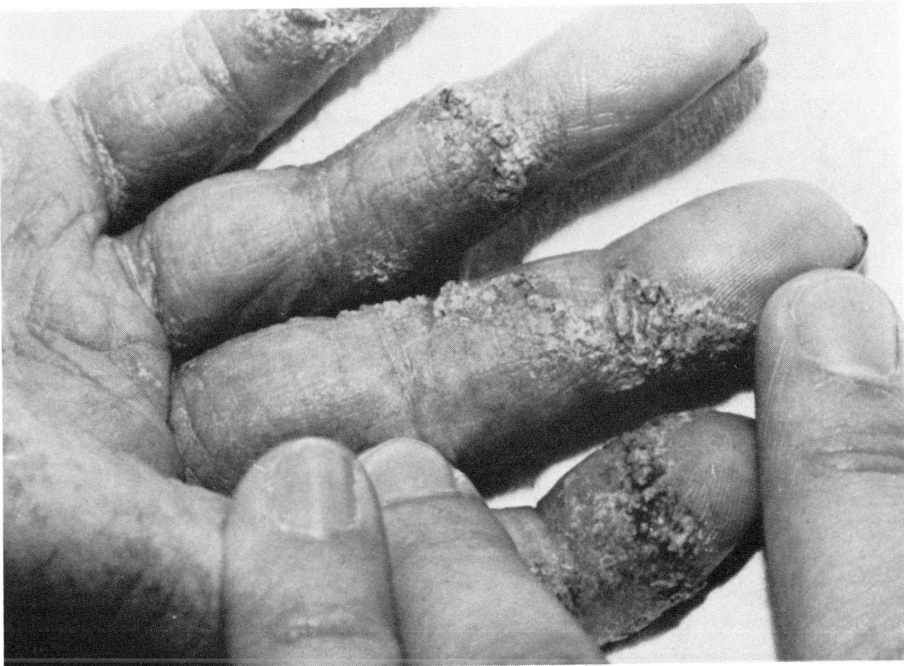

Figure 18–95. Tuberculosis verrucosa cutis. Same patient as in Figure 18–94. (Courtesy of Dr. Paul Lucky.)

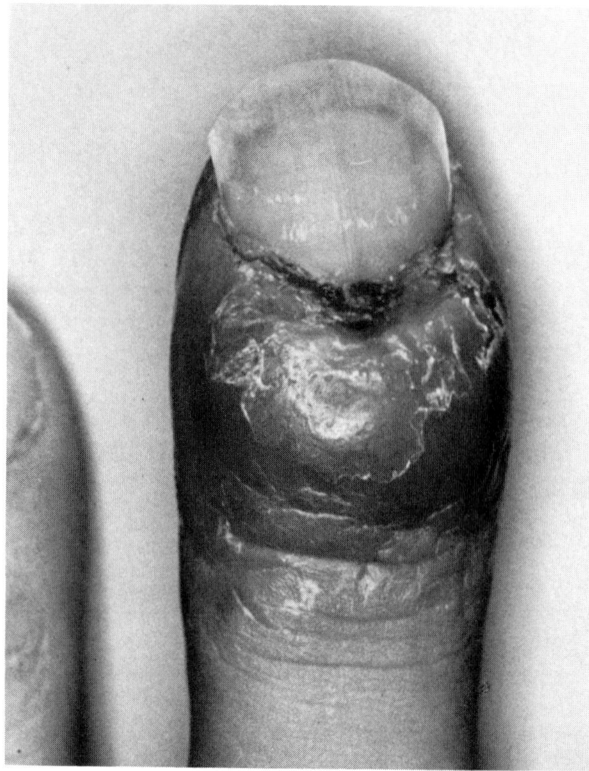

Figure 18–96. Syphilis. Paronychia as manifestation of primary inoculation site.

exposure.[102] Culture of lesions at suspected inoculation sites or along their lymphangitic spread will establish the correct diagnoses in all the above infections. The punch biopsy proves to be a simple and effective technique for this purpose.

Tuberculosis

In addition to the chancriform syndromes described above, *M. tuberculosis* produces three other important manifestations of infection. Individuals with lesser degrees of cell-mediated immunity to the tubercle bacillus can develop lupus vulgaris, a chronic progressive form of cutaneous tuberculosis. Affected individuals often have underlying active tuberculosis elsewhere. Lupus vulgaris involves the skin of the head and neck primarily, including the conjunctival, nasal, and oral mucosae. However, the extremities and trunk can be affected as well. The disease is less common in America than in England and Europe. Lupus vulgaris begins as a small reddish-brown papule that slowly spreads centrifugally to form a plaque with elevated papular borders (Fig. 18–97). It may remain as a solid plaque or it may produce a lesion with an active papular border and a central area of cutaneous atrophy and scarring, hyper- and hypopigmentation, and gross telangiectasia simulating radiodermatitis (Figs. 18–98 to 18–101). The centers may ulcerate and heal with scarring contractures. The lesions have varying degrees of adherent scale and produce a variety of appearances including ulcers, nodules, hypertrophic verrucous plaques, and annular lesions resembling sarcoid or syphilis. When the mucous membranes are affected, horrible disfigurement is produced, and nasal cartilage, if affected, is frequently destroyed.

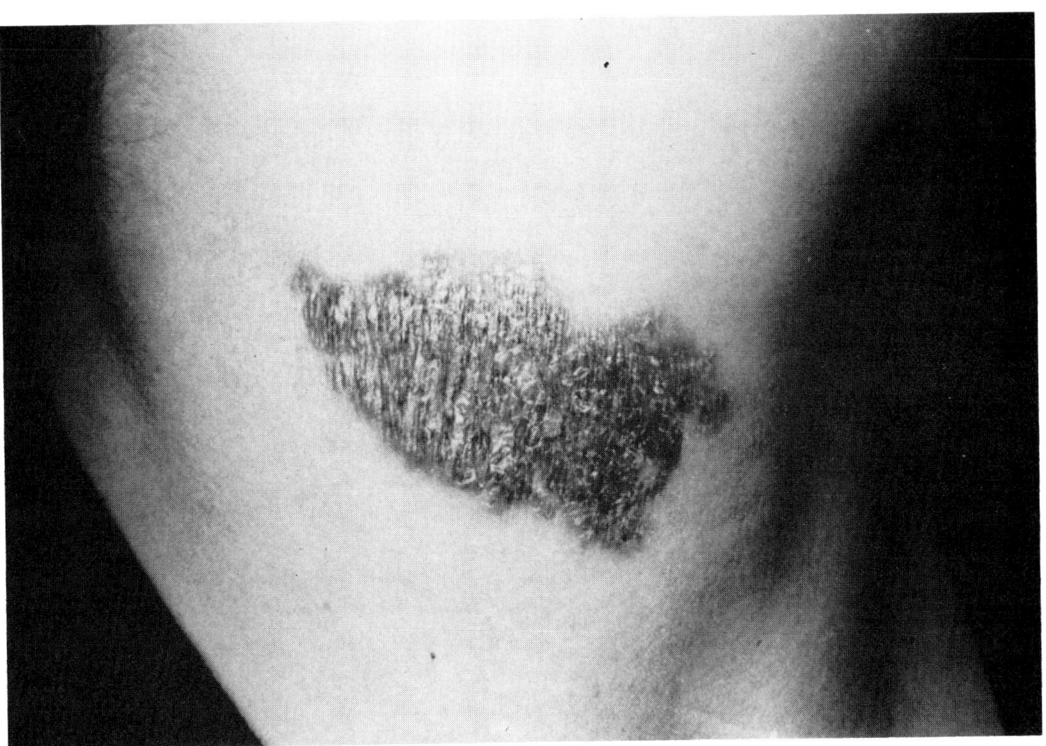

Figure 18–97. Lupus vulgaris. Plaque variety

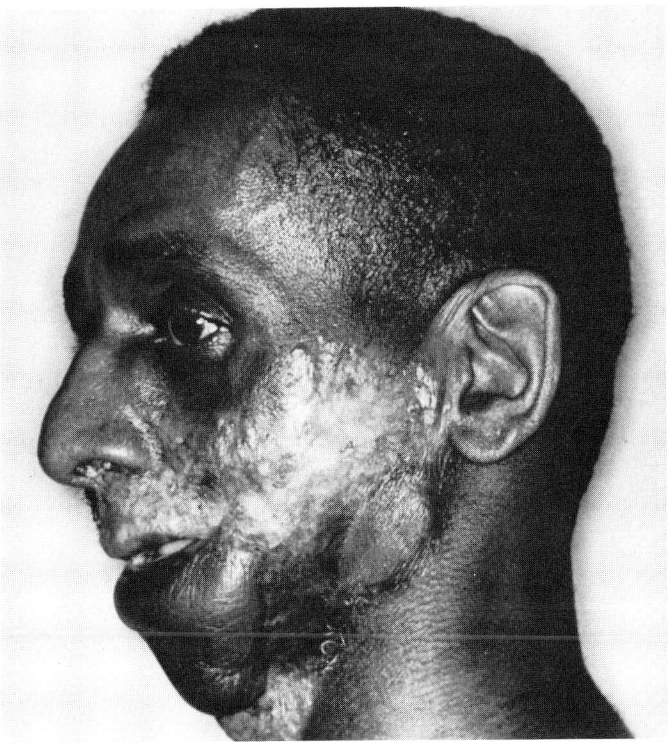

Figure 18–98. Lupus vulgaris. Scarring from several plastic procedures for treatment of multiple squamous cell carcinomas. Patient still has area of active disease on neck.

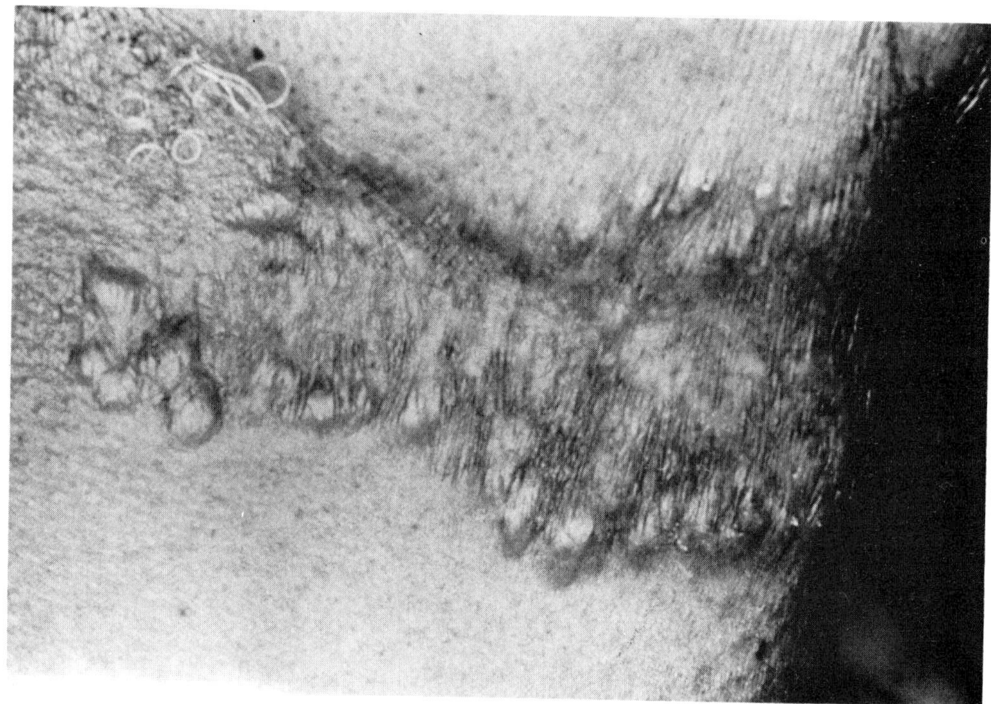

Figure 18–99. Lupus vulgaris. Plaque with active papular border and central scarring and depigmentation on neck of patient shown in Figure 18–98.

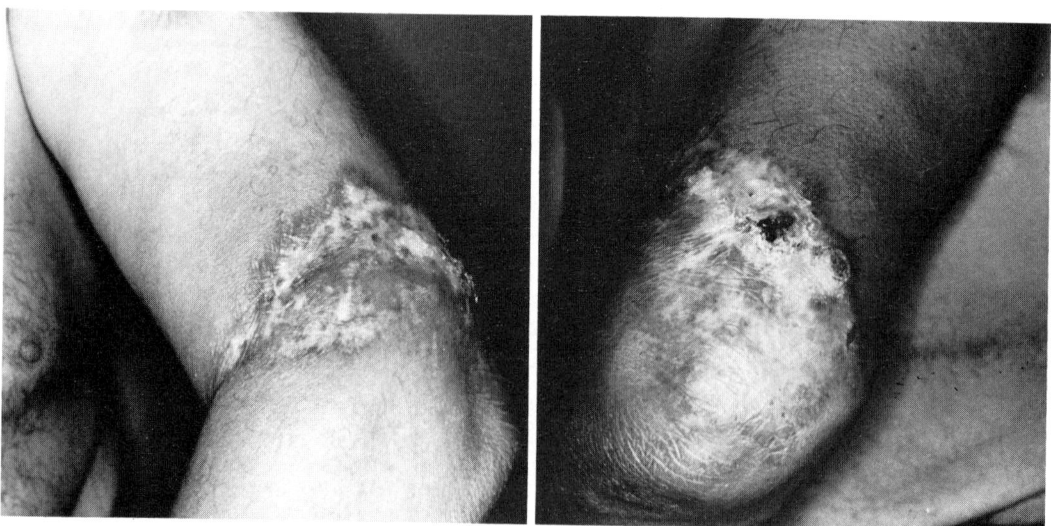

Figure 18–100. Lupus vulgaris on elbow.

Figure 18–101. Lupus vulgaris. Squamous cell carcinoma arising as crusted plaque. Same patient as in Figure 18–100.

If the reddish-brown plaque is pressed with a glass slide (diascopic examination), the blood vessels are compressed and the underlying tubercles appear as yellowish nodules (apple jelly). If not effectively treated, lupus vulgaris can increase in size indefinitely. A major complication of the infection besides horrible disfigurement is the development of highly invasive squamous cell carcinomas from the ulcerations and thick scars. In some patients, the clinical appearance of lupus vulgaris may be confused with LE, sarcoid, granuloma faciale, lymphadenosis benigna cutis, Bowen's disease, gumma, and blastomycosis. History, laboratory findings, and biopsy will distinguish one from the other.

Miliary tuberculosis in children and older persons can be associated with hematogenous spread of bacilli to the skin, resulting in papules, pustules, or purpura. Persons with severe pulmonary and gastrointestinal tuberculosis can develop oral and mucocutaneous lesions because of the large numbers of bacilli present in the mouth. The tip and lateral margins of the tongue and the hard and soft palates are primarily affected. The lesions appear as painful eroded papules and plaques that may be indistinguishable from the mucous patches of syphilis (Figs. 18–102 and 18–103). Mucocutaneous ulceration involving the lips can occur in advanced pulmonary and gastrointestinal tuberculosis; the perianal tissues in intestinal tuberculosis; and the vulvar region in genitourinary tuberculosis.[105, 106]

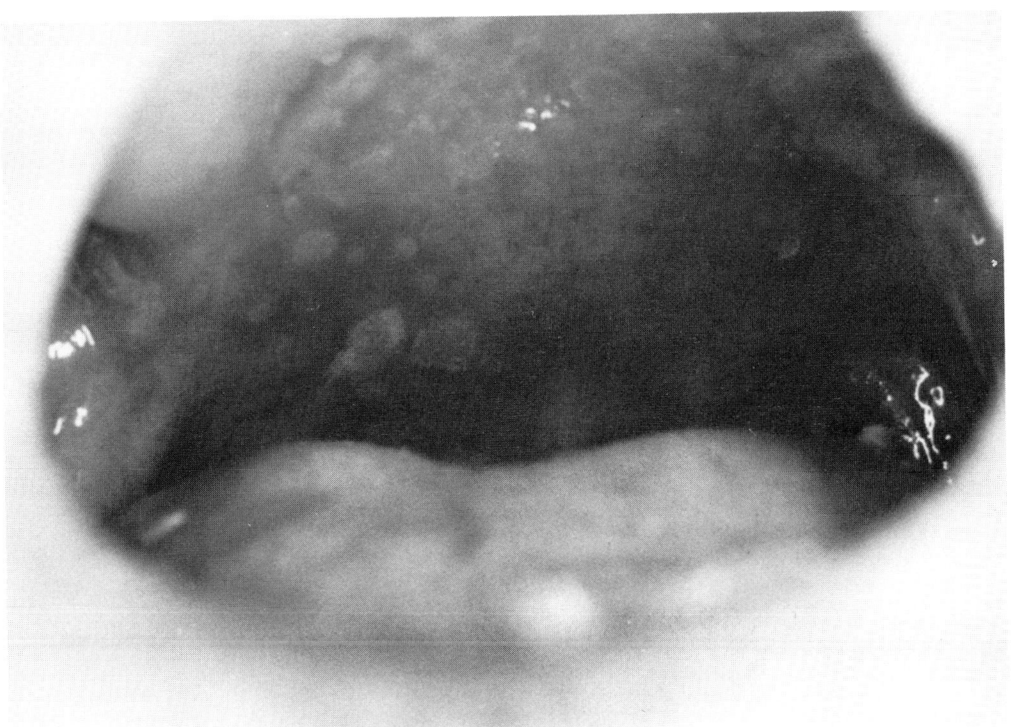

Figure 18–102. Miliary tuberculosis. Eroded plaques on mucosa of hard palate simulating mucous patches of syphilis.

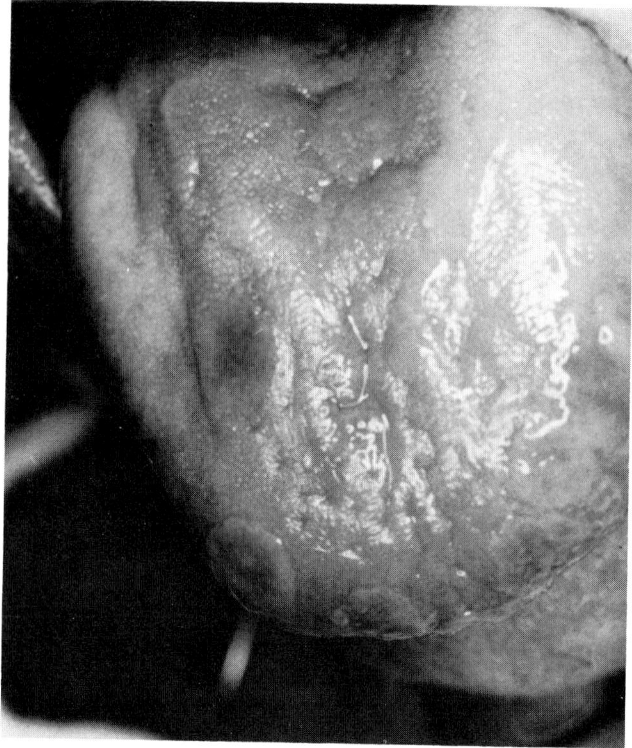

Figure 18–103. Miliary tuberculosis. Eroded plaques on tongue simulating mucous patches of syphilis.

Atypical Mycobacteria

The most common atypical mycobacteria producing cutaneous infections are *M. marinum*, discussed earlier, and *M. ulcerans* and *M. buruli*, responsible for ulcers of the legs in tropical countries and Australia. *M. fortuitum* can infect submaxillary cervical nodes to produce a picture resembling scrofula, and the skin to produce subcutaneous abscesses. *M. kansasii* is not considered to be a common pathogen, but it can produce chronic abscesses, verrucous nodular lesions, and papulopustules.[107] *M. kansasii* and *M. chelonei* have been isolated from patients with a sporotrichoid pattern similar to that produced by *M. marinum*.[108, 109] It is now becoming apparent that atypical mycobacteria can be significant pathogens in persons who are immunocompromised either by drugs, by underlying lymphomatous-leukemic disorders, or idiopathically.

Leprosy

Leprosy (Hansen's disease), which is caused by *Mycobacterium leprae*, exhibits a broad spectrum of clinical disease that is in large part determined by the patient's degree of cell-mediated immunity against the organism.[110-112] The disease can be divided into five major clinical groups that correlate reasonably well with the degree of bacterial proliferation in the tissues, the extent of granuloma formation, and the degree of cell-mediated immunity as measured by the reaction at three weeks to the

Table 18–1. CORRELATION OF FIVE-GROUP CLASSIFICATION OF LEPROSY WITH IMMUNOLOGIC REACTIVITY AND HISTOPATHOLOGIC FINDINGS

	TT	BT	BB	BL	LL
Lepromin reactivity (Mitsuda)	+	+/−	−	−	−
Bacilli in tissue	0	1+	2+	3+	4+
Granuloma formation	2+	1+	+/−	−	−
Macrophages with bacilli (foam cells)	−	−	+/−	+	4+

intradermal injection of lepromin (Mitsuda reaction) (Table 18–1). Tuberculoid leprosy (TT), characterized by well-developed cell-mediated immunity, is at one pole, and lepromatous leprosy (LL), in which there is anergy, is at the other. Both TT and LL are clinically stable conditions. In between, there are three clinical groups listed in the order of decreasing cellular immunity: BT (borderline tuberculoid), BB (borderline dimorphous), and BL (borderline lepromatous). For research purposes, two subpolar groups — TI (tuberculoid indefinite) and LI (lepromatous indefinite) — have been added, but as yet they have not improved the value of the basic five-group clinical classification. BT, BB, and BL are clinically unstable and patients with these forms can pass from lower to higher states and vice versa. Without therapy patients tend to develop weakening of their cell-mediated immunity and move toward LL. With therapy they tend to develop more cell-mediated immunity and progress toward TT. Although the reversal of disease activity toward greater cell-mediated immunity permits the host to contain and eradicate the bacilli better, this favorable change is accompanied by increased tissue destruction of affected nerves. This paradoxical reaction is responsible for the disabling neurological complications of leprosy. Currently, however, it is possible to modify these destructive reactions with corticosteroids, so that the patient can ultimately benefit from increased resistance while moderating the tissue destruction to some extent.

TT is usually a relatively benign, self-limited form of the disease in which there is eventual eradication of the infection by chemotherapy. The typical cutaneous lesions number one to a few, are asymmetric, and can appear as hypopigmented (partially depigmented) macules with well-defined borders and occasional scale (Figs. 18–104 and 18–105). The lesions can also be red to violaceous macules and plaques with clear centers. The borders of the plaques may be smooth or made up of papules. Clinically they can mimic sarcoidosis and mycosis fungoides. However, they are easily differentiated because eye lesions and hyperglobulinemia are not present in TT. The regional nerve trunk near the cutaneous lesion is usually thickened and palpable. The macule or plaque is also anesthetic: loss of sensation for light touch and heat. Sweating is also absent, so that the lesional skin feels dry and rough. The mucous membranes, nose, and upper respiratory tract are not affected. The nerves are involved early in the course of TT and are severely damaged as a result of the heightened tissue inflammation caused by cell-mediated hypersensitivity. (In LL, there is much less destructive inflammation directed against the nerves, which contain great quantities of bacilli, so that neural dysfunction is not as severe as in TT.) The nerves most commonly affected in TT are the greater auricular nerve (Fig. 18–106), the

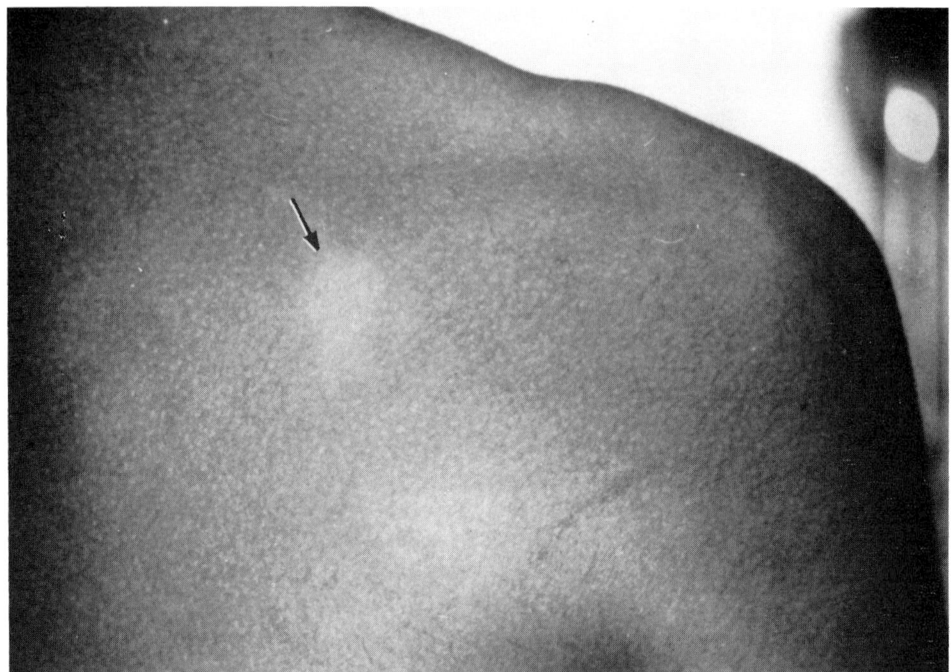

Figure 18–104. Hansen's disease. Hypopigmented anesthetic patch of tuberculoid leprosy (arrow). (Courtesy of Dr. Salvatore Romano.)

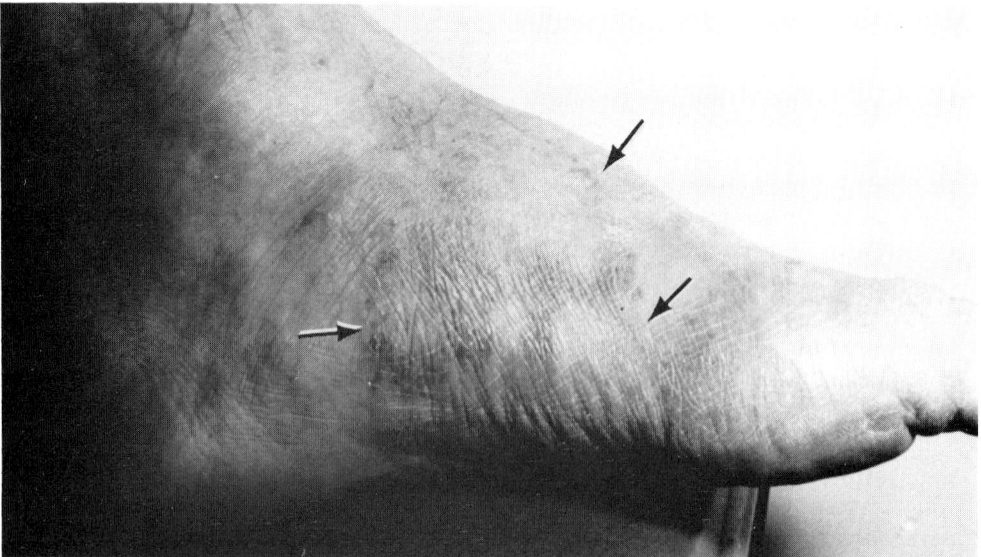

Figure 18–105. Hansen's disease. Oval patches with slightly scaly borders (arrows) producing a reticulated pattern. Tuberculoid leprosy acquired in South Pacific during World War II.

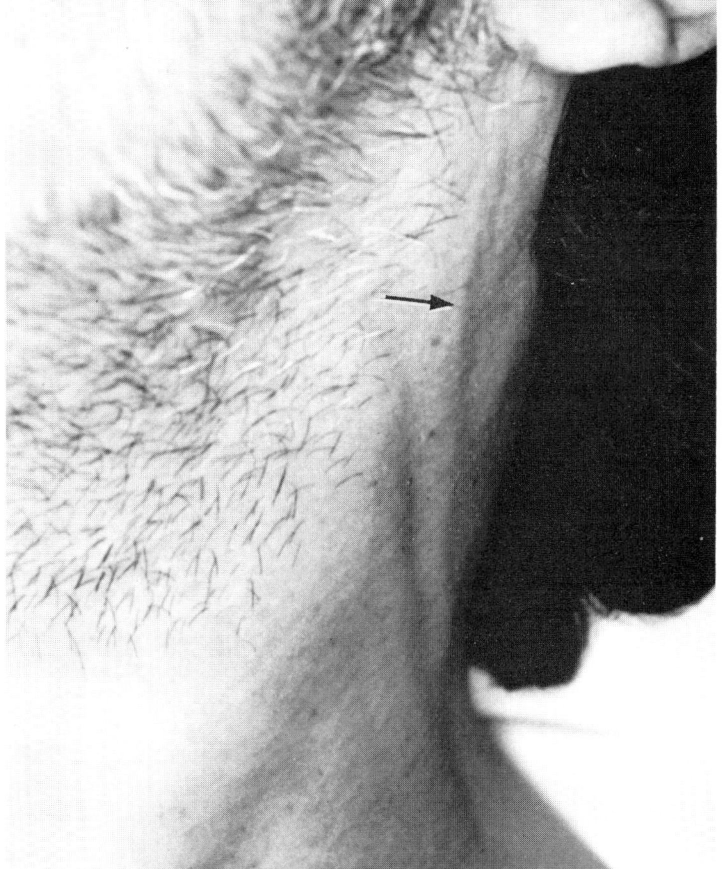

Figure 18–106. Hansen's disease. Lepromatous leprosy. Thickening of greater auricular nerve (arrow).

ulnar nerve, which is often associated with a claw hand (Fig. 18–107), and the sural, common peroneal, posterior tibial, radial, and supraorbital nerves. A patch of anesthesia may develop in normal-appearing skin because of involvement of an underlying nerve. Nerve involvement produces autonomic and sensory dysfunction, motor disturbances, and trophic changes in the skin. The skin may become dry, scaly, and atrophic. Perforating ulcers of the soles may develop, and the phalanges of the hands and feet and even the metatarsal bones can be resorbed, producing short, squatty fingers and toes. The fingers and toes do not drop off in leprosy; they shorten because of bone resorption. The eyelid muscles may become paralyzed, producing either keratitis or corneal exposure with ulceration. The testes and lymph nodes are unaffected in TT. There is more disability produced by "burned-out" TT than by LL.

In LL, the bacilli are able to multiply in the tissues without much restriction or containment. The bacilli are contained in macrophages (foam cells), which kill the organisms only very slowly. The macrophages proliferate in the skin to produce lesions that frequently mimic the lymphomatous diseases. The proliferating bacilli in the nerves produce clinically palpable cords and demonstrable neurologic dysfunction late in the course of LL, rather than early as in TT. Bacilli are also present in

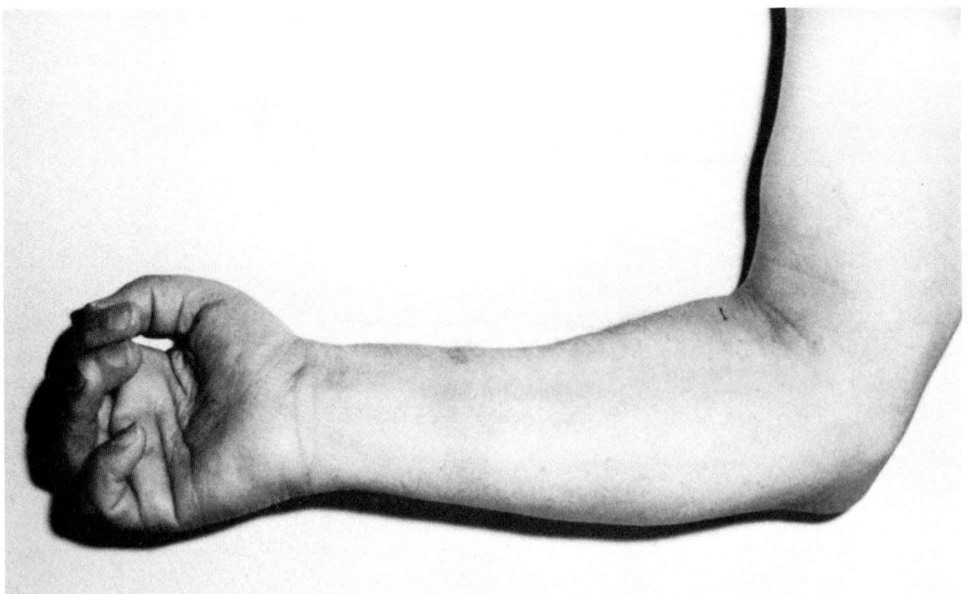

Figure 18–107. Hansen's disease. Tuberculoid leprosy producing claw hand because of involvement of ulnar nerve. Same patient as in Figure 18–105.

macrophages in lymph nodes, liver, spleen, bone marrow, and testes. The anterior portions of the eye are also affected: conjunctiva, cornea, sclera, iris, and ciliary body. The mucosae from the larynx to the nose are involved. However, areas of increased body temperature such as the flexures, axillae, and groin are unaffected. The cooler areas of the body are often involved: pinnae and lobes of the ears, nose, lips, and chin. The lesions of LL include macules, papules, plaques, and nodules (Figs. 18–108 to 18–111). The macules may be hypopigmented, red, or purplish and are not as sharply outlined as in TT. They are small, numerous, and often symmetrically distributed over the body. Neurological disturbances are usually not present in the macule and, if they are, they are not confined to it as in TT. The plaques and nodules are well defined and often red or purple. The plaques can have clear centers and be horseshoe shaped. The papules can simulate lichen planus. The nodules produce the typical leonine facies in far-advanced disease. In addition to the areas of increased skin temperature, the lesions of LL also appear to avoid the scalp, palms, soles, area between nasion and internal ocular canthi, and the midline of the back and intermammary zone — all sites where the skin is tightly bound down. Loss of eyebrows and eyelashes is characteristic of LL, but it does not occur in TT (Fig. 18–112). The cutaneous lesions of LL can be almost exact mimics of those of mycosis fungoides. In many cases it would be impossible to distinguish mycosis fungoides from LL by gross morphology alone.

In LL, the nasal mucosa is affected and the underlying cartilaginous septum may ulcerate, perforate, and eventually collapse to produce nasal deformities and a saddle nose (Fig. 18–113). Similarly, ulcerations can develop in the nasopharynx, pharynx, palate, and larynx. Tracheostomy may be required for laryngeal obstruction.

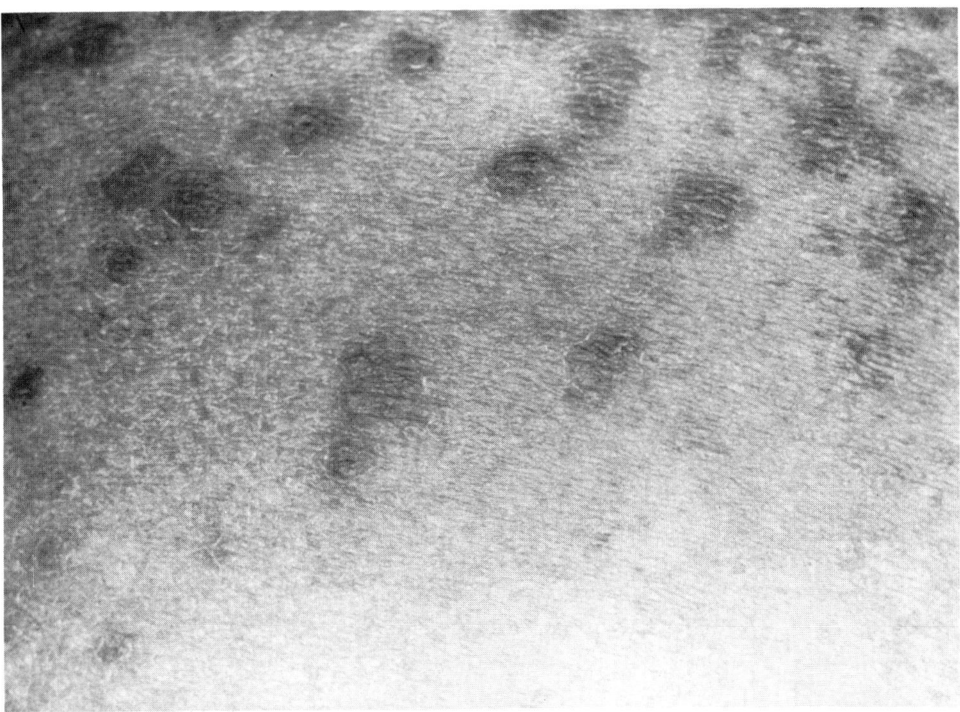

Figure 18–108. Hansen's disease. Lepromatous leprosy. Violaceous flat-topped papules and plaques suggestive of lichen planus. Same patient as in Figures 18–106, 18–109, and 18–110.

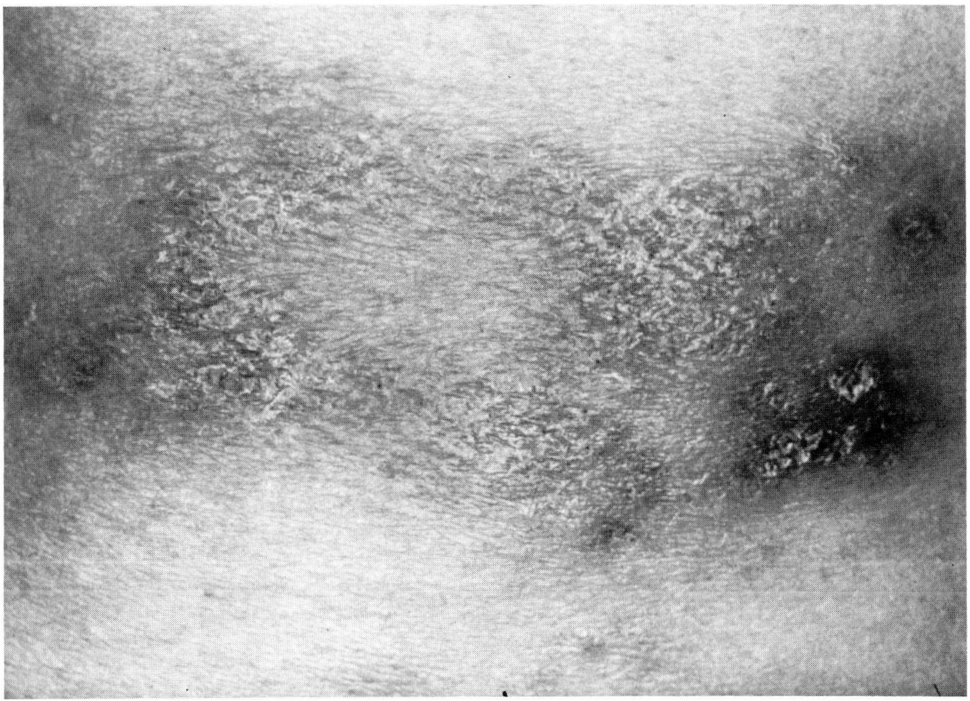

Figure 18–109. Hansen's disease. Lepromatous leprosy. Oval lesion with clear center and active scaly border.

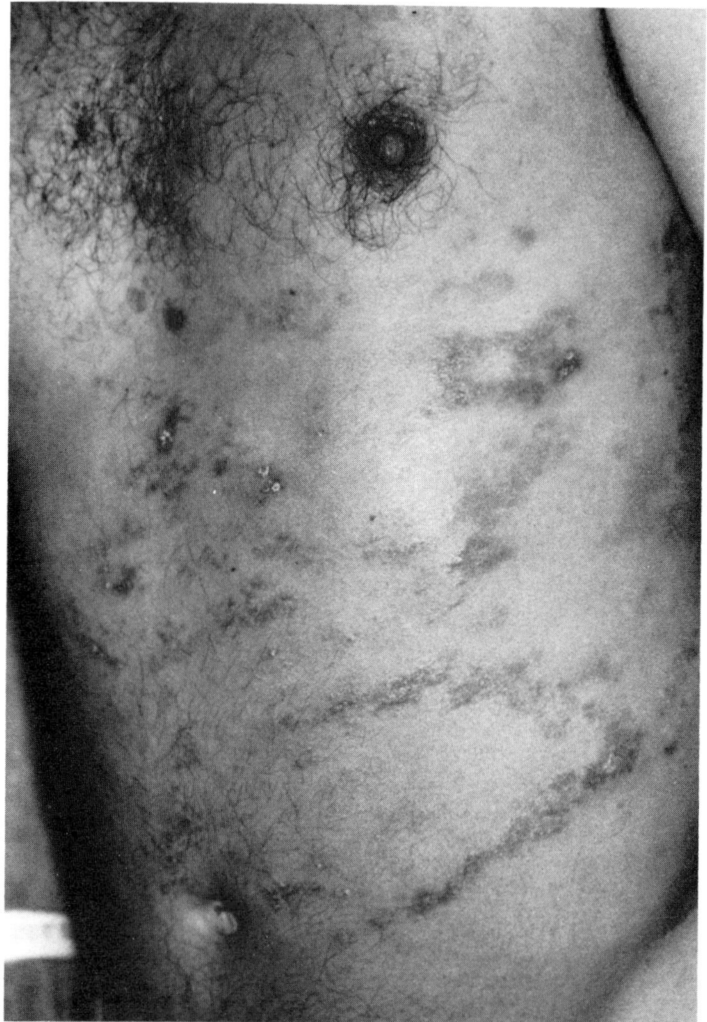

Figure 18–110. Hansen's disease. Lepromatous leprosy. Arciform lesions with active scaly borders.

Neural involvement is usually bilateral and symmetric in LL. The areas of anesthesia when they develop have a "stocking and glove" distribution, in contrast to TT, in which they are confined to the cutaneous lesions. The eventual nerve dysfunction in LL produces weakness and atrophy of muscles, resulting in widened palpebral fissures and drooping of upper and lower eyelids and oral commissures (Fig. 18–114). The finger tips may be tapered and the thenar and hypothenar muscles may be flat before the typical claw hand develops.

The skin lesions in BT, BB, and BL form a spectrum by becoming smaller, more numerous and symmetrical, and showing less correspondence between nerve dysfunction and skin lesion. The well-defined macules and plaques of TT begin to disappear, and the plaques and nodules of LL begin to become prominent. The diagnosis of BT, BB, and BL is based on the collective results of lepromin testing, numbers of bacilli and foam cells in the tissue, and the degree of granuloma formation and not just on the basis of the morphology of skin lesions.

Three reactional states occur in leprosy.[113] In the *reversal* lepra

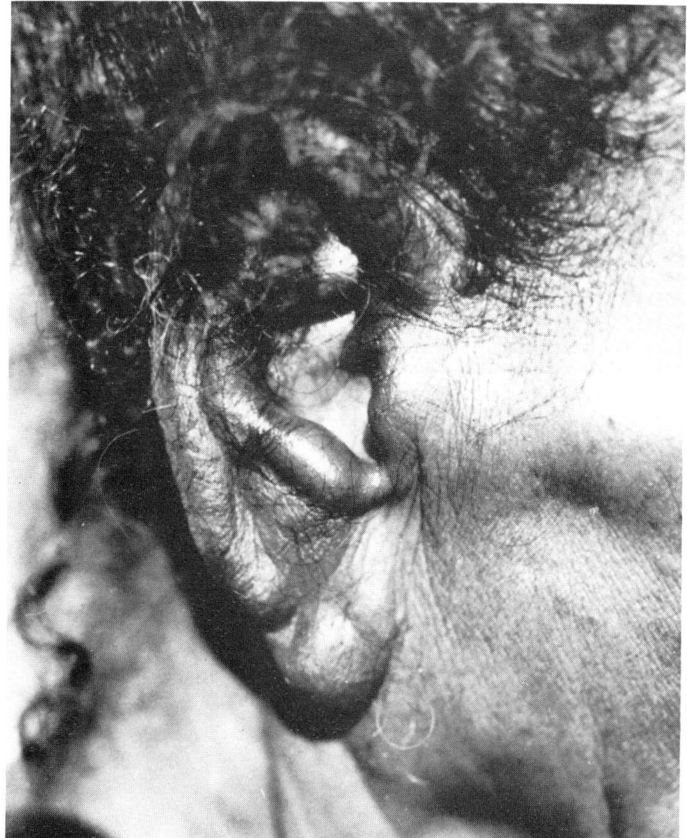

Figure 18–111. Hansen's disease. Lepromatous leprosy. Nodular formation on ear.

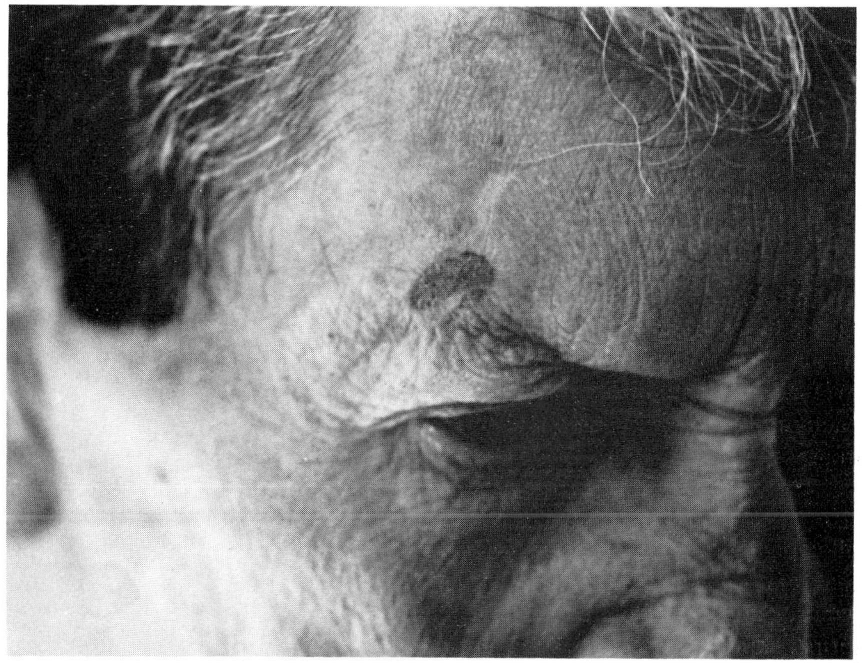

Figure 18–112. Hansen's disease. Lepromatous leprosy. Loss of eyebrows.

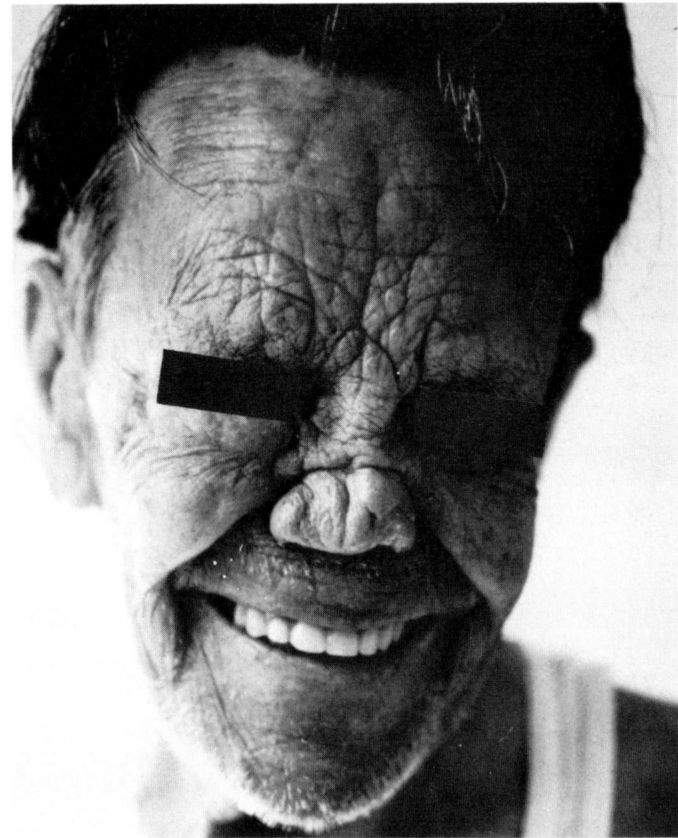

Figure 18–113. Hansen's disease. Lepromatous leprosy. Saddle nose and loss of eyebrows.

reaction, the patients develop increased cell-mediated immunity either spontaneously or following therapy, and they usually pass from the BB or BL state to BT. Clinically there is swelling of existing skin and nerve lesions. In severe reactions, ulcerations of cutaneous lesions develop accompanied by fever, malaise, and generalized edema. The reversal reaction usually develops during the first year of treatment. If not moderated by steroids, the sudden and severe nerve damage can result in profound loss of sensory and motor functions. The improved resistance to *M. leprae* is paid for at a high cost.

In the *downgrading* lepra reaction, there is a further depression of cell-mediated immunity. It may occur spontaneously or follow an intercurrent infection or disease. The clinical features are identical to the reversal reaction. Only by biopsy of the skin lesions and reevaluating skin reactivity to lepromin can one determine in which direction the disease is progressing.

The *erythema nodosum leprosum (ENL)* reaction occurs primarily in cases of LL and less commonly in BL. It can occur spontaneously or following therapy, intercurrent infections, pregnancy, childbirth, vaccination, and physical or mental stress. Clinically, patients have fever, malaise, and crops of tender, red papules and nodules that appear on normal skin in between existing lepromatous lesions that remain morphologically unchanged. Individual lesions last for one to seven days. In

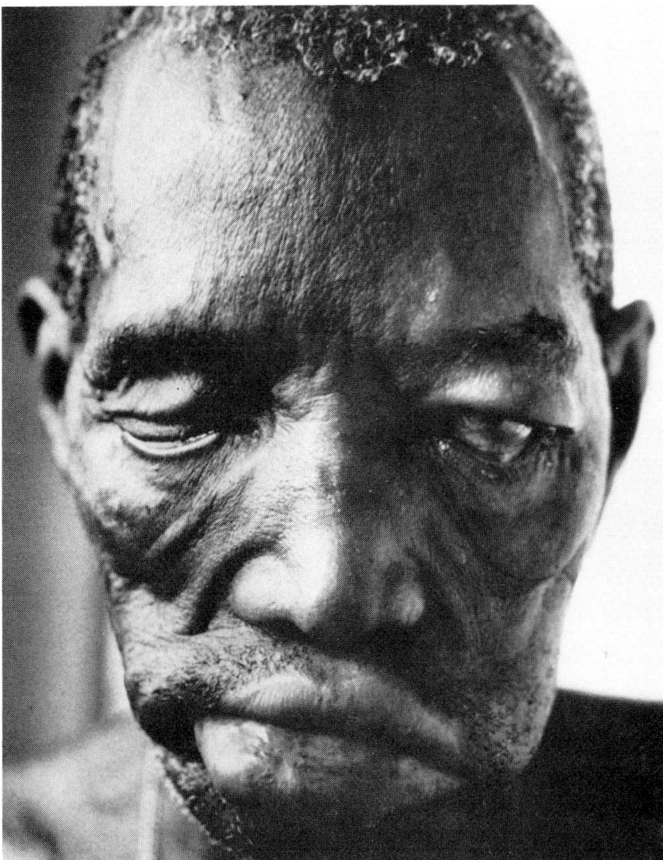

Figure 18–114. Hansen's disease. Lepromatous leprosy. Weakness and atrophy of facial muscles secondary to nerve dysfunction producing drooping of eyelids and lips.

severe attacks the lesions can develop into hemorrhagic blisters or ulcerations. The crops can continue for weeks, months, and, rarely, years. The basis of these lesions is a necrotizing vasculitis secondary to circulating immune complexes. Other features of ENL are generalized or dependent edema, neuritis, arthralgias, arthritis, epistaxis, iritis, lymphadenopathy, and orchitis. Without adequate treatment, iritis can lead to blindness and orchitis to sterility. Immune complex glomerulonephritis also occurs as part of ENL.

During these three reactions, chemotherapy should continue, with the addition of corticosteroids and clofazimine to control the lepra and ENL reactions or corticosteroids and thalidomide for ENL reactions.

LL leads to secondary amyloidosis of the kidney, spleen, liver, and adrenal glands because of its chronic inflammatory nature. It is also associated with polyclonal hypergammaglobulinemia and a variety of autoantibodies — rheumatoid factor, antinuclear antibody, and false positive serologic reactions — reflecting the disturbance in B and T cell interaction.

In Mexico and Central America a special manifestation of leprosy can be found — la lepra bonita, "the pretty leprosy."[114] In this form there is diffuse cutaneous infiltration without formation of plaques, nodules, or tumors. At first, the skin has a shiny or waxy appearance. Later facial features may thicken slightly and eyelashes, eyebrow, and body hair, except for scalp hair, are lost. The nasal septum may perforate, epistaxis may occur, and a saddle nose deformity may result. Symmetrical anesthesia of the distal extremities develops. Ocular involvement is rare. This form of leprosy is also called "pure and primitive" diffuse lepromatosis. It has also been seen occasionally in Spain and Asia. La lepra bonita exhibits a unique complication of leprosy, the Lucio phenomenon, which usually occurs three to four years after the onset of the disease.

The Lucio phenomenon is a severe necrotizing, ulcerating process that develops chiefly on the extremities but may also affect the buttocks, trunk, and rarely the face[114-116] (Fig. 18–115). The phenomenon begins as bluish, slightly infiltrated plaques with erythematous halos that evolve within 24 to 48 hours into cutaneous infarcts as large as 5 cm in diameter. The plaques may become bullous before they ulcerate. The ulcerations are often covered with crusts. The Lucio phenomenon can be recurrent — in one patient it was present only during pregnancy (four episodes in seven years), and in another, the attacks were precipitated by upper respiratory infections.[116] In most cases, the Lucio phenomenon is idio-

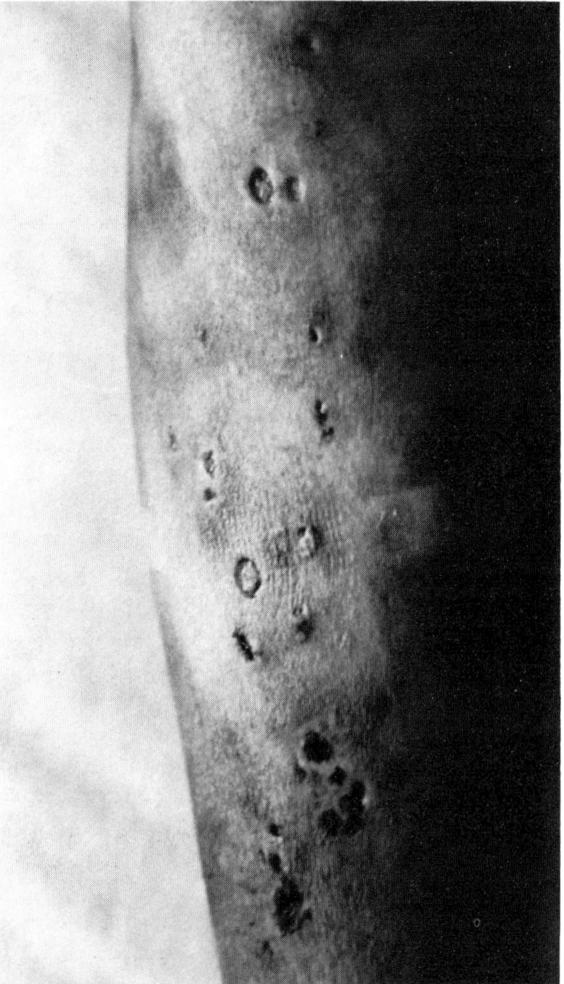

Figure 18–115. Hansen's disease. Lucio's phenomenon. Ulcerations on extremities are probably produced as a result of chronic disseminated intravascular coagulation.

pathic and not related to the institution of therapy. Fever and leukocytosis can be associated with the Lucio phenomenon. The process can last from two to four weeks to five months. Antileprosy therapy appears to exert no consistent effect on the initiation of healing.[116] Histologic study of the lesions in Lucio's phenomenon shows vascular changes of endothelial swellings, thromboses, and dermal necrosis. Acid-fast bacilli are present in the endothelial cells. Perivascular inflammation is mild and the infiltrate is composed primarily of lymphocytes.[115, 116] The histology is most compatible with chronic DIC and not leukocytoclastic angiitis, which had been thought to be present in some cases. It is possible that both mechanisms occur, but the infarctive appearance of the early lesions is more in favor of DIC or an arteritis of large vessels. The histology of the Lucio phenomenon is similar to that of acute meningococcemia. My interpretation is that the Lucio phenomenon represents DIC induced by bacteremia with *M. leprae*. The Lucio phenomenon needs to be reevaluated in terms of a presumptive underlying vasculitic process, because more stringent criteria are being applied to this diagnosis currently than were done in the early studies of the Lucio phenomenon.[114]

Indeterminate leprosy represents early disease that can evolve toward either pole or spontaneously heal. In this form of the disease, macules with ill-defined borders and varying degrees of hypopigmentation are present. Few bacilli are present in the lesions, histologically there is minimal involvement of nerves, and neurologically there is very little deficit. Indeterminate leprosy is most often diagnosed in contacts or endemic areas where the index of suspicion is high.

Syphilis

The syphilitic chancre begins as a papule at the point of inoculation of *Treponema pallidum* about three weeks after sexual contact.[117] It quickly breaks down to form a well-demarcated, punched-out, indurated nontender ulcer (Figs. 18–116 and 18–117). The chancre is tender if there is secondary infection. The regional lymph nodes are enlarged, firm, and nonsuppurating. Although chancres are usually single and appear on the glans, prepuce, coronal sulcus, or frenum, they may be multiple and may involve the shaft or base of the penis and scrotum.[118] Chancres can arise anywhere depending upon the patterns of sexual contact — lips, tongue, tonsils, eyelids, face, breast, fingers, and anus. In women, chancres are frequently present on the cervix, where they often pass unnoticed. They can also be found on the labia, fourchette, urethra, or anywhere on the perineum (Fig. 18–118).

Within one to 12 weeks (average three weeks) after the chancre has appeared, secondary syphilis develops. The chancre is usually healing as the secondary phase begins. Secondary syphilis can appear as long as six months after the infection begins but the usual duration is six to eight weeks. Secondary syphilis ought to be considered when the following features occur together: fever and malaise; generalized adenopathy; a widespread rash involving the face, trunk, genitals, palms, and soles and composed of lesions that are discrete and remain sharply demarcated rather than becoming confluent; and lesions involving the mucous membranes. The eruption in secondary syphilis is usually symmetrical and

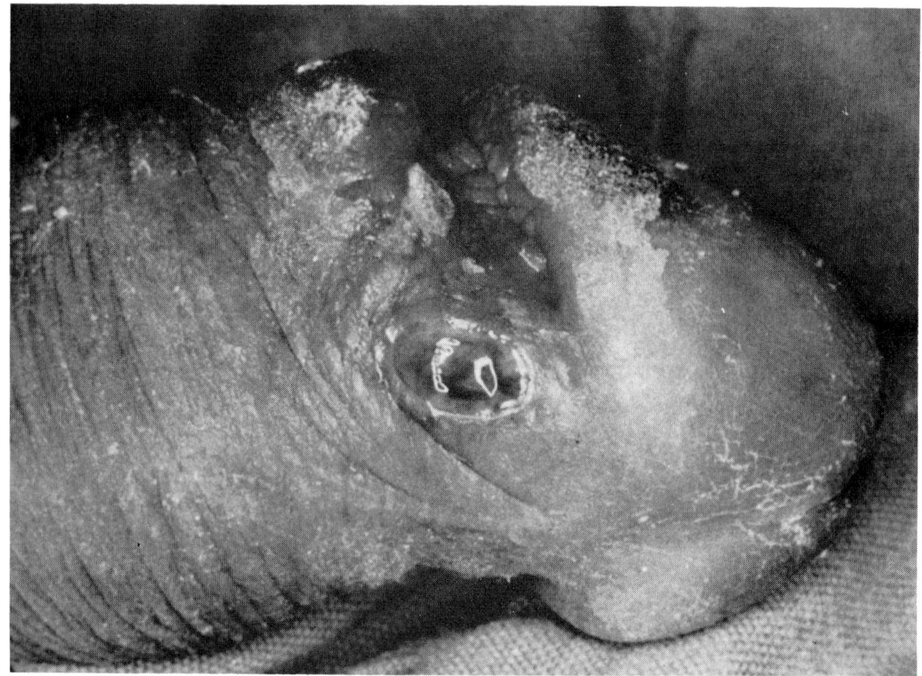

Figure 18–116. Syphilis. Penile chancre.

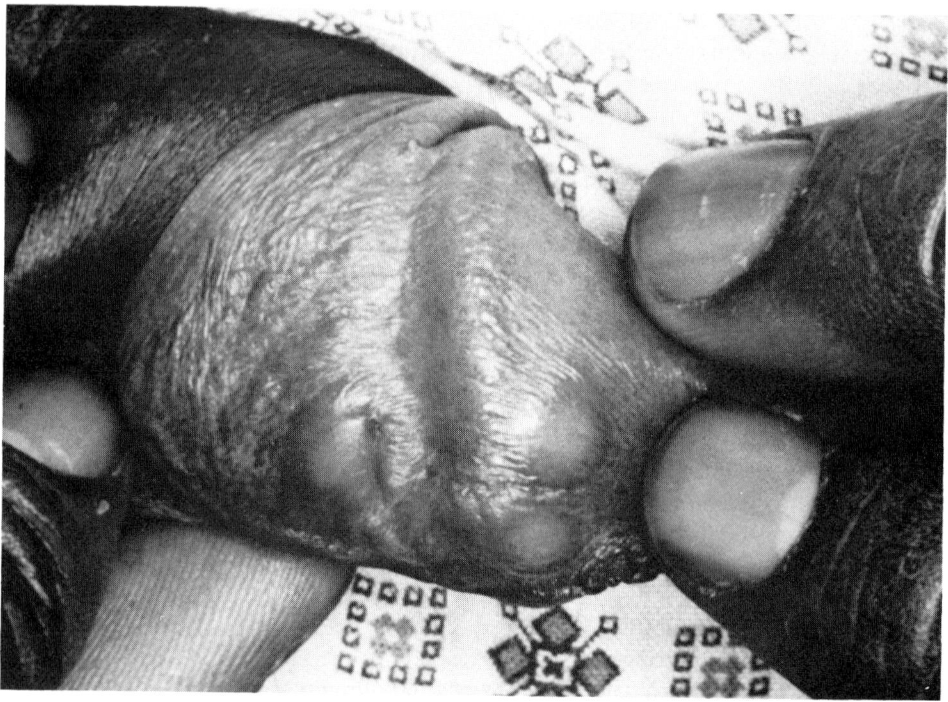

Figure 18–117. Syphilis. Multiple penile chancres.

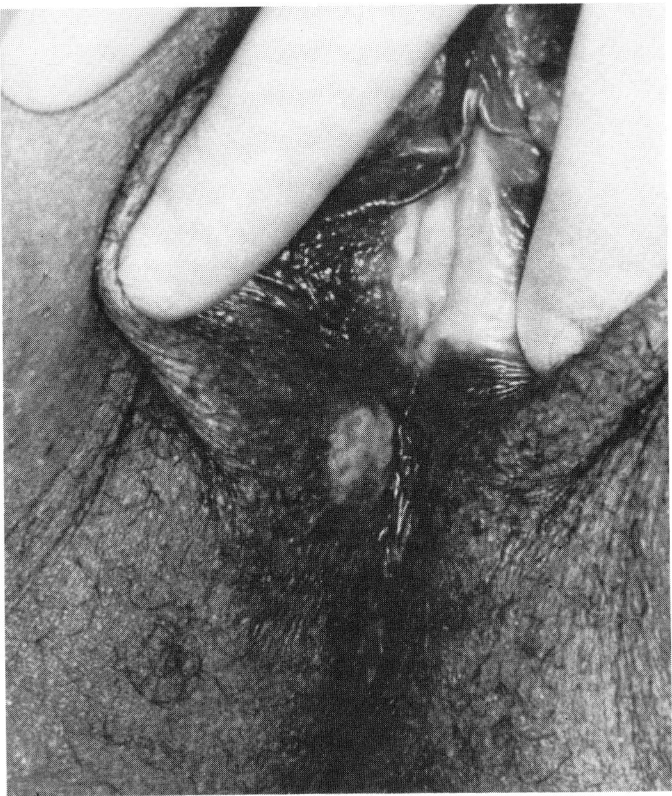

Figure 18–118. Syphilis. Chancre.

nonpruritic, but exceptions to this latter point do occur.[119] The cutaneous lesions of secondary syphilis can last for a few weeks or persist for as long as 12 months, but they usually heal spontaneously in two to ten weeks. In about 25 per cent of patients, the lesions can relapse and remit one to three times. Such relapsing lesions tend to be nodular, arciform, and asymmetric in morphology and location.

The lesions of secondary syphilis can be divided into macular, papular, and pustular types. Vesicular lesions are never a sign of syphilis in adults, but they can develop in congenital syphilis. The earliest rash of secondary syphilis is a red macular rash that arises on the trunk, shoulders, and extremities and only rarely affects the palms and soles. It lasts for one to two weeks before disappearing. It may be confused with measles, rubella, drug eruptions, tinea versicolor, and even seborrheic dermatitis if close attention is not paid to the eruption. The macular rash of syphilis remains discrete and is not scaly, thereby differentiating it from these other disorders. The macular rash does not always occur. The classic papular rash develops in the absence of a preceding macular rash or while the macular rash is present or fading. The papules are copper red and erupt on the face, palms, soles, chest, back, and abdomen (Figs. 18–119 and 18–120). They have a tendency to occur in groups or to spread peripherally to form annular, ring-shaped, or polycyclic patterns (Fig. 18–121). The annular lesions occur on the face in white patients, but are more commonly found on other areas of the body in black patients. The papules may be scaly and simulate psoriasis, but the scale is scanty and

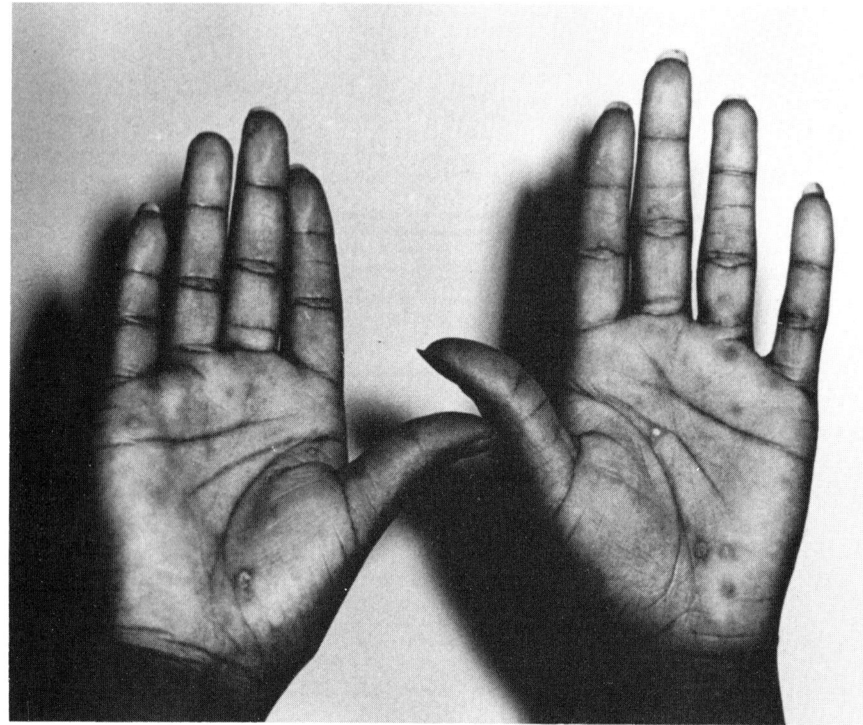

Figure 18–119. Syphilis. Palmar lesions of secondary syphilis.

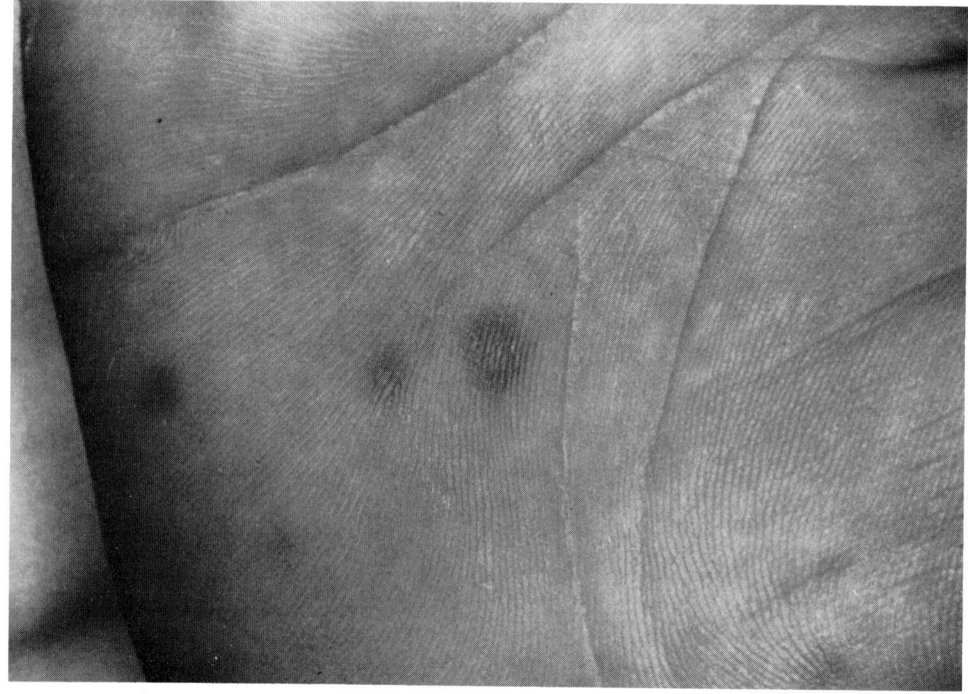

Figure 18–120. Syphilis. Palmar lesions of secondary syphilis.

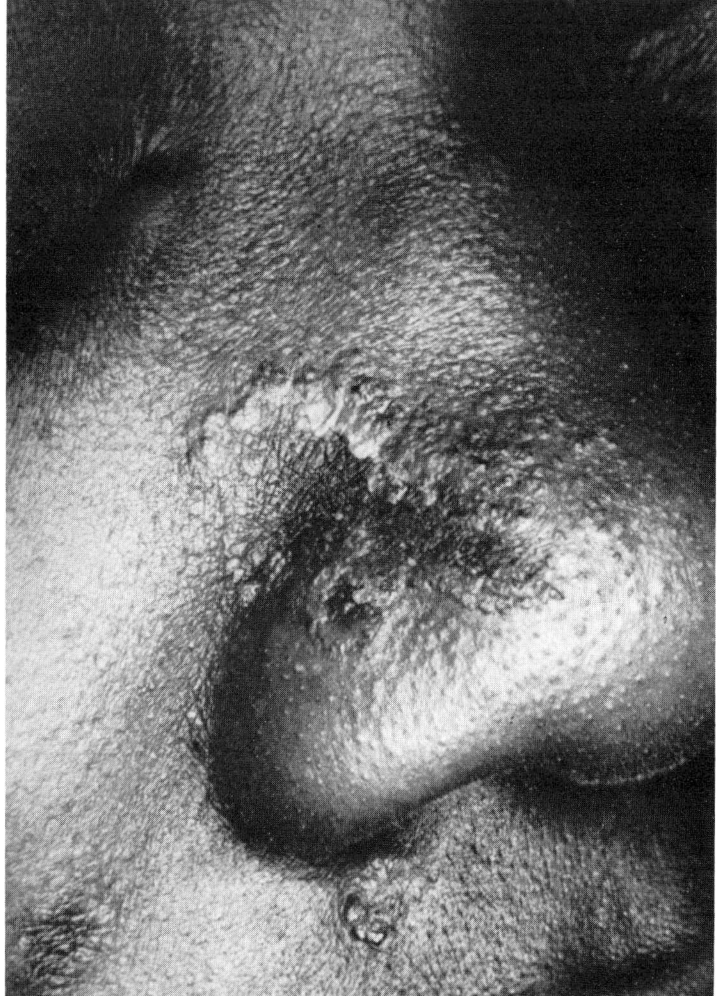

Figure 18–121. Syphilis. Annular lesion of secondary syphilis.

flakes off easily, unlike that found in typical psoriatic plaques. The papules may be lichenoid, simulating lichen planus,[120] but the involvement of the palms and soles is unusual in that disease. Minute papules can form around the openings of the follicles. These follicular papules are usually present in groups on the trunk, where they may be confused with an atypical pityriasis rosea and vice versa. However, the distribution of oval lesions along the lines of cleavage of the skin that is diagnostic of pityriasis rosea does not occur with the eruptions of secondary syphilis. Alopecia of the scalp and beard, usually described as "moth eaten" in appearance, and loss of eyebrows, eyelashes, and body hair are produced by these follicular papules, which represent infection around the hair bulbs. When the papules occur on the oral mucosal and the moist surfaces of the genitals, they form mucous patches — oval lesions with slightly raised borders that have superifical erosions or deeper ulcers covered by a grayish white membrane (Figs. 18–122 and 18–123). In warm moist areas of the body such as the labial folds, inner thighs, axillae, under the breasts, and even in the toe webs, the papules coalesce to form hyper-

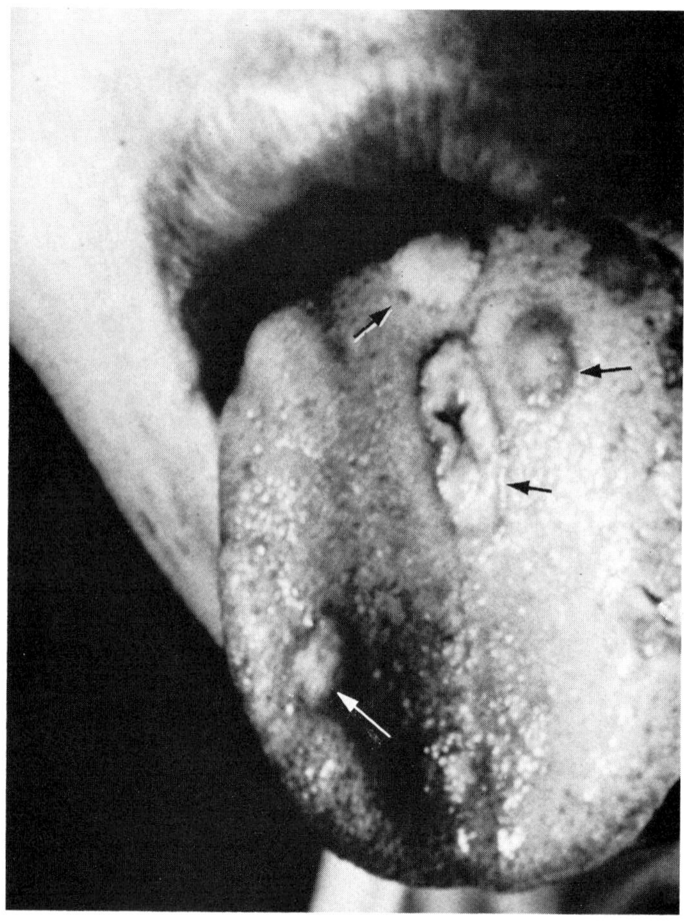

Figure 18–122. Syphilis. Mucous patches on tongue (arrows). (Courtesy of Dr. Hubert Merchant.)

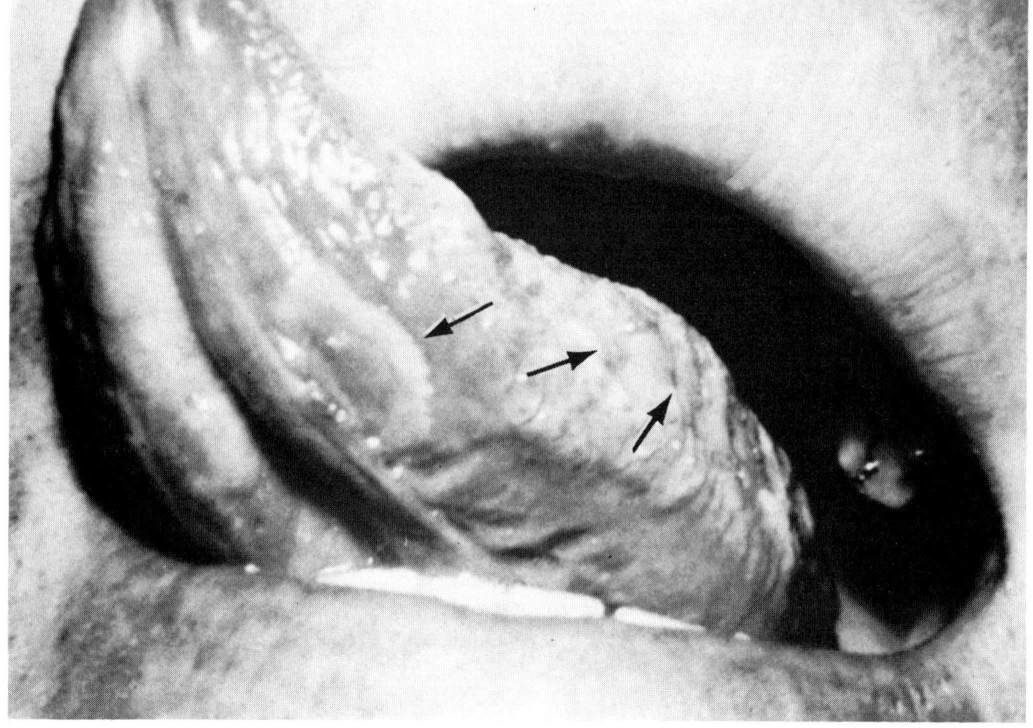

Figure 18–123. Syphilis. Mucous patches on tongue (arrows). (Courtesy of Dr. Hubert Merchant.)

trophic exuberant plaques that are moist with grayish, flat tops — condylomata lata. When they occur at the corners of the mouth they are called split papules (Fig. 18–124). The mucous patches and condylomata teem with spirochetes and are highly infectious. The papules may ulcerate and become crusted producing pustular lesions resembling impetigo or chickenpox. Persons with this type of lesion are generally sicker than those with the more common rashes of secondary syphilis. Rarely, the papules may enlarge or coalesce into nodules that break down to form large destructive ulcers.[121] The follicular and psoriasiform papules tend to be pruritic, in contrast to the other types, which are asymptomatic.

The nephrotic syndrome and hemorrhagic nephritis may be produced during secondary syphilis by circulating immune complexes composed of treponemal antigen–antitreponemal antibody complexes.[122]

Latent syphilis is a laboratory diagnosis. The patient is asymptomatic but has repeated positive blood serologies. The cerebrospinal fluid shows no evidence of syphilis.

The late (tertiary) stage is characterized by mucocutaneous, osseous, visceral, and cardiovascular lesions. The mucocutaneous and bony abnormalities often occur together. Cardiovascular syphilis characterized by aortitis leading to aortic insufficiency and aortic aneurysm is frequently associated with neurosyphilis. It is unusual for all four complications to occur together.

The cutaneous hallmark of late syphilis is the gumma, a granulomatous nodule that is thought to represent a hypersensitivity response to *T. pallidum*.[123] The gumma usually occurs one to ten years after infection in 15 per cent of untreated patients. The gumma in its simplest form begins as a small painless nodule, often at a site of trauma, especially over the

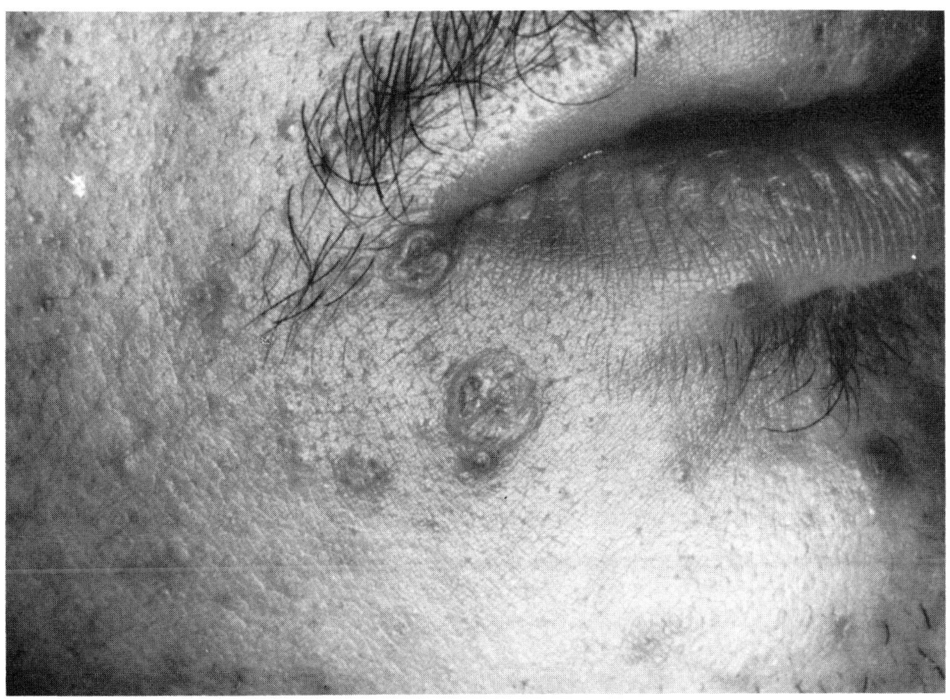

Figure 18–124. Syphilis. Split papule of secondary syphilis at oral commissure.

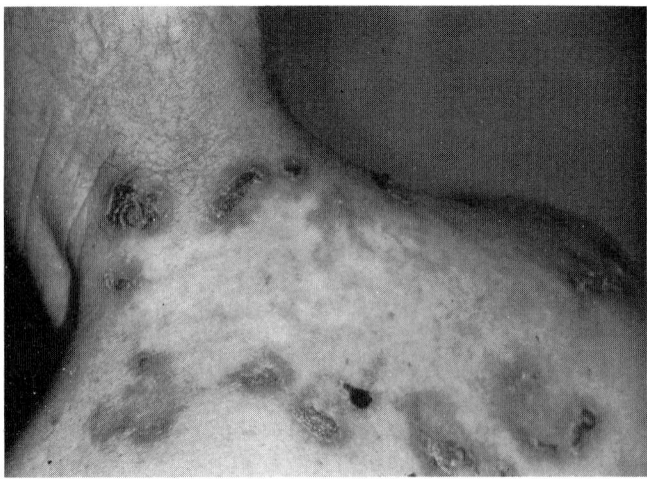

Figure 18–125. Syphilis. Nodulo-ulcerative lesions (gummas) of tertiary syphilis. (From Moschella, S. L., Pillsbury, D. M., and Hurley, H. J., Jr.: Dermatology. Philadelphia, W. B. Saunders Company, 1975, p. 715).

bones of the skull, sternum, clavicle, and tibia. The nodule increases in size, has a rubbery consistency, and is dusky in color. The gumma can resolve spontaneously, leaving a wrinkled scar, but it usually ulcerates, discharging a yellowish rubbery slough to produce a granulating base that heals with an atrophic wrinkled scar surrounded by a thin ring of hyperpigmentation. Gummas tend to occur in groups forming ringed, arciform, or polycyclic patterns (Fig. 18–125). The gummas expand centrifugally with punched out ulcerated borders. Healing with wrinkled, atrophic, noncontractile scars takes place behind the expanding borders. The noncontractile nature of the scar helps distinguish the gumma of late syphilis from similar-appearing lesions produced by tuberculosis of the skin, which usually have deforming contractile scars. Gummas affect mainly the skin and bones, but rarely they can involve the liver, stomach, larynx, and myocardium. Even rarer is their appearance during secondary syphilis.[124] Gummas of the nasal septum and hard palate can lead to perforation of these tissues. Gummas also can develop on the soft palate, tongue, lips, nasopharynx, and posterior pharyngeal wall. Gummas involving sites other than the skin often produce gross tissue destruction with scarring and deformities upon healing.

Congenital Syphilis

The cutaneous lesions of congenital syphilis usually develop before the age of three months in 50 per cent of cases, before six months in 80 per cent, and before age two years in the remainder.[125] Infants developing syphilis *in utero* before the fourth month develop a pattern of cutaneous lesions that is different from the pattern produced by an infection contracted in the last three months of pregnancy.

Infants who have been infected with syphilis early in pregnancy may have a weeping eczematous eruption around the mouth or over most of the face, except the nose. A similar eruption may be present around the anal region, in the groins and axillae, and about the neck (Figs. 18–126 and 18–127). Fissuring is present in these acute dermatitic areas and leads to

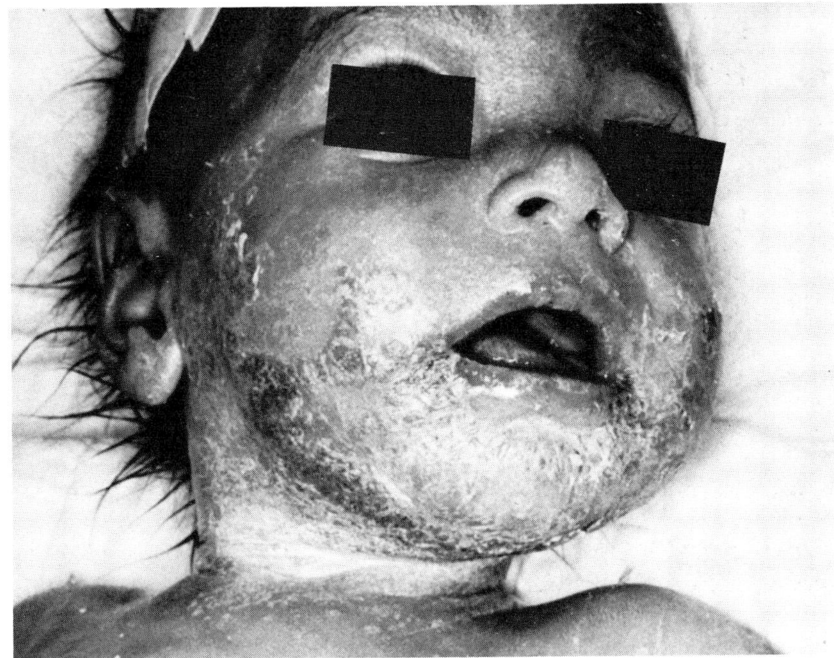

Figure 18–126. Congenital syphilis. Eczematous eruption around mouth.

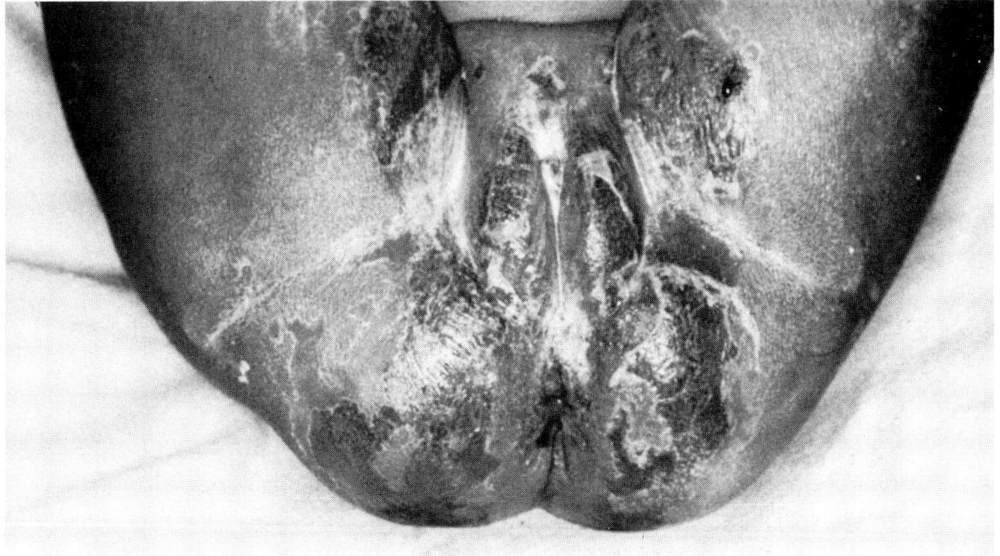

Figure 18–127. Congenital syphilis. Eczematous eruption with erosions on perineum.

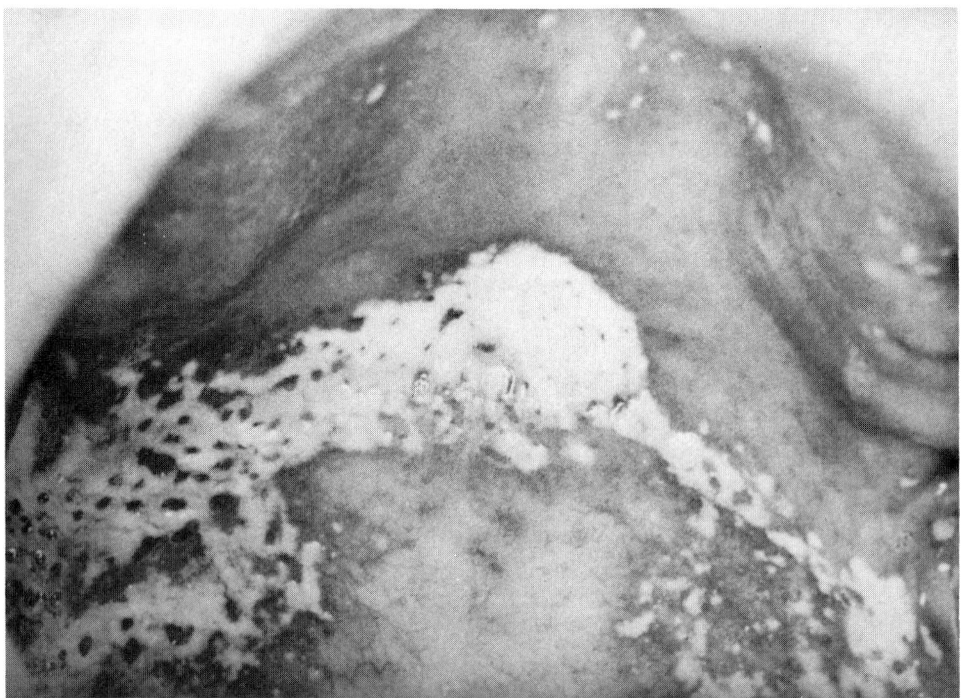

Figure 18–128. Candidiasis. Cheesy white exudate on erythematous base.

permanent linear scars around the mouth, called rhagades, after the skin has healed. *T. pallidum* can be demonstrated in the areas of weeping dermatitis. Other cutaneous signs may include bullae on the palms and soles as well as the other areas of the body; red palms and soles that have a shiny appearance and develop desquamation several days after birth; mucous patches in the mouth and throat and a roseola-like macular eruption. Almost every case exhibits "snuffles" — swelling of the nasal mucosa because of syphilitic involvement, producing nasal obstruction with a mucosanguinous discharge. The nasal cartilage and bone are often affected as well, leading to a saddle nose and underdevelopment of the maxillary bone. These children also have generalized lymphadenopathy, hepatosplenomegaly, and sometimes ascites.

The children who are infected late in pregnancy develop a pattern of lesions which is similar in every respect to that of the adult patient. A tertiary stage also occurs in congenital syphilis and the gumma is the characteristic lesion as in adults.

If the diagnosis of syphilis has been missed in early infancy or inadequately treated, various signs and symptoms may appear later in life. The best-known of these stigmata is Hutchinson's triad: interstitial keratitis that appears at any time from age 5 to 25 years; abnormalities of the permanent upper central incisors, in which there is thickening in the anterior-posterior dimension and central notching along the bite margin; and eighth nerve deafness, which develops at puberty. Other stigmata include abnormalities of the six year molars, which have four dwarfed cusps and are prone to rapid decay (mulberry molars); rhagades, the radiating scars around the mouth caused by the facial eczematoid eruption; frontal bossing produced by periostitis of the frontal and parietal bones; depressed saddle nose, shortened maxilla, and high arched palate related to the rhinitis ("snuffles"); perforation of the nasal septum and palate by gummas; thickening and anterior bowing of the tibia (sabre shins) and thickening of the sternoclavicular portion of the clavicle (Higouménakis's sign), both produced by periostitis; and painless hydrarthrosis of the knees and sometimes the elbows (Clutton's joints), which usually appears at puberty.

Candidiasis

Most instances of candidiasis develop because of an alteration in host defense by factors that are correctable. Repeated infections are often caused by recurrence of these predisposing factors. However, in a minority of patients candidiasis is a chronically persistent infection with frequent acute exacerbations. Most, but not all, of these latter individuals have a demonstrable defect in cell-mediated immunity to the antigens of *Candida albicans*.

Most instances of candidiasis take one of the following forms. The term *thrush* is commonly used to describe the cheesy white exudate of candidiasis which affects the tongue and oral mucosa (Fig. 18–128). Involvement of the commissures of the mouth is called *perlèche* or *angular stomatitis*. When the whitish exudate is gently scraped off the mucosal surfaces, the underlying tissue is intact and bright red with vascular congestion. If there are underlying ulcerations, then the correct diagnosis has not been made. In such cases, the presumed whitish exudate usually represents the nonviable epithelial roof of a blistering disorder such as erythema multiforme, primary herpes simplex, or pemphigus. It is extremely rare for candidiasis to produce erosions in the mouth. Microscopic examination of the cheesy exudate will show pseudohyphae and budding yeasts. Candidiasis commonly involves the inner thighs, perianal area, vagina, vulva, scrotum, umbilicus, axillae, and inframammary areas (Figs. 18–129 and 18–130). In extensive infections the buttocks, intergluteal folds, and lower back can be affected. The infection appears as bright red edematous plaques with irregular advancing borders. Erythematous papulopustules are present as satellite lesions just beyond the spreading margins. Dermatophyte infections, such as *Trichophyton rubrum* or *Epidermophyton floccosum*, which also produce infections in these sites, are not accompanied by satellite lesions, nor do they involve the scrotal skin. Psoriasis can also produce bright red, sharply marginated plaques without scale in the perineal and intertriginous areas (Figs. 18–131 and 18–132). Satellite lesions are absent in psoriasis. However, sometimes psoriatic plaques are secondarily infected by *C. albicans*.

The factors predisposing to these common forms of candidiasis include treatment with penicillin, broad-spectrum antibiotics, and birth control pills; increased temperature and moisture in the relatively occluded intertriginous and perineal areas, which can be made worse by hot, humid weather or urinary and fecal incontinence; diabetes mellitus; and chronic corticosteroid therapy. The diaper rash in infants is caused in large part by candidiasis. The vulvar itching in most cases of diabetes mellitus and pregnancy is produced by vaginal candidiasis. Angular stomatitis occurs because the upper lip overhangs the lower one to produce a pocket in which moisture is retained. This overhang may be an

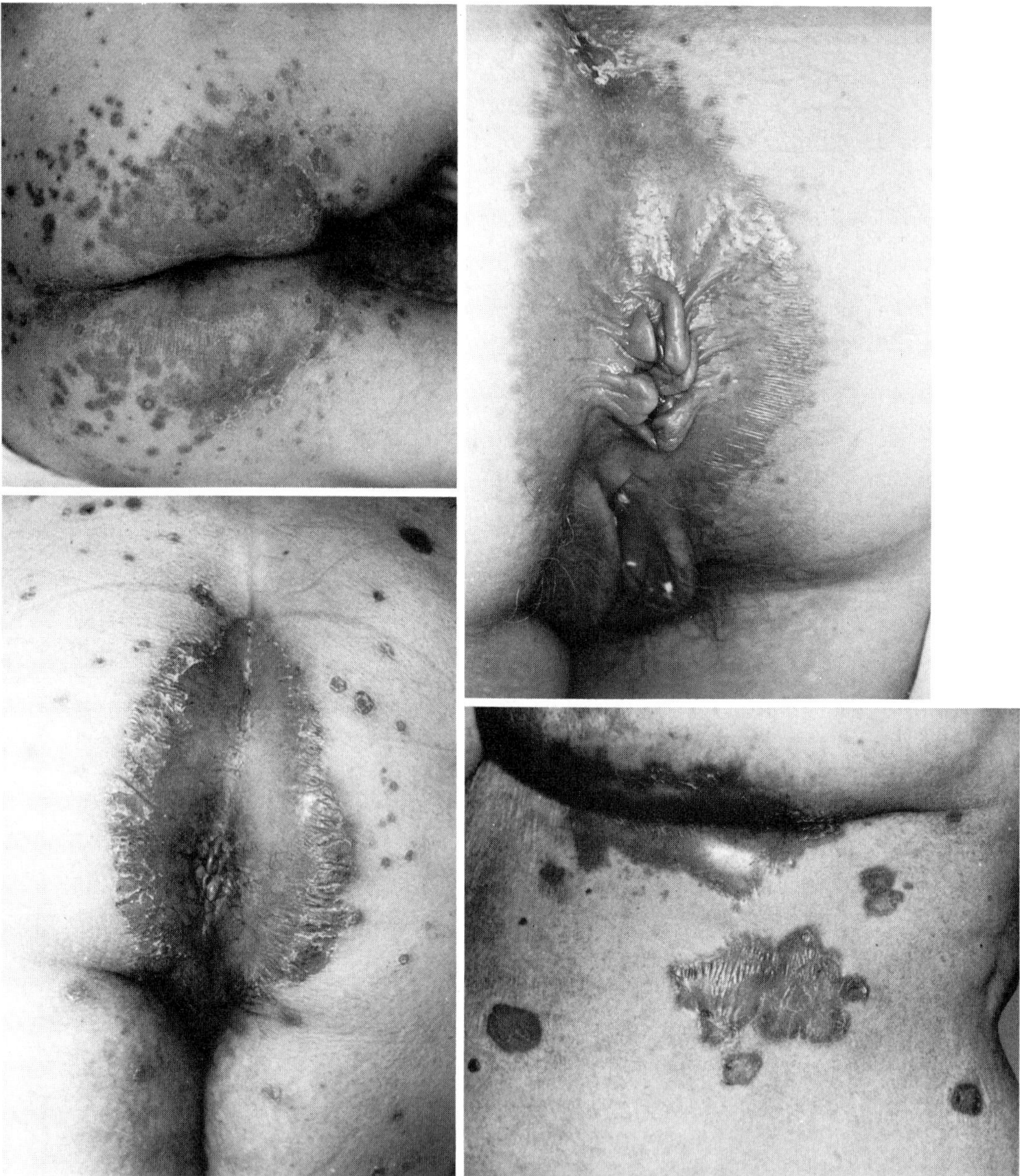

Figure 18–129. Top left. Candidiasis. Diffuse erythema with satellite lesions.

Figure 18–130. Top right. Candidiasis. Diffuse erythema with satellite lesions.

Figure 18–131. Bottom left. Psoriasis. Erythematous plaques with satellite lesions simulating candidiasis.

Figure 18–132. Bottom right. Psoriasis. Intertriginous involvement simulating candidiasis.

anatomical abnormality or may result from poorly fitted dentures. Correction of the overhang will often eradicate or lead to better control of the candidiasis. In some individuals with dentures, candidiasis develops on the hard palate under the appliance.

Bartenders, dishwashers, and others who constantly immerse their hands in water for long periods of time develop maceration, which predisposes them to candidiasis involving the second and third interdigital spaces and the periungual tissues (Figs. 18–133 and 18–134). Infection of the glans penis occasionally follows sexual intercourse, often with a partner who has an asymptomatic vaginal candidiasis. Candidal balanitis is characterized by patches of erythema studded with pustules (Fig. 18–135). The predisposing factors underlying these forms of mucocutaneous candidiasis are usually correctable or avoidable so that the infections can be successfully treated.

Chronic mucocutaneous candidiasis can be divided into four major clinical groups for purposes of discussion, without implying homogeneity for any group in terms of etiology and pathogenesis.[126, 127]

(1) Chronic candidiasis of the mouth, tongue, lips, nails, and vagina develops in children with the congenital polyendocrinopathy syndrome of hypoparathyroidism, hypothyroidism, adrenal insufficiency, and vitiligo. The candidiasis is limited to these sites and does not extend beyond them. Chronic infections of the tongue and buccal mucosa with *C. albicans* often produces a thickened white plaque instead of the easily dislodged cheesy exudate seen in acute infections (Fig. 18–136). A deficit in cell-mediated immunity to *C. albicans* appears to be responsible for the infection in some of these children (see p. 641).

(2) Chronic mucocutaneous candidiasis also develops in children older than age five in the absence of polyendocrinopathy. The yeast infection may be limited to the lips with chronic erythema and recurrent desquamation, as illustrated by one of our patients in Plate 41*F*. The chronic candidiasis may involve the mouth, tongue, lips, vagina, and nails as described in children with congenital hypoparathyroidism (Figs. 18–137 and 18–138). Another group of patients has the candidal granuloma syndrome. In addition to the multiple sites listed above, infections also occur on the scalp, face, extremities, and trunk (Figs. 18–138 to 18–141). These infections are unique in that marked hyperkeratotic papules and plaques develop at the cutaneous sites of infection. Mounds and columns of horny material arise from the skin of the scalp and face (Figs. 18–142 to 18–144). The nose and fingers can be encased by hyperkeratotic cocoons (Figs. 18–145 and 18–146). These particular cutaneous infections begin as erythematous macules that become boggy and elevated before developing massive hyperkeratotic horns on their surfaces. Treatment with intravenous amphotericin B is followed by disappearance of the lesions for six to 36 months in many cases. The initial response to treatment is a disappearance of the erythema and edema at the base of the horn followed by slow spontaneous separation of the hyperkeratotic horn from the underlying epidermis. In one of our patients whose thumb was affected, the horny growth separated as an intact outer casing. Scarring of the underlying skin is absent or minimal. Most but not all of these patients have an identifiable defect in cell-mediated immunity ranging from complete anergy to anergy only for candidal antigens.[127] Although this syndrome is not associated with polyendocrinopathy or isolated hypoparathyroidism, a few patients

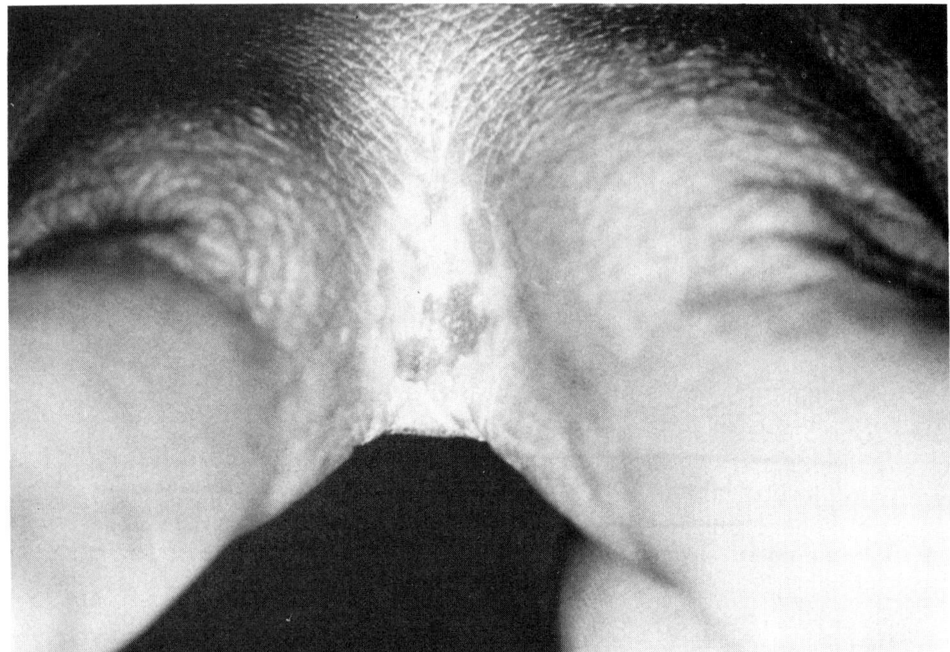

Figure 18–133. Candidiasis. Involvement of finger web producing maceration and fissuring.

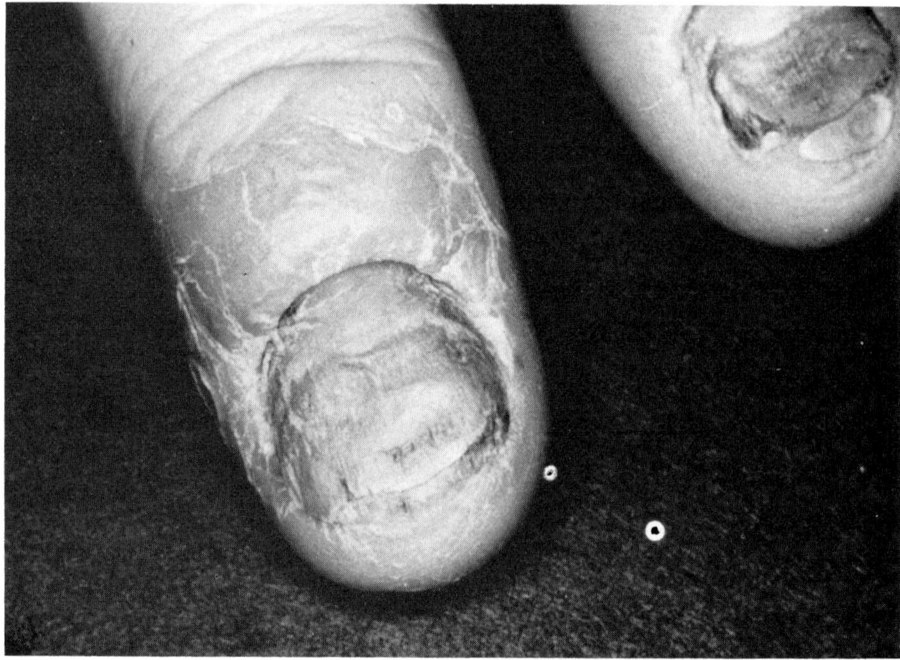

Figure 18–134. Candidiasis is usual cause of chronic paronychia.

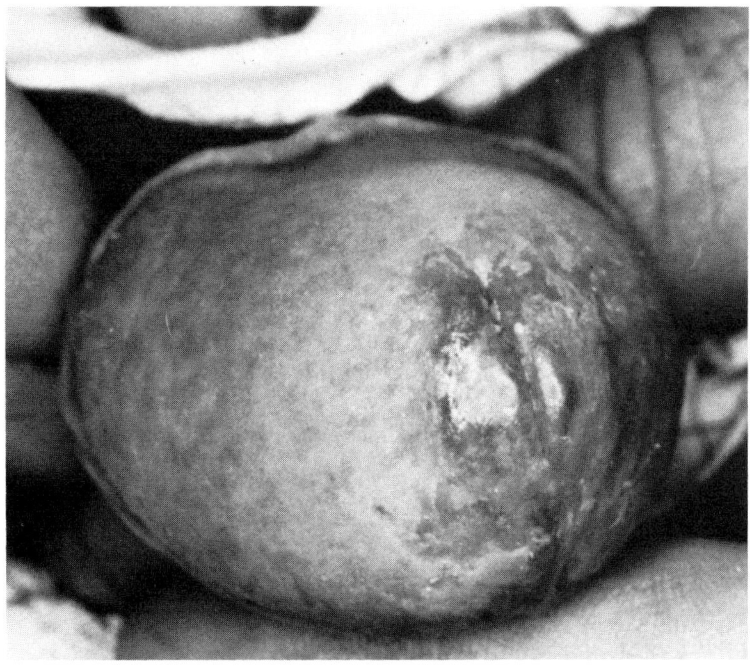

Figure 18–135. Candidal balanitis.

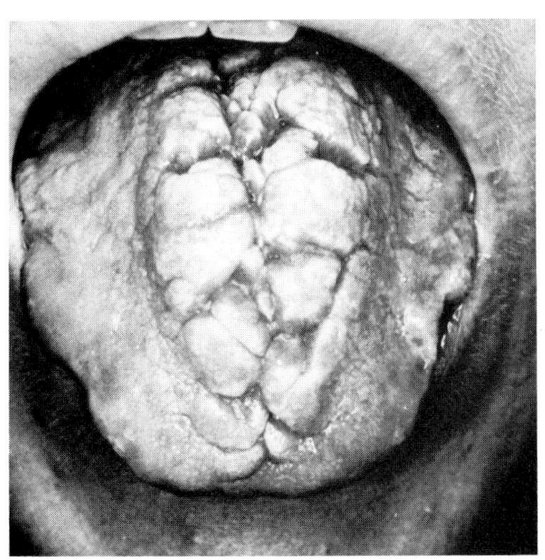

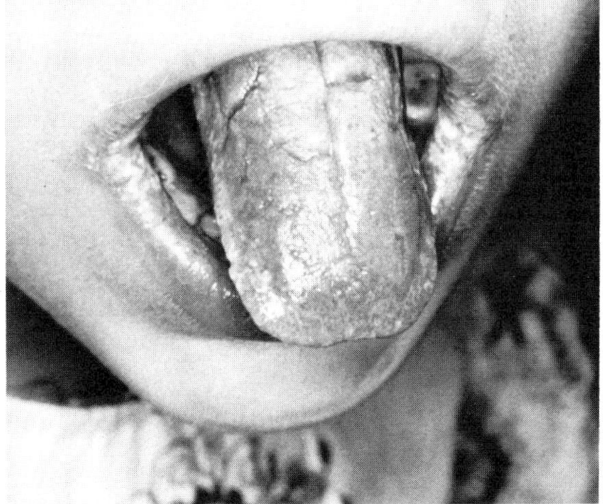

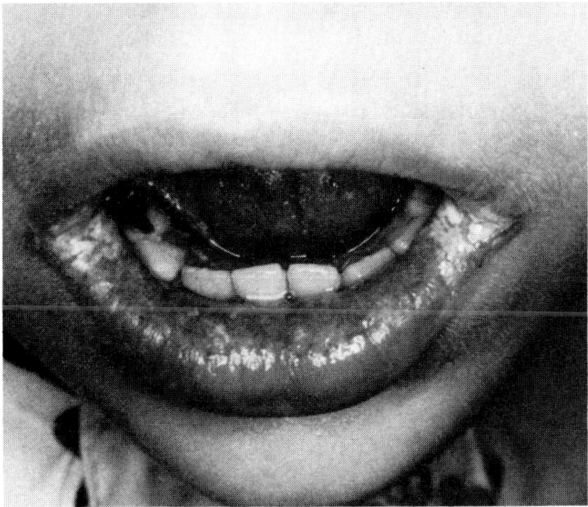

Figure 18–136. Top left. Chronic mucocutaneous candidiasis producing thickened white plaques on tongue.

Figure 18–137. Top right. Chronic mucocutaneous candidiasis involving tongue and lips.

Figure 18–138. Bottom. Chronic mucocutaneous candidiasis involving lips and oral commissures. Vermilion border of lower lip is red and edematous.

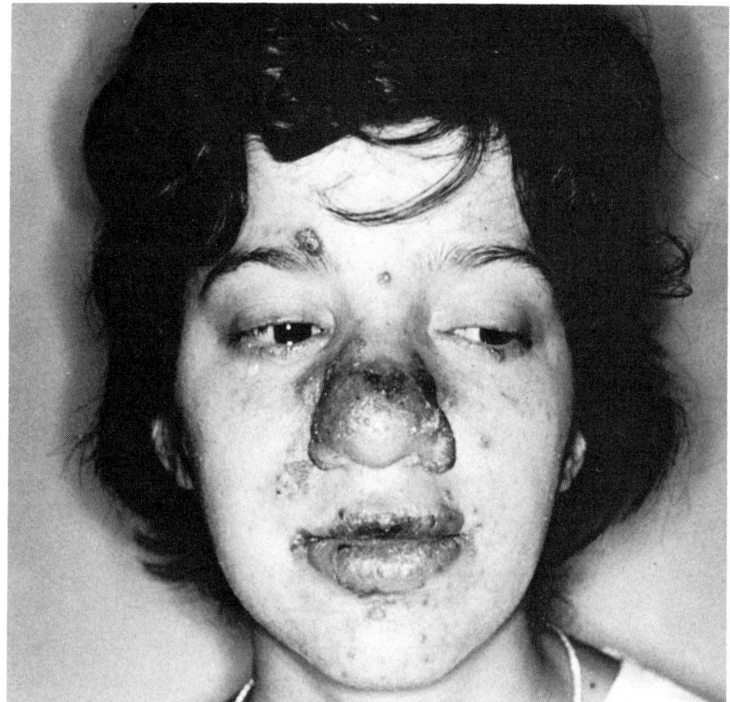

Figure 18–139. Chronic mucocutaneous candidiasis producing hyperkeratotic papules and plaques (Candidal granuloma syndrome). Pre-treatment.

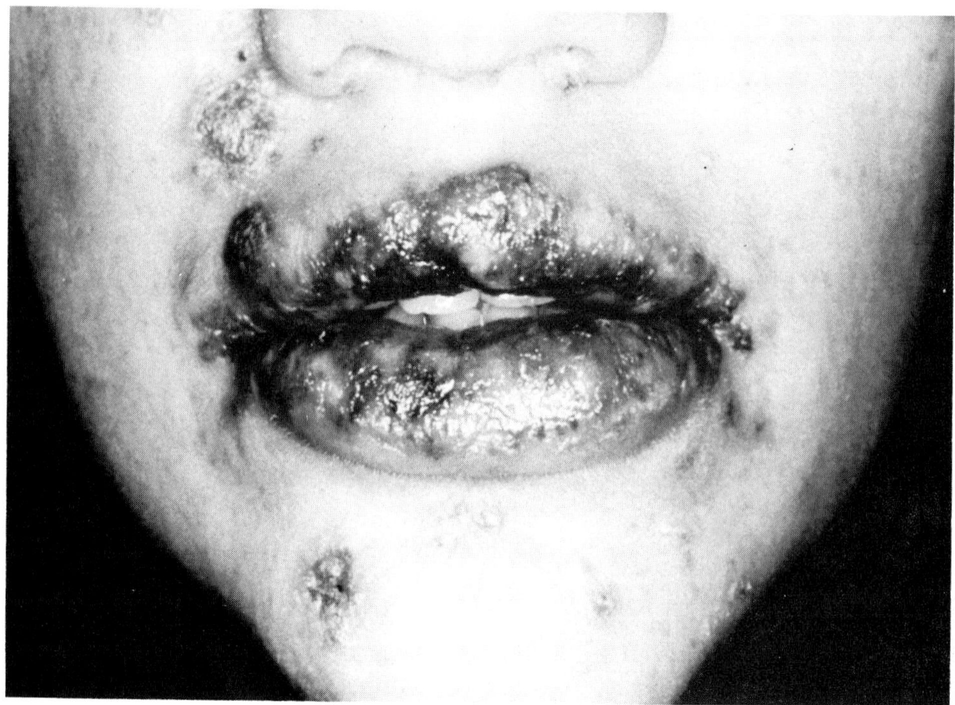

Figure 18–140. Candidal granuloma syndrome. Close-up of perioral hyperkeratotic plaques in patient shown in Figure 18–139.

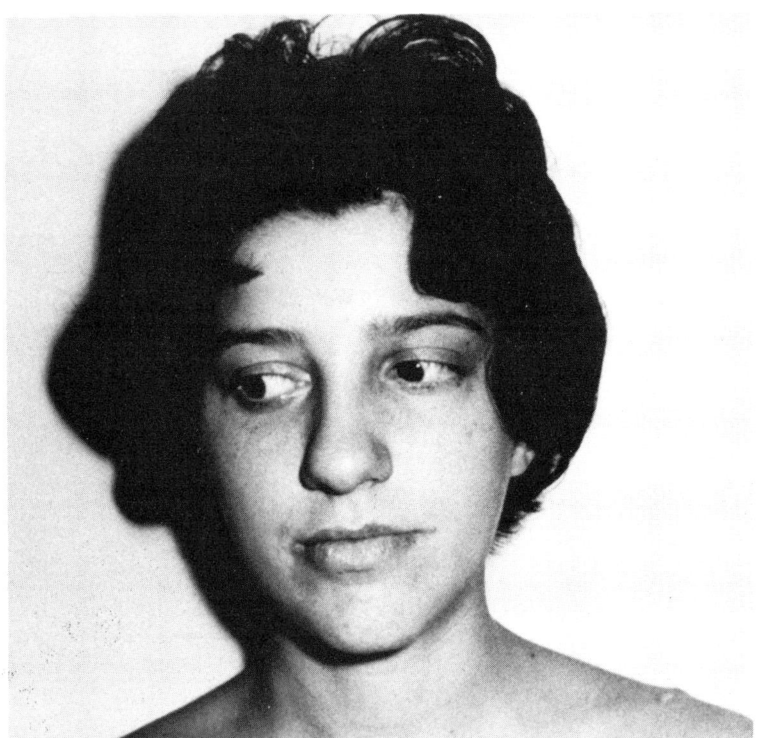

Figure 18–141. Candidal granuloma syndrome. Patient shown in Figures 18–139 and 18–140. Post–amphotericin B treatment.

have developed hypothyroidism, adrenal insufficiency, or diabetes mellitus several years after the candidiasis began.[127] This form of chronic candidiasis has never become systemic, but the infection has involved the esophagus and larynx when the mouth was extensively involved. Rarely the candidiasis may produce dry scaly plaques resembling ringworm on the trunk and extremities. In addition to candidiasis some of the patients have had recurrent staphylococcal boils[128] and cutaneous infections with other fungi such as *T. tonsurans*, *E. floccosum*,[127] and *M. audouini*.[128]

(3) Chronic mucocutaneous candidiasis has developed in children under five years of age in association with combined immunologic deficiency syndromes. These youngsters developed systemic candidiasis in addition to their mucocutaneous involvement.

(4) Chronic mucocutaneous candidiasis of the nails, skin, and mucous membranes has also been associated with absence of the thymus or presence of a thymoma. Correction of these thymic abnormalities, as well as effective therapy for associated endocrine disorders, has not produced any beneficial effects on the candidiasis.[127]

Septicemia with *C. albicans* occurs chiefly in individuals who are immunocompromised either by lymphomatous diseases or by drugs. Others at risk include heroin addicts and patients who have undergone cardiac surgery or who have had indwelling catheters and shunts for prolonged periods. The septicemic syndromes can take either the form of an endocarditis-like syndrome, as seen in heroin addicts (see p. 850), or the form of multiple septic emboli in the skin.[129-132] In most of the reported

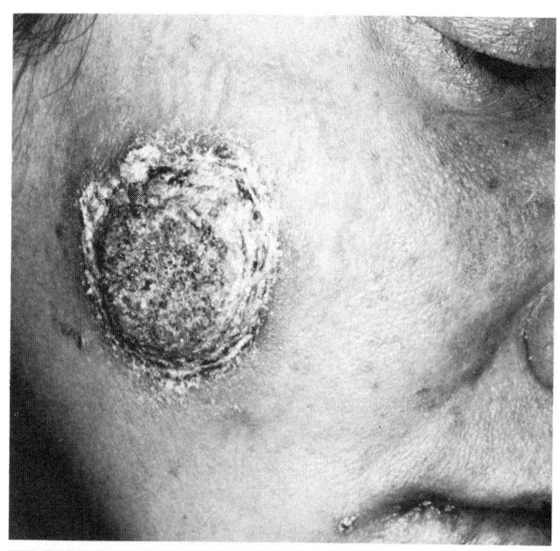

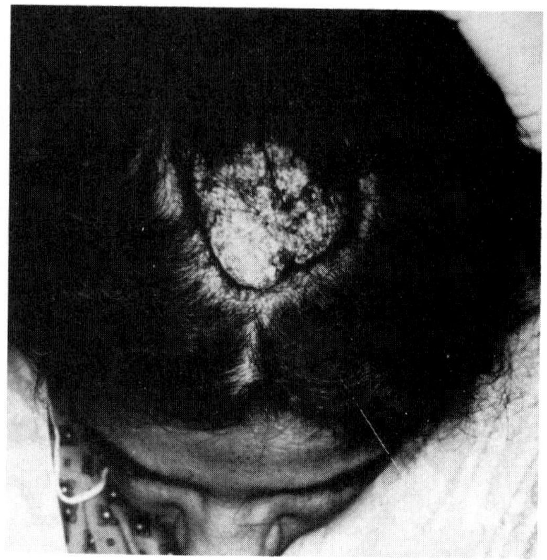

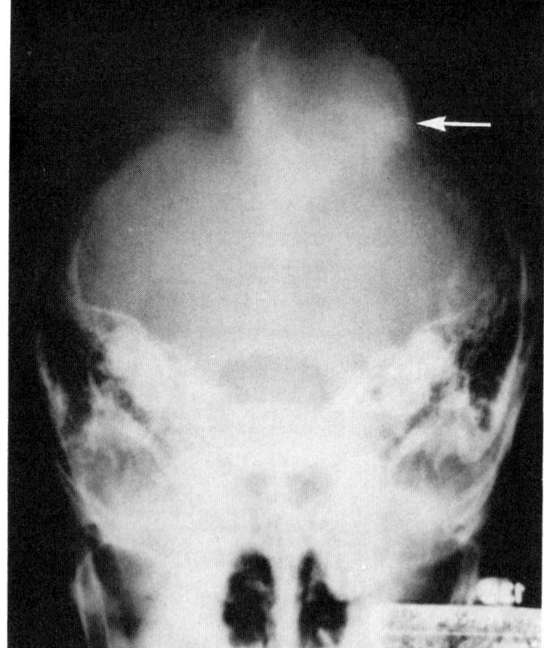

Figure 18–142. Top left. Candidal granuloma syndrome. Hyperkeratotic plaque on cheek.

Figure 18–143. Top right. Candidal granuloma syndrome. Hyperkeratotic plaque on scalp.

Figure 18–144. Bottom. Candidal granuloma syndrome. Cranial x-ray of patient in Figure 18–143 showing cutaneous horn formation on scalp (arrow).

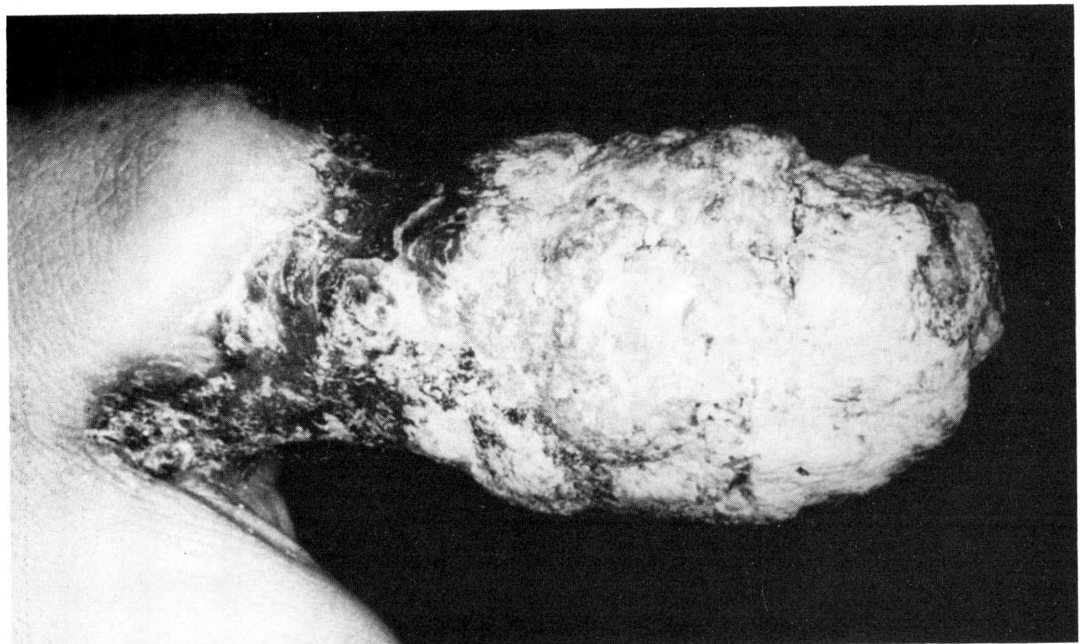

Figure 18–145. Candidal granuloma syndrome. Involvement of thumb. Pretreatment.

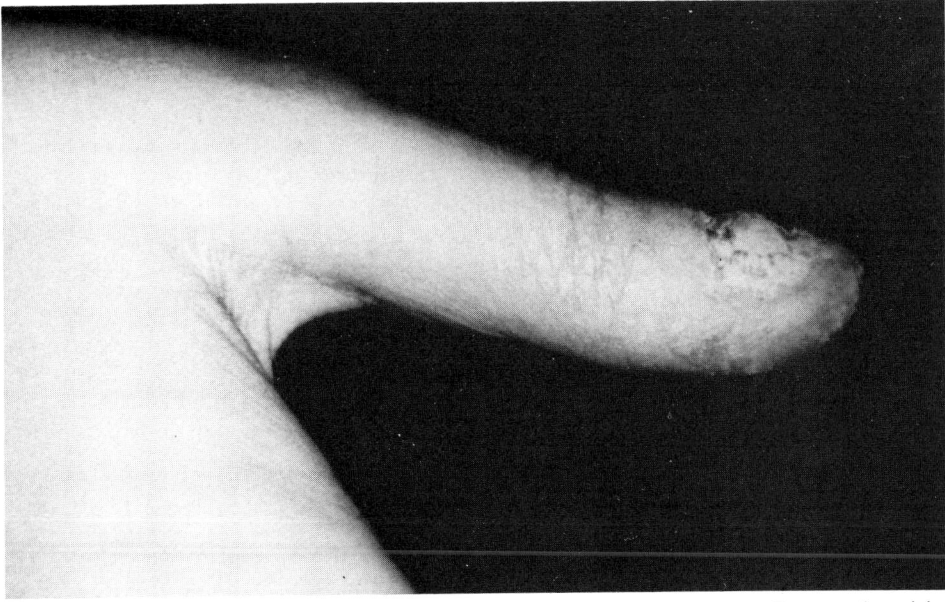

Figure 18–146. Candidal granuloma syndrome. Same patient shown in Figure 18–145. Post–amphotericin B treatment.

cases, the septic emboli have been described as red papules and nodules 0.2 to 1.0 cm in diameter surrounded by wide rings of erythema. They have appeared on the arms, face, chest, and abdomen. The nodules have been described as being uniformly red, having pale or yellowish centers, or becoming hemorrhagic if the patient had thrombocytopenia. In one series of 77 patients with candidal septicemia, 13 per cent of patients had septic emboli.[130] Less commonly, the red nodules have become necrotic, producing an ulceration resembling ecthyma gangrenosum — a sign of gram-negative bacterial sepsis.[131] The organisms are easily identified in biopsy specimens of these lesions. The most common species isolated have been *C. albicans,* following in decreasing order by *C. tropicalis, C. krusei,* and *C. parapsilosis.*

Cryptococcosis

The yeast-like fungus *Cryptococcus neoformans* is worldwide in distribution. It is found in pigeon droppings, in their resting and nesting areas, and in soil contaminated by their excreta. The pigeons are not infected by the cryptococcus, but other wild and domestic animals, e.g., the cat and the cow, can be. However, there is no proof that animal-to-man or man-to-man transmission has ever occurred.[133] Inhalation is thought to be the route of entry for the cryptococcus. Dissemination occurs from the lung primarily to the central nervous system, skin, and bones. Other sites of infection, which are rare, include the prostate, liver, endocardium, pericardium, kidney, and eye. Disseminated infection occurs most frequently in individuals who are immunocompromised or who otherwise have impaired host defenses. Persons primarily at risk include those with lymphomas, leukemia, myeloma, sarcoidosis, and other chronic debilitating illnesses. Individuals under prolonged therapy with corticosteroids and immunosuppressive drugs are similarly predisposed.

Cryptococcal meningitis behaves as a chronic infection closely simulating tuberculosis and is present in most patients with disseminated disease. Focal involvement of the brain can also occur, producing signs and symptoms suggestive of brain tumor. Pulmonary involvement can be asymptomatic or it can be accompanied by cough, sputum production, chest pain, weight loss, and radiologic findings that can mimic those of primary or metastatic lung carcinoma. Cryptococcal infection of bone produces osteolytic lesions.

Mucocutaneous involvement develops in 10 to 15 per cent of individuals with cryptococcosis and may be the first sign of dissemination. Primary cutaneous cryptococcal infection does occur but is very rare.[134] The cutaneous lesions may be acneiform — dome-shaped red papules and nodules that develop slightly depressed centers progressing to ulceration with the extrusion of thick pus (Fig. 18–147).[135] Cutaneous cryptococcosis may mimic a bacterial cellulitis (Plate 14*B*), or it may appear as a cellulitis, evolve into a vesicular phase, and then become hemorrhagic and ulcerate.[11] These three manifestations should make one think of cryptococcosis when they appear in a debilitated or immunocompromised patient. Other cutaneous manifestations include purpuric nodules and indurated plaques, sinus tracts, and subcutaneous swellings arising in the fat, bones, or joints which spontaneously ulcerate.[136-138] The

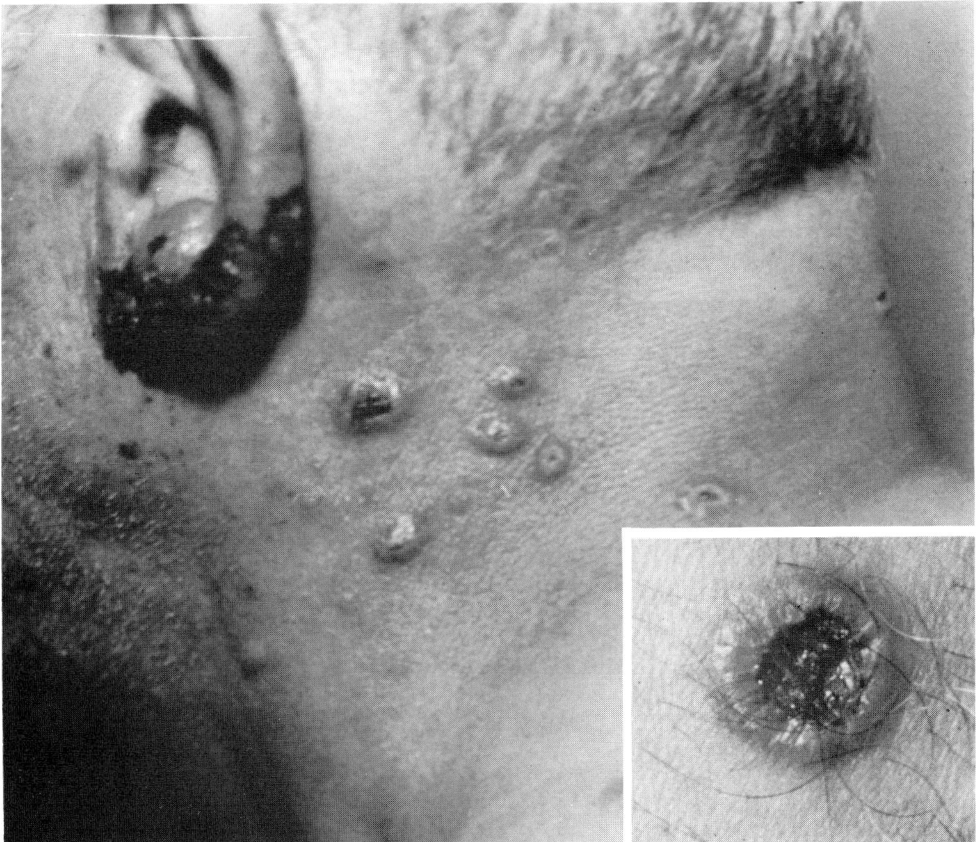

Figure 18–147. Cryptococcosis. *A*, Dome-shaped erythematous papules and nodules undergoing necrosis. *B*, Close-up of a necrotic papule. (*A* from Crounse, R. G., and Lerner, A. B.: Cryptococcosis. Case with unusual skin lesions and favorable response to amphotericin B therapy. Arch. Dermatol., *77*:210, 1958.)

acneiform papules and nodules may enlarge to form verrucous nodules and tumors and hyperkeratotic exudative plaques. Cutaneous cryptococcosis may begin as bullae or vesicles on normal-appearing skin and rapidly enlarge to form deeply punched-out ulcers with pearly edges and a smooth granulating base simulating basal cell carcinoma.

The oral mucosa is involved less often than the skin, but when present, the oral lesions may spread to involve the face. Violaceous nodules, tumors, and ulcers may arise on the gums, soft and hard palates, tonsillar pillars, nasal septum, and in the naso- and oropharynx.

The Deep Mycoses

North American blastomycosis, coccidioidomycosis, and histoplasmosis have several features in common even though each disorder has its own characteristic natural history and pattern of cutaneous manifestations. All three begin as pulmonary infections which can be acute and self-limited or chronic and progressive with cavity formation. The acute phase of the infection may be accompanied by erythema nodosum in all three and by erythema multiforme in the second and third. The soil is the main source of the fungal infection. The infection in adults affects men much more often than women. In each disorder the pulmonary infection serves as a source for the hematogenous spread of the organisms to the skin, mucous membranes, and visceral organs. Cutaneous lesions often are a sign of disseminated disease, which proves fatal in most cases. However, in each disorder, a minority of persons with cutaneous lesions will have a benign prognosis because the pulmonary focus has healed after the skin lesions have developed. The patient can be cured by excision of the pulmonary lesion and appropriate surgical therapy or chemotherapy of the cutaneous disease. Primary inoculation (chancriform) syndromes develop in all three disorders, but most commonly as laboratory accidents.

North American blastomycosis caused by *Blastomyces dermatitidis* is endemic in the southeastern United States — Kentucky, Tennessee, North and South Carolina, southern Ohio, and to a lesser degree in the adjacent areas.[139, 140] A focus is also present in the midwestern United States — Wisconsin and Minnesota. The cutaneous lesions can develop anywhere, but they are most frequently found on the face, wrists, hands, and feet. They begin as papules or nodules that develop a verrucous surface with minute pustules as they slowly enlarge. The lesions may remain as verrucous nodules and tumors, or they may expand peripherally, forming rings or horseshoe-shaped patterns (Fig. 18–148). The advancing elevated edges are erythematous or violaceous, verrucous, and studded with tiny pustules. The centers of the expanding lesions develop scars that are characteristically thick and somewhat contractile. However, in some cases, the scars have been described as thin or wrinkled. Less commonly, the initial papules produce nonspecific-appearing punched-out ulcers. Cutaneous infections may mimic hidradenitis suppurativa

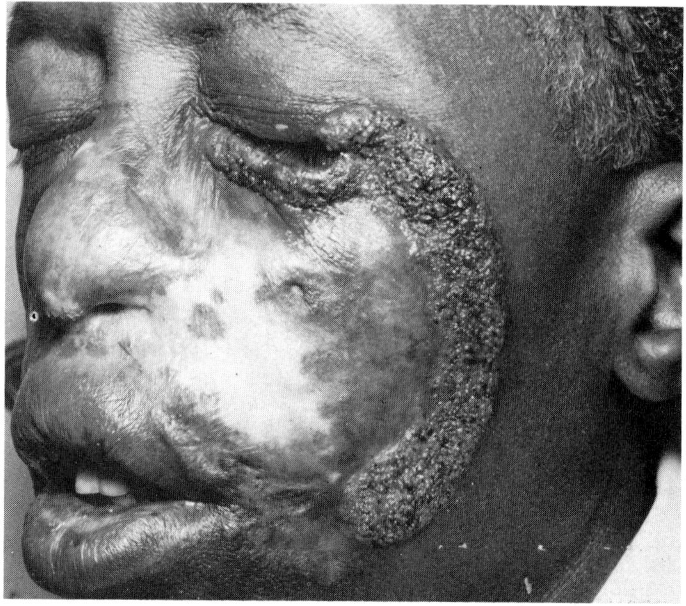

Figure 18–148. North American blastomycosis. Elevated advancing edges are erythematous and studded with tiny pustules. The centers of the lesions often become thick contractile scars. (From Moschella, S. L., Pillsbury, D. M., and Hurley, H. J., Jr.: Dermatology. Philadelphia, W. B. Saunders Company, 1975, p. 681).

when the axillae are affected. In some patients the infection begins in the subcutaneous fat as nodules that ulcerate. Mucosal involvement occurs but is uncommon.

Disseminated blastomycosis characteristically involves the bones. Osseous infections may drain directly into the overlying skin to form sinus tracts, or they may open into a joint and from there form a tract to the skin. The most commonly infected bones are the thoracic, lumbar, and sacral vertebrae, followed by the long bones of the lower extremities, pelvis, and ribs. In older men, the prostate, testis, and epididymis are commonly infected in disseminated disease, and the fungus is easily detected and recovered from the secretions of these organs. Uncommon sites of infection include the brain, liver, and spleen. The kidney and gastrointestinal tract are rarely affected.

The cutaneous lesions of blastomycosis can be confused with iododerma and bromoderma (Figs. 18–149 and 18–150), tuberculosis verruco-

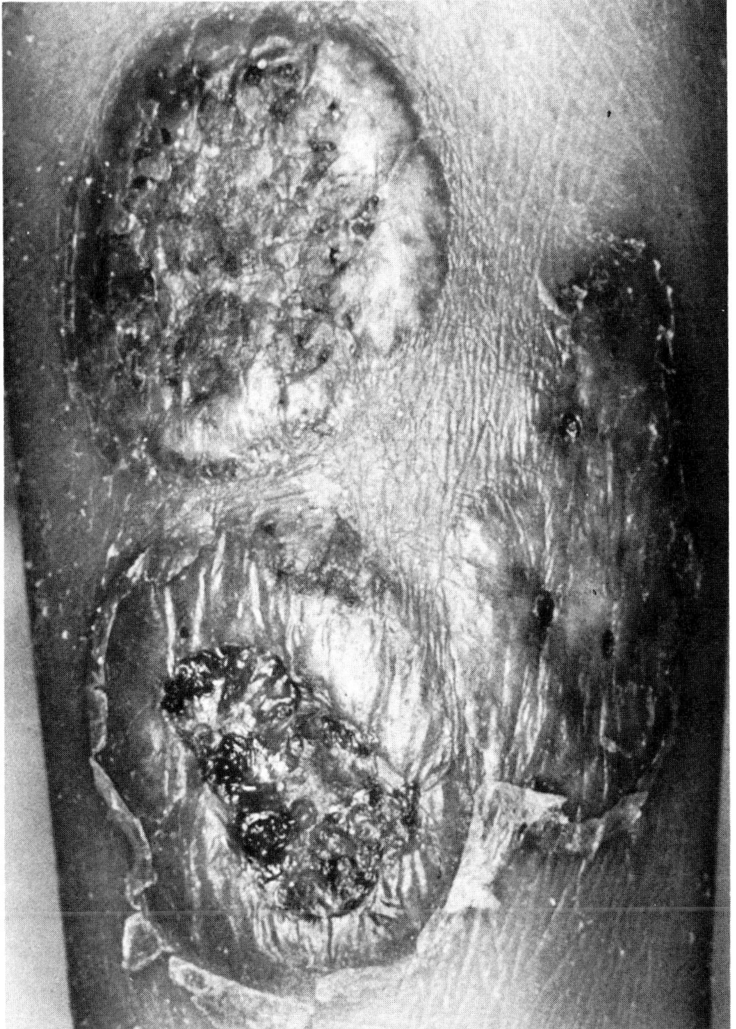

Figure 18–149. Iododerma on shin. Plaques with eroded surface and superficial pustules produced by reaction to saturated solution of potassium iodide.

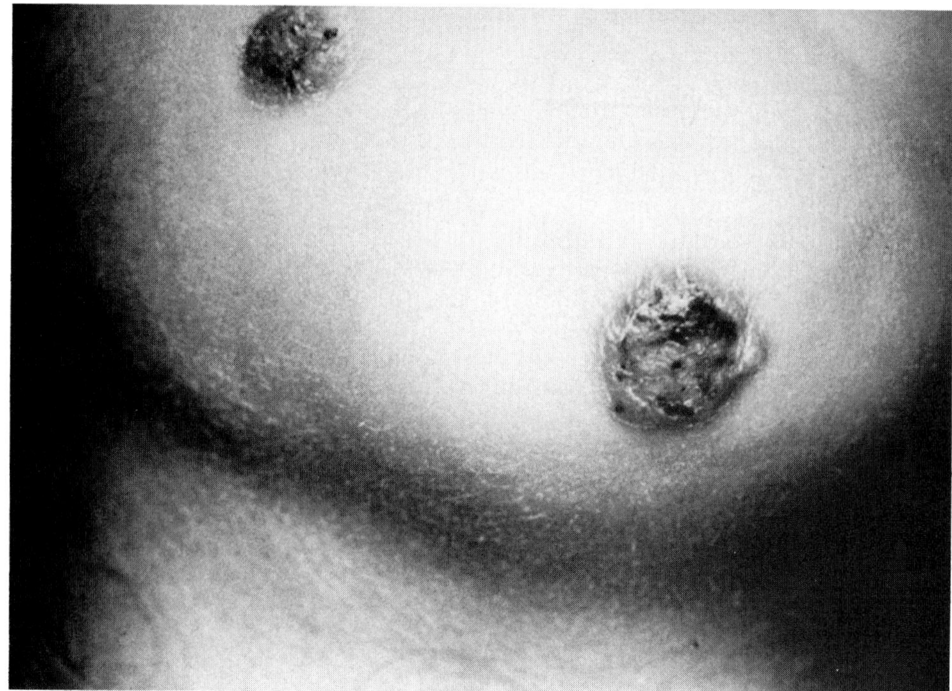

Figure 18–150. Iododerma on chin. Same patient as in Figure 18–149.

sa cutis, and disseminated coccidioidomycosis because of the verrucous surface studded with minute pustules.

Coccidioidomycosis is found in the southwestern United States — California, west Texas, Arizona, New Mexico, Utah, and Nevada — in areas where the climatic-geologic conditions are characterized by low altitude and semi-arid conditions with hot summers and infrequent freezing winters. Central America and northern Mexico are also endemic areas. The etiologic agent, *Coccidioides immitis,* produces disseminated disease within a few weeks after the primary pulmonary infection in predisposed persons. Males and black men are affected more than women and other ethnic groups, respectively. The cutaneous lesions may begin as subcutaneous nodules that suppurate to form chronic ulcers. Long-standing ulcers may become verrucous, clinically simulating blastomycosis. The lesions of coccidioidomycosis can also arise on the face and scalp as papules and nodules that become verrucous as they enlarge, again mimicking blastomycosis (Figs. 18–151 and 18–152). The type and distribution of osseous involvement in coccidioidomycosis are identical to those found in blastomycosis — osteolytic foci producing local tenderness and swelling of adjacent soft tissues with sinus tract formation. Involvement of the central nervous system and endocardium occurs but is not common. The gastrointestinal tract and adrenal glands are spared.[141, 142]

Histoplasmosis, caused by *Histoplasma capsulatum,* is endemic in the Mississippi and Ohio River valleys. The fungus is found primarily in soil contaminated by the excreta of birds and bats. In the disseminated phase of the disease, which develops chiefly in infants under age two years and in men over 50, the organism can be found in the reticuloen-

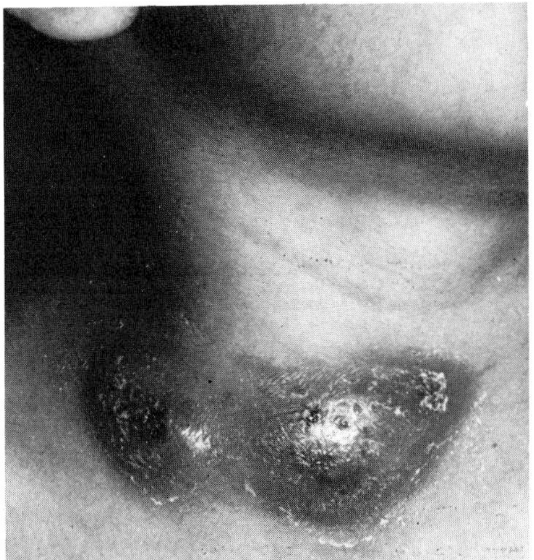

Figure 18–151. Coccidioidomycosis. Subcutaneous nodules suppurate to form chronic ulcers. (From Moschella, S. L., Pillsbury, D. M., and Hurley, H. J., Jr.: Dermatology. Philadelphia, W. B. Saunders Company, 1975, p. 678).

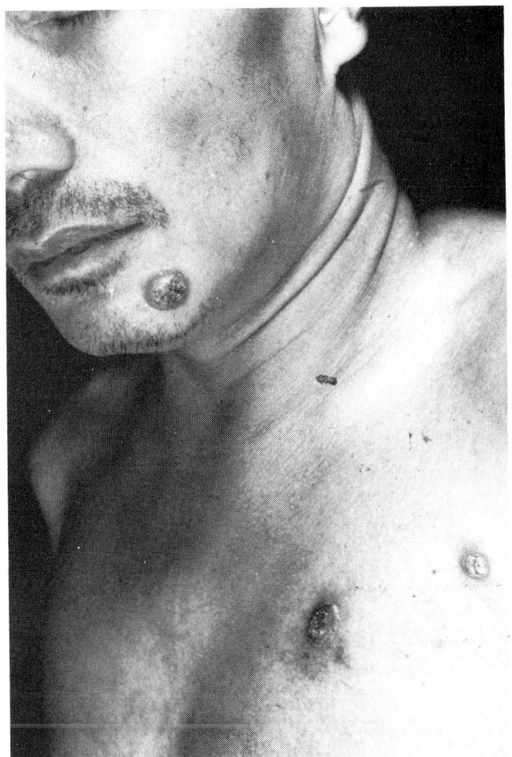

Figure 18–152. Coccidioidomycosis. Papules and nodules mimicking blastomycosis and iododerma. (From Moschella, S. L., Pillsbury, D. M., and Hurley, H. J., Jr.: Dermatology. Philadelphia, W. B. Saunders Company, 1975, p. 677).

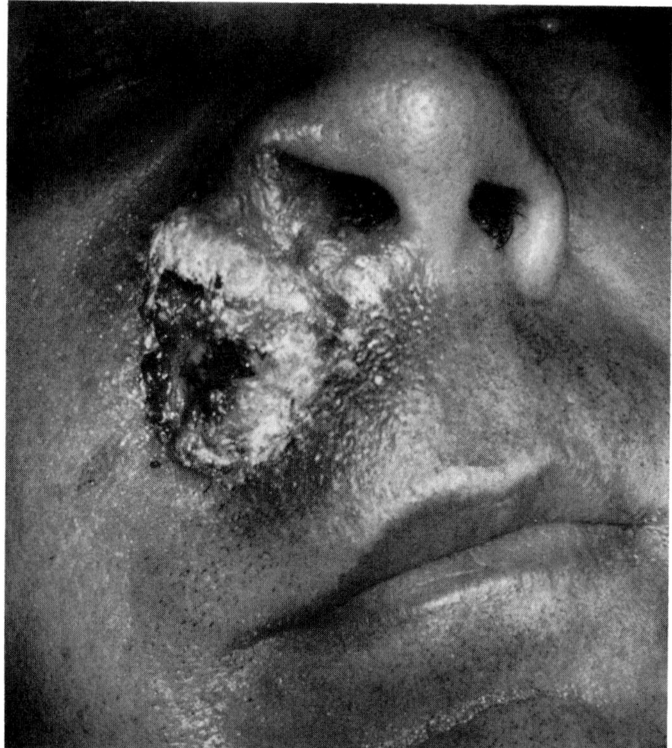

Figure 18–153. Histoplasmosis. Ulcerating nodules arising in nose and extending to facial skin.

dothelial tissues of the spleen, bone marrow, lymph nodes, liver, and intestinal mucosa.[143] The endocardium, adrenals, meninges, and bone can also be affected. In infants, disseminated histoplasmosis mimics lymphomatous disease with fever, lymphadenopathy, hepatosplenomegaly, and weight loss. In adults, disseminated histoplasmosis may present as endocarditis, meningitis, pericarditis, or adrenal insufficiency. Disseminated disease also declares its presence through mucocutaneous lesions that develop in one third to one half of affected individuals.[144] The most frequently encountered lesions are nodules with superficial ulcerations or nodules evolving into punched-out ulcers that arise in the mouth, tongue, pharynx, and larynx and lead to complaints of pain, hoarseness, and dysphagia (Fig. 18–153). Ulcers can also develop in the mucosa of the stomach, small intestine, and colon as a manifestation of disseminated histoplasmosis. In addition to oral ulcerations, gastrointestinal involvement may be accompanied by perianal ulcers. Histoplasmosis can also produce penile and vaginal ulcerations. Perforation of the nasal septum in a patient from an endemic area should suggest the possibility of histoplasmosis. Rare manifestations have included exfoliative dermatitis and verrucous pustular lesions resembling blastomycosis.

Actinomycosis

Actinomycosis is caused by an anaerobic gram-positive filamentous bacterium, *Actinomyces israelii*. It is normally present in the mouth, but does not become pathogenic or invasive until the tissues have been

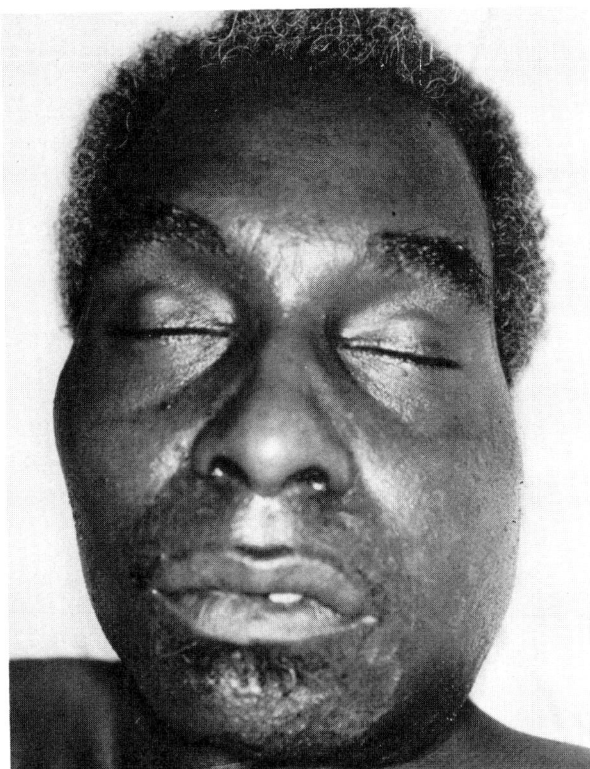

Figure 18–154. Actinomycosis. Painless indurated swelling in mandibular area.

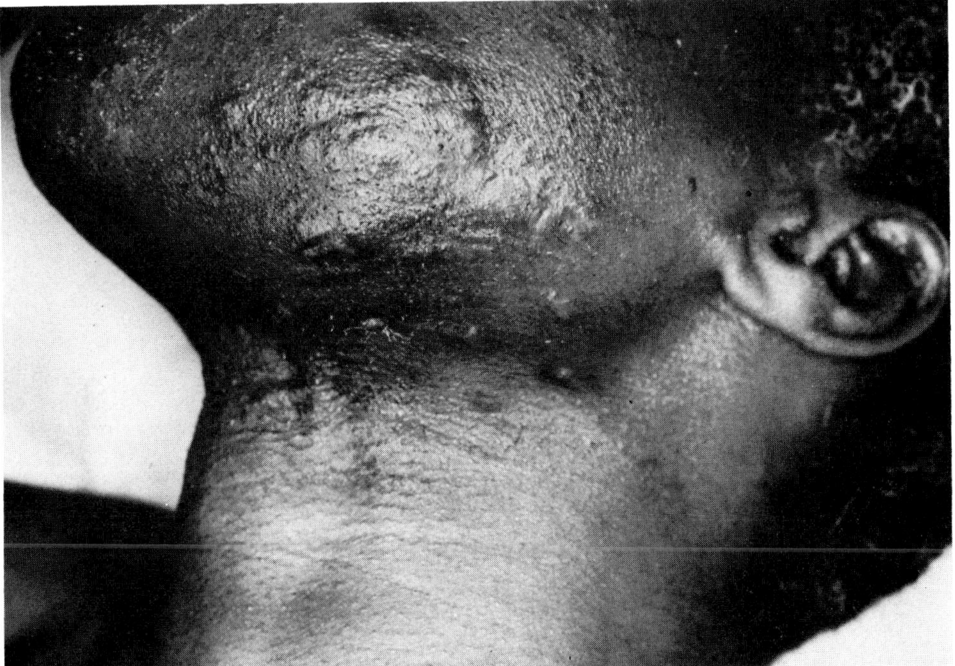

Figure 18–155. Actinomycosis. Sinus tracts discharged purulent material containing yellow grains called sulfur granules from the swollen mandibular area.

injured in some manner — infection, trauma, or surgical manipulations. The most common form of this infection is the *cervicofacial* variety, which usually follows dental infections and manipulations in individuals with poor oral hygiene. The infection begins in the soft tissues of the mouth and burrows along to reach the skin under the jaw. It begins as a painless reddish-blue swelling below the mandible that slowly enlarges, becomes indurated, and forms sinus tracts that discharge purulent material containing yellow grains the size of a pinpoint (Figs. 18–154 and 18–155). These so-called sulfur granules are colonies of the etiologic agent *A. israelii*. In *thoracic* actinomycosis, the organisms become pathogenic in the lung tissue because of underlying pulmonary disorders such as bronchiectasis, lung cancer, lung abscess, or any other process that allows the organisms to proliferate. Burrowing occurs here as well to produce multiple draining sinuses of the chest wall. In *abdominal* actinomycosis, the infection begins in the ileocecal area, and sinus tracts develop not only to the abdominal wall but also to internal viscera.

REFERENCES

1. Mandell, G. L., Douglas, R. G., Jr., and Bennett, J. E. (eds.): Principles and Practice of Infectious Diseases. John Wiley and Sons, New York, 1979.
2. Krugman, S., Ward, R., and Katz, S. L.: Infectious Diseases of Children. C. V. Mosby Company, St. Louis, 1977.
3. Ramsay, A. M., and Edmond, R. T. D.: Infectious Diseases, 2nd ed. Wm. Heinemann Medical Books, Ltd., London, 1978.
4. Hoeprich, P. D. (ed.): Infectious Diseases, 2nd ed. Harper and Row, Hagerstown, Md., 1977.
5. Top, F. H., Sr., and Wehrle, P. F. (eds.): Communicable and Infectious Diseases, 8th ed. C. V. Mosby Co., St. Louis, 1976.
6. Collins, R. N., and Nadel, M. S.: Gangrene due to the hemolytic streptococcus — a rare but treatable disease. N. Engl. J. Med., *272*:578, 1965.
7. Rea, W., and Wyrick, W.: Necrotizing fasciitis. Ann. Surg., *172*:957, 1970.
8. Feingold, M., and Gellis, S. S.: Cellulitis due to Haemophilus influenzae type B. N. Engl. J. Med., *272*:788, 1965.
9. Drapkin, M. S., Wilson, M. E., Shrager, S. M., and Rubin, R.: Bacteremic Hemophilus influenzae type B cellulitis in the adult. Am. J. Med., *63*:449, 1977.
10. Gauder, J. P.: Cryptococcal cellulitis. J.A.M.A., *237*:672, 1977.
11. Schupach, C. W., Wheeler, C. E., Jr., Briggaman, R. A., Warner, N. A., and Kanof, E. P.: Cutaneous manifestations of disseminated cryptococcosis. Arch. Dermatol., *112*:1734, 1975.
12. Klauder, J. V.: Erysipelothrix rhusiopathiae infection in swine and in human beings. Arch. Dermatol., *50*:151, 1944.
13. Nelson, E.: Five hundred cases of erysipeloid. Rocky Mt. Med. J., *52*:40, 1955.
14. Top, F. H., Sr., and Wehrle, P. F.: *op cit.*, p. 664.
15. Top, F. H., Sr., and Wehrle, P. F.: *op. cit.*, p. 659.
16. Stevens, F. A.: Occurrence of Staphylococcus aureus infection with scarlatiniform rash. J.A.M.A., *88*:1957, 1927.
17. Aranow, H., Jr., and Wood, W. B., Jr.: Staphylococcal infection simulating scarlet fever. J.A.M.A., *119*:1491, 1942.
18. McCloskey, R. V.: Scarlet fever and necrotizing fasciitis caused by coagulase positive Staphylococcus aureus, phage type 85. Ann. Intern. Med., *78*:85, 1973.
19. Ramsay, A. M., and Edmond, R. T. D.: *op. cit.*, p. 267.
20. Robboy, S. J., Mihm, M. C., Colman, R., and Minna, J. D.: The skin in disseminated intravascular coagulation. Br. J. Dermatol., *88*:221, 1973.
21. Lerner, A. M., Klein, J. O., Cherry, J. D., and Finland, M.: New viral exanthems. N. Engl. J. Med., *269*:678, 736, 1963.
22. Swierczewski, J. A., Mason, E. J., Cabrera, P. B., and Liber, M.: Fulminating meningitis with Waterhouse-Friderichsen syndrome due to Neisseria gonorrhoeae. Am. J. Clin. Pathol., *54*:202, 1970.
23. Nielsen, L. T.: Chronic meningococcemia. Arch. Dermatol., *102*:97, 1970.
24. Saslaw, S.: Chronic meningococcemia. N. Engl. J. Med., *266*:605, 1962.
25. Barr, J., and Danielsson, D.: Septic gonococcal dermatitis. Br. Med. J., *1*:482, 1971.
26. Shapiro, L., Teisch, J. A., and Brownstein, M. H.: Dermatohistopathology of chronic gonococcal sepsis. Arch. Dermatol., *107*:403, 1973.

27. Walker, L. C., Ahlin, T. D., Tung, K. S. K., and Williams, K. C., Jr.: Circulating immune complexes in disseminated gonnorrheal infection. Ann. Intern. Med., *89*:28, 1978.
28. Suringa, D. W. R., Bank, L. J., and Ackerman, A. B.: Role of measles virus in skin lesions and Koplik's spots. N. Engl. J. Med., *283*:1139, 1970.
29. Lachmann, P. J.: Immunopathology of measles. Proc. R. Soc. Med., *67*:1120, 1974.
30. Fulginiti, V. A., Eller, J. J., Downie, A. W., and Kempe, C. H.: Altered reactivity to measles virus. J.A.M.A., *202*:1075, 1967.
31. Bellanti, J. A., Sanga, R. L., Klutinis, B., Brandt, B., and Artenstein, M. S.: Antibody responses in serum and nasal secretions of children immunized with inactivated and attenuated measles-virus vaccines. N. Engl. J. Med., *280*:628, 1969.
32. Bayer, W. L., Sherman, F. E., Michaels, R. H., Szeto, I. L. F., and Lewis, J. H.: Purpura in congenital and acquired rubella. N. Engl. J. Med., *273*:1362, 1965.
33. Lauer, B. A., MacCormack, J. N., and Wilfert, C.: Erythema infectiosum. An elementary school outbreak. Am. J. Dis. Child., *130*:252, 1976.
34. Greenwald, P., and Bashe, W. J.: An epidemic of erythema infectiosum. Am. J. Dis. Child., *107*:30, 1964.
35. Balfour, H. H.: Erythema infectiosum (fifth disease). Clin. Pediatr., *8*:721, 1969.
36. Gianotti, F.: The Gianotti-Crosti syndrome. J. Contin. Edu. Dermatol., *18*:15, 1979.
37. Ishimaru, Y., Ishimaru, H., Toda, G., Baba, K., and Mayumi, M.: An epidemic of infantile papular acrodermatitis in Japan associated with hepatitis B surface antigen subtype ayw. Lancet, *1*:707, 1976.
38. Karzon, D. T.: Infectious mononucleosis. Adv. Pediatr., *22*:231, 1976.
39. Patel, B. M.: Skin rash with infectious mononucleosis and ampicillin. Pediatrics, *40*:910, 1967.
40. Sheon, R. P., and Van Ommen, R. A.: Fever of obscure origin. Am. J. Med., *34*:486, 1963.
41. Petersdorf, R. G., and Beeson, P. B.: Fever of unexplained origin. Medicine, *40*:1, 1961.
42. Deal, W. B.: Fever of unknown origin. Postgrad. Med., *50*:182, 1971.
43. Frayha, R., and Uwaydah, M.: Fever of unknown origin. Lab. Med. J., *26*:49, 1973.
44. Howard, P., Jr., Hahn, H. H., Palmer, P. L., and Hardin, W. J.: Fever of unknown origin: a prospective study of 100 patients. Tex. Med., *73*:56, 1977.
45. Aduan, R. P., Fauci, A. S., Dale, D. C., and Wolff, S. M.: Prolonged fever of unknown origin (FUO). A prospective study of 347 patients. Clin. Res., *26*:558A, 1978.
46. Melish, M. E., and Glasgow, L. A.: Staphylococcal scalded skin syndrome: the expanded clinical syndrome. J. Pediatr., *78*:958, 1971.
47. Rasmussen, J. E.: Toxic epidermal necrolysis. A review of 75 cases in children. Arch. Dermatol., *111*:1135, 1975.
48. Elias, P. M., Fritsch, P., and Epstein, E. H., Jr.: Staphylococcal scalded skin syndrome. Clinical features, pathogenesis and recent microbiological and biochemical developments. Arch. Dermatol., *113*:207, 1977.
49. Sturman, S. W., and Malkinson, F. D.: Staphylococcal scalded skin syndrome in an adult and a child. Arch. Dermatol., *112*:1275, 1976.
50. Levine, G., and Norden, C. W.: Staphylococcal scalded skin syndrome in an adult. N. Engl. J. Med., *287*:1339, 1972.
51. Reid, L. H., Weston, W. L., and Humbert, J. R.: Staphylococcal scalded skin syndrome. Adult onset in a patient with deficient cell mediated immunity. Arch. Dermatol., *109*:239, 1974.
52. Fritsch, P., Elias, P., and Varga, J.: The fate of staphylococcal exfoliation in newborn and adult mice. Br. J. Dermatol., *95*:275, 1976.
53. Peck, G. L., Hertzig, G. P., and Elias, P. M.: Toxic epidermal necrolysis in a patient with graft-vs-host reaction. Arch. Dermatol., *105*:561, 1972.
54. Billingham, R. E., and Streilen, J. W.: Toxic epidermal necrolysis and homologous disease in hamsters. Arch. Dermatol., *98*:528, 1968.
55. Wannamaker, L. W.: Differences between streptococcal infections of the throat and skin. N. Engl. J. Med., *282*:23, 78, 1970.
56. Farrior, J. B., III, and Silverman, M. E.: A consideration of the differences between a Janeway's lesion and an Osler's node in infectious endocarditis. Chest, *70*:239, 1976.
57. Alpert, J. S., Krous, H. F., Dalen, J. E., O'Rourke, R. A., and Bloor, C. M.: Pathogenesis of Osler's nodes. Ann. Intern. Med., *85*:471, 1976.
58. Von Gemmengen, G. R., and Winkelmann, R. K.: Osler's nodes of subacute bacterial endocarditis. Arch. Dermatol., *95*:91, 1967.
59. Weinstein, L., and Schlesinger, J. J.: Pathanatomic, pathophysiologic and clinical correlations in endocarditis. N. Engl. J. Med., *291*:832, 1122, 1974.
60. Kennedy, J. E., and Wise, G. N.: Clinicopathologic correlation of retinal lesions, subacute bacterial endocarditis. Arch. Ophthalmol., *74*:658, 1965.
61. Gutman, R. A., Striker, G. E., Gilliland, B. C., and Cutler, R. E.: The immune complex glomerulonephritis of bacterial endocarditis. Medicine, *51*:1, 1972.
62. Levy, R. L., and Hong, R.: The immune nature of subacute bacterial endocarditis (SBE) nephritis. Am. J. Med., *54*:645, 1973.

62a. Dowling, R. H.: Sub-ungual splinter haemorrhages. Postgrad. Med. J., *40*:595, 1964.

63. Braverman, I. M., and Yen, A.: Demonstration of immune complexes in spontaneous and histamine-induced lesions and in normal skin of patients with leukocytoclastic angiitis. J. Invest. Dermatol., *64*:105, 1975.

64. Nahmias, A. J., and Roizman, B.: Infection with herpes-simplex viruses 1 and 2. N. Engl. J. Med., *289*:667, 719, 781, 1973.

65. Baringer, J. R., and Swoveland, P.: Recovery of herpes-simplex virus from human trigeminal ganglions. N. Engl. J. Med., *288*:648, 1973.

66. Baringer, J. R.: Recovery of herpes simplex virus from human sacral ganglions. N. Engl. J. Med., *291*:828, 1974.

67. Finelli, P. F., and McDonald, S. D.: Herpes simplex virus in sensory ganglions. N. Engl. J. Med., *292*:51, 1975.

68. Warren, K. G., Brown, S. M., Wroblewska, Z., Golden, D., Koprowski, H., and Subak-Sharpe, J.: Isolation of latent herpes simplex virus from the superior cervical and vagus ganglions of human beings. N. Engl. J. Med., *298*:1068, 1978.

69. White, J. G.: Fulminating infection with herpes-simplex virus in premature and newborn infants. N. Engl. J. Med., *269*:454, 1963.

70. Honig, P. J., Holzwanger, J., and Leyden, J. J.: Congenital herpes simplex virus infections. Arch. Dermatol., *115*:1329, 1979.

71. Nahmias, A. J., Visintine, A. M., and Josey, W. E.: Cesarean section and genital herpes. N. Engl. J. Med., *296*:1359, 1977.

72. Weathers, D. R., and Griffin, J. W.: Intraoral ulcerations of recurrent herpes simplex and recurrent aphthae: Two distinct clinical entities. J. Am. Dent. Assoc., *81*:81, 1970.

73. Music, S. I., Fine, E. M., and Togo, Y.: Zoster-like disease in the newborn due to herpes-simplex virus. N. Engl. J. Med., *284*:24, 1971.

74. Mok, C. H.: Zoster-like disease in infants and young children. N. Engl. J. Med., *285*:294, 1971.

75. Hanke, C. W., III, and Huntley, D. W.: Zosteriform herpes simplex. Cutis, *16*:913, 1975.

76. Leider, W., Magoffin, R. L., Lennette, E. H., and Leonards, L. N. R.: Herpes-simplex-virus encephalitis. Its possible association with reactivated latent infection. N. Engl. J. Med., *273*:341, 1965.

77. Terni, M., Caccialanza, P., Cassai, E., and Kieff, E.: Aseptic meningitis in association with herpes progenitalis. N. Engl. J. Med., *285*:503, 1971.

78. Rosato, F. E., Rosato, E. F., and Plotkin, S. A.: Herpetic paronychia — an occupational hazard of medical personnel. N. Engl. J. Med., *283*:805, 1970.

79. Howard, W. R., Taylor, J. S., and Steck, W. D.: Lymphatic complications of manual herpes simplex infection. Cutis, *23*:580, 1979.

80. Selling, B., and Kibrick, S.: An outbreak of herpes simplex among wrestlers (herpes gladiatorum). N. Engl. J. Med., *270*:979, 1964.

81. Wheeler, C. E., Jr., and Abele, D. C.: Eczema herpeticum primary and recurrent. Arch. Dermatol., *93*:162, 1966.

82. Foley, F. D., Greenwald, K. A., Nash, G., and Pruitt, B. A., Jr.: Herpesvirus infection in burned patients. N. Engl. J. Med., *282*:652, 1970.

83. Logan, W. S., Tindall, J. P., and Elson, M. L.: Chronic cutaneous herpes simplex. Arch. Dermatol., *103*:606, 1971.

84. Muller, S. A., Herrmann, E. C., Jr., and Winkelmann, R. K.: Herpes simplex infections in hematologic malignancies. Am. J. Med., *52*:102, 1972.

85. Montgomerie, J. Z., Becroft, D. M. O., Croxson, M. C., Doak, P. B., and North, J. D. K.: Herpes-simplex-virus infection after renal transplantation. Lancet, *2*:867, 1969.

86. Kawasaki, T., Kosaki, F., Okawa, S., Shigematsu, I., and Yanagawa, H.: A new infantile acute febrile mucocutaneous lymph node syndrome (MLNS) prevailing in Japan. Pediatrics, *54*:271, 1974.

87. Melish, M. E., Hicks, R. M., and Larson, E.: Mucocutaneous lymph node syndrome (MLNS) in the U.S. Am. J. Dis. Child., *130*:599, 1976.

88. Shigematsu, I., Shibata, S., Tamashiro, H., Kawasaki, T., and Kusakawa, S.: Kawasaki disease continues to increase in Japan. Pediatrics, *64*:386, 1979.

89. Landing, B. H., and Larson, E. J.: Are infantile periarteritis nodosa with coronary artery involvement and fatal mucocutaneous lymph node syndrome the same? Comparison of 20 patients from North America with patients from Hawaii and Japan. Pediatrics, *59*:651, 1977.

90. Kusakawa, S., and Heiner, D. C.: Elevated levels of immunoglobulin E in the acute febrile mucocutaneous lymph node syndrome. Pediatr. Res., *10*:108, 1976.

91. Yanagisawa, M., Kobayashi, N., and Matsuya, S.: Myocardial infarction due to coronary thromboarteritis, following acute febrile mucocutaneous lymph node syndrome (MLNS) in an infant. Pediatrics, *54*:277, 1974.

92. Fetterman, G. H., and Hashida, Y.: Mucocutaneous lymph node syndrome (MLNS): a disease wide spread in Japan which demands our attention. Pediatrics, *54*:268, 1974.

93. Hirose, S., and Hamashima, Y.: Morphological observations on the vasculitis in the mucocutaneous lymph node syndrome. Eur. J. Pediatr., *129*:17, 1978.

93a. Marsh, W. L., Jr., Bishop, J. W., and Koenig, H. M.: Bone marrow and lymph node findings in a fatal case of Kawasaki's disease. Arch. Pathol. Lab. Med., *104*:563, 1980.

94. Schlossberg, D., Kandra, J., and Kreiser, J.: Possible Kawasaki disease in a 20-year-old woman. Arch. Dermatol., *115*:1435, 1979.
95. Lee, T. J., and Vaughan, D.: Mucocutaneous lymph node syndrome in a young adult. Arch. Intern. Med., *139*:104, 1979.
96. Caron, G. A.: Kawasaki disease in an adult. J.A.M.A., *243*:430, 1980.
97. Everett, E. D.: Mucocutaneous lymph node syndrome (Kawasaski disease) in adults. J.A.M.A., *242*:542, 1979.
98. Barbour, A. G., Krueger, G. G., Feorino, P. M., and Smith, C. B.: Kawasaki-like disease in a young adult. Association with primary Epstein-Barr virus infection. J.A.M.A., *241*:397, 1979.
99. Anderson, V. M., Bauer, H. M., and Kelly, A. P.: Mucocutaneous lymph node syndrome in an adult receiving diphenylhydantoin. Cutis, *23*:493, 1979.
100. Seehafer, J. R., Goldberg, N. C., Dicken, C. H., and Su, W. P. D.: Cutaneous manifestations of angioimmunoblastic lymphadenopathy. Arch. Dermatol., *116*:41, 1980.
101. Morens, D. M.: Thoughts on Kawasaki disease etiology. J.A.M.A., *241*:399, 1979.
102. Schwarz, J., and Kauffman, C. A.: Occupational hazards from deep mycoses. Arch. Dermatol., *113*:1270, 1977.
103. Cox, R. L., and Reller, L. B.: Auricular sporotrichosis in a brick mason. Arch. Dermatol., *115*:1229, 1979.
104. Philpott, J. A., Jr., Woodburne, A. R., Philpott, O. S., Schaefer, W. B., and Mollohan, C. S.: Swimming pool granuloma. A study of 290 cases. Arch. Dermatol., *88*:158, 1963.
105. Morrow, H., and Miller, H. E.: Tuberculosis of the tongue. J.A.M.A., *83*:1483, 1924.
106. Bryant, J. C.: Oral tuberculosis. Am. Rev. Tuberculosis, *39*:738, 1939.
107. Bolivar, R., Satterwhite, T. K., and Floyd, M.: Cutaneous lesions due to Mycobacterium kansasii. Arch. Dermatol., *116*:207, 1980.
108. Owens, D. W., and McBride, M. E.: Sporotrichoid cutaneous infection with Mycobacterium kansasii. Arch. Dermatol., *100*:54, 1969.
109. Greer, K. E., Gross, G. P., and Martensen, S. H.: Sporotrichoid cutaneous infection due to Mycobacterium chelonei. Arch. Dermatol., *115*:738, 1979.
110. Arnold, H. L., Jr., and Fasal, P.: Leprosy. Diagnosis and Management, 2nd ed. Charles C Thomas, Springfield, Ill., 1973.
111. Ridley, D. S., and Jopling, W. H.: Classification of leprosy according to immunity. A five-group system. Int. J. Leprosy, *34*:255, 1966.
112. Rea, T. H., and Levan, N. E.: Current concepts in the immunology of leprosy. Arch. Dermatol., *113*:345, 1977.
113. Jolliffe, D. S.: Leprosy reactional states and their treatment. Br. J. Dermatol., *97*:345, 1977.
114. Moschella, S. L.: The lepra reaction with necrotizing skin lesions. Arch. Dermatol., *95*:565, 1967.
115. Pursley, T. V., Jacobson, R. R., and Apisarnthanarax, P.: Lucio's phenomenon. Arch. Dermatol., *116*:201, 1980.
116. Rea, T. H., and Levan, N. E.: Lucio's phenomenon and diffuse nonnodular lepromatous leprosy. Arch. Dermatol., *114*:1023, 1978.
117. Fiumara, N. J.: The sexually transmissible diseases. Disease-A-Month, *25*:No. 3, 1978.
118. Wade, T. R., and Huntley, A.: Multiple penile chancres. An atypical manifestation of primary syphilis. Arch. Dermatol., *115*:227, 1979.
119. Cole, G. W., Amon, R. B., and Russell, P. S.: Secondary syphilis presenting as a pruritic dermatosis. Arch. Dermatol., *113*:488, 1977.
120. Lochner, J. C., and Pomeranz, J. R.: Lichenoid secondary syphilis. Arch. Dermatol., *109*:81, 1974.
121. Petrozzi, J. W., Lockshin, N. A., and Berger, B. J.: Malignant syphilis. Severe variant of secondary syphilis. Arch. Dermatol., *109*:387, 1974.
122. Gamble, C. N., and Reardan, J. B.: Immunopathogenesis of syphilitic glomerulonephritis. N. Engl. J. Med., *292*:449, 1975.
123. Stokes, J. H.: Modern Clinical Syphilology, 2nd ed. W. B. Saunders Company, Philadelphia, 1934, p. 771.
124. Pariser, H.: Precocious noduloulcerative cutaneous syphilis. Arch. Dermatol., *111*:76, 1975.
125. Dennie, C. C., and Pakula, S. F.: Congenital Syphilis. Lea and Febiger, Philadelphia, 1940, p. 119.
126. Kirkpatrick, C. H., Rich, R. R., and Bennett, J. E.: Chronic mucocutaneous candidiasis: model building in cellular immunity. Ann. Intern. Med., *74*:955, 1971.
127. Kirkpatrick, C. H., and Smith, T. K.: Chronic mucocutaneous candidiasis: immunologic and antibiotic treatment. Ann. Intern. Med., *80*:310, 1974.
128. Braverman, I. M.: Unpublished data.
129. Balandron, L., Rothschild, H., Pugh, N., and Seabury, J.: A cutaneous manifestation of systemic candidiasis. Ann. Intern. Med., *78*:400, 1973.
130. Bodey, G. P., and Luna, M.: Skin lesions associated with disseminated candidiasis. J.A.M.A., *229*:1466, 1974.
131. File, T. M., Jr., Marina, O. A., and Flowers, F. P.: Necrotic skin lesions associated with disseminated candidiasis. Arch. Dermatol., *115*:214, 1979.
132. Grossman, M. E., Silvers, D. N., and Walther, R. R.: Cutaneous manifestations

of disseminated candidiasis. J. Am. Acad. Dermatol., *2*:111, 1980.
133. Hoeprich, P. D.: Cryptococcosis. *In* Hoeprich, P. D. (ed.): Infectious Diseases. *op. cit.,* p. 902.
134. Iacobellis, F. W., Jacobs, M. I., and Cohen, R. P.: Primary cutaneous cryptococcosis. Arch. Dermatol., *115*:984, 1979.
135. Crounse, R. G., and Lerner, A. B.: Cryptococcosis. Case with unusual skin lesions and favorable response to amphotericin B therapy. Arch. Dermatol., *77*:210, 1958.
136. Cawley, E. P., Grekin, R. H., and Curtis, A. C.: Torulosis. A review of the cutaneous and adjoining mucous membrane manifestations. J. Invest. Dermatol., *14*:327, 1950.
137. Moore, M.: Cryptococcosis with cutaneous manifestations. J. Invest. Dermatol., *28*:159, 1957.
138. Rook, A., and Woods, B.: Cutaneous cryptococcosis. Br. J. Dermatol., *74*:43, 1962.
139. Witorsch, P.: North American blastomycosis: a study of 40 patients. Medicine, *47*:169, 1968.
140. Hildick-Smith, G., Blank, H., and Sarkany, I.: Fungus Diseases and Their Treatment. Little, Brown and Co., Boston, 1964, p. 222.
141. Hildick-Smith, G., Blank, H., and Sarkany, I.: *op. cit.,* p. 241.
142. Rippon, J. W.: Medical Mycology. The Pathogenic Fungi and the Pathogenic Actinomycetes. W. B. Saunders Company, Philadelphia, 1974, p. 356.
143. Rippon, J. W.: *op. cit.,* p. 321.
144. Baum, G. L., Schwarz, J., Slot, W. J. B., and Straub, M.: Mucocutaneous histoplasmosis. Arch. Dermatol., *76*:4, 1957.

Index

Page numbers in *italics* indicate illustrations. Page numbers in **bold type** indicate color plates. Page numbers followed by t indicate tables. vs. indicates differential diagnosis.

Progressive pigmented purpuric dermatoses

include Angioma Serpiginosum